Aulton's Pharmaceutics

The Design and Manufacture
of Medicines

Aulton's Pharmaceutics

The Design and Manufacture of Medicines

FIFTH EDITION

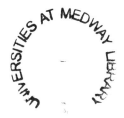

Edited by

Michael E. Aulton BPharm PhD FAAPS FSP FRPharmS

Emeritus Professor, De Montfort University, Leicester, UK

Kevin M. G. Taylor BPharm PhD FRPharmS

Professor of Clinical Pharmaceutics, UCL School of Pharmacy, London, UK

ELSEVIER

Edinburgh   London   New York   Oxford   Philadelphia   St Louis   Sydney   Toronto   2018

First edition 1988
Second edition 2002
Third edition 2007
Fourth edition 2013
Fifth edition 2018

Notices

Knowledge and best practice in this field are constantly changing. As new research and experience broaden our understanding, changes in research methods, professional practices, or medical treatment may become necessary.

Practitioners and researchers must always rely on their own experience and knowledge in evaluating and using any information, methods, compounds, or experiments described herein. In using such information or methods, they should be mindful of their own safety and the safety of others, including parties for whom they have a professional responsibility.

With respect to any drug or pharmaceutical products identified, readers are advised to check the most current information provided (1) on procedures featured or (2) by the manufacturer of each product to be administered to verify the recommended dose or formula, the method and duration of administration, and contraindications. It is the responsibility of practitioners, relying on their own experience and knowledge of their patients, to make diagnoses, to determine dosages and the best treatment for each individual patient, and to take all appropriate safety precautions.

To the fullest extent of the law, neither the publisher nor the authors, contributors, or editors assume any liability for any injury and/or damage to persons or property as a matter of product liability, negligence, or otherwise, or from any use or operation of any methods, products, instructions, or ideas contained in the material herein.

ISBN   978-0-7020-7005-1
International Edition   978-0-7020-7003-7

Printed in China
Last digit is the print number: 9   8   7   6   5   4   3   2   1

Content Strategist: Pauline Graham
Content Development Specialist: Fiona Conn
Project Manager: Andrew Riley
Design: Christian Bilbow
Illustration Manager: Amy Faith Heyden
Marketing Manager: Deborah Watkins

Contents

▶ **Self Assessment** *Please check your eBook at* ***https://studentconsult.inkling.com/*** *for self-assessment questions. See inside cover for registration details.*

This is the fifth edition of *Aulton's Pharmaceutics: The Design and Manufacture of Medicines*. The first edition was published in 1988, the second in 2002, the third in 2007 and the fourth in 2013. The pedigree of the book is, however, actually much older. It was originally known as *Tutorial Pharmacy* (which itself went to six editions) and was initially edited by John Cooper and Colin Gunn, and later by Sidney Carter. Professor Mike Aulton and Professor Kevin Taylor continue their editing role and have identified new authors and fresh subject matter for this new edition.

The philosophy of this fifth edition remains unchanged from that of previous editions, i.e. it is intentionally designed and written for newcomers to the design of dosage forms (drug products). Other expert texts can take you into much greater detail for each of the subject areas considered here, once you have mastered these basics. The subject matter of the book remains, in essence, the same but the detail has changed significantly, because pharmaceutics has changed. Since the last edition there have been changes in the way that dosage forms are designed and manufactured and drugs are delivered. These developments are reflected in this new edition.

The involvement of a wide range of authors continues in this edition, all authors being a recognized expert in the field on which they have written. Just as importantly, each author has experience of imparting that information to undergraduate pharmacy and pharmaceutical science students, and to practitioners in the pharmaceutical and associated industries and those working in technical services within hospital pharmacy who are new to the subject. Many authors from the previous edition remain as they are still world leaders in their field. Other chapters have been written by a new generation of experts. The new authorship reflects contemporary knowledge and thinking in pharmaceutics.

The fourth edition of this book saw major restructuring and revision of the text, with the addition of many new chapters and deletion of others. In this edition, the changes have been less radical, but necessary and important nonetheless. Every chapter has received detailed attention and has been revised and updated appropriately to reflect modern thinking and current university curricula worldwide. Some of the basic science remains virtually unchanged – and will always do so – but other areas, particularly biopharmaceutics and some areas of drug delivery, have changed significantly in recent years. Several new authors have been included in this edition to ensure the comprehensive nature and currency of this text.

All purchasers of the print version of this new edition receive the enhanced ebook, which can be used online or downloaded to their mobile device for convenient, any time access. The ebook includes more than 400 self-assessment questions, based on the book, to check understanding and to help with any examination preparation.

We wish you well in your studies if you are an undergraduate student, or with your career if you are working in industry, medicines regulation or the hospital service. We sincerely hope that this book helps you with your understanding of pharmaceutics – the science of the design and manufacture of medicines.

M. E. Aulton
K. M. G. Taylor

Contributors

Göran Alderborn PhD
Professor in Pharmaceutical Technology, Uppsala University, Uppsala, Sweden

Marianne Ashford BSc (Pharm), PhD
Associate Principal Scientist Drug Delivery, AstraZeneca, Macclesfield, UK

David Attwood BPharm, PhD, DSc, CChem, FRSC
Emeritus Professor, University of Manchester, Manchester, UK

Michael E. Aulton BPharm, PhD, FAAPS, FSP, FRPharmS
Emeritus Professor, De Montfort University, Leicester, UK

Susan A. Barker BPharm, PhD
Senior Lecturer in Pharmaceutics, UCL School of Pharmacy, London, UK

Andrew R. Barnes BSc (Pharm), PhD
Quality Assurance Specialist, Pharmacy Quality Assurance Specialist Services, Hellesdon Hospital, Norwich, UK

Abdul W. Basit BPharm, PhD
Professor of Pharmaceutics, UCL School of Pharmacy, London, UK

Steve Brocchini BA, PhD
Professor of Chemical Pharmaceutics, UCL School of Pharmacy, London, UK

Graham Buckton BPharm, PhD, DSc
Emeritus Professor of Pharmaceutics, UCL School of Pharmacy, London, UK

John H. Collett PhD, DSC, FRPharmS
Professor of Pharmaceutics, University of Manchester, Manchester, UK

Soraya Dhillon BPharm, PhD
Professor and Dean, Life and Medical Sciences, University of Hertfordshire, Hatfield, UK

Kalliopi Dodou BSc (Pharm), PhD
Reader, Pharmacy Health and Wellbeing, University of Sunderland, Sunderland, UK

Gillian M. Eccleston BSc, PhD
Professor of Pharmacy, University of Strathclyde, Glasgow, UK

Hala Fadda MPharm, PhD
Associate Professor of Pharmaceutics, College of Pharmacy and Health Sciences, Butler University, Indianapolis, USA

Josephine Ferdinando BSc, MSc, PhD
Senior Vice President, Nonclinical Development, Shire Research and Development, Basingstoke, UK

Ana Cristina Freire PhD
Development Manager, Kuecept, Potters Bar, UK

Göran Frenning
Professor in Pharmaceutical Physics, Uppsala University, Uppsala, Sweden

Simon Gaisford BSc, MSc, PhD
Professor in Pharmaceutics, UCL School of Pharmacy, London, UK

Geoffrey W. Hanlon BSc, PhD
Emeritus Professor of Pharmaceutical Microbiology, University of Brighton, Brighton, UK

Norman A. Hodges MPharm, PhD
Principal Lecturer in Pharmaceutical Microbiology, School of Pharmacy and Biomolecular Sciences, University of Brighton, Brighton, UK

Keith G. Hutchison BSc (Pharm), PhD
Senior Vice President Research and Development,
Capsugel, Bornem, Belgium

Brian E. Jones BPharm, MPharm
Scientific Advisor, Qualicaps Europe, Alcobendas, Spain
Honorary Senior Lecturer, Welsh School of Pharmacy,
Cardiff University, Cardiff, UK

Ashkan Khalili MD, PhD
Research Fellow, UCL School of Pharmacy, London, UK
NIHR Biomedical Research Centre, Moorfields Eye
Hospital and UCL Institute of Ophthalmology, London,
UK

Peng Tee Khaw PhD, FRCP, FRCS, FRCOphth, FRCPath,
FSB, FMedSci
Professor of Ophthalmology, NIHR Biomedical Research
Centre, Moorfields Eye Hospital and UCL Institute of
Ophthalmology, London, UK

Alison B. Lansley BSc (Pharm), PhD
Principal Lecturer, School of Pharmacy and
Biomolecular Sciences, University of Brighton, Brighton,
UK

G. Brian Lockwood BPharm, PhD, MRPharmS
Professor of Pharmaceutical Sciences, University of
Manchester, Manchester, UK

Robert Lowe BPharm
Director of Pharmacy, Quality Assurance Specialist
Services, East of England and Northamptonshire NHS
England, Norwich, UK

Jean-Yves Maillard BSc, PhD
Professor of Pharmaceutical Microbiology, School of
Pharmacy and Pharmaceutical Sciences, Cardiff
University, Cardiff, UK

Christopher Marriott PhD, DSc
Emeritus Professor of Pharmaceutics, King's College
London, London, UK

Paul Marshall BPharm, PhD
Principal Consultant, Integrated Product Development,
PAREXEL International, London, UK

Gary P. Martin BPharm, PhD, FRPharmS
Emeritus Professor of Formulation Science, King's
College London, London, UK

Emma L. McConnell MPharm, PhD, MRPharmS
Medical Writer, KnowledgePoint360 Group,
Macclesfield, UK

Sudaxshina Murdan BPharm, PhD
Reader in Pharmaceutics, UCL School of Pharmacy,
London, UK

Mine Orlu BD, MSc, PhD
Lecturer, UCL School of Pharmacy, London, UK

Yvonne Perrie BSc (Pharm), PhD
Professor of Drug Delivery, University of Strathclyde,
Glasgow, UK

Stuart C. Porter BPharm, PhD
Director and Senior Research Fellow Pharmaceutical
Research and Development, Ashland Specialty
Chemicals, Wilmington, USA

Andreas G. Schätzlein BVMS, DrMedVet
Professor of Translational Therapeutics, UCL School of
Pharmacy, London, UK

Satyanarayana Somavarapu MPharm, PhD
Lecturer in Pharmaceutics, UCL School of Pharmacy,
London, UK

Kevin M. G. Taylor BPharm, PhD, FRPharmS
Professor of Clinical Pharmaceutics, UCL School of
Pharmacy, London, UK

Catherine Tuleu DPharm, MSc, PhD
Reader, UCL School of Pharmacy, London, UK

Andrew M. Twitchell BSc, PhD
Pharmaceutical Assessor, Licensing, Medicines and
Healthcare products Regulatory Agency, London, UK

Ijeoma F. Uchegbu PhD
Professor of Pharmaceutical Nanoscience, UCL School
of Pharmacy, London, UK

Nkiruka Umaru MPharm, PhD
Principal Lecturer in Clinical Pharmacy, School of Life
and Medical Sciences Pharmacy, University of
Hertfordshire, Hatfield, UK

Susannah E. Walsh BSc, PhD, MBA
Principal Lecturer School of Pharmacy, De Montfort
University, Leicester, UK

Adrian C. Williams BSc, PhD
Professor of Pharmaceutics, University of Reading,
Reading, UK

Gareth R. Williams MChem, DPhil
Lecturer in Pharmaceutics, UCL School of Pharmacy,
London, UK

David Wright BPharm, PhD, PGCHE
Professor of Pharmacy, University of East Anglia,
Norwich, UK

Peter York BSc, PhD, DSc
Emeritus Professor, School of Pharmacy, University of
Bradford, Bradford, UK

Acknowledgements

The editors wish to take this opportunity to thank those who have assisted with the preparation of this text. We are extremely indebted to the following:

The authors for the time and quality of effort that they have put into their texts; always under pressure from numerous other commitments, and also from us. Modern life has few spare moments and so the time that they have spent in contributing so knowledgeably and professionally to this text is warmly appreciated.

The many academic and industrial pharmaceutical scientists who helped during the design of the contents and organization of this edition to ensure that it corresponds as closely as possible with modern practice and with the curricula of current pharmacy and pharmaceutical science courses internationally.

The publishing companies who have given their permission to reproduce material in this edition.

The many secretaries and artists who have assisted the authors, editors and publishers in the preparation of their work.

Christine Aulton for typing and other secretarial assistance, and for help in countless other ways that has enabled time to be spent on this edition of the book.

Pauline Taylor for her support and forbearance during the evenings, weekends and holidays spent in the preparation of this book.

Catherine Baumber (Pharmaceutics Department, UCL School of Pharmacy) for her considerable secretarial and administrative support throughout this book's preparation.

John Malkinson (UCL School of Pharmacy) for assistance in the checking of Chapter 7.

Fiona Conn (of Elsevier) for being efficient, pleasant and extremely helpful to the editors and authors during the chapter-creation and chapter-submission phases.

Andrew Riley of Elsevier Production.

On reaching the milestone of the fifth edition of *Aulton's Pharmaceutics*, the editors acknowledge the contribution of all previous authors to earlier editions. Each of the following has left their mark on the book today, and elements of their earlier contributions still remain.

Dr John Richards (Chapters 2 and 3)
Dr John Pugh (Chapter 7)
The late Professor John Staniforth (Chapters 9, 10, 12)
The late Dr Stuart Proudfoot (Chapters 18–22)
Dr Malcolm Summers (Chapter 28)
Dr Josef Tukker (Chapter 41)
Professor Sanjay Garg (Chapter 41)

Mike Aulton
Kevin Taylor

What is 'pharmaceutics'?

Welcome to 'Ceutics!

One of the earliest impressions that many new pharmacy and pharmaceutical science students have of their chosen subject is the large number of long and sometimes unusual-sounding names that are used to describe the various subject areas within pharmacy and the pharmaceutical sciences. The aim of this section is to explain to the reader what is meant by just one of them – *'pharmaceutics'*. It describes how the term has been interpreted for the purpose of this book and how pharmaceutics fits into the overall scheme of pharmaceutical science and the process of designing and manufacturing a new medicine. This note also leads the reader through the organization of this book and explains the reasons why an understanding of the material contained in its chapters is important in the design of modern drug delivery systems.

The word 'pharmaceutics' is used in pharmacy and the pharmaceutical sciences to encompass a wide range of subject areas that are all associated with the steps to which a drug is subjected towards the end of its development. It encompasses the stages that follow on from the discovery or synthesis of the drug, its isolation and purification, and its testing for beneficial pharmacological effects and absence of serious toxicological problems. Put at its simplest – *pharmaceutics converts a drug into a medicine.*

Just a comment here about the word 'drug'. This is the pharmacologically active ingredient in a medicine. 'Drug' is the correct word, but because the word has been somewhat hijacked as the common term for a substance of misuse, alternatives are frequently used, such as 'medicinal agent', 'pharmacological agent', 'active principle', 'active ingredient', or increasingly 'active pharmaceutical ingredient (API)', etc. The book uses the simpler and still correct word, 'drug'. Phrases like 'active ingredient' can suggest that the other ingredients of a medicine have no function at all. This book will teach you loud and clear that this is not the case.

Pharmaceutics, and therefore this book, is concerned with the scientific and technological aspects of the design and manufacture of dosage forms. Arguably, it is the most diverse of all the subject areas in the pharmaceutical sciences and encompasses:

- an understanding of the basic physical chemistry necessary for the effective design of dosage forms (physical pharmaceutics)
- an understanding of relevant body systems and how drugs arrive there following administration (biopharmaceutics)
- the design and formulation of medicines (dosage form design)
- the manufacture of these medicines on a small (compounding), intermediate (pilot-scale) and large (manufacturing) scale
- the avoidance and elimination of microorganisms in medicines (pharmaceutical microbiology, sterilization), and
- product performance testing (physical testing, drug release, stability testing).

Medicines are *drug-delivery systems*. That is, they are a means of administering drugs to the body in a safe, effective, accurate, reproducible and convenient manner. The book discusses the overall considerations that must be made so that the conversion of a drug

1

to a medicine can take place. It emphasizes the fact that medicines are very rarely drugs alone but require additives (termed excipients) to make them into dosage forms, and this in turn introduces the concept of formulation. The book explains that there are three major considerations in the design of dosage forms:

1. the physicochemical properties of the drug itself
2. biopharmaceutical considerations, such as how the administration route and formulation of a dosage form affect the rate and extent of drug absorption into the body, and
3. therapeutic considerations of the disease state and patient to be treated, which in turn determine the most suitable type of dosage form, possible routes of administration and the most suitable duration of action and dose frequency for the drug in question.

The first chapter provides an excellent introduction to the subject matter of the book as a whole and clearly justifies the need for the pharmacist and formulation scientist to understand the science contained in this text. New readers are encouraged to read this chapter first, thoroughly and carefully, so that they can grasp the basics of the subject before proceeding onto the more detailed information that follows.

The book is then divided into various Parts that group together chapters into related subject areas. Part 1 collects some of the more important physicochemical knowledge that is required to design and prepare dosage forms. The chapters have been designed to give the reader an insight into those scientific and physicochemical principles that are important to the formulation scientist. These chapters are not intended as a substitute for a thorough understanding of physical chemistry and many specific, more detailed, texts are available containing this information.

For many reasons, which are discussed in the book, the vast majority of dosage forms are administered via the mouth in the form of solid products, such as tablets and capsules. This means that one of the most important stages in drug administration is the dissolution of solid particles to form a solution in the gastrointestinal tract. The formulation scientist therefore needs knowledge of both liquid and solid materials, in particular the properties of drugs in solution and the factors influencing their dissolution from solid particles. Once solutions are formed, the formulation scientist must understand the properties

of these solutions. The reader will see later in the book how drug release from the dosage form and absorption of the drug into the body across biological barriers are strongly dependent on the properties of the drug in solution, such as the degree of ionisation and speed of diffusion of the drug molecules.

The properties of surfaces and interfaces are described next. These are important to an understanding of adsorption onto solid surfaces, and are involved in the dissolution of solid particles and the study of disperse systems, such as colloids, suspensions and emulsions. The scientific background to the systems mentioned is also discussed. Knowledge of the flow properties of liquids (whether solutions, suspensions or emulsions) and semisolids is useful in solving certain problems relating to the manufacture, performance and stability of liquid and semi-solid dosage forms. This Part ends with an explanation of the kinetics of many different processes. As the chapter explains, the mathematics of these processes has importance in a large number of areas of product design, manufacture, storage and drug delivery. Relevant processes include: dissolution, microbiological growth and destruction, biopharmaceutics (including drug absorption, distribution, metabolism and excretion), preformulation, the rate of drug release from dosage forms, and the decomposition of medicinal compounds and products.

Part 2 collects together those aspects of pharmaceutics associated with powdered materials. By far the majority of drugs are solid (mainly crystalline) powders and, unfortunately, most of these particulate solids have numerous adverse characteristics that must be overcome or controlled during the design of medicines to enable their satisfactory manufacture and subsequent performance in dosage forms.

The book therefore explains the concept of the solid state and how the internal and surface properties of solids are important and need to be characterized. This is followed by an explanation of the more macroscopic properties of powders that influence their performance during the design and manufacture of dosage forms – particle size and its measurement, size reduction, and the separation of powders with the desired size characteristics from those of other sizes. There follows an explanation of the many problems associated with the mixing and flow of powders. In large-scale tablet and capsule production, for example, powders must contain a satisfactory mix of all the ingredients in order to achieve uniformity of dosage in every dosage unit manufactured. The powder must have fast and uniform powder flow in high-speed tableting and encapsulation machines. For convenience, the mixing of liquids and semisolids is also discussed here as the basic theory is the same.

Another extremely important area that must be understood before a satisfactory dosage form can be designed and manufactured is the microbiological aspects of medicines development and production. It is necessary to control or eliminate viable micro-organisms from the product both before and during manufacture. Microbiology is a very wide-ranging subject. This book concentrates only on those aspects of microbiology that are directly relevant to the design, production and distribution of dosage forms. This mainly involves avoiding (asepsis) and eliminating (sterilization) the presence (contamination) of viable microorganisms in medicines, and preventing the growth of any microorganism which might enter the product during storage and use of the medicine (preservation). Techniques for testing that these intentions have been achieved are also described. The principles and practice of sterilization are also discussed. The relevant aspects of pharmaceutical microbiology and sterilization are considered in Part 3 of this book.

It is not possible to begin to design a satisfactory dosage form without knowledge and understanding of how drugs are absorbed into the body, the various routes that can be used for this purpose and the fate of the drugs once they enter the body and reach their site(s) of action. The terms 'bioavailability' and 'biopharmaceutics' are defined and explained in Part 4. The factors influencing the bioavailability of a drug and methods of its assessment are described. This is followed by a consideration of the manner in which the frequency of drug administration and the rate at which drug is released from a dosage form affect its concentration in the blood plasma at any given time. This book concentrates on the preparation, administration, release and absorption of drugs but stops there. It leaves to other texts the detail of how drugs enter individual cells, how they act and how they are metabolized and eliminated from the body.

Having gathered this understanding of the basics of pharmaceutics, the formulation scientist should now be equipped to begin a consideration of the design and manufacture of the most suitable dosage forms for the drug in question.

Superficially, the formulation and manufacture of dosage forms containing drugs may seem relatively straightforward. The chapters in Part 5 will demonstrate that this is not the case. The full potential of the active pharmaceutical ingredient, whether it is a small synthetic molecule, a plant extract or a biotechnology product can only be achieved by the involvement of the formulation scientist. Good formulation can enhance therapeutic efficacy and/or limit adverse effects. A couple of examples illustrate this:

- Whilst an immediate-release capsule of nifedipine has a dosing frequency of three times a day, formulation of the drug in a modified-release capsule permits once-daily dosing, with an improved drug plasma profile and increased patient convenience and adherence.
- A cream formulation of a sunscreen applied to the skin restricts the active component(s) to the skin surface, whilst a gel formulation of estradiol, also applied to the skin surface, is formulated so as to ensure effective penetration of drug through the skin and into the systemic circulation.

The first stage of designing and manufacturing a dosage form is known as preformulation. This, as the name implies, is a consideration of the steps that need to be performed before formulation proper can begin. Preformulation involves a full understanding of the physicochemical properties of drugs and other ingredients (excipients) in a dosage form and how they may interact. An early grasp of this knowledge is of great use to the formulation scientist as the data gathered in these early stages will influence strongly the design of the future dosage form. Results of tests carried out at this stage of development can give a much clearer indication of the possible (and indeed impossible) dosage forms for a new drug candidate.

Following, consideration of preformulation, the remaining chapters of Part 5 cover the formulation, small and large scale manufacture, and the advantages, disadvantages and characterization of the wide range of available dosage forms. The properties of these dosage forms can be modified dependent on the properties of the drug, excipients included, the route of drug administration and specific patient needs. Early chapters consider liquid dosage forms, namely solutions (drug dispersed as molecules or ions), suspensions (drug dispersed as particles) and emulsions (one liquid phase dispersed in another, with drug present in either phase, dependent upon its relative solubility). Appropriate formulation of emulsions results in more structured semi-solid creams, most frequently used for application to the skin.

These dosage forms may be administered by a number of routes, and their formulation requirements will vary dependent on the route of administration.

Whilst drugs in the solid state can be administered as simple powders, they are more usually formulated as solid dosage forms, namely tablets (currently the most commonly encountered solid dosage form) and capsules. Several chapters in this Part describe the various stages in the processing of a powder required to manufacture tablets: granulation (formation of drug-excipient aggregates), drying, compaction and coating. Tablet formulation and manufacture requires inclusion of several excipients, including fillers, disintegrants, binders, glidants, lubricants and anti-adherents. The purposes of these are described, together with their impact on product quality and performance. The strategies to modify the release of drug from solid dosage forms include: production of monolithic matrix systems, the use of a rate-controlling membrane or osmotic pump systems. These are described in a separate chapter, as are other solid dosage forms: hard and soft capsules. For all dosage forms, drug must be released at an appropriate rate at the appropriate site for drug action and/or absorption to occur. This is particularly pertinent for solid peroral dosage forms, which must permit dissolution of drug at an appropriate rate and at an appropriate site within the gastrointestinal tract. Bioavailability (i.e. the amount of drug that is absorbed into the bloodstream) may be limited by the rate of drug dissolution, whilst the pH range in the gastrointestinal tract (pH 1–8) may adversely affect the absorption of ionizable drugs. Consequently, dissolution testing is a key quality control test and is considered in detail here.

Solid dosage forms are administered predominantly (though not exclusively) by the oral route. Whilst the oral route is the most common way of administering drugs, many other routes for administration exist and are necessary. Each of these is considered in detail. Such routes include parenteral administration (injections, infusions, implants), pulmonary (aerosols), nasal (sprays, drops, semisolids, powders), ocular (drops, semisolids, injection, implants), topical and transdermal (semisolids, patches, liquids, powders), ungual (nail lacquers, liquids), rectal (suppositories, tablets, capsules, semisolids, liquids, foams) and vaginal (pessaries, semisolids, films, rings, tampons). For each route, consideration is given to the nature of the administration site and the formulation requirements either to localize drug action, or to control absorption, as appropriate. The dosage forms available

for delivering drugs by each route are outlined and particular aspects regarding their formulation and manufacture are highlighted. The methods used to characterize and test these dosage forms, for formulation development and quality assurance purposes are also detailed.

The final chapters of Part 5 reflect special considerations in dosage form design and manufacture. Drugs of natural (plant) origin are discussed. Unlike conventional dosage forms these comprise plant extracts that have many complex components with potentially variable composition.

Certain biotechnology products, for instance insulin, are long established, whilst others such as nucleic acids for gene therapy offer exciting therapeutic possibilities for the future. All are relatively large macromolecules and present particular formulation and drug delivery challenges. To meet some of the challenges associated with delivery of biotechnology products, pharmaceutical nanotechnology has become established in recent years as a means of improving solubility and dissolution rate, protecting drugs from hostile environments, minimizing adverse effects and delivering drugs to specific therapeutic targets. The preparation and properties of various nanomedicines, including antibodies, polymer-drug conjugates, liposomes, nanoparticles and dendrimers are considered.

Some specific patient groups (in particular the elderly and young children) have particular needs (difficulty swallowing, subdivision of commercially available doses, etc.) and the formulation consequences are discussed.

Before finalizing the formulation and packaging of the dosage form, there must be a clear understanding of the stability of the drug(s) and other additives in a pharmaceutical product with respect to the reasons why, and the rates at which, they may degrade during storage. Aspects of product stability, stability testing and the selection of appropriate packaging to minimize deterioration during storage are considered in Part 6.

The product pack and any possible interactions between it and the drug or medicine it contains are so vitally linked that the final pack should not be considered as an afterthought. Instead, packaging considerations should be uppermost in the minds of formulators as soon as they receive the drug substance on which to work. The technology of packaging and filling of products is discussed.

No product will be stable indefinitely, and so mechanisms (i.e. the fundamental chemistry) and kinetics of degradation must be understood so that a safe and realistic shelf-life for every product can be determined.

Possible routes of microbiological contamination of medicines and the ways in which this can be prevented or minimized are discussed. It is shown how the presence of antimicrobial preservatives in the medicine can minimize the consequences of such contamination. However, such preservatives must be nontoxic by the route of administration and should not interact with components of the drug product or its packaging.

Finally, the book explains how packaging considerations, chemical degradation and microbial contamination influence the stability of the final drug product.

At this point the product is considered to be of appropriate quality for patient use and, once approved by regulatory authorities, the pharmaceutical technologist passes the product on to another aspect of pharmacy – the interface with the patient, i.e. dispensing and pharmacy practice. These disciplines are dealt with in other texts.

1

Design of dosage forms

Peter York

Principles of dosage form design

Drugs are rarely administered as pure chemical substances alone and are almost always given as formulated preparations or medicines. These can range from relatively simple solutions to complex drug delivery systems through the use of appropriate additives or excipients in the formulations. The excipients provide varied and specialized pharmaceutical functions. It is the formulation additives that, amongst other things, solubilize, suspend, thicken, preserve, emulsify, modify dissolution, increase the compactability and improve the flavour

of drug substances to form various medicines or dosage forms.

The principal objective of dosage form design is to achieve a predictable therapeutic response to a drug included in a formulation which can be manufactured on a large scale with reproducible product quality. To ensure product quality, numerous features are required: chemical and physical stability, with suitable preservation against microbial contamination if appropriate, uniformity of the dose of the drug, acceptability to users, including both prescriber and patient, and suitable packaging and labelling. Ideally, dosage forms should also be independent of patient-to-patient variation, although in practice this feature remains difficult to achieve. However, recent developments are beginning to accommodate this requirement. These include drug delivery systems that rely on the specific metabolic activity of individual patients and implants that respond, for example, to externally applied sound or magnetic fields to trigger a drug delivery function.

Consideration should be given to differences in the bioavailability of drugs (the rate and extent to which they are absorbed) and their biological fate in patients between apparently similar formulations and possible causative reasons. In recent years, increasing attention has therefore been directed towards elimination of variation in bioavailability characteristics, particularly for medicinal products containing an equivalent dose of a drug substance, as it is recognized that formulation factors can influence their therapeutic performance. To optimize the bioavailability of drug substances, it is often necessary to carefully select the most appropriate chemical form of the drug. For example, such selection should address solubility requirements, drug particle size and drug physical

Table 1.1 Dosage forms available for different administration routes

Administration route	Dosage forms
Oral	Solutions, syrups, suspensions, emulsions, gels, powders, granules, capsules, tablets
Rectal	Suppositories, ointments, creams, powders, solutions
Topical	Ointments, creams, pastes, lotions, gels, solutions, topical aerosols, foams, transdermal patches
Parenteral	Injections (solution, suspension, emulsion forms), implants, irrigation and dialysis solutions
Respiratory	Aerosols (solution, suspension, emulsion, powder forms), inhalations, sprays, gases
Nasal	Solutions, inhalations
Eye	Solutions, ointments, creams
Ear	Solutions, suspensions, ointments, creams

form and should consider appropriate additives and manufacturing aids coupled with selection of the most appropriate administration route(s) and dosage form(s). Additionally, suitable manufacturing processes, labelling and packaging are required.

There are numerous dosage forms into which a drug substance can be incorporated for the convenient and efficacious treatment of a disease. Dosage forms can be designed for administration by a variety of delivery routes to maximize therapeutic response. Preparations can be taken orally or injected, as well as being applied to the skin or inhaled; Table 1.1 lists the range of dosage forms which can be used to deliver drugs by the various administration routes. However, it is necessary to relate the drug substance to the clinical indication being treated before the correct combination of drug and dosage form can be made, as each disease or illness often requires a specific type of drug therapy. In addition, factors governing the choice of administration route and the specific requirements of that route which affect drug absorption need to be taken into account when dosage forms are being designed.

Many drugs are formulated into several dosage forms of various strengths, each having selected pharmaceutical characteristics which are suitable for a specific application. One such drug is the glucocorticoid prednisolone used in the suppression of inflammatory and allergic disorders. Through the use of different chemical forms and formulation additives, a range of effective anti-inflammatory preparations are available, including tablets, gastro-resistant coated tablets, injections, eye drops and enemas. The extremely low aqueous solubility of the base prednisolone and its acetate salt makes these forms useful in tablet and slowly absorbed intramuscular suspension injection forms, whilst the soluble sodium phosphate salt enables preparation of a soluble tablet form and solutions for eye and ear drops, enemas and intravenous injections. The analgesic paracetamol is also available in a range of dosage forms and strengths to meet the specific needs of the user, including tablets, dispersible tablets, paediatric soluble tablets, paediatric oral solution, sugar-free oral solution, oral suspension, double-strength oral suspension and suppositories.

In addition, whilst many new drugs based on low molecular weight organic compounds continue to be discovered and transformed into medicinal products, the development of drugs from biotechnology is increasing and the importance of these therapeutic agents is growing. Such active compounds are macromolecular and of relatively high molecular weight, and include materials such as peptides, proteins and viral components. These drug substances present different and complex challenges in their formulation and processing into medicines because of their alternative biological, chemical and structural properties. Nevertheless, the underlying principles of dosage form design remain applicable.

At present, these therapeutic agents are principally formulated into parenteral and respiratory dosage forms, although other routes of administration are being considered and researched. Delivery of these biotechnologically based drug substances via these routes of administration imposes additional constraints on the selection of appropriate formulation excipients.

Another growing area of clinically important medicines is that of polymer therapeutics. These agents include designed macromolecular drugs, polymer–drug and polymer–protein conjugates as nanomedicines, generally in injection form. These agents can also provide drug-targeting features (e.g. treating specific cancers) as well as modified pharmacokinetic profiles (e.g. changed drug metabolism and elimination kinetics).

It is therefore apparent that before a drug substance can be successfully formulated into a dosage form, many factors must be considered. These can be broadly grouped into three categories:

1. biopharmaceutical considerations, including factors affecting the absorption of the drug substance from different administration routes;

2. drug factors, such as the physical and chemical properties of the drug substance; and

3. therapeutic considerations, including consideration of the clinical indication to be treated and patient factors.

High-quality and efficacious medicines will be formulated and prepared only when all these factors are considered and related to each other. This is the underlying principle of dosage form design.

Biopharmaceutical aspects of dosage form design

Biopharmaceutics can be regarded as the study of the relationship between the physical, chemical and biological sciences applied to drugs, dosage forms and drug action. Clearly, understanding the principles of this subject is important in dosage form design, particularly with regard to drug absorption, as well as drug distribution, metabolism and excretion. In general, a drug substance must be in solution before it can be absorbed via absorbing membranes and epithelia of the skin, gastrointestinal tract and lungs into body fluids. Drugs are absorbed in two general ways: by passive diffusion and by carrier-mediated transport mechanisms. In passive diffusion, which is thought to control the absorption of many drugs, the process is driven by the concentration gradient existing across the cellular barrier, with drug molecules passing from regions of high concentration to regions of low concentration. Lipid solubility and the degree of ionization of the drug at the absorbing site influence the rate of diffusion. Recent research into carrier-mediated transport mechanisms has provided much information and knowledge, providing guidance in some cases for the design of new drug molecules. Several specialized transport mechanisms are postulated, including active and facilitated transport. Once absorbed, the drug can exert a therapeutic effect either locally or at a site of action remote from the site of administration. In the latter case the drug has to be transported in body fluids (Fig. 1.1).

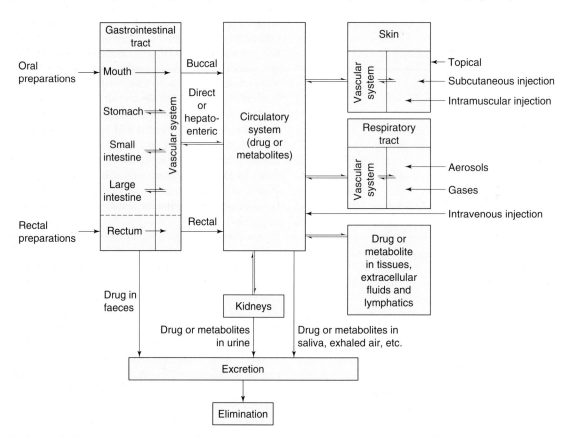

Fig. 1.1 • Pathways a drug may take following the administration of a dosage form by different routes.

When the dosage form is designed to deliver drugs via the buccal, respiratory, rectal, intramuscular or subcutaneous routes, the drug passes directly into the circulating blood from absorbing tissues, whilst the intravenous route provides the most direct route of all. When a drug is delivered by the oral route, onset of drug action will be delayed because of the required transit time in the gastrointestinal tract before absorption, the absorption process and factors associated with hepatoenteric blood circulation. The physical form of the oral dosage form will also influence the absorption rate and onset of action, with solutions acting faster than suspensions, which in turn generally act faster than capsules and tablets. Dosage forms can thus be listed in order of the time of onset of the therapeutic effect (Table 1.2). However, all drugs irrespective of their delivery route remain foreign to the human body, and distribution, metabolic and elimination processes commence immediately following drug absorption until the drug is eliminated from the body via the urine, faeces, saliva, skin or lungs in unchanged or metabolized form.

Routes of drug administration

The absorption pattern of drugs differs considerably between individual drug substances, as well as between the different administration routes. Dosage forms are designed to provide the drug in a suitable form for absorption from each selected route of administration. The following discussion considers briefly the routes of drug administration and, whilst dosage forms are mentioned, this is intended only as an introduction

since they will be dealt with in greater detail later in this book.

Oral route

The oral route is the most frequently used route for drug administration. Oral dosage forms are intended usually for systemic effects resulting from drug absorption through the various epithelia and mucosa of the gastrointestinal tract. A few drugs, however, are intended to dissolve in the mouth for rapid absorption or for local effect in the gastrointestinal tract because of poor absorption by this route or low aqueous solubility. Compared with other routes, the oral route is the simplest, most convenient and safest means of drug administration. However, disadvantages include the relatively slow onset of action and possibilities of irregular absorption and destruction of certain drugs by the enzymes and secretions of the gastrointestinal tract. For example, insulin-containing preparations are inactivated by the action of stomach fluids.

Whilst drug absorption from the gastrointestinal tract follows the general principles described later in this book, several specific features should be emphasized. Changes in drug solubility can result from reactions with other materials present in the gastrointestinal tract; for example, interference with absorption of tetracyclines through the formation of insoluble complexes with calcium, which can be available from foodstuffs or formulation additives.

Gastric emptying time is an important factor for effective drug absorption from the intestine. Slow gastric emptying can be detrimental to drugs inactivated by the gastric juices and can delay absorption of drugs more effectively absorbed from the intestine. In addition, since environmental pH can influence the ionization and lipid solubility of drugs, the pH change occurring along the gastrointestinal tract, from a pH as low as 1 in the stomach to approximately 7 or 8 in the large intestine, is important for both the degree and the site of drug absorption. Since membranes are more permeable to un-ionized forms than to ionized forms and since most drugs are weak acids or bases, it can be shown that weak acids, being largely un-ionized, are well absorbed from the stomach. In the small intestine (pH from approximately 4 to 6.5), with its extremely large absorbing surface, both weak acids and weak bases are well absorbed.

The most popular oral dosage forms are tablets, capsules, suspensions, solutions and emulsions. Tablets

Table 1.2 Variation in time of onset of action for different dosage forms

Time of onset of action	Dosage forms
Seconds	Intravenous injections
Minutes	Intramuscular and subcutaneous injections, buccal tablets, aerosols, gases
Minutes to hours	Short-term depot injections, solutions, suspensions, powders, granules, capsules, tablets, modified-release tablets
Several hours	Gastro-resistant coated formulations
Days to weeks	Depot injections, implants
Varied	Topical preparations

are prepared by compaction and contain drugs and formulation additives which are included for specific functions, such as disintegrants, which promote tablet break-up into granules and powder particles in the gastrointestinal tract, facilitating drug dissolution and absorption. Tablets are often coated, either to provide a protective barrier to environmental factors for drug stability purposes or to mask unpleasant drug taste, as well as to protect drugs from the acid conditions of the stomach (gastro-resistant coating). Increasing use is being made of modified-release tablet products such as fast-dissolving systems and controlled-release, delayed-release or sustained-release formulations. The benefits of controlled-release tablet formulations, achieved, for example, by the use of polymeric-based tablet cores or coating membranes, include reduced frequency of drug-related side effects and maintenance of steady levels of drug in the plasma for extended periods, which are important when medications are delivered for chronic conditions or where constant levels are required to achieve optimal efficacy, as in treatment of angina and hypertension.

Capsules are solid dosage forms containing the drug and, usually, appropriate filler(s), enclosed in a hard or soft shell composed primarily of gelatin or other suitable polymeric material. As with tablets, uniformity of dose can be readily achieved, and various sizes, shapes and colours of the shell are commercially available. The capsule shell readily ruptures and dissolves following oral administration, and in most cases drugs are released from capsules faster than from tablets. Recently, increased interest has been shown in the filling of hard capsules with semisolid and microemulsion formulations to provide rapidly dispersing dosage forms for poorly soluble drugs.

Suspensions, which contain finely divided drugs suspended in a suitable vehicle, are a useful means of administering large amounts of drugs that would be inconvenient if they were taken in tablet or capsule form. They are also useful for patients who experience difficulty in swallowing tablets and capsules and for paediatric use. Whilst dissolution of drugs is required before absorption, the fine solid particles in a suspension have a large surface area to present to the gastrointestinal fluids, and this facilitates drug dissolution, thus aiding absorption and thereby the onset of drug action. Not all oral suspensions, however, are formulated for systemic effects, and several are designed for local effects in the gastrointestinal tract. On the other hand, solutions, including formulations such as syrups and linctuses, are absorbed more rapidly than solid dosage forms or suspensions since drug dissolution is not required.

Rectal route

Drugs given rectally in solution, suppository or emulsion form are generally administered for local rather than systemic effects. Suppositories are solid forms intended for introduction into body cavities (usually rectal but also vaginal and urethral), where they melt, releasing the drug. The choice of suppository base or drug carrier can greatly influence the degree and rate of drug release. This route of drug administration is also indicated for drugs inactivated by the gastrointestinal fluids when given orally or when the oral route is precluded, for example when a patient is vomiting or unconscious. Drugs administered rectally enter the systemic circulation without passing through the liver, an advantage for drugs significantly inactivated by the liver following oral route absorption. Disadvantageously, the rectal route is inconvenient and drug absorption is often irregular and difficult to predict.

Parenteral routes

A drug administered parenterally is one injected via a hollow needle into the body at various sites and to various depths. The three main parenteral routes are subcutaneous, intramuscular and intravenous. Other routes, such as intracardiac and intrathecal, are used less frequently. The parenteral route is preferred when rapid absorption is essential, as in emergency situations or when patients are unconscious or unable to accept oral medication, and in cases when drugs are destroyed, inactivated or poorly absorbed following oral administration. In general, the blood levels attained are more predictable than those achieved by oral dosage forms.

Injectable preparations are usually sterile solutions or suspensions of drugs in water or other suitable physiologically acceptable vehicles. As referred to previously, drugs in solution are rapidly absorbed, and thus suspension injections act more slowly than solution injections. In addition, since body fluids are aqueous, by use of drugs suspended in oily vehicles, a preparation exhibiting slower absorption characteristics can be formulated to give a depot preparation, providing a reservoir of the drug, which is released slowly into the systemic circulation. Such preparations are administered by intramuscular injection deep into skeletal muscles (e.g. several penicillin-containing injections). Alternatively, depot preparations can be achieved by subcutaneous implants or pellets, which are compacted or moulded discs of drug placed in loose subcutaneous tissue under the outer layers of the skin. Such systems include solid microspheres and biodegradable polymeric microspheres (e.g. lactide and glycolic acid homopolymers and copolymers) containing proteins or peptides (e.g. human growth hormone and leuprolide). More generally, subcutaneous injections are aqueous solutions or suspensions which allow the drug to be placed in the immediate vicinity of blood capillaries. The drug then diffuses into the capillaries. Inclusion of vasoconstrictors or vasodilators in subcutaneous injections will clearly influence blood flow through the capillaries, thereby modifying the capacity for absorption. This principle is often used in the administration of local anaesthetics with the vasoconstrictor adrenaline, which delays drug absorption. Conversely, increased drug absorption can result when vasodilators are included. Intravenous administration involves injection of sterile aqueous solutions directly into a vein at an appropriate rate. The volumes delivered can range from a few millilitres, as in emergency treatment or for hypnotics, to litre quantities, as in replacement fluid treatment or parenteral nutrition.

Given the generally negative patient acceptance of this important route of drug delivery, primarily associated with pain and inconvenience, recent developments to help with self-injection by patients have focused on 'needle-free' injection systems and devices which propel the drug in aqueous solution or powder form at high velocity directly through the external layers of the skin.

Topical route

Drugs are applied topically (i.e. to the skin) mainly for local action. Whilst this route can also be used for systemic drug delivery, percutaneous absorption is often poor and erratic, although several transdermal patches delivering drugs for systemic distribution (e.g. fentanyl patches for severe pain management and nicotine patches for cessation of smoking) are available. The drugs applied to the skin for local effect include antiseptics, antifungals and anti-inflammatory agents, as well as skin emollients for protective effects.

Pharmaceutical topical formulations – ointments, creams and pastes – are composed of the drug in a suitable semisolid base which is either hydrophobic or hydrophilic. The bases play an important role in determining the character of drug release from the formulation. Ointments are hydrophobic, oleaginous-based dosage forms, whereas creams are semisolid emulsions. Pastes contain more solids than ointments and thus are stiffer. For topical application in liquid form other than solution, lotions, suspensions of solids in aqueous solution or emulsions are used.

Application of drugs to other topical surfaces such as the eye, ear and nose is common, and ointments, creams, suspensions and solutions are used. Ophthalmic preparations are required, amongst other features, to be sterile. Nasal dosage forms include solutions or suspensions delivered by drops or fine aerosol from a spray. Ear formulations, in general, are viscous to prolong contact with affected areas.

Respiratory route

The lungs provide an excellent surface for absorption when the drug is delivered in gaseous, aerosol mist or ultrafine solid particle form. For drug particles presented to the lungs as an aerosol, particle size largely determines the extent to which they penetrate the alveolar region, the zone of rapid absorption. Drug particles that have diameters in the region of $1\ \mu m$ to $5\ \mu m$ reach the deep lung. Particles smaller than $1\ \mu m$ are largely exhaled, and particles larger than $5\ \mu m$ are deposited on larger bronchial airways. This delivery route is particularly useful for the direct treatment of asthma, with use of both powder aerosols (e.g. salmeterol xinafoate) and pressurized metered-dose inhalers containing the drug in liquefied inert propellant (e.g. salbutamol sulfate inhaler). Importantly, this delivery route is being increasingly recognized as a useful means of administering the therapeutic agents emerging from biotechnology requiring systemic distribution and targeted delivery, such as peptides and proteins.

Drug factors in dosage form design

Each type of dosage form requires careful study of the physical and chemical properties of drug substances to achieve a stable, efficacious product. These properties, such as dissolution, crystal size and polymorphic form, solid-state stability and drug–additive interaction, can have profound effects on the physiological availability and physical and chemical stability of the drug. Through combination of such information and knowledge with that from pharmacological and biochemical studies, the most suitable drug form and additives can be selected for the formulation of chosen dosage forms.

Whilst comprehensive property evaluation will not be required for all types of formulations, those properties which are recognized as important in dosage form design and processing are listed in Table 1.3. The stresses to which the formulation might be exposed during processing and manipulation into dosage forms, as well as the procedures involved are also listed in Table 1.3. Variations in physicochemical properties, occurring, for example, between batches of the same material or resulting from alternative treatment procedures, can modify the formulation requirements, as well as processing and dosage form performance. For instance, the fine milling of poorly water-soluble drug substances can modify their wetting and dissolution characteristics, important properties during granulation and product performance respectively. Careful evaluation of these properties and understanding of the effects of these stresses on these parameters are therefore important in dosage form design and processing, as well as for product performance.

Particle size and surface area

Particle size reduction results in an increase in the specific surface area (i.e. surface area per unit weight)

of powders. Drug dissolution rate, drug absorption rate, drug content uniformity in dosage forms and stability are all dependent to various degrees on particle size, particle size distribution and particle interaction with solid surfaces. In many cases, for both drugs and additives, particle size reduction is required to achieve the desired physicochemical characteristics.

It is now generally recognized that poorly water-soluble drugs showing a dissolution-rate-limiting step in the absorption process will be more readily bioavailable when administered in a finely subdivided form with a larger surface than as a coarse material. Examples include griseofulvin, tolbutamide, indometacin and nifedipine. The fine material, often of micrometre or nanometre size, with large specific surface area, dissolves at a faster rate, which can lead to increased drug absorption by passive diffusion. With many of the new drugs being introduced exhibiting extremely low aqueous solubility, alternative formulation strategies to enhance drug dissolution are being used, such as coprecipitates of drug and adjuvant particles, complexation with hydrophilic polymers or oligosaccharides, or the formation of co-crystals with hydrophilic templating compounds.

The rate of drug dissolution can be adversely affected, however, by unsuitable choice of formulation additives, even though solids of appropriate particle size are used. Tableting lubricant powders, for example, can impart hydrophobicity to a formulation and inhibit drug dissolution. Fine powders can also increase air adsorption or static charge, leading to wetting or agglomeration problems. Micronizing drug powders can lead to changes in crystallinity and particle surface energy which cause reduced chemical stability. Drug particle size also influences content uniformity in solid dosage forms, particularly for low-dose formulations. It is important in such cases to have as many particles as possible per dose to minimize potency variation between dosage units. Other dosage forms are also affected by particle size, including suspensions (for controlling flow properties and particle interactions), inhalation aerosols (for optimal penetration of drug particles to absorbing mucosa) and topical formulations (for freedom from grittiness).

Solubility

All drugs, regardless of their administration route, must exhibit at least limited aqueous solubility for

Table 1.3 Properties of drug substances important in dosage form design and potential stresses occurring during processes, with a range of manufacturing procedures

Properties	Processing stresses	Manufacturing procedures
Particle size, surface area	Pressure	Precipitation
	Mechanical	Filtration
Particle surface chemistry	Radiation	Emulsification
	Exposure to liquids	Milling
Solubility		Mixing
Dissolution	Exposure to gases and liquid vapours	Drying
Partition coefficient		Granulation
	Temperature	Compaction
Ionization constant		Autoclaving
Crystal properties, polymorphism		Crystallization
		Handling
Stability		Storage
Organoleptic		Transport
Molecular weight		

therapeutic efficacy. Thus, relatively insoluble compounds can exhibit erratic or incomplete absorption, and it might be appropriate to use a more soluble salt or other chemical derivatives. Alternatively, micronizing, complexation or solid dispersion techniques might be used. Solubility, and especially the degree of saturation in the vehicle, can also be important in the absorption of drugs already in solution in liquid dosage forms, since precipitation in the gastrointestinal tract can occur, modifying bioavailability.

The solubilities of acidic or basic compounds are pH dependent and can be altered by their forming salts, with different salts exhibiting different equilibrium solubilities. However, the solubility of a salt of a strong acid is less affected by changes in pH than the solubility of a salt of a weak acid. In the latter case, when the pH is lower, the salt hydrolyses to an extent dependent on the pH and pK_a, resulting in decreased solubility. Reduced solubility can also occur for slightly soluble salts of drugs through the common-ion effect. If one of the ions involved is added as a different, more soluble salt, the solubility product can be exceeded and a portion of the drug precipitates.

Dissolution

As mentioned already, for a drug to be absorbed it must first be dissolved in the fluid at the site of absorption. For example, an orally administered drug in tablet form is not absorbed until drug particles are dissolved or solubilized by the fluids at some point along the gastrointestinal tract, depending on the pH–solubility profile of the drug substance. Dissolution describes the process by which the drug particles dissolve.

During dissolution, the drug molecules in the surface layer dissolve, leading to a saturated solution around the particles to form the diffusion layer. Dissolved drug molecules then pass throughout the dissolving fluid to contact absorbing mucosa and are absorbed. Replenishment of diffusing drug molecules in the diffusion layer is achieved by further drug dissolution, and the absorption process continues. If dissolution is fast or the drug remains in solution form, the rate of absorption is primarily dependent on the ability of the drug to traverse the absorbing membrane. If, however, drug dissolution is slow because of its physicochemical properties or formulation factors, then dissolution may be the rate-limiting step in absorption and impacts drug bioavailability.

The dissolution of a drug is described in a simplified manner by the Noyes–Whitney equation:

$$\frac{dm}{dt} = kA(C_s - C)$$

$$(1.1)$$

where dm/dt is the dissolution rate, k is the dissolution rate constant, A is the surface area of dissolving solid, C_s is the drug's solubility and C is the concentration of the drug in the dissolution medium at time t. The equation reveals that the dissolution rate can be raised by increase of the surface area (reducing particle size) of the drug, by increase of the solubility of the drug in the diffusion layer and by increase of k, which in this equation incorporates the drug diffusion coefficient and the diffusion layer thickness. During the early phases of dissolution, $C_s > C$, and if the surface area, A, and experimental conditions are kept constant, then k can be determined for compacts containing drug alone. The constant k is termed the intrinsic dissolution rate constant and is a characteristic of each solid drug compound in a given solvent under fixed hydrodynamic conditions.

Drugs with values of k less than 0.1 mg cm^{-2} usually exhibit dissolution-rate-limited absorption. This value is a helpful guide figure indicating the level below which drug dissolution becomes the rate-limiting step in absorption. Particulate dissolution can also be examined where an effort is made to control A, and formulation effects can be studied.

Dissolution rate data, when combined with solubility, partition coefficient and pK_a data, provide an insight into the potential in vivo absorption characteristics of a drug. However, in vitro tests have significance only when they are related to in vivo results. Once such a relationship has been established, in vitro dissolution tests can be used as a predictor of in vivo behaviour. The importance of dissolution testing, for quality control purposes, has been widely recognized by official compendia, as well as drug regulatory authorities, with the inclusion of dissolution specifications using standardized testing procedures for a range of preparations.

The Biopharmaceutics Classification System (BCS), established in 1995, is a guide for predicting the intestinal absorption of drugs for orally administered medicines on the basis of the solubility, dissolution ability, and permeation ability of drugs. This system has proved extremely useful in aiding the design of oral medicines and has recently been extended with the Biopharmaceutics Drug Disposition

Classification System (BDDCS) to incorporate drug absorption and transport, and the effects of metabolism.

Partition coefficient and pK_a

As pointed out earlier, for relatively insoluble compounds the dissolution rate is often the rate-determining step in the overall absorption process. Alternatively, for soluble compounds the rate of permeation across biological membranes is the rate-determining step. Whilst the dissolution rate can be changed by modification of the physicochemical properties of the drug and/or alteration of the formulation composition, the permeation rate is dependent on the size, relative aqueous and lipid solubilities and ionic charge of drug molecules, factors which can be altered through molecular modifications. The absorbing membrane acts as a lipophilic barrier to the passage of drugs, which is related to the lipophilic nature of the drug molecule. The partition coefficient, for example between oil and water, is a measure of lipophilic character.

Most low molecular weight drugs are weak acids or bases and, depending on the pH, exist in an ionized or un-ionized form. Membranes of absorbing mucosa are more permeable to un-ionized forms of drugs than to ionized species because of the greater lipid solubility of the un-ionized forms and the highly charged nature of the cell membrane, which results in the binding or repelling of the ionized drug, thereby decreasing penetration.

The dominating factors that therefore influence the absorption of weak acids and bases are the pH at the site of absorption and the lipid solubility of the un-ionized species. These factors, together with the Henderson–Hasselbalch equations for calculating the proportions of ionized and un-ionized species at a particular pH, constitute the pH-partition theory for drug absorption. However, these factors do not describe completely the process of absorption as certain compounds with low partition coefficients and/or which are highly ionized over the entire physiological pH range show good bioavailability, and therefore other factors are clearly involved.

Crystal properties: polymorphism

Practically all drug substances are handled in powder form at some stage during their manufacture into dosage forms. However, for those substances composed of or containing powders or compacted powders in the finished product, the crystal properties and solid-state form of the drug must be carefully considered. It is well recognized that drug substances can be amorphous (i.e. without regular molecular lattice arrangements), crystalline, anhydrous, in various degrees of hydration or solvated with other entrapped solvent molecules, as well as differing in crystal hardness, shape and size. In addition, many drug substances can exist in more than one form with different molecular packing arrangements in the crystal lattice. This property is termed polymorphism, and different polymorphs may be prepared by manipulation of the conditions of particle formation during crystallization, such as solvent, temperature and rate of cooling. It is known that only one form of a pure drug substance is stable at a given temperature and pressure, with the other forms, termed metastable, converting at different rates to the stable crystalline form. The different polymorphs differ in their physical properties such as dissolution ability and solid-state stability, as well as processing behaviour in terms of powder flow and compaction during tableting in some cases.

These different crystalline forms can be of considerable importance in relation to the ease or difficulty of formulation and as regards stability and biological activity. As might be expected, higher dissolution rates are obtained for metastable polymorphic forms; for example, the alternative polymorphic forms of rifaximin exhibit different in vitro dissolution rates and bioavailability. In some cases, amorphous forms are more active than crystalline forms.

The polypeptide hormone insulin, widely used in the regulation of carbohydrate, fat and protein metabolism, also demonstrates how differing degrees of activity can result from the use of different crystalline forms of the same agent. In the presence of acetate buffer, zinc combines with insulin to form an extremely insoluble complex of the proteinaceous hormone. This complex is an amorphous precipitate or crystalline product depending on the environmental pH. The amorphous form, containing particles of no uniform shape and smaller than 2 μm, is absorbed following intramuscular or subcutaneous injection and has a short duration of action, whilst the crystalline product, consisting of rhombohedral crystals of size 10 μm to 40 μm, is more slowly absorbed and has a longer duration of action. Insulin preparations which are intermediate in duration of action are prepared by use of physical mixtures of these two products.

Polymorphic transitions can also occur during milling, granulating, drying and compacting operations (e.g. transitions during milling for digoxin and spironolactone). Granulation can result in solvate formation, and during drying, a solvent or water molecule(s) may be lost to form an anhydrous material. Consequently, the formulator must be aware of these potential transformations which can result in undesirable modified product performance, even though routine chemical analyses may not reveal any changes. Reversion from metastable forms, if used, to the stable form may also occur during the lifetime of the product. In suspensions, this may be accompanied by changes in the consistency of the preparation, which affects its shelf life and stability. Such changes can often be prevented by additives, such as hydrocolloids and surface-active agents.

Stability

The chemical aspects of formulation generally centre on the chemical stability of the drug and its compatibility with the other formulation ingredients. In addition, the packaging of the dosage form is an important factor contributing to product stability and must be an integral part of stability testing programmes. It has been mentioned previously that one of the principles of dosage form design is to ensure that the chemical integrity of drug substances is maintained during the usable life of the product. At the same time, chemical changes involving additives and any physical modifications to the product must be carefully monitored to optimize formulation stability.

In general, drug substances decompose as a result of the effects of heat, oxygen, light and moisture. For example, esters such as aspirin and procaine are susceptible to solvolytic breakdown, whilst oxidative decomposition occurs for substances such as ascorbic acid. Drugs can be classified according to their sensitivity to breakdown:

1. stable in all conditions (e.g. kaolin)
2. stable if handled correctly (e.g. aspirin)
3. only moderately stable even with special handling (e.g. vitamins) and
4. very unstable (e.g. certain antibiotics in solution form).

Whilst the mechanisms of solid-state degradation are complex and often difficult to analyse, a full understanding is not a prerequisite in the design of a suitable formulation containing solids. For example, in cases where drug substances are sensitive to hydrolysis, steps such as minimization of exposure to moisture during preparation, low moisture content specifications for the final product and moisture-resistant packaging can be used. For oxygen-sensitive drugs, antioxidants can be included in the formulation and, as with light-sensitive materials, suitable packaging can reduce or eliminate the problem. For drugs administered in liquid form, the stability in solution, as well as the effects of pH over the physiological range of pH 1–8, should be understood. Buffers may be required to control the pH of the preparation to increase stability; where liquid dosage forms are sensitive to microbial attack, preservatives are required.

In these formulations, and indeed in all dosage forms incorporating additives, it is also important to ensure that the components, which may include additional drug substances as in multivitamin preparations, do not produce chemical interactions themselves. Interactions between the drug(s) and added excipients such as antioxidants, preservatives, suspending agents, colourants, tablet lubricants and packaging materials do occur and must be checked for during the design of formulations. In recent years, data from thermal analysis techniques, particularly microcalorimetry and differential scanning calorimetry (DSC), when critically examined, have been found useful in rapid screening for possible drug–additive and drug–drug interactions. For example, DSC has revealed that the widely used tableting lubricant magnesium stearate interacts with aspirin and should be avoided in formulations containing this drug.

Organoleptic properties

Modern medicines require that pharmaceutical dosage forms are acceptable to the patient. Unfortunately, many drug substances in use today are unpalatable and unattractive in their natural state, and dosage forms containing such drugs, particularly oral preparations, may require the addition of approved flavours and/or colours.

The use of flavours applies primarily to liquid dosage forms intended for oral administration. Available as concentrated extracts, solutions, adsorbed onto powders or microencapsulated, flavours are usually composed of mixtures of natural and synthetic materials. The taste buds of the tongue respond quickly to bitter, sweet, salt or acid elements of a flavour. Unpleasant taste can be overcome by use of water-insoluble derivatives of drugs which have little or no taste. An example is the use of amitriptyline pamoate, although other factors, such as bioavailability, must remain unchanged. If an insoluble derivative is unavailable or cannot be used, a flavour or perfume can be used. However, unpleasant drugs in capsules or prepared as coated particles or tablets may be easily swallowed, avoiding the taste buds.

Selection of flavour depends on several factors but particularly on the taste of the drug substance. Certain flavours are more effective at masking various taste elements; for example, citrus flavours are frequently used to combat sour or acid-tasting drugs. The solubility and stability of the flavour in the vehicle are also important. In addition, the age of the intended patient should also be considered, since children, for example, prefer sweet tastes, as well as the psychological links between colours and flavours (e.g. yellow is associated with lemon flavour). Sweetening agents may also be required to mask bitter tastes. Sucrose continues to be used, but alternatives, such as sodium saccharin, which is 200–700 times sweeter depending on the concentration, are available. Sorbitol is recommended for diabetic preparations.

Colours are used to standardize or improve an existing drug colour, to mask a colour change or complement a flavour. Whilst colours are obtained from natural sources (e.g. carotenoids) or are synthesized (e.g. amaranth), most of the colours used are synthetically produced. Dyes may be water soluble (e.g. amaranth) or oil soluble (e.g. Sudan IV) or insoluble in water and oil (e.g. aluminium lakes). Lakes, which are generally calcium or aluminium complexes of water-soluble dyes, are particularly useful in tablets and tablet coatings because of their greater stability to light than corresponding dyes, which also differ in their stability to pH and reducing agents. However, in recent years, the inclusion of colours in formulations has become extremely complex because of the banning of many traditionally used colours in many countries.

Other drug properties

At the same time as ensuring that dosage forms are chemically and physically stable and are therapeutically efficacious, one should also establish that the selected formulation can be efficiently manufactured and, in most cases, on a large scale. In addition to those properties previously discussed such as particle size and crystal form, other characteristics such as hygroscopicity, flowability and compactability are particularly important when solid dosage forms are being prepared where the drugs constitute a large percentage of the formulation. Hygroscopic drugs can require low moisture manufacturing environments and need to avoid water during preparation. Poorly flowing formulations may require the addition of flow agents (e.g. fumed silica). Studies of the compactability of drug substances are frequently undertaken with use of instrumented tablet machines in formulation laboratories to examine the tableting potential of the material so as to foresee any potential problems during compaction, such as lamination or sticking, which may require modification of the formulation or processing conditions.

Therapeutic considerations in dosage form design

The nature of the clinical indication, disease or illness for which the drug is intended is an important factor when one is selecting the range of dosage forms to be prepared. Factors such as the need for systemic or local therapy, duration of action required, and whether the drug will be used in emergency situations need to be considered. In the vast majority of cases, a single drug substance is prepared in a number of dosage forms to satisfy both the particular preferences of the patient or physician and the specific needs of a certain clinical situation. For example, many asthmatic patients use inhalation aerosols, from which the drug is rapidly available to the constricted airways following deep inhalation for rapid emergency relief, and oral products for chronic therapy.

Patients requiring urgent relief from angina pectoris, a coronary circulatory problem, place tablets of glyceryl trinitrate under their tongue (sublingual administration). This results in rapid drug absorption directly into the blood capillaries under the tongue. Thus, whilst systemic effects are generally obtained following oral and parenteral drug administration, other routes can be used as the drug and situation demand. Local effects are generally restricted to dosage forms applied directly, such as those applied to the skin, ear, eye, throat and lungs. Some drugs may be well absorbed by one route but not by another and must therefore be considered individually.

The age of the patient also plays a role in defining the types of dosage forms made available. Infants generally prefer liquid dosage forms, usually solutions and mixtures, given orally. In addition, with liquid preparations, the amount of drug administered can be readily adjusted by dilution to give the required dose for the particular patient, taking the patient's weight, age and condition into account. Children can have difficulty in swallowing solid dosage forms, and for this reason many oral preparations are prepared as pleasantly flavoured syrups or mixtures. Adults generally prefer solid dosage forms, primarily because of their convenience. However, alternative liquid preparations are usually available for those unable to take tablets and capsules.

Interest has grown in the design of drug-containing formulations which deliver drugs to specific 'targets' in the body (e.g. the use of liposomes and nanoparticles), as well as providing drugs over longer periods at controlled rates. Alternative technologies for preparing particles with the required properties – crystal engineering – provide new opportunities. Supercritical fluid processing using carbon dioxide as a solvent or antisolvent is one such method, allowing fine-tuning of crystal properties and particle design and fabrication. Undoubtedly, these new technologies and others, as well as sophisticated formulations, will be required to deal with the advent of gene therapy and the need to deliver such labile macromolecules to specific targets and cells in the body. Interest is also likely to be directed to individual patient requirements such as age, weight and physiological and metabolic factors, features which can influence drug absorption and bioavailability, and the increasing application of diagnostic agents will play a key role in this area.

Other areas of innovation in formulation science responding to drug regulatory agency requirements in applications for marketing authorization of medicines are emerging, such as the concept of 'computational pharmaceutics'. This topic incorporates (1) the use of in silico procedures to predict drug substance properties and (2) decision making and optimization tools, such as experimental design, artificial intelligence and neural computing. All these can facilitate faster and rational design of formulations and manufacturing processes.

Summary

This chapter has demonstrated that the formulation of drugs into dosage forms requires the interpretation and application of a wide range of information and knowledge from several study areas. Whilst the physical and chemical properties of drugs and additives need to be understood, the factors influencing drug absorption and the requirements of the disease to be treated also have to be taken into account when potential delivery routes are being identified. The formulation and associated preparation of dosage forms demand the highest standards, with careful examination, analysis and evaluation of wide-ranging information by pharmaceutical scientists to achieve the objective of creating high-quality, safe and efficacious dosage forms.

Bibliography

Blagden, N., de Matas, M., Gavan, P.T., et al., 2007. Crystal engineering of active pharmaceutical ingredients to improve solubility and dissolution rate. Adv. Drug Deliv. Rev. 59, 617–630.

Brayfield, A. (Ed.), 2014. Martindale: The Complete Drug Reference, thirty-eighth ed. Pharmaceutical Press, London.

British Pharmacopoeia Commission, 2017. British Pharmacopoeia. Stationery Office, London.

Byrn, S.R., Pfeiffer, R.R., Stowell, J.G., 1999. Solid State Chemistry of Drugs, second ed. SSCI, West Lafayette.

Colbourn, E., Rowe, R.C., 2005. Neural computing and formulation optimization. In: Swarbrick, J., Boylan, J. (Eds.), Encyclopedia of Pharmaceutical Technology, third ed. Marcel Dekker, New York.

Duncan, R., 2011. Polymer therapeutics as nanomedicines: new perspectives. Curr. Opin. Biotechnol. 22, 492–501.

Florence, A.T., Attwood, D., 2016. Physicochemical Principles of Pharmacy: In Manufacture, Formulation and Clinical Use, sixth ed. Pharmaceutical Press, London.

Shekunov, B.Yu, York, P., 2000. Crystallisation processes in pharmaceutical technology and drug delivery design. J. Cryst. Growth 211, 122–136.

Wu, C.Y., Benet, L.Z., 2005. Predicting drug disposition via application of BCS: transport/absorption/ elimination interplay and development of a biopharmaceutics drug disposition classification system. Pharm. Res. 22, 11–23.

2

Dissolution and solubility

Michael E. Aulton

CHAPTER CONTENTS

KEY POINTS

- Dissolution rate and solubility are two separate properties. While a solid with a fast dissolution rate often has a high solubility (and vice versa), this is not always the case. The differences are explained in this chapter.
- The process of dissolution involves a molecule, ion or atom of a solid entering a liquid phase in which the solid is immersed.
- The rate of dissolution is controlled either by the speed of removal of the molecule, ion or atom from the solid surface or by the rate of diffusion of that moiety through a boundary layer that surrounds the solid.
- Various factors influence the rate of diffusion of a solute through a boundary layer. Some of these may be manipulated by the formulator.
- It is important for the formulator to be aware of the parameters which affect the solubility of a solid in a liquid phase.
- The dissolution rate and solubility of solids in liquids, gases in liquids and liquids in liquids are each important in pharmaceutical science, and these are discussed.

Introduction

Solutions are encountered frequently in pharmaceutical development, either as a dosage form in their own right or as a clinical trials material. Additionally, almost all drugs function in solution in the body.

This chapter discusses the principles underlying the formation of solutions from a solute and a solvent and the factors that affect the rate and extent of the dissolution process. This process will be discussed particularly in the context of a solid dissolving in a liquid as this is the situation most likely to be encountered in the formation of a drug solution, either during manufacturing or during drug delivery.

Dissolution of gases in liquids, solids in semisolids, liquids in semisolids and liquids in liquids is also encountered pharmaceutically.

Further properties of solutions are discussed in Chapters 3 and 24. Because of the number of principles and properties that need to be considered, the contents of each of these chapters should only be regarded as introductions to the various topics. The student is encouraged, therefore, to refer to the bibliography at the end of each chapter to augment the present contents. The textbook written by Florence & Attwood (2016) is recommended particularly. The authors use a large number of pharmaceutical examples to aid the understanding of physicochemical principles.

Definition of terms

This chapter will begin by clarifying and defining some of the key terms relevant to solutions.

Solution, solubility and dissolution

A *solution* may be defined as a mixture of two or more components that form a single phase which is homogeneous down to the molecular level. The component that determines the phase of the solution is termed the *solvent*; it usually (but not necessarily) constitutes the largest proportion of the system. The other components are termed *solutes*, and these are dispersed as molecules or ions throughout the solvent, i.e. they are said to be *dissolved* in the solvent.

The transfer of molecules or ions from a solid state into solution is known as *dissolution*. Fundamentally, this process is controlled by the relative affinity between the molecules of the solid substance and those of the solvent.

The *extent* to which the dissolution proceeds under a given set of experimental conditions is referred to as the *solubility* of the solute in the solvent. The solubility of a substance is the *amount* of it that has passed into solution when *equilibrium* is established between the solute in solution and the excess (undissolved) substance.

The solution that is obtained under these conditions is said to be *saturated*. A solution with a concentration less than that at equilibrium is said to be *subsaturated*. Solutions with a concentration greater than that at equilibrium can be obtained in certain conditions; these are known as *supersaturated* solutions (see Chapter 8 for further information).

Since the above definitions are general ones, they may be applied to all types of solution involving any of the three states of matter (gas, liquid, solid) dissolved in any of the three states of matter, i.e. solid in liquid, liquid in solid, liquid in liquid, solid in vapour, etc. However, when the two components forming a solution are either both gases or both liquids, then it is more usual to talk in terms of *miscibility* rather than solubility. Other than the name, all principles are the same.

One point to emphasize at this stage is that the rate of solution (dissolution rate) and amount which can be dissolved (solubility) are not the same and are not necessarily related. In practice, high drug solubility is usually associated with a high dissolution rate, but there are exceptions; an example is the commonly used film-coating material hydroxypropyl methylcellulose (HPMC) which is very water soluble yet takes many hours to hydrate and dissolve.

Process of dissolution

Dissolution mechanisms

The majority of drugs are crystalline solids. Liquid, semisolid and amorphous solid drugs do exist but these are in the minority. For now, we will restrict our discussion to dissolution of crystalline solids in liquid solvents. In addition, to simplify the discussion, it will be assumed that the drug is molecular in nature. The same discussion applies to ionic drugs. Similarly, to avoid undue complication in the explanations that follow, it can be assumed that most solid crystalline materials, whether drugs or excipients, will dissolve in a similar manner.

The dissolution of a solid in a liquid may be regarded as being composed of two consecutive stages.

1. First is an *interfacial reaction* that results in the liberation of solute molecules from the solid phase to the liquid phase. This involves a phase change so that molecules of the solid become molecules of the solute in the solvent in which the crystal is dissolving.

2. After this, the solute molecules must migrate through the boundary layer surrounding the crystal to the bulk of solution.

These stages, and the associated solution concentration changes, are illustrated in Fig. 2.1.

These two stages of dissolution are now discussed in turn.

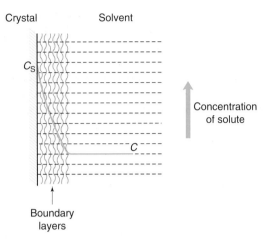

Fig. 2.1 • Boundary layer and concentration change surrounding a dissolving particle.

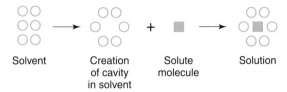

Fig. 2.3 • The theory of cavity creation in the mechanism of dissolution.

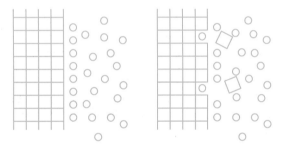

Fig. 2.2 • Replacement of crystal molecules with solvent molecules during dissolution.

Interfacial reaction

Leaving the surface. Dissolution involves the replacement of crystal molecules by solvent molecules. This is illustrated in Fig. 2.2.

The process of the removal of drug molecules from a solid, and their replacement by solvent molecules, is determined by the relative affinity of the various molecules involved. The solvent/solute forces of attraction must overcome the cohesive forces of attraction between the molecules of the solid.

Moving into the liquid. On leaving the solid surface, the drug molecule must become incorporated in the liquid phase, i.e. within the solvent. Liquids are thought to contain a small amount of so-called free volume. This can be considered to be in the form of 'holes' that, at a given instant, are not occupied by the solvent molecules themselves. Individual solute molecules are thought to occupy these holes, as shown in Fig. 2.3.

The process of dissolution may be considered, therefore, to involve the relocation of solute molecules from an environment where they are surrounded by other identical molecules, with which they undergo intermolecular attraction, into a cavity in a liquid where they are surrounded by nonidentical molecules, with which they may interact to different degrees.

Diffusion through the boundary layer

This step involves transport of the drug molecules away from the solid–liquid interface into the bulk of the liquid phase under the influence of diffusion or convection. Boundary layers are static or slow-moving layers of liquid that surround all solid surfaces that are surrounded by liquid (discussed further later in this chapter and in Chapter 6). Mass transfer occurs more slowly (usually by diffusion; see Chapter 3) through these static or slow-moving layers. These layers inhibit the movement of solute molecules from the surface of the solid to the bulk of the solution. The solution adjacent to the solid will be saturated (because it is in direct contact with undissolved solid). During diffusion, the solution in the boundary layer changes from being saturated (C_S) at the crystal surface to having a concentration equal to that of the bulk of the solution (C) at its outermost limit, as shown in Fig. 2.1.

Energy/work changes during dissolution

For the process of dissolution to occur spontaneously at a constant pressure, the accompanying change in free enthalpy (i.e. the change in Gibbs free energy, ΔG) must be negative. The free energy (G) is a measure of the energy available to the system to perform work. Its value decreases during a spontaneously occurring process until an equilibrium position is reached when no more energy can be made available, i.e. $\Delta G = 0$ at equilibrium.

In most cases heat is absorbed when dissolution occurs, and the process is usually defined as an *endothermic* one and the solution often cools. In some systems, where there is marked affinity between solute and solvent, the process is an *exothermic* one and heat may be evolved.

Dissolution rates of solids in liquids

Like any reaction that involves consecutive stages, the *overall* rate of dissolution will be dependent on which of the steps previously described is the slowest (the *rate-determining* or *rate-limiting step*). In dissolution, the interfacial step (as described earlier) is almost always virtually instantaneous, and so the rate of dissolution will most frequently be determined by the rate of the slower step of diffusion of dissolved solute through the static boundary layer of liquid that exists at a solid–liquid interface.

Interface-controlled dissolution rate

On the rare occasions when the release of the molecule from the solid into solution is slow and the transport across the boundary layer to the bulk solution is faster, dissolution is said to be *interfacially controlled*.

Diffusion-controlled dissolution rate

If the rate of diffusion of the solute molecules through the boundary layer is the slowest step, dissolution is said to be *diffusion controlled*. The movement of solute molecules through the boundary layer will obey Fick's first law of diffusion. This law states that the rate of change in the concentration of a dissolved material with time is directly proportional to the concentration difference between the two sides of the diffusion layer, i.e.

$$\frac{dC}{dt} \propto \Delta C$$

(2.1)

or

$$\frac{dC}{dt} = k\Delta C$$

(2.2)

where C is the concentration of solute in solution at any position and at time t, and the constant k is the *rate constant* (s^{-1}). The energy difference between the two concentration states provides the driving force for the diffusion.

In the present context, ΔC is the difference in the concentration of the solution at the solid surface (C_1) and the bulk of the solution (C_2). Thus $\Delta C = C_1 - C_2$. If C_2 is less than saturation, the molecules will move from the solid to the bulk of solution (as during dissolution). If the concentration of the bulk (C_2) is greater than saturation, the solution is referred to as being *supersaturated* and movement of solid molecules will be in the direction of bulk solution to the surface (as occurs during crystallization).

Noyes–Whitney equation

An equation known as the Noyes–Whitney equation was developed to define the dissolution from a single spherical particle. This equation has found great usefulness in the estimation or prediction of the dissolution rate of pharmaceutical particles. The rate of mass transfer of solute molecules or ions through a static diffusion layer (dm/dt) is directly proportional to the area available for molecular or ionic migration (A) and the concentration difference (ΔC) across the boundary layer and is inversely proportional to the thickness of the boundary layer (h). This relationship is shown in Eq. 2.3:

$$\frac{dm}{dt} = \frac{k_1 A \Delta C}{h}$$

(2.3)

The constant k_1 is known as the *diffusion coefficient*. It is commonly given the symbol D and has the units of $m^2\ s^{-1}$).

An alternative form of the Noyes-Whitney equation can be used when, at equilibrium, the solution in contact with the solid (C_1) will be saturated. In this case, the symbol C_S is used. It is also common practice to use the symbol C in place of C_2 (the bulk concentration). This gives Eq. 2.4:

$$\frac{dm}{dt} = \frac{k_1 A (C_S - C)}{h}$$

(2.4)

If the volume of the solvent is large, or solute is removed from the bulk of the dissolution medium by some process at a faster rate than it passes into solution, then C remains close to zero and the term $(C_S - C)$ in Eq. 2.4 may be approximated to C_S. In practice, if the volume of the dissolution medium is so large that C is not allowed to exceed 10% of the

Table 2.1 Factors affecting in vitro dissolution rates of solids in liquids

Term in the Noyes–Whitney equation (Eq. 2.4)	Affected by
A: surface area of undissolved solid (rate of dissolution increases proportionally with increasing A)	Size of solid particles (A increases with particle size reduction) Dispersibility of powdered solid in dissolution medium Porosity of solid particles
C_S: saturated solubility of solid in dissolution medium (Rate of dissolution increases proportionally with increasing difference between C_S and C. Thus high C_S speeds up dissolution rate)	Temperature Nature of dissolution medium Molecular structure of solute Crystalline form of solid Presence of other compounds
C: concentration of solute in solution at time t (Rate of dissolution increases proportionally with increasing difference between C_S and C. Thus low C speeds up dissolution rate)	Volume of dissolution medium (increased volume decreases C) Any process that removes dissolved solute from the dissolution medium (hence decreasing C)
k: dissolution rate constant	Diffusion coefficient D of solute in the dissolution medium Viscosity of medium
h: thickness of boundary layer (Rate of dissolution decreases proportionally with increasing boundary layer thickness)	Degree of agitation of dissolution medium (increased agitation decreases boundary layer thickness)

value of C_S, then the same approximation may be made. In either of these circumstances dissolution is said to occur under 'sink' conditions and Eq. 2.4 may be simplified to

$$\frac{dm}{dt} = \frac{k_1 A C_S}{h}$$

(2.5)

Sink conditions may arise in vivo when a drug is absorbed into the body from its solution in the gastrointestinal fluids at a faster rate than it dissolves in those fluids from a solid dosage form, such as a tablet. The phrase is illustrative of the solute molecules 'disappearing down a sink'!

If solute is allowed to accumulate in the dissolution medium to such an extent that the aforementioned approximation is no longer valid, i.e. when $C >$ ($C_S/10$), then 'nonsink' conditions are said to be in operation. When C builds up to such an extent that it equals C_S, i.e. the dissolution medium is saturated with solute, it is clear from Eq. 2.4 that the overall rate of dissolution will be zero.

Factors affecting the rate of dissolution of diffusion-controlled systems

The various factors that affect the in vitro rate of diffusion-controlled dissolution of solids in liquids can be predicted by examination of the Noyes–Whitney equation (Eq. 2.3 or Eq. 2.4). Most of the effects of these factors are included in the summary given in Table 2.1.

Clearly, increases in those factors in the numerator on the right-hand side of the Noyes–Whitney equation will increase the rate of diffusion (and therefore the overall rate of dissolution), and increases in factors in the denominator of the equation will result in a decreased rate of dissolution. The opposite situation obviously applies regarding a reduction in these parameters. Each of these is discussed in the following sections.

Surface area of undissolved solid (A)

Size of solid particles. The Noyes–Whitney equation (Eq. 2.4) shows that there is a directly proportional increase in dissolution rate with increasing area of solid available for dissolution. The surface area of a fixed mass of isodiametric particles is inversely proportional to the particle size, i.e. as the particle size is reduced, the area of solid surface available to the liquid phase increases. The effect can be visualized in Fig. 2.4, and the consequences are described in Box 2.1.

A further illustration of this property is shown in Table 2.2, with the increase in surface area as the particle size is decreased quantified mathematically. In each row of Table 2.2 the mass and volume of

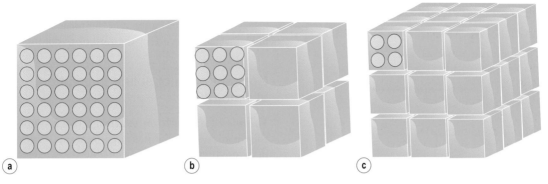

Fig. 2.4 • Visualization of increase in available surface area as the particle size of a fixed mass of powder is reduced.

  Box 2.1

Worked example

Consider the model size reduction shown in Fig. 2.4. The total surface area is equal to the surface area of each particle (approximated here as a cube) multiplied by the number of cubes in total. Considering the surface area in terms of the number of molecules available for dissolution (represented by light green spheres) that can fit around the surface, it can be seen that:

In Fig. 2.4a, $36 \times 6 = 216$ molecules can be accommodated on the surface of the single starting cube. These will be in contact with the dissolution medium and available for dissolution.

In Fig. 2.4b, $9 \times 6 = 54$ molecules can be accommodated on the surface of each cube. For all eight cubes this gives 432 molecules that will be in contact with the dissolution medium and available for dissolution.

In Fig. 2.4c, $4 \times 6 = 24$ molecules can be accommodated on the surface of each cube. For all 27 cubes this gives 648 molecules that will be in contact with the dissolution medium and available for dissolution.

Note that the total *mass* of the solid remains unchanged during the size reduction.

Table 2.2 Calculation of the surface area generated during size reduction of a single cube

Dimensions of one face of each cubic particle	Number of cubic particles (with same total mass)	Area of one face of each particle	Total surface area of one particle (i.e. all six faces)	Total surface area of all particles
100 μm × 100 μm	1	10 000 μm²	60 000 μm²	60 000 μm²
10 μm × 10 μm	1000 (10 × 10 × 10)	100 μm²	600 μm²	600 000 μm²
1 μm × 1 μm	1 000 000 (100 × 100 × 100)	1 μm²	6 μm²	6 000 000 μm²

solid material remain the same; however, the increase in surface area is dramatic as the size of the particles is reduced. In order to simplify the explanation, the particles are assumed to be cubes and remain as cubes during size reduction.

It can be seen that reducing the size of the same mass of powder from one 100 μm cube to 1000 10 μm cubes will increase the surface area by a factor of 10. Further size reduction to 1 000 000 1 μm cubes will result in a further tenfold increase in area. Thus there is an overall increase by a factor of 100.

There is much practical evidence to show that, in general, milling or other means of particle size reduction will increase the rate of dissolution of sparingly soluble drugs.

Dispersibility of powdered solid in dissolution medium. If solid particles form cohered masses in the dissolution medium, then the surface area available for dissolution is reduced. This effect may be overcome by the addition of a wetting agent to improve the dispersion of the solid into primary powder particles.

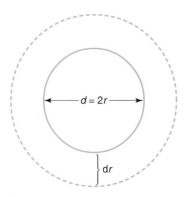

Fig. 2.5 • The reduction in surface area and volume during the dissolution of a spherical particle.

Porosity of solid particles. Pores in some materials, particularly granulated ones, may be large enough to allow access of the dissolution medium into these pores, dissolution to occur within the pores and then outward diffusion of dissolved solute molecules.

Changing area during dissolution. An added complication in practice is that the particle size will change during the dissolution process, because large particles will become smaller and will eventually disappear. This effect is shown in Fig. 2.5.

Compacted masses of solid may also disintegrate into smaller particles, thus increasing the surface area available for dissolution as the disintegration process progresses. (This effect is shown in Fig. 30.7 and explained further in the associated discussion).

Solubility of solid in dissolution medium (C_S)

Temperature. Dissolution may be an exothermic or an endothermic process. Temperature changes will influence the energy balance and thus the energy available to promote dissolution. These relationships are discussed later in this chapter in the section headed 'Factors affecting the solubility of solids in liquids'.

Nature of dissolution medium. Factors such as solubility parameters, pH and the presence of cosolvents will affect the rate of dissolution.

Molecular structure of solute. The use of salts of either weakly acidic or weakly basic drugs, or esterification of neutral compounds, can influence solubility and the dissolution rate.

Crystalline form of solid. The presence of polymorphs, hydrates, solvates or the amorphous form of the drug can have an influence on the dissolution rate and solubility (see later in this chapter and Chapter 8).

Presence of other compounds. The common-ion effect, complex formation and the presence of solubilizing agents can affect the rate of dissolution.

Concentration of solute in solution at time t (C)

Volume of dissolution medium. If the volume of the dissolution medium is large (whether in vitro or in vivo), then C may be negligible with respect to C_S and thus 'sink' conditions will operate. If the volume is small, C can rapidly increase during dissolution and approach C_S. The volume of the dissolution can be controlled easily in vitro but must be taken into account in vivo as the volume of the stomach contents can vary greatly. The common instruction 'To be taken with a glass of water' takes this into account. In addition, the volume of the fluid at other drug delivery sites, e.g. in the rectum and vagina, is small (see Chapter 41) and so this consideration can be important in drug delivery from suppositories and pessaries.

Any process that removes dissolved solute from the dissolution medium. Adsorption onto an insoluble adsorbent, partitioning into a second liquid that is immiscible with the dissolution medium, and removal of solute by dialysis or by continuous replacement of solution by fresh dissolution medium can all result in a decrease in C and thus an increased rate of dissolution. This can also occur in vivo in the case of a drug with a high gastrointestinal tract permeability, i.e. a high rate of absorption.

In the case of a drug that has very low aqueous solubility and poor absorption, the concentration of the drug in solution in the gastrointestinal tract (C) may rise until it is equal to C_S. At that point ($C_S - C$) will be zero, and hence from the Noyes–Whitney equation (Eq. 2.4) the rate of dissolution will be zero, i.e. dissolution will cease. This scenario is sometimes called *solubility-limited dissolution*.

Dissolution rate constant (k)

Thickness of the boundary layer. This is affected in vitro by the degree of agitation, which in turn depends on the speed of stirring or shaking, the shape, size and position of the stirrer, the volume of the dissolution medium, the shape and size of the container, and the viscosity of dissolution medium. Note the inverse relationship in the Noyes–Whitney equation (Eq. 2.4) between rate of dissolution ($dm/$

dt) and the thickness of the boundary layer (h). Decreasing the thickness of the boundary layer (e.g. by increased agitation) increases the rate of dissolution. It is beyond the control of the formulator to manipulate boundary layer thickness in vivo.

Diffusion coefficient of solute in the dissolution medium. The diffusion coefficient of the solute in the dissolution medium is affected by the viscosity of the dissolution medium, and the molecular characteristics and size of diffusing molecules.

It should be borne in mind that pharmaceutical scientists are often concerned with the rate of dissolution of a drug from a formulated product such as a tablet or a capsule, as well as with the dissolution rates of pure solids. In practice, the rate of dissolution can have zero-order, first-order, second-order or cube-root kinetics. These are discussed later in the book when they are relevant to particular dosage forms. Later chapters in this book can also be consulted for information on the influence of formulation factors on the rates of release of drugs into solution from various dosage forms.

Intrinsic dissolution rate

Since the rate of dissolution is dependent on so many factors, it is advantageous to have a measure of the rate of dissolution that is independent of some of these – rate of agitation and area of solute available in particular.

A useful parameter is the *intrinsic dissolution rate* (IDR). The IDR is the rate of mass transfer per unit area of dissolving surface and typically has the unit of mg mm^{-2} s^{-1}). The IDR should be independent of the boundary layer thickness and the volume of the solvent (i.e. it is assumed that sink conditions have been achieved). The IDR is given by

$$\text{IDR} = k_1 C_S$$

$$(2.6)$$

Thus the IDR measures the intrinsic properties of the drug only as a function of the dissolution medium, e.g. its pH, ionic strength, and presence of counterions, and is independent of many other factors.

Techniques for measuring the IDR

Rotating and static disc methods are used. In these methods, the compound to be assessed for the rate of dissolution is compacted into a nondisintegrating disc. This is mounted in a holder so that only one face of the disc is exposed to the dissolution medium

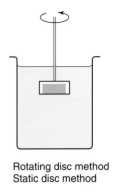

Rotating disc method
Static disc method

Fig. 2.6 • Measurement of intrinsic dissolution rate.

(Fig. 2.6). The holder and disc are immersed in the dissolution medium and either held in a fixed position in the static disc method or rotated at a given speed in the rotating disc method. Samples of dissolution medium are removed after known times, filtered and assayed for the dissolved substance. Further information on this method can be found in Chapter 23.

This design of the test attempts to ensure that the surface area, from which dissolution can occur, remains constant. Under these conditions, the amount of substance dissolved per unit time and unit surface area can be determined. This should be referred to as the *intrinsic dissolution rate* (IDR) and should be distinguished from the measurements obtained by other methods. In nondisc methods (see Chapter 35) the surface area of the drug that is available for dissolution changes considerably during the course of the determination because the dosage form usually disintegrates into many smaller particles and the size of these particles then decreases as dissolution proceeds and, generally, the area of dissolving surface is unknown at any particular time.

Measurement of dissolution rates of drugs from dosage forms

Many methods have been described in the literature, particularly in relation to the determination of the rate of release of drugs into solution from tablet and capsule formulations, because such release may have an important effect on the therapeutic efficacy of these dosage forms (see Chapter 20). In vitro dissolution tests for assessing the rates of dissolution of drugs from solid-unit dosage forms are discussed fully in Chapter 35. Other chapters in Part Five of this book should be referred to for information on the dissolution methods applied to other specific dosage forms.

Solubility

The solution produced when equilibrium is established between undissolved and dissolved solute in a dissolution process is termed a *saturated solution*. The amount of substance that passes into solution in order to establish this equilibrium at constant temperature and so produce a saturated solution is known as the *solubility* of the substance. It is possible to obtain *supersaturated solutions* but these are unstable and precipitation of the excess solute tends to occur readily and spontaneously.

Methods of expressing solubility and concentration

Solubilities may be expressed by any of the variety of concentration terms explained in the following sections. In general, solubility is expressed in terms of the maximum mass or volume of solute that will dissolve in a given mass or volume of solvent at a particular temperature and at equilibrium.

Expressions of concentration

Quantity per quantity

Concentrations are often expressed simply as the weight or volume of solute that is contained in a given weight or volume of the solution. Most solutions encountered in pharmaceutical practice consist of solids dissolved in liquids. Consequently, concentration is expressed most commonly by the weight of solute contained in a given volume of solution. Although the SI unit is kg m^{-3} the terms that are used in practice are based on more convenient or appropriate weights and volumes. For example, in the case of a solution with a concentration of 1 kg m^{-3} the strength may be denoted by any one of the following concentration terms, depending on the circumstances:

1 g L^{-1}, 0.1 g per 100 mL, 1 mg mL^{-1}, 5 mg in 5 mL or 1 µg µL^{-1}.

Percentage

Pharmaceutical scientists have a preference for quoting concentrations in percentages. The concentration of a solution of a solid in a liquid is given by

$$\text{concentration } (\% \text{ w/v}) = \frac{\text{weight of solute}}{\text{volume of solution}} \times 100$$

$$(2.7)$$

Equivalent percentages based on weight (w) and volume (v) ratios (expressed as % v/w, % v/v and % w/w) can also be used for solutions of liquids in liquids and solutions of gases in liquids.

It should be realized that if concentration is expressed in terms of the weight of solute in a given *volume* of solution, then changes in volume caused by temperature fluctuations will alter the concentration.

Parts

Pharmacopoeias give information on the approximate solubility of official substances in terms of the number of 'parts' of solute dissolved in a stated number of 'parts' of solution. Use of this method to describe the concentration of a solution of a solid in a liquid suggests that a certain number of parts by weight (g) of solid are contained in a given number of parts by volume (mL) of solution. In the case of solutions of liquids in liquids, parts by volume of solute in parts by volume of solution are intended, whereas with solutions of gases in liquids, parts by weight of gas in parts by weight of solution are inferred. The use of 'parts' in scientific work, or indeed in practice, is not recommended as there is the chance for some degree of ambiguity.

Molarity

This is the number of moles of solute contained in 1 dm^3 (more commonly expressed in pharmaceutical science as 1 L) of solution. Thus solutions of equal molarity contain the same number of solute molecules in a given volume of solution. The unit of molarity (M) is mol L^{-1} (equivalent to 10^3 mol m^{-3} if converted to the strict SI unit).

Molality

This is the number of moles of solute divided by the mass of the solvent, i.e. its SI unit is mol kg^{-1}. Although it is less likely to be encountered in pharmaceutical science than the other terms, it does offer a more precise description of concentration because it is unaffected by temperature.

Mole fraction

This is often used in theoretical considerations, and is defined as the number of moles of solute divided by the total number of moles of solute and solvent, i.e.

$$\text{mole fraction of solute } (x_1) = \frac{n_1}{n_1 + n_2}$$

$$(2.8)$$

Table 2.3 Descriptive solubility: *United States Pharmacopeia* **and** *European Pharmacopoeia* **terms for describing solubility**

Descriptive term	Approximate volume of solvent (mL) necessary to dissolve 1 g of solute (at a temperature between 15 °C and 25 °C)	Solubility range (mg mL^{-1})
Very soluble	<1	≥1000
Freely soluble	From 1 to 10	100–1000
Soluble	From 10 to 30	33–100
Sparingly soluble	From 30 to 100	10–33
Slightly soluble	From 100 to 1000	1–10
Very slightly soluble	From 1000 to 10 000	0.1–1
Practically insoluble[a]	>10 000	≤ 0.1

Some pharmacopoeias include the term 'partially soluble'. This refers to a mixture of components, of which only some dissolve.
[a]This term is absent from the *European Pharmacopoeia*.

where n_1 and n_2 are the numbers of moles of solute and solvent respectively.

Milliequivalents and normal solutions

The concentrations of solutes in body fluids and in solutions used as replacements for these fluids are usually expressed in terms of the number of millimoles (1 millimol = one-thousandth of a mol) in 1 L of solution. In the case of electrolytes, however, these concentrations may still be expressed in terms of milliequivalents per litre. A milliequivalent (mEq) of an ion is, in fact, one-thousandth of the gram equivalent of the ion, which is, in turn, the ionic weight expressed in grams divided by the valency of the ion. Alternatively,

$$1 \, mEq = \frac{ionic \, weight \, (mg)}{valency}$$

(2.9)

Knowledge of the concept of chemical equivalents is also required in order to understand the use of 'normality' as a means of expressing the concentration of solutions. A *normal solution*, i.e. one with a concentration of 1 N, is one that contains the equivalent weight of the solute, expressed in grams, in 1 L of solution. It was expected that this term would have disappeared following the introduction of SI units but it is still encountered in some volumetric assay procedures.

Qualitative descriptions of solubility

Pharmacopoeias also express approximate solubilities that correspond to descriptive terms such as 'freely soluble' and 'sparingly soluble'. The interrelationship between such terms and approximate solubility is shown in Table 2.3.

Prediction of solubility

Probably the most sought after information about solutions in formulation problems is 'what is the best solvent for a given solute?'. Theoretical prediction of precise solubility is an involved and occasionally unsuccessful operation but, from knowledge of the structure and properties of the solute and solvent, an educated guess is possible. This guess is best expressed in qualitative terms, such as 'very soluble' or 'sparingly soluble', as previously described. Often (particularly in preformulation or early formulation) this approximation is all that the formulator requires. A more precise value can be obtained later in the development process.

Speculation on what is likely to be a good solvent is usually based on the 'like dissolves like' principle. That is, a solute dissolves best in a solvent with similar chemical properties. The concept traditionally follows two rules:

1. Polar solutes will dissolve better in polar solvents.

2. Nonpolar solutes will dissolve better in nonpolar solvents.

Chemical groups that confer polarity to their parent molecules are known as *polar groups*. In the context of solubility, a *polar molecule* has a high dipole moment.

To rationalize these rules, you can consider the forces of attraction between solute and solvent molecules. The following section explains the basic physicochemical properties of solutions that lead to such observations.

Physicochemical prediction of solubility

Similar types of intermolecular force may contribute to solute–solvent, solute–solute and solvent–solvent interactions. The attractive forces exerted between polar molecules are much stronger, however, than those that exist between polar and nonpolar molecules or between nonpolar molecules themselves. Consequently, a polar solute will dissolve to a greater extent in a polar solvent (where the strength of the solute–solvent interaction will be comparable to that between solute molecules) than in a nonpolar solvent (where the solute–solvent interaction will be relatively weak). In addition, the forces of attraction between the molecules of a polar solvent will be too great to facilitate the separation of these molecules by the insertion of a nonpolar solute between them, because the solute–solvent forces will again be relatively weak. Thus solvents for nonpolar solutes tend to be restricted to nonpolar liquids.

These considerations thus follow the very general 'like dissolves like' principle. Such generalizations should be treated with caution in practice, because the intermolecular forces involved in the process of dissolution are influenced by factors that are not obvious from a consideration of the overall polarity of a molecule. For example, the possibility of intermolecular hydrogen bond formation between solute and solvent may be more significant than polarity.

Solubility parameters. Attempts have been made to define a parameter that indicates the ability of a liquid to act as a solvent. The most satisfactory approach, introduced by Hildebrand and Scott in 1962, is based on the concept that the solvent power of a liquid is influenced by its intermolecular cohesive forces and that the strength of these forces can be expressed in terms of a solubility parameter. The initial parameters, which are concerned with the behaviour of nonpolar, noninteracting liquids, are referred to as *Hildebrand solubility parameters*. Whilst these provide good quantitative predictions of the behaviour of a small number of hydrocarbons, they provide only a broad qualitative description of the behaviours of most liquids, because of the influence of factors such as hydrogen bond formation and ionization. The concept has been extended, however, by the introduction of *partial solubility parameters*,

e.g. Hansen parameters and interaction parameters. These have improved the quantitative treatment of systems in which polar effects and interactions occur.

Solubility parameters, in conjunction with the electrostatic properties of liquids, e.g. dielectric constant and dipole moment, have often been linked by empirical or semiempirical relationships either to these parameters or to solvent properties. Studies on solubility parameters are reported in the pharmaceutical literature. The use of dielectric constants as indicators of solvent power has also received attention but deviations from the behaviour predicted by such methods may occur in practice.

Mixtures of liquids are often used as solvents. If the two liquids have similar chemical structures, e.g. benzene and toluene, then neither tends to associate in the presence of the other and the solvent properties of a 50:50 mixture would be the mean of those of each pure liquid. If the liquids have dissimilar structures, e.g. water and propanol, then the molecules of one liquid tend to associate with each other and so form regions of high concentration within the mixture. The solvent properties of this type of system are not so simply related to its composition as in the previous case.

Solubility of solids in liquids

Solutions of solids in liquids are the most common type of solution encountered in pharmaceutical practice. A pharmaceutical scientist should therefore be aware of the general method of determining the solubility of a solid in a liquid and the various precautions that should be taken during such determinations.

Determination of the solubility of a solid in a liquid

The following points should be observed in all solubility determinations:

- The solvent and solute must be as pure as possible. The presence of small amounts of many impurities may either increase or decrease the measured solubility. This is a particular problem with early preformulation samples, which are often impure, and here special care must be taken. This point is discussed further in Chapter 23.
- A saturated solution must be obtained before any solution is removed for analysis and then all

undissolved material must be removed prior to analysis.

- The method of separating a sample of saturated solution from undissolved solute must be satisfactory.
- The method of analysing the solution must be sufficiently accurate and reliable.
- Temperature must be adequately controlled.

A saturated solution is obtained either by stirring excess powdered solute with solvent for several hours at the required temperature, until equilibrium has been attained, or by warming the solvent with an excess of the solute and allowing the mixture to cool to the required temperature. It is essential that some undissolved solid should be present at the completion of the cooling stage to ensure that the solution is saturated and not either subsaturated or supersaturated.

A sample of the saturated solution is obtained for analysis by separating out undissolved solid from the solution. Filtration is usually used, but precautions should be taken to ensure that:

- it is carried out at the temperature of the solubility determination in order to prevent any change in the equilibrium between dissolved and undissolved solute;
- loss of any volatile component does not occur; and
- adsorption of sample material onto surfaces within the filter is minimized.

Membrane filters that can be used in conjunction with conventional syringes fitted with suitable in-line adapters have proved to be successful.

The amount of solute contained in the sample of saturated solution may be determined by a variety of methods, e.g. gravimetric analysis, UV spectrophotometry and chromatographic methods (particularly high-performance liquid chromatography [HPLC]). The selection of an appropriate method is affected by the nature of the solute and the solvent and by the concentration of the solution.

Factors affecting the solubility of solids in liquids

Knowledge of these factors, together with their practical applications, as discussed in the following sections, is an important aspect of a pharmaceutical scientist's expertise. Additional information, which shows how some of these factors may be used to improve the solubility and bioavailability of drugs, is given in Chapters 20 and 24.

Temperature and heat input

The dissolution process is usually an endothermic one, i.e. heat is normally absorbed when dissolution occurs. In this type of system, supply of heat will lead to an increase in the solubility of a solid. Conversely, in the case of the less commonly occurring systems that exhibit exothermic dissolution, which attempt to evolve heat, an increase in supplied heat will result in a decrease in solubility.

Plots of solubility versus temperature, referred to as *solubility curves*, are often used to describe the effect of temperature on a given system. Some examples are shown in Fig. 2.7. Most of the curves are continuous. However, abrupt changes in slope may be observed with some systems if a change in the nature of the dissolving solid occurs at a specific transition temperature. For example, sodium sulfate exists as the decahydrate $Na_2SO_4 \cdot 10H_2O$ up to 32.5 °C and its dissolution in water is an endothermic process. Its solubility therefore increases with a rise in temperature until 32.5 °C is reached. Above this temperature the solid is converted into the anhydrous form (Na_2SO_4), and the dissolution of this compound is exothermic. The solubility therefore exhibits a change from a positive to a negative slope as the temperature exceeds the transition value, i.e. the solubility falls.

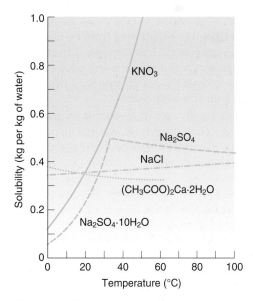

Fig. 2.7 • Solubility curves for various substances in water.

Molecular structure of solute

It should be appreciated from the previous comments in this chapter on the prediction of solubility that the nature of the solute and the solvent will be of paramount importance in determining the solubility of a solid in a liquid. It should also be realized that even a small change in the molecular structure of a compound can have a marked effect on its solubility in a given liquid. For example, the introduction of a hydrophilic hydroxyl group to a molecule can produce a large increase in water solubility. This is evidenced by the more than 100-fold greater aqueous solubility of phenol compared with benzene.

In addition, the conversion of a weak acid to its sodium salt leads to a much greater degree of ionic dissociation of the compound when it dissolves in water. The overall interaction between solute and solvent is increased markedly and the solubility consequently rises. An example of this effect is provided by a comparison of the aqueous solubility of salicylic acid and that of its sodium salt, which are 1 in 550 and 1 in 1 respectively.

The reduction in aqueous solubility of a parent drug by its esterification may also be cited as an example of the effects of changes in the chemical structure of the solute. Such a reduction in solubility may be beneficial to provide a suitable method for:

- masking the taste of a parent drug, e.g. chloramphenicol palmitate has been used in paediatric suspensions rather than the more soluble but very bitter tasting chloramphenicol base;
- protecting the parent drug from excessive degradation in the gastrointestinal tract, e.g. erythromycin propionate is less soluble and consequently less readily degraded than erythromycin base; and
- increasing the ease of absorption of drugs from the gastrointestinal tract, e.g. erythromycin propionate is also more readily absorbed than erythromycin base.

Nature of solvent: cosolvents

The importance of the nature of the solvent has already been discussed in terms of the statement 'like dissolves like' and in relation to solubility parameters. In addition, the point has been made that mixtures of solvents may be employed. Such mixtures are often used in pharmaceutical practice in order to obtain aqueous-based systems that contain solutes in excess of their individual solubility in pure water. This is achieved by using cosolvents such as ethanol or propylene glycol, which are miscible with water and which act as better solvents for the solute in question.

For example, the aqueous solubility of metronidazole is about 100 mg in 10 mL. The solubility of this drug can be increased markedly by the incorporation of one or more water-miscible cosolvents so that a solution containing 500 mg in 10 mL (and thus suitable for parenteral administration in the treatment of anaerobic infections) can be obtained.

Crystal characteristics: polymorphism and solvation

When the conditions under which crystallization is allowed to occur are varied, some substances produce crystals in which the constituent molecules are aligned in different ways with respect to one another in the lattice structure. These different crystalline forms of the same substance, which are known as polymorphs, consequently possess different lattice energies, and this difference is reflected by changes in other properties. For example, the polymorphic form with the lowest free energy will be the most stable and possess the highest melting point. Other less stable (or metastable) forms will tend to transform into the most stable one at rates that depend on the energy differences between the metastable and stable forms.

Many drugs exhibit polymorphism, e.g. steroid polymorphs are common. Polymorphs are explained more fully in Chapter 8 (which also includes an explanation of why polymorphs may have different solubilities) and Chapter 23. Examples of the importance of polymorphism with respect to the bioavailability of drugs are given in Chapter 20.

The effect of polymorphism on solubility is particularly important from a pharmaceutical point of view, because it provides a means of increasing the solubility of a crystalline material, and hence its rate of dissolution, by using a metastable polymorph.

Although the more soluble polymorphs are metastable and will convert to the stable form, the rate of such conversion is often slow enough for the metastable form to be regarded as being *sufficiently stable* from a pharmaceutical viewpoint. The degree of conversion should obviously be monitored during storage of the drug product to ensure that its efficacy is not altered significantly. There are products on the market containing a more soluble, but less stable, polymorph of the drug, where the chosen polymorph is *stable enough* to survive the approved storage conditions and declared shelf life.

Conversion to the less soluble and most stable polymorph may contribute to the growth of crystals in suspension formulations. Examples of the importance of polymorphism with respect to the occurrence of crystal growth in suspensions are given in Chapter 26.

The absence of a crystalline structure that is usually associated with an *amorphous* powder (discussed in Chapter 8) may also lead to an increase in the solubility of a drug when compared with that of its crystalline form.

In addition to the effect of polymorphism, the lattice structures of crystalline materials may be altered by the incorporation of molecules of the solvent from which crystallization occurred (discussed in Chapter 8). The resultant solids are called *solvates* and the phenomenon is referred to correctly as *solvation*. It is sometimes incorrectly and confusingly referred to as *pseudopolymorphism*. The alteration in crystal structure that accompanies solvation will affect the internal energetics of the solid such that the solubility of the solvated and unsolvated crystals will differ.

If water is the solvating molecule, i.e. a *hydrate* is formed, then the interaction between the substance and water that occurs in the crystal phase reduces the amount of energy liberated when the solid hydrate dissolves in water. Consequently, hydrated crystals tend to exhibit a lower aqueous solubility than their unhydrated forms. This decrease in solubility can lead to precipitation of drugs from solutions.

In contrast, the aqueous solubility of other, i.e. nonaqueous, solvates is often greater than that of the unsolvated forms. Examples of the effects of solvation and the attendant changes in solubilities of drugs on their bioavailabilities are given in Chapter 20.

Particle size of the solid

It has been postulated that the solubility of particles changes with the particle size. These changes arise from the presence of an electric charge on the particles. The effect of this charge becomes more important as the particle size decreases, particularly when the particles have a very small radius (less than about 1 μm). Thus such solubility changes are rarely an issue in conventional dosage forms but could be significant with nanotechnology products.

pH

If the pH of a solution of either a weakly acidic drug or a salt of such a drug is reduced, then the proportion of un-ionized acid molecules in the solution increases. Precipitation may occur, therefore, because the solubility of the un-ionized species is usually less than that of the ionized form. Conversely, in the case of solutions of weakly basic drugs or their salts, precipitation is favoured by an increase in pH. Such precipitation is an example of one type of chemical incompatibility that may be encountered in the formulation of liquid medicines.

This relationship between pH and solubility of ionized solutes is extremely important with respect to the ionization of weakly acidic and basic drugs as they pass through the gastrointestinal tract where they can experience pH changes of between about 1 and 8 pH units. This will affect the degree of ionization of the drug molecules, which in turn influences their solubility and their ability to be absorbed. This aspect is discussed elsewhere in this book in some detail, and the reader is referred in particular to Chapters 3 and 20.

The relationship between pH, pK_a and solubility of weakly acidic or weakly basic drugs is given by a modification of the Henderson–Hasselbalch equations. To avoid repetition here, the reader is referred to the relevant section of Chapter 3.

Common-ion effect

The equilibrium in a saturated solution of a sparingly soluble salt in contact with an undissolved solid may be represented by

$$\underset{\text{(ions)}}{A^+ + B^-} \Leftrightarrow \underset{\text{(solid)}}{AB}$$

$$(2.10)$$

From the law of mass action,

$$[A^+][B^-] = K[AB]$$

$$(2.11)$$

where the square brackets signify the concentrations of the respective components. Thus the equilibrium constant K for this reversible reaction is given by Eq. 2.12:

$$K = \frac{[A^+][B^-]}{[AB]}$$

$$(2.12)$$

Since the concentration of a solid may be regarded as being constant, the equation may be written as

$$K_S' = [A^+][B^-]$$

$$(2.13)$$

where K'_S is a constant known as the *solubility product* of compound AB.

If each molecule of the salt contains more than one ion of each type, e.g. $A_x^+ B_y^-$, then in the definition of the solubility product, the concentration of each ion is expressed to the appropriate power, i.e.

$$K'_S = [A^+]^x[B^-]^y$$

(2.14)

These equations for the solubility product are applicable only to solutions of sparingly soluble salts.

The presence of additional A^+ in the dissolution medium, i.e. where A^+ is a common ion, would push the equilibrium shown in Eq. 2.10 towards the right in order to restore the equilibrium. Solid AB will be precipitated and the solubility of this compound is therefore decreased. This is known as the *common-ion effect*. The addition of common B^- ions would have the same effect. An example is the reduced solubility of a hydrochloride salt of a drug in the stomach.

The precipitating effect of the presence of ions and other ingredients in the dissolution medium (as may be encountered in the gastrointestinal tract, for example) is often less apparent in practice than expected from this discussion. The reasons for this are explained in the following sections.

Effect of different electrolytes on the solubility product. The solubility of a sparingly soluble electrolyte may be increased by the addition of a second electrolyte that does not possess ions common to the first electrolyte, i.e. it is a different electrolyte.

Effective concentration of ions. The activity of a particular ion is related to its effective concentration. In general, this is lower than the actual concentration because some ions produced by dissociation of the electrolyte are strongly associated with other oppositely charged ions and do not contribute so effectively to the properties of the system as completely unallocated ions.

Effect of nonelectrolytes on the solubility of electrolytes. The solubility of electrolytes depends on the dissociation of dissolved molecules into ions. This dissociation is affected by the dielectric constant of the solvent, which is a measure of the polar nature of the solvent. Liquids with a high dielectric constant (e.g. water) are able to reduce the attractive forces that operate between oppositely charged ions produced by dissociation of an electrolyte.

If a water-soluble nonelectrolyte, such as alcohol, is added to an aqueous solution of a sparingly soluble electrolyte, the solubility of the latter is decreased because the alcohol lowers the dielectric constant of the solvent and ionic dissociation of the electrolyte becomes more difficult.

Effect of electrolytes on the solubility of nonelectrolytes. Nonelectrolytes do not dissociate into ions in aqueous solution, and in dilute solution the dissolved species therefore consists of single molecules. Their solubility in water depends on the formation of weak intermolecular bonds (hydrogen bonds) between their molecules and those of water. The presence of a very soluble electrolyte, the ions of which have a marked affinity for water, will reduce the solubility of a nonelectrolyte by competing for the aqueous solvent and breaking the intermolecular bonds between the nonelectrolyte and water. This effect is important in the precipitation of proteins.

Complex formation. The apparent solubility of a solute in a particular liquid may be increased or decreased by the addition of a third substance which forms an intermolecular complex with the solute. The solubility of the complex will determine the apparent change in the solubility of the original solute.

Solubilizing agents. These agents are capable of forming large aggregates or micelles in solution when their concentrations exceed certain values. In aqueous solution the centre of these aggregates resembles a separate organic phase, and organic solutes may be taken up by the aggregates, thus producing an apparent increase in their solubility in water. This phenomenon is known as *solubilization*. A similar phenomenon occurs in organic solvents containing dissolved solubilizing agents because the centre of the aggregates in these systems constitutes a more polar region than the bulk of the organic solvent. If polar solutes are taken up into these regions, their apparent solubility in the organic solvents is increased.

Solubility of gases in liquids

The amount of gas that will dissolve in a liquid is determined by the nature of the two components and by temperature and pressure.

Provided that no reaction occurs between the gas and the liquid, then the effect of pressure is indicated by Henry's law, which states that at constant temperature the solubility of a gas in a liquid is directly proportional to the pressure of the gas above the liquid. The law may be expressed by Eq. 2.15:

$$w = kp$$

(2.15)

where w is the mass of gas dissolved by unit volume of solvent at an equilibrium pressure p, and k is a proportionality constant. Although Henry's law is most applicable at high temperatures and low pressures, when solubility is low, it provides a satisfactory description of the behaviour of most systems at normal temperatures and reasonable pressures, unless the solubility is very high or a reaction occurs. Eq. 2.15 also applies to the solubility of each gas in a solution of several gases in the same liquid provided that p represents the partial pressure of a particular gas.

The solubility of most gases in liquids decreases as the temperature rises. This provides a means of removing dissolved gases. For example, water for injections free from either carbon dioxide or air may be prepared by boiling water with minimum exposure to air and preventing access of air during cooling. The presence of electrolytes may also decrease the solubility of a gas in water by a 'salting-out' process, which is caused by the marked attraction exerted between the electrolyte and water.

Solubility of liquids in liquids

The components of an ideal solution are miscible in all proportions. Such complete miscibility is also observed in some real binary systems, e.g. ethanol and water, under normal conditions. However, if one of the components tends to self-associate because the attractions between its own molecules are greater than those between its molecules and those of the other component, i.e. if a positive deviation from Raoult's law occurs, the miscibility of the components may be reduced (Raoult's law is discussed more fully in Chapter 3). The extent of the reduction in miscibility depends on the strength of the self-association and, therefore, on the degree of deviation from Raoult's law. Thus partial miscibility may be observed in some systems, whereas virtual immiscibility may be exhibited when the self-association is very strong and the positive deviation from Raoult's law is large.

In those cases where partial miscibility occurs under normal conditions, the degree of miscibility is usually dependent on the temperature. This dependency is indicated by the *phase rule*, introduced by J. Willard Gibbs. This is expressed quantitatively by Eq. 2.16:

$$F = C - P + 2$$

(2.16)

where P and C are the numbers of phases and components in the system respectively, and F is the number of degrees of freedom, i.e. the number of variable conditions such as temperature, pressure and composition, that must be stated in order to define completely the state of the system at equilibrium.

The overall effect of temperature variation on the degree of miscibility in these systems is usually described by means of phase diagrams, which are graphs of temperature versus composition at constant pressure. For convenience of discussion of their phase diagrams, the partially miscible systems may be divided into the following types.

Systems showing an increase in miscibility with rise in temperature

A positive deviation from Raoult's law arises from a difference in the cohesive forces that exist between the molecules of each component in a liquid mixture. This difference becomes more marked as the temperature decreases, and the positive deviation may then result in a decrease in miscibility sufficient to cause the separation of the mixture into two phases. Each phase consists of a saturated solution of one component in the other liquid. Such mutually saturated solutions are known as *conjugate solutions*.

The equilibria that occur in mixtures of partially miscible liquids may be followed either by shaking the two liquids together at constant temperature and analysing samples from each phase after equilibrium has been attained, or by observing the temperature at which known proportions of the two liquids, contained in sealed glass ampoules, become miscible (as indicated by the disappearance of turbidity).

Systems showing a decrease in miscibility with rise in temperature

A few mixtures, which probably involve compound formation, exhibit a lower critical solution temperature (CST), e.g. triethylamine plus water and paraldehyde plus water. The formation of a compound produces a negative deviation from Raoult's law, and miscibility therefore increases as the temperature falls.

Systems showing upper and lower critical solution temperatures

The decrease in miscibility with increase in temperature in systems having a lower CST is not indefinite. Above a certain temperature, positive deviations from Raoult's law become important and miscibility starts to increase again with further rise in temperature. This behaviour is shown by the nicotine–water system.

Table 2.4 The effects of additives on the critical solution temperature

Type of CST	Solubility of additive in each component	Effect on CST	Effect on miscibility
Upper	Approximately equally soluble in both components	Lowered	Increased
Upper	Readily soluble in one component but not in the other	Raised	Decreased
Lower	Approximately equally soluble in both components	Raised	Increased
Lower	Readily soluble in one component but not in the other	Lowered	Decreased

CST, critical solution temperature.

In some mixtures where an upper and a lower CST are expected, these points are not, in fact, observed since a phase change by one of the components occurs before the relevant CST is reached. For example, the ether–water system should exhibit a lower CST, but water freezes before the temperature is reached.

Effects of added substances on critical solution temperatures

CST is an invariant point at constant pressure, but this temperature is very sensitive to impurities or added substances. The effects of additives are summarized in Table 2.4.

Blending

The increase in miscibility of two liquids caused by the addition of a third substance is referred to as *blending*. An example is the use of propylene glycol as a blending agent to improve the miscibility of volatile oils and water. Full understanding of this interrelationship requires the use of a ternary-phase diagram. This diagram is a triangular plot which indicates the effects of changes in the relative proportions of all three components at constant temperature and pressure. The plot shows the areas (i.e. combinations of the three ingredients) that result in a single 'blended' phase.

Distribution of solutes between immiscible liquids

Partition coefficients

When a substance which is soluble in both components of a mixture of immiscible liquids is dissolved in such a mixture, when equilibrium is attained at constant temperature, it is found that the solute is distributed between the two liquids in such a way that the ratio of the activities of the substance in each liquid is a constant. This is known as the Nernst distribution law and may be expressed by Eq. 2.17:

$$\frac{a_A}{a_B} = \text{constant}$$

(2.17)

where a_A and a_B are the activities of the solute in solvent A and solvent B respectively. When the solutions are dilute or when the solute behaves ideally, the activities may be replaced by concentrations (C_A and C_B):

$$\frac{C_A}{C_B} = K$$

(2.18)

The constant K is known as the *distribution coefficient*, or *partition coefficient*. In the case of sparingly soluble substances, K is approximately equal to the ratio of the solubility (S_A and S_B) of the solute in each liquid. Thus

$$\frac{S_A}{S_B} = K$$

(2.19)

In most other systems, however, deviation from ideal behaviour invalidates Eq. 2.19. For example, if the solute exists as monomers in solvent A and as dimers in solvent B, the distribution coefficient is given by Eq. 2.20, in which the square root of the concentration of the dimeric form is used:

$$K = \frac{C_A}{\sqrt{C_B}}$$

(2.20)

If the dissociation into ions occurs in the aqueous layer, B, of a mixture of immiscible liquids, then the degree of dissociation (α) should be taken into account, as indicated by Eq. 2.21:

$$K = \frac{C_A}{C_B(1-\alpha)}$$

(2.21)

The solvents in which the concentrations of the solute are expressed should be indicated when partition coefficients are quoted. For example, a partition coefficient of 2 for a solute distributed between oil and water may also be expressed as a partition coefficient between water and oil of 0.5. This can be represented as $K_{water}^{oil} = 2$ and $K_{oil}^{water} = 0.5$. The abbreviation K_w^o is often used for the former, and this notation has become the most commonly used.

The determination of partition coefficients is important in preformulation, and so this is discussed further in Chapter 23.

Solubility of solids in solids

If two solids are either melted together and then cooled or dissolved in a suitable liquid solvent that is then removed by evaporation, the solid that is redeposited from the melt or the solution will either be a one-phase solid solution or a two-phase solid dispersion.

In a *solid solution*, as in other types of solution, the molecules of one component (the solute) are dispersed *molecularly* throughout the other component (the solvent). Complete miscibility of two solid components is only achieved if:

- the molecular size of the solute is similar to that of the solvent so that a molecule of the former can be substituted for one of the latter in its crystal lattice structure; or
- the solute molecules are much smaller than the solvent molecules so that the former can be accommodated in the spaces of the solvent lattice structure.

These two types of solvent system are referred to as *substitutional solid solutions* and *interstitial solid solutions* respectively, and are illustrated in Fig. 2.8. A typical pharmaceutical example of an interstitial solid solution would be when one of these solids is a drug and the other is a polymeric material with large spaces between its intertwined molecules that can accommodate solute molecules.

Since the criteria for a solid solution are only satisfied in relatively few systems, it is more common to observe *partial miscibility* of solids. Often (following coprecipitation is an example) the resulting matrix may contain undissolved particles or groups of matrix particles. In this case, the resulting system is known as a *solid dispersion*.

When the carrier solid (the polymer) is dissolved away, the molecules or small crystals of insoluble drug may dissolve more rapidly than a conventional powder because the contact area between the drug and water is increased. The rate of dissolution and, consequently, the bioavailability of poorly soluble drugs may be improved by the use of solid solutions or solid dispersions. Disperse systems are discussed more fully in Chapters 6 and 26.

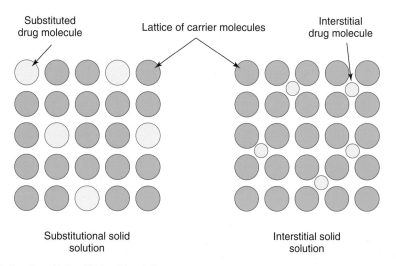

Fig. 2.8 • Substitutional and interstitial solid solutions.

Summary

This chapter has shown that the process of dissolution is a change in phase of a molecule or ion. Most often this is from solid to liquid. Simple diffusional mechanisms and equations usually define the rate and extent of this process. The concept of solubility in a pharmaceutical context has also been discussed. The chapter that follows will describe the properties of the solution thus produced.

Please check your eBook at **https://studentconsult. inkling.com/** for self-assessment questions. See inside cover for registration details.

Reference

Florence, A.T., Attwood, D., 2016. *Physicochemical* Principles of Pharmacy: In Manufacture, Formulation and Clinical Use, sixth ed. Pharmaceutical Press, London.

Bibliography

Barton, A.F.M., 1991. Handbook of Solubility Parameters and Other Cohesion Parameters. CRC Press, Boca Raton.

British Pharmacopoeia Commission, 2017. British Pharmacopoeia. Stationery Office, London.

European Pharmacopoeia Commission, 2017. European Pharmacopoeia, ninth ed. Council of Europe, Strasbourg.

Florence, A.T., Siepmann, J. (Eds.), 2009. Modern Pharmaceutics, vol. 1 and 2, fiveth ed. Informa, New York.

Noyes, A.A., Whitney, W.R., 1897. The rate of solution of solid substances in their own solutions. J. Am. Chem. Soc. 19, 930.

Rowe, R.C., Sheskey, P.J., Cook, W.G., et al., 2016. Handbook of Pharmaceutical Excipients, eighth ed. Pharmaceutical Press, London.

Troy, D.B. (Ed.), 2006. Remington: The Science and Practice of Pharmacy, twenty first ed. Lippincott Williams & Wilkins, Baltimore.

United States Pharmacopeial Convention, 2016. United States Pharmacopeia and National Formulary. United States Pharmacopeial Convention, Rockville.

Wichmann, K., Klamt, A., 2010. Drug solubility and reaction thermodynamics. In: am Ende, D.J. (Ed.), Chemical Engineering in the Pharmaceutical Industry: R&D to Manufacture. John Wiley & Sons (in conjunction with AIChE), Hoboken.

Properties of solutions

3

Michael E. Aulton

CHAPTER CONTENTS

KEY POINTS

- Once solutions are formed in the manner described in the previous chapter, they have various properties that are important in pharmaceutical science.
- There are various types of solution that need to be understood. This includes understanding the differences between theoretical, or 'ideal', solutions and the 'real' solutions found in practice.
- Of particular relevance to drug delivery via the gastrointestinal tract is the degree of ionization of solutes and the effect that changes in pH have on ionization.
- The concept of pH and pK_a and their interrelationship, and the link between the degree of ionization and solubility are key to an understanding of the delivery of drugs to the gastrointestinal tract. This is because the surrounding pH changes during the passage of the drug down the tract.
- Other solution properties of particular importance include vapour pressure, osmotic pressure and diffusibility.

Introduction

The aim of this chapter is to provide information on certain properties of solutions that relate to their applications in pharmaceutical science. This chapter deals mainly with the physicochemical properties of solutions that are important in pharmaceutical systems. These aspects are covered in sufficient detail to introduce the pharmaceutical scientist to these properties in order to allow an understanding of their importance in dosage form design and drug delivery. Much is published elsewhere in far greater detail, and any reader requiring this additional information can trace some of this by referring to the bibliography at the end of the chapter.

Types of solution

Solutions may be classified on the basis of the physical state (i.e. gas, liquid or solid) of the solute(s) and solvent. Although a variety of different types can exist, solutions of pharmaceutical interest virtually all possess liquid solvents. In addition, the solutes are predominantly solid substances. Consequently, most of the information in this chapter is relevant to solutions of solids in liquids.

Vapour pressures of solids, liquids and solutions

An understanding of many of the properties of solutions requires an appreciation of the concept of an *ideal solution* and its use as a reference system, to which the behaviours of real (nonideal) solutions can be compared. This concept is itself based on a consideration of vapour pressure. The present section serves as an introduction to the discussions later in this chapter on ideal and nonideal solutions.

The kinetic theory of matter indicates that the thermal motions of molecules of a substance in its gaseous state are more than adequate to overcome the attractive forces that exist between the molecules. The molecules will undergo completely random movement confined only by the container. The situation is reversed, however, when the temperature is lowered sufficiently so that a *condensed phase* is formed. Here the thermal motions of the molecules are now insufficient to overcome completely the intermolecular attractive forces, and some degree of order in the relative arrangement of molecules occurs. This condensed state may be either liquid or solid.

If the intermolecular forces are so strong that a high degree of order is brought about, when the structure is hardly influenced by thermal motions, then the substance is usually in the solid state.

In the liquid condensed state, the relative influences of thermal motion and intermolecular attractive forces are intermediate between those in the gaseous and solid states. Thus the effects of interactions between the permanent and induced dipoles, i.e. the so-called van der Waals forces of attraction, lead to some degree of coherence between the molecules of liquids. Consequently, liquids, unlike gases, occupy a definite volume *with a surface*, and whilst there is evidence of structure within liquids, such structure is much less apparent than in solids.

Although both solids and liquids are condensed systems with cohering molecules, some of the surface molecules in these systems will occasionally acquire sufficient energy to overcome the attractive forces exerted by adjacent molecules. The molecules can therefore escape from the surface to form a vapour phase. If temperature is maintained constant, equilibrium will be established eventually between the vapour phase and the condensed phase. The pressure exerted by the vapour at this equilibrium is referred to as the *vapour pressure* of the substance.

All condensed systems have the inherent ability to give rise to a vapour pressure. However, the vapour pressures exerted by solids are usually much lower than those exerted by liquids, because the intermolecular forces in solids are stronger than those in liquids. Thus the escaping tendency for surface molecules is higher in liquids. Consequently, surface loss of vapour from liquids by the process of evaporation is more common than surface loss of vapour from solids by sublimation.

In the case of a liquid solvent containing a dissolved solute, molecules of both the solvent and the solute may show a tendency to escape from the surface and so contribute to the vapour pressure. The relative tendencies to escape will depend on the relative numbers of the different molecules in the surface of the solution, and on the relative strengths of the attractive forces between adjacent solvent molecules on the one hand and between solute and solvent molecules on the other hand. Because the intermolecular forces between solid solutes and liquid solvents tend to be relatively strong, such solute molecules do not generally escape from the surface of a solution nor contribute to the vapour pressure. In other words, the solute is generally nonvolatile and the vapour pressure arises solely from the dynamic equilibrium that is set up between the rates of evaporation and condensation of solvent molecules contained in the solution. In a mixture of miscible liquids, i.e. a liquid-in-liquid solution, the molecules of both components are likely to evaporate and both will contribute to the overall vapour pressure exerted by the solution.

Ideal solutions: Raoult's law

The concept of an ideal solution has been introduced in order to provide a model system that can be used as a standard with which real or nonideal solutions can be compared. In the model, it is assumed that the strengths of all intermolecular forces are identical. Thus solvent–solvent, solute–solvent and solute–solute interactions are the same and are equal to the strength of the intermolecular interactions in either the pure solvent or the pure solute. Because of this equality, the relative tendencies of solute and solvent molecules to escape from the surface of the solution will be determined only by their relative numbers in the surface.

Since a solution is homogeneous by definition, the relative number of these surface molecules will be the same as the relative number in the whole of the solution. The latter can be expressed conveniently by the mole fractions of the components because for a binary solution (i.e. one with two components), $x_1 + x_2 = 1$, where x_1 and x_2 are the mole fractions of the solute and solvent respectively.

The total vapour pressure (P) exerted by a binary solution is given by Eq. 3.1:

$$P = p_1 + p_2$$

(3.1)

where p_1 and p_2 are the partial vapour pressures exerted above the solution by the solute and the solvent respectively. Raoult's law states that the partial vapour pressure (p) exerted by a volatile component in a solution at a given temperature is equal to the vapour pressure of the pure component at the same temperature ($p°$) multiplied by its mole fraction in the solution (x), i.e.

$$p = p°x$$

(3.2)

Thus from Eqs 3.1 and 3.2,

$$P = p_1 + p_2 = p_1°x_1 + p_2°x_2$$

(3.3)

where $p_1°$ and $p_2°$ are the vapour pressures exerted by pure solute and pure solvent respectively. If the total vapour pressure of the solution is described by Eq. 3.3, then Raoult's law is obeyed by the system.

One of the consequences of the preceding comments is that an ideal solution may be defined as one that obeys Raoult's law. In addition, ideal behaviour should be expected to be exhibited only by real systems composed of chemically similar components, because it is only in such systems that the condition of equal intermolecular forces between components (as assumed in the ideal model) is likely to be satisfied. Consequently, in reality Raoult's law is obeyed over an appreciable concentration range by relatively few systems.

Mixtures of, for example, benzene and toluene, n-hexane and n-heptane, ethyl bromide and ethyl iodide, and binary mixtures of fluorinated hydrocarbons are systems that exhibit ideal behaviour. Note the chemical similarity of the two components of the mixture in each example.

Real or nonideal solutions

The majority of real solutions do not exhibit ideal behaviour because solute–solute, solute–solvent and solvent–solvent forces of interaction are unequal. These inequalities alter the effective concentration of each component such that it cannot be represented by a normal expression of concentration, such as the mole fraction term x that is used in Eqs 3.2 and 3.3. Consequently, deviations from Raoult's law are often exhibited by real solutions, and the previous equations are not obeyed in such cases. These equations can be modified, however, by substituting for each concentration term (x) a measure of the effective concentration; this is provided by the so-called *activity* (or *thermodynamic activity*), a. Thus Eq. 3.2 becomes Eq. 3.4,

$$p = p°a$$

(3.4)

and the resulting equation is applicable to all systems, whether they are ideal or nonideal. It should be noted that if a solution exhibits ideal behaviour, then a equals x, whereas a will not equal x if deviations from such behaviour are apparent. The ratio of activity divided by the mole fraction is termed the *activity coefficient* (f) and it provides a measure of the deviation from the ideal. Thus when $a = x$, $f = 1$.

If the attractive forces between solute and solvent molecules are weaker than those between the solute molecules themselves or between the solvent molecules themselves, then the components will have little affinity for each other. The escaping tendency of the surface molecules in such a system is increased when compared with an ideal solution. In other words, p_1, p_2 and therefore P (Eq. 3.3) are greater than expected from Raoult's law, and the thermodynamic activities of the components are greater than their mole fractions, i.e. $a_1 > x_1$ and $a_2 > x_2$. This type of system is said to show a *positive deviation* from Raoult's law, and the extent of the deviation increases as the miscibility of the components decreases. For example, a mixture of alcohol and benzene shows a smaller deviation than the less miscible mixture of water and diethyl ether, whilst the virtually immiscible mixture of benzene and water exhibits a very large positive deviation.

Conversely, if the solute and solvent molecules have a strong mutual affinity (that sometimes may result in the formation of a complex or compound), then a negative deviation from Raoult's law occurs. Thus p_1, p_2 and therefore P are lower than expected, and $a_1 < x_1$ and $a_2 < x_2$. Examples of systems that show this type of behaviour include chloroform plus acetone, pyridine plus acetic acid and water plus nitric acid.

Although most systems are nonideal and deviate either positively or negatively from Raoult's law, such deviations are small when a solution is dilute. This is because the effect that a small amount of solute has on interactions between solvent molecules is minimal. Thus dilute solutions tend to exhibit ideal behaviour and the activities of their components approximate to their mole fractions, i.e. a_1 approximately equals x_1 and a_2 approximately equals x_2. Conversely, large deviations may be observed when the concentration of a solution is high.

Knowledge of the consequences of such marked deviations is particularly important in relation to the distillation of liquid mixtures. For example, the complete separation of the components of a mixture by fractional distillation may not be achievable if large positive or negative deviations from Raoult's law give rise to the formation of so-called azeotropic mixtures with minimum and maximum boiling points respectively.

Ionization of solutes

Many solutes dissociate into ions if the dielectric constant of the solvent is high enough to cause sufficient separation of the attractive forces between the oppositely charged ions. Such solutes are termed *electrolytes* and their ionization (or dissociation) has several consequences that are often important in pharmaceutical practice. Some of these consequences are indicated in the following sections.

Hydrogen ion concentration and pH

The dissociation of water can be represented by Eq. 3.5:

$$H_2O \leftrightarrow H^+ + OH^-$$

(3.5)

It should be realized that this is a simplified representation because the hydrogen and hydroxyl ions do not exist in a free state but combine with undissociated water molecules to yield more complex ions such as H_3O^+ and $H_7O_4^-$.

In pure water the concentrations of H^+ and OH^- ions are equal and at 25 °C both have the value of 1×10^{-7} mol L^{-1}. The Lowry–Brönsted theory of acids and bases defines an acid as a substance which donates a proton (or hydrogen ion), so it follows that the addition of an acidic solute to water will result in a hydrogen ion concentration that exceeds that of pure water. Conversely, the addition of a base, which is defined as a substance that accepts protons, will decrease the concentration of hydrogen ions in solution. The hydrogen ion concentration range decreases from 1 mol L^{-1} for a strong acid to 1×10^{-14} mol L^{-1} for a strong base.

To avoid the frequent use of inconvenient numbers that arise from this very wide range, the concept of pH has been introduced as a more convenient measure of hydrogen ion concentration; pH is defined as the negative logarithm of the hydrogen ion concentration ($[H^+]$) as shown by Eq. 3.6:

$$pH = -\log_{10}[H^+]$$

(3.6)

so the pH of a neutral solution and the pH of pure water are both 7. This is because, as mentioned previously, the concentration of H^+ ions (and thus OH^- ions) in pure water is 1×10^{-7} mol L^{-1}. The pH of acidic solutions is less than 7 and the pH of alkaline solutions is greater than 7.

The pH has several important implications in pharmaceutical practice. It has an effect on:

- The degree of ionization of drugs that are weak acids or weak bases.
- The solubility of drugs that are weak acids or weak bases.
- The ease of absorption of drugs from the gastrointestinal tract into the blood. For example, many drugs (about 75%) are weak bases or their salts. These drugs dissolve more rapidly in the low pH of the acidic stomach. However, there will be little or no absorption of the drug there as it will be too ionized. Drug absorption normally will have to wait until the drug reaches the more alkaline intestine, where the ionization of the dissolved weak base is reduced.
- The stability of many drugs.
- Body tissues (both extremes of pH are injurious).

These implications have great consequence during peroral drug delivery as the pH experienced by the drug could range from pH 1 to pH 8 at it passes down the gastrointestinal tract. The interrelationship between the degree of ionization, solubility and pH is discussed later in this chapter. The biopharmaceutical consequences are discussed in Chapter 20.

Dissociation (or ionization) constants; pK_a and pK_b

Many drugs are either weak acids or weak bases. In solutions of these drugs, equilibria exist between undissociated molecules and their ions. In a solution of a weakly acidic drug HA, the equilibrium may be represented by Eq. 3.7:

$$HA \leftrightarrow H^+ + A^-$$

(3.7)

Similarly, the protonation of a weakly basic drug B can be represented by Eq. 3.8:

$$B + H^+ \leftrightarrow BH^+$$

(3.8)

In solutions of most salts of strong acids or strong bases in water, such equilibria are shifted strongly to one side of the equation because these compounds are virtually completely ionized. In the case of aqueous solutions of weaker acids and bases, the degree of ionization is much more variable and indeed, as will be seen, controllable.

The *ionization constant* (or *dissociation constant*) K_a of a partially ionized weakly acidic species can be obtained by application of the law of mass action to yield Eq. 3.9:

$$K_a = \frac{[I^+][I^-]}{[U]}$$

(3.9)

where $[I^+]$ and $[I^-]$ represent the concentrations of the dissociated ionized species and $[U]$ is the concentration of the un-ionized species.

For the case of a weak acid, this can be written (from Eq. 3.7) as

$$K_a = \frac{[H^+][A^-]}{[HA]}$$

(3.10)

Taking logarithms of both sides of Eq. 3.10 yields

$$\log_{10} K_a = \log_{10}[H^+] + \log_{10}[A^-] - \log_{10}[HA]$$

(3.11)

The signs in this equation may be reversed to give Eq. 3.12:

$$-\log_{10} K_a = -\log_{10}[H^+] - \log_{10}[A^-] + \log_{10}[HA]$$

(3.12)

The symbol pK_a is used to represent the negative logarithm of the acid dissociation constant K_a in an analogous way that pH is used to represent the negative logarithm of the hydrogen ion concentration (as Eq. 3.6). Therefore

$$pK_a = -\log_{10} K_a$$

(3.13)

Eq. 3.12 may therefore be rewritten as Eq. 3.14:

$$pK_a = pH + \log_{10}[HA] - \log_{10}[A^-]$$

(3.14)

or

$$pK_a = pH + \log_{10} \frac{[HA]}{[A^-]}$$

(3.15)

or even

$$pH = pK_a + \log_{10} \frac{[A^-]}{[HA]}$$

(3.16)

Eqs 3.15 and 3.16 are known as the Henderson–Hasselbalch equations for a weak acid.

Ionization constants of both acidic and basic drugs are usually expressed in terms of pK_a. The equivalent acid dissociation constant (K_a) for the protonation of a weak base is given (from Eq. 3.8) by Eq. 3.17. Note the equation appears to be inverted, but it is written in terms of K_a rather than K_b (the base dissociation constant):

$$K_a = \frac{[H^+][B]}{[BH^+]}$$

(3.17)

Taking negative logarithms yields Eq. 3.18:

$$-\log_{10} K_a = -\log_{10}[H^+] - \log_{10}[B] + \log_{10}[BH^+]$$

(3.18)

or

$$pK_a = pH + \log_{10} \frac{[BH^+]}{[B]}$$

(3.19)

or

$$pH = pK_a + \log_{10} \frac{[B]}{[BH^+]}$$

(3.20)

Eqs 3.19 and 3.20 are known as the Henderson–Hasselbalch equations for a weak base.

Link between pH, pK_a, degree of ionization and solubility of weakly acidic or basic drugs

There is a direct link for most polar ionic compounds between the degree of ionization and aqueous solubility. As shown earlier, in turn, the degree of ionization is controlled by the pK_a of the molecule and the pH of its surrounding environment. This interrelationship is shown diagrammatically in Fig. 3.1.

Taking the weak acid line first, we can see that at high pH the drug is fully ionized and at its maximum solubility. Under low pH conditions the opposite is true. The shape of the curve is defined by the Henderson–Hasselbalch equation for weak acids (Eq. 3.15), which shows the link between pH, pK_a and degree of ionization for a weakly acidic drug. It can also be seen from Fig. 3.1 that when the pH is equal to the pK_a of the drug, the drug is 50% ionized. This is also predicted from the Henderson–Hasselbalch equation.

Eq. 3.16 shows that when $[A^-] = [HA]$, log ($[A^-]$/$[HA]$) will equal log 1 (i.e. zero) and thus pH = pK_a. Put another way, when the pH of the surrounding solution equals the pK_a, then the concentration of the ionized species $[A^-]$ will equal the concentration of the un-ionized species $[HA]$, i.e. the drug is 50% ionized. The Henderson–Hasselbalch equations also show that a drug is almost completely ionized or non-ionized (as appropriate) when it is 2 pH units away from its pK_a.

Examination of the equivalent line for a weak base will indicate that it is probably not a coincidence that most drugs for peroral delivery are weak bases. A weak base will be ionized and at its most soluble in the acidic stomach and non-ionized and therefore more easily absorbed in the more alkaline small intestine. The choice of the pK_a for a drug is thus of paramount importance in peroral drug delivery.

Use of the Henderson–Hasselbalch equations to calculate the degree of ionization of weakly acidic or basic drugs

Various analytical techniques, e.g. spectrophotometric and potentiometric methods, may be used to determine ionization constants, but the temperature at which the determination is performed should be specified because the values of the constants vary with temperature.

The degree of ionization of a drug in a solution can be calculated from rearranged Henderson–Hasselbalch equations for weak acids (Eq. 3.15) and weak bases (Eq. 3.19) if the pK_a of the drug and the pH of the solution are known. The resulting equations for weak acids and weak bases are Eqs 3.21 and 3.22 respectively:

$$\log_{10} \frac{[HA]}{[A^-]} = pK_a - pH$$

$$(3.21)$$

$$\log_{10} \frac{[BH^+]}{[B]} = pK_a - pH$$

$$(3.22)$$

Such calculations are particularly useful in determining the degree of ionization of drugs in various parts of the gastrointestinal tract and in the plasma. The examples shown in Box 3.1 are therefore related to this type of situation.

Buffer solutions and buffer capacity

Buffer solutions will maintain a constant pH even when small amounts of acid or alkali are added to the solution. Buffers usually contain mixtures of a weak acid and one of its salts, although mixtures of a weak base and one of its salts may also be used.

The action of a buffer solution can be appreciated by considering, as an example, a simple system such

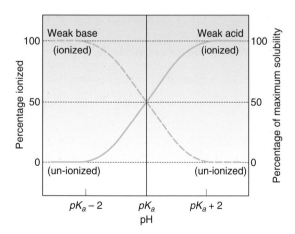

Fig. 3.1 • Change in degree of ionization and relative solubility of weakly acidic and weakly basic drugs as a function of pH.

Box 3.1

1. The pK_a of aspirin (acetylsalicylic acid), which is a weak acid, is about 3.5. If the pH of the gastric contents is 2.0, then from Eq. 3.21,

$$\log_{10}\frac{[HA]}{[A^-]} = pK_a - pH = 3.5 - 2.0 = 1.5$$

so the ratio of the concentration of un-ionized acetylsalicylic acid to acetylsalicylate anion is given by

$$[HA]:[A^-] = \text{antilog}\,1.5 = 31.6:1$$

2. The pH of plasma is 7.4, so the ratio of un-ionized to ionized acetylsalicylic acid in this medium is given by

$$\log_{10}\frac{[HA]}{[A^-]} = pK_a - pH = 3.5 - 7.4 = -3.9$$

and

$$[HA]:[A^-] = \text{antilog}(-3.9) = 1.26 \times 10^{-4}:1$$

3. The pK_a of the weakly *acidic* drug sulfapyridine is about 8.0, and if the pH of the intestinal contents is 5.0, then the ratio of un-ionized to ionized drug is given by

$$\log_{10}\frac{[HA]}{[A^-]} = pK_a - pH = 8.0 - 5.0 = 3.0$$

and

$$[HA]:[A^-] = \text{antilog}\,3.0 = 10^3:1$$

4. The pK_a of the *basic* drug amidopyrine is 5.0. In the stomach, the ratio of ionized to un-ionized drug is calculated from Eq. 3.22 as follows:

$$\log\frac{[BH^+]}{[B]} = pK_a - pH = 5.0 - 2.0 = 3.0$$

and

$$[BH^+]:[B] = \text{antilog}\,3.0 = 10^3:1$$

whilst in the intestine, the ratio is given by

$$\log\frac{[BH^+]}{[B]} = pK_a - pH = 5.0 - 5.0 = 0$$

and

$$[BH^+]:[B] = \text{antilog}\,0 = 1:1$$

---

as a solution of acetic acid and sodium acetate in water. The acetic acid, being a weak acid, will be confined virtually to its undissociated form because its ionization will be suppressed by the presence of common acetate ions produced by complete dissociation of the sodium salt. The pH of this solution can be described by Eq. 3.23:

$$pH = pK_a + \log\frac{[A^-]}{[HA]}$$

(3.23)

This is Eq. 3.16 in which $[A^-]$ is the concentration of acetate ions and $[HA]$ is the concentration of acetic acid in the buffer solution.

It can be seen from Eq. 3.23 that the pH will remain constant as long as the logarithm of the ratio of the acetate concentration to acetic acid concentration does not change. When a small amount of an acid is added to the solution, it will convert some of the salt into acetic acid, but when the concentrations of both acetate ion and acetic acid are reasonably large, then the effect of the change will be negligible and the pH will remain constant. Similarly, the addition of a small amount of base will convert some of the acetic acid into its salt but the pH will be virtually unaltered if the overall changes in the concentrations of the two species are relatively small.

If large amounts of acid or base are added to a buffer, then changes in the ratio of ionized to un-ionized species become appreciable and the pH will then alter. The ability of a buffer to withstand the effects of acids and bases is an important property from a practical point of view. This ability is expressed in terms of *buffer capacity* (β). It can be defined as being equal to the amount of strong acid or strong base, expressed as moles of H^+ or OH^- ion, required to change the pH of 1 L of the buffer by 1 pH unit. From the previous remarks, it should be clear that buffer capacity increases as the concentrations of the buffer components increase. In addition, buffer capacity is also affected by the ratio of the concentrations of weak acid and its salt, maximum capacity (β_{max}) being obtained when the ratio of acid to salt is 1:1, i.e. the pH equals the pK_a of the acid (as was shown in Eq. 3.16).

The components of various buffer systems and the concentrations required to produce different pHs are listed in several reference books, such as the pharmacopoeias. When one is selecting a suitable buffer, the pK_a of the acid should be close to the required pH and the compatibility of its components with other ingredients in the system should be considered. The toxicity of buffer components must also be taken into account if the solution is to be used for medicinal purposes.

Colligative properties

When a nonvolatile solute is dissolved in a solvent, certain properties of the resulting solution are largely independent of the nature of the solute and are determined by the concentration of solute particles. These properties are known as *colligative properties*. In the case of a nonelectrolyte, the solute particles will be molecules, but if the solute is an electrolyte, then its degree of dissociation will determine whether the particles will be ions only or a mixture of ions and undissociated molecules.

The most important colligative property from a pharmaceutical aspect is *osmotic pressure*. However, since all colligative properties are related to each other by virtue of their common dependency on the concentration of the solute molecules, other colligative properties (which include lowering of the vapour pressure of the solvent, elevation of its boiling point and depression of its freezing point) are of pharmaceutical interest. Observations of these other properties offer alternatives to osmotic pressure measurements as methods of comparing the colligative properties of different solutions.

Osmotic pressure

The osmotic pressure of a solution is the external pressure that must be applied to the solution in order to prevent it being diluted by the entry of solvent via a process known as *osmosis*. This is the spontaneous diffusion of solvent from a solution of low solute concentration (or a pure solvent) into a more concentrated one through a semipermeable membrane. Such a membrane separates the two solutions and is permeable only to solvent molecules (i.e. not solute ones).

Since the process occurs spontaneously at constant temperature and pressure, the laws of thermodynamics indicate that it will be accompanied by a decrease in the *free energy* (G) of the system. This free energy may be regarded as the energy available for the performance of useful work. When an equilibrium position is attained, then there is no remaining difference between the energies of the states that are in equilibrium. The rate of increase in free energy

of a solution caused by an increase in the number of moles of one component is termed the *partial molar free energy* ($\bar{G}$) or *chemical potential* (μ) of that component. For example, the chemical potential of the solvent in a binary solution is given by Eq. 3.24:

$$\left(\frac{\partial G}{\partial n_2} \right)_{T,P,n_1} = \bar{G_2} = \mu_2$$

(3.24)

The subscripts outside the bracket on the left-hand side indicate that the temperature, pressure and amount of component 1 (the solute in this case) remain constant.

Since (by definition) only solvent molecules can pass through a semipermeable membrane, the driving force for osmosis arises from the inequality of the chemical potentials of the solvent on opposing sides of the membrane. Thus the direction of osmotic flow is from the dilute solution (or pure solvent), where the chemical potential of the solvent is highest because of the higher concentration of solvent molecules, into the concentrated solution, where the concentration and consequently the chemical potential of the solvent are reduced by the presence of more solute. The chemical potential of the solvent in the more concentrated solution can be increased by forcing its molecules closer together under the influence of an externally applied pressure. Osmosis can be prevented by such means, hence the term *osmotic pressure*.

The relationship between osmotic pressure (π) and concentration of a nonelectrolyte is defined for dilute solutions, which may be assumed to exhibit ideal behaviour, by the van't Hoff equation (Eq. 3.25):

$$\pi V = n_2 RT$$

(3.25)

where V is the volume of the solution, n_2 is the number of moles of solute, T is the absolute temperature and R is the gas constant. This equation, which is similar to the ideal gas equation, was derived empirically but it corresponds to a theoretically derived equation if approximations based on low solute concentrations are taken into account.

If the solute is an electrolyte, Eq. 3.25 must be modified to allow for the effect of ionic dissociation, because this will increase the number of particles in the solution. This modification is achieved by insertion of the van't Hoff correction factor (i) to give

$$\pi V = i n_2 RT$$

(3.26)

where

$$i = \frac{\text{observed colligative property}}{\substack{\text{colligative property expected} \\ \text{if dissociation did not occur}}}$$

Osmolality and osmolarity

The amount of osmotically active particles in a solution is sometimes expressed in terms of osmoles or milliosmoles. These osmotically active particles may be either molecules or ions. Osmole values depend on the number of particles dissolved in a solution, regardless of charge. For substances that maintain their molecular structure when they dissolve (e.g. glucose), osmolarity and molarity are essentially the same. For substances that dissociate when they dissolve, the osmolarity is the number of free particles times the molarity. Thus a 1 molar solution of pure NaCl would be 2 osmolar (1 osmolar for Na^+ and 1 osmolar for Cl^-).

The concentration of a solution may therefore be expressed in terms of its *osmolarity* or its *osmolality*. Osmolarity is the number of osmoles per litre of solution and osmolality is the number of osmoles per kilogram of solvent.

Isoosmotic solutions

If two solutions are separated by a perfect semipermeable membrane, i.e. a membrane which is permeable only to solvent molecules, and no net movement of solvent occurs across the membrane, then the solutions are said to be *isoosmotic* and have equal osmotic pressures.

Isotonic solutions

Biological membranes do not always function as perfect semipermeable membranes and some solute molecules in addition to water are able to pass through them. If two isoosmotic solutions remain in osmotic equilibrium when separated by a biological membrane, they may be described as being *isotonic* with respect to that particular membrane.

Adjustment of isotonicity is particularly important for formulations intended for parenteral routes of administration (this is discussed in Chapter 36). Excessively hypotonic or hypertonic solutions can cause biological damage.

Diffusion in solution

The components of a solution, by definition, form a homogeneous single phase. This homogeneity arises from the process of diffusion, which occurs spontaneously and is consequently accompanied by a decrease in the free energy (G) of the system. *Diffusion* may be defined as the spontaneous transference of a component from a region in the system which has a high chemical potential into a region where its chemical potential is lower. Although such a gradient in chemical potential provides the driving force for diffusion, the laws that describe this phenomenon are usually expressed, more conveniently, in terms of concentration gradients. An example is Fick's first law of diffusion, which is discussed in Chapter 2.

The most common explanation of the mechanism of diffusion in solution is based on the lattice theory of the structure of liquids. Lattice theories postulate that liquids have crystalline or quasicrystalline structures. The concept of a crystal type of lattice is only intended to provide a convenient starting point and should not be interpreted as a suggestion that liquids possess rigid structures. The theories also postulate that a reasonable proportion of the volume occupied by the liquid is, at any moment, empty, i.e. there are 'holes' in the liquid lattice network (discussed in Chapter 2 in the context of dissolution), which constitute the so-called *free volume* of the liquid.

Diffusion can therefore be regarded as the process by which solute molecules move from hole to hole within a liquid lattice. In order to achieve such movement, a solute molecule must acquire sufficient kinetic energy at the right time so that it can break away from any bonds that tend to anchor it in one hole and then jump into an adjacent hole. If the average distance of each jump is δ (cm) and the frequency with which the jumps occur is ϕ (s^{-1}), then the *diffusion coefficient* (D) is given by

$$D = \frac{\delta^2 \phi}{6} \text{ cm}^2 \text{ s}^{-1}$$

(3.27)

The diffusion coefficient is assumed to have a constant value for a particular system at a given temperature. This assumption is only strictly true at infinite dilution, and the value of D may therefore exhibit some concentration dependency. In a given solvent, the value of D decreases as the size of the diffusing solute molecule increases. In water, for example, D is of the order of 2×10^{-5} cm^2 s^{-1} for solutes with molecular weights of approximately 50 Da and it decreases to about 1×10^{-6} cm^2 s^{-1} for molecular weight of a few thousand Da.

The value of δ for any given solute is reasonably constant. Differences in the diffusion coefficient of a substance in solution in various solvents arise mainly from changes in jump frequency (ϕ), which is determined, in turn, by the free volume or looseness of packing in the solvent.

When the size of the solute molecules is not appreciably larger than that of the solvent molecules, then it has been shown that the diffusion coefficient of the former is related to its molecular weight (M) by the relationship:

$$DM^{1/2} = \text{constant}$$

$$(3.28)$$

When the solute is much greater in size than the solvent, diffusion arises largely from transport of solvent molecules in the opposite direction, and the relationship becomes

$$DM^{1/3} = \text{constant}$$

$$(3.29)$$

This latter equation forms the basis of the Stokes–Einstein equation (Eq. 3.30) for the diffusion of spherical particles that are larger than surrounding liquid molecules. Since the mass (m) of a spherical particle is proportional to the cube of its radius (r), i.e. $r \propto m^{1/3}$, it follows from Eq. 3.29 that $Dm^{1/3}$ and consequently D and r are constants for such a system. The Stokes–Einstein equation is usually written in the form

$$D = \frac{kT}{6\pi r \eta}$$

$$(3.30)$$

where k is the Boltzmann constant, T is the absolute temperature and η is the viscosity of the liquid. The appearance of a viscosity term in this type of equation is not unexpected because the reciprocal of viscosity, which is known as the *fluidity* of a liquid, is proportional to the free volume in a liquid. Thus the jump frequency (ϕ) and diffusion coefficient (D) will increase as the viscosity of a liquid decreases or as the number of 'holes' in its structure increases.

The experimental determination of diffusion coefficients of solutes in liquid solvents is not easy because the effects of other factors that may influence the movement of solute in the system, e.g. temperature and density gradients, mechanical agitation and vibration, must be eliminated.

Summary

This chapter has outlined the key fundamental issues relating to the properties of solutions. The issues discussed are of relevance both to dosage forms, which themselves comprise solutions, and to the fate of the drug molecule once it is in solution following administration.

Please check your eBook at **https://studentconsult. inkling.com/** for self-assessment questions. See inside cover for registration details.

Bibliography

Allen, L.V., 2012. Remington: The Science and Practice of Pharmacy, twenty second ed. Pharmaceutical Press, London.

Cairns, D., 2012. Essentials of Pharmaceutical Chemistry, fourth ed. Pharmaceutical Press, London.

Florence, A.T., Attwood, D., 2016. Physicochemical Principles of Pharmacy: In Manufacture, Formulation and Clinical Use, sixth ed. Pharmaceutical Press, London.

Florence, A.T., Siepmann, J. (Eds.), 2009. Modern Pharmaceutics,

vol. 1 and 2, fifth ed. Informa, New York.

Martin, A., Bustamante, P., 1993. Physical Pharmacy: Physical Chemical Principles in the Pharmaceutical Sciences, fourth ed. Lea & Febiger, Philadelphia.

Surfaces and interfaces

4

Graham Buckton

KEY POINTS

- Solids and liquids have surfaces that define the outer limits. The contact between any two materials is an interface, which can be between two solids, two liquids, a solid and a liquid, a solid and a vapour, or a liquid and a vapour.
- Inevitably for materials to react and interact, interfacial contact must be made.
- The study of surfaces and their interfacial interactions is therefore important as it defines (at least the onset of) all interactions and reactions.
- The surfaces of liquids (liquid–vapour interfaces) are studied by use of surface tension measurements, and the magnitude of the surface tension is related to the strength of bonding pulling molecules at the surface towards the bulk. Hydrogen bonding (as in water) is stronger than van der Waals forces, so water has a higher surface tension than an alkane.
- The surfaces of solids can be studied by use of contact angle measurements, which define the extent to which a liquid wets the solid. If there is no wetting, then there is no interaction and a solid could not, for example, dissolve in the liquid. To aid drug dissolution in the gastrointestinal tract, good wetting is desirable.
- Adsorption is defined as a higher concentration at the surface than in the bulk, and can be related to solid–liquid and solid–vapour systems through adsorption isotherms. Amongst other uses, adsorption can be used to measure the surface area of a powder.
- Absorption is the movement of one phase into another. Water often absorbs into amorphous solids, but adsorbs onto crystalline solids.

Introduction

A surface is the outer boundary of a material. In reality, each surface is the boundary between two phases: an interface, which can be solid/liquid (SL), solid/vapour (SV) or liquid/vapour (LV); or a boundary between two immiscible phases of the same state, i.e. liquid/liquid or solid/solid interfaces. There cannot be vapour/vapour interfaces, as two vapours would mix, rather than form an interface.

Pharmaceutically we often think of materials in terms of their bulk properties, such as solubility, particle size, density and melting point. However, surface material properties often bear little relationship to bulk properties; for example, materials can be readily wetted by a liquid but not dissolve in it, i.e. they could have water-loving surfaces but not be soluble (an example of this is glass). As contact between materials occurs at interfaces, knowledge of surface properties is necessary if interactions between two materials are to be understood (or predicted). Every process, reaction, interaction, whatever it may be, either starts or fails to start due to the extent of interfacial contact.

Surface tension

If we compare the forces acting on a molecule in the bulk of a liquid with those acting on a molecule at the interface (Fig. 4.1), in the bulk the molecules are surrounded on all sides by other liquid molecules and will consequently have no net force acting on them (all attractive forces generally being balanced). At the surface, however, each liquid molecule is surrounded by other liquid molecules to the sides and below (essentially in a hemisphere below the molecule), whilst above the molecule the interactions will be with

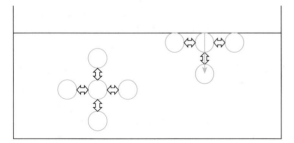

Fig. 4.1 • The balance of forces on molecules at the surface and in the bulk of a liquid. Molecules (depicted here as *large circles*) in the bulk of a liquid have neighbours on all sides and a net balance of forces. Molecules at the surface have neighbours to each side, but no balance for the attraction of molecules from below, giving a net inward force into the body of the liquid – this is the basis of surface tension.

gas molecules from the vapour; these will be much weaker than those between the liquid molecules. As the molecule at the liquid surface has balanced forces pulling sideways, the imbalance is a net inward attraction in a line perpendicular to the interface. Because of the net inward force exerted on liquids, the liquid surface will tend to contract, and to form a sphere (the geometry with minimum surface area to volume ratio). The contracted liquid surface is said to exist in a state of tension – known as *surface tension*. The value of surface tension for a liquid will be related to the strength of the pull between the liquid molecules. The interfacial interactions are a consequence of long-range forces which are electrical in nature and consist of three types: dipole, induced dipole and dispersion forces.

Dipole forces are due to an imbalance of charge across the structure of a molecule. This situation is quite common; most drugs are ionizable, and have such an asymmetric charge distribution, as do many macromolecules and proteins. Such materials are said to have permanent dipoles, and interactive forces are due to attraction between the negative pole of one molecule when it is in reasonably close contact with the positive pole of another. Hydrogen-bonding interactions are a specific sort of this type of bonding, occurring because hydrogen consists of only one proton and one electron, making it very strongly electronegative. When hydrogen bonds, its electron is 'lost', leaving an 'exposed' proton (i.e. one without any surrounding electrons). This unique situation causes a strong attraction between the proton and an electronegative region from another atom. The strength of the hydrogen bond results in drastically different properties of interaction, exemplified by the fact that water has such a high surface tension, melting point and boiling point (in comparison with non-hydrogen-bonded materials).

A bond between carbon and oxygen would be expected to be dipolar; however, if the molecule of carbon dioxide is considered ($O=C=O$), it can be seen that the molecule is in fact totally symmetrical, the dipole on each end of the linear molecule being in perfect balance with that on the other end. Even though these molecules do not carry a permanent dipole, if they are placed in the presence of a polarized material, a dipole will be induced on the (normally symmetrical) molecule, such that interaction can occur (dipole–induced dipole, or Debye, interactions).

London van der Waals forces are termed dispersion forces. These are interactions between molecules which do not have a charge imbalance, and which do not have the ability to have an induced dipole either. Essentially these are interactions between nonpolar materials. These dispersion forces occur between all materials, and thus even though the interaction forces are weak, they make a very significant contribution to the overall interaction between two molecules. Dispersion forces can be understood in a simplistic fashion by considering the fact that the electrons which spin around two neighbouring nonpolarized atoms will inevitably not remain equally spaced. This will result in local imbalances in charge that lead to transient induced dipoles. These induced dipoles, and the forces which result from them, will be constantly changing, and obviously the magnitude of these interactions is small compared with the permanent and induced dipole situations described previously. Dispersion forces are long range, of the order of 10 nm, which is significantly longer than a bond length.

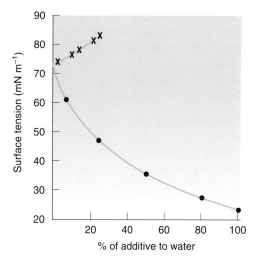

Fig. 4.2 • The surface tension of mixtures of methanol and water *(circles)* and sodium chloride and water *(crosses)*. Based on data from Weast, 1988.

Measurement of surface tension

The surface tension of a liquid is the combined strength of the polar and dispersion forces that are pulling on the molecules in the surface of the liquid. There are a number of methods by which surface tension can be measured, including the rise of a liquid in a capillary, but more usually the force experienced by the surface is measured using a microbalance. To do this, an object in the form of either a thin plate (Wilhelmy plate) or a ring (Du Nouy ring) is introduced to the surface and then pulled free, with the force at detachment being measured. For the Wilhelmy plate method, a plate (usually very clean glass or platinum) is positioned edge on in the surface whilst suspended from a microbalance arm; the force is then measured as the plate is pulled out of the liquid. The surface tension is obtained by dividing the measured force at the point of detachment by the perimeter of the plate.

Water is the liquid with the highest value for its surface tension of all commonly used liquids in the pharmaceutical field (although metals have much higher surface tensions than water, e.g. mercury with a surface tension of 380 mN m^{-1}). Water is also of great pharmaceutical interest, being the vehicle used for the large majority of liquid formulations, and being the essential component of all biological fluids. At the standard reporting temperature, the surface tension of water is 72.6 mN m^{-1}.

The addition of small quantities of impurities will alter the surface tension. In general, organic impurities are found to lower the surface tension of water significantly. Take, for example, the addition of methanol to water. The surface tension of methanol is 22.7 mN m^{-1}, but the surface tension of a 7.5% solution of methanol in water is 60.9 mN m^{-1} (Fig. 4.2). On the basis of a linear reduction in surface tension in proportion to the concentration of methanol added, the surface tension of this mixture would be expected to be about 68.9 mN m^{-1}; thus the initial reduction in surface tension on addition of an organic impurity is dramatic, and cannot be explained by the weighted mean of the surface tensions of the two liquids. Methanol has been used as the example here, as it is one of the more polar organic liquids, containing just one carbon, attached to a polar hydroxyl group. However, it is its hydrophobicity that causes the significant reduction in surface tension. The reason for the large effect on surface tension is that the water molecules have greater attraction to each other than to methanol; consequently the methanol is concentrated at the water–air interface, rather than in the bulk of the water. The methanol here is said to be surface active (surface-active agents are discussed elsewhere in this book; in particular in Chapters 4, 5 and 27). Water obtained directly from a tap can have a surface tension greater than 72.6 mN m^{-1}, because of the presence of ionic impurities, such as sodium chloride, which are concentrated preferentially in the bulk of water rather than at the surface. Inorganic additives also strengthen the bonding within water, so the surface tension is increased in their presence.

Solid wettability

The vast majority of pharmaceutically active compounds exist in the solid state at standard temperatures and pressures. Inevitably, the solid drug will come into contact with a liquid phase, either during processing, and/or in the formulation, and also ultimately during use in the body. Consequently, the solid/liquid interface is of great importance. Here the term *wettability* is used to assess the extent to which a solid will come into contact with a liquid. Obviously a material which is potentially soluble but which is not wetted by the liquid (i.e. the liquid does not spread over the solid) will have limited contact with the liquid and this will certainly reduce the rate at, and potentially the extent to, which the solid will dissolve. When formulating an active pharmaceutical ingredient, it is important that the powder ultimately becomes wetted by body fluids so that it will dissolve.

As with liquid surfaces, there is a net imbalance of forces in the surface of a solid, and so solids will have a surface energy. The surface energy of a solid is a reflection of the ease of making new surface, and in simple terms can be considered to be the same as surface tension for a liquid. With liquids, the surface molecules are free to move, and consequently surface levelling is seen, resulting in a consistent surface tension/energy over the entire surface. However, with solids the surface molecules are held much more rigidly, and are consequently less able to move. The shape of solids is dependent upon previous history (perhaps crystallization or milling techniques). These processes may yield rough surfaces with different regions of the same solid's surface having different surface energies. Certainly different crystal faces and edges can all be expected to have a different surface nature due to the local orientation of the molecules presenting different functional groups at the surface of different faces of the crystal – some more and some less polar, and therefore some regions more water loving and other regions less so.

Contact angle

The properties of solids raise many problems with respect to surface energy determination, not least

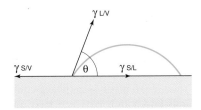

Fig. 4.3 • A contact angle – the angle (θ) between the tangent to the drop (drawn at the point where liquid, solid and vapour all coexist), measured through the liquid to the solid surface. The angle is a consequence of the interfacial energies of γ_{LV} (the surface tension of the liquid) and the interfacial tension between the solid and vapour (γ_{SV}), and the solid and liquid (γ_{SL}).

the fact that it is not possible to measure directly the forces exerted on the surface. The methods that are used for liquid surface tension measurement, such as immersing a Wilhelmy plate and measuring the force as it is pulled from the liquid, cannot be used as the plate cannot gain access to the solid. This means that surface properties of solids must be derived from techniques such as contact angle measurement. The tendency for a liquid to spread is estimated from the magnitude of the contact angle (θ), which is defined as the angle formed between the tangent drawn to the liquid drop at the three-phase interface and the solid surface, measured through the liquid (Fig. 4.3). The contact angle is a consequence of a balance of the three interfacial forces; γ_{SV} acting to aid spreading; γ_{SL} acting to prevent spreading and γ_{LV}, which acts along the tangent to the drop. The interfacial forces are related to the contact angle by Young's equation:

$$\gamma_{LV} \cos\theta = \gamma_{SV} - \gamma_{SL}$$

$$(4.1)$$

A low value for the contact angle indicates good wettability, with total spreading being described by an angle of 0°. Conversely, a high contact angle indicates poor wettability, with an extreme being total nonwetting with a contact angle of 180°. The contact angle provides a numerical assessment of the tendency of a liquid to spread over a solid, and as such is a measure of wettability.

If a contact angle were measured on an ideal (perfectly smooth, homogeneous and flat) surface with a pure liquid, then there would be only one value for the contact angle. In reality there are many contact angles that can be formed on a solid surface. The simplest analogy is water on glass. The contact angle of pure water on clean glass is zero, which provides the basis of surface tension experiments (as a finite contact angle would prevent such measurements). However, whenever raindrops are seen to form on a glass window, they do not spread, but rather form drops. The reason for this is that the window will not be clean and the liquid not pure. If raindrops fall onto a plate of glass which is horizontal, each drop will have the same contact angle all around its circumference. This value is termed the *equilibrium contact angle* (θ_E). If the glass plate is displaced from the horizontal, the drops will run down the surface, forming a tear shape. The leading edge of this drop will always have a larger contact angle than the trailing edge. The angle formed at the leading edge is termed the *advancing contact angle* (θ_A) and the other angle is termed *the receding contact angle* (θ_R). The difference between θ_A and θ_R defines the *contact angle hysteresis*. There are two possible reasons for contact angle hysteresis: surface roughness and contamination or variability of the composition of the surface, i.e. surface heterogeneity.

There are many different methods by which it is possible to measure a contact angle formed by a liquid on a solid. The vast majority of studies deal with smooth flat surfaces, such as polymer films, onto which it is comparatively simple to position a drop of liquid. The approaches for determination of the angle for such systems include direct measurement of the angle on a video image.

The Wilhelmy plate apparatus was described earlier as a method by which it is possible to measure surface tension. To do so it is necessary for the liquid to have zero contact angle on the plate. Conversely, it is possible to assess the contact angle (θ) between the solid plate and the liquid if the surface tension of the liquid (γ_{LV}) is known. The force detected by the balance (F) is

$$F = p\gamma_{LV}\cos\theta$$

(4.2)

where p is the perimeter of the plate, and from this the value of the contact angle can be determined.

As mentioned already, certain polymeric systems are readily formed into smooth flat plates for contact angle studies; however, most pharmaceutical materials exist as powders, for which such a physical state is not readily achievable. A full understanding of powder

surface energetics, and an ability to alter and control powder surface properties, would be a major advantage to the pharmaceutical scientist.

A drug crystal will consist of a number of different faces which may each consist of different proportions of the functional groups of the drug molecule; thus a contact angle for a powder will in fact be, at best, an average of the contact angles of the different faces, with contributions from crystal edges and defects. Also, impurities in the crystallizing solvent can cause an adjustment of habit, and crystals of the same drug can exist in different polymorphic forms; such changes in molecular packing will potentially alter the surface properties. A final complication is that despite the fact that most pharmaceutical powders have a very high degree of crystallinity (and are called crystals), in reality sometimes they will have a small degree of amorphous content which is likely to be present at the surface. Thus drug powders have heterogeneous surfaces of different shapes and sizes, which can readily change their surface properties. It is clear that all contact angle data for powders and the appropriate choice of methodology must be viewed in full knowledge of the inherent difficulties of the solid sample.

The most cited method of obtaining a contact angle for powders is to prepare a compact in order to produce a smooth surface, and then to place a drop on the surface in order to measure the contact angle that is formed. The first major problem with compacted samples is that the very process of compaction will potentially change the surface energy of the sample. Compacts form by processes of brittle fracture and plastic deformation; thus new surfaces will be formed during compaction, which can mask subtle differences in the original surface nature. In fact the formation of a compact is the conversion of the material from being individual particles into a single bonded mass (no longer individual particles), so a measurement of a contact angle on a compact gives information about the material generally, but cannot be expected to give information about the unique aspects of a type of particle of that material, as the compaction will have altered the material. The alternative is to not compact the powder; for example, sticking fine powder on a piece of doubled-sided adhesive tape. This presents a rough surface which gives rise to hysteresis and potentially also has a contribution from the surface property of the adhesive. There is no solution to these sample preparation difficulties, so a compromise has to be made in order to proceed with measurements.

Alternatives to placing a drop on the surface of a material exist for powder contact angle measurement, including making the powder into a plate and adapting the Wilhelmy plate method, and also measuring the rate at which liquid penetrates into a packed bed of the powder. These methods and their limitations have been reviewed elsewhere (Buckton, 1995). The different methods by which the contact angle is measured for powders gives rise to different results, so comparison of data should take this into account.

An alternative to contact angle measurement is to use inverse gas chromatography (IGC). Further discussion of IGC is presented later in this chapter.

Adsorption at interfaces

Adsorption is the presence of a greater concentration of a material at the surface than in the bulk. The material which is adsorbed is called the *adsorbate*, and that which does the adsorbing is the *adsorbent*. Adsorption can be due to physical bonding between the adsorbent and the adsorbate (*physisorption*) or chemical bonding (*chemisorption*). The differences between physisorption and chemisorption are that physisorption is by weak bonds (such as hydrogen bonding, with energies up to $40 \, kJ \, mol^{-1}$), whilst chemisorption is due to strong bonding ($> 80 \, kJ \, mol^{-1}$); physisorption is reversible, whilst chemisorption seldom is; physisorption may progress beyond a single-layer coverage of molecules on the surface (*monolayer formation* to *multilayer formation*), whilst chemisorption can only proceed to monolayer coverage.

Solid–liquid interfaces

The usual pharmaceutical situation is to have a liquid (solvent), particles of a solid dispersed in that liquid and another component dissolved in the liquid (solute). This forms the basis of stabilizing suspension formulations, where there may be water with suspended active pharmaceutical ingredient and in order to help stabilize the suspension (keep the solid particles from joining together) there may be a surface-active agent dissolved in the water. The surface-active agent will adsorb on the surface of the powder particles and help to keep them separated from each other (steric stabilization). It is also possible to use this surface interaction in the treatment of drug overdose, where charcoal of high surface area can be administered and the excess drug in the patient's gastrointestinal

tract can be adsorbed from solution onto the surface of the charcoal, which is then cleared from the patient. Kaolin is administered as a therapy to adsorb toxins in the stomach and so reduce gastrointestinal tract disturbances. A further example is analysis by high-performance liquid chromatography (HPLC) – where molecules in solution are adsorbed onto a column to achieve separation. As a final example, the loss of active pharmaceutical ingredient, or preservative, from a solution product to a container can be a damaging effect of adsorption from solution to a solid.

The quantity of solute which adsorbs will be related to its concentration in the liquid. The adsorption will proceed until equilibrium is reached between the solute that has been adsorbed at the interface and solute in the bulk.

Many factors will affect adsorption from solution onto a solid; these include temperature, concentration and the nature of the solute, solvent and solid. The effect of temperature is almost always that an increase in temperature will result in a decrease in adsorption. This can be viewed as a consequence of giving the solute molecules more energy, and thus allowing them to escape the forces of adsorption, or simply viewed as the fact that adsorption is almost always exothermic, and thus an increase in temperature will cause a decrease in adsorption.

The pH is important as many materials are ionizable, and the tendency to interact will vary greatly if they exist as polar ions, rather than a nonpolar un-ionized material. In most pharmaceutical examples (chromatographic separation being an obvious exception), adsorption will be from aqueous fluids, and for these, adsorption will tend to be greatest when the solute is in its un-ionized form, i.e. at low pH for weak acids, at high pH for weak bases, and at the isoelectric points for amphoteric compounds (those which exhibit acid and basic regions), although at other pH values the solubility in water will be higher (due to greater ionization favouring the interaction with water) and there will still be some un-ionized molecules present, which will usually adsorb on surfaces in preference to maintaining a disfavoured interaction with water.

The effect of solute solubility will influence adsorption as the greater the affinity of the solute for the liquid, the lower the tendency to adsorb to a solid. Thus adsorption from solution is approximately inversely related to solubility.

The nature of the solid (the adsorbent) will be very important, both in terms of its chemical composition and its physical form. The physical form is the easiest to deal with, as it relates largely to available surface area. Materials such as carbon black (a very finely divided form of carbon) have extremely large surface areas, and as such are excellent adsorbents, both from solution (e.g. as an antidote as mentioned earlier) and from the vapour state, where it has been used for gas masks. The chemical nature of the adsorbent solid is important, as it can be a nonpolar hydrophobic surface, or a polar (charged) surface. Obviously, adsorption to a nonpolar surface will be predominantly by dispersion force interactions, whilst charged materials can also interact by ionic or hydrogen-bonding processes.

Solid–vapour interfaces

When considering the solid–vapour interface, it is necessary to understand the processes of adsorption and absorption. Adsorption has already been defined as the presence of greater concentrations of a material at the surface than is present in the bulk. Pharmaceutically, *absorption* is usually considered as the passage of a molecule across a barrier membrane, and is the essential requirement for enteral drug delivery routes to the systemic circulation. However, absorption should be considered as the movement into something; for example, a gas or vapour can pass into the structure of an amorphous material, such that the uptake onto/into the solid is the sum of adsorption (to the surface) and absorption (into the bulk). If the uptake is thought to consist of both adsorption and absorption processes, it is often referred to by the general term *sorption*.

There are many processes at the solid–vapour interface which are of pharmaceutical interest, but two of the most important are water vapour–solid interactions, and surface area determination using nitrogen (or similar inert gas)–solid interactions.

Solid–vapour adsorption isotherms

As with adsorption at the solid–liquid interface, the process can be due to chemisorption or physisorption. Most usually we will be concerned with physisorption.

Adsorption isotherms for adsorption of vapours onto solids are representations of experimental data, usually plotted as the amount adsorbed as a function of the pressure of the gas, at a constant temperature. For such a plot, the pressure of the gas can be varied from zero to the saturated vapour pressure of the gas at that temperature (P_o), and in each case the amount adsorbed can be determined (often by monitoring of the change of weight of the sample). The concept of named adsorption isotherms (e.g. the Langmuir isotherm) is simply one of observing whether the experimental data fit to one of the existing mathematical models. If the data can be fitted, then there are several advantages: firstly, it becomes possible to define the adsorption process numerically, and thus exact comparisons can be made with similar data for other materials; secondly, the models provide clues as to the nature of the adsorption process that has occurred (e.g. indicating whether the process is monolayer or multilayer).

Langmuir (type I) isotherm

The Langmuir isotherm (one which fits the equation developed by Langmuir) is shown schematically in Fig. 4.4. It has a characteristic shape of fairly rapid adsorption at low pressures of gas/vapour, and reaches a plateau well below P_o, after which any further increases in pressure do not cause an increase in adsorption. This is the idealized model for monolayer adsorption, in that initially the surface is 'clean' and consists entirely of adsorption sites. Thus a small amount of vapour allows rapid and

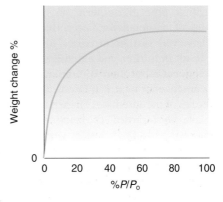

Fig. 4.4 • A Langmuir isotherm. Weight increases as the partial pressure of the vapour (P/P_o) is increased until a monolayer of molecules has formed on the surface of the solid, after which there is no further weight change as P/P_o is increased further. The mass uptake (no scale shown) will depend on the available surface area of the sample.

extensive adsorption. Subsequently, more and more of the available adsorption sites become occupied, and thus further increases in pressure result in comparatively little increase in the amount adsorbed. At a certain pressure, all the adsorption sites will be occupied, i.e. monolayer coverage has been achieved, after which adsorption stops, giving a plateau region in which further increases in pressure have no effect on the amount adsorbed.

The Langmuir isotherm can only occur in situations where the entire surface is covered with equally accessible, identical adsorption sites, and the presence of an adsorbed molecule on one site does not hinder (or encourage) adsorption to a neighbouring site. For a system to follow a Langmuir isotherm, there must be a strong nonspecific interaction between the adsorbate and the adsorbent (such that adsorption is desirable over the entire surface), and there must be little adsorbate–adsorbate interaction (in terms of attraction or repulsion).

Type II isotherms

The Langmuir isotherm (see Fig. 4.4) which describes adsorption of a monolayer only is often referred to as a type I physical adsorption isotherm. There are other common shapes for adsorption isotherms, each of which can be taken to give an indication of the nature of the adsorption process. The schematic shapes of some other isotherms are shown in Fig. 4.5. Type II isotherms are thought to correspond to a process which initially follows the Langmuir type of isotherm, in that there is a build-up of a monolayer; after this monolayer region, however, further increases in the vapour content result in further, and extensive, adsorption. This subsequent adsorption is multilayer coverage, and is a consequence of strong interactions between the molecules of the adsorbate. These post-monolayer regions can be regarded as being analogous to condensation, and the isotherm rises as the pressure approaches P_o.

Type III isotherms

Type III isotherms are typical of the situation where the interaction between adsorbate molecules is greater than that between the adsorbate and adsorbent molecules, i.e. the solid and the vapour have no great affinity for each other. This results in an isotherm

Type II

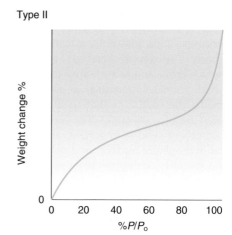

Type III

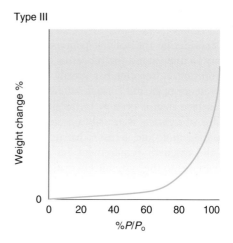

Fig. 4.5 • Type II and type III isotherms. The type II isotherm *(top)* shows weight gain as the partial pressure of the vapour (P/P_o) (which would be relative humidity for water) is increased, with rapid uptake at low P/P_o, passing through monolayer to multilayer coverage. The type III isotherm *(bottom)* shows little weight gain at low P/P_o, with mass gain accelerating at higher P/P_o.

shape for which it is necessary to have a significant presence of vapour before the adsorption process becomes significant, but once the surface starts to be covered with adsorbate, the favourable adsorbate–adsorbate interaction results in a dramatic increase in adsorption for limited further increases in vapour concentration.

Brunauer, Emmett and Teller isotherm

The isotherm derived by Brunauer, Emmett and Teller is eponymously known as the BET isotherm. It is widely used as a standard method of determining surface area for solids. Just as the Langmuir isotherm fits to the type I physical isotherm, the BET isotherm fits those situations which follow the type II isotherm. The type II isotherm is perhaps the most commonly encountered practically determined isotherm.

Interpretation of isotherm plots

With the Langmuir isotherm it can be assumed that the plateau region corresponds to monolayer formation; thus the quantity of gas adsorbed at the monolayer is known, and consequently, as the area of each molecule of gas is known, the surface area of the solid can be determined. With a type II isotherm, the system passes through monolayer coverage, at a region on the isotherm. This is rather difficult to define with any certainty from the graphical isotherm, but can easily be obtained from the BET equation:

$$(P/P_o)/[1-(P/P_o)]V = [1/(cV_{mon})] \\ + [(c-1)/(cV_{mon})](P/P_o)$$

$$(4.3)$$

where P is vapour pressure, P_o is saturated vapour pressure (note P/P_o for water is the relative humidity), V is the volume of gas adsorbed, V_{mon} is the volume of gas adsorbed at monolayer coverage and c is a constant.

If $(P/P_o)/[1-(P/P_o)]V$ is plotted as a function of P/P_o, the slope will be $(c-1)/(cV_{mon})$ and the intercept will be $1/(cV_{mon})$. From this it is possible to calculate V_{mon}, the volume of the adsorbed gas which covers a monolayer. If the volume of gas is known, the number of gas molecules can be calculated, and then if the area occupied by each gas molecule is known, the surface area of the solid is obtained.

The measured surface area can differ depending on the gas/vapour used to determine the isotherm. The most commonly used gas for surface area determination is nitrogen. The concept of fractal geometries brings into question all definitions of length, and consequently surface area. The standard typical illustration of fractals is shown in Fig. 4.6, in which it can be seen that the length of an irregular, rough object can be altered enormously depending on the resolution used in its measurement. For example, it is easy to consider the length of coastline at low magnification, but it becomes hard to know at what

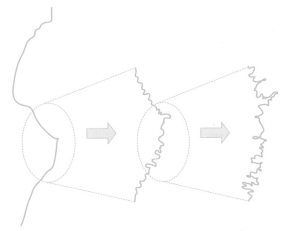

Fig. 4.6 • The same region of a surface seems to have a bigger surface area as the accuracy of measurement is increased. Expanding part of the line on the *left* gives a rougher surface *(middle)*, and expanding part of the *middle* gives further features *(right)*.

magnification one should reasonably stop, as with each magnification the length will increase by a factor proportional to that magnification. This caution is included, as the surface area of most solids is determined in relation to a nitrogen molecule as a probe. There will be many indentations in solids which may not be readily accessed by nitrogen gas, so a different probe gas (different size of molecule, e.g. krypton gas) can access different regions of the solid surface and the calculated surface area will change.

Isotherm models, other than Langmuir and BET models, exist which can also be used to understand powder–vapour interactions, but these will not be discussed here.

Interactions between powders and water vapour

The interaction between water and a product is a consideration for almost every pharmaceutical product. Water may be important during formulation/preparation (e.g. affecting powder flow, in a wet granulation process, in drying processes, for ease of compaction, as a film-coating solvent, and in aqueous liquid formulations), during storage (where it may influence chemical stability, physical transitions such as crystallization, or microbial spoilage), and during use (where there is a need to contact aqueous body fluids).

It is clear from the previous paragraph that interaction with water is essential at certain stages, but undesirable in other situations. Consequently, an understanding of how, why, where, when and how much water will associate with a solid is an important issue in the development of pharmaceutical products. Water may interact with surfaces by adsorption and condensation, with some solids by absorption, as well as by inclusion into crystal structures as hydrates.

Water adsorption

Water is able to adsorb to a wide range of different materials over a wide range of temperature and humidity. Most gases that have been mentioned so far, such as nitrogen, are thought to adsorb uniformly across surfaces, whilst water is thought to selectively bind to polar regions of a solid surface. Thus the extent of adsorption of water to a solid surface is related to the degree of polarity of the solid itself.

It has been reported (van Campen et al., 1983; Kontny et al., 1987) that the adsorption of water onto most crystalline solids is not able to cause the solids to dissolve. This is because only a few layers of water molecules form as a 'multilayer' on solids and this is a very small volume for dissolution. Furthermore, the structure of water adsorbed to the surface of a solid is different to the tetrahedral structure of bulk water, so the adsorbed material cannot be expected to have the same properties as a solvent, as would be expected of bulk water. Given the observation of Kontny et al. (1987) that the layer of water which is adsorbed to the surface is only a few molecules thick and is not acting as bulk liquid, the question must be asked as to why water can have such a huge influence on the properties of materials, and on their physical and chemical stability. It can easily be calculated that the quantities of water which are said to be associated with solids are greatly in excess of that which can be accommodated in a few layers around their surface. Water can also interact with powders by being condensed in capillaries (or at other regions), or can be absorbed in amorphous regions, which is water that has the properties of bulk water and the ability to cause instability and spoilage.

The water content can be divided into different regions by considering the shape of the isotherm. The standard type II isotherm (Fig. 4.7) has two inflection points, the first of which is termed W_m (the water content at the point which is thought to be the onset of monolayer coverage) and the

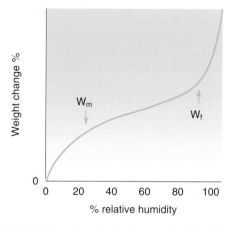

Fig. 4.7 • Water adsorption isotherm, showing W_m as the point where monolayer coverage will have occurred and W_f as the point above which the water is considered to be 'free' and to have the properties of bulk water.

second of which is termed W_f (the water content regarded as free). At all humidities below that which corresponds to W_m, the water can be regarded as tightly bound. At all points above W_f, the water is considered to be liquid at room temperature and freezable.

The condensation of water into capillaries is a consequence of the small pore sizes reducing the relative pressure at which condensation is possible. It can be estimated that the relative humidity at which water would condense would be 99% for pores of 100 nm, but only 50% for pores of 1.5 nm. It follows that materials which have surfaces which consist of many thousands of large-volume micropores will adsorb huge quantities of water by capillary condensation. Materials such as silica gel have this type of structure, but it is comparatively rare to find pharmaceuticals which have microporous surfaces.

Water absorption

It is incorrect to assume that most pharmaceuticals are fully crystalline, or that most water association with pharmaceuticals is by adsorption. It has already been stated that pharmaceuticals can have amorphous regions, and that even those which are regarded as crystalline can have amorphous surfaces. Amorphous surfaces result from physical treatment moving surface molecules, and there being no mechanism by which they can recrystallize rapidly. The amorphous regions can result in chemical instability and altered interactions between surfaces.

For amorphous materials, experimental evidence points to water uptake being due to absorption of water, as the quantity of water sorbed is related to the weight of materials present, and not the surface area (as would be the case for adsorption). It is also common for sorption and desorption isotherms for amorphous materials to show considerable hysteresis, despite the absence of microporous structure (the other main cause of such effects).

The interpretation of isotherms for systems which are suspected to have undergone absorption must be undertaken with care. The value W_m, for example, will still exist as a type II isotherm will be a common occurrence; however, it can no longer be expected to represent monolayer coverage. For amorphous materials, the value of W_m reflects the polarity of the solid: the higher the value, the more polar the solid. The second inflection point (W_f) for amorphous materials is believed to be the point at which the water has so plasticized the solid that the glass transition temperature (T_g) of the amorphous mass has fallen, such that it now equals the temperature of the experiment.

The *glass transition temperature* (T_g) of an amorphous material is the point at which it shows a change in properties. Below the T_g materials are brittle and are said to be in the glass (or glassy) state. For example, window glass has a T_g of about $1000\,^{\circ}C$, and as such is brittle at ambient conditions. Above the T_g a material becomes more rubbery. It is often desirable to have materials of a rubbery nature at room temperature, e.g. for the production of bottles which are less prone to shatter than glass. It is possible to mix another material with the main component; the minor component will fit between the molecules of the first component, and will allow greater molecular movement, thus lowering T_g. The additive is called a *plasticizer*. It is possible to estimate the effect of a plasticizer by use of the following simple equation:

$$1/T_{g12} = W_1/T_{g1} + W_2/T_{g2}$$

(4.4)

where W_1 is the weight fraction of material 1 (with $T_g = T_{g1}$), W_2 is the weight fraction of material 2 (with $T_g = T_{g2}$) and T_{g12} is the T_g of the mixture. Thus a plasticizer is a material which has a lower T_g than the material, and which can gain access to regions

within the molecules of the material. Water has a T_g of about $-138\,^{\circ}C$, and as such can efficiently plasticize many amorphous materials.

The process of amplification has been explained by Ahlneck & Zografi (1990), who regard absorption into amorphous regions as being the preferred form of interaction between powders and water vapour. It is argued that the amorphous regions are energetic 'hot spots', such that water would rather absorb than adsorb to the general surface. If we accept this hypothesis, which does seem entirely reasonable, then there must be great concern about materials which have a very small amorphous content and a small amount of associated water. It is quite usual for materials to contain 0.5% moisture, which sounds insignificant; however, if the material is 0.5% amorphous then it is likely that 0.5% moisture is in 0.5% of the solid, and is thus present in a 50:50 ratio of water to solid. This would provide a region of enormous potential for physical transition, chemical reaction or microbial spoilage. The example does not have to be as extreme as this; it has been calculated (Ahlneck & Zografi, 1990) that only 0.1% moisture content is needed in a sucrose sample which is 1% amorphous in order to plasticize the T_g of the amorphous sucrose to below room temperature.

It is clear then that the critical, drastic consequences of water–solid interaction are much more likely to result as a consequence of amplification of water into the minor regions of amorphous surface material than by surface adsorption. It follows that materials can be *expected* to change their properties as a consequence of any process which can reorder surface molecules, such as milling or spray-drying.

It is worth restating that the great increases in molecular mobility that accompany the transition from glass to rubber state will be sufficient to trigger physical changes and to initiate, or speed up, chemical degradation processes. This can occur in any amorphous material, which includes surface regions of 'crystalline' drugs and excipients.

The presence of high proportions of water in amorphous regions of solids is often enough to promote surface recrystallization. The surface need not have dissolved in the true dissolution sense of the word, but may simply have been plasticized to give sufficient reduction in viscosity to allow molecular realignment. It is now a matter of some commercial interest that surfaces will behave in totally different manners depending on whether they are partially amorphous or crystalline, and this will relate to ease

Table 4.1 The relative humidity that is produced in a sealed air space above certain saturated solutions at different temperatures

Salt	Relative humidity (%)						
	10°C	15°C	20°C	25°C	30°C	35°C	40°C
Potassium sulfate	98	97	97	97	96	96	96
Potassium chloride	88	87	86	85	84	83	82
Sodium chloride	76	76	76	75	75	75	75
Magnesium nitrate	57	56	55	53	52	50	49
Potassium carbonate	47	44	44	43	43	43	42
Magnesium chloride	34	34	33	33	33	32	32
Potassium acetate	24	23	23	22	22	21	20
Lithium chloride	13	13	12	12	12	12	11

Data from Wade (1980).

of use, stability on storage and ease of manufacture (see the examples in Chapter 8).

Deliquescence

Certain saturated solutions of salts are known to produce an atmosphere of a certain relative humidity above their surface. If any of these salts are stored in solid form at any humidity above the values that would be produced above their saturated solutions, then they will dissolve in the vapour. If they are stored below that critical humidity, then they will adsorb water vapour, but will not dissolve. Such materials which dissolve in water vapour are known as *deliquescent*.

A major characteristic of deliquescent materials is that they are very soluble, and have a large colligative effect on the solution formed, such that the vapour pressure of water is drastically reduced by the presence of the dissolved solute. The stage of events in deliquescence is that some water is adsorbed/absorbed. At a critical humidity, a small amount of the highly soluble solid dissolves and this lowers the vapour pressure of water, leading to extensive condensation, and an autocatalytic process develops (i.e. as more solid dissolves, the vapour pressure lowers, which causes more condensation to occur, which causes more solid to dissolve). The process will continue until all the material has dissolved, or until the relative humidity falls below that which is exhibited above

the saturated solution of the salt. The reason that different salts produce such a range of relative humidities above their saturated solution is due to the colligative action of their respective molecules reducing the activity of water. The relative humidity produced in the vapour space above saturated solutions of certain salts is reported in Table 4.1.

Inverse phase gas chromatography (IGC)

As mentioned earlier, there are practical issues with measuring the contact angle for powdered systems. An alternative is to study the interaction between the powder and a vapour. Gas chromatography is a well-established analytical method. A column is packed with a powder and a test sample is injected into a constant flow of gas that is passing through the column, which is held at constant temperature. A detector is positioned at the end of the column. The test sample will be carried through the column by the carrier gas; however, as it interacts with the powder in the column, components of the test sample will be slowed to different extents on the basis of the extent of interaction between them and the powder in the column. This achieves separation and good analysis. Inverse gas chromatography is where a known substance is injected and the test material is the powder packed into the column. For example, the known gas could be hexane vapour and the powder packed into the column is the material for which we wish to know the nature of its surface. It would be usual to inject vapours of a series of alkanes, say hexane, heptane, octane, nonane, and also to inject a number of polar vapours. From the retention times of the injected vapour it is possible to understand the dispersive surface energy (from the retention of the alkanes) and the polar surface energy (from the retention of polar probes) of the test solid. This allows the surface nature of different solids to be compared without the need to compact the sample and measure a contact angle.

Please check your eBook at **https://studentconsult. inkling.com/** for self-assessment questions. See inside cover for registration details.

References

Ahlneck, C., Zografi, G., 1990. The molecular basis of moisture effects on the physical and chemical stability of drugs in the solid state. Int. J. Pharm. 62, 87–95.

Buckton, G., 1995. Interfacial Phenomena in Drug Delivery and Targeting. Harwood Academic Press, Amsterdam.

Kontny, M.J., Grandolfi, G.P., Zografi, G., 1987. Water vapour sorption in water soluble substances: Studies of crystalline solids below their critical relative humidity. Pharm. Res. 4, 247–254.

van Campen, L., Amidon, G.L., Zografi, G., 1983. Moisture sorption kinetics for water-soluble substances. 1)

Theoretical considerations of heat transport control. J. Pharm. Sci. 72, 1381–1388.

Wade, A. (Ed.), 1980. Pharmaceutical Handbook. Pharmaceutical Press, London.

Weast, R.C. (Ed.), 1988. Handbook of Chemistry and Physics. CRC Press, Boca Raton.

5

Disperse systems

David Attwood

CHAPTER CONTENTS

KEY POINTS

- Disperse systems comprise one component, the disperse phase, dispersed as particles or droplets throughout another component, the continuous phase. They may be colloidal dispersions (1 nm to 1 μm), such as surfactant micelles, or coarse dispersions, such as emulsions, suspensions or aerosols.

- Colloids can be broadly classified as:
- *lyophobic* (solvent hating) (*hydrophobic* in aqueous systems); or
- *lyophilic* (*hydrophilic* in aqueous systems).
- The physical stability of disperse systems is determined by forces of interaction between the particles, including electrical double layer interaction, van der Waals attraction, solvation forces and steric repulsion arising from adsorbed polymeric material. The stability of lyophobic systems may be explained quantitatively by the Derjaguin–Landau–Verwey–Overbeek (DLVO) theory.

- Emulsions are usually dispersions of oil in water or water in oil, stabilized by an interfacial film of surfactant or hydrophilic polymer around the dispersed droplets. They are intrinsically unstable systems, and if droplet growth is unchecked, the emulsion will separate into two phases (i.e. crack).

- Suspensions may be stabilized if the flocculation of the dispersed particles is controlled by the addition of electrolytes or ionic surfactants.

- Aqueous surfactant solutions form micelles when the concentration of surfactant exceeds a critical value, termed the critical micelle concentration, determined by the chemical structure of the surfactant and the external conditions. Micellar solutions are stable dispersions within the true colloidal size range. Unlike other colloidal dispersions, there is a dynamic equilibrium between the micelles and the free surfactant molecules in solution; the micelles continuously break down and reform in solution. The interior core of typical micelles has properties similar to that of a liquid hydrocarbon, and is a site of solubilization of poorly soluble drugs.

Introduction

A disperse system consists essentially of one component, the *disperse phase*, dispersed as particles or droplets throughout another component, the *continuous phase*. By definition, those dispersions in which the size of the dispersed particles is within the range 10^{-9} m (1 nm) to about 10^{-6} m (1 μm) are termed *colloidal*. However, the upper size limit is often extended to include emulsions and suspensions which are very polydisperse systems in which the droplet size frequently exceeds 1 μm, but which show many of the properties of colloidal systems. Some examples of colloidal systems of pharmaceutical interest are shown in Table 5.1. Many natural systems such as suspensions of microorganisms, blood and isolated cells in culture are also colloidal dispersions.

This chapter will examine the properties of both coarse dispersions, such as emulsions, suspensions and aerosols, and fine dispersions, such as micellar systems, which fall within the defined size range of true colloidal dispersions.

Colloids can be broadly classified as those that are *lyophobic* (solvent hating) and those that are *lyophilic* (solvent liking). The terms *hydrophobic* and *hydrophilic* are used when the solvent is water. Surfactant molecules tend to associate in water into aggregates called micelles and these constitute hydrophilic colloidal dispersions. Proteins and gums also form lyophilic colloidal systems because of a similar affinity between the dispersed particles and the continuous phase. On the other hand, dispersions of oil droplets in water or water droplets in oil are examples of lyophobic dispersions.

It is because of the subdivision of matter in colloidal systems that they have special properties. A common feature of these systems is a large surface-to-volume ratio of the dispersed particles. As a consequence, there is a tendency for the particles to associate so as to reduce their surface area. Emulsion droplets, for example, eventually coalesce to form a macrophase, so attaining a minimum surface area and hence an equilibrium state. This chapter will examine how the stability of colloidal dispersions can be understood by a consideration of the forces acting between the dispersed particles. Approaches to the formulation of emulsions, suspensions and aerosols will be described, and the instability of these coarse dispersions will be discussed using a theory of colloid stability. The association of surface-active agents into micelles and the applications of these colloidal dispersions in the solubilization of poorly water-soluble drugs will also be considered.

Colloids

Preparation of colloidal systems

Lyophilic colloids

The affinity of lyophilic colloids for the dispersion medium leads to the spontaneous formation of colloidal dispersions. For example, acacia, tragacanth, methylcellulose and certain other cellulose derivatives readily disperse in water. This simple method of dispersion is a general one for the formation of lyophilic colloids.

Lyophobic colloids

The preparative methods for lyophobic colloids may be divided into those methods that involve the

Table 5.1 Types of disperse systems

Disperse phase	Dispersion medium	Name	Examples
Liquid	Gas	Liquid aerosol	Fogs, mists, aerosols
Solid	Gas	Solid aerosol	Smoke, powder aerosols
Gas	Liquid	Foam	Foam-on-surfactant solutions
Liquid	Liquid	Emulsion	Milk, pharmaceutical emulsions
Solid	Liquid	Sol, suspension	Silver iodide sol, aluminium hydroxide suspension
Gas	Solid	Solid foam	Expanded polystyrene
Liquid	Solid	Solid emulsion	Liquids dispersed in soft paraffin, opals, pearls
Solid	Solid	Solid suspension	Pigmented plastics, colloidal gold in glass, ruby glass

breakdown of larger particles into particles of colloidal dimensions (dispersion methods) and those in which the colloidal particles are formed by aggregation of smaller particles such as molecules (condensation methods).

Dispersion methods

The breakdown of coarse material may be carried out by the use of a colloid mill or ultrasonics.

Colloid mills. These mills cause the dispersion of coarse material by shearing in a narrow gap between a static cone (the stator) and a rapidly rotating cone (the rotor).

Ultrasonic treatment. The passage of ultrasonic waves through a dispersion medium produces alternating regions of cavitation and compression in the medium. The cavities collapse with great force and cause the breakdown of coarse particles dispersed in the liquid.

With both these methods, the particles will tend to reunite unless a stabilizing agent such as a surface-active agent is added.

Condensation methods

These involve the rapid production of supersaturated solutions of the colloidal material under conditions in which it is deposited in the dispersion medium as colloidal particles and not as a precipitate. The supersaturation is often obtained by means of a chemical reaction that results in the formation of the colloidal material. For example, colloidal silver iodide may be obtained by reacting together dilute solutions of silver nitrate and potassium iodide; colloidal sulphur is produced from sodium thiosulfate and hydrochloric acid solutions; and ferric chloride boiled with excess water produces colloidal hydrated ferric oxide.

A change of solvent may also cause the production of colloidal particles by condensation methods. If a saturated solution of sulphur in acetone is poured slowly into hot water, the acetone vaporizes, leaving a colloidal dispersion of sulphur. A similar dispersion may be obtained when a solution of a resin, such as benzoin in alcohol, is poured into water.

Purification of colloidal systems

Dialysis

Colloidal particles are not retained by conventional filter papers but are too large to diffuse through the pores of membranes such as those made from regenerated cellulose products, e.g. collodion (cellulose nitrate evaporated from a solution in alcohol and ether) and cellophane. The smaller molecules in solution are able to pass through these membranes. Use is made of this difference in diffusibility to separate micro-molecular impurities from colloidal dispersions. The process is known as *dialysis*. The process of dialysis may be hastened by stirring so as to maintain a high concentration gradient of diffusible molecules across the membrane and by renewing the outer liquid from time to time.

Ultrafiltration

By applying pressure (or suction), the solvent, solutes and small particles may be forced across a membrane, whilst the larger colloidal particles are retained. The process is referred to as *ultrafiltration*. It is possible to prepare membrane filters with known pore size, and use of these allows the particle size of a colloid to be determined. However, particle size and pore size cannot be properly correlated because the membrane permeability is affected by factors such as electrical repulsion, when both the membrane and the particle carry the same charge, and particle adsorption, which can lead to blocking of the pores.

Electrodialysis

An electric potential may be used to increase the rate of movement of ionic impurities through a dialysing membrane and so provide a more rapid means of purification. The concentration of charged colloidal particles at one side and at the base of the membrane is termed electrodecantation.

Properties of colloids

Size and shape of colloidal particles

Size distribution

Within the size range of colloidal dimensions specified earlier, there is often a wide distribution of sizes of the dispersed colloidal particles. The molecular weight or particle size is therefore an average value, the magnitude of which is dependent on the experimental technique used in its measurement. When determined by the measurement of colligative properties such as osmotic pressure, a number-average value, M_n, is obtained, which, in a mixture containing $n_1, n_2, n_3,$ ... moles of particle of mass $M_1, M_2, M_3,$ ..., respectively, is defined by

$$M_n = \frac{n_1M_1 + n_2M_2 + n_3M_3 + ...}{n_1 + n_2 + n_3 + ...} = \frac{\sum n_iM_i}{\sum n_i}$$

$$(5.1)$$

In the light-scattering method for the measurement of particle size, larger particles produce greater scattering and the weight rather than the number of particles is important, giving a weight-average value, M_w, defined by

$$M_w = \frac{m_1 M_1 + m_2 M_2 + m_3 M_3 + \ldots\ldots}{m_1 + m_2 + m_3 + \ldots\ldots} = \frac{\sum n_i M_i^2}{\sum n_i M_i}$$

(5.2)

In Eq. 5.2, m_1, m_2 and m_3 are the masses of each species, and m_i is obtained by multiplying the mass of each species by the number of particles of that species; that is, $m_i = n_i M_i$. A consequence is that $M_w > M_n$, and only when the system is monodisperse will the two averages be identical. The ratio M_w/M_n expresses the degree of polydispersity of the system.

Shape

Many colloidal systems, including emulsions, liquid aerosols and most dilute micellar solutions, contain spherical particles. Small deviations from sphericity are often treated using ellipsoidal models. Ellipsoids of revolution are characterized by their axial ratio, which is the ratio of the half-axis a to the radius of revolution b (Fig. 5.1). Where this ratio is greater than unity, the ellipsoid is said to be a prolate ellipsoid (rugby ball shaped), and when less than unity an oblate ellipsoid (discus shaped).

High molecular weight polymers and naturally occurring macromolecules often form random coils in aqueous solution. Clay suspensions are examples of systems containing plate-like particles.

Kinetic properties

In this section several properties of colloidal systems, which relate to the motion of particles with respect to the dispersion medium, will be considered. Thermal motion manifests itself in the form of Brownian motion, diffusion and osmosis. Gravity (or a centrifugal field) leads to sedimentation. Viscous flow

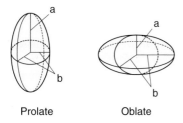

Prolate   Oblate

Fig. 5.1 • Model representation of ellipsoids of revolution.

is the result of an externally applied force. Measurement of these properties enables molecular weights or particle size to be determined.

Brownian motion

Colloidal particles are subject to random collisions with the molecules of the dispersion medium with the result that each particle pursues an irregular and complicated zigzag path. If the particles (up to about 2 μm diameter) are observed under a microscope or the light scattered by colloidal particles is viewed using an ultramicroscope, an erratic motion is seen. This movement is referred to as Brownian motion after Robert Brown, who first reported his observation of this phenomenon with pollen grains suspended in water.

Diffusion

As a result of Brownian motion, colloidal particles spontaneously diffuse from a region of higher concentration to one of lower concentration. The rate of diffusion is expressed by Fick's first law. One form of this relationship is shown in Eq. 5.3:

$$J = -D\frac{dC}{dx}$$

(5.3)

where J is the flux (flow of particles per unit time) across a plane of unit area under the influence of a concentration gradient dC/dx (the minus sign denotes that diffusion takes place in the direction of decreasing concentration). D is the diffusion coefficient and has the dimensions of area per unit time. The diffusion coefficient of a dispersed material is related to the frictional coefficient, f, of the particles by Einstein's law of diffusion:

$$Df = k_B T$$

(5.4)

where k_B is the Boltzmann constant and T temperature.

Therefore, as the frictional coefficient is given by the Stokes equation

$$f = 6\pi\eta a$$

(5.5)

where η is the viscosity of the medium and a the radius of the particle (assuming sphericity), then

$$D = \frac{k_B T}{6\pi\eta a} = \frac{RT}{6\pi\eta a N_A}$$

(5.6)

where N_A is the Avogadro constant, R is the universal gas constant and $k_B = R/N_A$. The diffusion coefficient may be obtained by an experiment measuring the change in concentration, via refractive index gradients, when the solvent is carefully layered over the solution to form a sharp boundary and diffusion is allowed to proceed. A more commonly used method is that of dynamic light scattering (photon correlation spectroscopy), which is discussed in the Optical properties section below. The diffusion coefficient can be used to obtain the molecular weight of an approximately spherical particle, such as egg albumin and haemoglobin, by use of Eq. 5.5 in the form

$$D = \frac{RT}{6\pi\eta N_A}\sqrt[3]{\frac{4\pi N_A}{3M\bar{v}}}$$

(5.7)

where M is the molecular weight and $\bar{v}$ is the partial specific volume of the colloidal material.

Sedimentation

Consider a spherical particle of radius a and density σ falling in a liquid of density ρ and viscosity η. The velocity v of sedimentation is given by Stokes law:

$$v = 2a^2 g(\sigma - \rho)/9\eta$$

(5.8)

where g is acceleration due to gravity.

If the particles are only subjected to the force of gravity then, because of Brownian motion, the lower size limit of particles obeying Eq. 5.8 is about 0.5 μm. A force stronger than gravity is therefore needed for colloidal particles to sediment, and use is made of a high-speed centrifuge, usually termed an ultracentrifuge, which can produce a force of about $10^6\ g$. In a centrifuge, g is replaced by $\omega^2 x$, where ω is the angular velocity and x the distance of the particle from the centre of rotation.

The ultracentrifuge is used in two distinct ways in investigating colloidal material. In the *sedimentation velocity* method, a high centrifugal field is applied, up to about $(4 \times 10^5)g$, and the movement of the particles, monitored by changes in concentration, is measured at specified time intervals. In the *sedimentation equilibrium* method, the colloidal material is subjected to a much lower centrifugal field until sedimentation and diffusion tendencies balance one another, and an equilibrium distribution of particles throughout the sample is attained.

Sedimentation velocity. The velocity dx/dt of a particle in a unit centrifugal force can be expressed in terms of the Svedberg coefficient s:

$$s = (dx/dt)/\omega^2 x$$

(5.9)

Under the influence of the centrifugal force, particles pass from position x_1 at time t_1 to position x_2 at time t_2. The differences in concentration with time can be measured using changes in refractive index and the application of the schlieren optical arrangement, whereby photographs can be taken showing these concentrations as peaks. The expression giving molecular weight M from this method is

$$M = \frac{RTs}{D(1-\bar{v}\rho)} = \frac{RT\ln x_2/x_1}{D(1-\bar{v}\rho)(t_2-t_1)\omega^2}$$

(5.10)

where $\bar{v}$ is the partial specific volume of the particle.

Sedimentation equilibrium. Equilibrium is established when sedimentation and diffusional forces balance.

Combination of sedimentation and diffusion equations is made in the analysis, giving

$$M = \frac{2RT\ln C_2/C_1}{\omega^2(1-\bar{v}\rho)(x_2^2 - x_1^2)}$$

(5.11)

where C_1 and C_2 are the sedimentation equilibrium concentrations at distances x_1 and x_2 from the axis of rotation. A disadvantage of the sedimentation equilibrium method is the length of time required to attain equilibrium, often as long as several days. A modification of the method in which measurements are made in the early stages of the approach to equilibrium significantly reduces the overall measurement time.

Osmotic pressure

The determination of molecular weights of dissolved substances from colligative properties such as the depression of the freezing point or the elevation of the boiling point is a standard procedure. However, of the available methods, only osmotic pressure has a practical value in the study of colloidal particles because of the magnitude of the changes in the properties. For example, the depression of freezing point of a 1% w/v solution of a macromolecule of molecular weight 70 000 is only 0.0026 K, far too small to be measured with sufficient accuracy by conventional methods and also very sensitive to the presence of low molecular weight impurities. In contrast, the osmotic pressure of this solution at 20 °C would be 350 N m^{-2}, or about 35 mm of water. Not only does the osmotic pressure provide an effect that is measurable, also the effect of any low molecular weight material, which can pass through a membrane, is virtually eliminated.

However, the usefulness of osmotic pressure measurement is limited to a molecular mass range of about 10^4–10^6 Da; below 10^4 Da the membrane may be permeable to the molecules under consideration and above 10^6 Da the osmotic pressure will be too small to permit accurate measurement.

If a solution and a solvent are separated by a semipermeable membrane, the tendency to equalize chemical potentials (and hence concentrations) on either side of the membrane results in a net diffusion of solvent across the membrane. The pressure necessary to balance this osmotic flow is termed the *osmotic pressure*.

For a colloidal solution the osmotic pressure, Π, can be described by

$$\Pi/C = RT/M + BC$$

(5.12)

where C is the concentration of the solution, M the molecular weight of the solute and B a constant depending on the degree of interaction between the solvent and solute molecules.

Thus a plot of Π/C versus C is linear, with the value of the intercept at $C \to 0$ giving RT/M, enabling the molecular weight of the colloid to be calculated. The molecular weight obtained from osmotic pressure measurements is a number-average value.

A potential source of error in the determination of molecular weight from osmotic pressure measurements arises from the *Donnan membrane effect*. The diffusion of small ions through a membrane will be affected by the presence of a charged macromolecule that is unable to penetrate the membrane because of its size. At equilibrium, the distribution of the diffusible ions is unequal, being greater on the side of the membrane containing the nondiffusible ions. Consequently, unless precautions are taken to correct for this effect or eliminate it, the results of osmotic pressure measurements on charged colloidal particles such as proteins will be invalid.

Viscosity

Viscosity is an expression of the resistance to flow of a system under an applied stress. An equation of flow applicable to colloidal dispersions of spherical particles was developed by Einstein:

$$\eta = \eta_o(1 + 2.5\phi)$$

(5.13)

where η_o is the viscosity of the dispersion medium and η the viscosity of the dispersion when the volume fraction of colloidal particles present is ϕ.

A number of viscosity coefficients may be defined with respect to Eq. 5.13. These include *relative viscosity*,

$$\eta_{rel} = \eta/\eta_o = 1 + 2.5\phi$$

(5.14)

and *specific viscosity*,

$$\eta_{sp} = \eta_{rel} - 1 = 2.5\phi \quad \text{or} \quad \eta_{sp}/\phi = 2.5$$

(5.15)

Since volume fraction is directly related to concentration, Eq. 5.15 may be written as

$$\eta_{sp}/C = k$$

(5.16)

where C is the concentration expressed as grams of colloidal particles per 100 mL of total dispersion, and k is a constant. If η is determined for a number of concentrations of macromolecular material in solution and η_{sp}/C is plotted versus C, then the intercept obtained on extrapolation of the linear plot to infinite dilution is known as the *intrinsic viscosity* $[\eta]$.

This constant may be used to calculate the molecular weight of the macromolecular material by use of the Mark–Houwink equation:

$$[\eta] = KM^{\alpha}$$

(5.17)

where K and α are constants characteristic of the particular polymer–solvent system. These constants are obtained initially by determining $[\eta]$ for a polymer fraction whose molecular weight has been determined by another method, such as sedimentation, osmotic pressure or light scattering. The molecular weight of the unknown polymer fraction may then be calculated. This method is suitable for use with polymers, such as dextrans used as blood plasma substitutes.

Optical properties

Light scattering

When a beam of light is passed through a colloidal sol (dispersion of very fine particles), some of the light may be absorbed (when light of certain wavelengths is selectively absorbed, a colour is produced), some is scattered and the remainder is transmitted undisturbed through the sample. Because of the light scattered, the sol appears turbid; this is known as the Tyndall effect. The turbidity of a sol is given by the expression

$$I = I_o \exp^{(-\tau l)}$$

(5.18)

where I_o is the intensity of the incident beam, I that of the transmitted light beam, l the length of the sample and τ the turbidity.

As most colloids show very low turbidities, instead of measuring the transmitted light (which may differ only marginally from the incident beam), it is more convenient and accurate to measure the scattered light, at an angle (usually 90 degrees) relative to the incident beam. The turbidity can then be calculated from the intensity of the scattered light, provided the dimensions of the particle are small compared to the wavelength of the incident light, by the expression

$$\tau = \frac{16\pi}{3} R_{90}$$

(5.19)

R_{90} is known as the Rayleigh ratio after Lord Rayleigh, who laid the foundations of the light-scattering theory. The light-scattering theory was modified for use in the determination of the molecular weight of colloidal particles by Debye, who derived the following relationship between turbidity and molecular weight:

$$HC/\tau = 1/M + 2BC$$

(5.20)

C is the concentration of the solute and B an interaction constant allowing for nonideality. H is an optical constant for a particular system depending on the refractive index change with concentration and the wavelength of light used. A plot of HC/τ against concentration results in a straight line of slope $2B$. The intercept on the HC/τ axis is $1/M$, allowing the molecular weight to be calculated. The molecular weight derived by the light-scattering technique is a weight-average value.

Light-scattering measurements are particularly suitable for finding the size of the micelles of surface-active agents and for the study of proteins and natural and synthetic polymers. For spherical particles, the upper limit of the Debye equation is a particle diameter of approximately one-twentieth of the wavelength λ of the incident light; that is, about 20 nm to 25 nm. The light-scattering theory becomes more complex when one or more dimensions exceed $\lambda/20$ because the particles can no longer be considered as point sources of scattered light. By measuring the light scattering from such particles as a function of both the scattering angle θ and the concentration C, and extrapolating the data to zero angle and zero concentration using a so-called Zimm plot, it is possible to obtain information on not only the molecular weight but also the particle shape. When the size of the particles of the colloidal dispersions approaches the wavelength of the incident light, as in the case of most emulsions (except microemulsions) and suspensions, the light scattering becomes more complex and should be treated using Mie scattering theory (see Chapter 9).

Because of developments of the light-scattering method, the technique described here is often referred to as static light scattering (SLS) to distinguish it from the dynamic light scattering method (DLS) described in the next section.

Light-scattering measurements are of great value for estimating particle size, shape and interactions, particularly of dissolved macromolecular materials, as the turbidity depends on the size (molecular weight) of the colloidal material involved. Measurements are simple in principle but experimentally difficult because of the need to keep the sample free from dust, the particles of which would scatter light strongly and introduce large errors. The essential components of the basic light-scattering instrument are a light source, usually a low-intensity laser, which provides a parallel beam of light of known wavelength, and a photomultiplier tube to measure the intensity of the light scattered by the particles of the colloidal dispersion. The incident light beam passes through a glass cell containing the dispersion, and the scattered light is detected by the photomultiplier tube mounted on a turntable which can be rotated to allow measurements at predetermined angles to the incident beam.

Because the intensity of the scattered light is inversely proportional to the fourth power of the wavelength of the light used, blue light ($\lambda = 450$ nm) is scattered much more than red light ($\lambda = 650$ nm). With incident white light, a scattering material will therefore tend to be blue when viewed at right angles to the incident beam, which is why the sky appears to be blue, the scattering arising from dust particles in the atmosphere.

Dynamic light scattering (photon correlation spectroscopy)

Colloidal particles undergo Brownian motion because of multiple collisions with neighbouring particles in solution. The intensity of the scattered light from these diffusing particles will fluctuate in time because there will be constructive and destructive interference of the scattered light from the particles as the distance between them is constantly changing with time. Analysis of these fluctuations can provide information about their diffusion coefficient and hence, from the Stokes–Einstein equation, their size and the distribution of sizes within the sample. This is the principle of the technique called dynamic light scattering (DLS) (also known as photon correlation spectroscopy [PCS]).

The timescale of the fluctuations in scattered light intensity is extremely rapid (10^{-6} s to 10^{-3} s) and requires high-speed detection and recording systems to extract information from them. The arrangement of the DLS measuring system is essentially the same as that of the static light scattering technique outlined in the previous section, i.e. a light source providing a beam of light of a selected wavelength, which, after passing through a narrow slit, is directed through the solution of colloidal material and the scattered light intensity is measured by a photomultiplier tube mounted on a turntable set at a predetermined angle (usually 90 degrees) to the beam. Whereas the static light scattering instrument measures only an average value of the fluctuating scattered light, refinement of the equipment in the DLS method allows the fluctuations in intensity to be analysed. A high-intensity laser is used as the light source, providing a narrow beam of intense coherent light which is directed through a very small aperture into the sample cell. The light scattered by the particles contained within this very small, well-defined, volume of the sample passes through a second small aperture and is measured using a high-speed detection system, the output of which is analysed using the appropriate software and displayed on a computer monitor. Essentially, the instrument compares scattering intensity at very short time intervals (time delays) and generates a correlation function which, if the sample is monodisperse, is in the form of an exponential decay curve. The numerical analysis of the correlation function to extract the particle size is complex and beyond the scope of this text. DLS is used to determine the properties of colloidal particles ranging in size from 0.002 μm to 2 μm, the lower size limit being dependent on the available laser power.

Ultramicroscopy

Colloidal particles are too small to be seen with an optical microscope. Light scattering is employed in the ultramicroscope first developed by Zsigmondy, in which a cell containing the colloid is viewed against a dark background at right angles to an intense beam of incident light. The particles, which exhibit Brownian motion, appear as spots of light against the dark background. The ultramicroscope is used in the technique of microelectrophoresis for measuring particle charge.

Electron microscopy

The electron microscope, capable of giving actual pictures of the particles, is used to observe the size, shape and structure of colloidal particles. The success of the electron microscope is due to its high resolving power, defined in terms of d, the smallest distance by which two objects are separated yet remain distinguishable. The shorter the wavelength of the radiation used, the smaller is d and the greater the resolving power. An optical microscope, using visible light as its radiation source, gives d of about 0.2 μm. The radiation source of the electron microscope is a beam of high-energy electrons having wavelengths in the region of 0.01 nm; d is thus about 0.5 nm. The electron beams are focused using electromagnets, and the whole system is under a high vacuum of about 10^{-3} Pa to 10^{-5} Pa to give the electrons a free path. With wavelengths of the order indicated, the image cannot be viewed directly, so the image is displayed on a monitor or computer screen.

A major disadvantage of the electron microscope for viewing colloidal particles is that normally only dried samples can be examined. Consequently, it usually gives no information on solvation or configuration in solution and, moreover, the particles may be affected by sample preparation. A development which overcomes these problems is environmental scanning electron microscopy (ESEM), which allows the observation of material in the wet state.

Electrical properties

Electrical properties of interfaces

Most surfaces acquire a surface electric charge when brought into contact with an aqueous medium, the principal charging mechanisms being as follows.

Ion dissolution. Ionic substances can acquire a surface charge by virtue of unequal dissolution of the oppositely charged ions of which they are composed. For example, the particles of silver iodide in a solution with excess I^- will carry a negative charge, but the charge will be positive if excess Ag^+ is present. Since the concentrations of Ag^+ and I^- determine the electric potential at the particle surface, they are termed potential-determining ions. In a similar way, H^+ and OH^- are potential-determining ions for metal oxides and hydroxides of, for example, magnesium and aluminium hydroxides.

Ionization. Here the charge is controlled by the ionization of surface groupings; examples include the model system of polystyrene latex, which frequently has carboxylic acid groups at the surface which ionize to give negatively charged particles. In a similar way, acidic drugs such as ibuprofen and nalidixic acid also acquire a negative charge.

Amino acids and proteins acquire their charge mainly through the ionization of carboxyl and amino groups to give $-COO^-$ and NH_3^+ ions. The ionization of these groups, and so the net molecular charge, depends on the pH of the system. At a pH below the pK_a of the COO^- group the protein will be positively charged because of the protonation of this group, $-COO^- \rightarrow COOH$, and the ionization of the amino group, $-NH_2 \rightarrow -NH_3^+$, which has a much higher pK_a. At higher pH, where the amino group is no longer ionized, the net charge on the molecule is negative because of the ionization of the carboxyl group. At a certain definite pH, specific for each individual protein, the total number of positive charges will equal the total number of negative charges and the net charge will be zero. This pH is termed the *isoelectric point* of the protein, and the protein exists as its zwitterion. This may be represented as follows.

$$R - NH_2 - COO^- \qquad \text{Alkaline solution}$$
$$\downarrow\uparrow$$
$$R - NH_3^+ - COO^- \qquad \text{Isoelectric point (zwitterion)}$$
$$\downarrow\uparrow$$
$$R - NH_3^+ - COOH \qquad \text{Acidic solution}$$

A protein is least soluble (the colloidal sol is least stable) at its isoelectric point and is readily desolvated by very water-soluble salts such as ammonium sulfate. Thus insulin may be precipitated from aqueous alcohol at pH 5.2.

Ion adsorption. A net surface charge can be acquired by the unequal adsorption of oppositely charged ions. Surfaces in water are more often negatively charged than positively charged, because cations are generally more hydrated than anions. Consequently, the former have the greater tendency to reside in the bulk aqueous medium, whereas the smaller, less hydrated and more polarizing anions have the greater tendency to reside at the particle surface. Surface-active agents are strongly adsorbed and have a pronounced influence on the surface charge, imparting either a positive or a negative charge depending on their ionic character.

The electrical double layer

Consider a solid charged surface in contact with an aqueous solution containing positive and negative ions. The surface charge influences the distribution of ions in the aqueous medium: ions of charge opposite to that of the surface, termed *counterions*, are attracted towards the surface; ions of like charge, termed *co-ions*, are repelled from the surface. However, the distribution of the ions will also be affected by thermal agitation, which will tend to redisperse the ions in solution. The result is the formation of an electrical double layer made up of the charged surface and a neutralizing excess of counterions over co-ions (the system must be electrically neutral) distributed in a diffuse manner in the aqueous medium.

The theory of the electrical double layer deals with this distribution of ions and hence with the magnitude of the electric potentials which occur in the locality of the charged surface. For a fuller explanation of what is a rather complicated mathematical approach, the reader is referred to a textbook on colloid science (e.g. Shaw, 1992). A somewhat simplified picture of what pertains from the theories of Gouy, Chapman and Stern follows.

The double layer is divided into two parts (Fig. 5.2a): the inner part, which may include adsorbed ions, and the diffuse part, where ions are distributed as influenced by electrical forces and random thermal motion. The two parts of the double layer are separated by a plane, the Stern plane, at about a hydrated ion radius from the surface; thus counterions may be held at the surface by electrostatic attraction, and the centre of these hydrated ions forms the Stern plane.

The potential changes linearly from ψ_o (the surface potential) to ψ_δ (the Stern potential) in the Stern layer and decays exponentially from ψ_δ to zero in the diffuse double layer (see Fig. 5.2b). A plane of shear is also indicated in Fig. 5.2. In addition to ions in the Stern layer, a certain amount of solvent will

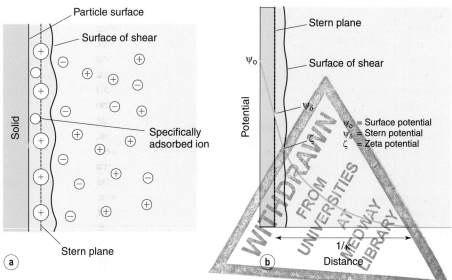

Fig. 5.2 • The electrical double layer. **(a)** Schematic representation. **(b)** Changes in potential with distance from the particle surface.

be bound to the ions and the charged surface. This solvating layer is held to the surface, and the edge of the layer, termed the surface or plane of shear, represents the boundary of relative movement between the solid (and attached material) and the liquid. The potential at the plane of shear is termed the zeta potential, ζ, or electrokinetic potential, and its magnitude may be measured using microelectrophoresis or any other of the electrokinetic phenomena. The thickness of the solvating layer is ill-defined, and the zeta potential therefore represents a potential at an unknown distance from the particle surface; its value, however, is usually taken as being slightly less than that of the Stern potential.

In the previous discussion, it was stated that the Stern plane existed at a hydrated ion radius from the particle surface; the hydrated ions are electrostatically attracted to the particle surface. It is possible for ions/molecules to be more strongly adsorbed at the surface, termed *specific adsorption*, than by simple electrostatic attraction. In fact, the specifically adsorbed ion/molecule may be uncharged as is the case with nonionic surface-active agents. Surface-active ions specifically adsorb by the hydrophobic effect and can have a significant effect on the Stern potential, causing ψ_o and ψ_δ to have opposite signs, as in Fig. 5.3a, or causing ψ_δ to have the same sign as ψ_o but be greater in magnitude, as in Fig. 5.3b.

Fig. 5.2b shows an exponential decay of the potential to zero with distance from the Stern plane. The distance over which this occurs is $1/\kappa$, referred to as the Debye–Hückel length parameter or the thickness of the electrical double layer. The parameter κ is dependent on the electrolyte concentration of the aqueous medium. Increasing the electrolyte concentration increases the value of κ and consequently decreases the value of $1/\kappa$, that is, it compresses the double layer. As ψ_δ stays constant, this means that the zeta potential will be lowered.

As indicated earlier, the effect of specifically adsorbed ions may be to lower the Stern potential and hence the zeta potential without compressing the double layer. Thus the zeta potential may be reduced by additives to the aqueous system in either (or both) of two different ways.

Electrokinetic phenomena

This is the general description applied to the phenomena that arise when attempts are made to shear off the mobile part of the electrical double layer from a charged surface. There are four such phenomena: namely, electrophoresis, sedimentation potential, streaming potential and electroosmosis. All of these electrokinetic phenomena may be used to measure the zeta potential but electrophoresis is the easiest to use and has the greatest pharmaceutical application.

Electrophoresis. The movement of a charged particle (plus attached ions) relative to a stationary liquid under the influence of an applied electric field is termed electrophoresis. When the movement of the particles is observed with a microscope, or the

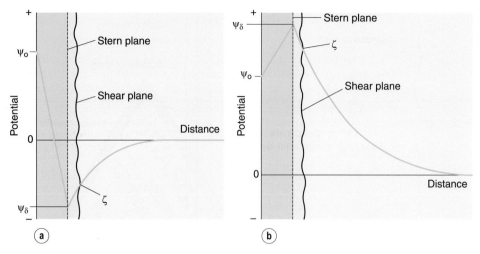

Fig. 5.3 • Changes in potential with distance from the solid surface. **(a)** Reversal of the charge sign of the Stern potential, ψ_δ, due to adsorption of surface-active or polyvalent counterion. **(b)** Increase in magnitude of the Stern potential, ψ_δ, due to adsorption of surface-active co-ions.

movement of light spots scattered by particles too small to be observed with the microscope is observed using an ultramicroscope, this constitutes microelectrophoresis.

A microscope equipped with an eyepiece graticule is used, and the speed of movement of the particle under the influence of a known electric field is measured. This is the electrophoretic velocity, v, and the electrophoretic mobility, u, is given by

$$u = v/E$$

(5.21)

where v is measured in m s^{-1}, and E, the applied field strength, is measured in V m^{-1}, so u has the dimensions of m^2 s^{-1} V^{-1}. Typically, a stable lyophobic colloidal particle may have an electrophoretic mobility of 4×10^{-8} m^2 s^{-1} V^{-1}. The equation used to convert the electrophoretic mobility, u, into the zeta potential depends on the value of κa (κ is the Debye–Hückel reciprocal length parameter described previously and a is the particle radius). For values of $\kappa a > 100$ (as is the case for particles of radius 1 μm dispersed in 10^{-3} mol dm^{-3} sodium chloride solution), the Smoluchowski equation can be used:

$$u = \varepsilon\zeta/\eta$$

(5.22)

where ε is the permittivity and η the viscosity of the liquid used. For particles in water at 25 °C, $\zeta = (12.85 \times 10^{-5})u$ V and, for the mobility given above, a zeta potential of 0.0514 V, or 51.4 mV, is obtained.

For values of $\kappa a < 100$, a more complex relationship which is a function of κa and the zeta potential is used.

The technique of microelectrophoresis finds application in the measurement of zeta potentials of model systems (e.g. polystyrene latex dispersions) to test colloid stability theory, in the measurement of coarse dispersions (e.g. suspensions and emulsions) to assess their stability, and in identification of charged groups and other surface characteristics of water-insoluble drugs and cells such as blood and bacteria.

Other electrokinetic phenomena. The other electrokinetic phenomena are as follows: *sedimentation potential*, the reverse of electrophoresis, is the electric field created when particles sediment; *streaming potential*, the electric field created when liquid is made to flow along a stationary charged surface, e.g. a glass tube or a packed powder bed; and *electroosmosis*, the opposite of streaming potential, the movement of liquid relative to a stationary charged surface, e.g. a glass tube, by an applied electric field.

Physical stability of colloidal systems

In colloidal dispersions, frequent encounters between the particles occur due to Brownian movement. Whether these collisions result in permanent contact of the particles (coagulation), which leads eventually to the destruction of the colloidal system as the large

Table 5.2 Comparison of properties of lyophobic and lyophilic sols

Property	Lyophobic	Lyophilic
Effect of electrolytes	Very sensitive to added electrolyte, leading to aggregation in an irreversible manner. Depends on: (a) Type and valency of counterion of electrolyte, e.g. with a negatively charged sol. $La^{3+} > Ba^{2+} > Na^+$ (b) Concentration of electrolyte. At a particular concentration, the sol passes from the disperse to the aggregated state. For the electrolyte types in (a), the concentrations are about 10^{-4} mol dm^{-3}, 10^{-3} mol dm^{-3}, and 10^{-1} mol dm^{-3} respectively. These generalizations, (a) and (b), form what is known as the Schulze–Hardy rule	Dispersions are generally stable in the presence of electrolytes. May be salted out by high concentrations of very soluble electrolytes. The effect is due to desolvation of the lyophilic molecules and depends on the tendency of the electrolyte ions to become hydrated. Proteins are more sensitive to electrolytes at their isoelectric points. Lyophilic colloids when salted out may appear as amorphous droplets known as a coacervate
Stability	Controlled by charge on particles	Controlled by charge and solvation of particles
Formation of dispersion	Dispersions usually of metals, inorganic crystals, etc., with a high interfacial surface-free energy due to a large increase in surface area on formation. For a positive ΔG of formation, a dispersion will never form spontaneously and is thermodynamically unstable. Sol particles remain dispersed because of electrical repulsion	Generally proteins, macromolecules, etc., which disperse spontaneously in a solvent. Interfacial free energy is low. There is a large increase in entropy when rigidly held chains of a polymer in the dry state unfold in solution. The free energy of formation is negative, a stable thermodynamic system
Viscosity	Sols of low viscosity, particles unsolvated and usually symmetric	Usually high. At sufficiently high concentration of disperse phase, a gel may be formed. Particles solvated and usually asymmetric

aggregates formed sediment out, or temporary contact (flocculation), or whether the particles rebound and remain freely dispersed (a stable colloidal system) depends on the forces of interaction between the particles.

These forces can be divided into three groups: electrical forces of repulsion, forces of attraction and forces arising from solvation. An understanding of the first two explains the stability of lyophobic systems, and all three forces must be considered in a discussion of the stability of lyophilic dispersions. Before considering the interaction of these forces, it is necessary to define the terms *aggregation, coagulation* and *flocculation* as used in colloid science.

Aggregation is a general term signifying the collection of particles into groups. Coagulation signifies that the particles are closely aggregated and difficult to redisperse – a primary minimum phenomenon of the Derjaguin–Landau–Verwey–Overbeek (DLVO) theory of colloid stability (see the next section). In flocculation, the aggregates have an open structure in which the particles remain a small distance from one another. This may be a secondary minimum phenomenon (see the DLVO theory) or a consequence

of bridging by a polymer or polyelectrolyte, as explained later in this chapter.

As a preliminary to discussion on the stability of colloidal dispersions, a comparison of the general properties of lyophobic and lyophilic sols is given in Table 5.2.

Stability of lyophobic systems (DLVO theory)

In considering the interaction between two colloidal particles, Derjaguin and Landau and, independently, Verwey and Overbeek in the 1940s produced a quantitative approach to the stability of hydrophobic sols. In what has come to be known as the *DLVO theory of colloid stability*, they assumed that the only interactions involved are electrical repulsion, V_R, and van der Waals attraction, V_A, and that these parameters are additive. Therefore the total potential energy of interaction V_T (expressed schematically in the curve shown in Fig. 5.4) is given by

$$V_T = V_A + V_R$$

$$(5.23)$$

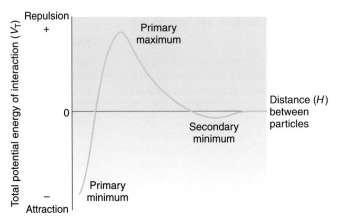

Fig. 5.4 • Total potential energy of interaction, V_T, versus distance of separation, H, for two particles. $V_T = V_R + V_A$.

Repulsive forces between particles. Repulsion between particles arises due to the osmotic effect produced by the increase in the number of charged species on overlap of the diffuse parts of the electrical double layer. No simple equations can be given for repulsive interactions; however, it can be shown that the repulsive energy that exists between two spheres of equal but small surface potential is given by

$$V_R = 2\pi\varepsilon a \psi_0^2 \exp(-\kappa H)$$

(5.24)

where ε is the permittivity of the polar liquid, a is the radius of the spherical particle of surface potential ψ_0, κ is the Debye–Hückel reciprocal length parameter and H is the distance between particles. An estimation of the surface potential can be obtained from zeta potential measurements. As can be seen, the repulsion energy is an exponential function of the distance between the particles and has a range of the order of the thickness of the double layer.

Attractive forces between particles. The energy of attraction, V_A, arises from van der Waals universal forces of attraction, the so-called dispersion forces, the major contribution to which are the electromagnetic attractions described by London. For an assembly of molecules, dispersion forces are additive, summation leading to long-range attraction between colloidal particles. As a result of the work of de Boer and Hamaker, it can be shown that the attractive interaction between spheres of the same radius, a, can be approximated to

$$V_A = -Aa/12H$$

(5.25)

where A is the Hamaker constant for the particular material derived from London dispersion forces. Eq. 5.25 shows that the energy of attraction varies as the inverse of the distance between particles, H.

Total potential energy of interaction. Consideration of the curve of total potential energy of interaction, V_T, versus the distance between particles, H (see Fig. 5.4), shows that attraction predominates at small distances, hence the very deep primary minimum. The attraction at large interparticle distances, which produces the secondary minimum, arises because the fall-off in repulsive energy with distance is more rapid than that of attractive energy. At intermediate distances, double layer repulsion may predominate, giving a primary maximum in the curve. If this maximum is large compared with the thermal energy $k_B T$ of the particles, the colloidal system should be stable, i.e. the particles should stay dispersed. Otherwise, the interacting particles will reach the energy depth of the primary minimum and irreversible aggregation, i.e. coagulation, occurs. If the secondary minimum is smaller than $k_B T$, the particles will not aggregate but will always repel one another, but if it is significantly larger than $k_B T$, a loose assemblage of particles will form which can be easily redispersed by shaking, i.e. flocculation occurs.

The depth of the secondary minimum depends on the particle size, and particles may need to be of radius 1 μm or greater before the attractive force is sufficiently great for flocculation to occur.

The height of the primary maximum energy barrier to coagulation depends on the magnitude of V_R, which is dependent on ψ_0 and hence the zeta potential. In

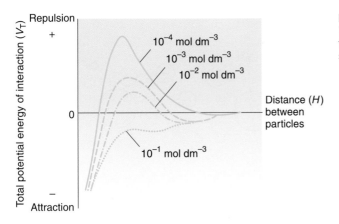

addition, it depends on electrolyte concentration via κ, the Debye–Hückel reciprocal length parameter. Addition of electrolyte compresses the double layer and reduces the zeta potential; this has the effect of lowering the primary maximum and deepening the secondary minimum (Fig. 5.5). This latter means that there will be an increased tendency for particles to flocculate in the secondary minimum, and this is the principle of the *controlled flocculation* approach to pharmaceutical suspension formulation described later. The primary maximum may also be lowered (and the secondary minimum deepened) by adding substances, such as ionic surface-active agents, which are specifically adsorbed within the Stern layer. Here ψ_δ is reduced and hence the zeta potential; the double layer is usually not compressed.

Stability of lyophilic systems

Solutions of macromolecules, lyophilic colloidal sols, are stabilized by a combination of electrical double layer interaction and solvation, and both of these stabilizing factors must be sufficiently weakened before attraction predominates and the colloidal particles coagulate. For example, gelatin has a sufficiently strong affinity for water to be soluble even at its isoelectric pH, where there is no double layer interaction.

Hydrophilic colloids are unaffected by the small amounts of added electrolyte which cause hydrophobic sols to coagulate. However, when the concentration of electrolyte is high, particularly with an electrolyte whose ions become strongly hydrated, the colloidal material loses its water of solvation to these ions and coagulates, i.e. a 'salting-out' effect occurs.

Variation in the degree of solvation of different hydrophilic colloids affects the concentration of soluble electrolyte required to produce their coagulation and precipitation. The components of a mixture of hydrophilic colloids can therefore be separated by a process of fractional precipitation, which involves the salting out of the various components at different concentrations of electrolyte. This technique is used in the purification of antitoxins.

Lyophilic colloids can be considered to become lyophobic by the addition of solvents such as acetone and alcohol. The particles become desolvated and are then very sensitive to precipitation by added electrolyte.

Coacervation and microencapsulation. Coacervation is the separation of a colloid-rich layer from a lyophilic sol as the result of the addition of another substance. This layer, which is present in the form of an amorphous liquid, constitutes the coacervate. Simple coacervation may be brought about by a salting-out effect on addition of electrolyte or addition of a nonsolvent. Complex coacervation occurs when two oppositely charged lyophilic colloids are mixed, e.g. gelatin and acacia. Gelatin at a pH below its isoelectric point is positively charged, and acacia above about pH 3 is negatively charged; a combination of solutions at about pH 4 results in coacervation. Any large ions of opposite charge, e.g. cationic surface-active agents (positively charged) and dyes used for colouring aqueous mixtures (negatively charged), may react in a similar way.

If the coacervate is formed in a stirred suspension of an insoluble solid, the macromolecular material will surround the solid particles. The coated particles can be separated and dried, and this technique forms the basis of one method of microencapsulation. A number of drugs, including aspirin, have been coated in this manner. The coating protects the drug from chemical attack, and microcapsules may be given orally to prolong the action of the medicament.

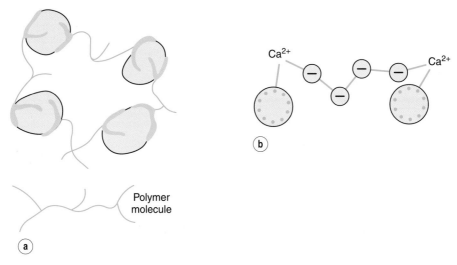

Fig. 5.6 • Flocs formed by **(a)** polymer bridging and **(b)** polyelectrolyte bridging in the presence of divalent ions of opposite charge.

Effect of addition of macromolecular material to lyophobic colloidal sols. When added in small amounts, many polyelectrolyte and polymer molecules (lyophilic colloids) can adsorb simultaneously onto two particles and are long enough to bridge the energy barrier between the particles. This can even occur with neutral polymers when the lyophobic particles have a high zeta potential (and would thus be considered a stable sol). A structured floc results (Fig. 5.6a).

With polyelectrolytes, where the particles and polyelectrolyte have charge of the same sign, flocculation can often occur when divalent and trivalent ions are added to the system (see Fig. 5.6b). These complete the 'bridge', and only very low concentrations of these ions are needed. Use is made of this property of small quantities of polyelectrolytes and polymers in removing colloidal material, resulting from sewage, in water purification.

On the other hand, if larger amounts of polymer are added, sufficient to cover the surface of the particles, then a lyophobic sol may be stabilized to coagulation by added electrolyte – the so-called steric stabilization or protective colloid effect.

Steric stabilization (protective colloid action)

It has long been known that nonionic polymeric materials such as gums, nonionic surface-active agents and methylcellulose adsorbed at the particle surface can stabilize a lyophobic sol to coagulation even in the absence of a significant zeta potential. The approach of two particles with adsorbed polymer layers results in a steric interaction when the layers overlap, leading to repulsion. In general, the particles do not approach each other closer than about twice the thickness of the adsorbed layer, and hence passage into the primary minimum is inhibited. An additional term has thus to be included in the potential energy of interaction for what is called steric stabilization, V_S:

$$V_T = V_A + V_R + V_s$$

(5.26)

The effect of V_S on the potential energy against distance between particles is seen in Fig. 5.7, showing that repulsion is generally seen at all shorter distances provided that the adsorbed polymeric material does not move from the particle surface.

Steric repulsion can be explained by reference to the free energy changes that occur when two polymer-covered particles interact. Free energy ΔG, enthalpy ΔH and entropy ΔS changes are related according to

$$\Delta G = \Delta H - T\Delta S$$

(5.27)

The second law of thermodynamics implies that a positive value of ΔG is necessary for dispersion stability, a negative value indicating that the particles have aggregated.

A positive value of ΔG can arise in a number of ways; for example, when ΔH and ΔS are both negative and $T\Delta S > \Delta H$. Here the effect of the entropy change opposes aggregation and outweighs the enthalpy term; this is termed *entropic stabilization*. Interpenetration

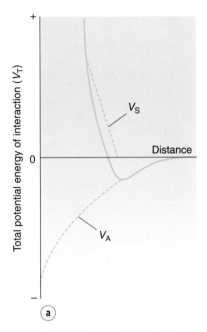

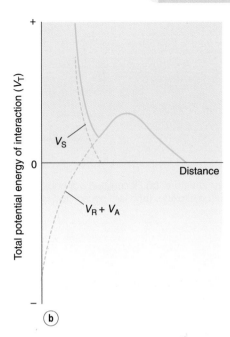

Fig. 5.7 • Total potential energy of interaction versus distance for two particles, showing the effect of the steric stabilization term V_S **(a)** in the absence of electrostatic repulsion, the *solid line* representing $V_T = V_A + V_S$, and **(b)** in the presence of electrostatic repulsion, the *solid line* representing $V_T = V_R + V_A + V_S$.

and compression of the polymer chains decrease the entropy as these chains become more ordered. Such a process is not spontaneous: 'work' must be expended to interpenetrate and compress any polymer chains existing between the colloidal particles, and this work is a reflection of the repulsive potential energy. The enthalpy of mixing of these polymer chains will also be negative. Stabilization by these effects occurs in nonaqueous dispersions.

Again, a positive ΔG occurs if both ΔH and ΔS are positive and $T\Delta S < \Delta H$. Here enthalpy aids stabilization, entropy aids aggregation. Consequently, this effect is termed *enthalpic stabilization* and is common with aqueous dispersions, particularly where the stabilizing polymer has polyoxyethylene chains. Such chains are hydrated in aqueous solution due to H-bonding between water molecules and the 'ether oxygens' of the ethylene oxide groups. The water molecules have thus become more structured and lost degrees of freedom. When interpenetration and compression of ethylene oxide chains occur, there is an increased probability of contact between ethylene oxide groups, resulting in some of the bound water molecules being released (Fig. 5.8). The released water molecules have greater degrees of freedom than those in the bound state. For this to occur, they must be supplied with energy, obtained from heat

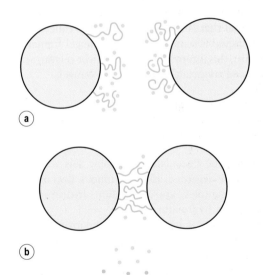

Fig. 5.8 • Enthalpic stabilization. **(a)** Particles with stabilizing polyoxyethylene chains and hydrogen-bonded water molecules. **(b)** Stabilizing chains overlap, water molecules released, resulting in positive ΔH.

absorption, i.e. there is a positive enthalpy change. Although there is a decrease in entropy in the interaction zone, as with entropic stabilization, this is overridden by the increase in the configurational entropy of the released water molecules.

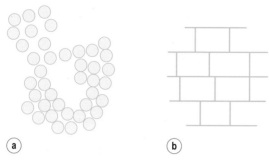

a   b

Fig. 5.9 • Gel structure. **(a)** Flocculated lyophobic sol, e.g. aluminium hydroxide. **(b)** 'Card house' floc of clays, e.g. bentonite.

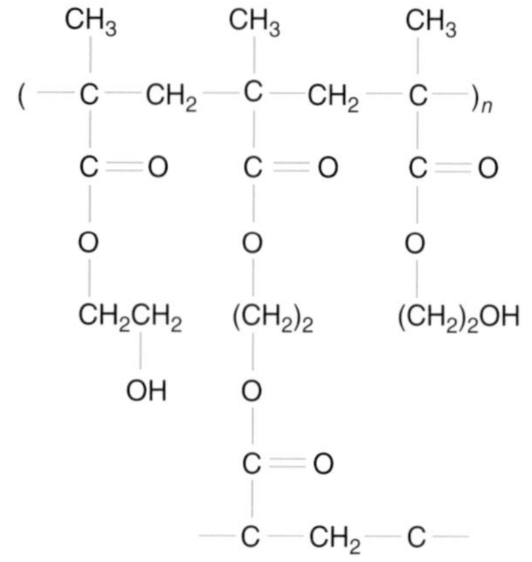

Gels

The majority of gels are formed by aggregation of colloidal sol particles; the solid or semisolid system so formed being interpenetrated by a liquid. The particles link together to form an interlaced network, thus imparting rigidity to the structure; the continuous phase is held within the meshes. Often only a small percentage of disperse phase is required to impart rigidity; for example, 1% agar in water produces a firm gel. A gel that is rich in liquid may be called a jelly; if the liquid is removed and only the gel framework remains, this is termed a xerogel. Sheet gelatin, acacia tears and tragacanth flakes are all xerogels.

Types of gel

Gelation of lyophobic sols

Gels may be flocculated lyophobic sols where the gel can be regarded as a continuous floccule (Fig. 5.9a). Examples are aluminium hydroxide and magnesium hydroxide gels.

Clays such as bentonite, aluminium magnesium silicate (Veegum) and to some extent kaolin form gels by flocculation in a special manner. They are hydrated aluminium (aluminium/magnesium) silicates whose crystal structure is such that they exist as flat plates. The flat part or 'face' of the particle carries a negative charge due to O^- atoms and the edge of the plate carries a positive charge due to Al^{3+}/Mg^{2+} atoms. As a result of electrostatic attraction between the face and the edge of different particles, a gel structure is built up, forming what is usually known as a 'card house floc' (see Fig. 5.9b).

The forces holding the particles together in this type of gel are relatively weak – van der Waals

Fig. 5.10 • Poly(2-hydroxyethyl methacrylate) cross-linked with ethylene glycol dimethacrylate.

forces in the secondary minimum flocculation of aluminium hydroxide, electrostatic attraction in the case of the clays. Because of this, these gels show the phenomenon of *thixotropy*, a nonchemical isothermal gel–sol–gel transformation. If a thixotropic gel is sheared (e.g. by simple shaking), these weak bonds are broken and a lyophobic sol is formed. On standing, the particles collide, flocculation occurs and the gel is reformed. Flocculation in gels is the reason for their anomalous rheological properties (see Chapter 6). This phenomenon of thixotropy is used in the formulation of pharmaceutical suspensions, e.g. bentonite in calamine lotion, and in the paint industry.

Gelation of lyophilic sols

Gels formed by lyophilic sols can be divided into two groups depending on the nature of the bonds between the chains of the network. Gels of *type I* are irreversible systems with a three-dimensional network formed by covalent bonds between the macromolecules. Typical examples of this type of gel are the swollen networks that have been formed by the polymerization of monomers of water-soluble polymers in the presence of a cross-linking agent. For example, poly(2-hydroxyethyl methacrylate) [poly(HEMA)], cross-linked with ethylene glycol dimethacrylate [EGDMA], forms a three-dimensional structure (Fig. 5.10) that swells in water but cannot dissolve because the cross-links are stable. Such polymers have been used in the fabrication of expanding implants that imbibe body fluids and swell to a predetermined volume. Implanted in the dehydrated state, these polymers swell to fill a body cavity or give form to surrounding tissues. They also find use

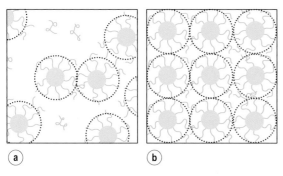

Fig. 5.11 • Polyoxyethylene-polyoxypropylene-polyoxyethylene block copolymers. **(a)** Micelle formation. **(b)** Formation of a cubic gel phase by packing of micelles.

in the fabrication of implants for the prolonged release of drugs, such as antibiotics, into the immediate environment of the implant.

Type II gels are held together by much weaker intermolecular bonds such as hydrogen bonds. These gels are heat reversible, a transition from the sol to gel occurring on either heating or cooling. Poly(vinyl alcohol) solutions, for example, gel on cooling to below a certain temperature referred to as the *gel point*. Because of their gelling properties, poly(vinyl alcohol)s are used as jellies for application of drugs to the skin. On application, the gel dries rapidly, leaving a plastic film with the drug in intimate contact with the skin. Concentrated aqueous solutions of high molecular weight polyoxyethylene-polyoxypropylene-polyoxyethylene block copolymers, commercially available as Pluronic™ or Synperonic™ surfactants, form gels on being heated. These compounds are amphiphilic and many form micelles with a hydrophobic core comprising the polyoxypropylene blocks, surrounded by a shell of the hydrophilic polyoxyethylene chains. Unusually, water is a poorer solvent for these compounds at higher temperatures, and consequently warming a solution with a concentration above the critical micelle concentration (CMC) leads to the formation of more micelles. If the solution is sufficiently concentrated, gelation may occur as the micelles pack so closely as to prevent their movement (Fig. 5.11). Gelation is a reversible process, the gels returning to the sol state on cooling.

Surface-active agents

Certain compounds, because of their chemical structure, have a tendency to accumulate at the boundary between two phases (see Chapter 4 for further information on surfaces and interfaces). Such compounds are termed amphiphiles, surface-active agents or surfactants. The adsorption at the various interfaces between solids, liquids and gases results in changes in the nature of the interface which are of considerable importance in pharmacy. Thus, the lowering of the interfacial tension between oil and water phases facilitates emulsion formation, the adsorption of surfactants on insoluble particles enables these particles to be dispersed in the form of a suspension, their adsorption on solid surfaces enables these surfaces to be more readily wetted, and the incorporation of insoluble compounds within micelles of the surfactant can lead to the production of clear solutions.

Surface-active compounds are characterized by having two distinct regions in their chemical structure, a hydrophilic (water-liking) region and a hydrophobic (water-hating) region. The existence of two such regions in a molecule is referred to as amphipathy and the molecules are consequently often referred to as amphipathic molecules. The hydrophobic portions are usually saturated or unsaturated hydrocarbon chains or, less commonly, heterocyclic or aromatic ring systems. The hydrophilic regions can be anionic, cationic or nonionic. Surfactants are generally classified according to the nature of the hydrophilic group. Typical examples are given in Table 5.3.

Many water-soluble drugs have also been reported to be surface active, this surface activity being a consequence of the amphipathic nature of the drugs. The hydrophobic portions of the drug molecules are usually more complex than those of typical surface-active agents, being composed of aromatic or heterocyclic ring systems. Examples include tranquillizers such as chlorpromazine which are based on the large tricyclic phenothiazine ring system; antidepressant drugs such as imipramine which also possess tricyclic ring systems; and antihistamines such as diphenhydramine which are based on a diphenylmethane group. Further examples of surface-active drugs are given in Attwood & Florence (1983).

Surface activity

The dual structure of amphipathic molecules is the unique feature that is responsible for the surface activity of these compounds. It is a consequence of their adsorption at the solution–air interface, the means by which the hydrophobic region of the molecule 'escapes' from the hostile aqueous

Table 5.3 Classification of surface-active agents

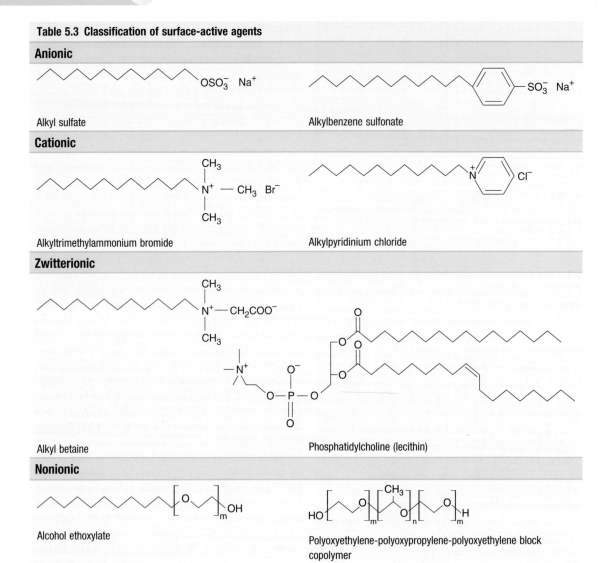

Anionic

Alkyl sulfate

Alkylbenzene sulfonate

Cationic

Alkyltrimethylammonium bromide

Alkylpyridinium chloride

Zwitterionic

Alkyl betaine

Phosphatidylcholine (lecithin)

Nonionic

Alcohol ethoxylate

Polyoxyethylene-polyoxypropylene-polyoxyethylene block copolymer

environment by protruding into the vapour phase above. Similarly, adsorption at the interface between water and an immiscible nonaqueous liquid occurs in such a way that the hydrophobic group is in solution in the nonaqueous phase, leaving the hydrophilic group in contact with the aqueous solution.

As discussed in Chapter 4, the molecules at the surface of a liquid are not completely surrounded by other like molecules as they are in the bulk of the liquid. As a result, there is a net inward force of attraction exerted on a molecule at the surface from the molecules in the bulk solution, which results in a tendency for the surface to contract. The contraction of the surface is spontaneous; that is, it is accompanied by a decrease in free energy. The contracted surface

thus represents a minimum free energy state, and any attempt to expand the surface must involve an increase in the free energy. The surface tension is a measure of the contracting power of the surface. Surface-active molecules in aqueous solution orient themselves at the surface in such a way as to remove the hydrophobic group from the aqueous phase and hence achieve a minimum free energy state. As a result, some of the water molecules at the surface are replaced by nonpolar groups. The attractive forces between these groups and the water molecules, or between the groups themselves, are less than those existing between water molecules. The contracting power of the surface is thus reduced and so therefore is the surface tension.

A similar imbalance of attractive forces exists at the interface between two immiscible liquids. The value of the interfacial tension is generally between those of the surface tensions of the two liquids involved except where there is interaction between them. Intrusion of surface-active molecules at the interface between two immiscible liquids leads to a reduction of interfacial tension, in some cases to such a low level that spontaneous emulsification of the two liquids occurs.

Micelle formation

The surface tension of a surfactant solution decreases progressively with increase of concentration as more surfactant molecules enter the surface or interfacial layer. However, at a certain concentration this layer becomes saturated, and an alternative means of shielding the hydrophobic group of the surfactant from the aqueous environment occurs through the formation of aggregates (usually spherical) of colloidal dimensions, called *micelles*. The hydrophobic chains form the core of the micelle and are shielded from the aqueous environment by the surrounding shell composed of the hydrophilic groups that serve to maintain solubility in water.

The concentration at which micelles first form in solution is termed the *critical micelle concentration* (CMC). This onset of micelle formation can be detected by a variety of experimental techniques. When physical properties such as surface tension, conductivity, osmotic pressure, solubility and light-scattering intensity are plotted as a function of concentration (Fig. 5.12), a change of slope occurs at the CMC, and such techniques can be used to measure its value. The CMC decreases with increase of the length of the hydrophobic chain. With nonionic surfactants, which are typically composed of a hydrocarbon chain and an oxyethylene chain (see Table 5.3), an increase of the hydrophilic oxyethylene chain length causes an increase of the CMC. Addition of electrolytes to ionic surfactants decreases the CMC and increases the micellar size. The effect is simply explained in terms of a reduction in the magnitude of the forces of repulsion between the charged head groups in the micelle, allowing the micelles to grow and also reducing the work required for their formation.

The primary reason for micelle formation is the attainment of a state of minimum free energy. The free energy change, ΔG, of a system is dependent on changes in both the entropy, S, and the enthalpy, H, which are related by the expression $\Delta G = \Delta H$

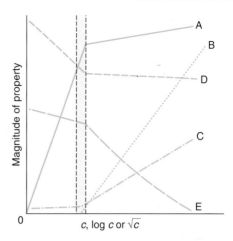

Fig. 5.12 • Solution properties of an ionic surfactant as a function of concentration, c: Osmotic pressure against c (A); solubility of a water-insoluble solubilizate against c (B); intensity of light scattered by the solution against c (C); surface tension against $\log c$ (D); molar conductivity against $\sqrt{c}$ (E).

$-T\Delta S$ (as previously discussed – see Eq. 5.27). For a micellar system at normal temperatures, the entropy term is by far the most important in determining the free energy changes ($T\Delta S$ constitutes approximately 90% to 95% of the ΔG value). The explanation most generally accepted for the entropy change is concerned with the structure of water. Water possesses a relatively high degree of structure due to hydrogen bonding between adjacent molecules. If an ionic or strongly polar solute is added to water, it will disrupt this structure, but the solute molecules can form hydrogen bonds with the water molecules that more than compensate for the disruption or distortion of the bonds existing in pure water. Ionic and polar materials thus tend to be easily soluble in water. No such compensation occurs with nonpolar groups, and their solution in water is accordingly resisted, the water molecules forming extra structured clusters around the nonpolar region. This increase in structure of the water molecules around the hydrophobic groups leads to a large negative entropy change. To counteract this, and achieve a state of minimum free energy, the hydrophobic groups tend to withdraw from the aqueous phase, either by orienting themselves at the interface with the hydrocarbon chain away from the aqueous phase or by self-association into micelles.

This tendency for hydrophobic materials to be removed from water, due to the strong attraction of water molecules for each other and not for the hydrophobic solute, has been termed *hydrophobic bonding*. However, because there is no actual bonding between the hydrophobic groups, the phenomenon is best described as the *hydrophobic effect*. When the nonpolar groups approach each other until they are in contact, there will be a decrease in the total number of water molecules in contact with the nonpolar groups. The formation of the hydrophobic bond in this way is thus equivalent to the partial removal of hydrocarbon from an aqueous environment and a consequent loss of the ice-like structuring which always surrounds the hydrophobic molecules. The increase in entropy and decrease in free energy which accompany the loss of structuring make the formation of the hydrophobic bond an energetically favourable process. An alternative explanation of the free energy decrease emphasizes the increase in internal freedom of the hydrocarbon chains which occurs when these chains are transferred from the aqueous environment, where their motion is restrained by the hydrogen-bonded water molecules, to the interior of the micelle. It has been suggested that the increased mobility of the hydrocarbon chains, and of course their mutual attraction, constitutes the principal hydrophobic factor in micellization.

It should be emphasized that micelles are in dynamic equilibrium with monomer molecules in solution, continuously breaking down and reforming. It is this factor that distinguishes micelles from other colloidal particles and the reason why they are called *association colloids*. The concentration of surfactant monomers in equilibrium with the micelles stays approximately constant at the CMC value when the solution concentration is increased above the CMC, i.e. the added surfactant all goes to form micelles.

A typical micelle is a spherical or near-spherical structure composed of some 50–100 surfactant molecules. Its shape is determined by the geometry of the surfactant molecule, which can be represented by a dimensionless parameter called the critical packing parameter (CPP), defined by the ratio v/la, where v is the volume of one chain, a is the cross-sectional area of the head group and l is the extended length of the alkyl chain of the surfactant. Spherical micelles are formed when CPP is less than or equal to one-third, which is the case for surfactants with a single hydrophobic chain and a simple ionic or nonionic head group. Most surfactants of pharmaceutical interest are of this type. Surfactants having a second alkyl chain have larger CPP values (approximating to 1) because of the increase in v, and form nonspherical structures such as bilayers from which vesicles may

be produced. Although in pharmaceutical formulation we are mainly concerned with surfactants in aqueous solution, it should be noted that micelles may also form in nonaqueous media. In these so-called reverse micelles, the hydrophilic groups form the micelle core and are shielded from the nonaqueous environment by the hydrophobic chains. The CPP associated with reverse micelles is usually greater than 1.

The radius of spherical micelles in aqueous solutions will be slightly less than that of the extended hydrocarbon chain (approximately 2.5 nm), with the interior core of the micelle having the properties of a liquid hydrocarbon. For ionic micelles, about 70% to 80% of the counterions will be attracted close to the micelle, thus reducing the overall charge. The compact layer around the core of an ionic micelle which contains the head groups and the bound counterions is called the *Stern layer* (Fig. 5.13a). The

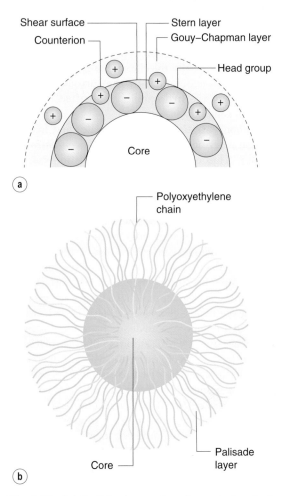

Fig. 5.13 • (a) Partial cross section of an anionic micelle and **(b)** a nonionic micelle.

outer surface of the Stern layer is the shear surface of the micelle. The core and the Stern layer together constitute what is termed the 'kinetic micelle'. Surrounding the Stern layer is a diffuse layer called the *Gouy–Chapman electrical double layer* that contains the remaining counterions required to neutralize the charge on the kinetic micelle. The thickness of the double layer is dependent on the ionic strength of the solution and is greatly compressed in the presence of electrolyte. Nonionic micelles have a hydrophobic core surrounded by a shell of oxyethylene chains which is often termed the *palisade layer* (see Fig. 5.13b). As well as the water molecules that are hydrogen bonded to the oxyethylene chains, this layer is also capable of mechanically entrapping a considerable number of water molecules. Micelles of nonionic surfactants tend, as a consequence, to be highly hydrated. The outer surface of the palisade layer forms the shear surface; that is, the hydrating molecules form part of the kinetic micelle.

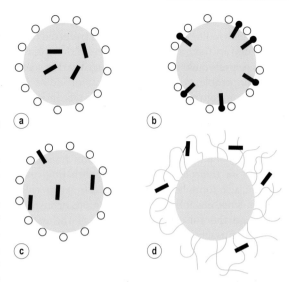

Fig. 5.14 • Sites of solubilization in ionic and nonionic micelles. **(a)** Nonpolar solubilizate; **(b)** amphipathic solubilizate; **(c)** slightly polar solubilizate; **(d)** polar solubilizate in polyoxyethylene shell of a nonionic micelle.

Solubilization

As outlined previously, the interior core of a micelle can be considered as having the properties of a liquid hydrocarbon and is thus capable of dissolving materials that are soluble in such liquids. This process, whereby water-insoluble or partly soluble substances are brought into aqueous solution by incorporation into micelles, is termed *solubilization*. The site of solubilization within the micelle is closely related to the chemical nature of the solubilizate. It is generally accepted that nonpolar solubilizates (e.g. aliphatic hydrocarbons) are dissolved in the hydrocarbon core (Fig. 5.14a). Water-insoluble compounds containing polar groups are oriented with the polar group at the surface of the ionic micelle amongst the micellar charged head groups, and the hydrophobic group buried inside the hydrocarbon core of the micelle (see Fig. 5.14b). Slightly polar solubilizates without a distinct amphiphilic structure are partitioned between the micelle surface and core (see Fig. 5.14c). Solubilization in nonionic polyoxyethylated surfactants can also occur in the polyoxyethylene shell (palisade layer) which surrounds the core (see Fig. 5.14d); thus *p*-hydroxybenzoic acid is solubilized entirely within this region hydrogen bonded to the ethylene oxide groups, whilst esters such as the parabens are located at the shell–core junction.

The maximum amount of solubilizate that can be incorporated into a given system at a fixed concentration is termed the *maximum additive concentration* (MAC). The simplest method of determining the MAC is to prepare a series of vials containing surfactant solution of known concentration. Increasing concentrations of solubilizate are added and the vials are then sealed and agitated until equilibrium conditions are established. The maximum concentration of solubilizate forming a clear solution can be determined by visual inspection or from turbidity measurements on the solutions. Solubility data are expressed as a solubility versus concentration curve or as phase diagrams. The latter are preferable since a three-component phase diagram completely describes the effect of varying all three components of the system: namely, the solubilizate, the solubilizer and the solvent.

Pharmaceutical applications of solubilization

A wide range of insoluble drugs have been formulated using the principle of solubilization, some of which will be considered here.

Phenolic compounds such as cresol, chlorocresol, chloroxylenol and thymol are frequently solubilized with a soap to form clear solutions which are widely used for disinfection. Pharmacopoeial solutions of chloroxylenol, for example, contain 5% v/v chloroxylenol with terpineol in an alcoholic soap solution.

Nonionic surfactants can be used to solubilize iodine; such iodine–surfactant systems (referred to as iodophors) are more stable than iodine–iodide systems. They are preferable in instrument sterilization since corrosion problems are reduced. Loss of iodine by sublimation from iodophor solutions is significantly less than from simple iodine solutions. There is also evidence of an ability of the iodophor solution to penetrate hair follicles of the skin, so enhancing the activity.

The low solubility of steroids in water presents a problem in their formulation for ophthalmic use. Because such formulations are required to be optically clear, it is not possible to use oily solutions or suspensions, and there are many examples of the use of nonionic surfactants as a means of producing clear solutions which are stable to sterilization. In most formulations, solubilization has been effected using polysorbates or polyoxyethylene sorbitan esters of fatty acids.

The polysorbate nonionics have also been employed in the preparation of aqueous injections of the water-insoluble vitamins A, D, E and K.

Whilst solubilization is an excellent means of producing an aqueous solution of a water-insoluble drug, it should be realized that it may well have effects on the drug's activity and absorption characteristics. As a generalization, it may be said that low concentrations of surface-active agents increase absorption, possibly due to enhanced contact of the drug with the absorbing membrane, whilst concentrations above the CMC either produce no additional effect or cause decreased absorption. In the latter case the drug may be held within the micelles such that the concentration available for absorption is reduced. For a wider appreciation of this topic, the review by Attwood & Florence (1983) can be consulted.

Solubilization and drug stability

Solubilization has been shown to have a modifying effect on the rate of hydrolysis of drugs. Nonpolar compounds solubilized deep in the hydrocarbon core of a micelle are likely to be better protected against attack by hydrolysing species than more polar compounds located closer to the micellar surface. For example, the alkaline hydrolysis of benzocaine and homatropine in the presence of several nonionic surfactants is retarded, the less polar benzocaine showing a greater increase in stability compared to homatropine because of its deeper penetration into the micelle. An important factor in considering the

breakdown of a drug located close to the micellar surface is the ionic nature of the surface-active agent. For base-catalysed hydrolysis, anionic micelles should give an enhanced protection due to repulsion of the attacking OH^- group. For cationic micelles there should be the converse effect. Whilst this pattern has been found, enhanced protection by cationic micelles also occurs, suggesting that in these cases the positively charged polar head groups hold the OH^- groups and thus block their penetration into the micelle.

Protection from oxidative degradation has also been found with solubilized systems.

As indicated earlier, drugs may be surface active. Such drugs form micelles and this self-association has been found in some cases to increase the drug's stability. Thus micellar solutions of penicillin G have been reported to be 2.5 times more stable than monomeric solutions under conditions of constant pH and ionic strength.

Detergency

Detergency is a complex process whereby surfactants are used for the removal of foreign matter from solid surfaces, be it removal of dirt from clothes or cleansing of body surfaces. The process includes many of the actions characteristic of specific surfactants. Thus, the surfactant must have good wetting characteristics so that the detergent can come into intimate contact with the surface to be cleaned. The detergent must have the ability to remove the dirt into the bulk of the liquid; the dirt–water and solid–water interfacial tensions are lowered and thus the work of adhesion between the dirt and solid is reduced, so that the dirt particle may be easily detached. Once removed, the surfactant can be adsorbed at the particle surface, creating charge and hydration barriers which prevent deposition. If the dirt is oily, it may be emulsified or solubilized.

Coarse disperse systems

Suspensions

A pharmaceutical suspension is a coarse dispersion in which insoluble particles, generally greater than 1 μm in diameter, are dispersed in a liquid medium, usually aqueous.

An aqueous suspension is a useful formulation system for administering an insoluble or poorly soluble drug. The large surface area of the dispersed drug ensures a high availability for dissolution and hence absorption. Aqueous suspensions may also be used for parenteral and ophthalmic use and provide a suitable form for the application of dermatological materials to the skin. Suspensions are used similarly in veterinary practice, and a closely allied field is that of pest control. Pesticides are frequently presented as suspensions for use as fungicides, insecticides, ascaricides and herbicides.

An acceptable suspension possesses certain desirable qualities, amongst which are the following: the suspended material should not settle too rapidly; the particles which do settle to the bottom of the container must not form a hard mass but should be readily dispersed into a uniform mixture when the container is shaken; and the suspension must not be too viscous to pour freely from the orifice of the bottle or to flow through a syringe needle.

Physical stability of a pharmaceutical suspension may be defined as the condition in which the particles do not aggregate and in which they remain uniformly distributed throughout the dispersion. Since this ideal situation is seldom realized, it is appropriate to add that if the particles do settle, they should be easily resuspended by a moderate amount of agitation.

The major difference between a pharmaceutical suspension and a colloidal dispersion is one of the size of the dispersed particles, with the relatively large particles of a suspension liable to sedimentation due to gravitational forces. Apart from this, suspensions show most of the properties of colloidal systems. The reader is referred to Chapter 26 for an account of the formulation of suspensions.

Controlled flocculation

A suspension in which all the particles remain discrete would, in terms of the DLVO theory, be considered to be stable. However, with pharmaceutical suspensions, in which the solid particles are very much coarser, such a system would sediment because of the size of the particles. The electrical repulsive forces between the particles allow the particles to slip past one another to form a close-packed arrangement at the bottom of the container, with the small particles filling the voids between the larger ones. The supernatant liquid may remain cloudy after sedimentation due to the presence of colloidal particles that will remain dispersed. Those particles lowermost in the sediment are gradually pressed together by the weight of the ones above. The repulsive barrier is thus overcome, allowing the particles to pack closely together. Physical bonding leading to 'cake' or 'clay' formation may then occur due to the formation of bridges between the particles resulting from crystal growth and hydration effects, forces greater than agitation usually being required to disperse the sediment. Coagulation in the primary minimum, resulting from a reduction in the zeta potential to a point where attractive forces predominate, thus produces coarse compact masses with a 'curdled' appearance, which may not be readily dispersed.

On the other hand, particles flocculated in the secondary minimum form a loosely bonded structure, called a *flocculate* or *floc*. A suspension consisting of particles in this state is said to be flocculated. Although sedimentation of flocculated suspensions is fairly rapid, a loosely packed, high-volume sediment is obtained in which the flocs retain their structure and the particles are easily resuspended. The supernatant liquid is clear because the colloidal particles are trapped within the flocs and sediment with them. Secondary minimum flocculation is therefore a desirable state for a pharmaceutical suspension.

Particles having a radius greater than 1 μm should, unless highly charged, show a sufficiently deep secondary minimum for flocculation to occur because the attractive force between particles, V_A, depends on particle size. Other contributing factors to secondary minimum flocculation are shape (asymmetric particles, especially those that are elongated, being more satisfactory than spherical ones) and concentration. The rate of flocculation depends on the number of particles present, so that the greater the number of particles, the more collisions there will be and flocculation is more likely to occur. However, it may be necessary, as with highly charged particles, to control the depth of the secondary minimum to induce a satisfactory flocculation state. This can be achieved by addition of electrolytes or ionic surface-active agents which reduce the zeta potential and hence V_R, resulting in the displacement of the whole of the DLVO plot to give a satisfactory secondary minimum, as indicated in Fig. 5.5. The production of a satisfactory secondary minimum leading to floc formation in this manner is termed *controlled flocculation*.

A convenient parameter for assessing a suspension is the sedimentation volume ratio, F, which is defined as the ratio of the final settled volume, V_u, to the original volume, V_o:

$$F = V_u/V_o$$

$$(5.28)$$

The ratio F gives a measure of the aggregated–deflocculated state of a suspension and may usefully be plotted, together with the measured zeta potential, against the concentration of the additive, enabling an assessment of the state of the dispersion to be made in terms of the DLVO theory. The appearance of the supernatant liquid should be noted and the redispersibility of the suspensions evaluated.

It should be pointed out that in using the controlled flocculation approach to suspension formulation, it is important to work at a constant, or narrow, pH range because the magnitude of the charge on the drug particle can vary greatly with pH.

Other additives such as flavouring agents may also affect particle charge.

Steric stabilization of suspensions

As described earlier in this chapter, colloidal particles may be stabilized against coagulation in the absence of a charge on the particles by the use of nonionic polymeric material – the concept of steric stabilization or protective colloid action. This concept may be applied to pharmaceutical suspensions where naturally occurring gums such as tragacanth and synthetic materials such as nonionic surfactants and cellulose polymers may be used to produce satisfactory suspensions. These materials may increase the viscosity of the aqueous vehicle and thus slow the rate of sedimentation of the particles, but they will also form adsorbed layers around the particles such that the approach of their surfaces and aggregation to the coagulated state is hindered.

Repulsive forces arise as the adsorbed layers interpenetrate and, as explained previously, these have an enthalpic component due to release of water of solvation from the polymer chains and an entropic component due to movement restriction. As a result, the particles will not usually approach one another closer than twice the thickness of the adsorbed layer.

However, as indicated in the discussion on controlled flocculation, from a pharmaceutical point of view an easily dispersed aggregated system is desirable. To produce this state, a balance between attractive and repulsive forces is required. This is not achieved by all polymeric materials, and the equivalent of deflocculated and caked systems may be produced. The balance of forces appears to depend on both the thickness and the concentration of the polymer in the adsorbed layer. These parameters determine the Hamaker constant and hence the attractive force,

which must be large enough to cause aggregation of the particles comparable to flocculation. The steric repulsive force, which depends on the concentration and degree of solvation of the polymer chains, must be of sufficient magnitude to prevent close approach of the uncoated particles, but low enough so that the attractive force is dominant, leading to aggregation at about twice the adsorbed layer thickness. It has been found, for example, that adsorbed layers of certain polyoxyethylene-polyoxypropylene block copolymers will product satisfactory flocculated systems, whilst many nonylphenyl ethoxylates will not. With both types of surfactant, the molecular moieties producing steric repulsion are hydrated ethylene oxide chains, but the concentration of these in the adsorbed layers varies, giving the results indicated previously.

Wetting problems

One of the problems encountered in dispersing solid materials in water is that the powder may not be readily wetted (explained in Chapter 4). This may be due to entrapped air or to the fact that the solid surface is hydrophobic. The wettability of a powder may be described in terms of the contact angle, θ, which the powder makes with the surface of the liquid. This is described by

$$\gamma_{LV} \cos\theta = \gamma_{SV} - \gamma_{SL}$$

or

$$\gamma_{SV} = \gamma_{SL} + \gamma_{LV} \cos\theta$$

or

$$\cos\theta = \frac{\gamma_{SV} - \gamma_{SL}}{\gamma_{LV}}$$

$$(5.29)$$

where γ_{SV}, γ_{SL} and γ_{LV} are the respective interfacial tensions.

For a liquid to completely wet a powder, there should be a decrease in the surface free energy as a result of the immersion process. Once the particle is submerged in the liquid, the process of *spreading wetting* becomes important. In most cases where water is involved, the reduction of contact angle may only be achieved by reducing the magnitude of γ_{LV} and γ_{SL} by the use of a wetting agent. The wetting agents are surfactants that not only reduce γ_{LV} but also adsorb onto the surface of the powder, thus reducing γ_{SL}. Both of these effects reduce the contact angle and improve the dispersibility of the powder.

Problems may arise because of the build-up of an adhering layer of suspension particles on the walls of the container just above the liquid line that occurs as the walls are repeatedly wetted by the suspension. This layer subsequently dries to form a hard, thick crust. Surfactants reduce this adsorption by coating both the container and particle surfaces such that they repel, reducing adsorption.

Rheological properties of suspensions

Flocculated suspensions tend to exhibit plastic or pseudoplastic flow, depending on the concentration, while concentrated deflocculated dispersions tend to be dilatant (see Chapter 6). This means that the apparent viscosity of flocculated suspensions is relatively high when the applied shearing stress is low, but it decreases as the applied stress increases and the attractive forces producing the flocculation are overcome. Conversely, the apparent viscosity of a concentrated deflocculated suspension is low at low shearing stress, but increases as the applied stress increases. This effect is due to the electrical repulsion that occurs when the charged particles are forced close together (see the DLVO plot of the potential energy of interaction between particles; Fig. 5.4), causing the particles to rebound, creating voids into which the liquid flows, leaving other parts of the dispersion dry. In addition to the rheological problems associated with particle charge, the sedimentation behaviour is also, of course, influenced by the rheological properties of the liquid continuous phase.

Emulsions

An emulsion is a system comprising two immiscible liquid phases, one of which is dispersed throughout the other in the form of fine droplets. A third component, the emulsifying agent, is necessary to stabilize the emulsion.

The phase that is present as fine droplets is called the *disperse phase* and the phase in which the droplets are suspended is the *continuous phase*. Most emulsions will have droplets with diameters of 0.1 μm to 100 μm and are inherently unstable systems; smaller globules exhibit colloidal behaviour and have the stability of a hydrophobic colloidal dispersion.

Pharmaceutical emulsions usually consist of water and an oil. Two main types of emulsion can exist, oil-in-water (o/w) and water-in-oil (w/o), depending on whether the continuous phase is aqueous or oily.

More complicated emulsion systems may exist; for example, an oil droplet enclosing a water droplet may be suspended in water to form a water-in-oil-in-water emulsion (w/o/w). Such systems, and their o/w/o counterparts, are termed *multiple emulsions* and are of interest as delayed-release drug delivery vehicles.

The pharmaceutical applications of emulsions as dosage forms are discussed in Chapter 27. Traditionally, emulsions have been used to render oily substances such as castor oil in a more palatable form. It is possible to formulate together oil-soluble and water-soluble medicaments in emulsions, and drugs may be more easily absorbed owing to the finely divided condition of emulsified substances.

A large number of bases used for topical preparations are emulsions, water-miscible ones being o/w type and greasy bases being w/o type. The administration of oils and fats by intravenous infusion, as part of a parenteral nutrition programme, has been made possible by the use of suitable nontoxic emulsifying agents such as lecithin. Here, the control of the particle size of emulsion droplets is of paramount importance in the prevention of the formation of emboli.

Microemulsions

Microemulsions are homogeneous, transparent systems which have a very much smaller droplet size (5 nm to 140 nm) than coarse emulsions, and unlike coarse emulsions are thermodynamically stable. Moreover, they form spontaneously when the components are mixed in the appropriate ratios. They are essentially swollen micellar systems, but obviously the distinction between a micelle containing solubilized oil and an oil droplet surrounded by an interfacial layer largely composed of surfactant is difficult to assess. They can be formed as dispersions of oil droplets in water or water droplets in oil, or as irregular bicontinuous structures consisting of areas of water separated by a connected amphiphile-rich interfacial layer. The type of microemulsion formed is determined by the nature of the surfactant, in particular its geometry, and the relative quantities of oil and water. If the critical packing parameter v/al (where v is the volume of the surfactant molecule, a is the cross-sectional area of its head group and l is the length), has values between 0 and 1, and small amounts of oil are present, then oil-in-water microemulsions are likely to be formed. When the critical packing parameter is greater than 1 and the amount of water is small, water-in-oil microemulsions are favoured. Values of critical packing parameter close to unity in systems containing almost equal amounts of oil and water can cause bicontinuous structures to form.

An essential requirement for their formation and stability is the attainment of a very low interfacial tension, γ. As a consequence of the small droplet size, the interfacial area, A, between oil and water is very large, giving rise to a high interfacial energy, γA. It is generally not possible to achieve a sufficiently low interfacial tension (approximately 0.03 mN m^{-1} is required for 10 nm droplets) to overcome this high interfacial energy with a single surfactant and it is necessary to include a second amphiphile in the formulation. The second amphiphile, referred to as the *cosurfactant*, is usually a medium-chain-length alcohol, which, although not generally regarded as a surfactant, nevertheless is able to reduce the interfacial tension by intercalating between the surfactant molecules in the interfacial film around the microemulsion droplets.

Although microemulsions have many advantages over coarse emulsions, particularly their transparency and stability, they require much larger amounts of surfactant for their formulation, which restricts the choice of acceptable components.

Theory of emulsion stabilization

Interfacial films

When two immiscible liquids, e.g. liquid paraffin and water, are shaken together, a temporary emulsion will be formed. The subdivision of one of the phases into small globules results in a large increase in the surface area and hence the interfacial free energy of the system. The system is thus thermodynamically unstable, which results, firstly, in the disperse phase being in the form of spherical droplets (the shape of the minimum surface area for a given volume) and, secondly, in coalescence of these droplets, causing phase separation, the state of minimum surface free energy.

The adsorption of a surface-active agent at the globule interface will lower the o/w interfacial tension, the process of emulsification will be made easier and the stability may be enhanced. However, if a surface-active agent such as sodium dodecyl sulfate is used, the emulsion, on standing for a short while, will still separate out into its constituent phases. On the other hand, substances such as acacia, which are only slightly surface active, produce stable emulsions. Acacia forms a strong viscous interfacial film around the globules, and it is thought that the characteristics of the interfacial film are most important in considering the stability of emulsions.

Pioneering work on emulsion stability by Schulman and Cockbain showed that a mixture of an oil-soluble alcohol such as cholesterol and a surface-active agent such as sodium cetyl (hexadecyl) sulfate was able to form a stable complex condensed film at the oil–water interface. This film was of high viscosity, sufficiently flexible to permit distortion of the droplets, resisted rupture and gave an interfacial tension lower than that produced by either component alone. The emulsion produced was stable, the charge arising from the sodium cetyl sulfate contributing to the stability as described for lyophobic colloidal dispersions. For complex formation at the interface, the correct 'shape' of molecule is necessary. Thus Schulman and Cockbain found that sodium cetyl sulfate stabilized an emulsion of liquid paraffin when elaidyl alcohol (the *trans* isomer) was the oil-soluble component but not when the *cis* isomer, oleyl alcohol was used.

In practice, the oil-soluble and water-soluble components are dissolved in the appropriate phases, and on mixing of the two phases, the complex is formed at the interface. Alternatively, an emulsifying wax may be used consisting of a blend of the two components. The wax is dispersed in the oil phase and the aqueous phase added at the same temperature. Examples of such mixtures are given in Table 5.4.

This principle is also applied with the nonionic emulsifying agents. For example, mixtures of sorbitan monooleate and polyoxyethylene sorbitan esters (e.g. polysorbate 80) have good emulsifying properties. Nonionic surfactants are widely used in the production of stable emulsions and have the advantage over ionic surfactants of being less toxic and less sensitive to electrolytes and pH variation. These emulsifying agents are not charged and there is no electrical repulsive force contributing to stability.

Table 5.4 Emulsifying waxes

Product	Oil-soluble component	Water-soluble component
Emulsifying wax (anionic)	Cetostearyl alcohol	Sodium lauryl sulfate (sodium dodecyl sulfate)
Cetrimide emulsifying wax (cationic)	Cetostearyl alcohol	Cetrimide (hexadecyltrimethylammonium bromide)
Cetomacrogol emulsifying wax (nonionic)	Cetostearyl alcohol	Cetomacrogol (polyoxyethylene monohexadecyl ether)

It is likely, however, that these substances, and the cetomacrogol emulsifying wax included in Table 5.4, sterically stabilize the emulsions as discussed under suspensions.

Hydrophilic colloids as emulsion stabilizers

A number of hydrophilic colloids are used as emulsifying agents in pharmaceutical science. These include proteins (gelatin, casein) and polysaccharides (acacia, cellulose derivatives and alginates). These materials, which generally exhibit little surface activity, adsorb at the oil–water interface and form multilayers. Such multilayers have viscoelastic properties, resist rupture and presumably form mechanical barriers to coalescence. However, some of these substances have chemical groups which ionize; for example, acacia consists of salts of arabic acid, and proteins contain both amino and carboxylic acid groupings, thus providing electrostatic repulsion as an additional barrier to coalescence. Most cellulose derivatives are not charged. However, there is evidence from studies on solid suspensions that these substances sterically stabilize, and it would appear probable that there will be a similar effect with emulsions.

Solid particles in emulsion stabilization

Emulsions may be stabilized by finely divided solid particles if they are preferentially wetted by one phase and possess sufficient adhesion for one another such that they form a film around the dispersed droplets.

Solid particles will remain at the interface as long as a stable contact angle, θ, is formed by the liquid–liquid interface and the solid surface. The particles must also be of sufficiently low mass for gravitational forces not to affect the equilibrium. If the solid is preferentially wetted by one of the phases, then more particles can be accommodated at the interface if the interface is convex towards that phase. In other words, the liquid whose contact angle (measured through the liquid) is less than 90 degrees will form the continuous phase (Fig. 5.15). Aluminium and magnesium hydroxides and clays such as bentonite are preferentially wetted by water and thus stabilize o/w emulsions, e.g. liquid paraffin and magnesium hydroxide emulsion. Carbon black and talc are more readily wetted by oils and stabilize w/o emulsions.

Emulsion type

When an oil, water and an emulsifying agent are shaken together, what decides whether an o/w

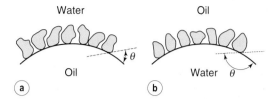

Fig. 5.15 • Emulsion stabilization by solid particles. **(a)** Preferential wetting of the solid by water, leading to an oil-in-water emulsion. **(b)** Preferential wetting of the solid by oil, leading to a water-in-oil emulsion.

emulsion or a w/o emulsion will be produced? A number of simultaneous processes have to be considered; for example, droplet formation, aggregation and coalescence of droplets, and interfacial film formation. When oil and water are shaken together, both phases initially form droplets. The phase that persists in droplet form for the longer time should become the disperse phase and it should be surrounded by the continuous phase formed from the more rapidly coalescing droplets. The phase volumes and interfacial tensions will determine the relative number of droplets produced and hence the probability of collision, i.e. the greater the number of droplets, the higher the chance of collision, so the phase present in greater amount should finally become the continuous phase. However, emulsions containing much more than 50% of disperse phase are common.

A more important consideration is the interfacial film produced by the adsorption of emulsifier at the o/w interface. Such films significantly alter the rates of coalescence by acting as physical and chemical barriers to coalescence. As indicated in the previous section, the barrier at the surface of an oil droplet may arise because of electrically charged groups producing repulsion between approaching droplets, or because of the steric repulsion, enthalpic in origin, from hydrated polymer chains. The greater the number of charged molecules present, or the greater the number of hydrated polymer chains at the interface, the greater will be the tendency to reduce oil droplet coalescence. On the other hand, the interfacial barrier for approaching water droplets arises primarily because of the nonpolar or hydrocarbon portion of the interfacial film. The longer the hydrocarbon chain length and the greater the number of molecules present per unit area of film, the greater is the tendency for water droplets to be prevented from coalescing. Thus, it may be said generally that it is the dominance of the polar or nonpolar characteristics of the emulsifying agent which plays a major part in the type of emulsion produced.

It would appear, then, that the type of emulsion formed, depending as it does on the polar/nonpolar characteristics of the emulsifying agent, is a function of the relative solubility of the emulsifying agent, the phase in which it is more soluble being the continuous phase. This is a statement of what is termed the Bancroft rule, an empirical observation.

The foregoing helps to explain why charged surface-active agents such as sodium and potassium oleates, which are highly ionized and possess strong polar groups, favour o/w emulsions, whereas calcium and magnesium soaps, which are little dissociated, tend to produce w/o emulsions. Similarly, nonionic sorbitan esters favour w/o emulsions, whilst o/w emulsions are produced by the more hydrophilic polyoxyethylene sorbitan esters.

By reason of the stabilizing mechanism involved, polar groups are far better barriers to coalescence than their nonpolar counterparts. It is thus possible to see why o/w emulsions can be made with greater than 50% disperse phase and w/o emulsions are limited in this respect and invert (change type) if the amount of water present is significant.

Hydrophile–lipophile balance

The fact that a more hydrophilic interfacial barrier favours o/w emulsions whilst a more nonpolar barrier favours w/o emulsions is used in the hydrophile–lipophile balance (HLB) system for assessing surfactants and emulsifying agents, which was introduced by Griffin. Here an HLB number is assigned to an emulsifying agent that is characteristic of its relative polarity. Although originally conceived for nonionic emulsifying agents with polyoxyethylene hydrophilic groups, it has since been applied with differing success to other surfactant groups, both ionic and nonionic.

By means of this number system, an HLB range of optimum efficiency for each class of surfactant is established, as seen in Fig. 5.16. This approach is empirical but it does allow comparison between different chemical types of emulsifying agent.

There are several formulae for calculating HLB values of nonionic surfactants. We can estimate values for polysorbates (Tween surfactants) and sorbitan esters (Span surfactants) from

$$HLB = (E + P)/5$$

$$(5.30)$$

where E is the percentage by weight of oxyethylene chains and P is the percentage by weight of polyhydric

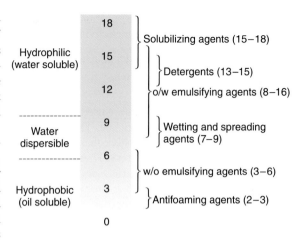

Fig. 5.16 • Hydrophile–lipophile balance scale showing classification of surfactant function. *o/w*, Water-in-oil; *w/o*, oil-in-water.

alcohol groups (glycerol or sorbitol) in the molecule. If the surfactant contains only polyoxyethylene as the hydrophilic group, then we can use a simpler form of the equation:

$$HLB = E/5$$

$$(5.31)$$

Alternatively, we can calculate HLB values directly from the chemical formula using empirically determined group numbers. The formula is then

$$HLB = \Sigma(\text{hydrophilic group numbers}) + \Sigma(\text{lipophilic group numbers}) + 7$$

$$(5.32)$$

Group numbers of some commonly occurring groups are given in Table 5.5. Finally, the HLB value of polyhydric alcohol fatty acid esters such as glyceryl monostearate may be obtained from the saponification value, S, of the ester and the acid number, A, of the fatty acid using:

$$HLB = 20(1 - S/A)$$

$$(5.33)$$

In addition, it has been suggested that certain emulsifying agents of a given HLB value appear to work best with a particular oil phase, and this has given rise to the concept of a *required HLB value* for any oil or combination of oils. However, this does not necessarily mean that every surfactant having the

Table 5.5 Group contributions to hydrophile–lipophile balance values

Group	Contribution
SO$_4$Na	+38.7
COOK	+21.1
COONa	+19.1
SO$_3$Na	+11.0
N (tertiary amine)	+9.4
Ester (sorbitan ring)	+6.8
Ester (free)	+2.4
COOH	+2.1
OH (free)	+1.9
–O– (ether)	+1.3
OH (sorbitan)	+0.5
CH, CH$_2$, etc.	0
OCH$_2$CH$_2$	+0.33
OCH(CH$_3$)CH$_2$	−0.15
Alkyl	−0.475
CF$_2$, CF$_3$	−0.870

required HLB value will produce a good emulsion; specific surfactants may interact with the oil, with another component of the emulsion or even with each other.

For reasons mentioned earlier, mixtures of surface-active agents give more stable emulsions than when used singly. The HLB value of a mixture of surfactants, consisting of fraction x of A and $(1 - x)$ of B, is assumed to be an algebraic mean of the two HLB numbers:

$$HLB_{mixt} = xHLB_A + (1-x)HLB_B$$

$$(5.34)$$

It has been found that, at the optimum HLB for a particular emulsion, the mean particle size of the emulsion is at a minimum and that this factor contributes to the stability of the emulsion system. The use of HLB values in the formulation of emulsions is discussed in Chapter 27.

Phase viscosity

The emulsification process and the type of emulsion formed are influenced to some extent by the viscosity of the two phases. Viscosity can be expected to affect interfacial film formation because the migration of molecules of emulsifying agent to the oil/water interface is diffusion controlled. Droplet movement prior to coalescence is also affected by the viscosity of the medium in which the droplets are dispersed.

Stability of emulsions

A stable emulsion may be defined as a system in which the globules retain their initial character and remain uniformly distributed throughout the continuous phase. The function of the emulsifying agent is to form an interfacial film around the dispersed droplets; the physical nature of this barrier controls whether or not the droplets will coalesce as they approach one another. If the film is electrically charged, then repulsive forces will contribute to stability.

Separation of an emulsion into its constituent phases is termed *cracking* or *breaking*. It follows that any agent that will destroy the interfacial film will crack the emulsion. Some of the factors that cause an emulsion to crack are as follows:

- The addition of a chemical that is incompatible with the emulsifying agent, thus destroying its emulsifying ability. Examples include surface-active agents of opposite ionic charge, e.g. the addition of cetrimide (cationic) to an emulsion stabilized with sodium oleate (anionic); addition of large ions of opposite charge, e.g. neomycin sulfate (cationic) to aqueous cream (anionic); addition of electrolytes such as calcium and magnesium salts to an emulsion stabilized with anionic surface-active agents.
- Bacterial growth – protein materials and nonionic surface-active agents are excellent media for bacterial growth.
- Temperature change – protein emulsifying agents may be denatured and the solubility characteristics of nonionic emulsifying agents change with a rise in temperature; heating above 70 °C destroys most emulsions. Freezing will also crack an emulsion; this may be because the ice formed disrupts the interfacial film around the droplets.

Other ways in which an emulsion may show instability are as follows.

Flocculation

Even though a satisfactory interfacial film is present around the oil droplets, secondary minimum flocculation, as described earlier in this chapter in the discussion on the DLVO theory of colloid stability, is likely to occur with most pharmaceutical emulsions. The globules do not coalesce and may be redispersed by shaking. However, due to the closeness of approach of droplets in the floccule, if any weaknesses in the interfacial films occur then coalescence may follow. Flocculation should not be confused with creaming (see later). The former is due to the interaction of attractive and repulsive forces and the latter is due to density differences in the two phases. Both may occur.

Phase inversion

As indicated in the section on emulsion type, the phase volume ratio is a contributory factor to the type of emulsion formed. Although it was stated there that stable emulsions containing more than 50% disperse phase are common, attempts to incorporate excessive amounts of disperse phase may cause cracking of the emulsion or phase inversion (conversion of an o/w emulsion to a w/o emulsion or vice versa). It can be shown that uniform spheres arranged in the closest packing will occupy 74% of the total volume irrespective of their size. Thus Ostwald suggested that an emulsion which resembles such an arrangement of spheres would have a maximum disperse phase concentration of the same order. Although it is possible to obtain more concentrated emulsions than this, because of the nonuniformity of the size of the globules and the possibility of deformation of the shape of the globules, there is a tendency for emulsions containing more than about 70% disperse phase to crack or invert.

Further, any additive that alters the HLB of an emulsifying agent may alter the emulsion type; thus addition of a magnesium salt to an emulsion stabilized with sodium oleate will cause the emulsion to crack or invert.

The addition of an electrolyte to anionic and cationic surfactants may suppress their ionization due to the common-ion effect, and thus a w/o emulsion may result even though normally an o/w emulsion would be produced. For example, pharmacopoeial white liniment is formed from turpentine oil, ammonium oleate, ammonium chloride and water. With ammonium oleate as the emulsifying agent, an o/w emulsion would be expected but the suppression of ionization of the ammonium oleate by the ammonium chloride (the common-ion effect) and a relatively large volume of turpentine oil produce a w/o emulsion.

Emulsions stabilized with nonionic emulsifying agents such as the polysorbates may invert on being heated. This is due to the breaking of the hydrogen bonds responsible for the hydrophilic characteristics of the polysorbate; its HLB value is thus altered and the emulsion inverts.

Creaming

Many emulsions cream on standing. The disperse phase, according to its density relative to that of the continuous phase, rises to the top or sinks to the bottom of the emulsion, forming a layer of more concentrated emulsion. The most common example is milk, an o/w emulsion, with cream rising to the top of the emulsion.

As mentioned earlier, flocculation may occur as well as creaming, but not necessarily. Droplets of the creamed layer do not coalesce, as may be found by gentle shaking which redistributes the droplets throughout the continuous phase. Although not so serious an instability factor as cracking, creaming is undesirable from a pharmaceutical point of view because a creamed emulsion is inelegant in appearance, provides the possibility of inaccurate dosage and increases the likelihood of coalescence since the globules are close together in the cream.

Those factors which influence the rate of creaming are similar to those involved in the sedimentation rate of suspension particles and are indicated by Stokes law (Eq. 5.8) as follows:

$$v = \frac{2a^2 g(\sigma - \rho)}{9\eta}$$

(as 5.8)

where v is the velocity of creaming, a is the globule radius, σ and ρ are the densities of the disperse phase and the dispersion medium respectively, and η is the viscosity of the dispersion medium. A consideration of this equation shows that the rate of creaming will be decreased by:

* a reduction in the globule size;
* a decrease in the density difference between the two phases; and
* an increase in the viscosity of the continuous phase.

A decrease of creaming rate may therefore be achieved by homogenizing the emulsion to reduce the globule size and by increasing the viscosity of the continuous phase, η, by the use of a thickening agent such as tragacanth or methylcellulose. It is seldom possible to satisfactorily adjust the densities of the two phases.

Assessment of emulsion stability

Approximate assessments of the relative stabilities of a series of emulsions may be obtained from estimations of the degree of separation of the disperse phase as a distinct layer, or from the degree of creaming. Whilst separation of the emulsion into two layers, i.e. cracking, indicates gross instability, a stable emulsion may cream, creaming being simply due to density differences and easily reversed by shaking. Some coalescence may, however, take place due to the close proximity of the globules in the cream; similar problems occur with flocculation.

However, instability in an emulsion results from any process which causes a progressive increase in particle size and a broadening of the particle size distribution, so that eventually the dispersed globules become so large that they separate out as free liquid. Accordingly, a more precise method for assessing emulsion stability is to follow the globule size distribution with time. An emulsion approaching the unstable state is characterized by the appearance of large globules as a result of the coalescence of others.

Foams

A foam is a coarse dispersion of a gas in a liquid which is present as thin films or lamellae of colloidal dimensions between the gas bubbles.

Foams find application in pharmacy as aqueous and nonaqueous spray preparations for topical, rectal and vaginal medication and for burn dressings. Equally important, however, is the destruction of foams and the use of antifoaming agents. These are of importance in manufacturing processes, preventing foam in, for example, liquid preparations. In addition, foam inhibitors, such as the silicones, are used in the treatment of flatulence, for the elimination of gas, air or foam from the gastrointestinal tract prior to radiography, and for the relief of abdominal distension and dyspepsia.

Because of their high interfacial area (and surface free energy), all foams are unstable in the thermodynamic sense. Their stability depends on two major factors: the tendency for the liquid films to drain and become thinner, and their tendency to rupture due to random disturbances such as vibration, heat and diffusion of gas from small bubbles to large bubbles. Gas diffuses from the small to the large bubbles because the pressure in the former is greater. This is a phenomenon of curved interfaces, the pressure difference, Δp, being a function of the interfacial tension, γ, and the radius, r, of the droplet according to $\Delta p = 2\gamma/r$.

Pure liquids do not foam. Transient or unstable foams are obtained with solutes such as short-chain acids and alcohols which are mildly surface active. However, persistent foams are formed by solutions of surfactants. The film in such foams consists of two monolayers of adsorbed surface-active molecules separated by an aqueous core. The surfactants stabilize the film by means of electrical double layer repulsion or steric stabilization as described for colloidal dispersions.

Foams are often troublesome, and knowledge of the action of substances that cause their destruction is useful. There are two types of antifoaming agent:

1. *Foam breakers* such as ether and *n*-octanol. These substances are highly surface active and are thought to act by lowering the surface tension over small regions of the liquid film. These regions are rapidly pulled out by surrounding regions of higher tension; small areas of film are therefore thinned out and left without the properties to resist rupture.

2. *Foam inhibitors*, such as polyamides and silicones. It is thought that these are adsorbed at the air–water interface in preference to the foaming agent, but they do not have the requisite ability to form a stable foam. They have a low interfacial tension in the pure state and may be effective by virtue of rapid adsorption.

Aerosols

Aerosols are colloidal dispersions of liquids or solids in gases. In general, mists and fogs possess liquid disperse phases, whilst smoke is a dispersion of solid particles in gases. However, no sharp distinction can be made between the two kinds because liquid is often associated with the solid particles. A mist comprises fine droplets of liquid that may or may not contain dissolved or suspended material. If the concentration of droplets becomes high, it may be called a *fog*.

While all the disperse systems mentioned previously are less stable than colloids that have a liquid as the dispersion medium, they have many properties in common with the latter and can be investigated in the same way. Particle size is usually within the colloidal range but if the particles are larger than

1 μm, the life of an aerosol is short because the particles settle out too quickly.

Preparation of aerosols

In common with other colloidal dispersions, aerosols may be prepared by either dispersion or condensation methods. The latter involve the initial production of supersaturated vapour of the material that is to be dispersed. This may be achieve by supercooling the vapour. The supersaturation eventually leads to the formation of nuclei, which grow into particles of colloidal dimensions. The preparation of aerosols by dispersion methods is of greater interest in pharmacy and may be achieved by the use of pressurized containers with, for example, liquefied gases used as propellants. If a solution or suspension of active ingredients is contained in the liquid propellant or in a mixture of this liquid and an additional solvent, then when the valve on the container is opened, the vapour pressure of the propellant forces the mixture out of the container. The large expansion of the propellant at room temperature and atmospheric pressure produces a dispersion of the active ingredients in air. Although the particles in such dispersions are often larger than those in colloidal systems, these dispersions are still generally referred to as aerosols.

Application of aerosols in pharmacy

The use of aerosols as a dosage form is particularly important in the administration of drugs via the respiratory system. In addition to local effects, systemic effects may be obtained if the drug is absorbed into the bloodstream from the lungs. Topical preparations (see Chapter 40) are also well suited for presentation as aerosols. Therapeutic aerosols for inhalation are discussed in more detail in Chapter 37.

Please check your eBook at **https://studentconsult.** **inkling.com/** for self-assessment questions. See inside cover for registration details.

References

Attwood, D., Florence, A.T., 1983. Surfactant Systems: Their Chemistry, Pharmacy and Biology. Chapman and Hall, London.

Shaw, D.J., 1992. Introduction to Colloid and Surface Chemistry, fourth ed. Butterworth-Heinemann, Oxford.

Bibliography

Florence, A.T., Attwood, D., 2016. Physicochemical Principles of Pharmacy: In Manufacture, Formulation and Clinical Use, sixth ed. Pharmaceutical Press, London.

Rosen, M.J., Kunjappu, J.T., 2012. Surfactants and Interfacial Phenomena, fourth ed. John Wiley & Sons, Hoboken.

Rheology

6

Christopher Marriott

CHAPTER CONTENTS

KEY POINTS

- The critical qualities of an excipient or a dosage form can be monitored by measurement of the appropriate viscosity coefficient based on Newton's law.
- The viscosity of a fluid will be modified by dissolved macromolecules, the nature of which in dilute solution can, in turn, be determined by simple viscometry: at higher concentrations the rheological properties will no longer be Newtonian.
- Measurement of the rheological properties of a material must be carried out with an instrument which is capable of producing meaningful results.

- The flow conditions within even a simple fluid can affect processes such as heat and mass transfer and the rate of dissolution of a dosage form.
- Knowledge of the types of non-Newtonian behaviour is often essential in the design of manufacturing processes or drug delivery systems.
- Assessment of rheological parameters of a medicine can be used to set product characteristics.
- Non-Newtonian materials are more properly considered as being viscoelastic in that they exhibit both liquid and solid characteristics simultaneously, the controlling parameter being time.

Viscosity, rheology and the flow of fluids

The *viscosity* of a fluid may be described simply as its resistance to flow or movement. Thus water, which is easier to stir than syrup, is said to have the lower viscosity. The reciprocal of viscosity is *fluidity*. *Rheology* (a term invented by Bingham and formally adopted in 1929) may be defined as the study of the flow and deformation properties of matter.

Historically the importance of rheology in pharmacy was merely as a means of characterizing and classifying fluids and semisolids. For example, all pharmacopoeias have included a viscosity standard to control substances such as liquid paraffin. However, the increased reliance on in vitro testing of dosage forms as a means of evaluating their suitability for the grant of a marketing authorization and the

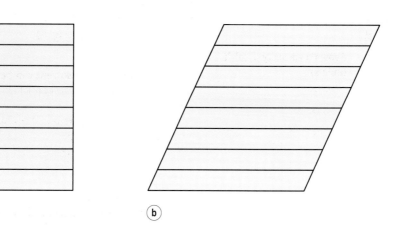

Force

Fig. 6.1 • The effect of shearing a 'block' of fluid. **(a)** unsheared **(b)** during shearing.

increased use of polymers in formulations and the construction of devices has given added importance to measurement of flow properties. Furthermore, advances in the methods of evaluation of the viscoelastic properties of semisolid materials have not only increased the amount and quality of the information that can be gathered but have also reduced the time required for its acquisition.

As a consequence, a proper understanding of the rheological properties of pharmaceutical materials is essential for the preparation, development, evaluation and performance of pharmaceutical dosage forms. This chapter describes rheological behaviour and techniques of measurement and will form a basis for the applied studies described in later chapters.

Newtonian fluids

Viscosity coefficients for Newtonian fluids

Dynamic viscosity

The definition of viscosity was put on a quantitative basis by Newton. He was the first to realize that the rate of flow (γ) is directly related to the applied stress (σ): the constant of proportionality is the *coefficient of dynamic viscosity* (η), more usually referred to simply as the viscosity. Simple fluids which obey this relationship are referred to as *Newtonian* fluids and those which do not are known as *non-Newtonian* fluids.

The phenomenon of viscosity is best understood by a consideration of a hypothetical cube of fluid made up of infinitely thin layers (laminae) which are able to slide over one another like playing cards in a pack or deck (Fig. 6.1a). When a tangential force is applied to the uppermost layer, it is assumed that each subsequent layer will move at progressively decreasing velocity and that the bottom layer will be stationary (see Fig. 6.1b). A velocity gradient will therefore exist and this can be calculated by dividing the velocity of the upper layer in m s^{-1} by the height of the cube in metres. The resultant gradient, which is effectively the rate of flow but is usually referred to as the *rate of shear* or *shear rate*, γ, and its unit is reciprocal seconds (s^{-1}). The applied stress, known as the *shear stress*, σ, is derived by dividing the applied force by the area of the upper layer, and its unit is N m^{-2}.

As Newton's law can be expressed as

$$\sigma = \eta\gamma$$

(6.1)

then

$$\eta = \frac{\sigma}{\gamma}$$

(6.2)

and η will take the unit of N s m^{-2}. Thus, by reference to Eq. 6.1, it can be seen that a Newtonian fluid of viscosity 1 N s m^{-2} will produce a velocity gradient of 1 m s^{-1} for a cube of 1 m dimensions if the applied force is 1 N. Because the derived unit of force per unit area in the SI system is the pascal (Pa), viscosity should be referred to in Pa s or, more practicably, mPa s (the dynamic viscosity of water is approximately 1 mPa s at 20 °C). The centipoise (cP) and poise (1 P

Table 6.1 Viscosities of some fluids of pharmaceutical interest

Fluid	Dynamic viscosity at 20 °C (mPa s)
Chloroform	0.58
Water	1.002
Ethanol	1.20
Fractionated coconut oil	30.0
Glyceryl trinitrate	36.0
Propylene glycol	58.1
Soya bean oil	69.3
Rape oil	163
Glycerol	1490

$= 1$ dyn cm^{-2}s $= 0.1$ Pa s) were units of viscosity in the now redundant cgs (centimetre–gram–second) system. These are no longer official and therefore are not recommended but still persist in the literature.

The values of the viscosity of water and some examples of other fluids of pharmaceutical interest are given in Table 6.1. Viscosity is inversely related to temperature (which should always be quoted alongside every measurement); in this case the values given are those measured at 20 °C.

Kinematic viscosity

The dynamic viscosity is not the only coefficient that can be used to characterize a fluid. The *kinematic viscosity* (v) is also used and may be defined as the dynamic viscosity divided by the density of the fluid (ρ)

$$v = \frac{\eta}{\rho}$$

(6.3)

and the SI unit will be m^2 s^{-1} or, more usefully, mm^2 s^{-1}. The cgs unit was the stoke (1 St $= 10^{-4}$ m^2 s^{-1}), which together with the centistoke (cS), may still be found in the literature.

Relative and specific viscosities

The *viscosity ratio* or *relative viscosity* (η_r) of a solution is the ratio of the viscosity of the solution to the viscosity of its solvent (η_o)

$$\eta_r = \frac{\eta}{\eta_o}$$

(6.4)

and the *specific viscosity* (η_{sp}) is given by

$$\eta_{sp} = \eta_r - 1$$

(6.5)

In these calculations the solvent can be of any nature, although in pharmaceutical products it is most usually water.

For a colloidal dispersion, the equation derived by Einstein may be used

$$\eta = \eta_o(1 + 2.5\phi)$$

(6.6)

where ϕ is the volume fraction of the colloidal phase (the volume of the dispersed phase divided by the total volume of the dispersion). The Einstein equation may be rewritten as

$$\frac{\eta}{\eta_o} = 1 + 2.5\phi$$

(6.7)

Since from Eq. 6.4 it can be seen that as the left-hand side of Eq. 6.7 is equal to the relative viscosity, it can be rewritten as

$$\frac{\eta}{\eta_o} - 1 = \frac{\eta - \eta_o}{\eta_o} = 2.5\phi$$

(6.8)

where the left-hand side equals the specific viscosity. Eq. 6.8 can be rearranged to produce

$$\frac{\eta_{SP}}{\phi} = 2.5$$

(6.9)

and as the volume fraction will be directly related to concentration, C, Eq. 6.9 can be rewritten as

$$\frac{\eta_{SP}}{C} = k$$

(6.10)

where k is a constant.

When the dispersed phase is a high molecular mass polymer, then a colloidal solution will result and, provided moderate concentrations are used, Eq. 6.10 can be expressed as a power series

$$\frac{\eta_{SP}}{C} = k_1 + k_2C + k_3C^2$$

(6.11)

Intrinsic viscosity

If η_{sp}/C, usually referred to as either the viscosity number or the reduced viscosity, is determined at a

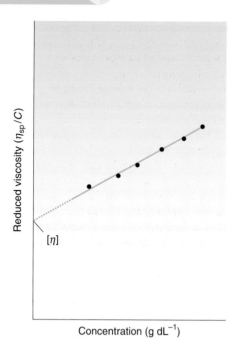

Fig. 6.2 • Reduced viscosity (η_{sp}/C), against concentration (g dL^{-1}) which by extrapolation gives the limiting viscosity number or intrinsic viscosity ($[\eta]$).

range of polymer concentrations (g dL^{-1}) and plotted as a function of concentration (Fig. 6.2), a linear relationship should be obtained. The intercept produced on extrapolation of the line to the ordinate will yield the constant k_1 (Eqn 6.11), which is referred to as the *limiting viscosity number* or the *intrinsic viscosity*, $[\eta]$.

The limiting viscosity number may be used to determine the approximate molecular mass (M) of polymers by use of the Mark–Houwink equation

$$[\eta] = KM^{\alpha}$$

(6.12)

where K and α are constants that must be obtained at a given temperature for the specific polymer–solvent system by means of another technique such as osmometry or light scattering. However, once these constants have been determined, viscosity measurements provide a quick and precise method for the viscosity-average molecular mass determination of pharmaceutical polymers such as dextrans, which are used as plasma extenders. Furthermore, the values of the two constants provide an indication of the shape of the molecule in solution: spherical molecules yield values of $\alpha = 0$, whereas extended rods have values greater than 1.0. A randomly coiled molecule will yield an intermediate value ($\sim$0.5).

The specific viscosity may be used in the following equation to determine the volume of a molecule in solution

$$\eta_{SP} = 2.5C\frac{NV}{M}$$

(6.13)

where C is concentration, N is Avogadro's number, V is the hydrodynamic volume of each molecule and M is the molecular mass. However, it does suffer from the obvious disadvantage that the assumption is made that all polymeric molecules form spheres in solution.

Huggins constant

The constant k_2 in Eq. 6.11 is referred to as the Huggins constant and is equal to the slope of the plot shown in Fig. 6.2. Its value gives an indication of the interaction between the polymer molecule and the solvent, such that a positive slope is produced for a polymer that interacts weakly with the solvent, and the slope becomes less positive as the interaction increases. A change in the value of the Huggins constant can be used to evaluate the interaction of drug molecules in solution with polymers.

Boundary layers

From Fig. 6.1 it can be seen that the rate of flow of a fluid over an even surface will be dependent on the distance from that surface. The velocity, which will be almost zero at the surface, increases with increasing distance from the surface until the bulk of the fluid is reached and the velocity becomes constant. The region over which such differences in velocity are observed is referred to as the *boundary layer*, which arises because the intermolecular forces between the liquid molecules and those of the surface result in a reduction of movement of the layer adjacent to the wall to zero. Its depth is dependent on the viscosity of the fluid and the rate of flow in the bulk fluid. High viscosity and a low flow rate will result in a thick boundary layer, which will become thinner as either the viscosity falls or the flow rate or temperature is increased. The boundary layer represents an important barrier to heat and mass transfer.

In the case of a capillary tube, the two boundary layers meet at the centre of the tube, such that the velocity distribution is parabolic (Fig. 6.3). With an increase in either the diameter of the tube or the

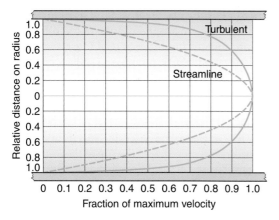

Fig. 6.3 • Velocity distributions across a pipe of circular cross section.

fluid velocity, the proximity of the two boundary layers is reduced and the velocity profile becomes flattened at the centre (see Fig. 6.3).

Laminar, transitional and turbulent flow

The conditions under which a fluid flows through a pipe, for example, can markedly affect the character of the flow. The type of flow that occurs can be best understood by reference to experiments conducted in 1883 by Reynolds, who used an apparatus (Fig. 6.4) which consisted of a horizontal, straight glass tube through which the fluid flowed under the influence of a force provided by a constant head of water. At the centre of the inlet of the tube, a fine stream of dye was introduced. At low flow rates the dye formed a coherent thread which remained undisturbed at the centre of the tube and increased very little in

thickness along the length. This type of flow is described as *streamline* or *laminar flow*, and the liquid is considered to flow as a series of concentric cylinders in a manner analogous to an extending telescope.

If the speed of the fluid is increased, a critical velocity is reached at which the thread begins to waver and then to break up, although no mixing occurs. This is known as *transitional flow*. When the velocity is increased to higher values, the dye instantaneously mixes with the fluid in the tube, as all order is lost and irregular motions are imposed on the overall movement of the fluid: such flow is described as *turbulent flow*. In this type of flow, the movement of molecules is totally haphazard, although the average movement will be in the direction of flow.

Reynolds experiments indicated that the flow conditions were affected by four factors: namely, the diameter of the pipe and the viscosity, density and velocity of the fluid. Furthermore, it was shown that these factors could be combined to give the following equation

$$Re = \frac{\rho u d}{\eta}$$

(6.14)

where ρ is the density, u is the velocity, η is the dynamic viscosity of the fluid and d is the diameter of the circular cross section of the pipe. Re is known as the Reynolds number and if compatible units are used, it will be dimensionless.

Values of Reynolds number in a circular cross-section pipe have been determined that can be associated with a particular type of flow. If it is below 2000, then laminar flow will occur, but if it is greater than 4000, then flow will be turbulent. In between these two values the nature of the flow will depend

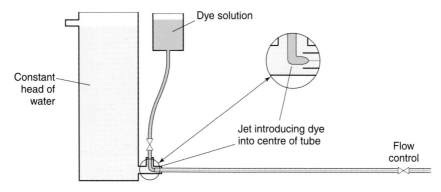

Fig. 6.4 • Reynolds apparatus.

on the surface over which the fluid is flowing. For example, if the surface is smooth, then laminar flow may not be disturbed and may exist at values of a Reynolds number greater than 2000. However, if the surface is rough or the channel tortuous, then flow may well be turbulent at values less than 4000, and even as low as 2000. Consequently, although it is tempting to state that a Reynolds number between 2000 and 4000 is indicative of transitional flow, such a statement would be correct only for a specific set of conditions. The fact that it is difficult to demonstrate transitional flow practically has led to the belief that it should be replaced by the critical Reynolds number (Re_c), which is 2100 and signifies the change from laminar to turbulent flow.

Nevertheless, the Reynolds number is still an important parameter and can be used to predict the type of flow that will occur in a particular situation. The reason why it is important to know the type of flow which is occurring is that whereas with laminar flow there is no component at right angles to the direction of flow and fluid cannot move across the tube, this component is strong for turbulent flow and interchange across the tube is rapid. Thus in the latter case, mass, for example, will be rapidly transported. In laminar flow the fluid layers will act as a barrier to such transfer, and therefore mass transfer can occur only by molecular diffusion, which is a much slower process.

Determination of the flow properties of simple fluids

A wide range of instruments exists that can be used to determine the flow properties of Newtonian fluids. However, only some of these are capable of providing data that can be used to calculate viscosities in fundamental units. The design of many instruments precludes the calculation of absolute viscosities as they are capable of providing data only in terms of empirical units.

In this chapter, the instruments described will be limited to those specified in various pharmacopoeias and will not include all of those available.

Capillary viscometers

A capillary viscometer can be used to determine viscosity provided that the fluid is Newtonian and the flow is laminar. The rate of flow of the fluid through the capillary is measured under the influence of gravity or an externally applied pressure.

Ostwald U-tube viscometer. Such instruments are described in pharmacopoeias and are the subject of a specification of the International Organization for Standardization (ISO). A range of capillary bores are available, and an appropriate one should be selected so that a flow time for the fluid of approximately 200 seconds is obtained; the wider-bore viscometers are thus for use with fluids of higher viscosity. For fluids where there is a viscosity specification in a pharmacopoeial monograph, the size of the instrument that must be used in the determination of their viscosity is stated.

In the viscometer shown diagrammatically in Fig. 6.5, liquid is introduced through arm V up to mark G by means of a pipette long enough to prevent wetting of the sides of the tube. The viscometer is then clamped vertically in a constant-temperature water bath and allowed to reach the required temperature. The level of the liquid is adjusted and it is then blown or sucked into tube W until the meniscus is just above mark E. The time for the meniscus to fall between marks E and F is then recorded, and determinations should be repeated until three readings all within 0.5 seconds are obtained. Care should be taken not to introduce air bubbles and to ensure that the capillary does not become partially occluded with small particles.

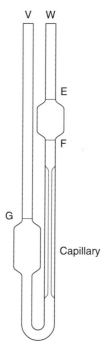

Fig. 6.5 • A U-tube viscometer.

The maximum shear rate, γ_m, is given by

$$\gamma_m = \frac{\rho g r_c}{2\eta}$$

(6.15)

where ρ is the density of the fluid, g the acceleration due to gravity, r_c the radius of the capillary and η the absolute viscosity. Consequently, for a fluid of viscosity 1 mPa s, the maximum shear rate is approximately 2×10^3 s^{-1} if the capillary has a diameter of 0.64 mm, but it will be of the order of 10^2 s^{-1} for a fluid of the same density with a viscosity of 1490 mPa s if the capillary has a diameter of 2.74 mm.

Suspended-level viscometer. This instrument is a modification of the U-tube viscometer which avoids the need to fill the instrument with a precise volume of fluid. It also addresses the fact that the pressure head in the U-tube viscometer is continually changing as the two menisci approach one another. This instrument is also described in pharmacopoeias and is shown in Fig. 6.6.

A volume of liquid which will at least fill bulb C is introduced via tube V. The only upper limit on the volume used is that it should not be so large as to block the ventilating tube Z. The viscometer is clamped vertically in a constant-temperature water bath and allowed to attain the required temperature.

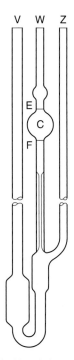

Fig. 6.6 • A suspended-level viscometer.

Tube Z is closed and fluid is drawn into bulb C by the application of suction through tube W until the meniscus is just above the mark E. Tube W is then closed and tube Z opened so that liquid can drain away from the bottom of the capillary. Tube W is then opened and the time the fluid takes to fall between marks E and F is recorded. If at any time during the determination the end of the ventilating tube Z becomes blocked by the liquid, the measurement must be repeated. The same criteria for reproducibility of timings described for the U-tube viscometer must be applied.

Because the volume of fluid introduced into the instrument can vary between the limits described, this means that measurements can be made at a range of temperatures without the need to adjust the volume.

Calculation of viscosity from capillary viscometers

Poiseuille's law states that for a liquid flowing through a capillary tube

$$\eta = \frac{\pi r^4 t P}{8LV}$$

(6.16)

where r is the radius of the capillary, t is the time of flow, P is the pressure difference across the ends of the tube, L is the length of the capillary and V is the volume of liquid. As the radius and length of the capillary, as well as the volume flowing, are constants for a given viscometer then

$$\eta = KtP$$

(6.17)

where K is equal to $\dfrac{\pi r^4}{8LV}$.

The pressure difference, P, depends on the density, ρ, of the liquid, the acceleration due to gravity, g, and the difference in the heights of the two menisci in the two arms of the viscometer. Because the value of g and the level of the liquids are constant, these can be included in a constant, and Eq. 6.17 can be written for the viscosities of an unknown and a standard liquid

$$\eta_1 = K't_1\rho_1$$

(6.18)

$$\eta_2 = K't_2\rho_2$$

(6.19)

Thus, when the flow times for two liquids are compared in the same viscometer, division of Eq. 6.18 by Eq. 6.19 gives

$$\frac{\eta_1}{\eta_2} = \frac{K't_1\rho_1}{K't_2\rho_2}$$

(6.20)

and reference to Eq. 6.4 shows that Eq. 6.20 will yield the viscosity ratio.

However, as Eq. 6.3 indicates that the kinematic viscosity is equal to the dynamic viscosity divided by the density, then Eq. 6.20 may be rewritten as

$$\frac{v_1}{v_2} = \frac{t_1}{t_2}$$

(6.21)

For a given viscometer a standard fluid such as water can be used for the purposes of calibration. Eq. 6.21 may then be rewritten as

$$v = ct$$

(6.22)

where c is the viscometer constant.

This equation justifies the continued use of the kinematic viscosity as it means that liquids of known viscosity but of differing density from the test fluid can be used as the standard. A series of oils of given viscosity are available commercially and are recommended for the calibration of viscometers if water cannot be used.

Falling-sphere viscometer

This viscometer is based on Stokes law (see Chapter 5). When a body falls through a viscous medium it experiences a resistance or viscous drag which opposes the downward motion. Consequently, if a body falls through a liquid under the influence of gravity, an initial acceleration period is followed by motion at a uniform terminal velocity when the gravitational force is balanced by the viscous drag. Eq. 6.23 will then apply to this terminal velocity when a sphere of density ρ_s and diameter d falls through a liquid of viscosity η and density ρ_1. The terminal velocity is u, and g is the acceleration due to gravity

$$3\pi\eta du = \frac{\pi}{6}d^3g(\rho_s - \rho_1)$$

(6.23)

The viscous drag is given by the left-hand side of the equation, whereas the right-hand side represents the force responsible for the downward motion of the sphere under the influence of gravity. Eq. 6.23 may be used to calculate viscosity by rearrangement to give

$$\eta = \frac{d^2g(\rho_s - \rho_1)}{18u}$$

(6.24)

Eq. 6.3 gives the relationship between η and the kinematic viscosity, such that Eq. 6.24 may be rewritten as

$$v = \frac{d^2g(\rho_s - \rho_1)}{18u\rho_1}$$

(6.25)

In the derivation of these equations it is assumed that the sphere falls through a fluid of infinite dimensions. However, for practical purposes the fluid must be contained in a vessel of finite dimensions and it is therefore necessary to divide the viscosity by a correction factor to account for the end and wall effects. The correction normally used is due to Faxen and may be given as

$$F = 1 - 2.104\frac{d}{D} + 2.09\frac{d^3}{D^3} - 0.95\frac{d^5}{D^5}$$

(6.26)

where D is the diameter of the measuring tube and d is the diameter of the sphere. The last term in Eq. 6.26 accounts for the end effect and may be ignored as long as only the middle third of the depth of the tube is used for measuring the velocity of the sphere. In practice, the middle half of the tube can be used if D is at least 10 times d, and the second and third terms, which account for the wall effects, can be replaced by $2.1d/D$.

The apparatus used to determine u is shown in Fig. 6.7. The liquid is placed in the fall tube, which is clamped vertically in a constant-temperature bath. Sufficient time must be allowed for temperature equilibration to occur and for any air bubbles to rise to the surface. A steel sphere which has been cleaned and brought to the temperature of the experiment is introduced into the fall tube through a narrow guide tube, the end of which must be below the surface of the fluid under test. The passage of the sphere is monitored by a method that avoids parallax, and the time it takes to fall between the etched marks A and B is recorded. It is usual to take the average of three readings, all of which must be within 0.5%, as the fall time, t, to calculate the viscosity. If

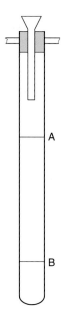

Fig. 6.7 • A falling-sphere viscometer.

the same sphere and fall tube are used, then Eq. 6.25 reduces to

$$v = Kt\left(\frac{\rho_S}{\rho_1} - 1\right)$$

(6.27)

where K is a constant that may be determined by the use of a liquid of known kinematic viscosity.

A number of pharmacopoeias specify the use of a viscometer of this type; it is sometimes referred to as a falling-ball viscometer. Like capillary viscometers, it should only be used with Newtonian fluids.

An inspired and very valuable application of Stokes law is the erythrocyte sedimentation rate test which is used as a non-specific means of assisting in the diagnosis and monitoring of a number of inflammatory disorders as it takes the form of a biological falling sphere viscometer. The test (known as the Westergren test, which has been used since the beginning of the 20th century) involves the use of fresh anticoagulated blood which is loaded into a 300 mm long glass or plastic tube with an internal diameter of 2.55 mm. The rate at which the erythrocytes (red blood cells) settle is measured, so they take the place of the steel sphere in the falling-sphere viscometer. The result is recorded as the volume that the cell sediment occupies after 60 minutes. The larger the volume, the more cells will have fallen to the bottom of the tube, which gives a direct indication of the degree of inflammation. However, the inclusion of the word

'rate' in the name of the test is misleading and is retained only because of traditional usage since obviously a rate cannot be calculated from a single measurement after 60 minutes. The reason why the red blood cells sediment more quickly is due to the elevation of the level of macromolecules in plasma, especially fibrinogen, which cause the red blood cells to aggregate in a stack (rather like a pile of coins) to form *rouleaux* which sediment more quickly as a result of their higher density. This happens even though an increased concentration of macromolecules in plasma will raise its viscosity (the measurement of which is another rheological test used in diagnosis of inflammatory states); this effect is more than countermanded by the increase in particle density. This simple rheological test, even after more than 100 years, continues to be a sensitive and quick way of diagnosing and monitoring the progress of inflammatory conditions such as rheumatoid arthritis, lupus and polymyalgia rheumatica.

Non-Newtonian fluids

The characteristics described in the previous sections apply only to fluids that obey Newton's law (Eqn 6.1) and which are consequently referred to as Newtonian. However, most pharmaceutical fluids do not obey this law as their viscosity varies with the shear rate. The reason for these deviations is that they are not simple fluids such as water and syrup, but may be disperse or colloidal systems, including emulsions, suspensions and gels. These materials are known as non-Newtonian, and with the increasing use of sophisticated polymer-based delivery systems, more examples of such behaviour are being found in pharmaceutical science.

Types of non-Newtonian behaviour

More than one type of deviation from Newton's law can be recognized, and the type of deviation that occurs can be used to classify the particular material.

If a Newtonian fluid is subjected to an increasing shear rate, γ, and the corresponding shear stress, σ, is recorded, then a plot of σ as a function of γ will produce the linear relationship shown in Fig. 6.8a. Such a plot is usually referred to as a flow curve or *rheogram*. The slope of this plot will give the viscosity of the fluid and its reciprocal will give the *fluidity*.

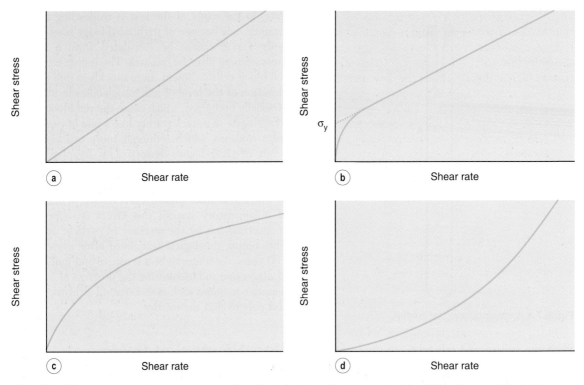

Fig. 6.8 • Flow curves or rheograms representing the behaviour of various materials: **(a)** Newtonian, **(b)** plastic, **(c)** pseudoplastic and **(d)** dilatant.

Eq. 6.1 predicts that this line will pass through the origin.

Plastic (or Bingham) flow

Fig. 6.8b indicates an example of *plastic* or *Bingham flow*, when the rheogram does not pass through the origin but intersects the shear stress axis at a point usually referred to as the yield value, σ_y. This implies that a plastic material does not flow until such a value of shear stress has been exceeded, and at lower stresses the substance behaves as a solid (elastic) material. Plastic materials are often referred to as Bingham bodies in honour of the worker who conducted many of the original studies on them. The equation he derived may be given as

$$\sigma = \sigma_y + \eta_P \gamma$$

(6.28)

where η_p is the plastic viscosity and σ_y the Bingham yield stress or Bingham value (see Fig. 6.8b). The equation implies that the rheogram is a straight line intersecting the shear stress axis at the yield value σ_y. In practice, flow will begin to occur at a shear stress lower than σ_y and the flow curve gradually approaches the extrapolation of the linear portion of the line shown in Fig. 6.8b. This extrapolation will also give the Bingham or apparent yield value; the slope is the plastic viscosity.

Plastic flow is exhibited by concentrated suspensions, particularly if the continuous phase is of high viscosity or if the particles are flocculated (see Chapter 26).

Pseudoplastic flow

The rheogram shown in Fig. 6.8c arises at the origin and, as no yield value exists, the material will flow as soon as a shear stress is applied; the slope of the curve gradually decreases with increasing shear rate, and since the viscosity is directly related to the slope, it therefore decreases as the shear rate is increased. Materials exhibiting this behaviour are said to be pseudoplastic and no single value of viscosity can be considered as characteristic. The viscosity, which can only be calculated from the slope of a tangent drawn to the curve at a specific point, is known as the apparent viscosity. It is only of any use if quoted in conjunction with the shear rate at which the determination was made. However, it would need several apparent viscosities to be determined in order to characterize a pseudoplastic material, so perhaps the most satisfactory representation is by means of the entire flow curve. However, it is frequently noted that at higher shear stresses the flow curve tends towards linearity, indicating that a minimum viscosity has been attained. When this is the case, such a viscosity can be a useful means of representation.

There is no completely satisfactory quantitative explanation of pseudoplastic flow; probably the most widely used is the power law, which is given as

$$\sigma = \eta' \gamma^n$$

(6.29)

where η' is a viscosity coefficient, and the exponent, n, is an index of pseudoplasticity. When $n = 1$, η' becomes the dynamic viscosity (η) and Eq. 6.29 becomes the same as Eq. 6.1, but as a material becomes more pseudoplastic then the value of n will increase. To obtain the values of the constants in Eq. 6.29, log σ must be plotted against log γ, from which the slope will produce n and the intercept η'. The equation may apply only over a limited range (approximately one decade) of shear rates, and so it may not be applicable for all pharmaceutical materials, and other models may have to be considered to fit the data. For example, the model known as Herschel–Bulkley can be given as

$$\sigma = \sigma_y + K\gamma^n$$

(6.30)

where K is a viscosity coefficient. This can be of use for flow curves that are curvilinear and which intersect with the stress axis.

The materials that exhibit this type of flow include aqueous dispersions of natural and chemically modified hydrocolloids, such as tragacanth, methylcellulose and carmellose, and synthetic polymers such as polyvinylpyrrolidone and polyacrylic acid. The presence of long, high molecular weight molecules in solution results in their entanglement with the association of immobilized solvent. Under the influence of shear, the molecules tend to become disentangled and align themselves in the direction of flow. They thus offer less resistance to flow and this, together with the release of some of the entrapped water, accounts for the lower viscosity. At any particular shear rate, equilibrium will be established between the shearing force and the molecular re-entanglement brought about by Brownian motion.

Dilatant flow

The opposite type of flow to pseudoplasticity is depicted by the curve in Fig. 6.8d: the viscosity increases with increase in shear rate. As such materials appear to increase in volume during shearing, they are referred to as *dilatant* and exhibit shear thickening. An equation similar to that for pseudoplastic flow (Eqn 6.29) may be used to describe dilatant behaviour, but the value of the exponent n will be less than 1 and will decrease as dilatancy increases.

This type of behaviour is less common than plastic or pseudoplastic flow but may be exhibited by dispersions containing a high concentration (~50%) of small, deflocculated particles; a suspension of 40% corn starch in water has been proposed as a good example. Under conditions of zero shear, the particles are able to pack closely together and the interparticulate voids will be at a minimum (Fig. 6.9), so there will be sufficient vehicle to fill them and the particles can slide over one another. Such materials can be poured slowly since the shear rates produced will be low. However, it has been shown that a large tank of corn starch suspension can support the weight of a fully grown person running across it, but if that person stops and stands still, they gradually sink to the bottom (videos can be found on YouTube, e.g. https://www.youtube.com/watch?v=S5SGiwS5L6I). It seems that this is not an example of shear thickening but that it is compression which is responsible. Waitukaitis & Jaeger (2012) demonstrated that when a solid metal rod is dropped onto the surface of a suspension of cornflour in water, on impact a deceleration equivalent to 100 times the acceleration due to gravity, g, is produced within 2 milliseconds. The impact compresses the suspension and rapidly produces a solid zone below the rod as the particles become jammed together. The surrounding material is dragged down with the solid zone and a conical raft is formed (van Hecke, 2012) which does not need to extend to the base of the container to support the weight

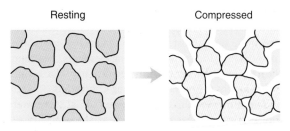

Resting   Compressed

Fig. 6.9 • Representation of the cause of dilatant behaviour in concentrated suspensions.

of the rod. Neither the rate at which the zone is formed nor its size is influenced by the viscosity of the continuous fluid. Fortunately, the behaviour is reversible, and removal of the shear stress results in the re-establishment of the fluid nature, although the reason why this happens is not understood.

This behaviour of particles suspended in fluids (e.g. silica in polyethylene glycol) has been put to good use in bullet-proof vests and body armour. This application depends on the rapid transformation from liquid to solid since it needs to occur sufficiently quickly to stop a bullet travelling at 1700 miles per hour. Some quicksands are also dilatant, although as they can equally well be pseudoplastic, they present a dilemma for anyone who accidentally walks on one!

It needs to be emphasized that these highly concentrated suspensions although quite properly described as dilatant are not examples of shear thickening. Chemically modified celluloses to which anionic surfactants have been added produce systems that can be truly considered to exhibit increased viscosity with an increase in shear rate.

Whatever the cause, dilatancy can be a problem during the processing of, for example, colloidal solutions and dispersions and in the granulation of tablet masses, when high-speed mills and mixers are employed. If the material being processed becomes dilatant in nature, then the resultant solidification could overload and damage the motor. Changing the batch or supplier of an ingredient could lead to processing problems that can only be avoided by rheological evaluation of the dispersions prior to their introduction in the production process.

Time-dependent behaviour

In the description of the different types of non-Newtonian behaviour it was implied that although the viscosity of a fluid might vary with shear rate it was independent of the length of time that the shear rate was applied and also that replicate determinations at the same shear rate would always produce the same viscosity. This must be considered as the ideal situation, since most non-Newtonian materials are colloidal in nature and the flowing elements, whether they are particles or macromolecules, may not adapt immediately to the new shearing conditions.

Therefore, when such a material is subjected to a particular shear rate, the shear stress and consequently the viscosity will decrease with time. Furthermore, once the shear stress has been removed,

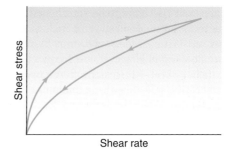

Fig. 6.10 • Rheogram produced by a thixotropic pseudoplastic material.

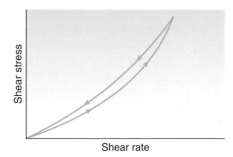

Fig. 6.11 • Rheogram produced by a thixotropic dilatant material.

even if the breakdown in structure is reversible, it may not return to its original condition (rheological ground state) instantly. The common feature of all these materials is that if they are subjected to a gradually increasing shear rate, which in turn is then decreased to zero, the down curve of the rheogram will be displaced with regard to the up curve and a hysteresis loop will be included (Fig. 6.10). In the case of plastic and pseudoplastic materials, the down curve will be displaced to the right of the up curve (see Fig. 6.10), whereas for dilatant substances the reverse will be true (Fig. 6.11). The presence of the hysteresis loop indicates that a breakdown in structure has occurred, and the area within the loop may be used as an index of the degree of breakdown.

The term that is used to describe such behaviour is *thixotropy*, which means 'to change by touch'. Although the term should only strictly be applied to an isothermal sol–gel transformation, it has become common to describe any material that exhibits a reversible time-dependent decrease in apparent viscosity as thixotropic. Such systems are usually composed of asymmetric particles or macromolecules that are capable of interacting by numerous secondary bonds to produce a loose three-dimensional structure, so that the material is gel-like when unsheared. The energy imparted during shearing disrupts these bonds, so that the flowing elements become aligned and the viscosity falls, as a gel–sol transformation has occurred. When the shear stress is eventually removed, the structure will tend to reform, although the process is not immediate but will increase with time as the molecules return to the original state under the influence of Brownian motion. Furthermore, the time taken for recovery, which can range from minutes to days depending on the system, will be directly related to the length of time the material was subjected to the shear stress, as this will affect the degree of this breakdown.

In some cases, the structure that has been destroyed is never recovered, no matter how long the system is left unsheared. Repeated determinations of the flow curve will then produce only the down curve which was obtained in the experiment that resulted in the destruction. It is suggested that such behaviour be referred to as 'shear destruction' rather than thixotropy, which, as will be appreciated from the discussion, is a misnomer in this case.

An example of such behaviour is the gels produced by high molecular weight polysaccharides, which are stabilized by large numbers of secondary bonds. Such systems undergo extensive reorganization during shearing such that the three-dimensional structure is reduced to a two-dimensional one; the gel-like nature of the original is then never recovered.

The occurrence of such complex behaviour creates problems in the quantification of the viscosity of these materials because not only will the apparent viscosity change with shear rate, but there will also be two viscosities that can be calculated for any given shear rate (i.e. from the up curve and the down curve). It is usual to attempt to calculate one viscosity for the up curve and another for the down curve but this requires each of the curves to achieve linearity over some of their length, otherwise a defined shear rate must be used; only the former situation is truly satisfactory. Each of the lines used to derive the viscosity may be extrapolated to the shear stress axis to give an associated yield value. However, only the one derived from the up curve has any significance, as that derived from the down curve will relate to the broken-down system.

Consequently, the most useful index of thixotropy can be obtained by integration of the area contained within the loop. This will not, of course, take into account the shape of the up and down curves, and

so two materials may produce loops of similar area but with completely different shapes, representing totally different types of flow behaviour. In order to prevent confusion, it is best to adopt a method whereby an estimate of area is accompanied by a yield value(s). This is particularly important when complex up curves exhibiting bulges are obtained, although it is now acknowledged that when these have been reported in the literature, they might well have been a consequence of the design of the instrument employed, rather than providing information on the three-dimensional structure of the material under investigation. The evidence for this is based on the flow curves produced using more modern instruments, which do not exhibit the same, if any, bulges.

Finally, there are some instances of materials that become more viscous with increased length of time that the shear stress is applied. The correct term for this behaviour is *rheopexy*. An everyday example is the thickening of cream with increased beating, and fluid pharmaceutical emulsions can become semisolid creams on being homogenized. Since these changes accompany a distinct change in the internal structure of the system, they are not reversible under normal conditions.

Determination of the flow properties of non-Newtonian fluids

With such a wide variety of rheological behaviour, it is extremely important to carry out measurements that will produce meaningful results. It is crucial therefore not to use a determination of viscosity at one shear rate which, although perfectly acceptable for a Newtonian fluid, would produce results which are useless for any comparative purposes. Fig. 6.12 shows rheograms that represent the four different types of flow behaviour, all of which intersect at point A, which is equivalent to a shear rate of 100 s^{-1}. Therefore, if a measurement was made at this one shear rate, all four materials would be shown to have the same viscosity ($\sigma/\gamma = 0.01$ Pa s) although they each exhibit different characteristics. Single-point determinations are quite obviously an extreme example, but are used here to emphasize the importance of properly designed experiments.

Rotational viscometers

These instruments rely on the viscous drag exerted on a body when it is rotated in a fluid to determine

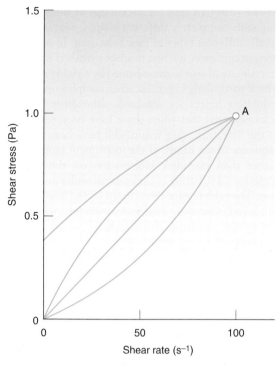

Fig. 6.12 • Explanation of the effect of single-point viscosity determination and the resultant errors.

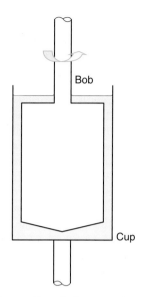

Fig. 6.13 • Concentric cylinder geometry.

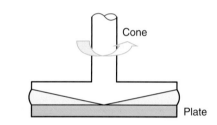

Fig. 6.14 • Cone–plate geometry.

its viscosity. They should really be referred to as rheometers since nowadays they are suitable for use with both Newtonian and non-Newtonian materials. Their major advantage is that wide ranges of shear rate can be achieved, and if a programme of shear rates can be selected automatically, then a flow curve or rheogram for a material may be obtained directly. A number of commercial instruments are available which range from those that can be used as simple in-line devices to sophisticated multifunction machines. However, all share a common feature in that various measuring geometries can be used; these include concentric cylinder (or Couette), cone–plate and parallel-plate geometries.

Concentric cylinder geometry. In this geometry there are two coaxial cylinders of different diameters, the outer forming the cup containing the fluid in which the inner cylinder or bob is positioned centrally (Fig. 6.13). In older types of instrument, the outer cylinder is rotated and the viscous drag exerted by the fluid is transmitted to the inner cylinder as a torque, inducing its rotation, which can be measured with a transducer or a fine torsion wire. The stress on this inner cylinder (when, for example, it is suspended on a torsion wire) is indicated by the angular deflection,

θ, once equilibrium (i.e. steady flow) has been attained. The torque, T, can then be calculated from

$$C\theta = T$$

(6.31)

where C is the torsional constant of the wire. The viscosity is then given by

$$\eta = \frac{\left(\dfrac{1}{r_1^2} - \dfrac{1}{r_2^2}\right)T}{4\pi h\omega}$$

(6.32)

where r_1 and r_2 are the radii of the inner and outer cylinders respectively, h is the height of the inner cylinder and ω is the angular velocity of the outer cylinder.

Cone–plate geometry. The cone–plate geometry comprises a flat circular plate with a wide-angle cone placed centrally above it (Fig. 6.14). The tip of the cone just touches the plate, and the sample is loaded into the included gap. When the plate is rotated, the

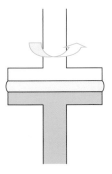

Fig. 6.15 • Parallel-plate geometry.

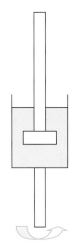

Fig. 6.16 • Representation of a controlled-rate rheometer.

cone will be caused to rotate against a torsion wire in the same way as the inner cylinder described earlier. Provided the gap angle is small (<1°), the viscosity will be given by

$$\eta = \frac{3\alpha T}{2\pi r^3 \omega}$$

(6.33)

where ω is the angular velocity of the plate, T is the torque, r is the radius of the cone and α is the angle between the cone and the plate.

Parallel-plate geometry. This only differs from cone–plate geometry in that the cone is replaced by a flat plate which is similar to the opposing part of the geometry (Fig. 6.15). The viscosity is given by

$$\eta = \frac{2hT}{\pi r^4 \omega}$$

(6.34)

where in this case r is the diameter of the plates and h the gap between them.

Rheometers

From Eq. 6.2 it can be seen that the viscosity of a fluid can be calculated by division of the shear stress by the shear rate. However, in order to do this, it is essential to have an instrument that is capable of imposing either a *constant shear rate* and measuring the resultant shear stress or a *constant shear stress* when measurement of the induced shear rate is required. The first type of instrument is referred to as controlled-rate (or strain) whereas the latter is known as a controlled-stress. As is the case with most scientific measurements, the history of the development of the instrumentation can be instructive in understanding the way in which they work. The MacMichael controlled-rate (or controlled-strain)

viscometer, which was patented in 1918, had a cup which contained the fluid under test and could be rotated at just one speed. A 5 mm thick disc suspended on a torsion wire was immersed in the fluid in the cup (Fig. 6.16). The viscous drag exerted by the fluid caused the disc to rotate, which in turn produced a deflection in the torsion wire to an equilibrium position which was inversely related to the viscosity. An early modification was to couple a gearbox to the synchronous electric motor so that a series of speeds (shear rates) could be employed. The change from a synchronous to a direct current motor and then a step (or stepper) motor has obviated the need to include a gearbox although these are still incorporated in some instruments as a means of extending the range of shear rates that can be applied.

The absolute viscosity could not be determined with these early instruments, but the incorporation of a calibrated torsion wire and a defined measuring geometry (such as concentric cylinder or cone–plate geometry) made this possible. Perhaps the most significant improvement made to the technology is the replacement of the torsion wire with more sophisticated torque measurement devices, sometimes referred to as dynamometers. Their introduction meant that the cup in Fig. 6.16 could be fixed and only the upper part of the geometry needed to be driven by the motor via a coiled spring (Fig. 6.17): the degree of flexure of the spring is, like that of the torsion wire that it replaced, inversely related to the resistance to flow (i.e. viscosity) of the fluid. Although this modification enabled the viscosity to be read directly off a scale and instruments to be automated,

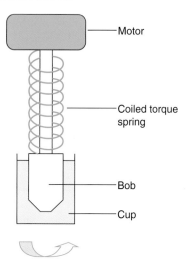

Fig. 6.17 • Representation of a controlled-rate rheometer with a coiled spring torque measuring device.

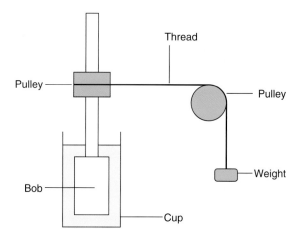

Fig. 6.18 • Representation of a controlled-stress rheometer.

the spring had to have a low elastic modulus and the weight of the measuring geometry needed to be kept to a minimum since it created inertia which had to be overcome when the motor was started. This resulted in a lag period before the bob began to rotate, followed by a rapid acceleration which, in turn, produced an overshoot. This type of behaviour was very apparent with the Ferranti–Shirley viscometer, which was widely used with pharmaceutical semisolids in the 1960s and 1970s. The instrument was highly automated for its time and produced a plot of a flow curve in real time on an X–Y recorder. However, the inertial overshoot was apparent as bulges in the flow curves that were obtained but, unfortunately, these artefacts were taken by some workers to represent rheological characteristics of the material. Advances in electronics meant that the spring could be replaced by a stiffer torsion strip or bar which is only deflected by a few degrees. The concomitant improvements in microprocessors enabled instrumental control and data collection to be integrated so that not only did measurements become automatic but also data processing was virtually instantaneous.

The first controlled-stress viscometer was described by Stormer in 1909 and was based on a cup and bob geometry where the outer cup was stationary and the inner one was immersed in the liquid under test. The inner cylinder was rotated at a constant stress produced by a weight attached to a length of thread which was wrapped around a horizontal pulley on the shaft of the cylinder and then passed over a vertical pulley so that it fell under the influence of gravity

(Fig. 6.18). The rate of rotation was measured with the aid of a stopwatch and an eagle-eyed operator. The most common way of using the instrument was to determine the weight that produced a predetermined rate of rotation: although this was useful for comparative purposes, it did not allow the calculation of absolute viscosities. Almost 60 years elapsed before workers attempted to adapt this instrument to operate at very low stresses and measure displacement over long times. Such experiments were known as creep tests, and once the technology became available, a similar enhancement in their application occurred as it did with controlled-rate instruments. In this instance, the most significant improvements were the use of air bearings to provide both lateral and axial support, the use of optical encoders to measure radial displacement and the addition of drag-cup motors to produce the torque. The latter not only allowed the smooth control of torque but also had very low inertia so that low stresses could be applied.

The design of instruments with the capacity to operate as controlled-strain or controlled-stress instruments has now advanced such that both types of test can be conducted with the same instrument. A generalized representation of the instruments is shown in Fig. 6.19. The air bearing supports the changeable measuring geometry and may be enclosed in a unit which also houses the motor and the displacement sensor. When used in the controlled-stress mode, the current to the motor generates a torque which rotates the measuring geometry against the resistance of the sample. The resultant displacement is measured by the sensor so that the speed can be calculated. The difference when the instrument is operated in

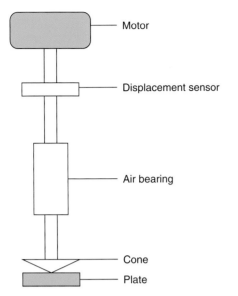

Fig. 6.19 • Schematic diagram of a rheometer that can operate in a variety of modes.

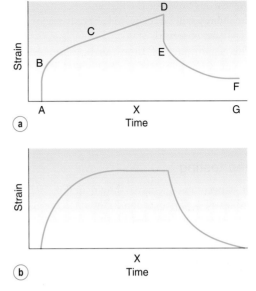

Fig. 6.20 • Creep (or compliance) curves for **(a)** an un-cross-linked system and **(b)** a cross-linked system.

controlled-strain mode is that there is feedback to the motor from the sensor so that instead of a predetermined stress being provided, the torque necessary to maintain a given strain is measured. In both cases, since the shear rate and shear stress are available, the viscosity can be calculated. Both instrumental designs can also be used for dynamic testing using forced oscillation, and thus to character-ize viscoelastic properties. As in many aspects of modern life, the developments in computing hardware and software have contributed significantly to advances in the design and use of rheometers.

Viscoelasticity

In experiments conducted with rotational viscometers, two observations are often made with pharmaceutical materials:

1. With cone–plate geometry, the sample appears to 'roll up' especially at high shear rates and is ejected from the gap.
2. With concentric cylinder geometry, the sample will climb up the spindle of the rotating inner cylinder (referred to as the Weissenberg effect).

The cause of both these phenomena is the same; that is, the liquids are not exhibiting purely viscous behaviour but are viscoelastic. Such materials display solid and liquid properties simultaneously, and the

factor that governs the actual behaviour is time. A whole spectrum of viscoelastic behaviour exists for materials that are predominantly either liquid or solid. Under a constant stress, all these materials will dissipate some of the energy in viscous flow and store the remainder, which will be recovered when the stress is removed. The type of response can be seen in Fig. 6.20a, where a small, constant stress has been applied to a 2% gelatin gel at 20 °C and the resultant change in shape (strain) is measured.

In the region A–B an initial elastic jump is observed, followed by a curved region B–C when the material is attempting to flow as a viscous fluid but is being retarded by its solid characteristics. At longer times, equilibrium is established, so for a system like this, which is ostensibly liquid, viscous flow will eventually predominate and the curve will become linear with a positive slope (C–D). If the concentration of gelatin in the gel had been increased to 30%, then the resultant material would be more solid-like and no flow would be observed at longer times, so the curve would level out as shown in Fig. 6.20b. In the case of the liquid system, when the stress is removed only the stored energy will be recovered, and this is represented by an initial elastic recoil (D–E, Fig. 6.20a) equivalent to region A–B and a retarded response E–F equivalent to B–C. There will be a displacement from the starting position (F–G) and this will be related to the amount of energy lost during viscous flow. For the higher-concentration gel, all the energy will be recovered, so only regions D–E and E–F are observed.

This significance of time can be observed from the point X on the time axis. Although both systems are viscoelastic, and, indeed, are produced by different concentrations of the same biopolymer, in Fig. 6.20a the sample is flowing like a high-viscosity fluid, whereas in Fig. 6.20b it is behaving like a solid.

Creep testing

Both experimental curves shown in Fig. 6.20 are examples of a phenomenon known as creep. If the measured strain is divided by the stress – which, it should be remembered, is constant – then a compliance will be derived. As compliance is the reciprocal of elasticity, its unit will be $m^2 N^{-1}$ or Pa^{-1}. The resultant curve, which will have the same shape as the original strain curve, then becomes known as a creep compliance curve. If the applied stress is below a certain limit (known as the linear viscoelastic limit), it will be directly related to the strain, and the creep compliance curve will have the same shape and magnitude regardless of the stress used to obtain it. This curve therefore represents a fundamental property of the material, and derived parameters are characteristic and independent of the experimental method. For example, although it is common to use either cone–plate or concentric cylinder geometries with viscoelastic pharmaceuticals, almost any measuring geometry can be used provided the shape of the sample can be defined and maintained throughout the experiment.

It is common to analyse the creep compliance curve in terms of a mechanical model, an example of which is shown in Fig. 6.21, which also indicates the regions on the curve shown in Fig. 6.20a to which the components of the model relate. Thus, the instantaneous jump can be described by a perfectly elastic spring and the region of viscous flow by a piston fitted into a cylinder containing an ideal Newtonian fluid (this arrangement is referred to as a dashpot). In order to describe the behaviour in the intermediate region, it is necessary to combine both these elements in parallel, such that the movement of the spring is retarded by the fluid in the dashpot; this combination is known as a Voigt unit. It is implied that the elements of the model do not move until the preceding one has become fully extended. Although it is not feasible to associate the elements of the model with the molecular arrangement of the material, it is possible to ascribe a viscosity to the

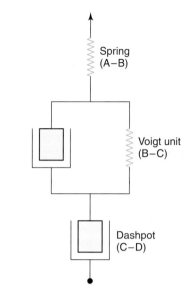

Fig. 6.21 • Mechanical model representation of a creep compliance curve.

fluids in each cylinder and elasticity (or compliance) to each spring.

Thus, a viscosity can be calculated for the single dashpot (see Fig. 6.21) from the reciprocal of the slope of the linear part of the creep compliance curve. This viscosity will be several orders of magnitude greater than that obtained by the conventional rotational techniques described previously. It may be considered to be that of the rheological ground state (η_0) as the creep test is non-destructive and should produce the same viscosity however many times it is repeated on the same sample as long as the environmental conditions remain constant. This is in direct contrast to continuous shear measurements, which destroy the structure being measured and with which it is seldom possible to obtain the same result in subsequent experiments on the same sample. The compliance (J_0) of the spring can be measured directly from the height of region A–B (see Fig. 6.20a) and the reciprocal of this value will yield the elasticity, E_0. It is fortunate that this value, together with η_0, often provides an adequate characterization of the material.

However, the remaining portion of the curve can be used to derive the viscosity and elasticity of the elements of the Voigt unit. The ratio of the viscosity to the elasticity is known as the retardation time, τ, and is a measure of the time taken for the unit to deform to $1/e$ of its total deformation. Consequently, more rigid materials will have longer retardation times and the more complex the material, the greater the number of Voigt units that are necessary to describe the creep curve.

It is also possible to use a mathematical expression to describe the creep compliance curve

$$J(t) = J_o - \sum_{i=1}^{n} J_i(1 - e^{t/\tau_i}) + t/\eta_o$$

(6.35)

where $J(t)$ is the compliance at time t, and J_i and τ_i are the compliance and retardation time respectively, of the ith Voigt unit. Both the model and the mathematical approach interpret the curve in terms of a line spectrum. It is also possible to produce a continuous spectrum in terms of the distribution of retardation times.

A stress relaxation test is essentially the reverse of a creep compliance test. The sample is subjected to a predetermined strain, and the stress required to maintain that strain is measured as a function of time. In this instance, a spring and dashpot in series (known as a Maxwell unit) can be used to describe the behaviour. Initially the spring will extend instantaneously, and will then contract more slowly as the piston flows in the dashpot. Eventually the spring will be completely relaxed but the dashpot will be displaced, and in this case the ratio of viscosity to elasticity is referred to as the relaxation time.

Dynamic testing

Both creep and relaxation experiments are considered to be static tests. Viscoelastic materials can also be evaluated by means of dynamic experiments, whereby the sample is exposed to a forced sinusoidal oscillation and the transmitted stress measured. If, once again, the linear viscoelastic limit is not exceeded, then the stress will also vary sinusoidally (Fig. 6.22). However, because of the nature of the material, energy will be lost, so the amplitude of the stress wave will be less than that of the strain wave, behind which it will also lag. If the amplitude ratio and the phase lag can be measured, then the elasticity, referred to as the *storage modulus*, G', is given by

$$G' = \left(\frac{\sigma}{\gamma}\right)\cos\delta$$

(6.36)

where σ is the stress, γ is the strain and δ is the phase lag. A further modulus, G'', known as the *loss modulus*, is given by

$$G'' = \left(\frac{\sigma}{\gamma}\right)\sin\delta$$

(6.37)

This can be related to viscosity, η', by

$$\eta' = \frac{G''}{\omega}$$

(6.38)

where ω is the frequency of oscillation in radians (s^{-1}). From Eqs 6.36 and 6.37 it can be seen that

$$\frac{G''}{G'} = \tan\delta$$

(6.39)

where $\tan\delta$ is known as the *loss tangent*. Thus, a perfectly elastic material would produce a phase lag of 0 degrees, whereas for a perfect fluid it would be 90 degrees.

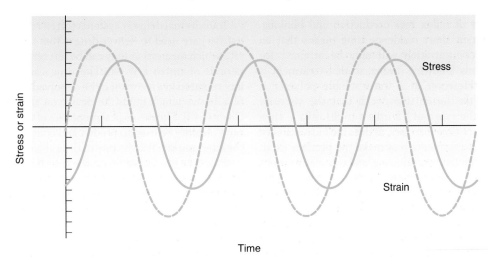

Fig. 6.22 • Sine waves showing the stress wave lagging behind the strain wave during dynamic testing.

Finally, the concepts of liquid-like and solid-like behaviour can be explained by the dimensionless *Deborah number* (*De*)

$$De = \frac{\tau}{T}$$

(6.40)

where τ is a characteristic time of the material and T is a characteristic time of the deformation process. For a perfectly elastic material (solid), τ will be infinite, whereas for a Newtonian fluid it will be zero. With any material, high Deborah numbers can be produced either by high values of τ or by small values of T. The latter will occur in situations where high rates of strain are experienced, e.g. slapping water with the hand. Also, even solid materials would flow if a high enough stress is applied for a sufficiently long time.

The applications of rheology in pharmaceutical formulation

The components used to make a formulation may not only affect the physical and release characteristics of the product but may also guide it to the site of absorption. In some cases, it may be possible to exploit the properties of the excipients such that the dosage form is retained at a specific location in the body. This approach is often necessary for locally acting products which are used to treat or prevent diseases of, for example, the eye and the skin. To treat conditions in the eye, an aqueous solution of the drug is delivered to the precorneal area by means of a dropper. If the solution is Newtonian and of low viscosity, then it will be rapidly cleared from the eye as a result of reflex tear production and blinking. The resultant short residence time means that an effective concentration will only be attained for brief periods following dosing, so that treatment is pulsatile. However, if a water-soluble polymer is added to the formulation, such that the viscosity is within the range of 15 mPa s to 30 mPa s, then the residence time increases, as does the bioavailability. Addition of excipients that make the product pseudoplastic will facilitate blinking, and this may improve acceptance and adherence by the patient. If the product can be made viscoelastic, then solutions of higher consistency may be tolerated. This can be achieved in the eye if a polymeric solution is designed to be Newtonian when it is instilled but then undergoes a sol–gel transition in situ in reaction to the change in environment such as temperature, pH or

ion content. Poly(vinyl alcohol), cellulose ethers and esters and sodium alginate are all examples of polymers which have been used as *viscolysers* in eye drops. Polyacrylic acid and cellulose acetate phthalate have been claimed to produce reactive systems. The formulation of eye drops and the importance of viscosity in the formulation of ocular delivery systems are discussed further in Chapter 39.

The ointments and creams which are applied to the skin to deliver a drug which has a local action, such as a corticosteroid or anti-infective agent, are usually semisolids. Their rheological properties need to be assessed after manufacture and during the shelf life in order to ensure that the product is physically stable; this is important because the rate of release of the drug and the concentration at the site of action are related to the apparent viscosity. Also, since these products are normally packaged in flexible tubes, rheological measurements will also indicate whether the product can be readily removed from the container (see also Chapter 40).

Knowledge of the flow properties of a product such as a gel for topical application can be used to predict patient acceptability, since humans can detect small changes in viscosity during activities such as rubbing an ointment on the skin, shaking ketchup from a bottle or squeezing toothpaste from a tube. Since the ability of the body to act as a rheometer involves the unconscious coordination of a number of senses, the term *psychorheology* has been adopted by workers in this field. All three situations provide examples of the advantages of designing a formulation which has a yield stress and exhibits plastic or pseudoplastic behaviour so that the patient only has to apply the appropriate shear rate.

Transdermal delivery systems (often referred to as *patches*) are used to deliver drug across the skin at a rate which means that they can be left on the skin for periods of up to a week. The drug can either be incorporated in a reservoir or be dissolved in the layer of adhesive which holds the device on the skin (see Chapter 40). The rheological properties of the adhesive can therefore be used to predict and control not only the adhesion but also the rate of drug absorption. The latter can be used to estimate the length of time that the device needs to be applied to the skin.

When a dosage form is intended to be administered perorally, so that the active ingredient can be absorbed from the gastrointestinal tract, then the gastrointestinal tract transit time plays a major role in the extent and amount of drug which appears in the bloodstream. The first phase of gastrointestinal tract transit is gastric emptying, which is in part dictated by the rise in viscosity of the stomach contents in the presence of food. The consequential increase in gastric residence time and decrease in the dissolution rate of the active ingredient can lead to a reduction in the rate, but not necessarily the extent, of absorption. Such effects can be exploited by the pharmaceutical formulator, for example, by including a gel-forming polymer in the formulation, since this can simulate in vivo the effect exerted by food. However, its use as a means of prolonging the duration of action of an orally administered medicine needs to be thoroughly understood particularly in relation to the effect of the presence and nature of food, since any benefit could be lost by, for example, administration of the dosage form following a high-fat meal. Many solid sustained-release dosage forms depend on the inclusion of high molecular weight polymers for their mode of action, and the viscosity of a particular polymer both in dilute solution and as a swollen gel is used to aid the selection of the most suitable candidate.

A final example of the application of rheology in the design and use of dosage forms is the administration of medicines by intramuscular injection. These are formulated as either aqueous or lipophilic (oily) solutions or suspensions. Following injection, the active ingredient is absorbed more quickly from an aqueous formulation than its lipophilic counterpart. The incorporation of the active ingredient as a suspension in either type of base offers a further opportunity of slowing the rate of release. The influence that the nature of the solvent has on the rate of drug release is in part due to its compatibility with the tissue, but its viscosity is also of importance. Although it may be possible to extend the dosing interval by further increasing the viscosity of the oil, it has to be borne in mind that the product needs to be able

to be drawn into a syringe via a needle, the diameter of which must not be so large as to alarm or discomfort the patient. Furthermore, adding other excipients such as polymers to the formulation or even just altering the particle size of the suspended particles can induce marked alterations in the rheological properties such that the injection may become plastic, pseudoplastic or dilatant. If it does become plastic, then provided that the yield value is not too high, it may be possible for it to pass through a syringe needle by application of a force which it is reasonable to achieve with a syringe. Quite obviously this will not be the case if the suspension becomes dilatant since as the applied force is increased the product will become more solid. Often the ideal formulation is one which is pseudoplastic because as the force is increased so the apparent viscosity will fall, making it easier for the injection to flow through the needle. Ideally the product should also be truly thixotropic because once it has been injected into the muscle, the reduction in shear rate will mean that the bolus will gel and thus form a depot, from which release of the drug may be expected to be delayed.

The use of appropriate rheological techniques in the development of such products can be beneficial not only to predict their performance in vivo but also to monitor changes in characteristics on storage. This is especially true for suspension formulations, since fine particles have a notorious and, sometimes, malevolent capacity for increasing in size on storage, and if as a result a pseudoplastic product becomes dilatant, then it will be impossible to administer it to the patient.

Please check your eBook at **https://studentconsult.**
inkling.com/ for self-assessment questions. See inside cover for registration details.

References

van Hecke, M., 2012. Running on cornflour. Nature 487, 174–175.

Waitukaitis, S.R., Jaeger, H.M., 2012. Impact-activated solidification of dense suspensions via dynamic

jamming fronts. Nature 487, 205–209.

Bibliography

Barnes, H.A., Hutton, J.F., Walters, K., 2014. An Introduction to Rheology. Elsevier Science, Amsterdam.

Barnes, H.A., Schimanski, H., Bell, D., 1999. 30 years of progress in viscometers and rheometers. Appl. Rheol. 9, 69–76.

Barnes, H.A., Bell, D., 2003. Controlled-stress rotational rheometry: an historical review. Korea-Aust. Rheol. J. 15, 187–196.

Lapasin, R., Pricl, S., 1999. Rheology of Industrial Polysaccharides: Theory

and Applications. Aspen Publishers, Gaithersburg.

Mezger, T.G., 2014. The Rheology Handbook. European Coatings Tech Files, Hanover.

7

Kinetics

Gareth R. Williams

CHAPTER CONTENTS

KEY POINTS

- Kinetics is the study of the rate at which processes occur. It is a 'how fast' concept, in contrast to thermodynamics, which describes 'how much'.
- The changes described may be chemical (decomposition of a drug, radiochemical decay) or physical (dissolution, transfer across a boundary such as the intestinal lining).

- For a process to occur, an energy barrier known as the activation energy must be overcome.
- Kinetic studies provide information that:
  - gives insight into the mechanisms of the changes involved; and
  - allows prediction of the amount of change that will occur after a given time.
- Processes can be classified as zero order, first order or second order depending on how many concentration terms are involved in determining the rate.
- In a zero-order reaction, the rate (e.g. of decomposition, dissolution or drug release) is constant and *independent* of the concentrations of the reactants. A constant rate of drug release from a dosage form is highly desirable to maintain a consistent plasma concentration.
- The rate of a first-order process is determined by one concentration term. These are by far the most common processes seen in pharmaceutical science. For instance, drug decomposition during storage and the movement of drugs from one body compartment to another follow first-order kinetics.
- The rates of second-order processes depend on the product of two concentration terms. These reactions are relatively rare in pharmaceutics.
- The half-life, $t_{1/2}$, is the time taken for the concentration (for instance of a drug in solution or in the body) to reduce by a half.
- Increasing the temperature increases the rate of reaction, with a 10 °C rise usually doubling the rate.
- The Arrhenius theory permits the influence of temperature on the reaction rate to be quantified.

Introduction

This chapter focuses on understanding and quantifying kinetics. The term *kinetics* refers to the rate at which processes occur. The concept can be applied equally to both chemical and physical changes, and kinetics are profoundly important in a number of aspects of formulation and product design, such as dissolution (see Chapter 2), microbial growth and death (see Part 3), drug absorption, distribution, metabolism and excretion (see Part 4), preformulation (see Chapter 23), the rate of drug release from dosage forms (see Part 5) and the decomposition of active ingredients (see Part 6). As a result, a thorough grounding in kinetics is very useful.

It is important to differentiate between the concepts of *kinetics* and *thermodynamics*. Kinetics relates to 'how fast', whereas thermodynamics concerns 'how much'. Both need to be taken into consideration in formulation science. For instance, when a patient is given a solid dosage form orally, the drug in the product needs to dissolve into solution before it can enter the systemic circulation. Two quantities need to be known to understand this process properly:

- The *dissolution rate*. This is a kinetic quantity, and refers to the rate at which the drug molecules transition from the solid state into solution.
- The *solubility*. This is a thermodynamic quantity, equal to the maximum amount of drug dissolved at equilibrium.

Both the dissolution rate and solubility will be crucially important in determining the efficacy of a formulation. If the drug dissolves very slowly, then very little drug will be able to pass into solution while the formulation is in the body. This is likely to result in drug concentrations too low to have a therapeutic effect. If the solubility is very low, it is less likely that a therapeutic concentration will be reached. Most often, drugs that are highly soluble also dissolve quickly, but this is not always true. These issues are discussed in more detail in Chapter 2.

The concepts of kinetics are equally useful in the consideration of chemical processes, in which there is a change in the molecular structure of the species being considered (e.g. decomposition of a drug, radioactive decay), and physical changes (e.g. dissolution, transfer across a boundary such as the intestinal epithelium). In kinetic studies, the change in the system is monitored as a function of time. Such experiments give information on the mechanisms of the changes involved, and also allow prediction of how much change will occur in a given time.

Energetics

For a chemical reaction to occur, it is necessary for the molecules involved to possess a certain minimum amount of energy, known as the *activation energy* (E_a; Fig. 7.1). Activation energy can be thought of as an energy barrier to a reaction. If the reactants do not have sufficient energy, then they will not be able to overcome this barrier, and hence no reaction will occur. The energies of a population of molecules are given by the Maxwell–Boltzmann distribution (Fig. 7.2).

As can be seen in Fig. 7.2, as the temperature rises the average energy of the molecules increases. The E_a for a reaction is a fixed quantity, and thus in general a reaction proceeds more quickly at higher temperatures (although this is not always true, it is in most cases).

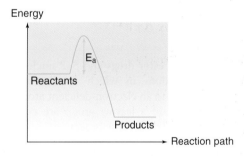

Fig. 7.1 • A plot showing the activation energy.

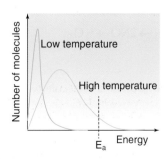

Fig. 7.2 • The Maxwell–Boltzmann distribution of molecular energies.

Homogeneous and heterogeneous processes

Homogeneous processes occur in one phase, most usually in the gas phase or in solution. Because molecular mobility is high in the liquid and gas phases, the processes are uniform throughout the whole reacting mass. *Heterogeneous processes* involve more than one phase: for instance, a solid dissolving into a liquid. These processes frequently can only occur at the phase boundary and their rates depend on the supply of fresh material to this boundary.

Molecularity

The *molecularity* of a reaction describes the number of reactant molecules involved in forming the product. This can be determined from the stoichiometry of the reaction. Some reactions, particularly decomposition processes, are *unimolecular*, in that only a single molecule is involved in the reaction. A generic example of such a process would be as follows:

$$A \rightarrow B$$

(7.1)

Many reactions involve two molecules reacting:

$$A + B \rightarrow C$$

(7.2)

The hydrolysis of ester drugs and S_N2 nucleophilic substitution reactions in which an electron-rich nucleophile bonds to an electron-deficient atom with simultaneous loss of a leaving group are common examples of such *bimolecular* processes.

As further examples,

$$CH_3CH_2Br + H_2O \rightarrow CH_3CH_2OH + HBr$$

(7.3)

is a bimolecular process, while

$$N_2O_5 \rightarrow 2NO_2 + \tfrac{1}{2}O_2$$

(7.4)

is unimolecular.

In a unimolecular process, a molecule will react if it has sufficient energy to overcome the activation energy barrier (i.e. the energy of the molecule must be greater than the activation energy). The number of high-energy molecules depends on how many molecules are present (their concentration in solution or pressure in a gas) and the temperature, in accordance with the Maxwell–Boltzmann distribution (see Fig. 7.2). In a bimolecular process, two molecules must collide with sufficient energy (and in an appropriate orientation) to react, and the likelihood of collision depends on the concentration of each species.

Rate laws and order of reaction

Much of the material in this chapter will be discussed in the context of chemical reactions, but the same principles apply equally to physical processes. Consider the reaction

$$2A + B \rightarrow C + 2D$$

(7.5)

The rate law is a function of the concentrations of the reacting species. This is because for them to react, molecules must collide, and the probability of collisions occurring increases with the concentration. The rate of formation of the product C is given by $d[C]/dt$ (the change in the concentration of C per unit time). Similarly, the rate of destruction of B is $-d[B]/dt$. A negative sign is used for the latter, because the rate is a positive quantity, and the change in the amount of B with time is negative. Given the stoichiometry of this reaction, expressions for the change in concentration of all the species involved can be written:

$$-\frac{1}{2}\frac{d[A]}{dt} = -\frac{d[B]}{dt} = \frac{d[C]}{dt} = \frac{1}{2}\frac{d[D]}{dt}$$

(7.6)

Most commonly, a simple rate law is written which allows a single rate term to be defined.

Consider the generic reaction

$$A + B \rightarrow C$$

(7.7)

The rate law can be expressed as

$$\text{rate} = k[A]^x[B]^y$$

(7.8)

where k is the rate constant, $[A]$ is the concentration of A, $[B]$ the concentration of B, x is the *order* of reaction with respect to A, y is the order of the reaction with respect to B, and $(x + y)$ is the *overall* reaction order. The higher the value of x (or y), the greater the influence of the concentration of A (or B) on the rate of reaction.

For the example reaction in Eq. 7.4 a rate equation can be written as follows:

$$rate = k[N_2O_5]$$

(7.9)

There is only a single concentration term here, and hence the reaction is *first order*. Similarly, for the reaction in Eq. 7.3,

$$rate = k[CH_3CH_2Br][H_2O]$$

(7.10)

There are two concentration terms in this equation, each raised to the first power. The reaction is first order with respect to each of CH_3CH_2Br and H_2O, but the sum of the powers is 2 and therefore the reaction is *second order* overall.

It is also possible to have *zero-order* processes, in which the rate is independent of the concentration:

$$rate = k$$

(7.11)

All three types of process arise in pharmaceutics, and thus will be discussed in turn. A quantitative treatment of rate laws and kinetics is usually needed, which requires the use of some simple concepts of calculus. Background information on these concepts can be found in the texts listed in the bibliography.

Zero-order processes

In a zero-order reaction, the rate is constant, regardless of the concentration(s) of species present. Zero-order drug release from a formulation can be highly desirable, because it allows the drug concentration in the blood plasma to be maintained at a constant level for prolonged periods. Many processes occurring at phase boundaries *appear* to be zero order; for instance, decomposition reactions in a suspension. Here it often seems that the rate of decay is constant, but on closer examination the rate may be correlated to the level of light in the container, or the presence of a catalyst (a nonreacting species that accelerates the rate of reaction). Zero-order can be seen where the concentration of reacting material at a surface remains constant either because reaction sites are saturated (enzyme kinetics, drug–receptor interactions) or because it is replenished constantly by diffusion of fresh material from within the bulk. The latter applies to the hydrolysis of drugs in suspensions and drug delivery from dosage forms such as transdermal patches.

For an example process A → products, the rate law can be written as follows:

$$\frac{d[A]}{dt} = -k$$

(7.12)

$d[A]/dt$ is what is referred to as a differential term: in essence, it describes very small changes in the concentration of A with respect to time. The minus sign denotes the fact that the concentration of A declines with time. Eq. 7.12 can then be rearranged to give

$$d[A] = -kdt$$

(7.13)

To describe real-world processes, all these tiny changes in concentration occurring during the period of interest need to be added together; to do this, the equation must be integrated. Eq. 7.13 can be integrated between $t = 0$ and t to yield

$$\int_{[A]_0}^{[A]_t} d[A] = -k\int_0^t d$$

(7.14)

$$[A]_t - [A]_0 = -k(t - 0)$$

(7.15)

$$[A]_t = [A]_0 - kt$$

(7.16)

A plot of $[A]_t$ versus t will thus give us a straight line of intercept $[A]_0$ and gradient $-k$ (see Box 7.1 and Fig. 7.3). k will have units of concentration time^{-1}, with concentration typically in mol dm^{-3} or alternatively in mol L^{-1}. Litre (L) and dm^3 are the same volume. They are used interchangeably.

Box 7.1

Worked example of a zero-order process

Data are collected on the decomposition of a drug, with the following results:

Time (min)	0	60	120	180	240
[A] (mol dm^{-3})	0.196	0.154	0.112	0.07	0.028

If this is a zero-order process, then a plot of $[A]_t$ versus time will give a straight line with gradient $-k$ and intercept on the vertical axis of $[A]_0$. This is shown in Fig. 7.3. From the plot, it can be found that the rate constant is 7×10^{-4} mol dm^{-3} min^{-1}. The intercept is $[A]_0 = 0.196$ mol dm^{-3}, which is in agreement with the initial concentration from the data in the table.

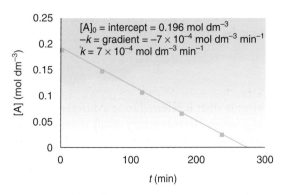

Fig. 7.3 • Concentration versus time for a zero-order reaction, produced with the data in Box 7.1.

First-order processes

These are processes in which the rate is determined by the concentration of a single reactant raised to the first power; that is, the rate of reaction is directly proportional to the concentration of a single species present. First-order processes are by a significant margin the most common processes in pharmaceutics. For instance, drug decomposition during storage is commonly a first-order reaction, and the passage of drugs from one body compartment to another (e.g. from the lumen of the intestine into the blood) is also typically first order.

For the generic reaction A → products, if the process is first order, then the rate law is written

$$\frac{d[A]}{dt} = -k[A]$$

(7.17)

As before, there is a negative sign in front of k because the concentration of A declines as time increases. The rate of constant, k, is thus a positive quantity.

Rearranging and integrating as previously:

$$\frac{1}{[A]}d[A] = -kdt$$

(7.18)

$$\int_{[A]_0}^{[A]_t} \frac{1}{[A]}d[A] = -k\int_0^t dt$$

(7.19)

$$\ln[A]_t - \ln[A]_0 = -k(t-0)$$

(7.20)

$$\ln[A]_t - \ln[A]_0 = -kt$$

(7.21)

$$\ln[A]_t = \ln[A]_0 - kt$$

(7.22)

From Eq. 7.22, if a graph of ln [A]$_t$ versus t is plotted, the result will be a straight line with intercept ln [A]$_0$ and gradient $-k$ (Fig. 7.4). The units on each side of Eq. 7.17 must balance, which means that the rate constant in a first-order process has units of time^{-1} (typically s^{-1}, min^{-1}, h^{-1}, etc.).

Conveniently, because k for a first-order process involves no concentration term, it is not necessary to convert experimental data to concentration in order to determine its value. For the zero-order processes discussed previously, concentration data are needed to determine k, but here any experimental measure which is directly proportional to concentration can be used. Concentrations are commonly measured using such properties as UV absorbance, solution conductivity, pressure or radioactivity. These values can be used directly to analyse first-order processes, whereas for zero-order (or indeed second or any other order) reactions it is necessary first to use these measurements to calculate the concentrations.

For example, the absorbance of light (Abs) by a drug solution is directly proportional to its concentration in accordance with the Beer–Lambert law. This states that Abs = εcl, where c is the concentration (in mol dm^{-3} or mol L^{-1}) and ε and l are the molar absorptivity and the length of solution the light must pass through respectively. This can be rearranged to $c = Abs/\varepsilon l$, and substitution into Eq. 7.22 gives

$$\ln\frac{Abs_t}{\varepsilon l} = \ln\frac{Abs_0}{\varepsilon l} - kt$$

(7.23)

Expanding the ln terms:

$$\ln Abs_t - \ln \varepsilon l = \ln Abs_0 - \ln \varepsilon l - kt$$

(7.24)

$$\ln Abs_t = \ln Abs_0 - kt$$

(7.25)

Hence the gradient in a plot of ln Abs versus t is the same as that in a plot of ln [A]$_t$ versus t. An example is given in Box 7.2 and Fig. 7.4.

Pseudo-first-order processes

It was identified earlier that the reaction in Eq. 7.3 is bimolecular, because there are two reacting species on the left of the equation:

Box 7.2

Worked example of a first-order process

A radiolabelled cardiac stimulant is administered by intravenous injection. Blood samples are taken and the following data (activity as counts per second; cps) are recorded:

Time (min)	0	30	60	90	120	150
Activity level (cps)	59.7	24.3	9.87	4.01	1.63	0.67
ln activity	4.09	3.19	2.29	1.39	0.49	−0.40

If this is a first-order process, then a plot of ln activity versus time will give a straight line, with gradient $-k$ and intercept ln (activity at time 0). This is shown in Fig. 7.4. From the plot, it can be found that the rate constant for elimination from the blood is 0.03 min^{-1}.

Box 7.3

Worked example of a pseudo-first-order process

For the reaction $CH_3CH_2Br + H_2O \rightarrow CH_3CH_2OH + HBr$, the following data are recorded:

Time (h)	0	1.0	2.0	4.0	6.0
$[CH_3CH_2Br]$ (mol dm^{-3})	0.020	0.017	0.014	0.009	0.006
ln $[CH_3CH_2Br]$	−3.912	−4.075	−4.269	−4.711	−5.116

Because the concentration of H_2O is essentially constant, this reaction can be treated like a first-order process, and a plot of ln $[CH_3CH_2Br]$ versus time will allow the determination of the rate constant (Fig. 7.5). A linear graph is obtained, and the rate constant determined to be k = −slope = 0.204 h^{-1}.

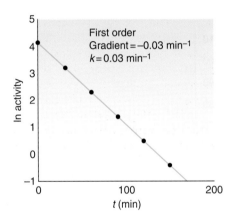

Fig. 7.4 • ln activity versus time for a first-order process, produced with the data in Box 7.2.

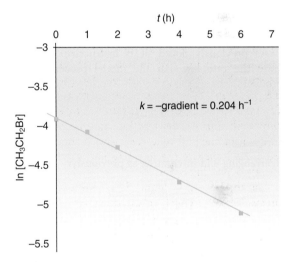

Fig. 7.5 • ln concentration versus time for a pseudo-first-order process, produced with the data in Box 7.3

$$CH_3CH_2Br + H_2O \rightarrow CH_3CH_2OH + HBr$$

$$(7.26)$$

This reaction is therefore expected to be second order, and the rate equation can be written as

$$rate = k[CH_3CH_2Br][H_2O]$$

$$(7.27)$$

However, this reaction is most likely to take place in an aqueous solution, where the concentration of CH_3CH_2Br will be much less than the concentration of water (1 dm^3 of water contains 55.6 mol of water!). Thus the concentration of water will barely change during the reaction: if the concentration of CH_3CH_2Br is, say, 0.1 mol dm^{-3} (a realistic value), then at most 0.1 mol dm^{-3} of water will be consumed if the

reaction goes to completion, leaving 55.5 mol dm^{-3}, or 99.8% of the original concentration.

In such situations, it is reasonable to make the assumption that the concentration of water is constant throughout the reaction, and thus the reaction will *appear to be first order*, with a rate constant k' (where $k' = k[H_2O]$). This gives

$$rate = k'[CH_3CH_2Br]$$

$$(7.28)$$

These processes are known as *pseudo-first-order* reactions, and many drug hydrolysis reactions in aqueous solution follow this type of kinetics. Some example data are given in Box 7.3 and Fig. 7.5.

Second-order processes

In second-order processes, the rate is dependent on either the concentration of one reactant raised to the second power, or the concentrations of two reactants each raised to the first power (i.e. second order overall). For the reaction $A \rightarrow$ products, the rate law would be

$$\text{rate} = k[A]^2$$

(7.29)

For a process $A + B \rightarrow$ products, the rate law would be

$$\text{rate} = k[A][B]$$

(7.30)

The units on both sides of the reaction must be the same, and thus for a second-order process k has units of concentration^{-1} time^{-1} (e.g. mol^{-1} dm^3 s^{-1}).

As previously noted, it is instructive to integrate the rate law. For the model process $A \rightarrow$ products,

$$\frac{d[A]}{dt} = -k[A]^2$$

(7.31)

Rearranging and integrating as previously:

$$\frac{1}{[A]^2}d[A] = -kdt$$

(7.32)

$$\int_{[A]_0}^{[A]_t} \frac{1}{[A]^2}d[A] = -k\int_0^t dt$$

(7.33)

$$\frac{-1}{[A]_t} - \frac{-1}{[A]_0} = -k(t-0)$$

(7.34)

$$\frac{1}{[A]_0} - \frac{1}{[A]_t} = -kt$$

(7.35)

$$\frac{1}{[A]_t} = \frac{1}{[A]_0} + kt$$

(7.36)

Here, a plot of $1/[A]_t$ versus t will yield a straight line with a positive gradient equal to the rate constant, k (see Box 7.4 and Fig. 7.6). The intercept on the vertical axis is equal to $1/[A]_0$.

Worked example of a second-order process

Suppose a pharmaceutical preparation contains an aqueous solution of a drug. To study potential decomposition in the bloodstream, a solution with concentration 0.02 mol dm^{-3} was prepared, and buffered to pH 7.4 at 37.5 °C. The drug concentration was monitored over time, and the following results were obtained:

Time (min)	0	30	60	90
[drug] (mol dm^{-3})	0.020	0.015	0.012	0.01
1/[drug] (mol^{-1} dm^3)	50.0	66.7	88.3	100.0

If the reaction is second order, a plot of reciprocal concentration versus time will give a straight line, as shown in Fig. 7.6. The gradient of this line gives the rate constant, 0.556 mol^{-1} dm^3 min^{-1}.

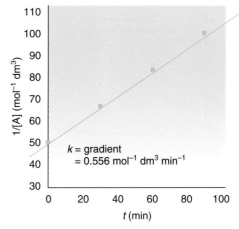

Fig. 7.6 • Reciprocal concentration versus time for a second-order drug decomposition process, produced with the data in Box 7.4.

The previous example assumes that there is a bimolecular decomposition process with two identical molecules colliding and reacting/decomposing. The situation is more complex if there are two different species reacting. For two species A and B, their initial concentrations are probably not the same (although they could be). This makes the mathematics more difficult. Considering this process, the rate law can be written as

$$\frac{d[A]}{dt} = \frac{d[B]}{dt} = -k[A][B]$$

(7.37)

Table 7.1 Equations for the half-life for zero-order, first-order and second-order processes of the form A → products

	Zero order	First order	Second order	Notes
$t =$	$\dfrac{[A]_0 - [A]_t}{k}$	$\dfrac{\ln([A]_0/[A]_t)}{k}$	$\dfrac{1/[A]_t - 1/[A]_0}{k}$	Rearrange Eqs 7.16, 7.22 and 7.36 so that t is the subject
$t_{1/2} =$	$\dfrac{[A]_0}{2k}$	$\dfrac{\ln 2}{k} = \dfrac{0.693}{k}$	$\dfrac{1}{[A]_0 k}$	Substitute $[A]_t = [A]_0/2$

Table 7.2 Summary of key parameters for processes of the form A → products

	Zero order	First order	Second order
Linear equation	$[A]_t = [A]_0 - kt$	$\ln [A]_t = \ln [A]_0 - kt$	$\dfrac{1}{[A]_t} = \dfrac{1}{[A]_0} + kt$
Intercept	$[A]_0$	$\ln [A]_0$	$1/[A]_0$
Gradient	$-k$	$-k$	k
Dimension of k	Concentration per unit time	Reciprocal time	Reciprocal concentration per unit time
Example units of k	$mol\ dm^{-3}\ s^{-1}$	s^{-1}	$mol^{-1}\ dm^3\ s^{-1}$
Half-life ($t_{1/2}$)	$\dfrac{[A]_0}{2k}$	$\dfrac{\ln 2}{k} = \dfrac{0.693}{k}$	$\dfrac{1}{[A]_0 k}$

d[A]/dt (or indeed d[B]/dt) can be integrated using partial fractions:

$$\frac{d[A]}{dt} = -k[A][B]$$

(7.38)

$$\ln\left(\frac{[A]_t}{[B]_t}\right) = \ln\left(\frac{[A]_0}{[B]_0}\right) + k([A]_0 - [B]_0)t$$

(7.39)

In such cases, a plot of $\ln([A]_t/[B]_t)$ against t will be linear, with a gradient of $k([A]_0 - [B]_0)$.

Half-life, $t_{1/2}$

The half-life ($t_{1/2}$) is the time taken for the concentration of a substance of interest to decline to half its initial value. For instance, for the process A → products, $t_{1/2}$ is the time taken for $[A]_0$ to decline to $[A]_0/2$. Half-life is a particularly useful concept when we are considering drug concentration in the blood, as it gives us an idea of the length of time for which the drug persists in the body. It also has uses in a range of other situations.

Equations for the half-life can easily be determined from the integrated rate equations. Rearrangement of these (Eqs 7.16, 7.22 and 7.36) in terms of t gives expressions in terms of concentration, and because $[A]_t = [A]_0/2$ when $t = t_{1/2}$, these can be further simplified (Table 7.1). For first-order reactions, $t_{1/2}$ is independent of concentration.

Summary of parameters

The key parameters for zero-order, first-order and second-order processes are given in Table 7.2.

Determination of order and rate constant

The order of a process and its rate constant are most easily determined by making three plots. For our exemplar process A → products, the following would be plotted:

- [A] against t – if this is a straight line, the reaction is zero order.
- ln [A] against t – if this is a straight line, the reaction is first order.
- 1/[A] against t – if this is a straight line, the reaction is second order.

Consider the data in Box 7.5; these are plotted in Fig. 7.7. The plot of [A] against t (Fig. 7.7a) is obviously not linear, so the reaction is not zero order. A

Box 7.5

Determining the reaction order and rate constant

The following data apply to the decomposition of a drug. This can be regarded as being a process of A → products.

Time (h)	0	10	20	30	40	50	60
[A] (mg dm^{-3})	10	6.2	3.6	2.2	1.3	0.8	0.6
ln [A]	2.30	1.82	1.28	0.788	0.262	−0.223	−0.511
1/[A] (mg^{-1} dm^3)	0.100	0.161	0.278	0.455	0.769	1.250	1.667

If the order of the reaction is not known, then it can be found simply by construction of the three graphs shown in Fig. 7.7.

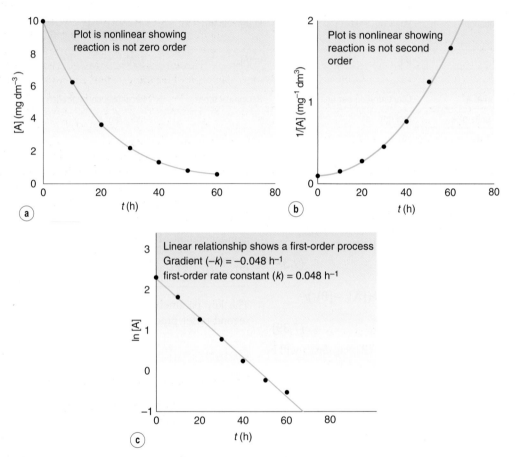

Fig. 7.7 • Determination of the reaction order for an experimental process. Plots of **(a)** [A] versus t, **(b)** 1/[A] versus t and **(c)** ln [A] versus t for the data in Box 7.5 are shown. The graphs in **(a)** and **(b)** are clearly nonlinear, demonstrating that the reaction is not **(a)** zero order or **(b)** second order. In contrast, the plot in **(c)** is linear, and thus the reaction is a first-order process.

plot of 1/[A] against t (Fig. 7.7b) is also nonlinear, and hence the reaction is not second order. The plot of ln [A] versus t (Fig. 7.7c) is linear, however, and thus the reaction is first order. From the graph, the gradient $-k = -0.048$ h^{-1} and $k = 0.048$ h^{-1}.

Complex reactions

The previous examples have all referred to simple reactions, in which only a single reaction is taking place and there is a straightforward progression from starting materials to products. However, often the situation is more complicated. On occasion, the product can itself affect the reaction process, and there may be multiple reactions occurring concurrently. Such processes are termed *complex reactions*, and there are three main types of these.

Consecutive reactions

This describes a situation in which one reaction follows another; for instance

$$A \rightarrow B \rightarrow C$$

$$(7.40)$$

These can be regarded as two separate reactions, with the process $A \rightarrow B$ described by a rate constant k_1 and the second process $B \rightarrow C$ by a second rate constant, k_2. If $k_2 > k_1$, then as soon as B forms it will be converted to C. Conversely, if $k_1 > k_2$, then A is converted to B more quickly than B is turned into C. This leads to an accumulation of B.

The slower step of a consecutive process is described as the *rate-determining step*. This is because it is this stage of the reaction which governs the overall rate at which the process can go to completion (i.e. the overall rate at which A can be converted to C in Eq. 7.40). The overall order of the reaction is also determined by this step: if the rate-limiting step is first order, the overall reaction will be first order.

Parallel (side) reactions

In this case, the reactant A can form a mixture of products. There are two reactions occurring at the same time:

$$A \rightarrow B \text{ (rate constant } k_1)$$

$$(7.41)$$

$$A \rightarrow C \text{ (rate constant } k_2)$$

$$(7.42)$$

In the synthesis of a new molecule, such parallel reactions are very common: usually, one of the products is the desired material, whereas the other is a by-product which is not required and must be removed by purification. If a drug decomposition process is considered, then both products are undesirable as they diminish the amount of active ingredient present. In such situations, the important quantity to consider is the rate at which the concentration of

A declines; this will be given by the sum of the rates of the parallel processes.

Reversible reactions

Reversible reactions arise where there is an *equilibrium* between the product(s) and the starting material(s), and the product(s) can reform into the reactant(s):

$$A \rightleftharpoons B + C$$

$$(7.43)$$

There are two reactions happening here. In one, A decomposes to give B and C. In the second, B and C combine to reform A. The forward reaction can be described by the rate constant k_1 and the reverse process with k_{-1}. Note that the '-1' subscript in k_{-1} simply means that it refers to the reversal of reaction 1: if the forward reaction (1) is $A + B \rightarrow C$, then the reverse reaction (-1) is $B + C \rightarrow A$. It is not true that if $k_1 = 0.5 \text{ s}^{-1}$ then $k_{-1} = -0.5 \text{ s}^{-1}$ as the rate constant cannot be negative.

In reversible reactions, the amount of products (B and C) present contributes to the rate of change in the concentration of A. To understand this, the rate equations can be written out in full. For the forward reaction,

$$\frac{d[A]}{dt} = -k_1[A]$$

$$(7.44)$$

For the reverse reaction,

$$\frac{d[A]}{dt} = k_{-1}[B][C]$$

$$(7.45)$$

The total rate of change in the amount of A is thus

$$\frac{d[A]}{dt} = k_{-1}[B][C] - k_1[A]$$

$$(7.46)$$

This makes the process complicated to unravel, and the overall reaction order can be very complex to interpret.

The Michaelis–Menten equation

A particularly important combination of consecutive and reversible reactions describes many processes that occur at interfaces. Such processes are widely observed in the life sciences, for instance in enzyme–substrate binding. Their kinetics are described by the *Michaelis–Menten* equation. This assumes that an enzyme, E, and a substrate, S, form an unstable complex, ES, which can either reform E and S or form a new product, P:

$$E + S \underset{k_2}{\overset{k_1}{\rightleftharpoons}} ES \xrightarrow{k_3} P + E$$

(7.47)

The enzyme is not consumed during this reaction. Its role is to bind the substrate and facilitate the conversion of the latter to the product. The overall rate of reaction is hence the rate at which P is formed – this is often referred to as the *velocity of reaction*, V. A first-order equation can be written for the change in concentration of ES with time:

$$\frac{d[P]}{dt} = V = k_3[ES]$$

(7.48)

The concentration of P *increases* with time, and thus there is no negative sign in this equation. There is a problem, however, because ES is a transient *intermediate* phase and, because it does not exist for very long, it is generally very difficult to measure its concentration directly. Looking at Eq. 7.47 though, the concentration of ES will depend on the rate of its formation through the combination of E and S minus the rate of its destruction, either back to E + S or to E + P. An equation can thus be written:

$$\frac{d[ES]}{dt} = k_1[E][S] - k_2[ES] - k_3[ES]$$

(7.49)

Collecting the terms of [ES] gives

$$\frac{d[ES]}{dt} = k_1[E][S] - (k_2 + k_3)[ES]$$

(7.50)

In practice, [ES] is small. This is because ES is a unstable intermediate, and when it forms it decomposes rapidly. A concept known as the *steady-state approximation* can therefore be used. This states that after an initial induction period where the concentration of the intermediate increases from zero, its concentration remains constant. Changes in [ES] are negligible compared with other concentration changes in the system, and thus it is reasonable to approximate

that $d[ES]/dt = 0$. Eq. 7.50 can therefore be rewritten as

$$\frac{d[ES]}{dt} = 0 = k_1[E][S] - (k_2 + k_3)[ES]$$

(7.51)

Rearranging this yields

$$k_1[E][S] = (k_2 + k_3)[ES]$$

(7.52)

$$[ES] = \frac{k_1[E][S]}{k_2 + k_3}$$

(7.53)

The Michaelis constant is helpfully defined as $K_M = (k_2 + k_3)/k_1$, which can be substituted into Eq. 7.53 to give

$$[ES] = \frac{[E]}{K_M/[S]}$$

(7.54)

K_M can be usefully conceptualized as the concentration of substrate at which the rate of reaction is half of the maximum rate. [ES] is not easily known, but the total concentration of enzyme, $[E]_0$, must be equal to [ES] + [E] as the enzyme must be present either in the free form or in a complex with the substrate. Substituting $[E] = [E]_0 - [ES]$ into Eq. 7.54 yields

$$[ES] = \frac{[E]_0 - [ES]}{K_M/[S]}$$

(7.55)

Eq. 7.55 now needs to be substituted into Eq. 7.48, such that V is expressed in terms of $[E]_0$ rather than [ES]. The mathematics is somewhat complex and not important here, but the key result is the Michaelis–Menten equation:

$$V = \frac{k_3[E]_0}{\left(\dfrac{K_M}{[S]}\right) + 1}$$

(7.56)

Full details of the underlying mathematics can be found in more specialized textbooks (additional information can be found in the texts listed in the bibliography). Examining the expression in Eq. 7.56, we see that the rate of reaction, V, is not linear, but will decline from its initial value as the substrate is consumed and [S] falls. This is because as [S] falls,

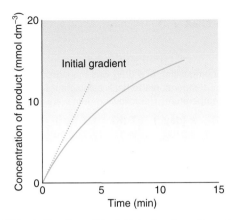

Fig. 7.8 • Estimation of the initial rate of reaction of an enzyme-catalysed reaction.

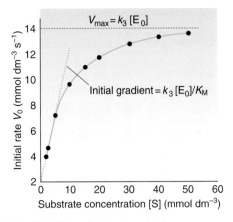

Fig. 7.9 • The Michaelis–Menten plot for an enzyme-catalysed reaction.

the value of $K_M/[S]$ will increase, and thus the value of the denominator increases. k_3 is a constant, and as the enzyme is not used up during the reaction, $[E]_0$ is also a constant value. Hence, as the denominator increases, the overall value for the rate declines. The initial rate of reaction can be determined from the initial gradient of a plot of [P] against t, as shown in Fig. 7.8.

If $[S] \ll K_M$, an approximation can be drawn that states

$$V_0 = \frac{k_3}{K_M}[E]_0[S]$$

(7.57)

Alternatively, if $[S] \gg K_M$,

$$V_{max} = k_3[E]_0$$

(7.58)

Eq. 7.58 gives us the maximum velocity possible for an enzyme-catalysed process (V_{max}). Under such concentrations, there are many more substrate molecules than there are enzymes present, and thus the enzyme sites are saturated by substrate. This results in a 'plateau' shape if the reaction velocity V is plotted against [S] (known as the Michaelis-Menten plot; see Fig. 7.9).

It is convenient to invert Eq. 7.56 to yield a linear relationship between $1/V$ and $1/[S]$:

$$\frac{1}{V_0} = \frac{1}{k_3[E]_0} + \frac{K_M}{k_3[E]_0}\left(\frac{1}{[S]}\right)$$

(7.59)

$$\frac{1}{V_0} = \frac{1}{V_{max}} + \frac{K_M}{V_{max}}\left(\frac{1}{[S]}\right)$$

(7.60)

This plot is known as a Lineweaver–Burke plot (Fig. 7.10). The intercept on the y-axis is given by $1/V_{max}$, meaning the maximum rate of reaction can easily be determined. K_M can then be calculated from the gradient (K_M/V_{max}), or alternatively is frequently estimated from the intercept at the x-axis. At the point at which the line crosses the x-axis, the y value is zero, hence $1/V_0 = 0$. As a result,

$$\frac{1}{[S]} = -\frac{1}{K_M}$$

(7.61)

From the data in Fig. 7.10, V_{max} is calculated to be 15.2 mmol dm^{-3} s^{-1} and $K_M = 5.7$ mmol dm^{-3}. The values of these parameters give further information on the nature of the enzyme-catalysed process.

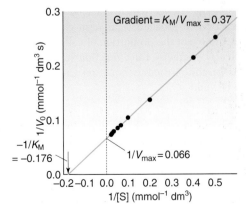

Fig. 7.10 • A Lineweaver–Burke plot for an enzyme-catalysed reaction.

Effect of temperature on reaction rate

In the vast majority of cases, increasing the temperature at which a reaction occurs will increase its rate. As a rule of thumb, a 10°C rise typically doubles the rate constant. More quantitative parameters can be extracted from a simple equation known as the Arrhenius equation. This builds on the ideas established at the start of the chapter, where it was noted that for them to react, two molecules must collide with sufficient energy to overcome the activation energy barrier. The Arrhenius equation states that

$$k = A \exp\left(\frac{-E_a}{RT}\right)$$

(7.62)

In this, k is the rate constant, A is a preexponential factor, E_a is the activation energy for the reaction, R is the ideal gas constant (8.314 J K^{-1} mol^{-1}) and T is the temperature in kelvin (K) (0°C = 273.15 K). The exact physical meaning of A is complex, but it can be thought of as the maximum possible rate constant if the reaction were infinitely hot. A is representative of the number of collisions occurring, and the orientation of these collisions (to react, it is not enough for two molecules to simply collide; they must collide in the correct orientation and with sufficient energy). Consider a simple S$_N$2 type process from organic chemistry, such as that shown in Eq. 7.3. For successful reaction, the incoming nucleophile must not only hit its target molecule, but must also collide with it at the $\delta+$ electrophilic centre where the reaction can occur.

As previously discussed, the activation energy, E_a, is the energy barrier which must be overcome for the reaction to proceed. The term $\exp(-E_a/RT)$ is representative of the proportion of collisions that are sufficiently energetic for a reaction to occur. Logarithms of the Arrhenius equation can usefully be taken to yield

$$\ln k = \ln A - \frac{E_a}{RT}$$

(7.63)

A plot of $\ln k$ versus $1/T$ will thus yield a straight line, with a gradient of $-E_a/R$. The activation energy can easily be determined from the graph, as R is known. The intercept at $1/T = 0$ will be $\ln A$, but because this occurs at infinite temperature (i.e. $1/T$

Box 7.6

Using the Arrhenius equation

The decomposition of a drug was monitored at a range of temperatures to back-calculate the rate at room temperature. The following data were obtained:

T (°C)	k (day⁻¹)	T (K)	1/T (K⁻¹)	ln k
70	0.0196	343	2.92×10^{-3}	−3.93
60	0.0082	333	3.00×10^{-3}	−4.80
50	0.0028	323	3.10×10^{-3}	−5.88
40	0.0011	313	3.20×10^{-3}	−6.81
25		298	3.36×10^{-3}	

The plot of $\ln k$ against $1/T$ (Fig. 7.11) is clearly linear. The equation of the line is found to be $\ln k = -10428/T + 26.474$. $\ln k$ at 25°C (298 K) can be calculated to be $\ln k_{25} = -10428/298 + 26.474 = -8.52$, and $k_{25} = 2.00 \times 10^{-4}$ day^{-1}. $\ln A$ is 26.474, and therefore A is found to be 3.14×10^{11} day^{-1}. It is normal for A to be such a large number because the molecules involved in the reaction are moving rapidly and randomly, leading to large numbers of collisions.

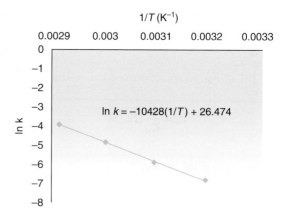

Fig. 7.11 • An Arrhenius plot of $\ln k$ versus $1/T$, showing the data from Box 7.6.

= 0), it is often impractical to determine $\ln A$ from a hand-drawn graph in this way. Typically to find $\ln A$, a point on the line is chosen, and the calculated gradient is used to evaluate $\ln A$ (and thus give A).

An exemplar set of data is given in Box 7.6, and a plot of these data presented in Fig. 7.11. The Arrhenius equation is very widely used in pharmaceutics, most commonly in determining the shelf life of medicines. In the early stages of development, it is necessary to obtain approximate data on this quickly so that the development process is not held up. To do this, formulations are commonly aged at elevated temperatures (much greater than the intended storage temperature) and the rate of reaction determined at these temperatures. Once E_a has been determined, it is possible to back-calculate the expected rate of decomposition at room temperature. As discussed in Chapter 49, there are some problems with this approach, but it is very useful for initial approximate studies.

Summary

This chapter has considered the fundamental points of reaction kinetics, illustrating these with examples.

This necessarily has required a significant amount of mathematics. The detailed mathematics are helpful to understand where equations come from, but the details of the derivations are not so important for our purposes – the applications are the real focus of this chapter. The most important equations are summarized in Table 7.2.

Please check your eBook at **https://studentconsult. inkling.com/** for self-assessment questions. See inside cover for registration details.

Bibliography

Atkins, P.W., De Paula, J., 2014. Atkins's Physical Chemistry, tenth ed. Oxford University Press, Oxford.

Campbell, M.K., Farrell, S.O., 2015. Biochemistry, eighth ed. Cengage Learning, Boston.

Croft, A., Davison, R., 2016. Foundation Maths, sixth ed. Pearson Education, New York.

Devlin, T.M., 2010. Textbook of Biochemistry with Clinical Correlations, seventh ed. Wiley, Hoboken.

Singh, U.K., Orella, C.J., 2010. Reaction kinetics and characterization. In: am Ende, D.J. (Ed.), Chemical Engineering in the Pharmaceutical Industry: R&D to Manufacture. John Wiley & Sons (in conjunction with AIChE), Hoboken.

Sinko, P.J., 2011. Martin's Physical Pharmacy and Pharmaceutical Sciences, sixth ed. Lippincott Williams & Wilkins, Baltimore.

Part 2: Particle science and powder technology

Solid-state properties

Graham Buckton

CHAPTER CONTENTS

KEY POINTS

- The three states of material are solid, liquid and gas (vapour).
- Solids may exist in crystal form, which means that there is repeating ordered packing of the molecules over a long range. They have a defined melting point.
- Amorphous solids (also known as supercooled liquids) do not have long-range packing order. They have no melting point, but have a glass transition temperature.
- Many materials can pack into more than one crystal form, and the different forms are called polymorphs.
- Polymorphs will convert to the stable form over time. They can have different properties, including dissolution rate, which can lead to changes in bioavailability for poorly soluble

drugs. This can have major consequences for patients. Regulatory authorities require control of polymorphs primarily for this reason.
- Many materials can include other materials in their crystal structure, resulting in hydrates, solvates and co-crystals. These too can have different physicochemical properties, requiring control to ensure consistent pharmaceutical performance.

Solid state

The three states of matter are solid, liquid and gas (or vapour). In a sealed container, vapours will diffuse to occupy the total space, liquids will flow to fill part of the container completely, whereas solids will retain their original shape unless a compressive force is applied to them. From this simple consideration it becomes clear that solids are unique. Importantly, their physical form (the packing of the molecules and the size and shape of the particles) can have an influence on the way the material will behave. At normal room temperature and pressure, most drugs and excipients exist as solids; thus the study of solid-state properties is of enormous pharmaceutical importance.

Solid particles are made up of molecules that are held in close proximity to each other by intermolecular forces. The strength of interaction between two molecules is due to the individual atoms within the molecular structure. For example, hydrogen bonds occur because of an electrostatic attraction involving one hydrogen atom and one electronegative atom, such as oxygen. For molecules which cannot hydrogen bond, attraction is due to van der Waals forces. The term *van der Waals forces* is generally taken to include dipole–dipole (Keesom), dipole–induced dipole (Debye) and induced dipole–induced dipole (London) forces. In this context a dipole is where the molecule has a small imbalance of charge from one end to the other, making it behave like a small bar magnet. When the molecules pack together to form a solid, these dipoles align and give attraction between the positive pole of one and the negative pole on the next. Induced dipoles are where the free molecule does not have an imbalance of charge, but an imbalance is caused by a second molecule being brought into close proximity with the first.

Crystallization

Materials in the solid state can be crystalline or amorphous (or a combination of both). Crystalline materials are those in which the molecules are packed in a defined order, and this same order repeats over and over again throughout the particle. In Fig. 8.1a, an ordered packing of a molecule is shown; here the shape of the molecule is shown as a 'hockey stick' style image, which is representing a planar structure with a functional group pointing up at the end. This is not a real molecule – it has been drawn to provide an easy representation of a possible crystal packing arrangement. A characteristic property of a crystal is that it has a melting point. The melting point is the temperature at which the crystal lattice breaks down, due to the molecules having gained sufficient energy from the heating process to overcome the attractive forces that hold the crystal together. It follows that crystals with weak forces holding the molecules together (such as paraffins, which have

only London van der Waals interactions) have low melting points, whereas crystals with strong lattices (i.e. those held together with strong attractive forces) have high melting points.

Crystals are produced by inducement of a change from the liquid to the solid state. There are two options: one is to cool a molten sample to below the melting point. Pharmaceutical examples of crystallizing through cooling include the formation of suppositories, creams and semisolid matrix oral dosage forms (although these will not always yield crystalline material). The other method of crystallization is to have a solution of the material and to change the system so that the solid is formed. At a given temperature and pressure, any *solute* (where the solute is the material that has been dissolved and the liquid is the *solvent*) has a certain maximum amount that can be dissolved in any liquid (called a *saturated solution*). If crystals are to be formed from a solution, it is necessary to have more solute present than can be dissolved, which is known as a *supersaturated solution*. As crystals form from a supersaturated solution, the systems will progress until there are solid particles in equilibrium with a saturated solution. To make a solid precipitate out of solution one can:

- remove the liquid by evaporation, thus making the concentration of solute rise in the remaining solvent (this is the way sea salt is prepared);
- cool the solution, as most materials become less soluble as the temperature is decreased; or
- add another liquid which will mix with the solution, but in which the solute has a low solubility. This second liquid is often called an *antisolvent*.

Many drugs are crystallized by addition of water as an antisolvent to a solution of the drug in an organic liquid. For example, if a drug is almost insoluble in water but freely soluble in ethanol, the drug could be crystallized by addition of water to a near-saturated solution of the drug in ethanol.

The processes by which a crystal forms are called nucleation and growth. Nucleation is the formation of a small mass onto which a crystal can grow. Growth is the addition of more solute molecules onto the nucleation site. To achieve nucleation and growth, it is necessary to have a supersaturated solution. As mentioned previously, a supersaturated solution is one where the amount of solute dissolved in the liquid is greater than the true solubility. Supersaturated solutions are not thermodynamically stable, so in these circumstances the system will adjust so as

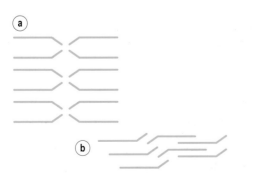

Figure 8.1 • A representation of two polymorphic forms of a crystal consisting of a molecule shown as a 'hockey stick' shape.

to move back to the true solubility, and to do this, the excess solute will precipitate. However, in some circumstances the process of nucleation can be slow. Many students will at some stage have had a super-saturated solution which has not crystallized but on their simply scratching the side of the beaker with a glass rod, crystallization was induced. The scratching action produces a small amount of rough surface that acts as a nucleation site and causes the supersaturated solute to precipitate rapidly.

Polymorphism

If the crystallization conditions are changed in any way, it is possible that the molecules may start to form crystals with a packing pattern different from that which occurred when the original conditions were used. The change in conditions could be a different solvent, a change in the stirring, or different impurities being present. In Fig. 8.1b, a packing arrangement is shown that is an alternative to that which occurred for the same molecule in Fig. 8.1a. As both packing arrangements in Fig. 8.1 are repeating ordered systems, they are both crystals; these would be called *polymorphic forms*.

By looking at the packing arrangements in Fig. 8.1, we can see that the molecules in Fig. 8.1a are more spaced out than those in Fig. 8.1b, which means that the two crystal forms would have different densities (i.e. the same mass of material would occupy different volumes). It looks as though it would be easier to physically pull a molecule off the structure in Fig. 8.1a than the structure in Fig. 8.1b, as the molecules in the structure in Fig. 8.1b are more interwoven into the structure. If this were the case, then the structure in Fig. 8.1a would have a lower melting point than the structure in Fig. 8.1b, and the structure in Fig. 8.1a may dissolve more easily. In addition, if an attempt were made to mill the two crystals, it looks as if the structure in Fig. 8.1a would break easily, as there are natural break lines (either vertically or horizontally), whereas the structure in Fig. 8.1b does not seem to have an obvious weak line to allow easy breakage. This could mean that the milling and compaction (tableting) properties of the two forms will differ. In summary, a change in the packing arrangement of the same molecule, giving two different crystal forms, could result in significant changes in the properties of the solid.

Many organic molecules, including drugs and excipients, exhibit polymorphism. Often this is of a form called *monotropic polymorphism*, which means that only one polymorphic form is stable and any other polymorph that is formed will eventually convert to the stable form. However, some materials exhibit *enantiotropic polymorphism*, which means that under different conditions (temperature and pressure) the material can reversibly transform between alternative stable forms; this type of behaviour will not be considered further here. Considering monotropic polymorphism, the true stable form has the highest melting point and all other forms are described as metastable. This means that the other forms exist for a period of time, and thus appear stable, but given a chance they will convert to the true stable form. Different metastable forms can exist for very short times or many months before they convert to the stable form, depending on the conditions under which they are stored.

In general, for poorly soluble materials there will be a correlation between the melting point of the different polymorphs and the rate of dissolution, because the one with the lowest melting point will most easily give up molecules to dissolve, whereas the most stable form (highest melting point) will not give up molecules to the solvent so readily. Freely soluble materials will dissolve rapidly and readily and therefore it is unlikely that there will be any significant impact of different melting points on the rate of dissolution.

High melting point = strong lattice
= hard to remove a molecule
= low dissolution rate

Low melting point = weak lattice
= easy to remove a molecule
= high dissolution rate

It is relatively easy to understand that changes in polymorphic form can cause changes in the rate at which a poorly soluble drug will dissolve. However, it is less easy to understand why this can lead to a change in the apparent solubility. Nonetheless, it is true that when a metastable polymorphic form is dissolved, it can give a greater amount of material in solution than the saturated solubility. In other words, metastable forms can dissolve to give supersaturated solutions. These supersaturated solutions will eventually return to the equilibrium solubility, due to the stable crystal form precipitating from solution, but that

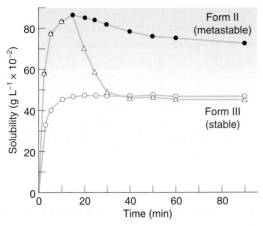

Figure 8.2 • The solubility–time relationship for sulfamethoxydiazine. *Open circles* represent the solubility of polymorphic form III, which rises to the drug's equilibrium solubility and plateaus. *Filled circles* represent the solubility of polymorphic form II, which dissolves to twice the extent of form III and then shows a gradual decline with time, as the stable form crystallizes from solution. *Triangles* represent the effect of addition of crystals of form III to the solution of form II at the peak of solubility. It can be seen that the amount dissolved falls rapidly from the supersaturated level to the true equilibrium solubility because the added crystals of form III act as nucleation sites. Adapted from Ebian et al., 1973, with permission.

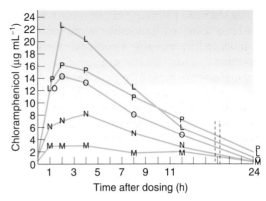

Figure 8.3 • Comparison of mean blood serum levels after administration of chloramphenicol palmitate suspensions with varying ratios of the stable (α) and the metastable (β) polymorphs. M, 100% α-polymorph; N, 25:75 β-polymorph to α-polymorph; O, 50:50 β-polymorph to α-polymorph; P, 75:25 β-polymorph to α-polymorph; L, 100% β-polymorph. Adapted from Aguiar et al., 1976, with permission.

process may not be instantaneous. In fact, the supersaturated solution can often exist long enough to cause an increase in bioavailability of a poorly soluble drug. In Fig. 8.2 the apparent solubility of two different polymorphs of sulfamethoxydiazine is shown. It can be seen that form II, a metastable form, has a higher apparent solubility than form III, a stable form, and that this lasts throughout the 90-minute experiment. However, if crystals of form III are added to the solution of form II, then the solubility reverts rapidly to that of form III, because the excess solute in the supersaturated solution will have seed crystals of form III on which to precipitate.

Polymorphism and bioavailability

Many drugs are hydrophobic and have very limited solubility in water. For drugs of this type, the rate at which they dissolve will be slow (slow dissolution rate), due to their limited aqueous solubility, and this can result in only a small percentage of the administered drug actually being available to the patient (low bioavailability). A classic example of the importance of polymorphism in bioavailability is that of chloramphenicol palmitate suspensions. In Fig. 8.3 the blood serum level is plotted as a function of time after dosing. It can be seen that the stable α-polymorph produces low serum levels, whereas the metastable β-polymorph yields much higher serum levels when the same dose is administered.

For drugs that are freely soluble in water, the bioavailability is not likely to be limited by the dissolution, so it would be surprising for polymorphism to influence bioavailability in this way. However, for drugs with low aqueous solubility, the polymorphic form must be well controlled to ensure that the bioavailability is the same each time the product is made, and throughout the shelf life of the product. It would be risky to deliberately make a product with anything other than the stable form of a drug, as other polymorphic forms could convert to the stable form during the shelf life of the product, which could result in a reduction in bioavailability and thus the therapeutic effect of certain products. This strategy is occasionally followed if the most soluble metastable form is 'stable enough' to survive the agreed shelf life of the product with insignificant change. The impact of polymorphism on drug dissolution and bioavailability is discussed further in Chapter 20.

In conclusion, the stable polymorphic form will have the slowest dissolution rate, so there may be occasions when it would be desirable to speed the dissolution by use of a metastable form. However, the risk associated with use of the metastable form is that it will convert back to the stable form during the product life, and give a consequent change in properties.

As polymorphism can have such serious consequences for bioavailability of drugs with low aqueous solubility, it is essential that manufacturers check for the existence of polymorphism and ensure that they use the same appropriate polymorphic form every time they make a product. New drugs are therefore screened to see how many polymorphs (and solvates and hydrates – see the next section) exist, and then to identify which one is the most stable. The screening process requires many crystallizations from numerous different solvent systems, with variations in method and conditions, to try to induce different polymorphs to form. The products are then checked with spectroscopy (e.g. Raman spectroscopy) and X-ray diffraction to see if they have different internal packing (see also Chapter 23). Sadly, there are examples of products being taken to market with what was believed to be the stable form, only for the stable form to be produced at a later stage. In these circumstances the stable form may have been inhibited from being formed by a certain impurity, which may have been lost because of an alteration in the method of chemical synthesis of the drug, so the stable form was suddenly produced. With the stable form having been produced, if the drug is poorly soluble, it is probable that the bioavailability will reduce. In addition, with the stable form having been made, it is often then very hard to stabilize the metastable form again. This can result in products having to be recalled from the market and reformulated and retested clinically. The fact that major pharmaceutical companies, all of which take the study of physical form very seriously, have seen the stable form arrive after product launch shows that it is difficult to be sure that you are working with the most stable form of the drug.

As mentioned earlier, many properties other than the rate of dissolution can change when a material is in a different polymorphic form. For example, paracetamol is a high-dose drug with poor compression properties, which can make it difficult to form into tablets. This is because there is an upper limit on the size of the tablet that can be swallowed easily, so for high-dose drugs the amount of compressible excipient that can be added is modest. Consequently, researchers have tried to experiment with different polymorphic forms of paracetamol to find one that is more compressible.

Hydrates and solvates

It is possible for materials to crystallize and in so doing to trap individual molecules of the solvent within the lattice. If the solvent used is water, the material will be described as a *hydrate*. This entrapment is often in an exact molar ratio with the crystallizing material; for example, a monohydrate will have one molecule of water for each molecule of the crystallizing material. It is possible to have different levels of hydrate; for example, some drugs can exist as a monohydrate, dihydrate and trihydrate (respectively one, two and three molecules of water to each molecule of the drug). Morris (1999) noted that approximately 11% (>16 000 compounds) of all structures recorded in the Cambridge Structural Database exist as hydrates. Of the classes of hydrate materials that were similar to drugs, approximately 50% were monohydrates, more than 20% were dihydrates, 8% were trihydrates and 8% were hemihydrates (one water molecule for two host molecules); other hydrate levels (up to 10 water molecules per host molecule) became progressively less common.

If solvents other than water are present in a crystal lattice, the material is called a *solvate*. For example, if ethanol is present, it would be an ethanolate. In general, it is undesirable to use solvates for pharmaceuticals as the presence of retained organic material would be regarded as an unnecessary impurity in the product, unless it was seen to possess advantageous properties and be safe for pharmaceutical use. If the organic solvent were toxic in any way, it would obviously be inappropriate for pharmaceuticals. For this reason, the discussion will be limited to hydrates.

Hydrates often have properties very different from those of the anhydrous form, in the same way as two different polymorphs have different properties with respect to each other. For this reason, the difference between hydrates and anhydrous forms is sometimes described inelegantly as *pseudopolymorphism*. With polymorphism the stable form will have the highest melting point and the slowest dissolution rate (see earlier). However, with hydrates it is possible for the hydrate form to have either a faster or a slower dissolution rate than the anhydrous form. The most usual situation is for the anhydrous form to have a faster dissolution rate than the hydrate; an example of this is shown in Fig. 8.4 for theophylline. In this situation, water could hydrogen bond between two drug molecules and tie the lattice together; this would give a much stronger, more stable lattice and thus a

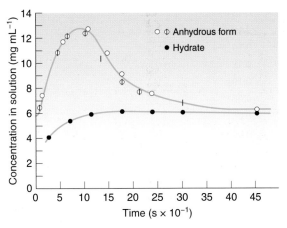

Figure 8.4 • The dissolution of theophylline monohydrate rising to an equilibrium solubility, compared with that for anhydrous theophylline, which forms a supersaturated solution with a peak more than twice that of the dissolving hydrate, before crystallizing to form the true equilibrium solubility. Adapted from Shefter & Higuchi, 1963, with permission.

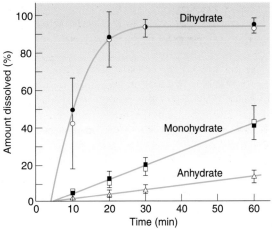

Figure 8.5 • The dissolution behaviour for erythromycin as the anhydrate, monohydrate and dihydrate, showing a progressively faster dissolution rate as the level of hydrate is increased. Adapted from Allen et al., 1978, with permission.

slower dissolution rate. It can be seen from Fig. 8.4 that the concentration of anhydrous theophylline rises to a high level in solution and then falls again until the amount dissolved is the same as that recorded for the hydrate. The reason for this is that the hydrate has come to the true equilibrium solubility, whereas the anhydrous form had initially formed a supersaturated solution (as described for metastable polymorphic forms earlier).

Although anhydrous forms are usually more rapidly soluble than the hydrate, there are examples of the opposite being true. In such circumstances one could think of water as a wedge pushing two molecules apart and preventing the optimum interaction between the molecules in the lattice. Here water would be weakening the lattice and would result in a more rapid dissolution rate. An example of the hydrate form speeding up dissolution is shown in Fig. 8.5 for erythromycin.

Amorphous state

When a material is in the solid state but the molecules are not packed in a repeating long-range ordered fashion, it is said to be *amorphous*. Amorphous solids have properties very different from those of the crystal form of the same material. For example, crystals have a melting point (the break-up of the crystal lattice), whereas the amorphous

form does not (as it does not have a crystal lattice to break!).

Polymeric materials (or other high molecular weight species) have molecules that are so large and flexible that it is not possible for them to align perfectly to form crystals. For these materials it will be usual to have ordered regions within the structure surrounded by disorder, so they are described as semicrystalline. For materials such as these, it will not be possible to produce a completely crystalline sample; however, the degree of crystallinity can vary depending on the processing conditions. This can affect the properties of the material and thus how it functions in pharmaceutical products.

For low molecular weight materials, the amorphous form may be produced if the solidification process was too fast for the molecules to have a chance to align in the correct way to form a crystal (this could happen, for example, when a solution is spray-dried). Alternatively, a crystal may be formed but then may be broken. This could happen if a crystal were exposed to energy, such as from milling. A simple analogy is that a crystal is like a brick wall, which has ordered long-range packing. If the wall is hit hard, perhaps as during demolition, the bricks will separate (Fig. 8.6). Unlike the brick wall, however, a disrupted crystal will be thermodynamically unstable and will revert to the crystal form. This conversion may be rapid or very slow and, as with polymorphism, its pharmaceutical significance will depend on how long the partially amorphous form survives.

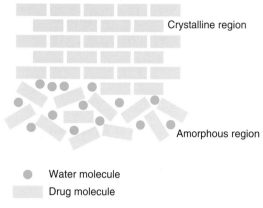

Crystalline region

Amorphous region

● Water molecule

▭ Drug molecule

Figure 8.6 • The disruption of a crystal (represented as a brick wall) giving the possibility for water vapour absorption in the amorphous region.

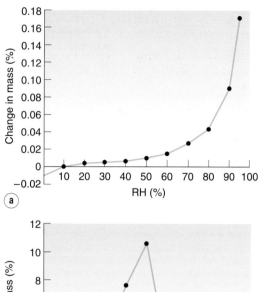

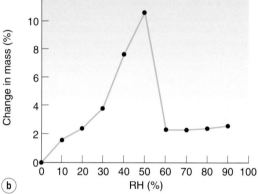

Figure 8.7 • (a) A water sorption isotherm for crystalline lactose monohydrate; the quantity of water adsorbed to the crystal surface is small. **(b)** A water sorption isotherm for amorphous lactose, showing a rise to approximately 11% water content due to absorption, followed by water loss as the sample crystallizes and the absorbed water is expelled. *RH*, Relative humidity.

Amorphous forms have a characteristic temperature at which there is a major change in properties. This is called the *glass transition temperature* (T_g). If the sample is stored below the glass transition temperature, the amorphous form will be brittle, described as being in the glassy state. If the sample is above its glass transition temperature, it becomes rubbery. The glass transition temperature, although not well understood, is a point at which the molecules in the glass exhibit a major change in mobility. The lack of mobility when the sample is glassy allows the amorphous form to exist for a longer time, whereas when the glass transition temperature is below the storage temperature, the increased molecular mobility allows rapid conversion to the crystalline form.

The glass transition temperature of an amorphous material can be lowered by addition of a small molecule, called a plasticizer, that fits between the glassy molecules, giving them greater mobility. Water has a good plasticizing effect on many materials, so the glass transition temperature will usually reduce when the material is in the presence of water vapour.

Most amorphous materials are able to absorb large quantities of water vapour. Absorption is a process whereby one molecule passes into the bulk of another material, and should not be confused with adsorption, which is where something concentrates at the surface of another material (see Chapter 4). The way in which water can access amorphous regions is shown in Fig. 8.6. Fig. 8.7 shows the amount of water that is adsorbed to a crystalline material (Fig. 8.7a) in comparison with that absorbed into an amorphous form of the same material (Fig. 8.7b). It can be seen that the amount absorbed is many times greater than

that adsorbed. This large difference in water content at any selected relative humidity is important in many materials. For example, it is possible that certain drugs can degrade by hydrolysis when amorphous, but remain stable when crystalline. The extent of hydrolysis of an antibiotic which had been processed to yield different levels of crystalline to amorphous forms is shown in Table 8.1; the extent of degradation is greater when the amorphous content is increased. This concept is also discussed in Chapter 8.

In Fig. 8.7 it can be seen that the amorphous form absorbs a very large amount of water until 50% relative humidity, after which there is a weight loss. The reason for the loss is that the sample has crystallized. Crystallization occurs because the absorbed water has plasticized the sample to such an extent that the

Table 8.1 The chemical stability of cephalothin sodium related to the amorphous content of the sample

Sample	Amorphous content (%)	Amount of stable drug (%) after storage at 31% relative humidity and 50 °C
Crystalline	0	100
Freeze-dried	12	100
Freeze-dried	46	85
Spray-dried	53	44

Data derived from Pikal et al. (1978).

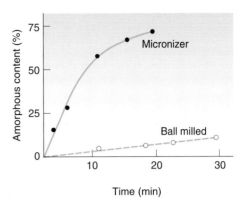

Figure 8.9 • The amorphous content of a model drug substance following milling in a ball mill and a micronizer. Adapted from Ahmed et al., 1996, with permission.

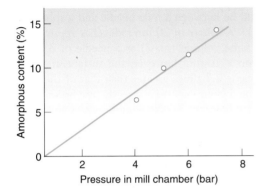

Figure 8.8 • The amorphous content induced in crystalline lactose as a consequence of milling in an air-jet mill at different air pressures. Adapted from Briggner et al., 1994, with permission.

glass transition temperature has dropped below room temperature and allowed sufficient molecular mobility that the molecules are able to align and crystallize. The water is lost during this process as absorption can occur only in the amorphous form, so it cannot endure into the crystalline state. However, some water is retained in this example (see Fig. 8.7), because lactose is able to form a monohydrate. The amount of water required to form a monohydrate with lactose is 5% w/w (calculated from the molecular weight of lactose and water), which is much less than the 11% that was present in the amorphous form (Fig. 8.7b).

In Fig. 8.8 the amorphous content of lactose is seen to increase in proportion to the length of time it was left in an air-jet mill (micronizer). In Fig. 8.9 it can be seen that a drug substance became partially amorphous when treated in a simple ball mill, and extensively amorphous when micronized. Although the example in Fig. 8.9 is an extreme behaviour, it

is not unusual for highly processed materials to become partially amorphous. Although milling does not necessarily make all materials partially amorphous, the chance of seeing disruption to the crystalline lattice will increase with the amount of energy used in the milling.

The fact that processing can make crystalline materials partially amorphous means that it is possible that very complex materials can be formed that contain different metastable states. For example, in Fig. 8.3 the plasma levels of two polymorphs of chloramphenicol palmitate are shown; if the β-polymorph were milled, it is possible that it may also become partially amorphous, which could make the plasma level even higher than when the crystalline form was used. However, milling the β-polymorph could also provide the necessary energy to convert it to the stable α-polymorph, which would reduce the effective plasma level. Equally, milling could disrupt the α-polymorph, giving a partially amorphous form that may have a higher bioavailability than the crystal. In other words, the effect of processing on the physical form can be very complicated, and often unpredictable. It is possible to produce a physical form that is partially amorphous and partially crystalline. The crystalline component could then be stable or metastable. Inevitably, with time (for low molecular weight species) the sample will revert to contain only the stable crystalline form, with no amorphous content and none of the metastable polymorph(s), but as this does not necessarily happen instantly, the physical form and its complexity are of great importance.

Crystal habit

All the previous discussion has related to the internal packing of molecules. It has been shown that they may have no long-range order (amorphous) or different repeating packing arrangements (polymorphic crystals) or have solvent molecules included in the crystal (solvates and hydrates). Each of these changes in internal packing of a solid will give rise to changes in properties. However, it is also possible to change the external shape of a crystal. The external shape is called the crystal habit, and this is a consequence of the rate at which different faces grow. Changes in internal packing usually (but not always) give an easily distinguishable change in habit. However, for the same crystal packing, it is possible to change the external appearance by changes in the crystallization conditions.

With any crystalline material, the largest face is always the slowest growing. The reason for this is shown in Fig. 8.10, where it can be seen that if drug is deposited on two faces of the hexagonal crystal habit, then the first consequence is that the face where drug is deposited actually becomes a smaller part of the crystal, whereas the other faces get larger. Eventually, the fastest growing faces will no longer exist (see Fig. 8.10). The growth on different faces will depend on the relative affinities of the solute for the solvent and the growing faces of the crystal. Every molecule is made up of different functional groups – some are relatively polar (such as carboxylic acid groups), whereas others are nonpolar (such as a methyl group). Depending on the geometry of the packing of the molecules into the lattice, some crystal faces may have more exposed polar groups and others may be relatively nonpolar. If the crystal were growing from an aqueous solution, drug would deposit on the faces that make the crystal more polar (i.e. the nonpolar faces would grow, making the more polar faces dominate). If, however, the same crystal form were growing from a nonpolar solvent, then the opposite would be true.

Obviously the external shape can alter the properties of drugs and excipients. For example, the dissolution rate of a drug can change if the surface area to volume ratio is altered. An extreme difference would be between a long needle and a sphere (Fig. 8.11). A sphere of 20 μm radius has approximately the same volume (mass) as a needle of 335 μm × 10 μm × 10 μm; however, the surface area of the needle is 2.7 times greater than that of the sphere. As the dissolution rate is directly proportional to the surface area, the needle would dissolve much faster than the sphere. Crystals do not grow to make spheres, although through milling, crystals can develop rounded geometries; the closest to a sphere would be a cube, which would still have less than half the surface area of the needle shown in Fig. 8.11.

As well as changes in the dissolution rate, different crystal habits can cause changes in powder flow (which is important as, for example, the die of a tableting machine is filled by volume and requires good powder flow to guarantee content uniformity of the product) and sedimentation and caking of suspensions.

It is technically possible to engineer changes in crystal habit by deliberate manipulation of the rate of growth of different faces of the crystal. This is done by the intentional addition of a small amount of impurity to the solution. The impurity must preferentially

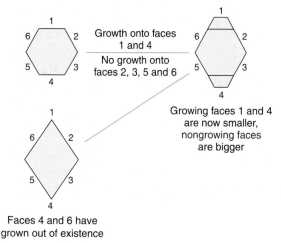

Faces 4 and 6 have grown out of existence

Figure 8.10 • Demonstration of how growth onto faces 1 and 4 of a hexagonal crystal results in the formation of a diamond.

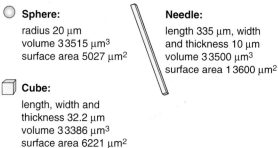

Sphere:
radius 20 μm
volume 33515 μm³
surface area 5027 μm²

Cube:
length, width and thickness 32.2 μm
volume 33386 μm³
surface area 6221 μm²

Needle:
length 335 μm, width and thickness 10 μm
volume 33500 μm³
surface area 13600 μm²

Figure 8.11 • The relative surface areas of a sphere, cube and needle that have similar volumes of material.

interact with one face of the growing crystal, and in so doing it will stop growth on that face, so the remaining faces grow more rapidly. The impurity would either be a molecule very similar to that of the crystallizing material, so that part of the molecule is included in the lattice but the remainder of the molecule blocks further layers from attaching, or it may be a surfactant that adsorbs to one growing face.

Surface nature of particles

Dry powder inhalers

Dry powder inhalers (see Chapter 37) often have a micronized drug, which has to be small enough to be inhaled, mixed with a larger carrier particle which is often lactose. The carrier particle is there to make the powder suitable for handling and dosing, as micronized particles have poor flow properties. The shape and surface properties of the drug and/or carrier particles can be critical parameters in controlling the dose of drug that is delivered. It may be necessary to adjust the surface roughness of carrier particles. Fig. 8.12a shows a cartoon of a rough carrier particle; this would hold the micronized drug too strongly, essentially trapped within the rough regions of the

carrier, so the inhaled dose would be very low. A smooth carrier particle with the same micronised drug is seen in Fig. 8.12b. Here the drug will easily be displaced from the carrier during inhalation but it may not stay mixed with the carrier during filling of the inhaler and dosing. In Fig. 8.12c, a rough carrier particle has first been mixed with micronized carrier and then with micronized drug. By this approach, the drug is free to detach from the carrier, as the micronized carrier is trapped in all the crevices on the carrier surface.

The hypothesis relating to the use of fine carrier particles to enhance the delivery of micronized drug from large carrier particles is not proved beyond doubt. It remains possible that interactions between the fine carrier and fine drug may be the reason for the enhanced delivery.

It should, of course, be noted that the diagrams in Fig. 8.12 simplify the real situation greatly. In Fig. 8.13 a real lactose particle is shown along with added micronized particles. It can be seen that the large lactose particle (lactose particles are often described as 'tomahawk' shaped) has rough ridges on its surface and there are some very fine particles aligned to some extent in the rough areas. It is also clear that many fine particles are not on the surface of the lactose and that some fine particles are on smooth regions of the lactose.

For products such as these (discussed more fully in Chapter 37), it is becomingly increasingly important

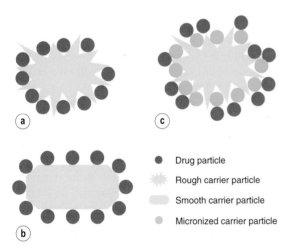

Drug particle

Rough carrier particle

Smooth carrier particle

Micronized carrier particle

Figure 8.12 • A hypothesis that surface roughness may relate to drug release from carrier particles in dry powder inhalers. **(a)** Drug trapped in the rough regions of the carrier particle giving a low inhaled dose. **(b)** Micronized drug can be readily removed from a smooth carrier particle. **(c)** Micronized drug may be removed readily (resulting in a high inhaled dose) if the carrier is first treated with micronized carrier particles, to fill the rough voids.

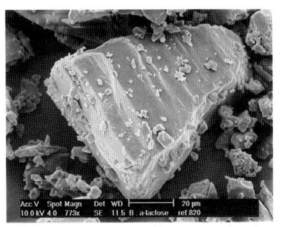

Figure 8.13 • An electron micrograph showing a large lactose carrier particle with added fine lactose, some of which is seen to be at rough spots on the large carrier, but there is also a lot of nonadsorbed fine lactose content. This shows that Fig. 8.12 is an enormous simplification of the real system.

to first measure the surface nature of samples and then to control the form to achieve the desired delivery of drug. The shape of the carrier is an important consideration for the design of this type of product. The presence of water can also be critical, as condensed water can alter the adhesion between the active pharmaceutical ingredient (API) and the carrier, which can give rise to variability in the detachment of the API particles during inhalation, which in turn can give a variable fine particle dose of API to the lungs. This means that the humidity used for filling (and hence the water content of the system) must be strictly controlled. A further concern is the surface energy, as this can influence the way in which the drug and carrier are attached to each other.

Surface energy

Surfaces and surface energy are discussed in Chapter 4, and a summary of those aspects relevant to the solid state is presented here. Molecules at the surface of a material have a net inward force exerted on them from the molecules in the bulk; this is the basis of surface energy. Surface energy is important as every interaction (except the mixing of two gasses) starts by an initial contact between two surfaces. If this surface interaction is favoured, then the process will probably proceed, whereas if it is not favoured, then the process will be limited. A good example of the role of surface energy is the wetting of a powder by a liquid; here the powder cannot dissolve until the liquid makes good contact with it. A practical example is instant coffee, where some brands are hard to wet and dissolve, whereas others dissolve easily. Changes in the wetting of powders can affect the processes of wet granulation, suspension formation, film coating and drug dissolution.

The measurement and understanding of surface energy for solid powders is complex. Even on the same crystal form, it would be expected that every crystal face, edge and defect could experience different forces pulling from the bulk and thus could have a different surface energy. It would be reasonable to assume that different physical forms of the same drug could have quite different surface energies. Thus for the same drug it is possible that changes in habit and/or polymorphic form and/or the presence of a solvate or hydrate would change the surface energy. For amorphous forms the molecules at the surface have greater freedom to move and reorient than do molecules in crystal surfaces, so the amorphous form

could have changes in surface energy with time (and with physical state in relation to the glass transition temperature).

The conventional way of determining the surface energy of a solid is to place a drop of liquid onto the solid surface and measure the contact angle as discussed in Chapter 4. Perfect wetting of a solid by a liquid will result in a contact angle of 0°.

For smooth solid surfaces, contact angles are an ideal way of assessing surface energy. However, powders present problems as it is not possible to place a drop of liquid on the surface. Consequently, a compromise will always be required when one is measuring a contact angle for powdered systems. An example of such a compromise would be to make a compact of the powder so as to produce a smooth flat surface. However, the disadvantage of this is that the process of compaction may well change the surface energy of the powder, as the compaction process will deform the particles, by fracture or flow, yielding a compact which is no longer individual particles but a single coherent structure. This new bonded compact will most probably have surfaces with properties different from those of the particles used to make it.

A preferred option by which to assess the surface energy of powders would be vapour sorption.

Vapour sorption

Adsorption, absorption and deliquescence are discussed fully in Chapter 4. When a powder is exposed to a vapour, or gas, the interaction will take one of the following forms:

- adsorption of the vapour to the powder surface;
- absorption into the bulk;
- deliquescence; or
- hydrate/solvate formation.

Absorption into the bulk can occur if the sample is amorphous, whereas the interaction will be limited to adsorption if the powder is crystalline. The extent and energetics of interaction between vapours and powder surfaces allow the surface energy to be calculated. The other processes listed are deliquescence, which is where the powder dissolves in the vapour, and hydrate formation, which is discussed in Chapter 4.

It is possible therefore to use adsorption and/or absorption behaviour as a method by which the powder surface energy can be determined. There are three basic approaches to this: gravimetric (measuring weight change), calorimetric (measuring heat change) and chromatographic (measuring retention to a solid with analysis such as flame ionization of the carrier eluted from a column). Each of these techniques has found application in studies of batch-to-batch variability of materials. An example of a critical case could be that a certain drug shows extensive variability in respirable dose from a dry powder inhaler. Assuming that the size distribution was acceptable in all cases, it would be necessary to understand why some batches yielded unacceptable doses. These vapour sorption techniques could then be used to assess the surface energy and then define values that would be acceptable to achieve good drug dosing, and equally to define batches of drug that will give unacceptable products.

Gravimetric methods use sensitive microbalances as a means of determining the extent of vapour sorption to a powder surface. The calorimetric approaches measure the enthalpy change associated with vapour–powder interaction, which gives clear information on the nature of the powder surface. By use of the principles of gas chromatography, it is possible to pack the powder, for which the surface energy is required, into a column and then to inject different vapours into the column with a carrier gas. Obviously, the time taken for the vapour to come out of the other end of the column is a measure of how favourable the interaction was between the powder and the vapour. Inverse gas chromatography, as this is called, is described in Chapter 4.

Please check your eBook at **https://studentconsult.inkling.com/** for self-assessment questions. See inside cover for registration details.

References

Ahmed, H., Buckton, G., Rawlins, D.A., 1996. The use of isothermal microcalorimetry in the study of small degrees of amorphous content of a hydrophobic powder. Int. J. Pharm. 130, 195–201.

Allen, P.V., Rahn, P.D., Sarapu, A.C., et al., 1978. Physical characterization of erythromycin: anhydrate, monohydrate and dihydrate crystalline solids. J. Pharm. Sci. 67, 1087–1093.

Briggner, L.-E., Buckton, G., Bystrom, K., et al., 1994. The use of isothermal microcalorimetry in the study of changes in crystallinity induced during processing of powders. Int. J. Pharm. 105, 125–135.

Ebian, A.R., Moustafa, M.A., Khalil, S.A., et al., 1973. Effect of additives on the kinetics of interconversion of suphamethoxydiazine crystal forms. J. Pharm. Pharmacol. 25, 13–20.

Morris, K.R., 1999. Structural aspects of hydrates and solvates. In: Brittain, H.G. (Ed.), Polymorphism in Pharmaceutical Solids. Marcel Dekker, New York.

Pikal, M.J., Lukes, A.L., Lang, J.E., et al., 1978. Quantitative crystallinity determinations for β-lactam antibiotics by solution calorimetry: correlations with stability. J. Pharm. Sci. 67, 767–773.

Shefter, E., Higuchi, T., 1963. Dissolution behavior of crystalline solvated and nonsolvated forms of some pharmaceuticals. J. Pharm. Sci. 52, 781–791.

Bibliography

Aguiar, A.J., Krc, J. Jr., Kinkel, A.W., et al., 1976. Effect of polymorphism on the absorption of chloramphenicol from chloramphenicol palmitate. J. Pharm. Sci. 56, 847–853.

Brittain, H.G. (Ed.), 1999. Polymorphism in Pharmaceutical Solids. Marcel Dekker, New York.

Buckton, G., 1995. Interfacial Phenomena in Drug Delivery and Targeting. Harwood Academic Press, Amsterdam.

Florence, A.T., Attwood, D., 2016. Physicochemical Principles of Pharmacy: In Manufacture, Formulation and Clinical Use, sixth ed. Pharmaceutical Press, London.

Mersmann, A. (Ed.), 1994. Crystallization Technology Handbook. Marcel Dekker, New York.

Particle size analysis

Kevin M. G. Taylor

CHAPTER CONTENTS

KEY POINTS

- The size of particulate solids and liquid droplets is a key factor for achieving optimal formulation and manufacture of pharmaceutical products.
- Equivalent sphere diameters are used by pharmaceutical scientists as a means of describing the size of irregularly shaped particles.
- In general, the method used to measure particle size determines the type of equivalent sphere diameter measured.
- A population of particles may be monodisperse, though pharmaceutical systems are more usually polydisperse.
- Several methods exist for measuring particle sizes, in the range from a few nanometres to thousands of micrometres.
- The most commonly used size analysis methods encountered within pharmaceutics are described here, including sieve analysis, microscopy, sedimentation techniques, the electrical sensing zone method, laser diffraction and dynamic light scattering.

Introduction

The appropriate size of particulate solids is important to achieve the optimal formulation and production of safe and effective medicines. Fig. 9.1 presents an outline of the lifetime of a drug, from synthesis to elimination from the body. During stages 1 and 2, when a drug is synthesized and formulated, the particle size of the drug and other powders in the formulation is determined. This will ultimately impact the physical performance of the drug product (medicine) and the subsequent pharmacological effects of the drug.

Particle size influences the production of many formulated medicines (stage 3, Fig. 9.1) as discussed in the chapters in Part 5 of this book. For instance, both tablets and capsules are manufactured with use of equipment that controls the mass of drug (and other

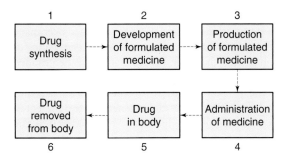

Fig. 9.1 • The lifetime of a drug.

solid excipients) by volumetric filling. Therefore any interference with the uniformity of fill volumes may alter the mass of drug incorporated into the tablet or capsule, adversely affecting the content uniformity of the product. Powders with different particle sizes have different flow and packing properties, which alter the volumes of powder during each encapsulation or tablet compression event. To avoid such problems, the particle sizes of drugs and other powders may be defined, and controlled, during formulation so that problems during production are avoided.

Following administration of the medicine (stage 4, Fig. 9.1), the dosage form should release the drug into solution at the optimal rate. This depends on several factors, one of which will be the dissolution rate of the drug, which is inversely related to particle size as described by the Noyes–Whitney equation, outlined in detail in Chapter 2. Thus reducing the size of particles will generally increase the rate of dissolution, which can have a direct impact on bio-availability and subsequent drug handling by the body (stages 5 and 6). For example, the drug griseofulvin has a low solubility by oral administration, but is rapidly distributed following absorption; reducing the particle size increases the rate of dissolution and consequently the amount of drug absorbed. However, a reduction in particle size to improve the dissolution rate and hence bioavailability is not always beneficial. For example, reducing the particle size of nitrofuran-toin increases its dissolution rate, which may consequently produce adverse effects because of its more rapid absorption. The effect of particle size on bio-availability is discussed more fully in Chapter 20.

It is clear from considerations of the lifetime of a drug, outlined previously, that knowledge and the control of particle size are important for both the production of drug products containing particulate solids and the efficacy/safety of such products following administration.

In practice, the pharmaceutical scientist may not need to know the precise size of particles intended for a particular purpose, rather a size range may be sufficient, and consequently powders are frequently graded on the basis of the size of the particles of which they comprise. The size or 'fineness' of a powder may be expressed by reference to the passage/nonpassage of the powder through sieves of defined mesh size, or to specific descriptive terms, for instance:

- coarse powder: median size (X_{50}): greater than 355 μm;
- moderately fine powder: median size (X_{50}): 180 μm to 355 μm;
- fine powder: median size (X_{50}): 125 μm to 180 μm;
- very fine powder: median size (X_{50}): 125 μm or less; and
- micronized powder: median size (X_{50}): less than 10 μm (most <5 μm).

Pharmacopoeial definitions of grades of powders, and the methods used to separate particles, by size, are discussed in detail in Chapter 10.

Whilst this chapter refers to 'particle size' and 'particle size analysis' and the previous discussion relates particularly to solid particles, many of the concepts discussed in this chapter apply equally to pharmaceutical systems where it is necessary to determine the size of a dispersed liquid, rather than the solid phase; for instance, in emulsions and aerosol sprays.

Particle size

Dimensions

Describing the size of irregularly shaped particles, as usually encountered in pharmaceutical systems, is a challenge. To describe adequately such a particle would require measurement of no fewer than three dimensions. Frequently, though, it is advantageous to have a single number to describe the size of particles. For instance, when milling powders for inclusion in a pharmaceutical formulation, production and quality assurance staff will want to know if the mean size is approximately the same as, larger than or smaller than that for previous milling procedures of the same material. To overcome the problem of describing a three-dimensional particle with a single number, we use the concept of the equivalent sphere.

In this approach, a particle is considered to approximate to a sphere: some property of the particle is measured and related to a sphere, the diameter of which can then be quoted. Because the measurement is then based on a hypothetical sphere, which represents only an approximation to the true size and shape of the particle, the dimension is referred to as the *equivalent sphere diameter* or *equivalent diameter* of the particle.

Equivalent sphere diameters

It is possible to generate more than one sphere which is equivalent to a given irregular particle shape. Fig. 9.2 shows the two-dimensional projection of a particle with two different diameters constructed about it.

The *projected area diameter* is based on a circle of area equivalent to that of the projected image of a particle; the *perimeter diameter* is based on a circle having the same perimeter as the particle. Unless the particles are unsymmetrical in three dimensions, these two diameters will be independent of particle orientation.

This is not true for *Feret's* and *Martin's diameters* (Fig. 9.3), the values of which are dependent on both the orientation and the shape of the particles. These are statistical diameters which are averaged over many different orientations to produce a mean value for each particle diameter. Feret's diameter is determined from the mean distance between two parallel tangents to the projected outline of the particle. Martin's diameter is the mean chord length of the projected particle perimeter, which can be considered as the boundary separating equal particle areas (A and B in Fig. 9.3).

It is also possible to determine the equivalent sphere diameters of particles based on other factors such as volume, surface area, sieve aperture and sedimentation characteristics. Some of the more commonly used equivalent sphere diameters are defined in Table 9.1. In general, the method used to determine particle size dictates the type of equivalent sphere diameter that is measured. This is explained for each particle size analysis method described later in this chapter. Interconversion of the various equivalent particle sizes may be done, mathematically or automatically as part of the size analysis. Clearly, then, a given particle may have a number of different values for its 'size' depending on the parameter measured and the method used for its measurement and/or calculation.

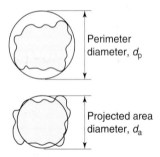

Fig. 9.2 • Different equivalent diameters constructed around the same particle.

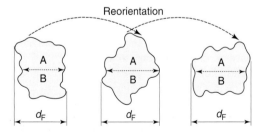

Fig. 9.3 • Influence of particle orientation on statistical diameters. The change in Feret's diameter is shown by the distances, d_F; Martin's diameter, d_M, corresponds to the *dotted lines* in the mid part of each image.

Particle size distribution

A particle population which consists of spheres or equivalent spheres of the same diameter is said to be *monodisperse* or *monosized*, and its characteristics can be described by a single diameter or equivalent sphere diameter.

However, it is unusual for particles to be completely monodisperse, and such a sample will rarely, if ever, be encountered in a pharmaceutical system. Most powders contain particles with a range of different equivalent diameters, i.e. they are *polydisperse* or *heterodisperse*. To be able to define a size distribution or compare the characteristics of two or more powders comprising particles with many different diameters, the size distribution can be broken down into different size ranges, which can be presented in the form of a histogram plotted from data such as those given in Table 9.2.

Such a histogram presents an interpretation of the particle size distribution and enables the percentage of particles having a given equivalent diameter to be determined. A histogram allows different particle size distributions to be compared. For example, the histogram in Fig. 9.4a is a representation of particles

Table 9.1 Equivalent sphere diameters of irregular particles

Equivalent sphere diameter	Symbol	Definition	Equation
Drag diameter (or frictional drag diameter)	d_d	Diameter of a sphere having the same resistance to motion in a fluid as the particle in a fluid of the same density (ρ_f) and same viscosity (η), and moving at the same velocity (v) (d_d approximates to d_s when the particle Reynolds number, Re_p, is small and particle motion is streamlined. i.e. $Re_p < 0.2$)	$F_D = C_D A \rho t \dfrac{v^2}{2}$, where C_D $A = f(d_d)$ (i.e. $F_D = 3\pi d_d \eta v$)
Feret's diameter	d_F	The mean value of the distance between pairs of parallel tangents to the projected outline of the particle. This can be considered as the boundary separating equal particle areas (see the text and Fig. 9.3)	None
Free-falling diameter	d_f	Diameter of a sphere having the same density and same free-falling speed as the particle in a fluid of the same density and viscosity	None
Hydrodynamic diameter	d_h	Diameter calculated from the diffusion coefficient according to the Stokes–Einstein equation (see the text)	$D = \dfrac{1.38 \times 10^{-12} T}{3\pi \eta d}\,\mathrm{m^2\,s^{-1}}$
Martin's diameter	d_M	The mean chord length of the projected outline of the particle (see the text and Fig. 9.3)	None
Projected-area diameter	d_a	Diameter of a circle having the same area (A) as the projected area of the particle resting in a stable position (see the text and Fig. 9.2)	$A = \dfrac{\pi}{4} d_a^2$
Perimeter diameter	d_p	Diameter of a circle having the same perimeter as the projected outline of the particle (see the text and Fig. 9.2)	None
Sieve diameter	d_A	The width of the minimum square aperture through which the particle will pass (see the text and Fig. 9.8)	None
Stokes diameter	d_{St}	The free-falling diameter (d_f, see above) of a particle in the laminar flow region ($Re_p < 0.2$)	Under these conditions, $d_{St}^2 = \dfrac{d_v^3}{d_d}$
Surface diameter	d_s	Diameter of a sphere having the same external surface area (S) as the particle	$S = \pi d_s^2$
Surface volume diameter	d_{sv}	Diameter of a sphere having the same external surface area to volume ratio as the particle	$d_{sv} = \dfrac{d_v^3}{d_s^2}$
Volume diameter	d_v	Diameter of a sphere having the same volume (V) as the particle	$V = \dfrac{\pi}{6} d_v^3$

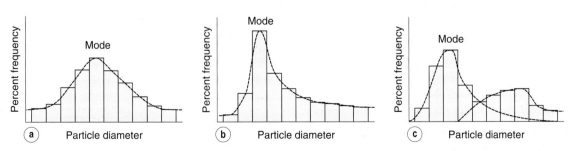

Fig. 9.4 • Size-frequency distribution curves and histograms corresponding to **(a)** a normal distribution, **(b)** a positively skewed distribution and **(c)** a bimodal distribution.

Table 9.2 Frequency and cumulative *frequency* distribution data for a nominal particle size analysis procedure

Range of equivalent diameters of particles measured *(known as the size fraction)* (μm)	Mean diameter of each size fraction (μm)	Number of particles in each size fraction *(frequency)*	Percentage of particles in each size fraction *(% frequency)*	Number of particles in the sample smaller than the mean diameter of each size fraction	Cumulative percent frequency smaller than the mean diameter of each size fraction *(cumulative percent undersize)*	Number of particles in the sample larger than the mean diameter of each size fraction	Cumulative percent frequency larger than the mean diameter of each size fraction *(cumulative percent oversize)*
≤9.9	–	0	0.0	0	0	2200	100.0
10–29.9	20	100	4.5	50	2.3	2150	97.7
30–49.9	40	200	9.1	200	9.1	2000	90.9
50–69.9	60	400	18.2	500	22.7	1700	77.3
70–89.9	80	800	36.4	1100	50.0	1100	50.0
90–109.9	100	400	18.2	1700	77.3	500	22.7
110–129.9	120	200	9.1	2000	90.9	200	9.1
130–149.9	140	100	4.5	2150	97.9	50	2.3
≥150		0	0.0	2200	100.0	0	0.0

that are *normally distributed* symmetrically about a central value. The peak frequency value, known as the *mode*, separates the *normal curve* into two identical halves, because the size distribution is fully symmetrical, i.e. the data in Table 9.2 are normally distributed.

Not all particle populations are characterized by symmetrical, 'normal' size distributions, and the frequency distributions of such populations are said to be skewed. The size distribution shown in Fig. 9.4b contains a large proportion of fine particles. A frequency curve such as this, with an elongated tail towards higher size ranges, is said to be *positively skewed*; the reverse case exhibits *negative skewness*. These skewed distributions can sometimes be normalized by the replotting of the equivalent particle diameters with use of a logarithmic scale, and are thus usually referred to as *log-normal distributions*.

In some size distributions more than one mode occurs: Fig. 9.4c shows a bimodal frequency distribution for a powder which has been subjected to milling. Some of the coarser particles from the unmilled population remain unbroken and produce a mode towards the largest particle size, whereas the fractured (size-reduced) particles have a new mode lower down the size range.

An alternative to the histogram or frequency curve representations of particle size distribution is obtained by sequential addition of the percent frequency values, as shown in Table 9.2, to produce a cumulative percent frequency distribution. If the addition sequence begins with the coarsest particles, the values obtained will be *cumulative percent frequency undersize* (or more commonly *cumulative percent undersize*); the reverse case produces a *cumulative percent oversize*.

It is possible to compare two or more particle populations by means of the cumulative distribution representation. Fig. 9.5 shows two cumulative percent frequency distributions. The size distribution in Fig. 9.5a shows that this powder has a larger range or spread of diameters (less steep gradient) than the powder represented in Fig. 9.5b. The median particle diameter corresponds to the point that separates the cumulative frequency curve into two equal halves, above and below which 50% of the particles lie (point *a* in Fig. 9.5).

Summarizing size distribution data

As we have seen, the mode and median are measures of central tendency, providing a single value near the middle of the size distribution that attempts to

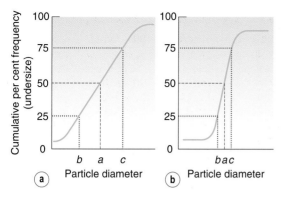

(a)   **(b)**

Fig. 9.5 • Cumulative-frequency distribution curves. Point *a* corresponds to the median diameter; *b* is the lower quartile point and *c* is the upper quartile point. Plot **(a)** is for particles having a wide size distribution and **(b)** is for a narrow size distribution.

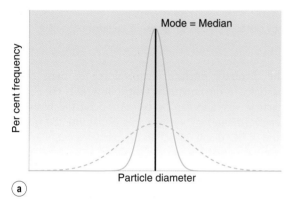

(a)

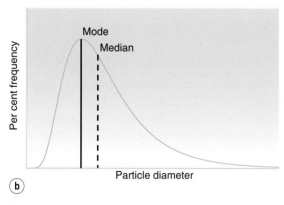

(b)

Fig. 9.6 • Size-frequency distribution curves, showing mean and mode values for **(a)** normal distributions for two populations of particles and **(b)** a positively skewed distribution.

represent a central particle diameter. For a normal distribution, the median and mode have the same value (Fig. 9.6a), whereas for skewed distributions the values will be different (Fig. 9.6b). However, from comparison of the two frequency curves shown

in Fig. 9.6a, it is clear that whilst both curves have the same values for the mode and median, the shapes of the curves differ, with one population of particles having a much wider size distribution, with both smaller and larger particles, than the other. Although it is possible to describe particle size distributions qualitatively, it is more useful to express particle size distribution data quantitatively. Thus log-normal distributions are frequently characterized by the median diameter and the geometric standard deviation of the size distribution.

An established method is to use a three-point size distribution, based on the diameters below which 90%, 50% and 10% of the particles lie. This is shown in Fig. 9.7, with values most readily calculated from a cumulative percent undersize plot. The values for the diameters may be written as

X_{90}, D90, d_{90}, or $D[0.90]$;

X_{50}, D50, d_{50}, or $D[0.50]$; and

X_{10}, D10, d_{10}, or $D[0.10]$.

It is also possible to summarize, mathematically, the symmetry of size distributions.

Just as the median divides a symmetrical cumulative size distribution curve into two equal halves, so the lower and upper quartile points at 25% and 75% divide the upper and lower ranges of a symmetrical curve into equal parts (points *b* and *c* respectively in Fig. 9.5).

To quantify the degree of skewness of a particle population, the *interquartile coefficient of skewness* (IQCS) can be determined as follows:

$$IQCS = \frac{(c-a)-(a-b)}{(c-a)+(a-b)}$$

(9.1)

where *a* is the median diameter and *b* and *c* are the lower and upper quartile points (see Fig. 9.5).

The IQCS can take any value between −1 and +1. If the IQCS is 0, then the size distribution is practically symmetrical between the quartile points. To avoid ambiguity in interpreting values for the IQCS, a large number of size intervals are required.

The degree of symmetry of a particle size distribution may also be quantified by calculation of a property known as *kurtosis*. The symmetry of a distribution is based on a comparison of the height or thickness of the tails and the 'sharpness' of the peaks of a frequency distribution with those of a normal distribution. 'Thick'-tailed, 'sharp' peaked curves are described

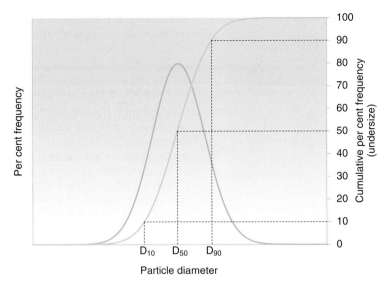

Fig. 9.7 • Size-frequency distribution and cumulative-frequency distribution curves, showing determination of triple-point size distribution parameters.

as *leptokurtic*, whereas 'thin'-tailed, 'blunt' peaked curves are *platykurtic* and the normal distribution is *mesokurtic*.

The coefficient of kurtosis, k (Eqn 9.2), has a value of 0 for a normal curve, a negative value for curves showing platykurtosis and positive values for leptokurtic size distributions:

$$k = \frac{N \sum (d-x)^4}{\left[\sum (d-x)^2 \right]^2} - 3$$

$$(9.2)$$

where d is any particle diameter, x is the mean particle diameter and N is the number of particles. Again, a large number of data points are required to provide an accurate analysis.

Mean particle sizes

As outlined already, it is impossible for any single number to fully describe the size distribution of particles in a real pharmaceutical system. However, for simplicity, pharmaceutical scientists wish to use a single number to represent the mean size of a powder sample. It is possible to define and calculate the 'mean' particle size in several ways.

Arithmetic means are obtained by summation of a particular parameter for all the individual particles in a sample and division of the value obtained by the total number of particles. Means can be related to

the diameter, surface area, volume or mass of a particle. In the equations that follow, D is the mean particle size and can be calculated on the basis of length (diameter), surface area or volume, Σd is the sum of the diameters of all the particles and n is the number of particles in the sample:

number-length mean: $D[1, 0] = \dfrac{\sum d}{n}$

$$(9.3)$$

number-surface mean: $D[2, 0] = \sqrt{\dfrac{\sum d^2}{n}}$

$$(9.4)$$

number-volume mean: $D[3, 0] = \sqrt[3]{\dfrac{\sum d^3}{n}}$

$$(9.5)$$

Such means are strictly referred to as *number mean* or *number average* particle sizes as they are based on the number of particles. Mean particle sizes based on length (radius/diameter) are smaller than the equivalent mean sizes based on volume or weight, as the latter are related to the radius cubed.

When one is sizing many particles, as occurs with modern, automated sizing techniques, such as laser diffraction described later in the chapter, equations may be used to calculate mean sizes in which the number of particles do not appear. For instance, the following may be calculated:

$$\text{volume-surface mean:} \quad D[3,2] = \frac{\sum d^3}{\sum d^2}$$

(9.6)

volume-moment or mass-moment mean:

$$D[4,3] = \frac{\sum d^4}{\sum d^3}$$

(9.7)

The volume-moment mean diameter is calculated by the software associated with a number of instruments and is often simply quoted as the $D[4,3]$. This is also sometimes referred to as the volume mean diameter or VMD, which for a given population of particles is likely to differ numerically from the volume median diameter (X_{50}), which may confusingly also be abbreviated to VMD.

Box 9.1 shows how such equations may be used to calculate the mean of a sample of particles.

Interconversion of mean sizes

For powders exhibiting a log-normal distribution of particle size, a series of relationships, sometimes known as the Hatch–Choate equations, link the different mean diameters of a size distribution. There are numerous combinations of these, and the interested reader is referred to Allen (1997) for further details.

Influence of particle shape

The techniques discussed so far for representing particle size distributions are all based on the assumption that particles can be adequately represented by an equivalent circle or sphere. Whilst this is usually the case, in some pharmaceutically relevant cases, particles may deviate markedly from sphericity, and the use of a single equivalent sphere diameter measurement may be inappropriate. For example, a powder consisting of monosized, needle-like, acicular particles would appear to have a wide size distribution according to statistical diameter measurements. However, the use of an equivalent diameter based on projected area would also be misleading. The shape of such particles may simply be characterized by calculation of the *aspect ratio* (A_R):

Box 9.1

Worked example calculating mean particle size

You measure the size of three spherical particles using a light microscope; one has a diameter of 1 μm, the second a diameter of 2 μm and the third a diameter of 3 μm. What is the mean diameter of these three particles?

The answer is self-evidently 2 μm. One does not need to be studying at degree level to add up the diameters and divide the total by the number of particles, and you are, of course, correct. You have intuitively calculated the number-length mean, expressed mathematically by Eq. 9.3 as $\frac{\sum d}{n}$, i.e. you summed the diameters (d) of the particles, then divided the sum by the number of particles (n). However, sometimes pharmaceutical scientists are particularly interested in the surface area of drug particles (e.g. in dissolution processes), which is related to d^2, or the volume of drug particles (dose is dependent on the mass of particles, which is a function of volume), which is related to d^3. More pharmaceutically useful means can thus be calculated by Eqs 9.4–9.7.

Considering our three particles with diameters of 1 μm, 2 μm and 3 μm, you can now calculate the following means, all of which are correct!

$$D[1,0] = \frac{\sum d}{n} = 2.00 \ \mu m$$

$$D[2,0] = \sqrt{\frac{\sum d^2}{n}} = 2.16 \ \mu m$$

$$D[3,0] = \sqrt[3]{\frac{\sum d^3}{n}} = 2.29 \ \mu m$$

$$D[3,2] = \frac{\sum d^3}{\sum d^2} = 2.57 \ \mu m$$

$$D[4,3] = \frac{\sum d^4}{\sum d^3} = 2.72 \ \mu m$$

$$A_R = X_{min} / X_{max}$$

(9.8)

where X_{min} and X_{max} are the minimum dimension and the maximum dimension respectively.

Another shape factor is circularity, sometimes termed sphericity, which seeks to quantify how closely the shape of a particle approximates to a sphere. Confusingly, a number of formulae exist for this parameter. One common approach is to calculate circularity (f_{circ}), from the perimeter (p) and area (A) of a particle:

$$f_{circ} = 4\pi A / p^2$$

(9.9)

Particle size analysis methods

To obtain equivalent sphere diameters with which to characterize the particle size of a powder, it is necessary to perform a size analysis with use of one or more different methods. Particle size analysis methods can be divided into different categories based on several different criteria: size range of analysis; wet or dry methods; manual or automated methods; cost or speed of analysis. The specialist area of sizing aerosolized particles using cascade impactor techniques is described in Chapter 37. Particle size instrumentation is developing quickly, but a summary of the principles of the methods most commonly encountered in pharmaceutics is presented here, based on the key features of each technique.

Sieve methods

Equivalent sphere diameter

Sieve diameter, d_A, as defined in Table 9.1 and shown diagrammatically in Fig. 9.8 for different-shaped particles.

Range of analysis

The International Organization for Standardization sets a lowest sieve diameter of 45 μm and, as powders are usually defined as having a maximum diameter of 1000 μm, this could be considered to be the upper limit. In practice, sieves can be obtained for size analysis over a range from 5 μm to 125 000 μm. These ranges are shown diagrammatically in Fig. 9.9.

Sample preparation and analysis conditions

Sieve analysis is usually performed with powders in the dry state, although for powders in liquid suspension or for those which agglomerate during dry sieving, a process of wet sieving can be used.

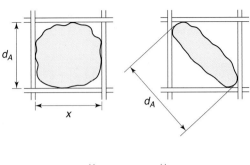
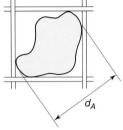

Fig. 9.8 • Sieve diameter d_A for particles of various shapes. x is the size of the sieve aperture.

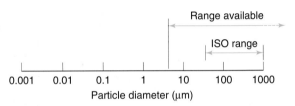

Fig. 9.9 • Size range of analysis using sieves. *ISO*, International Organization for Standardization.

Principles of measurement

Sieve analysis uses a woven, punched or electroformed mesh, often made from stainless steel or brass, with known aperture dimensions which forms a physical barrier to the particles. Most sieve analyses use a series, stack or 'nest' of sieves, which has the smallest mesh above a collection tray, above which are meshes that become progressively coarser towards the top of the stack of sieves. A sieve stack usually comprises six to eight sieves with an aperture progression based on a $\sqrt{2}$ change in area between adjacent sieves. Powder is loaded onto the coarsest sieve at the top of the assembled stack, and the nest is subjected to mechanical agitation. After a suitable time, the sieve diameter of a particle is the length of the side of the minimum square aperture through which it has passed. The weight of material collected on each stage is determined and used to plot a cumulative-undersize plot. Sieving is rarely complete as some particles can take a long time to orient themselves over the sieve apertures and pass through. Thus sieving times, which are usually 5–30 minutes for dry sieving, should not be arbitrary and should be defined; hence it is recommended when standard-sized sieves (200 mm diameter) are used that sieving be continued until the mass on any sieve does not change by more than 5% or 1 g of the previous mass on that sieve.

Alternative techniques

Another form of sieve analysis, called *air-jet sieving*, uses individual sieves rather than a complete nest of sieves. The process starts with the finest-aperture sieve and progressively removes the undersize particle fraction by sequentially increasing the apertures of each sieve, encouraging particles to pass through each aperture under the influence of a partial vacuum applied below the sieve mesh. A reverse air jet circulates beneath the sieve mesh, blowing oversize particles away from the mesh to prevent blockages. Air-jet sieving is often more efficient and reproducible than conventional mechanically vibrated sieve analysis, although with finer particles, agglomeration can become a problem. In the related method, *sonic-sifter sieving*, relatively small powder samples are lifted in a vertically oscillating column of air, such that particles are carried against a sieve mesh at a set number of pulses per minute.

Microscope methods

Equivalent sphere diameters

Projected area diameter, d_a, perimeter diameter, d_p, Feret's diameter, d_F, and Martin's diameter, d_M (all defined in Table 9.1).

Range of analysis

This is shown diagrammatically in Fig. 9.10.

Sample preparation and analysis conditions

Specimens prepared for light microscopy must be adequately dispersed on a microscope slide to avoid analysis of agglomerated particles. Specimens for scanning electron microscopy are prepared by their being fixed to aluminium stubs before being sputter coated with a film of gold a few nanometres in thickness. Specimens for transmission electron microscopy are often set in resin, sectioned by a microtome and supported on a metal grid before they are stained.

Light microscopy

Principles of measurement

Size analysis by light microscopy is performed on two-dimensional images of particles which are generally assumed to be randomly oriented in three dimensions. In many cases, this assumption is valid, although for crystal dendrites, fibres or flakes, it is very improbable that the particles will orient with their minimum dimensions in the plane of measurement. Under such conditions, size analysis is performed accepting that such particles are viewed in their most stable orientation. This will lead to an overestimation of size because the larger dimensions of the particle will be observed, as the smallest dimension will most often orient vertically.

The two-dimensional images are analysed according to the desired equivalent diameter. With use of a conventional light microscope, particle size analysis can be performed with an eyepiece graticule which has previously been calibrated. One can also use a graticule which has a series of opaque and transparent circles of different diameters, usually in a $\sqrt{2}$ progression. Particles are compared with the two sets of circles and are sized according to the circle that corresponds most closely to the equivalent particle

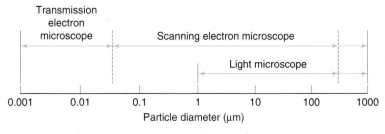

Fig. 9.10 • Size range of analysis using microscopy.

diameter being measured. The field of view is divided into segments to facilitate measurement of different numbers of particles.

Electron microscopy

Alternatives to light microscopy include scanning electron microscopy (SEM) and transmission electron microscopy. SEM is particularly appropriate when a three-dimensional particle image is required; in addition, the very much greater depth of field of an SEM compared with a light microscope may also be beneficial. Both scanning electron microscopy analysis and transmission electron microscopy analysis allow the lower particle sizing limit to be greatly extended over that possible with a light microscope.

Image analysis

With manual microscopy, only a few particles can be examined and sized in a reasonable time. This risks selection of an unrepresentative sample, operator subjectivity and operator fatigue. Automated image analysis, for light and electron microscopy, has the advantages of being more objective and much faster than manual analysis, and it also enables a much wider variety of size and shape parameters to be processed. Image acquisition is usually achieved by digital imaging, with a charge-coupled device (CCD) sensor placed in the optical path of the microscope to generate high-resolution images. This allows both image analysis and image processing to be performed. Image analysis may be static, whereby particles on a microscope slide are inspected with use of a microscope and digital camera, or dynamic (flow-image analysis), whereby images of particles dispersed in a liquid are captured by a camera as they pass through a flow cell. Each particle passing through the cell is counted and imaged, with information provided about the particle's size, morphology (shape parameters) and transparency.

Sedimentation methods

Equivalent sphere diameters

(Frictional) drag diameter, d_d, and Stokes diameter, d_{St} (Table 9.1).

Range of analysis

This is shown diagrammatically in Fig. 9.11.

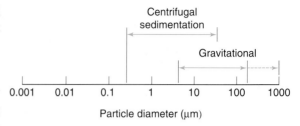

Fig. 9.11 • Size range of analysis using sedimentation methods.

Sample preparation and analysis conditions

Particle size distributions can be determined by examination of a powder as it sediments in a liquid. In cases where the powder is not uniformly dispersed in a fluid, it can be introduced as a thin layer on the surface of the liquid. If the powder is hydrophobic, it may be necessary to add a dispersing agent to aid wetting. In cases where the powder is soluble in water, it will be necessary to use nonaqueous liquids or perform the analysis in a gas.

Principles of measurement

The techniques of size analysis by sedimentation can be divided into two main categories according to the method of measurement used. One type is based on the measurement of particles in a retention zone; a second type uses a nonretention measurement zone.

An example of a nonretention zone measurement method is known as the pipette method. In this method, known volumes of suspension are withdrawn and the concentration differences are measured with respect to time.

One of the most popular of the pipette methods is that developed by Andreasen and Lundberg and is commonly called the Andreasen pipette (Fig. 9.12). The Andreasen fixed-position pipette comprises a graduated cylinder which can hold approximately 500 mL of suspension fluid. A pipette is located centrally in the cylinder and is held in position by a ground-glass stopper so that its tip coincides with the zero level. A three-way tap allows fluid to be drawn into a 10 mL reservoir, which can then be emptied into a beaker or centrifuge tube. The amount of powder can be determined by weight following drying or centrifuging; alternatively, chemical analysis of the collected particles can be performed.

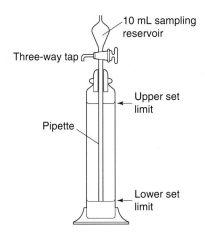

Fig. 9.12 • Representation of an Andreasen pipette.

The largest size present in each sample is then calculated from Stokes's equation. Stokes's law is an expression of the drag factor in a fluid and is linked to the flow conditions characterized by the Reynolds number. Drag is one of three forces acting on a particle sedimenting in a gravitational field. A drag force, F_d, acts upwards, as does a buoyancy force, F_b; a third force is gravity, F_g, which acts as the driving force of sedimentation. At the constant terminal velocity, which is rapidly achieved by sedimenting particles, the drag force becomes synonymous with particle motion. Thus for a sphere of diameter d and density ρ_s, falling in a fluid of density ρ_f, the equation of motion is

$$F_d = \frac{\pi}{6}(\rho_s - \rho_f)F_g d^3$$

(9.10)

According to Stokes,

$$F_d = 3\pi d_h \eta v_{St}$$

(9.11)

where v_{St} is the Stokes terminal velocity, i.e. sedimentation rate. That is,

$$v_{St} = \frac{(\rho_s - \rho_f)F_g d^2}{18\eta}$$

(9.12)

as $v_{St} = h/t$, where h is the sedimentation height or distance and t is the sedimentation time. By rearrangement, Stokes's equation is obtained:

$$d_{St} = \sqrt{\frac{18\eta h}{(\rho_s - \rho_f)F_g t}}$$

(9.13)

Stokes's equation for determining particle diameters is based on the following assumptions:

- near-spherical particles;
- motion equivalent to that in a fluid of infinite length;
- terminal velocity conditions;
- low settling velocity so that inertia is negligible;
- large particle size relative to fluid molecular size, so that diffusion is negligible;
- no particle aggregation; and
- laminar flow conditions, characterized by particle Reynolds numbers ($Re_p = \rho_s v_{St} d_{st}/\eta$) of less than approximately 0.2.

The second type of sedimentation size analysis, using retention zone methods, also uses Stokes's law to quantify particle size. One of the most common retention zone methods uses a sedimentation balance. In this method the amount of sedimented particles falling onto a balance pan suspended in the fluid is recorded. The continual increase in the weight of sediment is recorded with respect to time.

Alternative techniques

One of the limitations of gravitational sedimentation is that below a diameter of approximately 5 μm, particle settling becomes prolonged and is subject to interference from convection, diffusion and Brownian motion. One can minimize these effects by increasing the driving force of sedimentation by replacing gravitational forces with a larger centrifugal force. Once again, sedimentation can be monitored by retention or nonretention methods, although Stokes's equation requires modification because particles are subjected to different forces according to their distance from the axis of rotation. To minimize the effect of distance on the sedimenting force, a two-layer fluid system can be used. A small quantity of concentrated suspension is introduced onto the surface of a bulk sedimentation liquid known as the spin fluid. With use of the technique of disc centrifugation, all particles of the same size are in the same position in the centrifugal field and hence move with the same velocity. An adaptation of a retention zone gravity sedimentation method is known as a *micromerograph* and measures sedimentation of particles in a gas rather than a fluid. The advantages of this method are that sizing and analysis are achieved relatively rapidly.

Electrical sensing zone (electrozone sensing) method (Coulter Counter®)

Equivalent sphere diameter

Volume diameter, d_v (Table 9.1).

Range of analysis

This is shown diagrammatically in Fig. 9.13.

Sample preparation and analysis conditions

Powder samples are dispersed in an electrolyte to form a very dilute suspension, which is usually subjected to ultrasonic agitation, for a period, to break up any particle aggregates. A dispersant may also be added to aid particle deaggregation.

Principles of measurement

The particle suspension is drawn through an aperture/orifice (Fig. 9.14) accurately drilled through a sapphire crystal set into the wall of a hollow glass tube. Electrodes, which are situated on either side of the aperture and surrounded by an electrolyte solution, monitor the change in electrical signal that occurs when a particle momentarily occupies the orifice and displaces its own volume of electrolyte. The volume of suspension drawn through the orifice is determined by the suction potential created by mercury rebalancing in a convoluted U-tube (Fig. 9.15). The volume of electrolyte fluid which is displaced in the

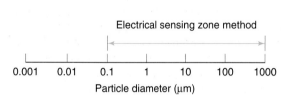

Fig. 9.13 • Size range of analysis using the electrical sensing zone method.

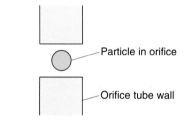

Fig. 9.14 • Particle passing through the measuring aperture of electrical sensing zone apparatus.

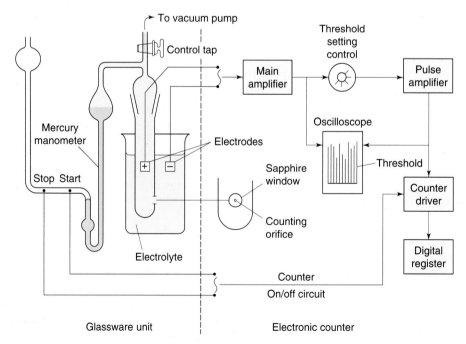

Fig. 9.15 • Electrical sensing zone apparatus.

orifice by the presence of a particle causes a change in electrical resistance between the electrodes that is proportional to the volume of the particle. The change in resistance is converted into a voltage pulse, which is amplified and processed electronically. Pulses falling within precalibrated limits or thresholds are used to split the particle size distribution into many different size ranges. To perform size analysis over a wide diameter range, it will be necessary to change the orifice diameter (and hence tube) used, to prevent coarser particles blocking a small-diameter orifice. Conversely, finer particles in a large-diameter orifice will cause too small a relative change in volume to be accurately quantified. Dispersions must be sufficiently dilute to avoid the occurrence of *coincidence*, whereby more than one particle may be present in the orifice at any one time. This may result in a loss of count (i.e. two particles counted as one) and inaccurate measurement as the equivalent sphere diameter calculated is based on the volume of two particles, rather than one.

Since the electrical sensing zone method principle was first described, there have been some modifications to the basic method, such as the use of alternative orifice designs and hydrodynamic focusing, but in general the particle sizing technique remains the same.

Another type of stream-sensing analyser uses the attenuation of a light beam by particles drawn through the sensing zone. Some instruments of this type use the change in reflectance, whereas others use the change in transmittance of light. It is also possible to use ultrasonic waves generated and monitored by a piezoelectric crystal at the base of a flow-through tube containing particles in fluid suspension.

Laser diffraction (low-angle laser light scattering)

Equivalent sphere diameters

Fraunhofer-diffraction models are based on the projected area diameter, d_a, and Mie theory assumes a volume model. Following computation, data are presented as the volume diameter, d_v (defined in Table 9.1).

Range of analysis

This is shown diagrammatically in Fig. 9.16.

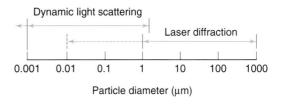

Fig. 9.16 • Size range of analysis using laser-light-scattering methods: laser diffraction and dynamic light scattering.

Sample preparation and analysis conditions

Depending on the type of measurement to be performed and the instrument used, particles can be presented to the instrument dispersed in either a liquid or a gas. Adequate dispersion is required to ensure aggregates of particles are dispersed into primary particles if that is the purpose of the assay. For particles dispersed in liquid, a dispersing agent (e.g. a surfactant) and/or mechanical agitation may be required. Dry powders may be dispersed with use of compressed gas at a pressure sufficient to ensure adequate dispersion, without causing undue attrition and consequent size reduction.

Principles of measurement

Monochromatic light from a helium–neon laser is incident on the sample of particles, dispersed at the appropriate concentration in a liquid or gas, and diffraction occurs. The scattered light pattern is focused by a Fourier lens directly onto a photodetector, comprising a series of detectors (Fig. 9.17). The light flux signals occurring on the photodetector are converted into electric current, which is digitized and processed into size-distribution data, based on an optical model using the principles of Fraunhofer diffraction or Mie theory. The measured scattering of the population of particles is taken to be the sum of the scattering of the individual particles within that sample.

Fraunhofer diffraction and Mie theory

For particles that are much larger than the wavelength of light, any interaction with particles causes light to be scattered in a forward direction with only a small change in angle. This phenomenon is known as Fraunhofer diffraction and produces light intensity patterns that occur at regular angular intervals, with the angle of scatter inversely proportional to the

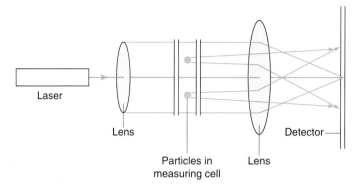

Fig. 9.17 • Laser diffraction particle sizer.

diameter of the particle producing it. The composite diffraction pattern produced by different-diameter particles may be considered to be the sum of all the individual patterns produced by each particle in the size distribution, at low to medium particle concentrations. The Fraunhofer model was used in early instruments and has the advantage that the refractive indices of samples and the dispersing medium do not need to be known, i.e. the model assumes particles are opaque and transmit no light.

As the size of particles approaches the dimension of the wavelength of the light, some light is still scattered in the forward direction, according to *Mie scatter theory*, but there is also some side scatter at different wavelengths and polarizations. Use of the Mie theory requires consideration of the optical properties of the dispersed particles and the dispersion medium, i.e. knowledge of their respective refractive indices is required for calculation of particle size distributions, but is superior for accurate determination of size distributions of smaller particles.

Dynamic light scattering (photon correlation spectroscopy)

Equivalent sphere diameter

Hydrodynamic diameter, d_h, defined in Table 9.1.

Range of analysis

This is shown diagrammatically in Fig. 9.16.

Sample preparation and analysis conditions

Particles are presented, suspended in a liquid of known viscosity. Mechanical agitation/sonication may be required to achieve adequate dispersion of particles.

Principles of measurement

In dynamic light scattering (DLS), also called photon correlation spectroscopy and quasielastic light scattering, the intensity of scattered light at a given angle is measured as a function of time for a population of particles. The rate of change of the scattered light intensity is a function of the movement of the particles by Brownian motion. Brownian motion is the random movement of a small particle or macromolecule caused by collisions with the smaller molecules of the fluid in which it is suspended. It is independent of external variations, except the viscosity of the suspending fluid and its temperature, and as it randomizes particle orientations, any effects of particle shape are minimized. Brownian motion is independent of the suspending medium, and although an increase in the viscosity does slow down the motion, the amplitude of the movements is unaltered. Because the suspended, small particles are always in a state of motion, they undergo diffusion. Diffusion is governed by the mean free path of a molecule or particle, which is the average distance of travel before diversion by collision with another molecule. DLS analyses the constantly changing patterns of laser light scattered or diffracted by particles undergoing Brownian motion, and monitors the rate of change of scattered light during diffusion. In most instruments, monochromatic light from a helium–neon laser is focused onto the measurement zone, containing particles dispersed in a liquid medium (Fig. 9.18). Light is scattered at all angles, and is often detected by a detector placed at an angle of 90°, although other angles may be chosen, depending on the instrument used. The detection

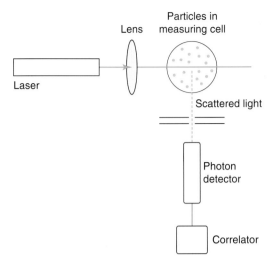

Lens   Particles in
         measuring cell

Laser

Scattered light

Photon
detector

Correlator

Fig. 9.18 • Dynamic light scattering particle sizer.

and spatial resolution of the fluctuations in the intensity of the scattered light, are used to calculate size distribution.

Brownian diffusion causes three-dimensional random movement of particles, where the mean distance travelled, $\bar{x}$, does not increase linearly with time, t, but according to the following relationship:

$$\bar{x} = \sqrt{Dt}$$

(9.14)

where D is the diffusion coefficient.

Eq. 9.15, known as the Stokes–Einstein equation, is the basis for calculating particle diameters by DLS:

$$D = \frac{1.38 \times 10^{-12} T}{3\pi\eta d_h} \, m^2\,s^{-1}$$

(9.15)

where d_h is the hydrodynamic diameter, η the fluid viscosity and T the absolute temperature (kelvins).

This calculation assumes that particles are spherical, and a very low particle concentration is required. The technique determines the hydrodynamic diameter. As colloidal particles in a liquid dispersion have an adsorbed layer of ions/molecules from the dispersion medium that moves with the particles, the hydrodynamic diameter is larger than the physical size of the particle. Most instruments also yield a polydispersity index (PDI), determined by cumulant analysis as described in the international standard on particle size analysis by DLS. The PDI, a dimensionless term, gives information regarding the width of

the size distribution, with values ranging between 0 and 1. For monodisperse samples, the PDI is theoretically zero, although values from 0 to 0.08 are taken as indicative of nearly monodisperse systems, whilst values from 0.08 to 0.2 represent particles having a relatively narrow size distribution.

Available instruments differ according to their ability to characterize different particle size ranges, produce complete size distributions, measure dispersions of both solid and liquid particles and determine the molecular weights of macromolecules. Some instruments combine DLS to determine particle size with electrophoretic light scattering to measure the electrophoretic movement of dispersed particles. The velocity of particles moving between two electrodes is measured by laser Doppler velocimetry and can be used to determine their zeta potential.

Particle counting

Sometimes it is necessary to know not only the size of particles but also their number or concentration. Pharmaceutically, this is most frequently encountered in tests to determine the subvisible particulate contamination of injections and infusions.

In the past, the electrical zone sensing method was used to count and size particles in a known volume of liquid as it is drawn through the orifice. Nowadays, the method of choice is *light obscuration*. Light obscuration requires a very dilute sample of particles in a liquid which is passed between a light source (laser) and a detector. The presence of particles in the beam causes blockage/obscuration of light, and the resultant signal is processed to give a number and size range of particles in a given volume. Alternatively, microscopy can be used to size and count particles retained on a filter following filtration of a known volume of liquid-dispersed particles. Microscopy combined with flow-image analysis is gaining acceptance as a method for counting and sizing small particles, whilst providing information on their morphology. This has shown particular application in the identification and sizing of aggregates in protein solutions.

Selection of a particle size analysis method

The selection of a particle size analysis method may be constrained by the instruments available in a laboratory, but wherever possible the choice of

Table 9.3 Summary of particle size analysis instrument characteristics

Analysis method		Sample measurement environment			Rapid analysis	Approximate size range (µm)				Initial cost	
		Gas	Aqueous liquid	Nonaqueous liquid		0.001–1	1–10	10–100	100–1000	High	Low
Sieve		√	√	√				√	√		√
Light microscopy	Manual	√	√	√			√	√	√		√
	Image analysis	√	√	√	√		√	√	√	√	
Electron microscopy						√	√	√	√	√	
Electrical sensing zone			√		√		√	√	√	√	
Laser diffraction		√	√	√	√	√	√	√	√	√	
Dynamic light scattering			√	√	√	√					
Sedimentation	Gravitational	√	√	√	√		√	√			√
	Centrifugal		√	√	√	√	√	√		√	

method should be governed by the properties of the sample being investigated and the type of size information required. For example, size analysis over a very wide range of particle diameters may preclude the use of a gravitational sedimentation method; alternatively, size analysis of tablet granules would not be done by DLS. As a general guide, it is often most appropriate to determine the particle size distribution of a powder in an environment that most closely resembles the conditions in which the powder will be processed or handled. There are many different factors influencing the selection of an analysis method: these are summarized in Table 9.3

and should be considered together with information from a preliminary microscopy analysis and any other known physical properties of the powder, such as solubility, density and cohesiveness. Further analysis requirements should then be considered, such as speed of measurement, particle size data processing, initial and ongoing costs of equipment, and the physical separation of powders of different particle size for subsequent processing.

Please check your eBook at **https://studentconsult. inkling.com/** for self-assessment questions. See inside cover for registration details.

Reference

Allen, T., 1997. Particle Size Measurement, vol. 1 and 2, fifth ed. Chapman and Hall, London.

Bibliography

Ahuja, S., Scypinski, S. (Eds.), 2010. Handbook of Modern Pharmaceutical Analysis, second ed. Academic Press, Amsterdam.

Allen, T., 2003. Powder Sampling and Particle Size Determination. Elsevier, Amsterdam.

American Society for Testing and
Materials Standards (1985) Manual
on Test Sieving Methods. ASTM
Special Technical Publication.
American Society for Testing and
Materials Standards, West
Conshohocken.

Barnett, M.I., Nystrom, C., 1982.
Coulter counters and microscopes
for the measurement of particles in
the sieve range. Pharmaceutical
Technology 6, 49–50.

de Boer, G.B.J., de Weerd, C.,
Thoenes, D., et al., 1987. Laser
diffraction spectrometry: Fraunhofer
diffraction versus Mie scattering.
Part Part Syst Charact 4,
14–19.

Kaye, B.H., 2006. Particle-size
characterization. In: Swarbrick, J.
(Ed.), Encyclopedia of
Pharmaceutical Technology, third ed.
Informa Healthcare, New York.

Masuda, H., Higashitani, K., Yoshida,
H. (Eds.), 2006. Powder Technology
Handbook, third ed. CRC Press,
Boca Raton.

Merkus, H.G., 2009. Particle Size
Measurements: Fundamentals,
Practice, Quality. Springer, New
York.

Rhodes, M. (Ed.), 1990. Principles of
Powder Technology. John Wiley &
Sons, Chichester.

Xu, R., 2000. Particle Characterization:
Light Scattering Methods. Particle
Technology Series, vol. 13. Springer,
New York.

Particle size reduction and size separation

Michael E. Aulton

CHAPTER CONTENTS

KEY POINTS

- The particle size of solid drugs and excipients has a significant effect on many of their properties, including the rate of dissolution and powder flow characteristics.

- During raw material manufacture, the solid produced is often of a larger size than that required pharmaceutically, and thus size reduction is a key process prior to incorporation of the material into a finished product.

- Solid particles possess a range of mechanical properties and consequently a number of different mechanisms of size reduction exist, dependent upon these properties for the material in question. In turn, this influences the design of the commercial equipment for efficient size reduction.

- The correct choice of the most efficient commercial size reduction machinery will depend upon knowledge of these properties and mechanisms.

- The method of size reduction not only affects the mean particle size but also the distribution of the sizes of the powdered material. Methods of determining and representing mean size and size distribution are discussed.

- It is often necessary to separate out from a widely distributed range of sizes the single size or narrow range of sizes that is best suited for the application in hand. This required size will depend on the subsequent use of the material. For example, a drug used in a dry powder inhalation formulation will need to be of a very different size than that required in an oral solid dosage form.

- Many different commercial size separation methodologies and apparatus exist – their designs are dependent on the final required particle size and the size of the commercial batch. These methods include sedimentation, sieving elutriation and cyclone methods.

- As with size reduction, the pharmaceutical scientist must understand the parameters for the selection of the best method for the material in question.

Introduction to size reduction

The significance of particle size in drug delivery has been discussed in Chapter 9, and some of the reasons for performing a size reduction operation have already been noted. In addition, the function of size reduction (also called *comminution*) may be to aid efficient processing of solid particles by facilitating powder mixing or the production of suspensions. There are also some special functions of size reduction, such as exposing cells in plant tissue prior to extraction of the active principles or reducing the bulk volume of a material to improve transportation efficiency.

Influence of material properties on size reduction

Crack propagation and toughness

Size reduction, or comminution, is carried out by a process of *crack propagation*, whereby localized stresses produce strains in the particles that are large enough to cause bond rupture and thus propagate the crack. In general, cracks are propagated through regions of a material that possess the most flaws or discontinuities. Crack propagation is related to the strain energy in specific regions according to Griffith's theory. The stress in a material is concentrated at the tip of a crack, and the stress multiplier can be calculated from an equation developed by Inglis:

$$\sigma_K = 1 + 2\left(\frac{L}{2r}\right)$$

(10.1)

where σ_K is the multiplier of the mean stress in a material around a crack, L is the length of the crack and r is the radius of curvature of the tip of the crack. For a simple geometric structure such as a circular discontinuity, $L = 2r$ and the stress multiplier σ_K will have a value of 3.

In the case of a thin disc-shaped crack, shown in cross section in Fig. 10.1, the crack is considered to have occurred at a molecular level between atomic surfaces separated by a distance of 2×10^{-10} m for a crack 3 μm long, which gives a stress multiplier of approximately 245. The stress concentration diminishes towards the mean stress according to the distance from the crack tip (Fig. 10.1). Once a crack has been initiated, the crack tip propagates at a velocity

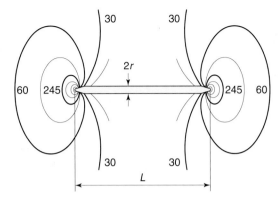

Fig. 10.1 • Stress concentrations at the edges of a disc-shaped crack; *r* is the radius of curvature of the crack tip and *L* is the crack length.

approaching 40% of the speed of sound in the solid. This crack propagation is so rapid that excess energy from strain relaxation is dissipated through the material and concentrates at other discontinuities, where new cracks are propagated. Thus a cascade effect occurs and almost instantaneous brittle fracture occurs.

Not all materials exhibit this type of brittle behaviour, and some can resist fracture at much larger stresses. This occurs because these tougher materials can undergo *plastic flow*, which allows strain energy relaxation without crack propagation. When plastic flow occurs, atoms or molecules slip over one another, and this process of deformation requires energy. Brittle materials can also exhibit plastic flow, and Irwin and Orowan suggested a modification of Griffiths' crack theory to take this into account. This relationship has a fracture stress, σ, which varies inversely with the square root of the crack length, L:

$$\sigma = \frac{E_p}{\sqrt{L}}$$

(10.2)

where E_p is the energy required to form unit area of double surface.

It can therefore be seen that the ease of comminution depends on the brittleness or plasticity of the material because of their relationship with crack initiation and crack propagation.

Surface hardness

In addition to the toughness of the material described in the previous section, size reduction may also be influenced by the hardness of the material. Hardness can be described empirically by its position on a scale devised by a German mineralogist called Mohs. The Mohs scale is a table of minerals; at the top of the table is diamond, with Mohs hardness >7, and this has a surface that is so hard that it can scratch anything below it. At the bottom of the table is talc, with Mohs hardness <3, and this is soft enough to be scratched by anything above it.

A quantitative measurement of surface hardness was devised by Brinell. This involves placing a hard spherical indenter (e.g. hardened steel or sapphire) in contact with the test surface and applying a known constant load to the sphere. The indenter will penetrate into the surface, and when the sphere is removed, the permanent deformation of the sample is measured. From this, the hardness of the material can be calculated. Hardness has the dimensions of stress (force applied to the indenter divided by the area of test material that will support the load, example units are MPa). A similar Vickers hardness test employs a square-pyramidal diamond as the indenter tip.

Such determinations of hardness are useful as a guide to the ease with which size reduction can be carried out because, while it appears to be a surface assessment, the test actually quantifies the deformation characteristics of the bulk solid. In general, harder materials are more difficult to comminute and can lead to abrasive wear of metal mill parts, which can then result in product contamination. Conversely, materials with a large elastic component, such as rubber, are extremely soft yet difficult to size-reduce.

Materials such as rubber that are soft under ambient conditions, waxy substances such as stearic acid that soften when heated, and 'sticky' materials such as gums are capable of absorbing large amounts of energy through elastic and plastic deformation without crack initiation and propagation. This type of material, which resists comminution at ambient or elevated temperatures, can be more easily size-reduced when temperatures are lowered below the glass transition point of the material. At these lower temperatures the material undergoes a transition from plastic to brittle behaviour, and crack propagation is facilitated.

Other factors that influence the process of size reduction include the moisture content of the material. In general, a material with a moisture content less than 5% is suitable for dry grinding and one with a moisture content greater than 50% will generally require wet grinding to be carried out.

Energy requirements of the size reduction process

Only a very small amount of the energy put into a comminution operation actually effects size reduction. This has been estimated to be as little as 2% of the total energy consumption, the remainder being lost in many ways, including:

- elastic deformation of particles;
- plastic deformation of particles without fracture;
- deformation to initiate cracks that cause fracture;
- deformation of metal machine parts;
- interparticulate friction;
- particle–machine wall friction;
- heat;
- sound; and
- vibration.

A number of hypotheses and theories have been proposed in an attempt to relate energy input to the degree of size reduction produced.

Rittinger's hypothesis relates the energy, E, used in a size reduction process to the new surface area produced, S_n, or

$$E = \kappa_R (S_n - S_i)$$

(10.3)

where S_i is the initial surface area and κ_R is Rittinger's constant, expressing energy per unit area.

Kick's theory states that the energy used in deforming or fracturing a set of particles of equivalent shape is proportional to the ratio of the change in size, or

$$E = \kappa_k \log\left(\frac{d_i}{d_n}\right)$$

(10.4)

where κ_k is Kick's constant of energy per unit mass, d_i is the initial particle diameter and d_n is the new particle diameter.

Bond's theory states that the energy used in crack propagation is proportional to the new crack length produced, which is often related to the change in particle dimensions according to the following equation:

$$E = 2\kappa_B \left(\frac{1}{d_n} - \frac{1}{d_i}\right)$$

(10.5)

Here κ_B is known as Bond's work index and represents the variation in material properties and size reduction methods, with dimensions of energy per unit mass.

Walker proposed a generalized differential form of the energy–size relationship that can be shown to link the theories of Rittinger and Kick, and in some cases that of Bond:

$$\partial E = -\kappa_W \frac{\partial d}{d^n}$$

$$(10.6)$$

where κ_W is Walker's constant, d is a size function that can be characterized by an integrated mean size or by a weight function, and n is an exponent. When $n = 1$ for particles defined by a weight function, integration of Walker's equation corresponds to a Kick-type theory, when $n = 2$, a Rittinger-type solution results and when $n = 1.5$, Bond's theory is given.

When designing a milling process for a given particle, the most appropriate energy relationship will be required in order to calculate energy consumptions. It has been considered that the most appropriate values for n are 1 for particles larger than 1 μm, where Kick-type behaviour occurs, and 2 for Rittinger-type milling of smaller particles of less than 1 μm. The third value of $n = 1.5$ is the average of these two extremes and indicates a possible solution where neither Kick's nor Rittinger's theory is appropriate. Other workers have found that n cannot be assumed to be constant, but varies with particle size.

Influence of size reduction on size distribution

In Chapter 9, several different size distributions are discussed, with some based on either a normal or a log-normal distribution of particle sizes. During a size reduction process the particles of feed material will be broken down and particles in different size ranges undergo different amounts of breakage. This uneven milling leads to a change in the size distribution, which is superimposed on the general movement of the normal or log-normal curve towards smaller particle diameters. Changes in size distributions that occur as milling proceeds have been demonstrated experimentally, and this showed that an initial normal particle size distribution was transformed through a size-reduced bimodal population into a much finer powder with a positively skewed, leptokurtic particle population (Fig. 10.2) as milling continued. The initial,

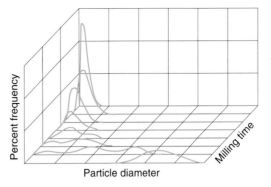

Fig. 10.2 • Changes in particle size distributions with increased milling time.

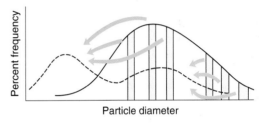

Fig. 10.3 • Transformation of an approximately normal particle size distribution into a finer bimodal population following milling.

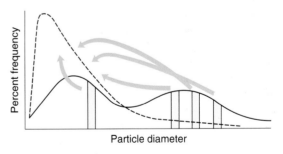

Fig. 10.4 • Transformation of a fine bimodal particle population into a finer unimodal distribution following prolonged milling.

approximately normal, size distribution was transformed into a size-reduced bimodal population through differences in the fracture behaviour of coarse and fine particles (Fig. 10.3). If milling is continued, a unimodal population reappears, as the energy input is not great enough to cause further fracture of the finest particle fraction (Fig. 10.4).

The lower particle size limit of a milling operation is dependent on the energy input and on material properties. With particle diameters smaller than approximately 5 μm, interactive cohesive forces between the particles generally predominate over comminution stresses as the comminution forces are distributed over increasing surface areas. This eventually results in particle agglomeration as opposed to particle fracture, and size reduction ceases. In some cases, particle agglomeration occurs to such a degree that subsequent milling actually causes size enlargement.

Size reduction methods

There are many different types of size reduction techniques, and the apparatus available for size reduction of pharmaceutical powders continue to develop. This chapter illustrates the principles associated with techniques that are classified according to the milling process employed to subdivide the powder particles. The chapter does not catalogue all existing milling equipment but instead illustrates the various principles involved – examples of each type are given below. The approximate size reduction range achievable with each technique is illustrated, although it should be remembered that the extent of size reduction is always related to milling time.

Cutting methods

Size reduction range

This is indicated in Fig. 10.5. The dotted line in this, and in other subsequent size-range diagrams, refers to the size range where the technique is used less often.

Cutter mill

A cutter mill (Fig. 10.6) consists of a series of knives attached to a horizontal rotor which act against a series of stationary knives attached to the mill casing. During milling, size reduction occurs by fracture of particles between the two sets of knives, which have a clearance of a few millimetres. A screen is fitted in the base of the mill casing and acts to retain material in the mill

until a sufficient degree of size reduction has been effected; thus it is self-classifying.

The shear rates present in cutter mills are useful in producing a coarse degree of size reduction of dried granulations prior to tableting.

Compression methods

Size reduction range

This is indicated in Fig. 10.7.

Runner mills

Size reduction by compression can be carried out on a small laboratory scale during development using a mortar and pestle.

Roller mill

A form of compression mill uses two cylindrical rollers mounted horizontally and rotated about their long axes. In roller mills, one of the rollers is driven directly

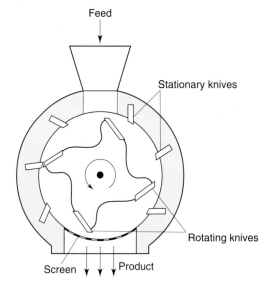

Fig. 10.6 • Cutter mill.

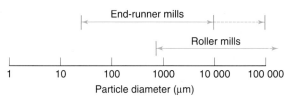

Fig. 10.7 • Size reduction range for compression methods.

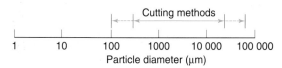

Fig. 10.5 • Size reduction range for cutting methods.

while the second is rotated by friction as material is drawn through the gap between the rollers.

Impact methods

Size reduction range

This is shown in Fig. 10.8.

Hammer mill

Size reduction by impact can be carried out using a hammer mill (Fig. 10.9). Hammer mills consist of a series of four or more hammers, hinged on a central shaft which is enclosed within a rigid metal case. During milling the hammers swing out radially from the rotating central shaft. The angular velocity of the hammers produces a strain rate up to 80 s^{-1}, which is so high that most particles undergo brittle fracture. As size reduction continues, the inertia of particles hitting the hammers reduces markedly (as particle mass is reduced) and subsequent fracture is less probable, so hammer mills tend to produce powders with narrow size distributions. Particles are retained within the mill by a screen that allows only adequately comminuted particles to pass through. Particles passing

through a given mesh can be much finer than the mesh apertures, as particles are carried around the mill by the hammers and approach the mesh tangentially. For this reason, square, rectangular or herringbone slots are often used. Depending on the purpose of the operation, the hammers may be square faced, tapered to a cutting edge or have a stepped form.

Vibration mill

An alternative to hammer milling which produces size reduction is vibration milling (Fig. 10.10). Vibration mills are filled to approximately 80% total volume with porcelain or stainless steel balls. During milling the whole body of the mill is vibrated and size reduction occurs by repeated impact. Comminuted particles fall through a screen at the base of the mill. The efficiency of vibratory milling is greater than that of conventional ball milling described later.

Attrition methods

Size reduction range

This is indicated in Fig. 10.11.

Roller mill

Roller mills use the principle of attrition to produce size reduction of solids in suspensions, pastes or ointments. Two or three porcelain or metal rollers

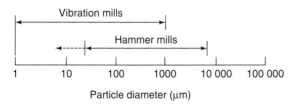

Fig. 10.8 • Size reduction range for impact methods.

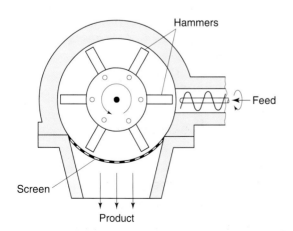

Fig. 10.9 • Hammer mill.

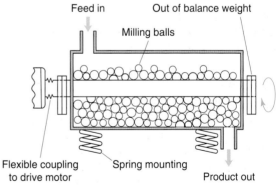

Fig. 10.10 • Vibration mill.

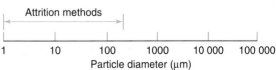

Fig. 10.11 • Size reduction range for attrition methods.

are mounted horizontally with an adjustable gap, which can be as small as 20 μm. The rollers rotate at different speeds so that the material is sheared as it passes through the gap and is transferred from the slower to the faster roller, from which it is removed by means of a scraper.

Combined impact and attrition methods

Size reduction range

This is indicated in Fig. 10.12.

Ball mill

A ball mill is an example of a comminution method which produces size reduction by both impact and attrition of particles. Ball mills consist of a hollow cylinder mounted such that it can be rotated on its horizontal longitudinal axis (Fig. 10.13). The cylinder contains balls that occupy 30% to 50% of the total volume, the ball size being dependent on the feed and mill size. Mills may contain balls with many different diameters as this helps to improve the process, as the large balls tend to break down the

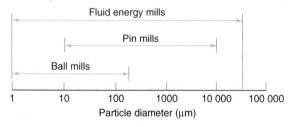

Fig. 10.12 • Size reduction range for combined impact and attrition methods.

coarse feed materials and the smaller balls help to form the fine product by reducing void spaces between balls.

The amount of material in a mill is of considerable importance: too much feed produces a cushioning effect, and too little causes loss of efficiency and abrasive wear of the mill parts.

The factor of greatest importance in the operation of the ball mill is the speed of rotation. At low angular velocities (see Fig. 10.13a) the balls move with the drum until the force due to gravity exceeds the frictional force of the bed on the drum, and the balls then slide back en masse to the base of the drum. This sequence is repeated, producing very little relative movement of the balls, so size reduction is minimal. At high angular velocities (see Fig. 10.13b), the balls are thrown out to the mill wall, where they remain due to centrifugal force, and no size reduction occurs. At approximately two-thirds of the critical angular velocity where centrifuging occurs (see Fig. 10.13c), a cascading action is produced. Balls are lifted on the rising side of the drum until their dynamic angle of repose is exceeded. At this point, they fall or roll back to the base of the drum in a cascade across the diameter of the mill. By this means, the most efficient size reduction occurs by impact of the particles with the balls and by attrition. The optimum rate of rotation is dependent on the mill diameter but is usually of the order of 0.5 revolutions per second.

Fluid energy mill

Fluid energy milling is another form of size reduction method that acts by particle impaction and attrition. A form of fluid energy or jet mill or micronizer is shown in Fig. 10.14. Both circular designs and oval-path designs (as shown in Fig. 10.14) are available.

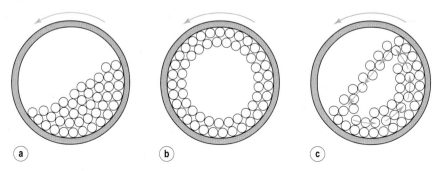

Fig. 10.13 • Ball mill in operation. (a) shows rotation speed too slow, (b) too fast and (c) the correct cascade action.

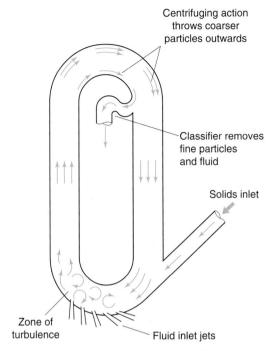

Fig. 10.14 • Fluid energy mill.

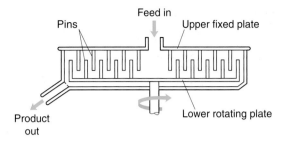

Fig. 10.15 • Pin mill.

The circular design is now the most common. This consists of a hollow toroid which has a diameter of 20 mm to 200 mm. A fluid, usually air, is injected as a high-pressure jet through nozzles at the bottom of the loop. The high velocity of the air gives rise to zones of turbulence into which solid particles are fed. The high kinetic energy of the air causes the particles to impact with other particles and with the sides of the mill with sufficient momentum for fracture to occur. Turbulence ensures that the level of particle–particle collisions is high enough to produce substantial size reduction by impact and some attrition.

A particle size classifier is incorporated in the design so that particles are retained in the toroid until sufficiently fine and are then entrained in the air stream that exhausts from the mill.

Pin mill

In addition to ball mills and fluid energy mills, there are other methods of comminution that act by producing particle impact and attrition. These include *pin mills* in which two discs with closely spaced pins rotate against one another at high speeds (Fig. 10.15). Particle size reduction occurs by impaction with the pins and by attrition between pins as the

particles travel outwards under the influence of centrifugal force.

Selection of the particle size reduction method

Different mills can produce differing end products from the same starting material. For example, particle shape may vary according to whether size reduction occurs as a result of impact or attrition. In addition, the proportion of fine particles in the product may vary, so that other properties of the powder will be altered.

The subsequent usage of a powder usually controls the degree of size reduction needed, but in some cases the precise particle size required is not critical. In these circumstances, because the cost of size reduction increases as the particle size decreases, it is economically undesirable to mill particles to a finer degree than is necessary. Once the particle size required has been established, the selection of mills capable of producing that size may be modified from knowledge of the particle properties, such as hardness and toughness. The influences of various process and material variables on the selection of a size reduction method are summarized in Table 10.1.

Introduction to size separation

Objectives of size separation

The significance of particle size and the principles involved in differentiating a powder into fractions of known particle size have been considered in Chapter 9. Methods for achieving the required size range on a manufacturing scale have been discussed in this chapter. Here the methods by which size separation can be achieved are discussed.

Table 10.1 Selection of size reduction mills according to particle properties and product size required

Mohs 'hardness'	Tough	Sticky	Abrasive	Friable
Fine powder product (<50 μm)				
1–3 (soft)	Ball, vibration (under liquid nitrogen)	Ball, vibration		Ball, vibration, pin, fluid energy
3–5 (intermediate)	Ball, vibration			Ball, vibration, fluid energy
5–10 (hard)	Ball, vibration, fluid energy		Ball, vibration, fluid energy	
Coarse powder product (50 μm to 1000 μm)				
1–3 (soft)	Ball, vibration, roller, pin, hammer, cutter (all under liquid nitrogen)	Ball, pin		Ball, roller, pin, hammer, vibration
3–5 (intermediate)	Ball, roller, pin, hammer, vibration, cutter			Ball, roller, pin, vibration, hammer
5–10 (hard)	Ball, vibration		Ball, vibration, roller	
Very coarse product (>1000 μm)				
1–3 (soft)	Cutter	Roller, hammer	Roller, hammer	
3–5 (intermediate)	Roller, hammer			Roller, hammer
5–10 (hard)	Roller		Roller	

Solid separation is a process by which powder particles are removed from gases or liquids, and has two main aims:

1. to recover valuable products or by-products; and

2. to prevent environmental pollution.

An important difference exists between the procedures known as *size analysis* and *size separation*. The former is designed to provide information on the size characteristics of a powder, whereas the latter is an integral part of a production process and results in a product powder of a given particle size range that is available for separate handling or subsequent processing. Thus a particle size analysis method such as microscopy would be of no use as a size separation method. However, sieving can be used for both purposes.

Size separation efficiency

The efficiency with which a powder can be separated into different particle size ranges is related to the particle and fluid properties and the separation method used. *Separation efficiency* is determined as a function of the effectiveness of a given process in separating particles into oversize and undersize fractions.

In a continuous size separation process, the production of oversize and undersize powder streams from a single feed stream can be represented by the following equation:

$$f_f = f_o + f_u$$

(10.7)

where f_f, f_o and f_u are functions of the mass flow rates of the feed material, oversize product and undersize product streams respectively. If the separation process is 100% efficient, then all oversize material will end up in the oversize product stream and all undersize material will end up in the undersize product stream. Invariably, industrial particle separation processes produce an incomplete separation, so that some undersize material is retained in the oversize stream and some oversize material may find its way into the undersize stream.

Considering the oversize material, a given powder feed stream will contain a certain proportion of true oversize material, δ_f; the outgoing oversize product stream will contain a fraction, δ_o, of true oversize particles, and the undersize product stream will contain a fraction, δ_u, of true oversize material (Fig. 10.16). The efficiency of the separation of oversize material can be determined by considering the relationship between the mass flow rates of feed and product streams and the fractional contributions

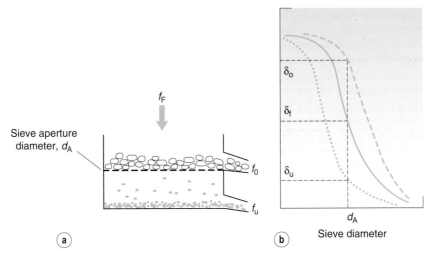

Fig. 10.16 • Size separation efficiency determination. **(a)** Separation operation. **(b)** Size distributions of feed, oversize material and undersize material to obtain values for δ_o, δ_f and δ_u.

of true size grade in the streams. For example, the efficiency E_o of a size separation process for oversize material in the oversize stream is given by

$$E_o = \frac{f_o \delta_o}{f_f \delta_f}$$

(10.8)

and the separation efficiency for undersize material in the undersize stream is given by

$$E_u = \frac{f_u (1 - \delta_o)}{f_f (1 - \delta_f)}$$

(10.9)

The total efficiency, E_t, for the whole size separation process is given by

$$E_t = E_u E_o$$

(10.10)

Separation efficiency determination can be applied to each stage of a complete size classification and is often referred to as *grade efficiency*. In some cases, knowledge of grade efficiency is insufficient, e.g. where a precise particle size cut is required. A *sharpness index* can be used to quantify the sharpness of the cut-off in a given size range. A sharpness index, S, can be determined in several different ways; for example, by taking the percentage values from a grade efficiency curve at the 25% and 75% levels (L_{25} and L_{75} respectively),

$$S_{25/75} = \frac{L_{25}}{L_{75}}$$

(10.11)

or at other percentile points, e.g. at the 10% and 90% levels:

$$S_{10/90} = \frac{L_{10}}{L_{90}}$$

(10.12)

Size separation methods

Some of the types of size separation equipment are discussed briefly in the following sections. These have been chosen to illustrate the basic principles of size separation. The actual equipment in use in pharmaceutical processing continues to develop, yet remains based on the principles illustrated.

Size separation by sieving

Separation ranges

These are shown in Fig. 10.17.

Principles of operation

The principles of sieving in order to achieve particle size analysis are described in Chapter 9. There are

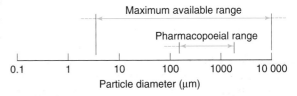

Fig. 10.17 • Separation range for sieving.

some differences in the methods used to achieve size separation rather than size analysis. The use of sieving in size separation usually requires the processing of larger volumes of powder than are commonly found in size analysis operations. For this reason the sieves used for size separation are often larger in area and of more robust construction than those used for size analysis.

There are several techniques for encouraging particles to separate into their appropriate size fractions efficiently. In dry sieving processes these are based on mechanical disturbances of the powder bed and include the following methods.

Agitation methods. Size separation is achieved by electrically induced oscillation, mechanically induced vibration of the sieve meshes or gyration in which sieves are fitted to a flexible mounting which is connected to an out-of-balance flywheel. In the last case, the eccentric rotation of the flywheel imparts a rotary movement of small amplitude and high intensity to the sieve and causes the particles to spin, thereby continuously changing their orientation and increasing their potential to pass through a given sieve aperture. The output efficiency of gyratory sieves is usually greater than that of oscillation or vibration methods.

Agitation methods can be made continuous by inclination of the sieve and the use of separate outlets for the undersize and oversize powder streams.

Brushing methods. A brush is used to reorient particles on the surface of a sieve and prevent apertures becoming blocked. A single brush can be rotated about the midpoint of a circular sieve or, for large-scale processing, a horizontal cylindrical sieve is employed with a spiral brush rotating about its longitudinal axis. It is important, however, that the brush does not force the particles through the sieve by distorting either the particles or the sieve mesh.

Centrifugal methods. In this type of equipment, particles are thrown outwards onto a vertical cylindrical sieve under the action of a high-speed rotor inside the cylinder. The current of air created by the rotor movement also assists the sieving process, especially where very fine powders are being processed.

Wet sieving can also be used to effect size separation and is generally more efficient than dry sieving methods.

Standards for powders based on sieving

Standards for the size of powders used pharmaceutically are sometimes provided in pharmacopoeias. These may indicate how the degree of coarseness or fineness of a powder is differentiated and expressed

Table 10.2 Example of powder grades as specified in pharmacopoeias

Description of grade of powder	Coarsest sieve diameter (μm)	Sieve diameter through which no more than 40% of powder must pass (μm)
Coarse	1700	355
Moderately coarse	710	250
Moderately fine	355	180
Fine	180	–
Very fine	125	–

Some pharmacopoeias define another size fraction, known as *ultrafine powder*, in which the maximum diameter of at least 90% of the particles must be no greater than 5 μm and none of the particles should have diameters greater than 50 μm.

by reference to the nominal mesh aperture size of the sieves used. Grades of powder are specified and defined in general terms by most pharmacopoeias. An example is shown in Table 10.2.

It should be noted that the term 'sieve number' has been used as a method of quantifying particle size in pharmacopoeias and is still favoured in some parts of the world. However, various monographs use the term differently, and in order to avoid confusion it is strongly recommended to always refer to particle sizes according to the appropriate equivalent diameters expressed in millimetres, micrometres or nanometres, as appropriate.

Size separation by sedimentation

Separation ranges

These are shown in Fig. 10.18.

Principles of operation

The principles of particle sizing using sedimentation methods are described in Chapter 9. Size separation

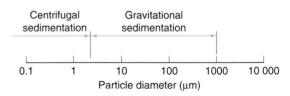

Fig. 10.18 • Separation range for sedimentation techniques.

by sedimentation utilizes the differences in settling velocities of particles with different diameters, and these can be related according to the Stokes equations (see Eqns 9.11–9.13).

One of the simplest forms of sedimentation classification uses a chamber containing a suspension of solid particles in a liquid, which is usually water. After predetermined times, particles less than a given diameter can be recovered from a fixed distance below the surface of the liquid. Size fractions can be collected continuously using a pump mechanism.

Alternatively, a single separation can be performed simply by removing the upper layer of suspension fluid after the desired time. Disadvantages of these simple methods are that they are batch processes and discrete particle fractions cannot be collected.

Size separation by elutriation

Separation ranges

These are shown in Fig. 10.19.

Principles of operation

In sedimentation methods the fluid is stationary and the separation of particles of various sizes depends solely on particle velocity. Therefore the division of particles into size fractions depends on the *time* of sedimentation.

Elutriation is a technique in which the fluid flows in an opposite direction to the sedimentation movement, so that in gravitational elutriators particles move vertically downwards while the fluid travels vertically upwards. If the upward velocity of the fluid is less than the settling velocity of the particle, sedimentation still occurs and the particles move slowly downwards against the flow of fluid. Conversely, if the upward fluid velocity is greater than the settling velocity of the particle, the particle moves upwards with the fluid flow. Therefore, in the case of elutriation, particles can be divided into different size fractions depending on the velocity of the fluid.

Elutriation and sedimentation methods are compared diagrammatically in Fig. 10.20, where the arrows are vectors; that is, they show the direction and magnitude of particle movement. This figure may indicate that if particles are suspended in a fluid moving up a column, there will be a clear cut into two fractions of particle size. In practice this does not occur, as there is a distribution of velocities across the tube in which a fluid is flowing – the highest velocity is found in the centre of the tube and the lowest velocity at the tube walls. Therefore the size of particles that will be separated depends on their position in the tube: the largest particles in the centre, the smallest towards the outside. In practice, particles may rise with the fluid in the centre of the apparatus and then move outwards to the tube wall, where the velocity is lower and they then fall. A separation into two size fraction occurs, but the size cut is not clearly defined. Assessing the sharpness of size cuts was discussed previously.

Separation of powders into several size fractions can be achieved by using a number of elutriators connected in series. The suspension is fed into the bottom of the narrowest column, overflowing from the top into the bottom of the next widest column and so on. Because the mass flow remains the same, as the column diameter increases, the fluid velocity decreases and therefore particles of decreasing size will be separated.

Adaptations of this technique in which the liquid is replaced by air are available. Air is used as the counterflow fluid in place of water for elutriation of

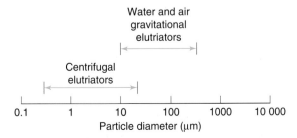

Fig. 10.19 • Separation range for elutriation methods.

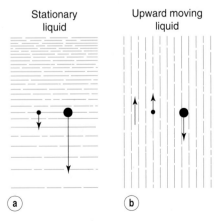

Fig. 10.20 • Comparison of **(a)** sedimentation and **(b)** elutriation.

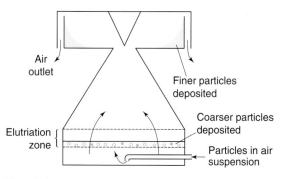

Fig. 10.21 • Upward airflow elutriator.

soluble particles into different size ranges. There are several types of air elutriator, which differ according to the airflow patterns used. An example of an upward airflow elutriator is shown in Fig. 10.21. Particles are held on a supporting mesh through which air is drawn. Classification occurs within a very short distance of the mesh and any particles remaining entrained in the air stream are accelerated to a collecting chamber by passage through a conical section of the tube. Further separation of any fine particles still entrained in the airflow may be carried out subsequently using different air velocities.

Size separation by cyclone methods

Separation range

This is shown in Fig. 10.22.

Principles of operation

Probably the most common type of cyclone used to separate particles from fluid streams is the reverse-flow cyclone (Fig. 10.23). In this system, particles in air or liquid suspension are often introduced tangentially into the cylindrical upper section of the cyclone, where the relatively high fluid velocity produces a vortex that throws solid particles out onto the walls of the cyclone. The particles are forced

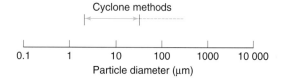

Fig. 10.22 • Separation ranges for cyclone methods.

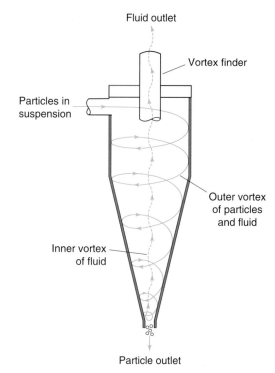

Fig. 10.23 • Reverse-flow cyclone separation.

down the conical section of the cyclone under the influence of the fluid flow – gravity interactions are a relatively insignificant mechanism in this process. At the tip of the conical section, the vortex of fluid is above the critical velocity at which it can escape through the narrow outlet and forms an inner vortex which travels back up the cyclone and out through a central outlet or vortex finder. Coarser particles separate from the fluid stream and fall out of the cyclone through the dust outlet, whereas finer particles remain entrained in the fluid stream and leave the cyclone through the vortex finder. In some cases, the outer vortex is allowed to enter a collector connected to the base of the cyclone, but the coarser particles still appear to separate from the fluid stream and remain in the collector. A series of cyclones having different flow rates or different dimensions could be used to separate a powder into different particle size ranges.

Selection of a size separation process

Selection of a specific size separation method may be limited by pharmacopoeial requirements, but for general cases the most efficient method should be selected based on particle properties. Of these, size is particularly important, as each separation method is most efficient over a particular size range, as indicated in the foregoing text.

Particles that have just undergone size reduction will already be in suspension in a fluid, whether air or water, and can be separated quickly by elutriation or cyclone separation methods, so that oversize material can be returned to the mill.

Alternatively, many powders used pharmaceutically are soluble in water, and size separation may have to be restricted to air classification methods.

Please check your eBook at **https://studentconsult. inkling.com/** for self-assessment questions. See inside cover for registration details.

Bibliography

Allen, T., 1997. Particle Size Measurement, vols. 1 and 2, fifth ed. Chapman and Hall, London.

Florence, A.T., Siepmann, J. (Eds.), 2009. Modern Pharmaceutics, vols. 1 and 2, fifth ed. Informa, New York.

Gotoh, K., Masuda, H., Higashitan, K., 1997. Powder Technology Handbook, second ed. Marcel Dekker, New York.

Lieberman, H., Lachman, L., Schwartz, J.B., 1990. Pharmaceutical Dosage Forms: Tablets, vol. 2, second ed. Marcel Dekker, New York.

Niazi, S.K. (Ed.), 2004. Handbook of Pharmaceutical Manufacturing Formulations, vol. 2. Uncompressed Solid Products. CRC Press, Boca Raton.

Rhodes, M. (Ed.), 1990. Principles of Powder Technology. John Wiley & Sons, Chichester.

Salmon, A.D., Hounslow, M.J., Seville, J.P.K. (Eds.), 2007. Handbook of Powder Technology, vol. 11, first ed. Elsevier, Amsterdam.

Schweitzer, P.A. (Ed.), 1997. Handbook of Separation Techniques for Chemical Engineers. McGraw-Hill Professional, New York.

Seibert, K.D., Collins, P.C., Fisher, E., 2010. Milling operations in the pharmaceutical industry. In: am Ende, D.J. (Ed.), Chemical Engineering in the Pharmaceutical Industry: R&D to Manufacture. John Wiley & Sons (in conjunction with AIChE), Hoboken.

Swarbrick, J., Boylan, J.C., 2002. Encyclopedia of Pharmaceutical Technology. Marcel Dekker, New York.

11

Mixing

Andrew M. Twitchell

CHAPTER CONTENTS

KEY POINTS

- A mixing operation is involved at some stage in the production of practically every pharmaceutical preparation.
- Mixing operations aim to distribute the components of the mix evenly so that a drug product possessing the required quality attributes is manufactured.
- Each dosage unit produced from a pharmaceutical mixture should have an active substance content within an acceptably narrow range around the label claim.
- There will always be some variation in the composition of samples taken from a powder mix. An understanding of the mechanisms by which mixing occurs and careful selection of powder properties, dosage form size and mixing procedures during formulation and processing is necessary to minimize this variation to acceptable levels.
- The factors which influence powder segregation should be appreciated so that a mix of the required quality can be produced and the occurrence of segregation minimized during subsequent handling and production processes.
- The choice of the mixer and how it is operated should be based on the physical characteristics of the materials that are to be mixed and the required properties of the mixed product.

Mixing principles

Importance of mixing

There are very few pharmaceutical products that contain only one component. In the vast majority of cases, several ingredients are needed to ensure that the dosage form functions as required. If, for example, a pharmaceutical company wishes to produce a tablet dosage form containing a drug which is active at a dose of 1 mg, other components (e.g. a diluent, binder, disintegrant and lubricant) will be needed both to enable the product to be manufactured and for it to be handled by the patient.

Whenever a product contains more than one component, a mixing or blending stage will be required in the manufacturing process. This may be to ensure an even distribution of the active component(s), an even appearance or that the dosage form releases the drug at the correct site and at the desired rate. The unit operation of mixing is therefore involved at some stage in the production of practically every pharmaceutical preparation, and control of mixing processes is of critical importance in ensuring the quality of pharmaceutical products. The importance of mixing is illustrated by the following list of products for which invariably mixing processes of some kind are used:

- tablets, capsules, sachets and dry powder inhalers – mixtures of solid particles;
- linctuses – mixtures of miscible liquids;
- emulsions and creams – mixtures of immiscible liquids; and
- pastes and suspensions – dispersions of solid particles.

Mixing and its control are also important in unit operations such as granulation, drying and coating.

This chapter considers the objectives of the mixing operation, how mixing occurs and the ways in which a satisfactory mix can be produced and maintained.

Definition and objectives of mixing

Mixing may be defined as a unit operation that aims to treat two or more components, initially in an unmixed or partially mixed state, so that each unit (particle, molecule, etc.) of the components lies as nearly as possible in contact with a unit of each of the other components.

If this is achieved, it produces a theoretical 'ideal' situation, i.e. a *perfect mix*. As will be shown, however, this situation is not normally practicable, is actually unnecessary and, indeed, is sometimes undesirable.

How closely it is attempted to approach the 'ideal' situation depends on the product being manufactured and the objective of the mixing operation. For example, when mixing a small amount of a potent drug in a powder mix, the degree of mixing must be of a high order to ensure a consistent dose. Similarly, when dispersing two immiscible liquids or dispersing a solid in a liquid, a well-mixed product is required to ensure product quality/stability. In the case of mixing lubricants with granules during tablet production, however, there is a danger of 'overmixing' and the subsequent production of a weak tablet with an increased disintegration time (discussed in Chapter 30).

Types of mixtures

Mixtures may be categorized into three types that differ fundamentally in their behaviour.

Positive mixtures

Positive mixtures are formed from materials such as gases or miscible liquids which mix *spontaneously* and *irreversibly* by diffusion and tend to approach a perfect mix. There is no input of energy required with positive mixtures if the time available for mixing is unlimited, although input of energy will shorten the time required to obtain the desired degree of mixing. In general, materials which mix by positive mixing do not present any problems during product manufacture.

Negative mixtures

With negative mixtures, the components will tend to separate out. If this occurs quickly, then there must be a continuous input of energy to keep the components adequately dispersed, e.g. with a suspension formulation where there is a dispersion of solids in a liquid of low viscosity. With other negative mixtures, the components tend to separate very slowly, e.g. emulsions, creams and viscous suspensions. Negative mixtures are generally more difficult to form and to maintain and require a higher degree of mixing efficiency than do positive mixtures.

Neutral mixtures

Neutral mixtures are said to be static in behaviour, i.e. the components have no tendency to mix spontaneously or segregate spontaneously once there has been input of work to mix them. Examples of this type of mixture include mixed powders, pastes and ointments. Neutral mixes are capable of demixing, but this requires energy input (as discussed in relation to powder segregation later in this chapter).

It should be noted that the type of mixture can change during processing. For example, if the viscosity increases sufficiently, a mixture may change from a negative to a neutral mixture. Similarly, if the particle size, degree of wetting or liquid surface tension changes, the mixture type may also change.

The mixing process

To discuss the principles of the mixing process, a situation will be considered where there are equal quantities of two powdered components of the same size, shape and density that are required to be mixed, the only difference between them being their colour. This situation will not, of course, occur practically but it will serve to simplify the discussion of the mixing process and allow some important considerations to be illustrated with the help of statistical analysis.

If the components are represented by coloured cubes, then a two-dimensional representation of the initial unmixed or completely segregated state can be shown as Fig. 11.1a.

From the definition of mixing, the ideal situation or *perfect mix* in this case would be produced when each particle lies adjacent to a particle of the other component (i.e. each particle lies as closely as possible in contact with a particle of the other component). This is shown in Fig. 11.1b, where it can be seen that the components are as evenly distributed as

possible. If this mix was viewed in three dimensions, then behind and in front of each coloured particle would be a white particle and vice versa. Powder mixing, however, is a 'chance' process, and while the situation shown in Fig. 11.1b could arise, the odds against it are so great that for practical purposes it can be considered impossible. For example, if there are only 200 particles present, the chance of a perfect mix occurring is approximately 1 in 10^{60} and is similar to the chance of the situation in Fig. 11.1a occurring after prolonged mixing. In practice, the best type of mix likely to be obtained will have the components under consideration distributed as indicated in Fig. 11.1c. This is referred to as a *random mix*, which can be defined as a mix where the *probability* of selecting a particular type of particle is the *same* at all positions in the mix and is equal to the *proportion* of such particles in the total mix.

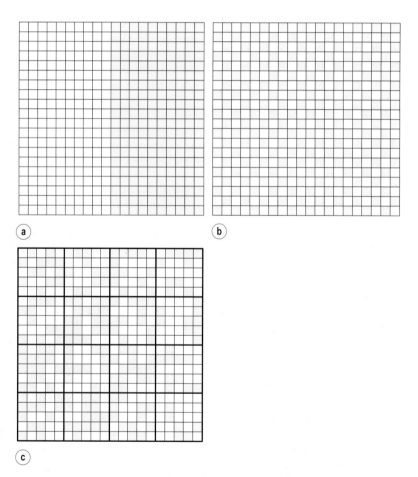

Fig. 11.1 • Different states of powder mixing. **(a)** Complete segregation. **(b)** An ideal or 'perfect' mix. **(c)** A random mix.

If any two adjacent particles are selected from the random mix shown:

- the chance of picking two coloured particles = 1 in 4 (25%)
- the chance of picking two white particles = 1 in 4 (25%)
- and the chance of picking one of each = 2 in 4 (50%).

If any two adjacent particles are selected from the perfect mix shown in Fig. 11.1b, there will always be one coloured particle and one white particle.

Thus if the samples taken from a random mix contain only two particles, then in 25% of cases the sample will contain no white particles and in 25% of cases it will contain no coloured particles. It may help in this and subsequent discussions to imagine the coloured particles as being the active drug and the white particles the inert excipient.

It can be seen that, in practice, the components will not be perfectly evenly distributed, i.e. there will not be full mixing. But if an overall view is taken, the components can be described as being mixed as in the total sample (Fig. 11.1c) the amount of each component is approximately similar (48.8% coloured and 51.2% white). If, however, Fig. 11.1c is considered as 16 different blocks of 25 particles, then it can be seen that the number of coloured particles in the blocks ranges from 6 to 19 (24% to 76% of the total number of particles in each block). Careful examination of Fig. 11.1c shows that as the number of particles in the sample increases, then the closer will be the proportion of each component to that which would occur with a perfect mix. This is a very important consideration in powder mixing, and is discussed in more detail in the following sections.

Scale of scrutiny

Often a mixing process produces a large 'bulk' of mixture that is subsequently subdivided into individual dose units (e.g. a tablet, capsule or 5 mL spoonful), and it is important that each dosage unit contains the correct amount/concentration of active component(s). It is the weight/volume of the *dosage unit* which dictates how closely the mix must be examined/analysed to ensure it contains the correct dose/concentration. This weight/volume is known as the *scale of scrutiny* and is the amount of material within which the quality of mixing is important. For example, if the unit weight of a tablet is 200 mg, then a 200 mg sample from the mix should be

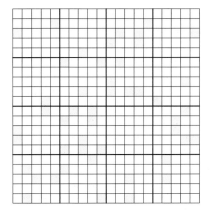

Fig.11.2 • Particle distribution in a representative random mix containing 10% active ingredient.

analysed to see if mixing is adequate; the scale of scrutiny therefore being 200 mg. If a larger sample size than the scale of scrutiny is analysed, this may mask important micro-nonuniformities such as those caused by agglomerates and may lead to the acceptance of an inadequate mix. Conversely, analysing too small a sample size may lead to the rejection of an acceptable mix.

The number of *particles* contained in the scale of scrutiny will depend on the sample weight, particle size and particle density, and will increase as the sample weight increases and the particle size and density decrease. This number should be sufficient to ensure an acceptably small deviation from the required dose in the dosage forms.

Another important factor to consider when carrying out a mixing process is the proportion of the active component in the dosage form/scale of scrutiny. This is illustrated in Fig. 11.2 and Table 11.1, the latter also demonstrating the importance of the number of particles in the scale of scrutiny.

Fig. 11.2 shows a random mix containing only 10% coloured particles (active ingredient). If the blocks of 25 particles are examined, it can be seen that the number of coloured particles varies from 0 to 8, or 0% to 32%. Thus the number of coloured particles as a percentage of the theoretical content varies from 0% to 320%. This is considerably greater than the range of 48% to 152% when the proportion of coloured particles was 0.5 or 50% (see Fig. 11.1c).

Table 11.1 shows how the content of a minor (potent) active constituent (present in a proportion of 1 part in a 1000, i.e. 0.1%) typically varies with the number of particles in the scale of scrutiny, when sampling a random mix. In the example shown, when

Table 11.1 Number of particles of a minor active constituent present in samples taken from a 1:1000 random powder mix with different numbers of particles in the scale of scrutiny

Sample number	Number of particles in scale of scrutiny		
	1000	10 000	100 000
1	1	7	108
2	0	10	91
3	1	15	116
4	2	8	105
5	0	13	84
6	1	10	93
7	1	6	113
8	2	5	92
9	0	12	104
10	1	13	90

The figures in the table are the numbers of particles of the minor constituent in the samples.

there are 1000 particles in the scale of scrutiny, three samples contain no active constituent and two have twice the amount that should be present. With 10000 particles in the scale of scrutiny, the deviation is reduced but samples may still deviate from the theoretical content of 10 particles by ±50%. Even with 100 000 particles, deviation from the theoretical content may exceed ±15% which is generally unacceptable for a pharmaceutical mixture. The difficulty in mixing potent substances can be appreciated if it is realized that there may only be approximately 75000 particles of diameter 150 μm in a tablet weighing 200 mg.

The information in Figs 11.1 and 11.2 and Table 11.1 leads to two important conclusions:

1. The lower the proportion of active component present in the mixture, the more difficult it is to achieve an acceptably low deviation in active content.

2. The more particles there are present in a unit dose/scale of scrutiny, the lower the likely deviation in content.

One way of reducing the deviation, therefore, would be to increase the number of particles in the unit dose by decreasing the particle size. This may, however, lead to particle agglomeration due to the increased cohesion and adhesion that occurs with smaller particles, which in turn may reduce the ease of mixing.

It should be noted that with liquid solutions, even very small samples are likely to contain many million 'particles'. Deviation in content is therefore likely to be very small with miscible liquids even if they are randomly mixed. Diffusion effects in miscible liquids arising from the existence of concentration gradients in an unmixed system mean that they tend to approach a perfect mix.

Mathematical treatment of the mixing process

It should be appreciated that there will always be some variation in the composition of samples taken from a pharmaceutical mix or a random mix. The aim during formulation and processing is to minimize this variation to acceptable levels by selecting an appropriate scale of scrutiny, particle size and mixing procedure (the latter involving the correct choice of mixer, rotation speed, etc.). The following section uses a simplified statistical approach to illustrate some of the factors that influence dose variation within a batch of a dosage form and demonstrates the difficulties encountered with drugs that are active in low doses (potent drugs).

Consider the situation where samples are taken from a random mix in which the particles are all of the same size, shape and density. The variation in the proportion of a component in samples taken from the random mix can be calculated from Eq. 11.1:

$$SD = \sqrt{\frac{p(1-p)}{n}}$$

(11.1)

where SD is the standard deviation in the proportion of the component in the samples (content SD), p is the proportion of the component in the total mix and n is the total number of particles in the sample.

Eq. 11.1 shows that as the number of particles present in the sample increases, the content SD decreases (i.e. there is less variation in sample content), as illustrated by the data in Fig. 11.2 and Table 11.1. The situation with respect to the effect of the proportion of the active component in the sample is not as clear from Eq. 11.1. As p is decreased, the value of content SD decreases, and this may lead to the incorrect conclusion that it is beneficial to have a low proportion of the active component. A more useful parameter to determine is the percentage coefficient of variation (% CV), which indicates the average deviation as a percentage of the mean amount of active component in the samples. Thus, % CV = (content standard deviation /mean content) × 100. The value of % CV will increase as p decreases, as illustrated in Box 11.1.

It might be considered that the variation in content could be reduced by increasing the unit dose size (increasing the scale of scrutiny), as this would increase the number of particles in each unit dose. The dose of a drug will, however, be fixed, and any increase in the unit dose size will cause a reduction in the proportion of the active component in the unit dose. The consequence of increasing the unit dose size depends on the initial proportion of the active component. If p is relatively high initially, increasing the unit dose size causes the %CV in content to increase. If p is small, increasing the unit dose size has little effect. Inserting appropriate values into Eq. 11.1 can substantiate this.

In a true random mix, the content of samples taken from the mix will follow a normal distribution. With a normal distribution, 68.3% of samples will be within ±1SD of the overall proportion of the component (p), 95.5% will be within ±2SD of p and 99.7% of samples will be within ±3SD of p. For example, if $p = 0.5$ and the standard deviation in content = 0.02, then for 99.7% of samples the

proportion of the component will be between 0.44 and 0.56. In other words, if 1000 samples were analysed, 997 samples would contain between 44% and 56% of drug (mean 50%).

Ideally, for a pharmaceutical product the active component should not deviate by more than ±5% of the mean or specified content. Thus the acceptable deviation is $p × (5/100)$, or $p × 0.05$ (note that this is not the same as a standard deviation of 5%). Based on the previous information, the number of particles that are required in a dosage form in order to achieve a drug product that meets defined quality criteria may be estimated. An illustrative calculation is shown in Box 11.2.

Estimation of the particle size required when formulating a dosage form

Using the preceding information, it is possible to estimate the particle size required so that a formulation may meet a desired specification. The worked

Box 11.2

Worked example

If a product contains an active component which makes up half of the weight of the dosage form ($p = 0.5$) and it is required that 99.7% of samples contain within ±5% of p, then the number of particles required in the product can be estimated as follows.

As 99.7% of samples will be within ±3SD and ±5% of p, Eq. 11.2 can be used to calculate the SD required:

$$3 × SD = p × (\text{percentage acceptable deviation}/100).$$

$$(11.2).$$

In this case, $3 × SD = 0.5 × 0.05$, so

$$\frac{0.5 × 0.05}{3} = \sqrt{\frac{p(1-p)}{n}}$$

Thus

$$6.94 × 10^{-5} = 0.5(1-0.5)/n$$

and therefore $n = 3600$.

This calculation indicates that 3600 particles are required in each sample or dosage form in order to be 99.7% sure that the content is within ±5% of the theoretical amount. If, however, the product contains a potent drug where $p = 1 × 10^{-3}$, the number of particles needed to meet the same criteria can be estimated to be $3.6 × 10^{6}$.

Box 11.1

Worked example

Consider the situation where $n = 100\,000$ and $p = 0.5$. With Eq. 11.1 it can be calculated that

$$SD = 1.58 × 10^{-3} \text{ and } \%CV = (1.58 × 10^{-3}/0.5) × 100$$
$$= 0.32\%$$

where %CV is the percentage coefficient of variation. Thus, on average, the content will deviate from the mean content by 0.32%, which is an acceptably low value for a pharmaceutical product.

If, however, p is reduced to 0.001 and n remains at 100 000, there is a reduction in SD to $9.99 × 10^{-5}$ but

$$\%CV = (9.99 × 10^{-5}/0.001) × 100 = 10\%$$

Thus in this latter case, the content will deviate from the theoretical content on average by 10%, which would be unacceptable for a pharmaceutical product.

Box 11.3

Worked example

Imagine it is necessary to produce a tablet weighing 50 mg which contains 50 µg of a potent steroid, and that the product specification requires 99.7% of tablets to contain between 47.5 µg and 52.5 µg of the steroid. If the mean particle density of the components is 1.5 g cm⁻³ (1500 kg m⁻³), what particle size should the steroid and excipients be?

As there is 50 µg of the steroid in a 50 mg tablet, the proportion of active component $p = 1 \times 10^{-3}$. The specification allows the content to vary by ±2.5 µg, and so the percentage deviation allowed = (2.5/50) × 100 = 5%. Under these circumstances the calculations described in the previous section (see Box 11.2) show that, providing a random mix is achieved, the number of particles required in the tablet = 3.6×10^6. The 50 mg tablet must therefore contain at least 3.6×10^6 particles, and each particle must weigh less than

$$50/3.6 \times 10^8 \text{ mg} = 1.39 \times 10^{-5} \text{ mg} = 1.39 \times 10^{-11} \text{ kg}$$

As the density of a particle = particle mass/particle volume, the volume of each particle must be less than

$$1.39 \times 10^{-11}/1500 \text{ m}^3 = 9.27 \times 10^{-15} \text{ m}^3$$

The volume of a particle (assuming it is spherical) = $4\pi r^3/3$, and so

$$r^3 \text{ must be} < 9.27 \times 10^{-15} \times 3/4\pi \text{ m}^3$$

i.e. $r^3 < 2.21 \times 10^{-15}$ m³ and $r < 1.30 \times 10^{-5}$ m

and therefore $d < 26$ µm.

---

example in Box 11.3 indicates that in order to meet the product specification, the particle size of the components needs to be of the order of 26 µm. There would therefore be practical difficulties in making this product, as particles of this size tend to become very cohesive, flow poorly (see Chapter 12) and are difficult to mix.

In order to appreciate the effect of changing the scale of scrutiny, it is suggested that the reader calculate in a similar manner what particle size would be required if the tablet weight was increased to 250 mg. It should be remembered that the tablet weight or scale of scrutiny will affect both the number of particles present and the proportion of active component.

In summary, the previous calculations illustrate the difficulty in mixing potent (low-dose) substances and the importance of both the number of particles

in the scale of scrutiny and proportion of the active component.

Evaluation of the degree of mixing

Manufacturers require some means of monitoring a mixing process for a variety of reasons. These could be to:

- indicate the degree/extent of mixing;
- follow a mixing process;
- indicate when sufficient mixing has occurred;
- assess the efficiency of a mixer; or
- determine the mixing time required for a particular process.

One evaluation method involves the generation of a *mixing index* that compares the content standard deviation of samples taken from a mix under investigation (S_{ACT}) with the content standard deviation of samples from a fully random mix (S_R). Comparison with a random mix is made because this is theoretically likely to be the best mix that is practically achievable. The simplest form of a mixing index (M) can be calculated as

$$M = \frac{S_R}{S_{ACT}}$$

(11.3)

At the start of the mixing process the value of S_{ACT} will be high so that M will be low. As mixing proceeds, S_{ACT} will tend to decrease as the mix approaches a random mix (Fig. 11.3). If the mix becomes random,

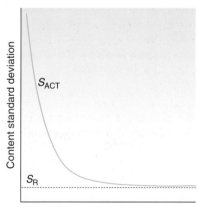

Fig. 11.3 • The reduction in content standard deviation as a random mix is approached. S_{ACT} represents the content standard deviation of samples taken from the mix and S_R represents the standard deviation expected from a random mix.

$S_{ACT} = S_R$ and $M = 1$. There is typically an exponential decrease in S_{ACT} as the mixing time or number of mixer rotations increases, although the shape of the curve will depend on the powder properties and mixer design and utilization. Other more complicated equations for calculating the mixing index have been used but they all tend to rely on similar principles to those described.

In order to evaluate a mixing process in this way, there are two basic requirements. First, a sufficient number of samples which are representative of the mix as a whole must be analysed. A minimum of 10 samples is usually analysed, these being removed from different depths into the mixer and from the middle and sides. Areas where blending may potentially be poor should also be included in the sampling. Samples are often taken with a 'sampling thief', which is a device that can be inserted into the mix and samples withdrawn with minimum disruption to the powder bed. Venables & Wells (2001) have discussed some of the problems associated with removing representative samples and analysing powder blends. Second, a suitable analytical technique must be available so that the value of S_{ACT} is a true reflection of the variation in content in the samples and not due to variation arising from the method of analysis.

When mixing formulations where the proportion of active component is high, it is possible to achieve an acceptably low variation in content without obtaining a random mix. Thus it may be possible to stop the mixing process before a random mix is achieved and therefore reduce manufacturing costs.

The quality of a mixture may be assessed by its ability to meet predefined specification limits. These could include assay limits for individual samples taken from the mix (e.g. 90% to 110% of the target content) and for the variation in content of these samples (e.g. % CV ≤3%).

An alternative method for monitoring and controlling powder blending is to use near-infrared (NIR) analysis. As most pharmaceutical active ingredients and excipients absorb NIR radiation, this technique has the potential advantage of providing homogeneity information on all of the mixture components. NIR spectroscopic methods may also be used noninvasively, which can eliminate the problems associated with the use of a sampling thief. Other potential advantages include the speed and nondestructive nature of the analysis. The reader is referred to texts by Bakeev (2010) and Ciurczak & Igne (2014) for further information.

Mechanisms of mixing and demixing

Powders

In order that powders may be mixed, the powder particles need to move relative to each other. There are three main mechanisms by which powder mixing occurs: namely, *convection*, *shear* and *diffusion*.

Convective mixing arises when there is the transfer of relatively large groups of particles from one part of the powder bed to another, e.g. as might occur when a mixer blade or paddle moves through the mix. This type of mixing contributes mainly to the macroscopic mixing of powder mixtures and tends to produce a large degree of mixing fairly quickly (as evidenced by a rapid drop in S_{ACT}). Mixing does not, however, occur *within* the group of particles moving together as a unit, and thus in order to achieve a random mix, an extended mixing time is required.

Shear mixing occurs when a 'layer' of material flows over another 'layer', resulting in the layers moving at different speeds and therefore mixing at the layer interface. This might occur when the removal of a mass by convective mixing creates an unstable shear/slip plane which causes the powder bed to collapse, or in high-shear or tumbling mixers, where the action of the mixer induces velocity gradients within the powder bed and hence 'shearing' of one layer over another.

In order to achieve a true random mix, movement of individual particles is required. This occurs with *diffusive mixing*. When a powder bed is forced to move or flow, it will 'dilate', i.e. the volume occupied by the bed will increase. This arises because the powder particles become less tightly packed and there is an increase in the air spaces or voids between them. Under these circumstances there is the potential for the powder particles to pass through the void spaces created either under gravitational forces (e.g. in a tumbling mixer) or by forced movement (e.g. in a fluidized bed). Mixing of individual particles in this way is referred to as diffusive mixing.

All three mixing mechanisms are likely to occur in a mixing operation. Which mechanism predominates and the extent to which each occurs will depend on the mixer type, mixing process conditions (mixer load, speed, etc.), particle characteristics and flowability of the components of the powder.

Liquids

The three main mechanisms by which liquids are mixed are *bulk transport*, *turbulent mixing* and *molecular diffusion*.

Bulk transport is analogous to the convective mixing of powders and involves the movement of a relatively large amount of material from one position in the mix to another, e.g. due to a mixer paddle. It too tends to produce a large degree of mixing fairly quickly, but leaves the liquid within the moving material unmixed.

Turbulent mixing arises from the haphazard movement of molecules when forced to move in a turbulent manner. The constant changes in speed and direction of movement mean that induced turbulence is a highly effective mechanism for mixing. Within a turbulent fluid there are, however, small groups of molecules moving together as a unit, referred to as eddies. These eddies tend to reduce in size and eventually break up, being replaced by new eddies. Turbulent mixing alone may therefore leave small unmixed areas within the eddies and in areas near the container surface, which will exhibit streamlined flow (see Chapter 6). Mixing of individual molecules in these regions will occur by the third mechanism, which is *molecular diffusion* (analogous to diffusive mixing in powders). This will occur with miscible fluids wherever a concentration gradient exists, and will eventually produce a well-mixed product, although considerable time may be required if this is the only mixing mechanism. In most mixers all three mechanisms will occur, bulk transport and turbulence arising from the movement of a stirrer or mixer paddle set at a suitable speed.

Powder segregation (demixing)

Segregation is the opposite effect to mixing, i.e. components tend to separate out. This is very important in the preparation of pharmaceutical products because if it occurs, an already formed random mix may change to a nonrandom mix, or a random mix may never be achieved. Care must be taken to avoid segregation occurring during handling after powders have been satisfactorily mixed, e.g. during transfer to filling machines or in the hopper of a tablet/capsule/sachet filling machine. Segregation will cause an increase in content variation in samples taken from the mix, i.e. it will result in a reduction in the quality of the mix and may cause a batch to fail a test for uniformity of content or uniformity of

dosage units. If segregation of granules occurs in the hopper of a filling machine, an unacceptable variation in weight may result.

Segregation arises because powder mixes encountered in practice are not composed of monosized spherical particles but contain particles that differ in size, shape, density and surface properties. These variations in particle properties mean that the particles will tend to behave differently when forced to move and hence tend to separate. Particles exhibiting similar properties tend to congregate together, giving regions in the powder bed which have a higher concentration of a particular component. Segregation is more likely to occur, or may occur to a greater extent, if the powder bed is subjected to vibration and when the particles have greater flowability.

Particle size effects

Differences in the particle sizes of components of a formulation are the main cause of segregation in powder mixes in practice. Smaller particles tend to fall through the voids between larger particles and thus move to the bottom of the mass. This is known as *percolation segregation*. It may occur in static powder beds if the percolating particles are small enough to fall into the void spaces between larger particles, but occurs to a greater extent as the bed 'dilates' on being disturbed. Domestically, percolation segregation is often observed in cereal packets or jars of coffee, where the smaller 'particles' congregate towards the bottom of the container.

Percolation can occur whenever a powder bed containing particles of different sizes is disturbed in such a way that particle rearrangement occurs, e.g. during vibration, stirring or pouring.

During mixing, larger particles will tend to have greater kinetic energy imparted to them (owing to their larger mass) and therefore move greater distances than smaller particles before they come to rest. This may result in separation of particles of different size, an effect referred to as *trajectory segregation*. This effect, along with percolation segregation, accounts for the occurrence of the larger particles at the edge of a powder heap when it is poured from a container.

During mixing, or when a material is discharged from a container, very small particles ('dust') in a mix may tend to be 'blown' upwards by turbulent air currents as the mass tumbles, and remain suspended in the air. When the mixer is stopped or material discharge is complete, these particles will sediment and subsequently form a layer on top of the coarser particles. This is called *elutriation segregation* and is also referred to as *dusting out* or *fluidization segregation*.

Particle density effects

If the components are of different density, the denser particles will have a tendency to move downwards, even if their particle sizes are similar. Trajectory segregation may also occur with particles of the same size but different densities due to their difference in mass. The effect of density on percolation segregation may be potentiated if the denser particles are also smaller. Often materials used in pharmaceutical formulations have similar densities and density effects are not generally too important. An exception to this is in fluidized beds, where density differences often have a greater adverse effect on the quality of the mix than particle size differences.

Particle shape effects

Spherical particles exhibit the greatest flowability and therefore are more easily mixed, but they also segregate more easily than nonspherical particles. Irregular or needle-shaped particles may become interlocked, decreasing the tendency to segregate once mixing has occurred. Nonspherical particles will also have a greater surface area to weight ratio (specific surface area), which will tend to decrease segregation by increasing any cohesive effects (greater contact surface area) but will increase the likelihood of 'dusting out'.

It should be remembered that the particle size distribution and particle shape may change during processing (due to attrition, aggregation, etc.) and therefore the tendency to segregate may also change.

Non-segregating mixes will improve with continued increases in mixing time, as shown in Fig. 11.3. This may not, however, occur for segregating mixes, where there is often an optimum mixing time. This arises because the factors causing segregation generally require a longer time to take effect than the time needed to produce a reasonable degree of mixing. During the initial stages of the process, the rate of mixing is greater than the rate of demixing. After a period of time, however, the rate of demixing may predominate, until eventually an equilibrium situation will be reached where the two effects are balanced. This is illustrated in Fig. 11.4, which demonstrates that, if factors exist which may cause segregation, then a random mix will

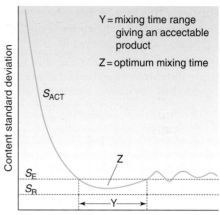

Fig.11.4 • Possible effect of extended mixing time on the content standard deviation of samples taken from a mix prone to segregation. S_{ACT} represents the content standard deviation of samples taken from the mix, S_E represents the estimated acceptable standard deviation and S_R represents the standard deviation expected from a random mix.

not be achieved and there may be both an optimum mixing time and a time range over which an acceptable mix can be produced.

Approaches to minimize segregation

If segregation is a problem with a formulation, there are a number of approaches that may be attempted to rectify the situation. These include the following:

- selection of particular size fractions (e.g. by sieving to remove fines or lumps) to achieve drug and excipients of the same narrow particle size range;
- milling of components (size reduction) either to reduce the particle size range (this may need to be followed by a sieving stage to remove fines) or to ensure all particles are smaller than approximately 30 μm, at which size segregation does not tend to cause serious problems (but may give rise to aggregation);
- controlled crystallization during production of the drug/excipients to give components of a particular crystal shape or size range;
- selection of excipients which have a density similar to that of the active component(s) – there is usually a range of excipients which will produce a product of the required properties;

- granulation of the powder mix (size enlargement) so that large numbers of different particles are evenly distributed in each segregating 'unit'/granule (see Fig. 28.1);
- reducing the extent to which the powder mass is subjected to vibration or movement after mixing (e.g. avoid the use of pneumatic transfer systems);
- using filling machine hoppers designed so that the powder residence time is minimized;
- using equipment where several operations can be carried out without transferring the mix, e.g. a fluidized-bed dryer or high-speed mixer/granulator for mixing and granulating; and
- production of an 'ordered' mix – this technique is also referred to as *adhesive* or *interactive* mixing and is described in more detail hereafter.

Ordered mixing

It would be expected that a mix composed of very small and much larger particles would segregate because of the size differences. Sometimes, however, if one powder is sufficiently small (micronized), it may become adsorbed onto 'active sites' on the surface of a larger 'carrier' particle and exhibit a great resistance to being dislodged. This has the effect of minimizing segregation while maintaining good flow properties. It was first noticed by Travers & White (1971) during the mixing of micronized sodium bicarbonate with sucrose crystals when the mixture was found to exhibit minimal segregation. The phenomenon is referred to as ordered mixing, as the particles are not independent of each other and there is a degree of order to the mix. If a carrier particle is removed, then some of the adsorbed smaller particles will automatically be removed with it. Ordered mixing has also been used in the production of dry antibiotic formulations to which water is added before use to form a liquid or syrup product. In these cases, the antibiotic in fine powder form is blended with, and adsorbed onto the surface of, larger sucrose or sorbitol particles (Nikolakakis & Newton, 1989).

Ordered mixing probably occurs to a certain extent in every pharmaceutical powder mix due to interactions and cohesive/adhesive forces between constituents. It is most likely to occur when smaller particles exist, as these have a high specific surface area and thus the attractive forces holding the particles to the adsorption site are more likely to be greater than the gravitational forces trying to separate the components.

Pharmaceutical powder mixes are therefore likely to be partly ordered and partly random, the extent of each depending on the component properties. With an ordered mix, it may be possible to achieve a degree of mixing which is superior to that of a random mix, which may be beneficial for potent drugs.

Ordered mixing has been shown to be important in direct-compression tablet formulations (see Chapter 30) in preventing segregation of the drug from direct compression bases.

Dry powder inhaler formulations also utilize ordered mixing to deliver drugs to the lungs (see Chapter 37). In this case the drug needs to be in a micronized form in order to reach its site of action. By adsorbing the drug onto larger carrier particles (usually lactose), it is possible to manufacture a product which will provide an even dosage on each inhalation.

Segregation in ordered mixes

Although ordered mixes can reduce or prevent segregation, it may still occur if, for example,

- *The carrier particles vary in size* – different-sized particles will have different surface area to weight ratios and will contain different amounts of adsorbed material per unit mass. If the different-sized carrier particles separate (e.g. by percolation segregation), drug-rich areas where the smaller carrier particles congregate may result. This is referred to as *ordered unit segregation*
- *There is competition for the active sites on the carrier particle* – if another component competes for sites on the carrier, it may displace the original adsorbed material, which may then segregate due to its small size. This is known as *displacement segregation* and has been shown to occur under certain circumstances with the addition of the lubricant magnesium stearate to tablet formulations
- *There are insufficient carrier particles* – each carrier particle can only accommodate a certain amount of adsorbed material on its surface. If there is any excess small-sized material that is not adsorbed onto the carrier particles, this may quickly separate. This is referred to as *saturation segregation* and may limit the proportion of the active component that can be used in the formulation.

With an ordered mix, particles may be dislodged if the mix is subjected to excessive vibration. The extent to which this occurs depends on the forces of attraction between the components and therefore on how tightly the adsorbed particles are attached to the surface. The orientation of the particles is also important, particles protruding out from the surface being more likely to be dislodged than those lying parallel to the surface.

Mixing of powders

Practical considerations

When mixing formulations in which there is a relatively low proportion of active ingredient(s), a more even distribution may be obtained by sequentially building up the amount of material in the mixer. This may be achieved by initially mixing the active component(s) with an approximately equal volume of diluent(s). Further amounts of diluents, equal to the amount of material in the mixer, can then be added and mixed, the process being continued until all material has been added. It may be more appropriate to preblend the active component with a diluent in a smaller mixer prior to transferring it to the main mixer in cases where the amount of active ingredient is very low.

Care must be taken to ensure that the volume of powder in the mixer is appropriate, as both over and underfilling may significantly reduce mixing efficiency. In the case of overfilling, for example, sufficient bed dilation may not take place for diffusive mixing to occur to the required extent or the material may not be able to flow in a way that enables shear mixing to occur satisfactorily. Underfilling may mean the powder bed does not move in the required manner in the mixer or that an increased number of mixing operations may be needed for a batch of material.

The mixer used should produce the mixing mechanisms appropriate for the formulation. For example, diffusive mixing is generally preferable if potent drugs are to be mixed, and high shear is needed to break up aggregates of cohered material and ensure mixing at a particulate level. The impact or attrition forces generated if too-high shear forces are used may, however, damage fragile material and thus produce fines. The mixer design should be such that it is dust tight, it can be easily cleaned and the product can be fully discharged. These features reduce the risk of cross-contamination between batches and protect the operator from the product.

In order to determine the appropriate mixing time, the process should be checked by removing and analysing representative samples after different mixing intervals. This may also indicate if segregation is occurring within the mixer and whether problems could occur if the mixing time is extended.

When particles rub past each other as they move within the mixer, static charges will be produced. These tend to result in 'clumping' and a reduction in diffusive mixing, and cause material to adhere to machine or container surfaces. To avoid this, mixers should be suitably earthed to dissipate the static charge and the process should be carried out at a relative humidity greater (although not excessively) than approximately 40%.

Powder-mixing equipment

Tumbling mixers/blenders

Tumbling mixers are commonly used for mixing/blending granules or free-flowing powders. There are many different designs of tumbling mixer, e.g. double-cone, twin-shell, cube, Y-cone and drum mixers, some of which are shown diagrammatically in Fig. 11.5. It is now common to use *intermediate bulk containers* (IBCs) as both the mixer bowl and to either feed

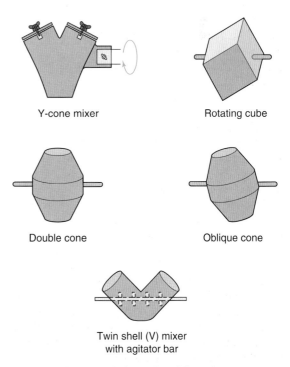

Y-cone mixer   Rotating cube

Double cone   Oblique cone

Twin shell (V) mixer
with agitator bar

Fig. 11.5 • Different designs of tumbling mixers.

the hopper of a tablet or a capsule machine, or act as the hopper itself. The shape of an IBC used for this purpose is illustrated in Fig. 11.6.

Mixing containers are generally mounted so that they can be rotated about an axis. When operated at the correct speed, the tumbling action indicated in Fig. 11.7 is achieved. Shear mixing will occur as a velocity gradient is produced, the top layer moving with the greatest velocity and the velocity decreasing as the distance from the surface increases. When the bed tumbles, it dilates, allowing particles to move downwards under gravitational force, and so diffusive mixing occurs. Most mixing will occur towards the surface of the bed, where the velocity gradients are highest and the bed is most dilated. Too high a rotation speed will cause the material to be held on the mixer walls by centrifugal force and too low a speed will

generate insufficient bed expansion and little shear mixing. Addition of 'prongs', baffles or rotating bars will also cause convective mixing (e.g. the V-mixer with agitator bar in Fig. 11.5).

Tumbling mixers are available to mix from approximately 50 g (e.g. for laboratory-scale development work) to over 100 kg (at a production scale). The material typically occupies approximately a half to two-thirds of the mixer volume. The rate at which the product is mixed will depend on the mixer geometry and rotation speed because they influence the movement of the material in the mixer.

Tumbling mixers are good for free-flowing powders/granules but are less effective for cohesive/poorly flowing powders because the shear forces generated are usually insufficient to break up any aggregates. Care also needs to be taken if there are significant differences in particle size as segregation is likely to occur. A common use of tumbling mixers is in the blending of lubricants, glidants or external disintegrants with granules prior to tableting.

Tumbling mixers can also be used to produce ordered mixes, although the process is often slow because of the cohesiveness of the adsorbing particles.

The Turbula shaker–mixer (Willy A. Bachofen, Muttenz, Switzerland) is a more sophisticated form of tumbling mixer which utilizes inversional motion in addition to the rotational and translational motion of traditional tumbling mixers. This leads to more efficient mixing and makes it less likely that material of different size and density will segregate.

High-speed mixer-granulators

In pharmaceutical product manufacture it is often preferable to use one piece of equipment to carry out more than one function. An example of this is the use of a mixer–granulator (one design of which is shown diagrammatically in Fig. 11.8). As the name suggests, it can both mix and granulate a product, thus removing the need to transfer the product between pieces of

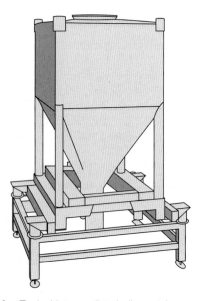

Fig.11.6 • Typical intermediate bulk container.

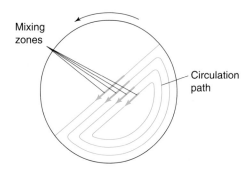

Fig.11.7 • Movement of the powder bed in a tumbling mixer.

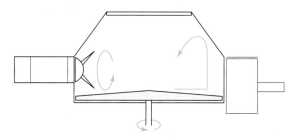

Fig.11.8 • A high-speed mixer–granulator.

equipment and thereby reducing the opportunity for segregation to occur. The centrally mounted impeller blade at the bottom of the mixer rotates at high speed, throwing the material towards the mixer bowl wall by centrifugal force. The material is then forced upwards before dropping back down towards the centre of the mixer. The particle movement within the bowl tends to mix the components quickly owing to high shear forces (arising from the high velocity) and the expansion in bed volume, which allows diffusive mixing. Once the material has been mixed, granulating agent can be added, and granules are formed in situ using a slower impeller speed and the action of the side-mounted chopper blade. Further details of granule production using this method can be found in Chapter 28.

Because of the high-speed movement within a mixer–granulator, care needs to be taken if the material being mixed fractures easily. This, and the problems associated with overmixing of lubricants, means that this type of mixer is not normally used for blending lubricants.

Fluidized-bed mixers

The main use of fluidized-bed equipment is in the drying of granules (see Chapter 29) or the coating of multiparticulates (see Chapter 32). Fluidized-bed equipment can, however, be used to mix powders prior to granulation in the same bowl. This is discussed in Chapter 28.

Agitator mixers

This type of mixer depends on the motion of a blade or paddle through the product, and hence the main mixing mechanism is convection. Examples include the ribbon mixer and the planetary mixer.

In the *ribbon mixer* (Fig. 11.9), mixing is achieved by the rotation of helical blades in a hemispherical trough. 'Dead spots' are difficult to eliminate in this type of mixer, and the shearing action caused by the movement of the blades may be insufficient to break up drug aggregates. The mixer does, however,

mix poorly flowing material and is less likely to cause segregation than a tumbling mixer.

A drawing of an industrial *planetary mixer* is shown in Fig. 11.10. Similar designs are used for both powder and semisolid mixing. The mixing bowl is shown in the lowered position for filling and emptying. The bowl is raised up to the mixing blade for the mixing process. The mixing blade is set off centre and is carried on a rotating arm. It therefore travels round the circumference of the mixing bowl while simultaneously rotating around its own axis (Fig. 11.11). This

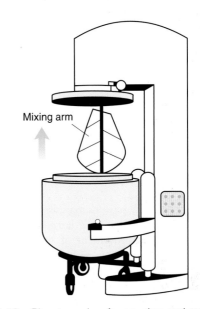

Fig.11.10 • Planetary mixer for powders and semisolids.

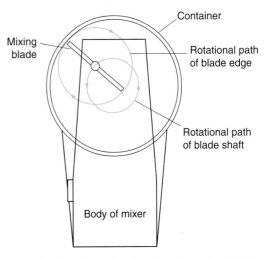

Fig.11.11 • Top view of a planetary mixer, showing the path of the paddle.

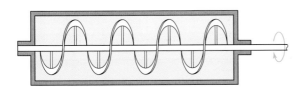

Fig.11.9 • Ribbon agitator powder mixer.

is therefore a double rotation similar to that of a spinning planet around the sun – hence the name – and is designed so that the blade covers all the volume of the mixer.

Scale-up of powder mixing

The extent of mixing achieved at a small laboratory scale during development work may not necessarily be mirrored when the same formulation is mixed at a full production scale, even if the same mixer design is used for both. Often, mixing efficiency and the extent of mixing are improved on scale-up owing to increased shear forces. This is likely to be beneficial in most cases, although when blending lubricants care is needed to avoid overlubrication, which may, for example, lead to soft tablets and delayed disintegration and dissolution.

Problems associated with a deficiency of some of the components of a formulation, which have been encountered at a production scale but not in development work, have been traced to adsorption of a minor constituent (e.g. a drug or colourant) onto the mixer wall or mixing blade.

Drug particle characteristics may also change when the drug is manufactured on a large scale. This in turn may affect the movement of the particles in the mixer and the interaction with other components and hence the tendency to mix and segregate.

The optimum mixing time and conditions should therefore be established and validated at a production scale so that the appropriate degree of mixing is obtained without segregation, overlubrication or damage to component particles. Minimum and maximum mixing times which give a satisfactory product should be determined, if appropriate, so that the 'robustness' of the mixing process is established.

Mixing of miscible liquids and suspensions

Mobile liquids with a low viscosity are easily mixed with each other. Similarly, solid particles are readily suspended in mobile liquids, although the particles are likely to settle rapidly when mixing is discontinued. Viscous liquids are more difficult to stir and mix but they reduce the sedimentation rate of suspended particles (discussed further in Chapter 26).

Mixers for miscible liquids and suspensions

Propeller mixers

A common arrangement for medium-scale fluid mixing is a propeller-type stirrer which is often used clamped to the edge of a vessel. A propeller has angled blades, which cause the circulation of the fluid in both an axial and a radial direction. An off-centre mounting discourages the formation of a vortex, which may form when the stirrer is mounted centrally. A vortex forms when the centrifugal force imparted to the liquid by the propeller blades causes it to back up round the sides of the vessel and form a depression around the shaft. As the speed of rotation is increased, air may be sucked into the fluid due to the formation of a vortex; this can cause frothing and possible oxidation (Fig. 11.12a). Another method of suppressing a vortex is to fit vertical baffles into the vessel. These divert the rotating fluid from its circular path into the centre of the vessel, where the vortex would otherwise form (see Fig. 11.12b).

The ratio of the diameter of a propeller stirrer to the diameter of the vessel is commonly $1:10$ to $1:20$, and it typically operates at speeds of 1 to 20 revolutions per second. The propeller stirrer depends for its action on a satisfactory axial and radial flow pattern, which will not occur if the fluid is too viscous. There must be a fast flow of fluid towards the propeller, which can only occur if the fluid is mobile.

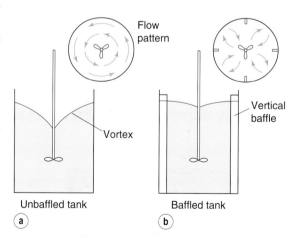

Fig. 11.12 • Propeller mixer with **(a)** an unbaffled tank and **(b)** a baffled tank.

Turbine mixers

A turbine mixer may be used for more viscous fluids, and a typical construction is shown in Fig. 11.13. The impeller has four flat blades surrounded by perforated inner and outer diffuser rings. The rotating impeller draws the liquid into the mixer 'head' and forces the liquid through the perforations with considerable radial velocity, sufficient to overcome the viscous drag of the bulk of the fluid. One drawback is the absence of an axial component, but a different head with the perforations pointing upwards can be fitted if this is desired. As the liquid is forced through the small orifices of the diffuser rings at high velocity, large shear forces are produced. When mixing immiscible liquids, if the orifices are sufficiently small and velocity sufficiently high, the shear forces produced enable the generation of droplets of the dispersed phase which are small enough to produce stable dispersions (water-in-oil or oil-in-water dispersions). Turbine mixers of this type (homogenizers) are therefore often fitted to vessels used for the large-scale production of emulsions and creams.

Turbine-type mixes will not cope with liquids of very high viscosity because the material will not be drawn into the mixer head. These liquids are best

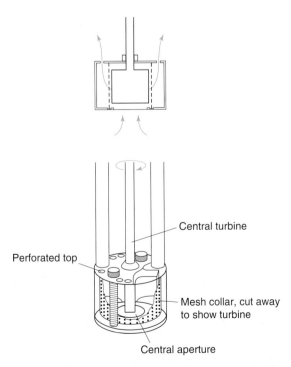

Fig.11.13 • Turbine mixer.

treated as semisolids and handled in the same equipment as used for such materials (see later).

In-line mixers

As an alternative to mixing fluids in batches in vessels, mobile miscible components may be fed through an 'inline' mixer designed to create turbulence in a flowing fluid stream. In this case, a continuous mixing process is possible.

Mixing of semisolids

The problems that arise during the mixing of semisolids (ointments and pastes) stem from the fact that, unlike liquids, semisolids will not flow easily. Material that finds its way to a 'dead spot' will remain there. For this reason, suitable mixers must have rotating elements with narrow clearances between themselves and the mixing vessel wall, and they must produce a high degree of shear mixing as diffusion mixing cannot occur.

Mixers for semisolids

Planetary mixers

This type of mixer is commonly found in the domestic kitchen (e.g. Kenwood-type mixers), and larger machines which operate on the same principle are used in the pharmaceutical industry (see Fig. 11.10). When used for the mixing of semisolids, they are designed so that there is only a small clearance between the vessel and the paddle in order to ensure sufficient shear. However, 'scraping down' of the bowl is usually necessary several times during a run to mix the contents well because some materials are forced to the top of the bowl.

Double planetary mixers that move material by rotating two identical blades (either rectangular or helical) on their own axes as they orbit on a common axis are often used for mixing highly viscous semisolid materials. As the blades continuously advance along the periphery of the mixer vessel, they remove material from the walls and transport it towards the interior.

Sigma blade mixers

This robust mixer will deal with stiff pastes and ointments and depends for its action on the close intermeshing of the two blades which resemble the Greek letter Σ in shape – hence the name. The clearance between the blades and the mixing trough is kept small by the design shown in Fig. 11.14.

Further treatment of semisolid dispersions

It is very difficult, when using primary mixers, to completely disperse powder particles in a semisolid base so that they are invisible to the eye. The mix is usually subjected to the further action of a roller mill or colloid mill so as to 'rub out' these particles by the intense shear generated by rollers or cones set with a very small clearance between them.

 Please check your eBook at **https://studentconsult. inkling.com/** for self-assessment questions. See inside cover for registration details.

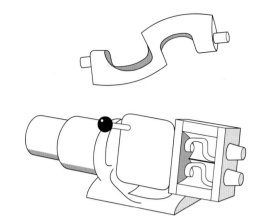

Fig.11.14 • Sigma blade mixer.

References

Bakeev, K.A., 2010. Process Analytical Technology. John Wiley & Sons, Chichester.

Ciurczak, E.W., Igne, B., 2014. Pharmaceutical and Medical Applications of Near-Infrared Spectroscopy, 2nd ed. CRC Press, Boca Raton.

Nikolakakis, N., Newton, J.M., 1989. Solid state adsorption of antibiotics onto sorbitol. J Pharm Pharmacol 41, 145–148.

Travers, D.N., White, R.C., 1971. The mixing of micronized sodium bicarbonate with sucrose crystals. J Pharm Pharmacol 23, 260S–261S.

Venables, H.J., Wells, J.I., 2001. Powder mixing. Drug Dev. Ind. Pharm. 27, 599–612.

Bibliography

Cullen, P.J., Romariach, R.J., Abatzoglou, N., et al., 2015. Pharmaceutical Blending and Mixing. John Wiley & Sons, Chichester.

Harnby, N., Edwards, M.F., Nienow, A.W., 1997. Mixing in the Process Industries, 2nd ed. Butterworth-Heinemann, Oxford.

Kaye, B.H., 1997. Powder Mixing. Chapman and Hall, London.

Levin, M., 2011. Pharmaceutical Process Scale-up, 3rd ed. Informa Healthcare, London.

Miyanami, K., 2006. Mixing. In: Masuda, H., Higashitani, K.Yoshida, H. (Eds.), Powder Technology Handbook, 3rd ed. Marcel Dekker, New York.

Paul, E.L., Atiemo-Obeng, V.A., Kresta, S.M., 2004. Handbook of Industrial Mixing – Science and

Practice. John Wiley & Sons, Hoboken.

Staniforth, J.N., 1982. Advances in powder mixing and segregation in relation to pharmaceutical processing. Int. J. Pharm. Tech. & Prod. Manuf. 3 (Suppl.), 1–12.

Powder flow

12

Michael E. Aulton

KEY POINTS

- The flow of powders and granules (a very common pharmaceutical operation) is much more difficult than that of liquids. The flow is often variable and unpredictable.
- These difficulties are caused by the adhesive and cohesive characteristics of the powder. These are surface properties and thus their magnitude is greatly influenced by particle and surface characteristics, such as particle size, roughness, surface free energy and shape.
- A thorough knowledge of powder flow can assist in the design of efficient equipment for powder handling.
- It is important that, even in the early stages of formulation development, the pharmaceutical scientist is aware of how the intended formulation will perform; for example, on a high-speed tableting machine.
- Because of the importance of powder flow, many laboratory tests have been developed to help predict how a material (or more often a mix of materials) will perform during manufacture. The Hausner ratio and Carr's index have proved to be particularly useful in this context.
- It is an important aspect in formulation design for the pharmaceutical scientist to make every effort to improve the flow of the powders in a particular product, rather than just accepting the material supplied, in order to minimize production problems. The scientist can help to set the specification of size, shape, size distribution, etc., or make formulation changes, e.g. by adding flow activators or glidants.

Introduction

Powders are generally considered to be composed of a collection of solid particles of the same or different chemical compositions having equivalent diameters less than 1000 μm. Granules are aggregated groups of small particles or individual larger particles which may have overall dimensions greater than 1000 μm. Chapter 28 discusses the differences between powders and granules in greater detail but, as far as powder flow is concerned, powders and granules will be discussed together here and the word 'powder' is used here to describe either system.

Powders exist as a dosage form in their own right, but the largest pharmaceutical use of powders is to produce tablets and capsules. Together with mixing and compaction properties, the flowability of a powder is of critical importance in the production of pharmaceutical dosage forms. Some of the reasons for producing free-flowing pharmaceutical powders include:

- uniform flow from bulk storage containers or hoppers into the feed mechanisms of tableting or capsule-filling equipment, allowing uniform particle packing and a constant volume-to-mass ratio in order to maintain tablet weight uniformity;
- reproducible filling of tablet dies and capsule dosators to improve weight uniformity and allow tablets to be produced with more consistent physicomechanical properties;
- uneven powder flow can result in excess entrapped air within powders, which in some high-speed tableting conditions may promote capping or lamination; and
- uneven powder flow can result from excess fine particles in a powder, which increases particle–die-wall friction, causing lubrication problems, and increased dust contamination risks during powder transfer.

There are many industrial processes that require powders to be moved from one location to another, and this is achieved by many different methods, such as gravity feeding, mechanically assisted feeding, pneumatic transfer, fluidization in gases and liquids and hydraulic transfer. In each of these examples, powders are required to flow and, as with other operations described earlier, the efficiency with which they do so is dependent on both process design and particle properties.

Particle properties

Adhesion and cohesion

The presence of molecular forces produces a tendency for individual solid particles to stick to each other and to other surfaces. Adhesion and cohesion can be considered as two aspects of the same phenomenon. *Cohesion* occurs between like surfaces, such as the same component particles in a bulk solid, whereas *adhesion* occurs between two different objects, e.g. between two different particles, or between a particle and a container wall.

Adhesive and cohesive forces acting between particles in a powder bed are composed mainly from short-range nonspecific van der Waals forces, which increase as particle size decreases and vary with changes in relative humidity. Other attractive forces contributing to interparticulate adhesion and cohesion may be produced by surface tension forces between adsorbed liquid layers at the particle surfaces and by electrostatic forces arising from contact or frictional charging. These may have short duration but increase adhesion and cohesion through improving interparticulate contacts and hence increasing the quantity of van der Waals interactions. Cohesion provides a useful method of characterizing the drag or frictional forces acting within a powder bed to prevent powder flow.

Angle of repose

Angle of repose is a simple measure of powder flow but it is based on scientific principles. An object, such as a particle, will begin to slide under gravitational forces when the angle of inclination is large enough to overcome frictional forces. Conversely, an object in motion will stop sliding when the angle of inclination is below that required to overcome adhesion/cohesion. This balance of forces causes a powder poured from a container onto a horizontal surface to form a heap. Initially the particles stack until the approach angle for subsequent particles joining the stack is large enough to overcome friction. They then slip and roll over each other until the gravitational forces balance with the interparticulate forces. The sides of the heap formed in this way make an angle with the horizontal. This angle is called the *angle of repose* and is a characteristic of the internal friction or cohesion of the particles.

The value of angle of repose will be high if a powder is cohesive and low if a powder is noncohesive. If the powder is very cohesive, the heap may be characterized by more than one angle of repose. Initially, the interparticulate cohesion causes a very steep cone to form, but on the addition of further powder, this tall stack may suddenly collapse, causing air to be entrained between particles and partially fluidizing the bed, thus making it more mobile. The resulting heap has two angles of repose: a large angle

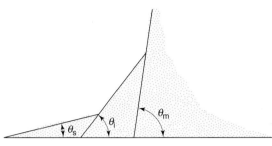

Fig. 12.1 • Cohesive powder poured in a heap and showing different angles of repose: θ_m maximum angle formed by cohesive particles; θ_s shallowest angle formed by collapse of the cohesive particle heap, resulting in flooding. In some cases, a third angle, θ_i, is identifiable as an intermediate slope produced by cohesive particles stacking on flooded powder.

remaining from the initial heap and a shallower angle formed by the powder flooding from the initial heap (Fig. 12.1).

Particle properties and bulk flow

In the previous discussion concerning adhesion/cohesion it is clear that an equilibrium exists between forces responsible for promoting powder flow and those preventing powder flow, i.e. at equilibrium:

$$\sum f(\text{driving forces}) = \sum f(\text{drag forces})$$
$$(12.1)$$

that is,

$$\sum f(\text{gravitational force, particle mass, angle of inclination of power bed, static head of powder, mechanical force, etc.}) = \sum f(\text{adhesive forces, cohesive forces, other surface forces, mechanical interlocking, etc.})$$
$$(12.2)$$

Some of these forces are modified or controlled by external factors related to particle properties, such as size, shape and density.

Particle size effects

Because adhesion and cohesion are surface phenomena, particle size will influence the flowability of a powder. In general, fine particles with a very high surface-to-mass ratio are more adhesive/cohesive than coarser particles. The latter are influenced more by gravitational forces. Particles larger than 250 μm are

usually relatively free flowing, but as the size falls below 100 μm, powders become more adhesive/cohesive and flow problems are likely to occur. Powders having a particle size of less than approximately 10 μm are usually extremely adhesive/cohesive and resist flow under gravity.

An important exception to this reduction in flowability with decrease in size is when the very small particles become adhered/cohered to larger ones and the flowability of the powder as a whole becomes controlled by the larger particles. This phenomenon is important in the concept of ordered mixing (see Chapter 11) and is exploited in the formulation of dry powder inhalers (see Chapter 37).

Particle shape

Powders with similar particle sizes but dissimilar shapes can have markedly different flow properties due to differences in interparticulate contact area. For example, a group of spheres has minimum interparticulate contact and generally optimal flow properties, whereas a group of particle flakes or dendritic particles have a very high surface-to-volume ratio, a larger area of contact and thus poorer flow properties. Irregularly shaped particles may experience mechanical interlocking in addition to adhesive and cohesive forces.

Particle density (true density)

Because powders normally flow under the influence of gravity, higher-density particles are generally less adhesive/cohesive than less dense particles of the same size and shape.

Packing geometry

A set of particles can be filled into a volume of space to produce a powder bed that is in static equilibrium due to the interaction of gravitational and adhesive/cohesive forces. By slight vibration of the bed, particles can be mobilized; if the vibration is stopped, the bed is once more in static equilibrium but occupies a different spatial volume than before. The change in bulk volume has occurred by rearrangement of the packing geometry of the particles. In general, such geometric rearrangements result in a transition from loosely packed particles to more tightly packed ones, so that the equilibrium balance moves from left to right in Eqs 12.1 and 12.2 and adhesion/cohesion increases. This also means that more tightly packed powders require a higher driving force to induce powder flow than more loosely packed particles of the same powder.

Characterization of packing geometry by porosity and bulk density

A set of monosized spherical particles can be arranged in many different geometric configurations. At one extreme, when the spheres form a cubic arrangement, the particles are most loosely packed and have a porosity of 48% (Fig. 12.2a). At the other extreme, when the spheres form a rhombohedral arrangement, they are most densely packed and have a porosity of only 26% (see Fig. 12.2b). The porosity used to characterize packing geometry is linked to the bulk density of the powder.

Bulk density, ρ_B, is a characteristic of the powder bulk rather than individual particles. It is calculated by dividing the mass, M, of powder by the volume, V, that it occupies (Eqn 12.3):

$$\rho_B = \frac{M}{V} \text{ kg m}^{-3}$$

(12.3)

The bulk density of a powder is always less than the true density of its component particles because the powder contains interparticulate voids and intraparticulate pores (intraparticulate voids) that are filled with air. Thus whereas a powder particle can only possess a single true density, it can have many different bulk densities, depending on the way in which the particles are packed and the bed porosity. However, a high bulk density value does not necessarily imply a close-packed low-porosity bed, as bulk density is directly proportional to true density:

bulk density ∝ true density

i.e. bulk density = k × true density

(12.4)

or:

$$k = \frac{\text{bulk density}}{\text{true density}}$$

(12.5)

The constant of proportionality, k, is known as the *packing fraction* or *fractional solids content*. For example, the packing fraction for dense, randomly packed spheres is approximately 0.65, whereas the packing fraction for a set of dense, randomly packed discs is 0.83. Also,

$$1 - k = e$$

(12.6)

where e is the *fractional voidage* of the powder bed, which is usually expressed as a percentage and termed the *bed porosity*. Another way of expressing fractional voidage is to use the ratio of particle volume, V_p, to bulk powder volume, V_B, i.e.

$$e = \frac{1 - V_p}{V_B}$$

(12.7)

A simple ratio of void volume, V_v, to particle volume, V_p, represents the voids ratio:

$$\frac{V_v}{V_p} = \frac{e}{(1 - e)}$$

(12.8)

which provides information about the stability of the powder mass.

For powders having comparable true densities, an increase in bulk density means a decrease in porosity. This increases the number of interparticulate contacts and contact areas and causes an increase in adhesion/cohesion. For very coarse particles, this may still be insufficient to overcome the gravitational influence on particles. Conversely, a decrease in bulk density may be associated with a reduction in particle size and produce a loose-packed powder bed which, although porous, is unlikely to flow because of the inherent adhesiveness/cohesiveness of the fine particles.

In powders where the particle shape or cohesiveness promotes arch or bridge formation, two equilibrium states could have similar porosities but widely different packing geometries. In such conditions, interparticulate pore size distributions can be useful for comparing packing geometry.

For example, Fig. 12.3a shows a group of particles in which arching has occurred and Fig. 12.3b shows a similar group of particles in which arch formation

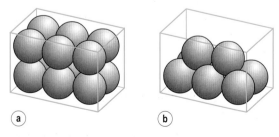

Fig. 12.2 • Different geometric packings of spherical particles. **(a)** Cubic packing. **(b)** Rhombohedral packing.

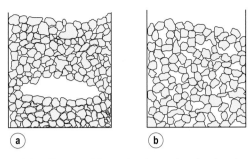

Fig. 12.3 • Two equidimensional powders having the same porosity but different packing geometries.

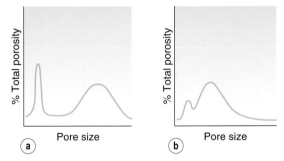

Fig. 12.4 • **(a)** Interparticulate pore size distribution corresponding to a close-packed bed containing a powder arch. **(b)** Interparticulate pore size distribution corresponding to a loosely packed bed.

is absent. The total porosity of the two systems can be seen to be similar, but the pore size distributions (Fig. 12.4) reveal that the powder in which arch formation has occurred is generally more tightly packed than that in which arching is absent.

Measurements of packing geometry by an assessment of percentage compressibility and changes in bulk density have proved to be useful indirect methods to estimate powder flow in an industrial manufacturing process (see later in this chapter).

Process conditions: hopper design

Flow through an orifice

There are many examples of this type of flow to be found in the manufacture of pharmaceutical solid dosage forms, e.g. when granules or powders flow through the opening in a hopper or bin used to feed powder to a tableting machine, capsule-filling machine or sachet-filling machine. Because of the importance of such flow in the production of unit solid dosage

forms, and the importance of flow behaviour in other industries, the behaviour of particles being fed through orifices has been extensively studied. A major goal is to achieve uniformity of flow to ensure that each single tablet, capsule, sachet, etc., contains the same or very similar powder masses. This work has led to the design of a hopper now used in most industrial pharmaceutical powder applications.

A hopper or bin can be modelled as a tall cylindrical container having a closed orifice in the base and initially full of a free-flowing powder which has a horizontal upper surface (Fig. 12.5a). When the orifice at the base of the container is opened, flow patterns develop as the powder discharges (Fig. 12.5).

The observed sequence is as follows:

1. On opening the orifice, there is no instantaneous movement at the surface but particles just above the orifice fall freely through it (Fig. 12.5b).

2. A depression forms at the upper surface of the powder and spreads outwards to the sides of the hopper (Fig. 12.5c, d).

3. Provided that the container is tall and not too narrow, the flow pattern illustrated in Fig. 12.5e and shown schematically in Fig. 12.6 is rapidly established. Particles in zone A move rapidly over the slower-moving particles in zone B, whereas those in zone E remain stationary. The particles in zone A feed into zone C, where they move quickly downwards and out through the orifice. The more slowly moving particles in zone B do not enter zone C.

4. Both powder streams in zones B and C converge to a 'tongue' just above the orifice, where the movement is most rapid and the particle packing is least dense. In a zone just above the orifice, the particles are in free flight downwards.

Important practical consequences of this flow pattern are that if a square-bottomed hopper or bin is repeatedly refilled and partially emptied, the particles in the zone towards the base and sides of the container (Fig. 12.5f) will never be discharged and may eventually degrade. Thus process hoppers are designed to have a conical lower section, in effect eliminating zone E in Fig. 12.6.

Factors affecting flow rates through orifices

The flow patterns described in the preceding section, together with the rates of powder flow through

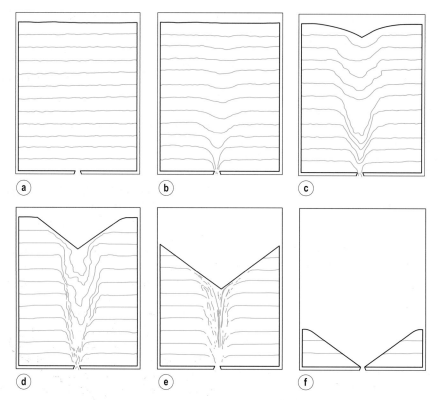

Fig. 12.5 • Development of flow through an orifice. The *horizontal lines* are formed by indicator particles to show the course of the discharge.

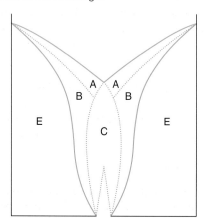

Fig. 12.6 • Fully developed flow of a free-flowing powder through an orifice.

orifices, are dependent on many different factors, some of which are particle related and some process related. Particle-related effects, notably particle size, were discussed earlier.

Orifice diameter. The rate of powder flow through an orifice is proportional to a function of orifice diameter, D_O. Flow rate is directly proportional to $D_O{}^A$, where A is a constant with a value of approximately 2.6. Provided that the height of the powder bed, called the *head of powder*, remains considerably greater than the orifice diameter, flow rate is virtually independent of powder head. This situation is unlike that relating to liquid flow through an orifice, where the flow rate falls off continuously as the head diminishes. The constant rate of flow for powders is a useful property as it means that if a bulk powder is filled into dies, sachets, capsules or other enclosures, they will receive equal weights if filled for equal times.

Hopper width, height of powder in the hopper and hopper wall angle also influence the rate of discharge of powder or granules from a hopper.

Characterization of powder flow

When examining the flow properties of a powder, it is useful to be able to quantify the type of behaviour in terms of speed and (possibly more importantly) uniformity of flow. Many different methods are available, either directly, using dynamic or kinetic methods, or indirectly, generally by measurements carried out on static beds. These tests attempt to correlate the various measures of powder flow to manufacturing properties. A wide range of equipment is available to cater for the wide range of powder types and particle sizes encountered in pharmaceutical applications.

The apparatus and techniques described in the following sections are illustrative of the principles on which most equipment is based. It is well established that no single, simple test will truly characterize the flow properties during large-scale manufacture but, with careful control, the tests can give a good estimate. This is particularly useful in the early stages of preformulation, formulation and scale-up.

In general, methods of measuring powder flow must be practical, useful, reproducible and sensitive, and must yield meaningful results. An appropriate strategy is to use multiple standardized test methods to characterize the various aspects of powder flow that need to be understood by the pharmaceutical scientist. Pharmacopoeias are making an effort to standardize the procedures and equipment used to assess powder flow. Currently, the preferred assessments are (1) angle of repose, (2) compressibility index and Hausner ratio, (3) flow rate through an orifice and (4) shear cell. Each of these is described later in this chapter.

Indirect methods

Measurement of cohesive/adhesive properties

Adhesive or cohesive forces (acting between particles of different substances or between particles of the same substance respectively) can, in practice, be determined by studying the adhesion/cohesion characteristics of a bed of powder. This avoids delicate and difficult experimentation to determine the attractive forces between, say, two individual particles.

Shear strength

Shear stress. This can be defined as the stress (force per unit area) necessary to shear a powder bed under conditions of zero normal load. Using this criterion, the shear strength of a powder can be determined from the resistance to flow caused by adhesion, cohesion or friction and can be measured using a shear cell.

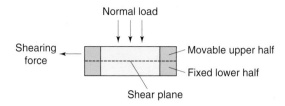

Fig. 12.7 • Representation of Jenike shear cell.

The shear cell (Fig. 12.7) is a relatively simple piece of apparatus which is designed to measure shear stress, τ, at different values of normal stress, σ. There are several types of shear cell which use different methods of applying the stresses and measuring the shear strengths, the most common being based on the original Jenike principle. In order to carry out a shear stress determination, powder is packed into the two halves of the cell and a normal stress is applied to the lid of the assembled cell. A shearing stress across the two halves of the cell is applied and the shear stress is determined by dividing the shear force by the cross-sectional area of the powder bed. The measured shear stress will increase as the normal stress is increased. Shear cell experiments are rather time-consuming and require a well-trained operator.

In order to calculate the cohesion in a powder bed using the shear cell method, the shear stress is plotted against normal stress and extrapolated back to zero normal stress, as the shear stress at zero normal stress is, by definition, equal to the cohesion of the powder. The higher the intercept the greater are the adhesive/cohesive forces. For a completely noncohesive powder, the extrapolated shear stress will pass through the origin, equivalent to zero shear stress.

Tensile strength

The tensile strength of a powder bed is also a characteristic of the internal friction, adhesion or cohesion of the particles. In tensile strength determinations, the powder bed is caused to fail in tension by splitting, rather than failing in shear by sliding, as is the case with shear stress determinations. The powder is packed into a split plate, one half of which is fixed and the other half free to move (Fig. 12.8). The table is then tilted towards the vertical until the angle is reached at which the powder cohesion is overcome and the mobile half-plate breaks away from the static half-plate. The tensile strength, σ_t, of the powder can then be determined from Eq. 12.9:

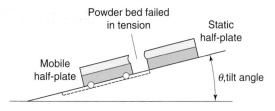

Fig. 12.8 • Measurement of tensile strength of a powder bed using the tilting table method.

$$\sigma_t = \frac{Mg\sin\theta}{A}$$

$$(12.9)$$

where M is the mass of the mobile half-plate plus powder, θ is the angle of the tilted table to the horizontal at the point of failure and A is the cross-sectional area of the powder bed.

The tensile strength values of different powders have been found to correlate reasonably well with another measurement of powder flowability – angle of repose.

Angle of repose

Angles of repose have been used as indirect methods of quantifying powder flowability, because of their relationship with interparticulate cohesion. There are many different methods of determining angles of repose, and some of these are shown in Table 12.1. The different methods may produce different values for the same powder, although these may be self-consistent. It is also possible that different angles of repose could be obtained for the same powder, owing to differences in the way the samples were handled prior to measurement. For these reasons, angles of repose tend to be variable and are not always representative of flow under specific conditions.

It is particularly difficult to determine this angle with very poor flowing material (see the discussion of Fig. 12.1). In order to overcome this problem, it is suggested that determinations of angles of repose be carried out using different concentrations of a very adhesive/cohesive powder and a nonadhesive/non-cohesive powder. The angles of repose are plotted against mixture concentration and extrapolated to 100% of the more adhesive/cohesive powder content so as to obtain the appropriate angle of repose that would be unobtainable in practice (Fig. 12.9).

As a general guide, powders with angles of repose greater than 45° have unsatisfactory flow properties, whereas minimum angles close to 25° will have

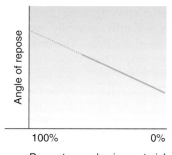

Fig.12.9 • Determination of angle of repose for very cohesive powders.

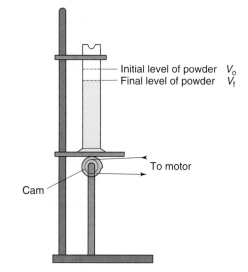

Fig. 12.10 • Mechanical tapping device (jolting volumeter).

excellent flow properties. A more detailed correlation was suggested by Carr. This is shown in Table 12.2.

Determinations based on bulk density

Bulk density measurements

The bulk density of a powder is dependent on particle packing and changes as the powder consolidates. A consolidated powder is likely to have a greater arch strength than a less consolidated one and may therefore be more resistant to powder flow. The ease with which a powder consolidates can be used as an indirect method of quantifying powder flow.

Fig. 12.10 shows a mechanical tapping device or jolting volumeter which can be used to follow the change in packing volume that occurs when void space

Table 12.1 Methods of measuring angle of repose

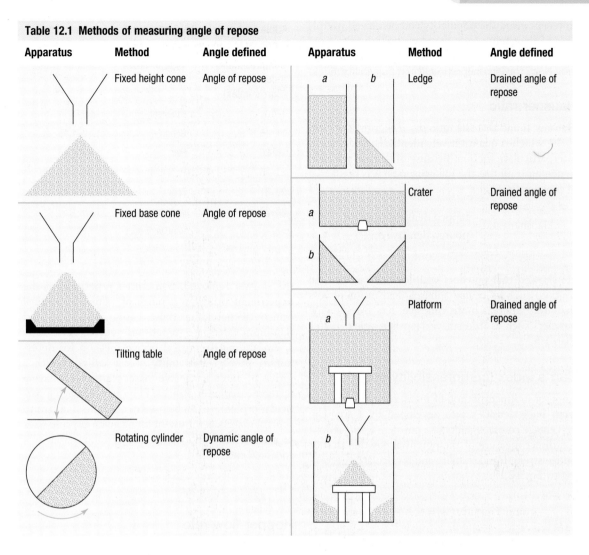

Apparatus	Method	Angle defined	Apparatus	Method	Angle defined
	Fixed height cone	Angle of repose	a b	Ledge	Drained angle of repose
	Fixed base cone	Angle of repose	a b	Crater	Drained angle of repose
	Tilting table	Angle of repose	a b	Platform	Drained angle of repose
	Rotating cylinder	Dynamic angle of repose			

Table 12.2 Angle of repose as an indication of powder flow properties (based on Carr)

Angle of repose (°)	Type of flow
25–30	Excellent
31–35	Good
36–40	Fair (flow aid not needed)
41–45	Passable (may hang up, flow aid might be needed)
46–55	Poor (agitation or vibration needed)
56–65	Very poor
>65	Very, very poor

diminishes and consolidation occurs. The powder contained in the measuring cylinder is mechanically tapped by means of a constant-velocity rotating cam. The volume decreases from its original state (V_o) to a final state (V_f). The initial bulk density ρ_{Bmin} (also known as fluff or poured bulk density) and the final bulk density ρ_{Bmax} (also known as equilibrium, tapped or consolidated bulk density when it has attained its most stable, i.e. unchanging, arrangement) are calculated from the mass (m) and bulk volume of the powder (Eqns 12.10 and 12.11):

$$\rho_{Bmin} = m/V_0$$

$$(12.10)$$

$$\rho_{Bmax} = m/V_f$$

$$(12.11)$$

In recent years the popularity and perceived useful-ness of flowability tests based on bulk density have increased. The two most useful and best characterized indices are the Hausner ratio and compressibility index.

Hausner ratio

Hausner found that the ratio ρ_{Bmax}/ρ_{Bmin} (or the ratio V_o/V_f, which is quantitatively identical) is related to interparticulate friction. Because of this, he was able to demonstrate that the following ratio was predictive of powder flow.

$$\text{Hausner ratio} = \frac{\text{tapped density }(\rho_{Bmax})}{\text{poured density }(\rho_{Bmin})} \times 100$$

(12.12)

He showed that powders with low interparticulate friction, such as coarse spheres, had ratios of less than 1.2, whereas more cohesive, less free-flowing powders such as flakes have Hausner ratios greater than 1.5.

Carr's index (compressibility index)

Another indirect method of measuring powder flow from bulk densities was developed by Carr. The percentage compressibility of a powder (Carr's index) is a direct measure of the potential powder arch or bridge strength and stability and is calculated accord-ing to Eq. 12.13:

$$\text{compressibility (\%)} = \frac{\rho_{Bmax} - \rho_{Bmin}}{\rho_{Bmax}} \times 100$$

(12.13)

Table 12.3 shows the generalized relationship between descriptions of powder flow and percent compress-ibility according to Carr. It also includes the equivalent Hausner ratios.

Critical orifice diameter

The critical orifice diameter is a measure of powder cohesion and arch strength. In order to carry out measurements of critical orifice diameter, powder is filled into a shallow tray to a uniform depth with near-uniform packing. The base of the tray is perfo-rated with a graduated series of holes, which are blocked either by resting the tray on a plane surface or by the presence of a simple shutter. The critical orifice diameter is the size of the smallest hole through which powder discharges when the tray is lifted or

Table 12.3 Relationship between powder flowability, percentage compressibility and Hausner ratio

Compressibility index (%) (Carr's index)	Type of flow	Hausner ratio
1–10	Excellent	1.00–1.11
11–15	Good	1.12–1.18
16–20	Fair	1.19–1.25
21–25	Passable	1.26–1.34
26–31	Poor	1.35–1.45
32–37	Very poor	1.46–1.59
>37	Very, very poor	>1.59

the shutter removed. Sometimes repetition of the experiment produces a range of values for critical orifice diameter; in these cases, maximum and minimum values are sometimes quoted.

An alternative critical orifice method for deter-mining powder flowability uses a cylinder with a series of interchangeable base plate discs having different-diameter orifices. Flow rate through a par-ticular orifice size can be used as a simple standard to specify materials for use in filling given capsule sizes or sachets or producing particular tablet sizes at a specified rate.

Direct measurements of flow

Hopper flow rate

A simple direct method of determining powder flowability is to measure the rate at which powder discharges from a hopper. A simple shutter is placed over the hopper outlet and the hopper is filled with powder. The shutter is then removed and the time taken for the powder to discharge completely is recorded. By dividing the discharged powder mass by this time, a mass flow rate is obtained which can be used for quantitative comparison of different powders.

Hopper or discharge tube outlets should be selected to provide a good model for a particular flow application. For example, if a powder discharges well from a hopper into a tablet machine feed frame but does not flow reproducibly into the tablet die, then it is likely that more useful information will be generated by selecting experimental conditions to model those occurring in flow from the feeder to the die, rather than those in flow from the hopper to the feeder.

Recording flowmeter

A recording flowmeter is essentially similar to the method described in the previous section for measurement of the hopper flow rate except that powder is allowed to discharge from a hopper or container onto a balance. The digital signal from the balance records the increase in powder mass with time. Recording flowmeters allow mass flow rates to be determined and also provide a means of quantifying uniformity of flow.

Improvement of powder flowability

Alteration of particle size and particle size distribution

Because coarse (larger) particles are generally less cohesive than fine (smaller) particles and an optimum size for free flow exists, there is a distinct processing disadvantage in using a finer grade of powder than is necessary.

The size distribution can also be altered to improve flowability by removing a proportion of the fraction of fine particles or by increasing the proportion of coarser particles, such as may be achieved through granulation.

Alteration of particle shape or texture

In general, for a given particle size, more spherical particles have better flow properties than more irregular particles. The process of spray-drying can be used to produce near-spherical excipients (e.g. spray-dried lactose). Under certain circumstances, drug particles that are normally acicular (needle shaped) can be made more spherical by spray-drying or by temperature-cycling crystallization.

The surface texture of particles may also influence powder flowability, as particles with very rough surfaces will have a greater tendency to interlock than smooth-surfaced particles. The shape and texture of particles can also be altered by control of production methods, such as crystallization conditions.

Alteration of surface forces

Reduction of electrostatic charges can improve powder flowability, and this can be achieved by altering process conditions to reduce frictional contacts. For example, where powder is poured down chutes or conveyed along pipes pneumatically, the speed and length of transportation should be minimized. Electrostatic charges in powder containers can be prevented or discharged by efficient earth connections.

The moisture content of particles is also of importance for powder flowability, as adsorbed surface moisture films tend to increase bulk density and reduce porosity. In cases where moisture content is excessive, powders should be dried, and if hygroscopic, stored and processed under low-humidity conditions.

Formulation additives: flow activators

Flow activators are commonly referred to pharmaceutically as 'glidants', although some also have lubricant or antiadherent properties. Flow activators improve the flowability of powders by reducing adhesion and cohesion.

A flow activator with an exceptionally high specific surface area is colloidal silicon dioxide, which may act by reducing the bulk density of tightly packed powders. Colloidal silicon dioxide also improves flowability of formulations, even those containing other glidants, although if used excessively it can cause flooding.

Where powder flowability is impaired through increased moisture content, a small proportion of very fine magnesium oxide may be used as a flow activator. Used in this way, magnesium oxide appears to disrupt the continuous film of adsorbed water surrounding the moist particles.

The use of silicone-treated powder, such as silicone-coated talc or sodium bicarbonate, may also be beneficial in improving the flowability of a moist or hygroscopic powder.

Alteration of process conditions

Use of vibration-assisted hoppers

In cases where the powder arch strength within a bin or hopper is greater than the stresses in it due to gravitational effects, powder flow will be interrupted or prevented. If the hopper cannot be redesigned to provide adequate downward stresses and if the physical properties of the particles cannot be adjusted or the formulation altered, then extreme measures are required. One method of encouraging powder flow where arching or bridging has occurred within a hopper is to add to the flow-inducing stresses by vibrating the hopper mechanically. Both the amplitude and the frequency of vibration can be altered to produce the desired effect. This may vary from a single cycle or shock, produced by a compressed-air device or hammer, to continuous high frequencies produced, for example, by out-of-balance electric motors mounted on a hopper frame.

Use of force feeders

The flow of powders that discharge irregularly or flood out of hoppers can be improved by fitting vibrating baffles at the base of the conical section within a hopper.

The outflowing stream from a hopper can be encouraged to move towards its required location using a slightly sloping moving belt or, in the case of some tableting machines, the use of mechanical force feeders. Force feeders are usually made up of a single or two counterrotating paddles at the base of the hopper just above the die table in place of a feed frame. The paddles act by preventing powder arching over dies and thereby improve die filling, especially at high turret speeds.

Summary

In most pharmaceutical technology operations, it is difficult to alter one process without adversely influencing another. In the case of alterations made in order to improve powder flow, relative particle motion will be promoted but this could lead to demixing or segregation. In extreme cases, improving powder flow to improve weight uniformity may reduce content uniformity through increased segregation.

Please check your eBook at **https://studentconsult. inkling.com/** for self-assessment questions. See inside cover for registration details.

Bibliography

Florence, A.T., Siepmann, J. (Eds.), 2009. Modern Pharmaceutics, vol. 1 and 2, fifth ed. Informa Healthcare, New York.

Gotoh, K., Masuda, H., Higashitan, K., 1997. Powder Technology Handbook, second ed. Marcel Dekker, New York.

Lieberman, H., 1996. Pharmaceutical Dosage Forms: Disperse Systems, vol. 2, second ed. Marcel Dekker, New York.

Lieberman, H., 1998. Pharmaceutical Dosage Forms: Disperse Systems, vol. 3, second ed. Marcel Dekker, New York.

Lieberman, H., Lachman, L., Schwartz, J.B., 1990. Pharmaceutical Dosage Forms: Tablets, vol. 2, second ed. Marcel Dekker, New York.

Niazi, S.K. (Ed.), 2004. Handbook of Pharmaceutical Manufacturing Formulations, vol. 2. Uncompressed Solid Products. CRC Press, Boca Raton.

Rhodes, M., 1990. Principles of Powder Technology. John Wiley & Sons, Chichester.

Salmon, A.D., Hounslow, M.J., Seville, J.P.K. (Eds.), 2007. Handbook of Powder Technology, vol. 11, first ed. Elsevier, Amsterdam.

Swarbrick, J., Boylan, J.C., 2002. Encyclopedia of Pharmaceutical Technology. Marcel Dekker, New York.

Part 3: Pharmaceutical microbiology and sterilization

Fundamentals of microbiology

13

Geoffrey W. Hanlon

KEY POINTS

- Microorganisms have the capacity to cause disease and to contaminate and spoil pharmaceutical products, but they can also be used to produce materials such as antibiotics and steroids for use in medicine.
- Viruses are not cellular structures but are packages of protein and nucleic acid. They have no independent existence and are obligate intracellular parasites.
- Bacteria are prokaryotic cells and the main focus of interest in pharmaceutical microbiology. They are found everywhere in the environment and are broadly divided into Gram-positive and Gram-negative cells based upon their cell wall structure.
- Fungi are eukaryotic organisms and as such their cells resemble mammalian cells in their general structure. They are primarily saprophytes but a small number of species are capable of causing disease. Many fungi are capable of producing materials which are of use industrially.

Introduction

Microorganisms are ubiquitous in nature and are vital components in the cycle of life. The majority are free-living organisms growing on dead or decaying matter whose prime function is the turnover of organic materials in the environment. Pharmaceutical microbiology, however, is concerned with the relatively small group of biological agents that cause human disease, spoil prepared medicines or can be used to produce compounds of medical interest.

In order to understand microorganisms more fully, living organisms of similar characteristics have been grouped together into taxonomic units. The most fundamental division is between prokaryotic and eukaryotic cells, which differ in a number of respects (Table 13.1) but particularly in the arrangement of their nuclear material. Eukaryotic cells contain chromosomes, which are separate from the cytoplasm and contained within a limiting nuclear membrane, i.e. they possess a true nucleus. Prokaryotic cells do not possess a true nucleus, and their nuclear material

Table 13.1 Differences between prokaryotic and eukaryotic organisms

Structure	Prokaryotes	Eukaryotes
Cell wall structure	Usually contains peptidoglycan	Peptidoglycan absent
Nuclear membrane	Absent	Present. Possess a true nucleus
Nucleolus	Absent	Present
Number of chromosomes	1	More than 1
Mitochondria	Absent	Present
Mesosomes	Present	Absent
Ribosomes	70S	80S

is free within the cytoplasm, although it may be aggregated into discrete areas called nuclear bodies. Prokaryotic organisms make up the lower forms of life and include Eubacteria and Archaeobacteria. Eukaryotic cell types embrace all the higher forms of life, of which only the fungi will be dealt with in this chapter.

One characteristic shared by all microorganisms is the fact that they are small; however, it is a philosophical argument whether all infectious agents can be regarded as living. Some are little more than simple chemical entities incapable of any free-living existence. Viroids, for example, are small circular, single-stranded RNA molecules not complexed with protein. One particularly well-studied viroid has only 359 nucleotides (1/10 the size of the smallest known virus) and yet causes a disease in potatoes. Prions are small, self-replicating proteins devoid of any nucleic acid. The prion associated with Creutzfeldt–Jakob disease in humans, scrapie in sheep and bovine spongiform encephalopathy in cattle has only 250 amino acids and is highly resistant to inactivation by normal sterilization procedures.

Viruses are more complex than viroids or prions, possessing both protein and nucleic acid. Despite being among the most dangerous infectious agents known, they are still not regarded as living. Table 13.2 shows the major groups of viruses infecting humans.

Viruses

Viruses are obligate intracellular parasites with no intrinsic metabolic activity, being devoid of ribosomes

and energy-producing enzyme systems. They are thus incapable of leading an independent existence and cannot be cultivated on cell-free media, no matter how nutritious. The size of human viruses ranges from the largest poxviruses, measuring approximately 300 nm, to the picornaviruses, such as poliovirus, which is approximately 20 nm. When one considers that a bacterial coccus measures 1000 nm in diameter, it can be appreciated that only the very largest virus particles may be seen under the light microscope, and electron microscopy is required for visualizing the majority. It will also be apparent that few of these viruses are large enough to be retained on the 200 nm (0.2 μm) membrane filters used to sterilize thermolabile liquids.

Viruses consist of a core of nucleic acid (either DNA as in vaccinia virus or RNA as in poliovirus) surrounded by a protein shell, or capsid. Most DNA viruses have linear, double-stranded DNA but in the case of the parvoviruses it is single stranded. The majority of RNA-containing viruses contain one molecule of single-stranded RNA, although in reoviruses it is double stranded. The protein capsid constitutes 50% to 90% of the weight of the virus and, as nucleic acid can only synthesize approximately 10% its own weight of protein, the capsid must be made up of a number of identical protein molecules. These individual protein units are called capsomeres and are not in themselves symmetrical but are arranged around the nucleic acid core in characteristic symmetrical patterns. Additionally, many of the larger viruses possess a lipoprotein envelope surrounding the capsid arising from the membranes within the host cell. In many instances the membranes are virus modified to produce projections outwards from the envelope, such as haemagglutinins or neuraminidase as found in influenza virus. The enveloped viruses are often called ether sensitive, as ether and other organic solvents may dissolve the membrane.

The arrangement of the capsomeres can be of a number of types.

- Helical. The classic example is tobacco mosaic virus (TMV), which resembles a hollow tube with capsomeres arranged in a helix around the central nucleic acid core
- Icosahedral. Such viruses often resemble spheres on cursory examination but when studied more closely, they are seen to be made up of icosahedra that have 20 triangular faces, each containing an identical number of

Table 13.2 The major groups of viruses that infect humans

Family	Capsid	Nucleic acid	Envelope	Example
Adenoviridae	Icosahedral	dsDNA	No	Human adenovirus
Arenaviridae	Helical	ssRNA	Yes	Lassa fever virus
Flaviviridae	Icosahedral	ssRNA	Yes	Yellow fever virus Hepatitis C virus
Hepadnaviridae	Icosahedral	dsDNA	No	Hepatitis B virus
Herpesviridae	Icosahedral	dsDNA	Yes	Herpes simplex virus Cytomegalovirus Varicella zoster virus
Orthomyxoviridae	Helical	ssRNA	Yes	Influenza virus
Papovaviridae	Icosahedral	dsDNA	No	Papillomavirus
Paramyxoviridae	Helical	ssRNA	Yes	Respiratory syncytial virus Measles virus Mumps virus
Picornaviridae	Icosahedral	ssRNA	No	Rhinovirus Poliovirus Coxsackie virus
Poxviridae	Complex	dsDNA	Yes	Molluscum contagiosum Vaccinia virus Variola virus
Reoviridae	Icosahedral	dsRNA	No	Rotavirus Colorado tick fever virus
Retroviridae	Icosahedral	ssRNA	Yes	HIV
Rhabdoviridae	Helical	ssRNA	Yes	Rabies virus
Togaviridae	Icosahedral	ssRNA	Yes	Rubella virus

dsDNA, Double-stranded DNA; dsRNA, double-stranded RNA; HIV, human immunodeficiency virus; ssRNA, single-stranded RNA.

capsomeres. Examples include the poliovirus and adenovirus.

- Complex. The poxviruses and bacterial viruses (bacteriophages) make up a group whose members have a geometry that is individual and complex.

Reproduction of viruses

Because viruses have no intrinsic metabolic capability, they require the functioning of the host cell machinery in order to manufacture and assemble new virus particles. It is this intimate association between the virus and its host that makes the treatment of viral infections so complex. Any chemotherapeutic approach which damages the virus will almost inevitably cause injury to the host cells and hence lead to side effects. An understanding of the life cycle of

the virus is, therefore, vital in determining suitable target sites for antiviral chemotherapy. The replication of viruses within host cells can be broken down into a number of stages.

Adsorption to the host cell

The first step in the infection process involves virus adsorption onto the host cell. This usually occurs via an interaction between protein or glycoprotein moieties on the virus surface with specific receptors on the host cell outer membrane. Different cells possess receptors for different viruses. For example, the human immunodeficiency virus (HIV) possesses two proteins involved in adsorption to T lymphocytes; these are known as gp41 and gp120. There are receptors on the lymphocyte surface to which HIV will bind. The main receptor is CD4, to which the protein gp120 attaches. Other receptors are CXCR4 and CCR5, to which the protein gp41 binds. Both attachments are necessary for infection and lead to conformational changes in the HIV envelope proteins, resulting in membrane fusion.

Penetration

Enveloped viruses fuse the viral membrane with the host cell membrane and release the nucleocapsid directly into the cytoplasm. Naked virions generally penetrate the cell by phagocytosis. Bacteriophages are viruses which specifically attack bacteria, and they inject their DNA into the host cell, while the rest of the virus remains on the outside.

Uncoating

In this stage the capsid is removed as a result of attack by cellular proteases, and this releases the nucleic acid into the cytoplasm. These first three stages are similar for both DNA viruses and RNA viruses.

Nucleic acid and protein synthesis

The detailed mechanisms by which DNA- and RNA-containing viruses replicate inside the cell are outside the scope of this chapter and the reader is referred to the bibliography for further information. After nucleic acid replication, early viral proteins are produced, the function of which is to switch off host cell metabolic activity and direct the activities of the cell towards the synthesis of proteins necessary for the assembly of new virus particles.

Assembly of new virions

Again, there are differences in the detail of how the viruses are assembled within the host cell, but construction of new virions occurs at this stage, and up to 100 new virus particles may be produced per cell.

Release of virus progeny

The newly formed virus particles may be liberated from the cell as a burst, in which case the host cell ruptures and dies. Infection with influenza virus results in a lytic response. Alternatively, the virions may be released gradually from the cell by budding of the host cell plasma membrane. These are often called 'persistent' infections, an example being hepatitis B.

Latent infections

In some instances, a virus may enter a cell but not go through the replicative cycle outlined in the previous sections and the host cell may be unharmed. The genome of the virus is conserved and may become integrated into the host cell genome, where it may be replicated along with the host DNA during cell division. At some later stage the latent virus may become reactivated and progress through a lytic phase, causing cell damage/death and the release of new virions. Examples of this type of infection are those which occur with the herpes simplex viruses associated with cold sores, genital herpes and also chickenpox, where the dormant virus may reactivate to give shingles later in life.

Oncogenic viruses

Oncogenic viruses have the capacity to transform the host cell into a cancer cell. In some cases, this may lead to relatively harmless, benign growths, such as warts caused by papovavirus, but in other cases more severe, malignant tumours may arise. Cellular transformation may result from viral activation or mutation of normal host genes, called protooncogenes, or the insertion of viral oncogenes.

Bacteriophages

Bacteriophages (phages) are viruses that attack bacteria but not animal cells. It is generally accepted that the interaction between a phage and a bacterium is highly specific, and there is probably at least one phage for each species of bacterium. In many cases the infection of a bacterial cell by a phage results in lysis of the bacterium; such phages are termed virulent. Some phages, however, can infect a bacterium without causing lysis. In this case the phage DNA becomes incorporated within the bacterial genome. The phage DNA can then be replicated along with the bacterial cell DNA; this is then termed a prophage. Bacterial cells carrying a prophage are called lysogenic, and phages capable of inducing lysogeny are called temperate. Occasionally some of the prophage genes may be expressed, and this will confer on the bacterial cell the ability to produce new proteins. The ability to produce additional proteins as a result of prophage DNA is termed lysogenic conversion.

The discovery of bacteriophages in the early 20th century is attributed to two workers, Frederick Twort and Felix d'Herelle. In 1896 Ernest Hankin had made an observation that the waters of the Ganges River possessed antibacterial properties which may have led to a reduction in cases of dysentery and cholera in the areas surrounding the river. Twort and d'Herelle independently came to the conclusion that this effect must be due to a virus. Twort did not continue with his research, but d'Herelle quickly established the potential of bacteriophages in antibacterial therapy 10 years before the advent of antibiotics. It was the discovery of penicillin by Alexander Fleming in 1928 that led to the demise of bacteriophage therapy, but interest is now increasing again due to the emergence of antibiotic-resistant strains of bacteria.

Archaea

Archaea are a fascinating group of prokaryotic microorganisms that are frequently found living in hostile environments. They differ in a number of respects from Eubacteria, particularly in the composition of their cell walls. They comprise methane producers, sulfate reducers, halophiles and extreme thermophiles. However, at present they have not been found to be of any value from a pharmaceutical or clinical standpoint and so will not be considered further.

Eubacteria

Eubacteria constitute the major group of prokaryotic cells that have pharmaceutical and clinical significance. They include a diverse range of microorganisms, from the primitive parasitic rickettsias that share some of the characteristics of viruses, through the more typical free-living bacteria to the branching, filamentous actinomycetes, which at first sight resemble fungi rather than bacteria.

Atypical bacteria

Rickettsiaceae, Coxiellaceae and Bartonellaceae

The families *Rickettsiaceae*, *Coxiellaceae* and *Bartonellaceae* include a number of clinically important genera, *Rickettsia*, *Coxiella* and *Bartonella*. Although these are prokaryotic cells, they differ from most other bacteria both in their structure and in the fact that the majority of species lead an obligate intracellular existence. This means that, with a few exceptions, they cannot be grown on cell-free media, although unlike many viruses they do possess some independent enzymes. They have a pleomorphic appearance, ranging from coccoid through to rod-shaped cells; multiplication is by binary fission. Their cell wall composition bears similarities to that of Gram-negative bacteria (see later in this chapter) and in general they stain this way. The genus *Rickettsia* has a number of species that give rise to human diseases, in particular epidemic typhus (*Rickettsia prowazekii*), murine typhus (*Rickettsia typhi*) and spotted fevers (various species). These are characterized by transmission via insect vectors, particularly mites, ticks, fleas and lice.

The mode of transmission by these vectors varies depending on the insect concerned. In the case of lice and fleas, the microorganisms multiply within the insect and get into the faeces. These insects then colonize humans and transmit the microorganism when the faeces or the insect itself is crushed onto the skin. No bite is necessary, and the faeces may also be inhaled. Mites and ticks pick up the microorganism when they take a blood meal from an infected animal. They then pass on the infection to humans when they accidentally bite us.

Coxiella burnetii is the only species in the genus *Coxiella* and it gives rise to a disease called Q fever. Although the source of the disease is infected animals, usually no insect vector is involved, and the most common route of transmission is by inhalation of infected dust. *Bartonella quintana* is the causative agent of trench fever, which, as the name suggests, occurs typically under conditions of war and deprivation. Each of the infections described here can be treated with the antibiotic doxycycline, although the duration of therapy may vary depending upon the nature of the disease and its severity.

Chlamydiae

These are obligate intracellular parasitic bacteria that possess some independent enzymes but lack the ability to generate ATP. Two cellular forms are identified: a small (0.3 μm) highly infectious elementary body, which, after infection, enlarges to give rise to the replicative form called the initial or reticulate body (0.8 μm to 1.2 μm). This divides by binary fission within membrane-bound vesicles in the cytoplasm of infected cells. Insect vectors are not required for the transmission of infection. Chlamydiae lack peptidoglycan in their cell walls and have weak Gram-negative characteristics.

Chlamydia trachomatis is a clinically important member of the group, being responsible for the disease trachoma, characterized by inflammation of the eyelids, which can lead to scarring of the cornea. This is the most common cause of infectious blindness worldwide. It is estimated that 400 million people are infected, with at least 6 million totally blind. The same species is also recognized as one of the major causes of sexually transmitted disease. *Chlamydophilia psittaci* and *Chlamydophilia pneumoniae* are responsible for respiratory tract infections. Chlamydial infections are responsive to treatment with tetracyclines, administered either topically or systemically as appropriate.

Mycoplasmas

The mycoplasmas are a group of very small (0.3 μm to 0.8 μm) prokaryotic microorganisms that are capable of growing on cell-free media but which lack cell walls. The cells are surrounded by a double-layered plasma membrane that contains substantial amounts of phospholipids and sterols. This structure has no rigidity owing to the absence of peptidoglycan, and so the cells are susceptible to osmotic lysis. The lack of peptidoglycan is also the reason for these bacteria being resistant to the effects of cell-wall-acting antibiotics such as the penicillins, and also the enzyme lysozyme. Members of this group are called pleomorphic, which means they can vary in shape, and these cells range from coccoid to filamentous. Most are facultative anaerobes capable of growth at 35 °C, and on solid media produce colonies with a characteristic 'fried egg' appearance. They contain a number of genera, of which the most important from a clinical point of view are *Mycoplasma* and *Ureaplasma*. *Mycoplasma pneumoniae* is a major cause of respiratory tract infections in children and young adults, whereas *Ureaplasma urealyticum* has been implicated in nonspecific genital infections. Despite being resistant to the β-lactam antibiotics, these infections can be effectively treated using either tetracyclines or erythromycin.

Actinomycetes

Many of the macroscopic features of the actinomycetes are those that are more commonly found among the filamentous fungi but they are indeed prokaryotic cells. They are a diverse group of Gram-positive bacteria morphologically distinguishable from other bacteria because they have a tendency to produce branching filaments and reproductive spores. *Actinomyces israelii* is the most common cause of actinomycosis, which can manifest itself as abscesses in the oral cavity or gastrointestinal tract. It may also cause endocarditis. The genus *Nocardia* contains a number of species that have been shown to be pathogenic to humans, but they are of low virulence and infect mainly immunocompromised patients. Reproduction in this genus is by fragmentation of the hyphal strands into individual cells, each of which can form a new mycelium. The genus *Streptomyces* contains no human pathogens, and most species are saprophytic bacteria found in the soil. They are aerobic microorganisms producing a nonfragmenting, branching mycelium that may bear spores. The reason for their pharmaceutical importance is their ability to produce a wide range of therapeutically useful antibiotics, including streptomycin, chloramphenicol, oxytetracycline, erythromycin and neomycin.

Typical bacteria

Shape, size and aggregation

Bacteria occur in a variety of shapes and sizes, determined not only by the nature of the organisms themselves but also by the way in which they are grown (Fig. 13.1). In general, bacterial dimensions lie in the range from 0.75 μm to 5 μm. The most common shapes are the sphere (coccus) and the rod (bacillus).

Some bacteria grow in the form of rods with a distinct curvature, e.g. vibrios are rod-shaped cells with a single curve resembling a comma, whereas a spirillum possesses a partial rigid spiral; spirochaetes are longer and thinner, exhibit a number of turns and are also more flexible. Rod-shaped cells occasionally grow in the form of chains but this is dependent on growth conditions rather than being a characteristic of the species.

Cocci, however, show considerable variation in aggregation, which is characteristic of the species. The plane of cell division and the strength of adhesion of the cells determine the extent to which they aggregate after division. Cocci growing in pairs are called diplococci, those growing in groups of four are called tetrads and those growing in groups of eight are called sarcina. If a chain of cells is produced resembling a string of beads this is termed a

Genus		Approximate dimensions (µm)
Staphylococcus Irregular clusters of spherical cells. Resemble bunch of grapes. Nonmotile	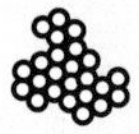	0.5–1.5
Streptococcus Spherical or ovoid cells occurring in pairs or in chains. Nonmotile	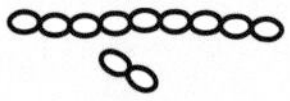	<2.0
Neisseria Small Gram-negative cocci. Occur in pairs with adjacent sides flattened. Nonmotile	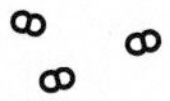	0.6–1.0
Lactobacillus Shape variable between long and slender to short coccobacillus. Nonmotile, chain formation common	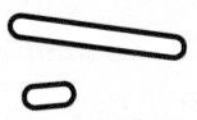	0.5–0.8 × 2–9
Escherichia Short rods, motile by peritrichous flagella	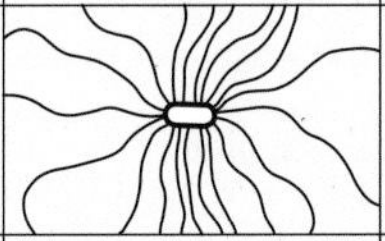	1.1–1.5 × 2–6
Bacillus Large endospore-forming rods. Motile by lateral flagella (not shown). Gram positive	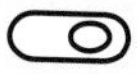	0.3–2.2 × 1.2–7.0
Vibrio Short curved or straight rods. Sometimes 'S' shaped. Motile by single polar flagella	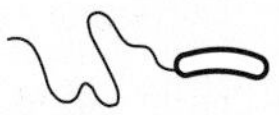	0.5 × 1.5–3.0
Spirochaeta Thin, flexible, helically coiled cells. Motile, possess axial fibrils (not shown)	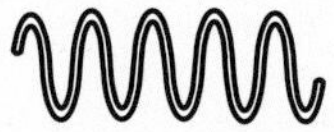	0.2–0.75 × 5–500
Spirillum Long, slender cells in rigid spirals. Number of turns differs. Motile bipolar flagellation	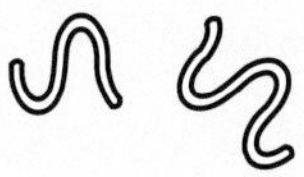	0.2–1.7 × 0.5–60
Streptomyces Slender, nonseptate branching filaments. Form reproductive spores. Nonmotile	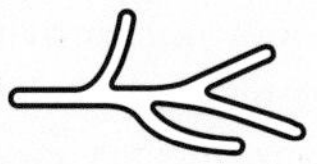	0.5–2.0 (diameter)

Fig. 13.1 • Morphology of different bacterial genera.

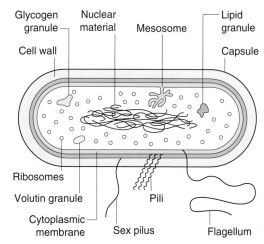

Fig. 13.2 • A typical bacterial cell.

Anatomy

Fig. 13.2 shows a diagrammatic representation of a typical bacterial cell. The various components are described in the following section.

Capsule

Many bacteria produce extracellular polysaccharides, which may take the form of either a discrete capsule, firmly adhered to the cell, or a more diffuse layer of slime. Not all bacteria produce a capsule, and even those that can will only do so under certain circumstances. For instance, many encapsulated pathogens, when first isolated, give rise to colonies on agar which are smooth (S) but subculturing leads to the formation of rough colonies (R). This S to R transition is due to loss of capsule production. Reinoculation of the R cells into an animal results in the resumption of capsule formation, indicating that the capacity has not been lost and that the cell can determine when production is required.

The function of the capsule is generally regarded as protective, as encapsulated cells are more resistant to disinfectants, desiccation and phagocytic attack. In some organisms, however, it serves as an adhesive mechanism; for example, *Streptococcus mutans* is an inhabitant of the mouth that metabolizes sucrose to produce a polysaccharide capsule enabling the cell to adhere firmly to the teeth. This is the initial step in the formation of dental plaque, which is a complex array of microorganisms and organic matrix that adheres to the teeth and ultimately leads to decay. The substitution of sucrose by glucose prevents capsule formation and hence eliminates plaque.

streptococcus and demonstrates division in one plane only and adhesion between cells after division. An irregular cluster similar in appearance to a bunch of grapes is called a staphylococcus and shows division in a number of different directions, as well as adhesion between cells after division. In many cases the aggregation of cells is sufficiently characteristic to give rise to the name of the bacterial genus, e.g. *Staphylococcus aureus* or *Streptococcus pneumoniae*.

A similar picture emerges with *Staphylococcus epidermidis*. This bacterium forms part of the normal microflora of the skin and was originally thought of as nonpathogenic. With the increased use of indwelling medical devices, coagulase-negative staphylococci, in particular *S. epidermidis*, have emerged as the major cause of device-related infections. The normal microbial flora has developed the ability to produce extracellular polysaccharide, which enables the cells to form resistant biofilms attached to the devices. These biofilms are very difficult to eradicate and have profound resistance to antibiotics and disinfectants. It is now apparent that the dominant mode of growth for aquatic bacteria is not planktonic (free swimming) but sessile, i.e. attached to surfaces and covered with protective extracellular polysaccharide or glycocalyx.

Cell wall

Bacteria can be divided into two broad groups by the use of the Gram-staining procedure (see later in this chapter for details), which reflects differences in cell wall structure. The classification is based on the ability of the cells to retain the dye methyl violet after they have been washed with a decolourizing agent such as absolute alcohol. Gram-positive cells retain the stain, whereas Gram-negative cells do not. As a *very rough* guide, the majority of small rod-shaped cells are Gram negative. Most large rods, such as the *Bacillaceae*, lactobacilli and actinomycetes, are Gram positive. Similarly, most cocci are Gram positive, although there are notable exceptions, such as the *Neisseriaceae*.

Bacteria are unique in that they possess peptidoglycan in their cell walls. This is a complex molecule with repeating units of *N*-acetylmuramic acid and *N*-acetylglucosamine (Fig. 13.3). This extremely long molecule is wound around the cell and cross-linked by polypeptide bridges to form a structure of great rigidity. The degree and nature of cross-linking vary between bacterial species. Cross-linking imparts to the cell its characteristic shape and has principally a protective function. Peptidoglycan (also called murein or mucopeptide) is the site of action of a number of antibiotics, such as penicillin, bacitracin, vancomycin and cycloserine. The enzyme lysozyme is also capable of hydrolysing the β-1–4 linkages between *N*-acetylmuramic acid and *N*-acetylglucosamine.

Fig. 13.4 shows simplified diagrams of a Gram-positive and a Gram-negative cell wall. The Gram-positive cell wall is much simpler in layout, containing peptidoglycan interspersed with teichoic

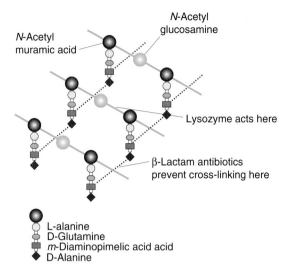

Fig. 13.3 • Peptidoglycan.

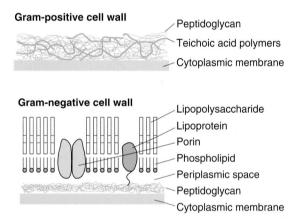

Fig. 13.4 • Structural components of bacterial cell walls.

acid polymers. These latter compounds are highly antigenic but do not provide structural support. Functions attributed to teichoic acids include the regulation of enzyme activity in cell wall synthesis, sequestration of essential cations, cellular adhesion and mediation of the inflammatory response in disease. In general, proteins are not found in Gram-positive cell walls. Gram-negative cell walls are more complex, comprising a much thinner layer of peptidoglycan surrounded by an outer bilayered membrane. This outer membrane acts as a diffusional barrier and is the main reason why many Gram-negative cells are much less susceptible to antimicrobial agents than are Gram-positive cells.

The lipopolysaccharide component of the outer membrane can be shed from the wall on cell death.

It is a highly heat-resistant molecule known as endotoxin, which has a number of toxic effects on the human body, including fever, shock and even death. For this reason, it is important that solutions for injection or infusion are not just sterile but are also free from endotoxins.

Cytoplasmic membrane

The cytoplasmic membranes of most bacteria are very similar and are composed of protein, lipids, phospholipids and a small amount of carbohydrate. The components are arranged in a bilayer structure with a hydrophobic interior and a hydrophilic exterior. The cytoplasmic membrane has a variety of functions:

- It serves as an osmotic barrier.
- It is selectively permeable and is the site of carrier-mediated transport.
- It is the site of ATP generation and cytochrome activity.
- It is the site of cell wall synthesis.
- It provides a site for chromosome attachment.

The cytoplasmic membrane has very little tensile strength, and the internal hydrostatic pressure of up to 20 bar forces it firmly against the inside of the cell wall. Treatment of bacterial cells with lysozyme may remove the cell wall and, as long as the conditions are isotonic, the resulting cell will survive. These cells are called protoplasts and, as the cytoplasmic membrane is now the limiting structure, the cell assumes a spherical shape. Protoplasts of Gram-negative bacteria are difficult to obtain because the layer of lipopolysaccharide protects the peptidoglycan from attack. In these cases, mixtures of EDTA and lysozyme are used, and the resulting cells, which still retain fragments of the cell envelope, are termed spheroplasts.

Nuclear material

The genetic information necessary for the functioning of the cell is contained within a single circular molecule of double-stranded DNA. When unfolded, this would be approximately 1000 times as long as the cell itself and so exists within the cytoplasm in a considerably compacted state. It is condensed into discrete areas called chromatin bodies that are not surrounded by a nuclear membrane. Rapidly dividing cells may contain more than one area of nuclear material but these are copies of the same chromosome, not different chromosomes, and arise because DNA replication proceeds ahead of cell division.

In addition to the main chromosome, cells may contain extra pieces of circular double-stranded DNA which are called plasmids. These can encode a variety of products which are not necessary for the normal functioning of the cell but confer some sort of selective advantage. For example, the plasmids may contain genes conferring antibiotic resistance or the ability to synthesize toxins or virulence factors. Plasmids replicate autonomously (i.e. independent of the main chromosome) and in some cases are able to be transferred from one cell to another (maybe of a different species).

Mesosomes

These are irregular invaginations, or infoldings, of the cytoplasmic membrane which are quite prominent in Gram-positive bacteria but less so in Gram-negative bacteria. It has been proposed that they have a variety of functions, including cross-wall synthesis during cell division and furnishing an attachment site for nuclear material, facilitating the separation of segregating chromosomes during cell division. They have also been implicated in enzyme secretions and may act as a site for cell respiration. However, it has also been suggested that they are simply artefacts which arise as a result of preparing samples for electron microscopy.

Ribosomes

The cytoplasm of bacteria is densely populated with ribosomes, which are complexes of RNA and protein in discrete particles 20 nm in diameter. They are the sites of protein synthesis within the cell, and the numbers present reflect the degree of metabolic activity of the cell. They are frequently found organized in clusters called polyribosomes or polysomes. Prokaryotic ribosomes have a sedimentation coefficient of 70 svedberg units ($1 S = 1 \times 10^{-13}$ s), compared with 80 S for ribosomes of eukaryotic cells. This distinction aids the selective toxicity of a number of antibiotics. The 70S ribosome is made up of RNA and protein, and can dissociate into one 30S subunit and one 50S subunit.

Inclusion granules

Certain bacteria tend to accumulate reserves of materials after active growth has ceased, and these become incorporated within the cytoplasm in the form of granules. The most common are glycogen granules, volutin granules (containing polymetaphosphate) and lipid granules (containing poly(β-hydroxybutyric acid)). Other granules, such as sulphur and iron, may also be found in the more primitive bacteria.

Flagella

A flagellum is made up of protein called flagellin and it operates by forming a rigid helix that turns rapidly like a propeller. This can propel a motile cell a distance up to 200 times its own length in 1 second. Under the microscope, bacteria can be seen to exhibit two kinds of motion: swimming and tumbling. When tumbling, the cell stays in one position and spins on its own axis, but when swimming, it moves in a straight line. Movement towards or away from a chemical stimulus is referred to as chemotaxis. The flagellum arises from the cytoplasmic membrane and is composed of a basal body, hook and filament. The number and arrangement of flagella depend on the organism and vary from a single flagellum (monotrichous) to a complete covering (peritrichous).

Pili and fimbriae

These terms are often used interchangeably but in reality these structures are functionally distinct from each other. Fimbriae are smaller than flagella and are not involved in motility. They are found all over the surface of certain bacteria (mainly Gram-negative cells) and are believed to be associated with adhesiveness and pathogenicity. They are also antigenic. Pili (of which there are different types) are larger and of a different structure to fimbriae and can be involved in the transfer of genetic information from one cell to another. This is of major importance in the transfer of drug resistance between cell populations. Other types of pili have been shown to be involved in a form of movement known as twitching. *Pseudomonas aeruginosa*, for example, exhibits three types of motility; swimming, swarming and twitching. Swimming and swarming are interlinked and are brought about by the use of flagella. Swimming is a characteristic of individual cells, whereas swarming is a coordinated migration of groups of cells. Twitching occurs on solid substrates when the cells are attaching to a surface during biofilm formation. It results from the repeated extension and retraction of type IV pili allowing the cells to translocate across the surface and thus form discrete microcolonies.

Endospores

Under conditions of specific nutrient deprivation, some genera of bacteria, in particular *Bacillus* and *Clostridium*, undergo a differentiation process at the end of logarithmic growth and change from an actively metabolizing vegetative form to a resting spore form. The process of sporulation is not a reproductive mechanism, as found in certain actinomycetes and filamentous fungi, but serves to enable the organism to survive periods of hardship. A single vegetative cell differentiates into a single spore. Subsequent encounter with favourable conditions results in germination of the spore and the resumption of vegetative activities.

Endospores are very much more resistant to heat, disinfectants, desiccation and radiation than are vegetative cells, making them difficult to eradicate from foods and pharmaceutical products. Heating at 80°C for 10 minutes would kill most vegetative bacteria, whereas some spores will resist boiling for several hours. The sterilization procedures now routinely used for pharmaceutical products are thus designed specifically with reference to the destruction of the bacterial spore.

The mechanism of this extreme heat resistance was a perplexing issue for many years. At one time it was thought to be due to the presence of a unique spore component, dipicolinic acid (DPA). This compound is found only in bacterial spores, where it is associated in a complex with calcium ions. The isolation of heat-resistant DPA-less mutants, however, led to the demise of this theory. Spores do not have a water content appreciably different from that of vegetative cells, but the distribution within the different compartments is unequal, and this is thought to generate the heat resistance. The central core of the spore houses the genetic information necessary for growth after germination, and this becomes dehydrated by expansion of the cortex against the rigid outer protein coats. Water is thus squeezed out of the central core. Osmotic pressure differences also help to maintain this water imbalance. Endospores are also highly unusual because of their ability to remain dormant and ametabolic for prolonged periods of time. Bacterial spores have been isolated from lake sediments where they were deposited 1000 years previously, and there have even been claims of spores revived from geological specimens up to 40 million years old.

The sequence of events involved in sporulation is illustrated in Fig. 13.5. It is a continuous process, although for convenience it may be divided into six stages. The complete process takes approximately 8 hours, although this may vary depending on the species and the conditions used. Occurring simultaneously with the morphological changes are a number of biochemical events that have been shown to be

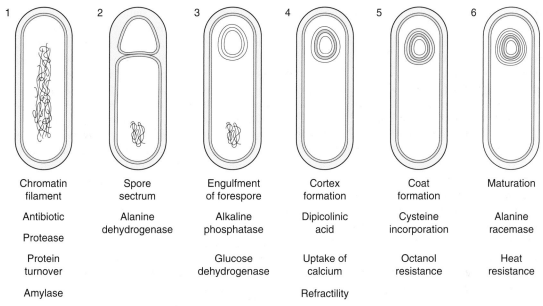

1	2	3	4	5	6
Chromatin filament	Spore sectrum	Engulfment of forespore	Cortex formation	Coat formation	Maturation
Antibiotic	Alanine dehydrogenase	Alkaline phosphatase	Dipicolinic acid	Cysteine incorporation	Alanine racemase
Protease					
Protein turnover		Glucose dehydrogenase	Uptake of calcium	Octanol resistance	Heat resistance
Amylase			Refractility		

Fig. 13.5 • Morphological and biochemical changes during spore formation.

associated with specific stages and occur in an exact sequence. One important biochemical event is the production of antibiotics. Peptides possessing anti-microbial activity have been isolated from the majority of *Bacillus* species and many of these have found pharmaceutical applications. Examples of antibiotics include bacitracin, polymyxin and gramicidin. Similarly, the proteases produced by *Bacillus* species during sporulation are used extensively in a wide variety of industries.

Microscopy and staining of bacteria

Bacterial cells contain approximately 80% water by weight and this accounts for their very low refractility, i.e. they are transparent when viewed under ordinary transmitted light. Consequently, in order to visualize bacteria under the microscope, the cells must be killed and stained with some compound that scatters the light or, if live preparations are required, special adaptations must be made to the microscope. Such adaptations are found in phase-contrast, dark-ground and differential-interference contrast microscopy.

The microscopic examination of fixed and stained preparations is a routine procedure in most laboratories, but it must be appreciated that not only are the cells dead but they may also have been altered morphologically by the often quite drastic staining process. The majority of stains used routinely are basic dyes, i.e. the chromophore has a positive charge and this readily combines with the abundant negative charges present both in the cytoplasm in the form of nucleic acids and on the cell surface. These dyes remain firmly adhered even after the cells have been washed with water. This type of staining is called simple staining, and all bacteria and other biological material are stained the same colour. Differential staining is a much more useful process as different organisms or even different parts of the same cell can be stained distinctive colours.

To prepare a film ready for staining, the glass microscope slide must be carefully cleaned to remove all traces of grease and dust. If the culture of bacteria is in liquid form, then a loopful of suspension is transferred directly to the slide. Bacteria from solid surfaces require suspension with a small drop of water on the slide to give a faintly turbid film. A common fault with inexperienced workers is to make the film too thick. The films must then be allowed to dry in air. When thoroughly dry, the film is fixed by passing the back of the slide through a small Bunsen flame until the area is just too hot to touch on the palm of the hand. The bacteria are killed by this procedure and are also stuck onto the slide. Fixing also makes the bacteria more permeable to the stain and inhibits lysis. Chemical fixation is commonly carried out using formalin or methyl alcohol; this causes less damage to the specimen but tends to be used principally for blood films and tissue sections.

Differential stains

A large number of differential stains have been developed, and the reader is referred to the bibliography for more details. Only a few of those available will be discussed here.

Gram stain. By far the most important in terms of use and application is the Gram stain, developed by Christian Gram in 1884 and subsequently modified. The fixed film of bacteria is flooded initially with a solution of methyl violet. This is followed by a solution of Gram's iodine, which is an iodine–potassium iodide complex acting as a mordant, fixing the dye firmly in certain bacteria and allowing easy removal in others. Decolourization is achieved with either alcohol or acetone or mixtures of the two. After treatment, some bacteria retain the stain and appear dark purple and these are called Gram positive. Others do not retain the stain and appear colourless (Gram negative). The colourless cells may be stained with a counterstain of contrasting colour, such as 0.5% safranin, which is red.

This method, although extremely useful, must be used with caution as the Gram reaction may vary with the age of the cells and the technique of the operator. For this reason, known Gram-positive and Gram-negative controls should be stained alongside the specimen of interest.

Ziehl–Neelsen acid-fast stain. The bacterium responsible for the disease tuberculosis (*Mycobacterium tuberculosis*) contains within its cell wall a high proportion of lipids, fatty acids and alcohols, which render it resistant to normal staining procedures. The inclusion of phenol in the dye solution, together with the application of heat, enables the dye (basic fuchsin) to penetrate the cell and, once attached, to resist vigorous decolourization by strong acids, e.g. 20% sulphuric acid. These organisms are therefore called acid fast. Any unstained material can be counterstained with a contrasting colour, e.g. methylene blue.

Fluorescence microscopy

Certain materials when irradiated by short-wave radiation (e.g. UV light) become excited and emit visible light of a longer wavelength. This phenomenon is termed fluorescence and will persist only for as long as the material is irradiated. A number of dyes have been shown to fluoresce and are useful in that they tend to be specific to various tissues, which can then be demonstrated by UV irradiation and subsequent fluorescence of the attached fluorochrome. Coupling antibodies to the fluorochromes can enhance specificity, and this technique has found wide application in microbiology. As with the staining procedures described earlier, this technique can only be applied to dead cells. The three following techniques have been developed for the examination of living organisms.

Dark-ground microscopy

The usual function of the microscope condenser is to concentrate as much light as possible through the specimen and into the objective lens. The dark-ground condenser performs the opposite task, producing a hollow cone of light that comes to a focus on the specimen. The rays of light in the cone are at an oblique angle, such that after passing across the specimen, they continue without meeting the front lens of the objective, resulting in a dark background. Any objects present at the point of focus scatter the light, which then enters the objective and shows up as a bright image against the dark background.

Specimen preparation is critical, as very dilute bacterial suspensions are required, preferably with all the objects in the same plane of focus. Air bubbles must be absent from both the film and the immersion oil, if used. Dust and grease also scatter light and destroy the uniformly black background required for this technique. With this technique it is not possible to see any real detail but it is useful to study motility.

Phase-contrast microscopy

This technique allows us to see transparent objects well contrasted from the background in clear detail and is the most widely used image-enhancement method in microbiology. In essence, an annulus of light is produced by the condenser of the microscope and focused on the back focal plane of the objective, where a phase plate, comprising a glass disc containing an annular depression, is situated. The direct rays of the light source annulus pass through the annular groove and any diffracted rays pass through the remainder of the disc. Passage of the diffracted light through this thicker glass layer results in retardation of the light. This alters its phase relationship to the direct rays and increases contrast.

Differential-interference contrast microscopy

This method uses polarized light and has other applications outside the scope of this chapter, such as detecting surface irregularities in opaque specimens. It offers some advantages over phase-contrast microscopy, notably the elimination of haloes around the object edges, and enables extremely detailed observation of specimens. It does, however, tend to be more difficult to set up.

Electron microscopy

The highest magnification available using a light microscope is approximately ×1500. This limitation is imposed not by the design of the microscope itself, as much higher magnifications are possible, but by the wavelength of light. An object can only be seen if it causes a ray of light to deflect. If a particle is very small, then no deflection is produced and the object is not seen. Visible light has a wavelength between 0.3 μm and 0.8 μm, and objects less than 0.3 μm will not be clearly resolved, i.e. even if the magnification were increased no more detail would be seen. In order to increase the resolution it is necessary to use light of a shorter wavelength, such as UV light. This has been done and resulted in some useful applications but generally, for the purposes of increased definition, electrons are used and they can be thought of as behaving like very short wavelength light. Transmission electron microscopy requires the preparation of ultrathin (50 nm to 60 nm) sections of material mounted on grids for support. Because of the severe conditions applied to the specimen during preparation, and the likelihood of artefacts, care must be taken in the interpretation of information from electron micrographs.

Growth and reproduction of bacteria

The growth and multiplication of bacteria can be examined in terms of individual cells or populations of cells. During the cell division cycle a bacterium assimilates nutrients from the surrounding medium and increases in size. When a predetermined size has been reached, the DNA duplicates itself and a

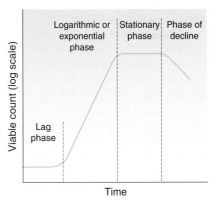

Fig. 13.6 • Phases of bacterial growth.

cross-wall will be produced, dividing the large cell into two daughter cells, each containing a copy of the parent chromosome. The daughter cells part, and the process is known as binary fission. In a closed environment, such as a culture in a test tube, the rate at which cell division occurs varies according to the conditions, and this manifests itself in characteristic changes in the population concentration. When fresh medium is inoculated with a small number of bacterial cells, the number remains static for a short time while the cells undergo a period of metabolic adjustment. This period is called the lag phase (Fig. 13.6) and its length depends on the degree of readjustment necessary. Once the cells have adapted to the environment, they begin to divide in the manner described previously, and this division occurs at regular intervals. The numbers of bacteria during this period increase in an exponential fashion (i.e. 2, 4, 8, 16, 32, 64, 128, etc.), and this is therefore termed the exponential or logarithmic phase. When cell numbers are plotted on a log scale against time, a straight line results for this phase.

During exponential growth (see Fig. 13.6) the medium undergoes continuous change, as nutrients are consumed and metabolic waste products excreted. The fact that the cells continue to divide exponentially during this period is a tribute to their physiological adaptability. Eventually, the medium becomes so changed, due to either substrate exhaustion or excessive concentrations of toxic products, that it is unable to support further growth. At this stage cell division slows and eventually stops, leading to the stationary phase. During this period some cells lyse and die, whereas others sporadically divide, but the cell numbers remain more or less constant. Gradually all the cells lyse and the culture enters the phase of decline.

It should be appreciated that this sequence of events is not a characteristic of the cell but a consequence of the interaction of the organisms with the nutrients in a closed environment. It does not necessarily reflect the way in which the organism would behave in vivo.

Genetic exchange

In addition to mutations, bacteria can alter their genetic make-up by transferring information from one cell to another, either as fragments of DNA or in the form of small extrachromosomal elements (plasmids). Transfer can be achieved in three ways: by transformation, transduction or conjugation.

Transformation. When bacteria die, they lyse and release cell fragments, including DNA, into the environment. Several bacterial genera (e.g. *Bacillus, Haemophilus, Streptococcus*) are able to take up these DNA fragments and incorporate them into their own chromosome, thereby inheriting the characteristics carried on that fragment. Cells able to participate in transformation are called competent. The development of competence has been shown in some cases to occur synchronously in a culture under the action of specific inducing proteins.

Transduction. Some bacteriophages can infect a bacterial cell and incorporate their nucleic acid into the host cell chromosome, with the result that the viral genes are replicated along with the bacterial DNA. In many instances this is a dormant lysogenic state for the phage but sometimes it is triggered into action and lysis of the cell occurs with liberation of phage particles. These new phage particles may have bacterial DNA incorporated into the viral genome, and this will infect any new host cell. On entering a new lysogenic state, the new host cell will replicate the viral nucleic acid in addition to that portion received from the previous host. Bacteria in which this has been shown to occur include members of the genera *Mycobacterium, Salmonella, Shigella* and *Staphylococcus*.

Conjugation. Gram-negative bacteria such as *Salmonella* species, *Shigella* species and *Escherichia coli* have been shown to transfer genetic material conferring antibiotic resistance by cellular contact. This process is called conjugation and is controlled by an R-factor plasmid, which is a small circular strand of duplex DNA replicating independently from the bacterial chromosome. R factor comprises a region containing resistance transfer genes that control the formation of sex pili, together with a variety of genes that code for the resistance to drugs. Conjugation is initiated when the resistance transfer genes stimulate the production of a sex pilus and random motion brings about contact with a recipient cell. One strand of the replicating R factor is nicked and passes through the sex pilus into the recipient cell. On receipt of this single strand of plasmid DNA, the complementary strand is produced and the free ends are joined. For a short time afterwards this cell has the ability to form a sex pilus itself and so transfer the R factor further.

This is by no means an exhaustive discussion of genetic exchange in bacteria, and the reader is referred to the bibliography for further information.

Bacterial nutrition

Bacteria require certain elements in fairly large quantities for growth and metabolism, including carbon, hydrogen, oxygen and nitrogen. Sulphur and phosphorus are also required but not in such large amounts. Only low concentrations of iron, calcium, potassium, sodium, magnesium and manganese are needed. Some elements, such as cobalt, zinc and copper, are required only in trace amounts, and an actual requirement may be difficult to demonstrate.

The metabolic capabilities of bacteria differ considerably, and this is reflected in the form in which nutrients may be assimilated. Bacteria can be classified according to their requirements for carbon and energy.

Lithotrophs (synonym: autotrophs). These utilize carbon dioxide as their main source of carbon. Energy is derived from different sources within this group:

* chemolithotrophs (chemosynthetic autotrophs) obtain their energy from the oxidation of inorganic compounds; and
* photolithotrophs (photosynthetic autotrophs) obtain their energy from sunlight.

Organotrophs (synonym: heterotrophs). Organotrophs utilize organic carbon sources and can similarly be divided into:

* chemoorganotrophs, which obtain their energy from oxidation or fermentation of organic compounds; and
* photoorganotrophs, which utilize light energy.

Oxygen requirements

As mentioned already, all bacteria require elemental oxygen in order to build up the complex materials necessary for growth and metabolism, but many organisms also require free oxygen as the final electron acceptor in the breakdown of carbon and energy sources. These organisms are called aerobes. If the organism will only grow in the presence of air, it is called a strict aerobe, but most organisms can either grow in its presence or its absence and are called facultative anaerobes. A strict anaerobe cannot grow and may even be killed in the presence of oxygen, because some other compound replaces oxygen as the final electron acceptor in these organisms. A fourth group of microaerophilic organisms has also been recognized which grow best in only trace amounts of free oxygen and usually prefer an increased carbon dioxide concentration.

Influence of environmental factors on the growth of bacteria

The rate of growth and metabolic activity of bacteria is the sum of a multitude of enzyme reactions. It follows that those environmental factors that influence enzyme activity will also affect growth rate. Such factors include temperature, pH and osmolarity.

Temperature. Bacteria can survive wide limits of temperature but each organism will exhibit minimum, optimum and maximum growth temperatures and on this basis bacteria fall into three broad groups:

- *Psychrophiles*. These grow best below 20°C but have a minimum growth temperature of approximately 0°C and a maximum growth temperature of 30°C. These organisms are responsible for low-temperature spoilage.
- *Mesophiles*. These exhibit a minimum growth temperature of 5°C to 10°C and a maximum growth temperature of 45°C to 50°C. Within this group, two populations can be identified: saprophytic mesophiles, with an optimum temperature of 20°C to 30°C, and parasitic mesophiles, with an optimum temperature of 37°C. The vast majority of pathogenic organisms are in this latter group.
- *Thermophiles*. These can grow at temperatures up to 70°C to 90°C but have an optimum of 50°C to 55°C and a minimum of 25°C to 40°C.

Organisms kept below their minimum growth temperature will not divide but can remain viable. As a result, very low temperatures (–70°C) are used to preserve cultures of organisms for many years. Temperatures in excess of the maximum growth temperature have a much more injurious effect, and this is considered in more detail in Chapter 16.

pH. Most bacteria grow best at around neutral pH, in the pH range from 6.8 to 7.6. There are, however, exceptions, such as the acidophilic organism lactobacillus, a contaminant of milk products, which grows best at pHs between 5.4 and 6.6. *Helicobacter* species have been associated with gastric ulcers and are found in the stomach growing at pHs of 1–3. At the other extreme, *Vibrio cholera* is capable of growing at pHs between 8 and 9. Yeasts and moulds prefer acid conditions with an optimum pH range of 4–6. The difference in pH optima between fungi and bacteria is used as a basis for the design of media permitting the growth of one group of organisms at the expense of others. Sabouraud medium, for example, has a pH of 5.6 and is a fungal medium, whereas nutrient broth, which is used routinely to cultivate bacteria, has a pH of 7.4. The adverse effect of extremes of pH has for many years been used as a means of preserving foods against microbial attack, e.g. by pickling in acidic vinegar.

Osmotic pressure. Bacteria tend to be more resistant to extremes of osmotic pressure than other cells owing to the presence of a very rigid cell wall. The concentration of intracellular solutes gives rise to an osmotic pressure equivalent to between 5 bar and 20 bar, and most bacteria will thrive in a medium containing approximately 0.75% w/v sodium chloride. Staphylococci have the ability to survive higher than normal salt concentrations. This has enabled the formulation of selective media, such as mannitol salt agar containing 7.5% w/v sodium chloride, which will support the growth of staphylococci but restrict the growth of other bacteria. Halophilic organisms can grow at much higher osmotic pressures but these are all saprophytic and are not pathogenic to humans. High osmotic pressures generated by either sodium chloride or sucrose have for a long time been used as preservatives. Syrup BP contains 66.7% w/w sucrose and is of sufficient osmotic pressure to resist microbial attack. This is used as a basis for many oral pharmaceutical preparations.

Handling and storage of microorganisms

Because microorganisms have such a diversity of nutritional requirements, there has arisen a bewildering array of media for the cultivation of bacteria, yeasts and moulds. Media are produced either as liquids or solidified with agar. Agar is an extract of seaweed, which at concentrations between 1% and 2% sets to form a firm gel below 45 °C. Unlike gelatin, bacteria cannot use agar as a nutrient, and so even after growth on the medium, the gel remains firm. Liquid media are stored routinely in test tubes or flasks, depending on the volume, both secured with either loose-fitting caps or plugs of sterile cotton wool. Small amounts of solid media are stored in Petri dishes or slopes (also known as slants), whereas larger volumes may be incorporated in Roux bottles or Carrell flasks.

Bacteria may only be maintained on agar in Petri dishes for a short time (days) before the medium dries out. For longer storage periods the surface of an agar slope is inoculated, and after growth the culture may be stored at 4 °C for several weeks. If even longer storage periods are required, then the cultures may be stored at low temperatures (−70 °C), usually in the presence of a cryoprotectant such as glycerol. Alternatively, they may be freeze-dried (lyophilized) before being stored at 4 °C. Some vegetative cells can survive lyophilization and may retain their viability for many years.

When a single cell is placed on the surface of an overdried agar plate, it becomes immobilized but can still draw nutrients from the substrate, and consequently grows and divides. Eventually the numbers of bacterial cells are high enough to become visible and a colony is formed. Each of the cells in that colony is a descendant from the initial single cell or group of cells, and so the colony is assumed to be a pure culture, with each cell having identical characteristics. The formation of single colonies is one of the primary aims of surface inoculation of solid media and allows the isolation of pure cultures from specimens containing mixed flora.

Inoculation of agar surfaces by streaking

The agar surface must be smooth. The surface should also be without moisture as this could cause the bacteria to become motile and the colonies to merge together. To dry the surface of the agar, the plates are placed in an incubator or drying cabinet for a short time. Inoculating loops are traditionally made of either platinum or nichrome wire twisted along its length to form a loop 2 mm to 3 mm in diameter at the end. Nichrome wire is cheaper than platinum but has similar thermal properties. The wire is held in a handle with an insulated grip, and the entire

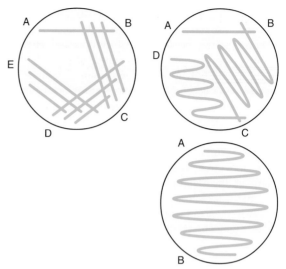

Fig. 13.7 • Typical streaking methods for obtaining isolated colonies.

length of the wire is heated in a Bunsen flame to red heat to sterilize it. The first few centimetres of the holder are also flamed before the loop is set aside in a rack to cool. Alternatively, disposable presterilized plastic loops are now frequently used.

The loop is used to remove a small portion of liquid from a bacterial suspension and this is then drawn across the agar surface from A to B, as indicated in Fig. 13.7. The loop is then resterilized (or replaced if plastic) and without reinoculating is streaked over the surface again, ensuring a small area of overlap with the previous streak line. The procedure is repeated as necessary. The pattern of streaking (other examples are shown in Fig. 13.7) is dictated largely by the concentration of the original bacterial suspension. The object of the exercise is to dilute the culture such that, after incubation, single colonies will arise in the later streak lines where the cells were sufficiently separated. All plates are incubated in an inverted position to prevent condensation from the lid falling on the surface of the medium and spreading the colonies.

Inoculation of slopes

A wire needle may be used to transfer single colonies from agar surfaces to the surface of slopes for maintenance purposes. The needle is similar to the loop except that the wire is single and straight, not terminating in a closed end. This is flamed and cooled as before, and a portion of a single colony is picked off the agar surface. The needle is then drawn upwards along the surface of the slant. Before incubation, the screw cap of the bottle should be loosened slightly to prevent oxygen starvation during growth. Some slopes are prepared with a shallower slope and a deeper butt to allow the needle to be stabbed into the agar when testing for gas production.

Transference of liquids

Graduated pipettes and Pasteur pipettes may be used for this purpose, the latter being short glass tubes one end of which is drawn into a fine capillary. Both types should be plugged with sterile cotton wool and filled via pipette fillers of appropriate capacity. Mouth pipetting should *never* be permitted. Automatic pipettes have generally replaced glass graduated pipettes in most areas of science for the measurement of small volumes of liquid. Provided they are properly maintained and calibrated, they have the advantage of being easy to use and reliable in performance.

Release of infectious aerosols

During all of these manipulations two considerations must be borne in mind. First, the culture must be transferred with the minimum risk of contamination from outside sources. To this end all pipettes, tubes, media, etc., are sterilized and the manipulations carried out under aseptic conditions. Second, the safety of the operator is paramount. During operations with microorganisms, it must be assumed that all organisms are capable of causing disease and that any route of infection is possible.

Most infections acquired in laboratories cannot be traced to a specific incident but arise from the inadvertent release of infectious aerosols. Two types of aerosols may be produced. The first kind produces large droplets (> 5 μm), containing many organisms, which settle locally and contaminate surfaces in the vicinity of the operator. These may initiate infections if personnel touch the surfaces and subsequently transfer the organisms to the eyes, nose or mouth. The second type of aerosol contains droplets smaller than 5 μm, which dry instantly to form droplet nuclei that remain suspended in the air for considerable periods. This allows them to be carried on air currents to places far removed from the site of initiation. These particles are so small that they are not trapped by the usual filter mechanisms in the nasal passages and may be inhaled, giving rise to infections of the lungs.

The aerosols described previously may be produced by a variety of means, such as heating wire loops, placing hot loops into liquid cultures, splashing during pipetting, rattling loops and pipettes inside test tubes and opening screw-capped tubes and ampoules. All microbiologists should have an awareness of the dangers of aerosol production and learn the correct techniques to minimize them.

Cultivation of anaerobes

Anaerobic microbiology is a much neglected subject owing principally to the practical difficulties involved in growing organisms in the absence of air. However, with the increasing implication of anaerobes in certain disease states and improved cultivation systems, the number of workers in this field is growing.

A common liquid medium for the cultivation of anaerobes is thioglycollate medium. In addition to sodium thioglycollate, the medium contains methylene blue as a redox indicator, and it permits the growth of aerobes, anaerobes and microaerophilic organisms. When in test tubes, the medium may be used after sterilization until not more than one-third of the liquid is oxidized, as indicated by the colour of the methylene blue indicator. Boiling and cooling of the medium just prior to inoculation are recommended for maximum performance. In some cases, the presence of methylene blue poses toxicity problems, and under these circumstances the indicator may be removed.

Anaerobic jars have improved considerably in recent years, making the cultivation of even strict anaerobes now relatively simple. A common system consists of a clear polycarbonate jar designed to be used with disposable oxygen absorbants and CO_2 generators such as the AnaeroGen® sachet. Once opened, the sachet will rapidly absorb atmospheric oxygen from the jar and simultaneously generate carbon dioxide. It is important therefore to open the sachet, place it within the jar and seal the lid of the jar within 1 minute. The oxygen level will be reduced to below 1% within 30 minutes and the final carbon dioxide level will be between 9% and 11%. Carbon dioxide is produced to allow the growth of many fastidious anaerobes, which fail to grow in its absence. The absence of oxygen can be demonstrated by the action of a redox indicator, which in the case of methylene blue will be colourless.

Counting bacteria

Estimates of bacterial numbers in a suspension can be evaluated from a number of standpoints, each equally valid, depending on the circumstances and the information required. In some cases, it may be necessary to know the total amount of biomass produced within a culture, irrespective of whether the cells are actively metabolizing. In other instances, only an assessment of living bacteria may be required. Bacterial counts can be divided into total counts and viable counts.

Total counts

These counts estimate the total number of bacteria present within a culture, both dead and living cells. A variety of methods are available for the determination of total counts, and the one chosen will depend largely on the characteristics of the cells being studied, i.e. whether they aggregate.

Microscope methods. Microscope methods employ a haemocytometer counting chamber (Fig. 13.8), which has a platform engraved with a grid of small squares each 0.0025 mm^2 in area. The platform is depressed 0.1 mm and a glass coverslip is placed over the platform, enclosing a space of known dimensions. The volume above each square is 0.00025 mm^3. For motile bacteria the culture is fixed by adding two to three drops of 40% formaldehyde solution per 10 mL of culture to prevent the bacteria from moving across the field of view. A drop of the suspension is then applied to the platform at the edge of the coverslip. The liquid is drawn into the space by capillary action. It is important to ensure that liquid does not enter a trench that surrounds the platform; the liquid must fill the whole space between the coverslip and the platform. This slide is examined using phase-contrast or dark-ground microscopy and, if necessary, the culture is diluted to give 2–10 bacteria per small square. A minimum of 300 bacterial cells should be counted to give statistically significant results (Box 13.1).

Spectroscopic methods. These methods are simple to use and very rapid but require careful calibration if meaningful results are to be obtained. Either opacity or light scattering may be used but both methods may only be used for dilute, homogeneous suspensions as at higher concentrations the cells obscure each other in the light path and the relationship between optical density and concentration is not linear. Simple colorimeters and nephelometers can be used but more accurate results are obtained using a spectrophotometer.

Electronic methods. A variety of automated methods are available for bacterial cell counting, including electronic particle counting, microcalorimetry, changes in impedance or conductivity, and radiometric and infrared systems for monitoring CO_2 production.

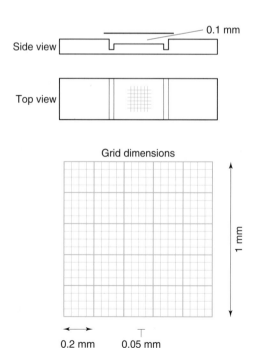

Grid dimensions

1 mm

0.2 mm   0.05 mm

Fig. 13.8 • Counting chamber for microscope method estimation of cell numbers.

Side view — 0.1 mm

Top view

Box 13.1

Example calculation for the haemocytometer method

Assume the mean cell count per small square is 6.

The volume above each small square $= 2.5 \times 10^{-4}$ mm^3

$= 2.5 \times 10^{-7}$ cm^3

As the volume above each square contains six cells, there are

$$\frac{6}{2.5 \times 10^{-7}} = 2.4 \times 10^{7} \text{ cells per millilitre}$$

Other methods. If an organism is prone to excessive clumping, or if a measure of biomass is needed rather than numbers, then estimates may be made by performing dry weight or total nitrogen determinations. For dry weight determinations, a sample of suspension is centrifuged and the pellet washed free of culture medium by further centrifugation in water. The pellet is collected and dried to a constant weight in a desiccator. Total nitrogen measures the total quantity of nitrogenous material within a cell population. A known volume of suspension is centrifuged and washed as before and the pellet digested using sulphuric acid in the presence of a $CuSO_4–K_2SO_4–$ selenium catalyst. This produces ammonia, which is removed using boric acid and estimated either by titration or colorimetrically.

Viable counts

These are counts to determine the number of bacteria in a suspension that are capable of division. In all these methods, the assumption is made that a colony arises from a single cell, although clearly this is often not the case, as cells frequently clump or grow as aggregates, e.g. *S. aureus*. For this reason, viable counts are usually expressed as colony-forming units (cfu) per mL rather than cells per mL.

Spread plates. A known volume, usually no more than 0.2 mL, of a suitably diluted culture is pipetted onto an overdried agar plate and distributed evenly over the surface using a sterile spreader made of glass or plastic. All the liquid must be allowed to soak in before the plates are inverted. A series of 10-fold dilutions should be made in a suitable sterile diluent and replicates plated out at each dilution in order to ensure that countable numbers of colonies (30–300) are obtained per plate.

The viable count is calculated from the average colony count per plate, knowing the dilution and the volume pipetted onto the agar (Box 13.2).

Pour plates. A series of dilutions of original culture are prepared as before, ensuring that at least one is in the range of 30–300 organisms/mL. One-millilitre quantities are placed into empty sterile Petri dishes. Molten agar, cooled to 45°C, is poured onto the suspension and mixed by gentle swirling. After setting of the agar, the plates are inverted and incubated. Because the colonies are embedded within the agar, they do not exhibit the characteristic morphology seen with surface colonies. In general, they assume a lens shape and are usually smaller. Because the oxygen tension below the surface is reduced, this

---

Box 13.2

Example calculation of a serial dilution scheme

Stock bacterial suspension, 1 mL added to 99 mL of sterile diluent – *call dilution A*. At this point the stock suspension has therefore been diluted by a factor of 100 (10^2).

1 mL of dilution A added to 99 mL of sterile diluent – *call dilution B* (dilution B has been diluted by a factor of 10^4).

1 mL of dilution B added to 9 mL of sterile diluent – *call dilution C* (dilution C has been diluted by a factor of 10^5).

1 mL of dilution C added to 9 mL of sterile diluent – *call dilution D* (dilution D has been diluted by a factor of 10^6).

1 mL of dilution D added to 9 mL of sterile diluent – *call dilution E* (dilution E has been diluted by a factor of 10^7).

0.2 mL of each dilution plated in triplicate.

The mean colony counts for each dilution after incubation at 37°C are as follows:

Dilution A	Too many to count
Dilution B	Too many to count
Dilution C	400 colonies
Dilution D	45 colonies
Dilution E	5 colonies

The result for dilution C is unreliable, as the count is too high. If the colony count exceeds 300, errors arise because the colonies become very small and some may be missed. This is why the colony count for dilution C does not exactly correspond to 10 times that found for dilution D. Similarly, the count for dilution E is unreliable because at counts below approximately 30 small variations introduce high percentage errors.

The result from dilution D is therefore taken for the calculation, as the colony count lies between 30 and 300.

45 colonies in 0.2 mL, therefore

45×5 colonies per millilitre

$= 225$ cfu mL^{-1} in dilution D.

This was diluted by a factor of 10^6 ($100 \times 100 \times 10 \times 10$) and so the count in the stock suspension was $225 \times 10^6 = 2.25 \times 10^8$ cfu mL^{-1}.

---

method is not suitable for strict aerobes. Calculations are similar to that given in the previous paragraph, except that no correction is necessary for the volume placed on the plate.

Membrane filtration. This method is particularly useful when the level of contamination is very low, such as in water supplies. A known volume of sample is passed through a membrane filter, typically made of cellulose acetate/nitrate, of sufficient pore size to retain bacteria (0.2 μm to 0.45 μm). The filtrate is discarded and the membrane placed bacteria uppermost on the surface of an overdried agar plate, avoiding trapped air between the membrane and the surface. On incubation, the bacteria draw nutrients through the membrane and form countable colonies.

ATP determination. There are sometimes instances when viable counts are required for clumped cultures or for bacteria adhered to surfaces, e.g. in biofilms. Conventional plate count techniques are not appropriate here, and ATP determinations can be used. The method assumes that viable bacteria contain a relatively constant level of ATP but that this falls to zero when the cells die. ATP is extracted from the cells using a strong acid such as trichloroacetic acid, and the extract is then neutralized by dilution with buffer. The ATP assay is based on the quantitative measurement of a stable level of light produced as a result of an enzyme reaction catalysed by firefly luciferase.

$$ATP + luciferin + O_2 \xrightarrow{\text{luciferase}} oxyluciferin + AMP$$
$$+ PP_i + CO_2 + light$$
$$(13.1)$$

where PP_i is pyrophosphate.

The amount of ATP is calculated by reference to light output from known ATP concentrations and the number of bacterial cells is calculated by reference to a previously constructed calibration plot.

Isolation of pure bacterial cultures

Mixed bacterial cultures from pathological specimens or other biological materials are isolated first on solid media to give single colonies. The resultant pure cultures can then be subjected to identification procedures. The techniques used for isolation depend on the proportion of the species of interest compared to the background contamination. Direct inoculation can only be used when an organism is found as a pure culture in nature. Examples include bacterial infections of normally sterile fluids such as blood or cerebrospinal fluid.

Streaking is the most common method employed. If the proportions of bacteria in the mixed culture are roughly equal, then streaking on an ordinary

nutrient medium should yield single colonies of all microbial types. More usually, the organism of interest is present only as a very small fraction of the total microbial population, necessitating the use of selective media.

A selective enrichment broth is initially inoculated with the mixed population of cells and this inhibits the growth of the majority of the background population. At the same time the growth of the organism of interest is encouraged. After incubation in this medium, the cultures are streaked out onto solid selective media, which frequently contain indicators to further differentiate species on the basis of fermentation of specific sugars.

Classification and identification

Taxonomy is the ordering of living organisms into groups on the basis of their similarities. In this way we can construct a hierarchy of interrelationships such that species with similar characteristics are grouped within the same genus, genera which have similarities are grouped within the same family, families grouped into orders, orders into classes and classes into divisions. The classification of bacteria does pose a problem because a species is defined as a group of closely related organisms that reproduce sexually to produce fertile offspring. Of course, bacteria do not reproduce sexually, and so a bacterial species is simply defined as a population of cells with similar characteristics.

Nomenclature

The total number of different bacterial species on the planet can only be speculated and probably runs into tens of millions; however, the number of known, named species is just over 6000. It is therefore extremely important to be sure there is no confusion when describing any one particular bacterial species. Although we are familiar with the use of trivial names in ornithology and botany (we understand what we mean when we describe a sparrow or a daffodil), such an approach could have disastrous consequences in clinical microbiology. For this reason, we use the binomial system of nomenclature developed by Carolus Linnaeus in the 18th century. In this system every bacterium is given two names, the first being the genus name and the second the species name. By convention, the name is italicized, and the genus name always begins with a capital letter, whereas the species name begins in lower case.

Identification

The organization of bacteria into groups of related microorganisms is based on the similarity of their chromosomal DNA. Although this provides a very accurate indicator of genetic relatedness, it is far too cumbersome a tool to use for the identification of an unknown bacterium isolated from a routine sample. In this instance, a series of rapid and simple tests is required that probe the phenotypic characteristics of the microorganism. The tests are conducted in a logical series of steps, the results from each test providing information for the next stage of the investigation. An example of such a procedure is given:

Morphology	Microscope investigations using a wet mount to determine cell size, shape, formation of spores, aggregation, motility, etc.
Staining reactions	Gram stain, acid-fast stain, spore stain
Cultural reactions	Appearance on solid media (colony formation, shape, size, colour, texture, smell, pigments, etc.), aerobic/anaerobic growth, temperature requirements, pH requirements
Biochemical reactions	Enzymatic activities are probed to distinguish between closely related bacteria. This can be performed in traditional mode or with kits

Biochemical tests

These are designed to examine the enzymatic capabilities of the organism. As there are a large number of biochemical tests that can be performed, the preliminary steps help to narrow down the range to those that will be most discriminatory. A few examples of commonly used biochemical tests are given hereafter. It should be noted that the methods described here are those traditionally used in the laboratory in order to convey the basic principles of the tests.

Sugar fermentation is very frequently used and examines the ability of the organism to ferment a range of sugars. A number of tubes of peptone water are prepared, each containing a different sugar. An acid–base indicator is incorporated into the medium, which also contains a Durham tube (a small inverted tube filled with medium) capable of collecting any gas produced during fermentation. After inoculation and incubation, the tubes are examined for acid production (as indicated by a change in the colour of the indicator) and gas production (as seen by a bubble of gas collected in the inverted Durham tube).

Proteases are produced by a number of bacteria, e.g. *Bacillus* and *Pseudomonas* species, and they are responsible for the breakdown of protein into smaller units. Gelatin is a protein that can be added to liquid media to produce a stiff gel similar to agar. Unlike in the case of agar, which cannot be utilized by bacteria, those organisms producing proteases will destroy the gel structure and liquefy the medium. A medium made of nutrient broth solidified with gelatin is traditionally incorporated in boiling tubes or small bottles and inoculated by means of a stab wire. After incubation, it is important to refrigerate the gelatin prior to examination; otherwise false positives may be produced. Proteases can also be detected using milk agar, which is opaque. Protease producers form colonies with clear haloes around them where the enzyme has diffused into the medium and digested the casein.

Oxidase is produced by *Neisseria* and *Pseudomonas* and can be detected using 1% tetramethyl-*p*-phenylene diamine. The enzyme catalyses the transport of electrons between electron donors in the bacteria and the redox dye. A positive reaction is indicated by the deep purple colour of the reduced dye. The test is carried out by placing the reagent directly onto an isolated colony on an agar surface. Alternatively, a filter paper strip impregnated with the dye is moistened with water and, using a platinum loop, a bacterial colony is spread across the surface. If the test is positive, a purple colour will appear within 10 seconds. Note that the use of iron loops may give false-positive reactions.

The indole test distinguishes those bacteria capable of decomposing the amino acid tryptophan to indole. Any indole produced can be tested for by a colorimetric reaction with *p*-dimethylaminobenzaldehyde. After incubation in peptone water, 0.5 mL Kovacs reagent is placed on the surface of the culture, the culture is shaken, and a positive reaction is indicated by a red colour. Organisms giving positive indole reactions include *E. coli* and *Proteus vulgaris*.

Catalase is responsible for the breakdown of hydrogen peroxide into oxygen and water. The test may be performed by addition of 1 mL of 10 vol hydrogen peroxide directly to the surface of colonies growing on an agar slope. A vigorous frothing of the surface liquid indicates the presence of catalase. *Staphylococcus* and *Micrococcus* are catalase positive, whereas *Streptococcus* is catalase negative.

Urease production enables certain bacteria to break down urea to ammonia and carbon dioxide:

$$NH_2\text{-}CO\text{-}NH_2 + H_2O \xrightarrow{\text{Urease}} 2NH_3 + CO_2$$

$$(13.2)$$

This test is readily carried out by growing the bacteria on a medium containing urea and an acid–base indicator. After incubation the production of ammonia will be shown by the alkaline reaction of the indicator. Examples of urease-negative bacteria include *E. coli* and *Enterococcus faecalis*.

Simmons citrate agar was developed to test for the presence of organisms that can utilize citrate as the sole source of carbon and energy and ammonia as the main source of nitrogen. It is used to differentiate members of the *Enterobacteriaceae*. The medium, containing bromothymol blue as indicator, is surface inoculated on slopes and citrate utilization is demonstrated by an alkaline reaction and a change in the indicator colour from a dull green to a bright blue. *E. coli*, *Shigella*, *Edwardsiella* and *Yersinia* do not utilize citrate, whereas *Serratia*, *Enterobacter*, *Klebsiella* and *Proteus* do and so give a positive result.

The methyl red test is used to distinguish organisms that, during metabolism of glucose, produce and maintain a high level of acidity from those that initially produce acid but restore neutral conditions with further metabolism. The organism is grown on glucose phosphate medium and, after incubation, a few drops of methyl red are added and the colour is immediately recorded. A red colour indicates acid production (positive), whereas a yellow colour indicates alkali (negative).

Some organisms can convert carbohydrates to acetyl methyl carbinol (CH_3–CO–CHOH–CH_3). This may be oxidized to diacetyl (CH_3–CO–CO–CH_3), which will react with guanidine residues in the medium under alkaline conditions to produce a colour. This is the basis of the Voges–Proskauer test, which is usually carried out at the same time as the methyl red test. The organism is again grown in glucose phosphate medium and, after incubation, 40% KOH is added together with 5% α-naphthol in ethanol. After mixing, a positive reaction is indicated by a pink colour in 2–5 minutes, gradually becoming darker red within 30 minutes. Organisms giving positive Voges–Proskauer reactions usually give negative methyl red reactions, as the production of acetyl methyl carbinol is accompanied by low acid production. *Klebsiella* species typically give a positive Voges–Proskauer reaction.

Rapid identification systems

With the increasing demand for quick and accurate identification of bacteria, a number of micromethods have been developed combining a variety of biochemical tests selected for their rapidity of reading and high discrimination. The API bacterial identification system is an example of such a micromethod and comprises a plastic tray containing dehydrated substrates in a number of wells. Culture is added to the wells, dissolving the substrate and allowing the fermentation of carbohydrates or the presence of enzymes similar to those just described to be demonstrated. In some cases, incubation times of 2 hours are sufficient for accurate identification. Kits are available with different reagents, permitting the identification of *Enterobacteriaceae*, *Streptococcaceae*, staphylococci, anaerobes, yeasts and moulds. Accurate identification is made by reference to a table of results.

Matrix-assisted laser desorption/ionization time of flight (MALDI-TOF) mass spectrometry is used increasingly. Here a bacterial sample is transferred to a MALDI target plate and overlaid with matrix solution. The sample is loaded into the mass spectrometer and a profile acquired. This profile is a unique fingerprint of the microorganism and is compared with the library of electronic mass spectra held within the software database. Although the equipment cost is high, this procedure is ideal for those laboratories that have a high throughput of microbial samples that require rapid processing.

The tests described so far will enable differentiation of an unknown bacterium to species level. However, it is apparent that not all isolates of the same species behave in an identical manner. For example, *E. coli* isolated from the intestines of a healthy person is relatively harmless compared with the well-publicized *E. coli* O157.H7, which causes intense food poisoning and haemolytic uraemic syndrome. On occasions it is therefore necessary to distinguish further between isolates from the same species. This can be performed using, among other things, serological tests and phage typing. The use of DNA profiling has now become a much more accessible tool for bacterial identification, but it is beyond the scope of the current chapter to describe this further.

Serological tests

Bacteria have antigens associated with their cell envelopes (O antigens), with their flagella (H antigens) and with their capsules (K antigens). When injected into an animal, antibodies will be produced directed specifically towards those antigens and able to react with them. Specific antisera are prepared by immunizing an animal with a killed or attenuated bacterial suspension and taking blood samples. Serum containing the antibodies can then be separated. If a sample of bacterial suspension is placed on a glass slide and mixed with a small amount of specific antiserum, then the bacteria will be seen to clump when examined under the microscope. The test can be made more quantitative by using the tube dilution technique, where a given amount of antigen is mixed with a series of dilutions of specific antisera. The highest dilution at which agglutination occurs is called the agglutination titre.

Phage typing. Many bacteria are susceptible to lytic bacteriophages whose action is very specific. Identification may be based on the susceptibility of a culture to a set of such type-specific lytic bacteriophages. This method enables very detailed identification of the organisms to be made, e.g. one serotype of *Salmonella typhi* has been further subdivided into 80 phage types using this technique.

Fungi

'Fungus' is a general term used to describe all yeasts and moulds, whereas a mould is a filamentous fungus exhibiting a mycelial form of growth. The study of fungi is called mycology. Yeasts and moulds are eukaryotic microorganisms possessing organized demonstrable nuclei enclosed within an outer membrane, a nucleolus and chromatin strands that become organized into chromosomes during cell division. Fungal cell walls are composed predominantly of polysaccharide. In most cases this is chitin mixed with cellulose, glucan and mannan. Proteins and glycoproteins are also present but peptidoglycan is absent. The polysaccharide polymers are cross-linked to provide a structure of considerable strength which gives the cell osmotic stability. The fungal membrane contains sterols such as ergosterol and zymosterol not found in mammalian cells, and this provides a useful target for antifungal antibiotics. The role of fungi in nature is predominantly a scavenging one and in this respect fungi are vital for the decomposition and recycling of organic materials. Of the more than 100 000 species of known fungi, fewer than 100 are human pathogens and most of these are facultative and not obligate parasites.

Fungal morphology

Fungi can be divided into five broad groups on the basis of their morphology.

Yeasts

These are spherical or ovoid unicellular bodies 2 μm to 4 μm in diameter which typically reproduce by budding. In liquid cultures and on agar they behave very much like bacteria. Examples include *Saccharomyces cerevisiae*, strains of which are used in baking and in the production of beers and wines. *Cryptococcus neoformans* is the only significant pathogen and this gives rise to a respiratory tract disease called cryptococcosis, which in most cases is relatively mild. However, the microorganism may disseminate, leading to multiorgan disease, including meningitis. Cryptococcosis is of particular significance in immunocompromised patients. If left untreated, 80% of patients with disseminated cryptococcosis will die within 1 year.

Yeast-like fungi

These organisms normally behave like typical budding yeasts but under certain circumstances the buds do not separate, and they become elongated. The resulting structure resembles a filament and is called a pseudomycelium. It differs from a true mycelium in that there are no interconnecting pores between the cellular compartments comprising the hyphae.

The most important member of this group is *Candida albicans*, which is usually resident in the mouth, intestines and vagina. Under normal conditions *C. albicans* does not cause problems but if the environmental balance is disturbed, then problems can arise. These include vaginal thrush (vaginitis) and oral thrush. Overgrowth of *C. albicans* within the gut can lead to symptoms of inexplicable fatigue and malaise that is difficult to diagnose. Predisposing factors may include poor diet, diabetes, alcoholism and long-term treatment with steroids.

Dimorphic fungi

These grow as yeasts or as filaments depending on the culture conditions. At 22 °C, either in the soil or in culture media, filamentous mycelial forms and reproductive spores are produced, whereas at 37 °C in the body, the microorganisms assume a yeast-like appearance. *Histoplasma capsulatum* is an important pathogen that gives rise to respiratory illness. The infectious form is the spore that is borne on the wind and is inhaled. It has been postulated that a single spore can elicit an infection. On entering the body, the spores germinate to give rise to the yeast form. Primary infections are often mild but progressive disseminated histoplasmosis is a very severe disease that can affect many organs of the body.

Filamentous fungi

This group comprises those multicellular moulds that grow in the form of long, slender filaments 2 μm to 10 μm in diameter called hyphae. The branching hyphae, which constitute the vegetative or somatic structure of the mould, intertwine and gradually spread over the entire surface of the available substrate, extracting nutrients and forming a dense mat or mycelium. The hyphae may be nonseptate (coenocytic) or septate, but in each case the nutrients and cellular components are freely diffusible along the length of the filament. This is facilitated by the presence of pores within the septa.

Mushrooms and toadstools

This group is characterized by the production of large reproductive fruiting bodies of complex structure. They also possess elaborate propagation mechanisms. Some of these fungi are edible and are used in cooking but others, such as *Amanita phalloides* (death cap), produce potent mycotoxins that may result in death if eaten.

Reproduction of fungi

In the somatic portion of most fungi the nuclei are very small and the mechanism of nuclear division is uncertain. Under the correct environmental conditions, the organisms will switch from the somatic or vegetative growth phase to a reproductive form, so that the fungus may propagate the species by producing new mycelia on fresh food substrates. Two types of reproduction are found: asexual and sexual.

Asexual reproduction

Asexual reproduction is, in general, more important for the propagation of the species. Mechanisms include binary fission, budding, hyphal fragmentation and spore formation. Each progeny is an exact replica of the parent and no species variation can occur. Some yeasts (e.g. *Schizosaccharomyces pombe*) reproduce by binary fission in the same way as bacteria. The parent cell enlarges, its nucleus divides and, when a cross-wall is produced across the cell, two identical daughter cells form.

Budding occurs in the majority of yeasts and is the production of a small outgrowth or bud from the parent cell. As the bud increases in size, the nucleus divides and one of the pair migrates into the bud. The bud eventually breaks off from the parent to form a new individual. A scar is left behind on the parent cell, and each parent can produce up to 24 buds.

Fungi growing in a filamentous form may employ hyphal fragmentation as a means of asexual propagation. The hyphal tips break up into component segments (called arthroconidia or arthrospores), each of which can disperse on the wind to other environments and fresh food substrates.

The formation of specialized spore-bearing structures containing reproductive spores is the most common method of asexual reproduction (Fig. 13.9). The spores can be borne in a sporangium, supported on a sporangiophore. A limiting membrane surrounds the sporangium, and the spores contained within it are called sporangiospores. The spores are released when the sporangium ruptures. This type of reproduction is found in the lower fungi possessing nonseptate hyphae (e.g. *Mucor* and *Rhizopus*). Separate spores produced at the tips of specialized conidiophores are called conidiospores. A diverse range of structures is found in nature, and Fig. 13.9 illustrates some of the different types of asexual spores found in fungi.

Sexual reproduction

Sexual reproduction involves the union of two compatible nuclei and allows variation of the species. Mycology is made much more complex because individual fungi are given different names depending on whether they are in the sexual or the asexual stage. Not all fungi have been observed to carry out sexual reproduction. Some species produce distinguishable male and female sex organs on the same mycelium and are therefore hermaphroditic, i.e. a single colony can reproduce sexually by itself. Others produce mycelia which are either male or female (called dioecious) and can therefore reproduce only when two dissimilar organisms come together.

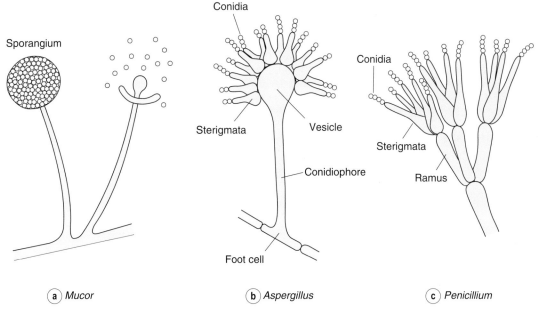

Conidia

(a) *Mucor*   (b) *Aspergillus*   (c) *Penicillium*

Fig. 13.9 • Spore-bearing structures of selected fungi **(a)** Mucor, **(b)** Aspergillus and **(c)** Penicillium.

Fungal classification

The pharmaceutically important fungi can be found within four main taxonomic classes.

Zygomycetes

These are terrestrial saprophytes possessing nonseptate hyphae and are sometimes referred to as the lower fungi. Apart from their hyphae, they can be distinguished from other filamentous fungi by the presence of sporangia. Examples are *Mucor* and *Rhizopus*, which are important in the manufacture of organic acids and the biotransformation of steroids. They are also common spoilage organisms.

Ascomycetes

Ascomycetes possess septate hyphae, and the sexual or perfect stage is characterized by the presence of a sac-like reproductive structure called an ascus. This typically contains eight ascospores. The asexual or imperfect stage involves conidiospores. An example is *Claviceps purpurea*, which is a parasite of rye and is important as a source of ergot alkaloids used to control haemorrhage and in treating migraine. The Ascomycetes include the yeasts, such as Saccharomyces and Cryptococcus, together with Candida yeasts such as *Saccharomyces* and *Cryptococcus*, together with *Torulopsis* and *Candida*.

Deuteromycetes

Sometimes called the Fungi Imperfecti, this group includes those fungi in which the sexual stage of reproduction has not been observed. *Penicillium* and *Aspergillus* are ascomycetes but are classified among the Deuteromycetes as the perfect stage is apparently absent. *Penicillium chrysogenum* is important in the production of the antibiotic penicillin, whereas *Aspergillus* species have found widespread industrial use owing to their extensive enzymic capabilities. Some *Aspergillus* species also produce mycotoxins and can cause serious infections in humans. The Deuteromycetes contain most of the human pathogens, such as *Blastomyces* and *Coccidioides*, and some of the dermatophyte fungi.

Basidiomycetes

This is the most advanced group, containing the mushrooms and toadstools. Sexual reproduction is by basidiospores. The group also includes the rusts (cereal parasites) and smuts.

Please check your eBook at **https://studentconsult. inkling.com/** for self-assessment questions. See inside cover for registration details.

Bibliography

Berg, J., Tymoczko, J., Gatto, G., et al., 2015. Biochemistry, eighth ed. Freeman, New York.

Collins, C.H., Lyne, P.M., Grange, J.M., et al., 2004. Microbiological Methods, eighth ed. Hodder Arnold, London.

Denyer, S.P., Hodges, N.A., Gorman, S.P., et al., 2011. Hugo and Russell's Pharmaceutical Microbiology, eighth ed. Wiley-Blackwell, Chichester.

Fraise, A., Maillard, J.Y., Sattar, S.A., 2013. Russell, Hugo and Ayliffe's Principles and Practice of Disinfection, Preservation and Sterilization, fifth ed. Wiley-Blackwell, Chichester.

Gillespie, S.H., Bamford, K., 2007. Medical Microbiology and Infection at a Glance, third ed. Blackwell, Oxford.

Hanlon, G.W., Hodges, N.A., 2013. Essential Microbiology for Pharmacy and Pharmaceutical Science. Wiley-Blackwell, Chichester.

Russell, A.D., Chopra, I., 1996. Understanding Antibacterial Action and Resistance, second ed. Ellis Horwood, London.

Pharmaceutical applications of microbiological techniques

14

Norman A. Hodges

CHAPTER CONTENTS

KEY POINTS

- Two of the major aspects of microbiology relevant to pharmacy are the measurement of activity of antimicrobial chemicals and the control of the microbiological quality of manufactured medicines.
- In order to obtain reliable and reproducible results in the measurement of antimicrobial activity it is necessary to rigorously control factors associated with both the test organism and the conditions of the test itself.
- Antibiotics can be assayed by conventional chemical methods or by biological (agar diffusion) methods. High-performance liquid chromatography (HPLC) is usually the method of choice, but it cannot be used in all situations.
- The minimum inhibitory concentration (MIC) is a commonly used measure of the sensitivity of a particular microorganism to an antimicrobial

chemical. The concentration of an antibiotic at an infection site in the body must exceed the MIC for the infecting organism.
- Preservative efficacy (challenge) tests are used to assess the adequacy with which a manufactured medicine is protected against microbial spoilage.
- Chemical assays of the preservative present in the medicine cannot accurately predict product vulnerability to microbial spoilage because the activity of preservatives is influenced by their interactions with other components of the formulation.
- Pharmaceutical products may be either sterile or nonsterile. Sterile products contain no living microorganisms at all, whereas the microbiological quality of nonsterile products is controlled by pharmacopoeial standards that specify the maximum permitted concentrations in different product types. Some hazardous organisms are specifically excluded from selected product categories.
- Sterility tests cannot be relied on to detect the low levels of microorganisms that might survive an inadequate sterilization process, so rigorous control of the manufacturing process is a major factor in assurance of sterility.

Introduction

The purpose of this chapter is to bring together those microbiological methods and procedures that are relevant to the design and production of medicines and medical devices. These are methods used (1) to determine the potency or activity of antimicrobial chemicals, e.g. antibiotics, preservatives and disinfectants, and (2) as part of the microbiological quality control of manufactured sterile and nonsterile products.

The chapter describes the experimental procedures that are unique or particularly relevant to pharmacy, rather than those that are common to microbiology as a whole. In the latter category, for example, are procedures used to identify and enumerate microorganisms. These, together with staining and microscopical techniques, are described in Chapter 13.

Several of the methods and tests discussed here are the subject of monographs or appendices in pharmacopoeias or they are described in national and international standards or other recognized reference works. It is not the intention to reproduce these official testing procedures in detail, but rather to explain the principles of the tests, to draw attention to difficult or important aspects, and to indicate the advantages, problems or shortcomings of the various methods.

Measurement of antimicrobial activity

In most of the methods used to assess the activity of antimicrobial chemicals, an inoculum of the test organism is added to a solution of the chemical under test, samples are removed over a period of time, the chemical is inactivated and the proportion of surviving cells is determined. Alternatively, culture medium is present together with the chemical, and the degree of inhibition of growth of the test organism is measured. In each case it is necessary to standardize and control such factors as the concentration of the test organism, its origin, i.e. the species and strain employed, together with the culture medium in which it was grown, the phase of growth from which the cells were taken, and the temperature and time of incubation of the cells after exposure to the chemical. Because such considerations are common to several of the procedures described here, e.g. antibiotic assays, preservative efficacy (challenge) tests and determinations of the minimum inhibitory concentration (MIC), it is appropriate that they should be considered first, both to emphasize their importance and to avoid repetition.

Factors to be controlled in the measurement of antimicrobial activity

Origin of the test organism

Although two cultures may bear the same generic and specific name, i.e. they may both be called *Escherichia coli*, this does not mean that they are identical. Certainly, they would normally be similar in many respects, e.g. morphology (appearance), cultural requirements and biochemical characteristics, but they may exhibit slight variations in some of these properties; such variants are described as strains of *E. coli*. A variety of strains of a single species may normally be obtained from a culture collection, e.g. the National Collection of Industrial, Food and Marine Bacteria (now managed by NCIMB) or the National Collection of Type Cultures (NCTC). Different strains may also occur in hospital pathology laboratories by isolation from swabs taken from infected patients or by isolation from contaminated food, cosmetic or pharmaceutical products, and many other sources. Strains obtained in these ways are likely to exhibit variations in resistance to antimicrobial chemicals. Strains from human or animal infections are frequently more resistant to antimicrobial chemicals, particularly antibiotics, than those from other sources. Similarly, strains derived from contaminated medicines may be more resistant to preservative chemicals than those obtained from culture collections. Therefore, in order to achieve results that are reproducible by a variety of laboratories, it is necessary to specify the strain of the organism used for the determination.

Many official testing methods now limit the number of times the culture collection specimen may be regrown in fresh medium (called the number of subcultures or passages) before it must be replaced. This is because the characteristics of the organism (including its resistance to antimicrobial chemicals) may progressively change as a result of mutation and natural selection through the many generations that might arise during months or years of laboratory cultivation.

Composition and pH of the culture medium

There are several methods of assessing antimicrobial activity which all have in common the measurement of inhibition of growth of a test organism when the antimicrobial chemical is added to the culture medium. In such cases the composition and pH of the medium may influence the result. The medium may contain substances that antagonize the action of the test compound, e.g. high concentrations of thymidine or *p*-aminobenzoic acid will interfere with trimethoprim and sulfonamide activity.

The antimicrobial activities of several groups of chemicals are influenced by the ease with which they cross the cell membrane and interfere with the metabolism of the cell. This, in turn, is influenced by the lipid solubility of the substance, because the membrane contains a high proportion of lipid and tends to permit the passage of lipid-soluble substances. Many antimicrobial chemicals are weak acids or weak bases, which are more lipid soluble in the un-ionized form. The pH of the environment therefore affects their degree of ionization, hence their lipid solubility and so, ultimately, their antimicrobial effect. Benzoic acid, for example, is a preservative used in several oral mixtures which has a much greater activity in liquids buffered to an acidic pH value than in those which are neutral or alkaline. Conversely, the aminoglycoside antibiotics, e.g. amikacin, neomycin and gentamicin, which are weak bases, are more active at slightly alkaline pH values, although this is more a consequence of the transport systems by which the molecules enter the bacterial cell working better at alkaline pH than of enhanced lipid solubility. The presence of organic matter, e.g. blood, pus or serum, is likely to have a marked protective effect on the test organism, and so antimicrobial chemicals may appear less active in the presence of such material. The activity of several antibiotics, notably tetracyclines and aminoglycosides, is reduced by the presence of high concentrations of divalent or trivalent cations, e.g. calcium, magnesium or iron, in the medium.

Exposure and incubation conditions

The temperature, duration and redox conditions of exposure to the antimicrobial chemical (or incubation of survivors after exposure) may all have a significant effect on its measured activity. Increasing the temperature of exposure of the test organism to the chemical increases the antimicrobial activity by a factor which is quantified by the temperature coefficient (Q_{10} value: the factor by which the effect increases for a 10 °C rise in temperature). Phenols and alcohols, for example, may respectively exhibit Q_{10} values of 3–5 and more than 10, and so a variation of 5 °C in the temperature of exposure (which is permitted by pharmacopoeial preservative efficacy tests) may lead to a markedly different rate of kill of the organism in question.

The time for which the test organism is exposed to the antimicrobial chemical may influence the recorded result because it is possible for the organism to adapt and become resistant to the presence of the chemical. In preservative efficacy tests, the exposure period is normally 28 days, which is sufficient time

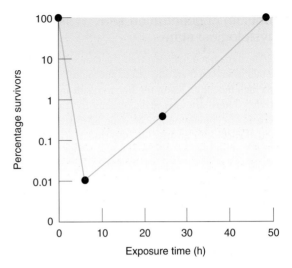

Fig. 14.1 • The survival and recovery of *Pseudomonas aeruginosa* exposed to benzethonium chloride during a preservative efficacy test.

for any cells that are not killed during the first 24–48 hours to recover and start to reproduce, so the final bacterial concentration may be much higher than that at the start. This is illustrated in Fig. 14.1, which shows the effect of the quaternary ammonium preservative benzethonium chloride on *Pseudomonas aeruginosa*. The concentration of bacteria was reduced to approximately 0.01% of the initial value during the first 6 hours, but the bacteria that survived this early period recovered to the original level within 2 days. There is the potential for a similar phenomenon to arise in other situations, e.g. in MIC determinations of bacteriostatic agents (those that do not kill but merely inhibit the growth of the test organism), although it is not common in MIC determinations because the exposure (incubation) time is much shorter than that in preservative testing.

The effect of some antibiotics may be influenced by the redox conditions during their period of contact with the test organism. Aminoglycosides, for example, are far less active, and metronidazole is far more active, under conditions of low oxygen availability. Such effects may even be seen during agar diffusion antibiotic assays, in which the antibiotic diffuses from a well into an agar gel inoculated with the test organism; the diameter of the zone of growth inhibition that surrounds a well filled with neomycin solution, for example, may be significantly greater at the surface of the agar (where there is abundant oxygen) than at its base, where the oxygen concentration is lower.

Inoculum concentration and physiological state

It is perhaps not surprising that the concentration of the inoculum can markedly affect antimicrobial action, with high inoculum levels tending to result in reduced activity. There are two main reasons for this. First, there is the phenomenon of drug adsorption onto the cell surface or absorption into the interior of the cell. If the number of drug molecules in the test tube is fixed yet the number of cells present is increased, this obviously results in fewer molecules available per cell and consequently the possibility of a diminished effect. In addition to this there is the second, more specialized case, again concerning antibiotics, where it is frequently observed that certain species of bacteria can synthesize antibiotic-inactivating enzymes, the most common of which are the various types of β-lactamases (those destroying penicillin, cephalosporin and related antibiotics). Thus a high inoculum means a high carryover of enzyme with the inoculum cells, or at least a greater potential synthetic capacity.

Perhaps less predictable than the inoculum concentration effect is the possibility of the inoculum history influencing the result. There is a substantial amount of evidence to show that the manner in which the inoculum of the test organism has been grown and prepared can significantly influence its susceptibility to toxic chemicals. Features such as the nature of the culture medium, e.g. nutrient broth or a defined glucose–salts medium, the metal ion composition of the medium and hence of the cells themselves, and the physiological state of the cells, i.e. 'young' actively growing cells from the logarithmic growth phase or 'old' nondividing cells from the stationary phase, all have the potential to influence the observed experimental values. Generally, antimicrobial chemicals are more effective against actively growing cells than slowly growing or dormant ones, e.g. bacterial spores.

Antibiotic assays

Methods of assaying antibiotics may be broadly divided into three groups:

- conventional chemical assays, e.g. titrations, spectrophotometry and high-performance liquid chromatography (HPLC);
- enzyme-based and immunoassays, where the antibiotic is, respectively, the substrate for a specific enzyme or the antigen with which a specific antibody combines; and
- biological assays in which biological activity, in this case bacterial growth inhibition, of the 'test' (sometimes referred to as the 'unknown') solution is compared with that of a reference standard.

Biological methods offer the advantage that the parameter being measured in the assay (growth inhibition) is the property for which the drug is used, and so inactive impurities or degradation products will not interfere and lead to an inaccurate result. Biological methods also offer other advantages (Table 14.1) but they have several significant limitations, and nonbiological methods are now generally preferred.

Enzyme-based and immunoassay kits (commonly referred to as enzyme-linked immunosorbent assays [ELISA]) are used in hospitals, notably for therapeutic

Table 14.1 Relative merits of different antibiotic assay methods

Assay method	Advantages	Disadvantages
Biological methods	Inactive impurities or degradation properties do not interfere	Slow, usually requiring overnight incubation
	Easily scaled up for multiple samples	Relatively labour intensive
	Do not require expensive equipment	Relatively inaccurate and imprecise, particularly with inexperienced operators
Nonbiological methods	Usually rapid, accurate and precise. May be more sensitive than biological assays	May require expensive equipment (e.g. HPLC) or expensive reagents or assay kits (enzyme and immunological methods)
	Enzyme and immunological methods usually use assay kits, which give reliable results with inexperienced operators	HPLC can assay samples only sequentially, so unusually large sample numbers may cause problems

HPLC, High-performance liquid chromatography.

monitoring of toxic antibiotics (e.g. aminoglycosides and vancomycin), whereas HPLC tends to be preferred in the pharmaceutical industry, particularly for quality assurance applications. Biological assays are most likely to be used when the alternatives are inappropriate, especially when the active antibiotic cannot readily be separated from inactive impurities, degradation products or interfering substances, or it cannot easily be assayed by HPLC without derivatization to enhance ultraviolet absorption (e.g. aminoglycosides). These situations may arise:

- when the antibiotic is present in a solution containing a wide variety of complex substances that would interfere with a chemical assay, e.g. fermentation broth, serum, or urine;
- when the antibiotic is present together with significant concentrations of its breakdown products, e.g. during stability studies as part of product development;
- when it has been extracted from a formulated medicine, e.g. a cream or linctus, when excipients might cause interference; and
- where the commercially available product is a mixture of isomers that have inherently different antimicrobial activities, which cannot easily be distinguished chemically and which may differ in proportion from batch to batch (e.g. neomycin and gentamicin).

Biological antibiotic assays, or bioassays as they are frequently known, may be of two main types: agar diffusion and turbidimetric. Despite bioassays having been superseded by HPLC in many situations, they are still used and the *European Pharmacopoeia* (PhEur) (European Pharmacopoeia Commission, 2017) describes experimental details for 19 diffusion and 15 turbidimetric methods; these details include test microorganisms, solvents, buffers, culture media and incubation conditions. In each case, a reference material of known activity must be available. When antibiotics were in their infancy, few could be produced in the pure state free from contaminating material, and specific chemical assays were rarely available. Thus the potency or activity of reference standards was expressed in terms of (international) units of activity. There are few antibiotics for which dose is still normally expressed in units: nystatin and colistin are two of the remaining examples. More commonly, potencies are recorded in terms of μg mL^{-1} of solution or μg antibiotic mg^{-1} of salt, with doses expressed in mg. The term potency ratio is used in pharmacopoeias to describe the assay result

and this is simply the ratio of the antibiotic concentration in the unknown or test solution divided by that in the standard solution.

Agar diffusion assays

In this technique the agar medium in a Petri dish or a larger assay plate is inoculated with the test organism, wells are created by removal of circular plugs of agar, and these wells are filled with a solution of the antibiotic or chemical under test (Fig. 14.2); alternatively, absorbent paper discs soaked in antibiotic solution are placed on the surface of the agar.

The chemical diffuses through the gel from A towards B and the concentration falls steadily in that direction. The concentration in the region from A to X is sufficiently high to prevent growth, i.e. it is an inhibitory concentration. Between X and B the concentration is subinhibitory and growth occurs. The concentration at X at the time the zone edge is formed is known as the critical inhibitory concentration. After incubation, the gel between A and X is clear and that between X and B is opaque as a result of microbial growth, which, with the common test organisms, is usually profuse. A zone of inhibition is therefore created, the diameter of which will increase as the concentration of the chemical in the well increases.

A graph may be constructed which relates zone diameter to the logarithm of the concentration of the solution in the well or paper disc (Fig. 14.3). It is normally found to be linear over a small concentration range, but the square of the diameter must be plotted to achieve linearity over a wide range. A plot such as that in Fig. 14.3 may, quite correctly, be used to calculate the concentration of a test solution of

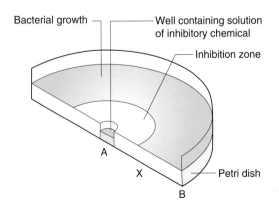

Fig. 14.2 • Assessment of antimicrobial activity by agar diffusion.

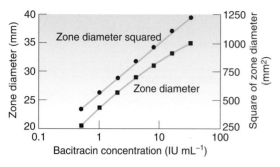

Fig. 14.3 • Calibration plots for agar diffusion assays.

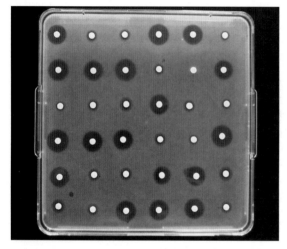

Fig. 14.4 • Antibiotic agar diffusion assay conducted with a 6 × 6 assay design in a 300 mm square assay plate.

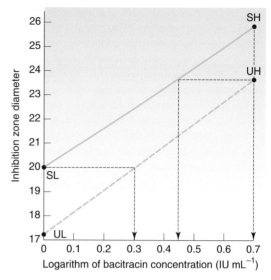

Fig. 14.5 • Four-point agar diffusion assay for bacitracin. *SH*, Standard high dose; *SL*, standard low dose; *UH*, unknown high dose; *UL*, unknown low dose.

antibiotic. In practice, however, it is found to be more convenient to obtain reliable mean zone diameters for the standard at just two or three concentrations rather than somewhat less reliable values for six or seven concentrations. There is no reason why an assay should not be based on a two- or three-point line, provided that those points are reliable and that preliminary experiments have shown that the plotted relationship over the concentration range in question is linear.

It is not common to conduct antibiotic assays in Petri dishes because too few zones may be accommodated on a standard-sized dish to permit the replication necessary to obtain the required accuracy and precision. Antibiotic assays, when performed on a large scale, are more often conducted with large assay plates 300 mm or more square (Fig. 14.4). The wells are created in a square design, and the number that may be accommodated will depend on the anticipated zone diameters: 36 or 64 wells are

common (6 × 6 or 8 × 8 respectively). The antibiotic standard material may be used in solution at three known concentrations (frequently referred to as 'doses'), and the antibiotic solution of unknown concentration is treated likewise; alternatively, each may be used at two concentrations. A randomization pattern known as a Latin square is used to ensure that there is a suitable distribution of the solutions over the plate, thereby minimizing any errors due to uneven agar thickness.

In the case of an assay based on standard solutions used at two concentrations, the potency ratio may be calculated directly from the graph (as shown in Fig. 14.5) or by use of the following formula:

$$\log X = \text{LDR} \times \frac{(\text{UH} + \text{UL}) - (\text{SH} + \text{SL})}{(\text{SH} - \text{SL}) + (\text{UH} - \text{UL})}$$

$$(14.1)$$

where X is the potency ratio, LDR is the logarithm of the dose ratio (i.e. ratio of concentrations of standard solutions) and UH, UL, SH and SL are the mean zone diameters for the unknown and standard high and low doses. The derivation of this is described in detail by Wardlaw (2000), who deals extensively with the subject of antibiotic assays. The tests for acceptable limits of parallelism between the line joining the standards and that joining the test points, together with confidence limits applicable to the calculated potency ratios, are described in the current PhEur.

In calculating the potency ratio directly from Fig. 14.5, the zone diameters for the standard and unknown high concentrations are plotted at the same abscissa values, and those for the low concentrations similarly. Two zone diameters are considered which are as widely separated on the ordinate as possible while still being covered by the standard and the test lines. The ratio of the concentrations required to achieve the selected diameter is thus an estimate of the potency ratio. The mean of the two estimates taken at the extremes of the range of common zone diameters should be identical to the value obtained by calculation from the formula. Thus, in Fig. 14.5, at a zone diameter of 23.75 mm, the first estimate of the potency ratio is 0.557 (antilog of 0.445 divided by the antilog of 0.699); the second is 0.507 (antilog of 0 divided by the antilog of 0.295). The mean value of 0.53 indicates the unknown solution has approximately half the activity of the standard.

Practical aspects of the conduct of agar diffusion assays

The agar may be surface inoculated or inoculated throughout while in the molten state prior to pouring. In the latter case, zones may arise which are different in diameter at the agar surface than at the base of the Petri dish; this may complicate the recording of zone diameters. Zones which are not perfectly circular may be disregarded, although it may be appropriate to record the mean of the long and short axes. Such zones may result from noncircular wells, careless filling or uneven drying of the agar gel owing to a poorly fitting plate cover. The zones may be read directly with callipers or, more conveniently, after enlargement by projection onto a screen. Automatic zone readers incorporating a series of photocells that detect opacity changes at the zone edge are available, and may be linked to a personal computer which rapidly calculates the result together with the appropriate statistical analyses. The size of the zone is determined by the relative rates of diffusion of the drug molecule and growth of the test organism. If the assay plates are left at room temperature for 1–4 hours prior to incubation, growth is retarded, whereas diffusion proceeds. This procedure, known as prediffusion, may result in larger zones and improved precision.

The zone diameter is affected by most of the factors previously stated to influence antimicrobial activity and, in addition, gel strength and the presence of other solutes in the antibiotic solution, e.g. buffer salts. If the antibiotic has been extracted from a formulated medicine, e.g. cream, lotion or mixture, excipients may be simultaneously removed and influence the diffusion of the antibiotic in the gel; sugars are known to have this effect. Because antibiotic assays involve a comparison of two solutions that are similarly affected by changes in experimental conditions, day-to-day variations in, for example, inoculum concentration will not have a great effect on the accuracy of the potency ratio obtained. However, the precision may be affected. The volume of liquid in the well is of minimal importance; it is usually of the order of 0.1 mL and is delivered by a semiautomatic pipette. For many antibiotics, the test organism is a *Bacillus* species and the inoculum is in the form of a spore suspension, which is easy to prepare, standardize and store. Alternatively, frozen inocula from liquid nitrogen may be used as a means of improving reproducibility.

Careful storage and preparation of the reference standards are essential. The reference antibiotic is usually stored at low temperature in a freeze-dried condition.

Turbidimetric assays

In this case, antibiotic standards at several concentrations are incorporated into liquid media and the extent of growth inhibition of the test organism is measured turbidimetrically using a nephelometer or spectrophotometer. The unknown or test antibiotic preparation is run simultaneously, again at several concentrations, and the degree of growth inhibition is compared. Such assays are less commonly used than agar diffusion methods because their precision is rather inferior, but they have the advantage of speed: the result may be available after an incubation period as short as 3–4 hours. They may also be more sensitive than diffusion assays and consequently may be applied to low-activity preparations.

The shape and slope of the dose–response plot for a turbidimetric assay may be more variable than that for agar diffusion, and nonlinear plots are common. Typical dose–response plots are shown in Hewitt & Vincent (1989). The plotted points are usually the mean turbidity values obtained from replicate tubes, and the assay may be conducted using a Latin square arrangement of tubes incubated in a shaker, which is necessary to ensure adequate aeration and uniform growth throughout the tube.

Practical aspects of the conduct of turbidimetric assays

The incubation time is critical in two respects. First, it is necessary to ensure that the culture in each of the many tubes in the incubator has exactly the same incubation period, because errors of a few minutes become significant in a total of only 3–4 hours' incubation. Care must therefore be taken to ensure that the tubes are inoculated in a precise order, and that growth is stopped in the same order by the addition of formalin, heating or other means.

The incubation period must be appropriate to the inoculum level so that the cultures do not achieve maximal growth. At the concentrations used for such assays, the antibiotics usually reduce the growth rate but do not limit total growth. Therefore, if the incubation period is sufficiently long, all the cultures may achieve the same cell density regardless of the antibiotic concentration.

There are certain other limitations to the use of turbidimetric assays. Because it is the 'cloudiness' of the culture that is measured, the standard and test solutions in which the organisms are suspended should, ideally, be clear before inoculation. Cloudy or hazy solutions which may result from the extraction of the antibiotic from a cream, for example, can be determined only after compensation of the standards in a similar manner or elimination of the error by other means. Test organisms that produce pigments during the course of the incubation should be avoided; so too should those that normally clump in suspension.

The rate of growth of the test organism may vary significantly from one batch of medium to another. Thus it is important to ensure that all the tubes in the assay contain medium from the same batch, and were prepared and sterilized at the same time. Many liquid media become darker brown on prolonged heating, and so samples from the same batch may differ in colour if the sterilizing time is not strictly controlled.

Minimum inhibitory concentration determinations

The MIC is the lowest concentration of an antimicrobial chemical found to inhibit the growth of a particular test organism. It is therefore a fundamental measure of the intrinsic antimicrobial activity (potency) of a chemical, which may be an antiseptic, disinfectant, preservative or antibiotic. MIC determinations are applied to chemicals in the pure state,

i.e. they are particularly relevant to raw materials rather than to the final formulated medicines; the latter are usually subject to preservative efficacy (challenge) tests to assess their antimicrobial activity. MICs values are usually expressed in terms of μg mL^{-1} or, less commonly %w/v (in the case of disinfectants, antiseptics or preservatives) or units mL^{-1} (for a few antibiotics). It is important to recognize that the test organism is not necessarily killed at the MIC. Whether or not the cells die or merely cease growing depends on the mode of action of the antimicrobial agent in question. MICs are commonly used to indicate the sensitivity of a particular organism to an antibiotic, so for the antibiotic to be effective in treating an infection its concentration at the infection site must comfortably exceed the MIC for the organism in question.

An MIC is an absolute value which is not based on a comparison with a standard/reference preparation, as in the case of antibiotic assays and certain disinfectant tests. For this reason, inadequate control of experimental conditions is particularly likely to have an adverse effect on results. Discrepancies in MICs measured in different laboratories are often attributable to slight variations in such conditions, and care must be taken to standardize all the factors previously stated to influence the result. It is important also to state the experimental details concerning an MIC determination. A statement such as 'the MIC for phenol against *E. coli* is 0.1% w/v' is not, by itself, very useful. It has far more value if the strain of *E. coli*, the inoculum concentration, the culture medium, etc., are also stated.

MIC test methods

The most common way to conduct MIC determinations is to incorporate the antimicrobial chemical at a range of concentrations into a liquid medium, the containers of which are then inoculated, incubated and examined for growth.

Test tubes may be used, but microtitre plates (small rectangular plastic trays with, usually, 96 wells each holding approximately 0.1 mL liquid) and other miniaturized systems are more common. It is also possible to incorporate the chemical into molten agar, which is then poured into Petri dishes and allowed to set. An advantage of using a microtitre plate or series of Petri dishes is that several organisms can be tested at the same time using a multipoint inoculator; there is also a greater chance of detecting contaminating organisms (as uncharacteristic colonies) on the agar surface than in liquid media. Usually the presence or absence of growth is easier to distinguish on the surface of agar than in liquid media. In tubes showing only faint turbidity, it is often difficult to decide whether growth has occurred or not. Regardless of the method used, the principle is the same and the MIC is the lowest concentration at which growth is inhibited.

In addition to the other experimental details that should be described in order to make the measured result meaningful, it is necessary to specify the increment by which the concentration of the test chemical changes from one container to the next. The operator could, for example, change the concentration 10-fold from one tube to the next in the rare circumstance where even the likely order of magnitude of the MIC is not known. Far more commonly, however, the concentration changes by a factor of 2, and this is almost invariably the case when antibiotic MIC values are determined; thus reference is made to 'doubling dilutions' of the antibiotic. If, for example, an MIC were to be measured using test tubes, an aqueous solution of the chemical would normally be mixed with an equal volume of *double*-strength growth medium in the first tube in the series, then half the contents of the first tube would be added to an equal volume of *single*-strength medium in the second, and so on. In this case half the contents of the last tube in the series would have to be discarded prior to inoculation in order to maintain the same volume in each tube. Control tubes may be included to demonstrate (1) that the inoculum culture was viable and that the medium was suitable for its growth (a tube containing medium and inoculum but no test chemical) and (2) that the operator was not contaminating the tubes with other organisms during preparation (a tube with no test chemical or added inoculum). It is possible to use an arithmetic series of concentrations of the test chemical, e.g. $0.1 \mu g \, mL^{-1}$, $0.2 \mu g \, mL^{-1}$, $0.3 \mu g \, mL^{-1}$, $0.4 \mu g \, mL^{-1}$, ... rather than $0.1 \mu g \, mL^{-1}$, $0.2 \mu g \, mL^{-1}$, $0.4 \mu g \, mL^{-1}$, $0.8 \mu g \, mL^{-1}$, ... The potential problem with this approach is that there may be merely a gradation in growth inhibition rather than a sharp point of demarcation with obvious growth in one tube in the series and no growth in the next.

All the solutions used must be sterilized; it must not be assumed that the test chemical is self-sterilizing. Most disinfectants, antiseptics and preservatives are bactericidal but they are unlikely to kill bacterial spores. Also, several antibiotics act by inhibiting growth and so would not necessarily kill vegetative cells with which they might be contaminated. If the experiment is conducted in tubes, all the tube contents must be mixed before inoculation as well as after, otherwise there is the possibility of the inoculum cells being killed by an artificially high concentration of the test chemical towards the top of the tube. If there is any risk of precipitation of the test chemical or the medium components during incubation, a turbidity comparison must be available for each concentration (same tube contents without inoculum); alternatively, in the case of bactericidal chemicals, the liquid in each tube may be subcultured into pure medium to see whether the inoculum has survived. Each of the tubes in the series may be prepared in duplicate or triplicate if it is considered desirable. This is the case where the incremental change in concentration is small.

Distinction between MICs determined in agar and the assessment of sensitivity using agar diffusion methods

It is important to understand that when MICs are determined by *agar dilution* methods in Petri dishes, the antimicrobial chemical is *dissolved* in the agar and is uniformly distributed through the gel when the test organism is inoculated into the surface. This is a fundamental difference from the test procedure used for antibiotic bioassays, where the antibiotic *diffuses* through the agar to create a growth inhibition zone. When MICs are determined by agar dilution, there is no diffusion and no zones of growth inhibition; the result merely depends on the presence or absence of growth of the test organism.

If the agar diffusion method were used, as in an antibiotic assay, to measure the size of the inhibition zones from a series of solutions of progressively decreasing concentration, it would obviously be possible to identify the concentration that just fails to produce an inhibition zone. This is sometimes incorrectly described as the MIC value for the antibiotic in question; such a procedure, however, gives the critical inhibitory concentration, not the MIC. Critical inhibitory concentrations usually exceed MIC values by a factor of 2–4. Not only is this misconception about agar diffusion methods giving MIC values commonly found in the pharmaceutical and chemical literature but misinterpretations of agar diffusion data are, unfortunately, also common. The diameter of a growth inhibition zone depends on several factors. Whilst the sensitivity of the test organism, its concentration and that of the chemical are paramount, the incubation conditions, the physicochemical composition of the gelled culture medium and the properties of the diffusing molecule are also important. It is tempting to take the simplistic view that if two chemicals are used at the same concentration and one produces a larger zone of growth inhibition than the other, that is a direct reflection of their intrinsic antimicrobial activities. Unfortunately, that is often not the case because it fails to take into account both the diffusion coefficients of the different molecules and their concentration exponents (see Chapter 15). To diffuse well in agar, a molecule should be small, water soluble and of a charge that does not interact with the components of the gel. There are several very effective antimicrobial chemicals that either do not diffuse well in agar or possess a high concentration exponent, both of which are properties that would predispose to small zones. If these agents were to be assessed purely on the basis of the inhibition zone diameter, they would be incorrectly dismissed as virtually inactive. Parabens and phenols are prime examples. Even saturated solutions of parabens in water can fail to give inhibition zones by agar diffusion (Fig. 14.6) but they are, nevertheless, amongst the most effective and widely used antimicrobial preservatives. Likewise, phenols, with their high concentration exponents, only give small inhibition zones, and this has led to misleading comparisons; manuka honey, for example, has been claimed to possess antibacterial activity equivalent to 10% phenol on the basis that the inhibition zone diameters are similar. This fundamental limitation of agar diffusion as a method of assessing antimicrobial potency is all too frequently overlooked.

There is, however, one MIC test method for antibiotics that *does* depend on diffusion: the Etest™ consists of a paper strip that is impregnated with a predefined antibiotic gradient which is placed on the surface of a plate inoculated with the test organism. After incubation, a zone of inhibition is formed which gives a reading of the MIC where the narrow end of the zone intersects with the paper strip. In Fig. 14.7, the vancomycin MIC would be recorded as $1.5 \ \mu g \ mL^{-1}$.

Preservative efficacy tests (or challenge tests)

These are tests applied to the formulated medicine in its final container to determine whether it is adequately protected against microbial spoilage; they are normally used only during product development and are not part of the routine quality control applied to batches of manufactured medicines. Preservative efficacy tests (rather than chemical assays of preservatives) are used to assess vulnerability to spoilage because it is not normally possible to predict how the activity of a preservative chemical will be influenced by the active ingredients, the excipients and the container itself.

Certain products may contain no added preservative, either because the active ingredients have sufficient antimicrobial activity themselves or because

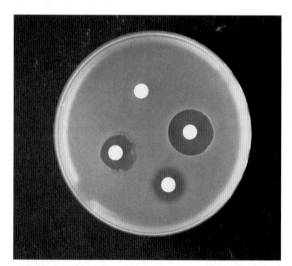

Fig. 14.6 • Zones of growth inhibition resulting from preservative chemicals. The disc at the top was soaked in a saturated solution of parabens but failed to produce an inhibition zone because parabens have a high concentration exponent.

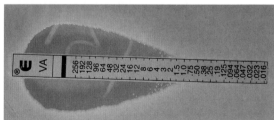

Fig. 14.7 • An Etest determination of vancomycin minimum inhibitory concentration for *Staphylococcus aureus*. From https://commons.wikimedia.org/wiki/File:Etest_Vancomycin_S_aureus.jpg; accessed 30 December 2016.

they already contain high concentrations of sugar or salts which restrict the growth of microorganisms. However, such products are rare; multidose injections or eye drops, the majority of oral mixtures, linctuses and similar preparations, together with creams and lotions, all contain preservatives. They are not normally required in anhydrous products, e.g. ointments, or in single-dose injections.

Again, it must not be assumed that products containing antimicrobial agents as the active ingredients are self-sterilizing. It is quite possible for an antibiotic cream, for example, to be active against certain bacteria yet fail to restrict the growth of contaminating yeasts or moulds.

The basic principle of a preservative test is to inoculate separate containers of the product with known concentrations of a variety of test organisms, then to remove samples from each container over a period of time and determine the proportion of the inoculum that has survived. When first introduced into national pharmacopoeias, preservative efficacy tests differed to some extent in experimental detail and differed markedly in the required performance criteria for preservatives to be used in different product categories. In the late 1990s, moves towards international harmonization of preservative testing procedures in the European, United States and Japanese pharmacopoeias meant that many (but not all) of the discrepancies in experimental detail were eliminated. The differences in performance criteria remain, however, with the PhEur generally requiring a greater degree of microbial inactivation for the preservative to be considered satisfactory than the *United States Pharmacopeia* (USP) and the *Japanese Pharmacopoeia*, which, in this respect, are very similar.

The PhEur (European Pharmacopoeia Commission, 2017) recommends the routine use of four test organisms, each at a final concentration of 10^5–10^6 cells mL^{-1} or g^{-1} in the product. Counts are performed on samples removed at O h, 6 h, 24 h, 48 h, 7 days, 14 days and 28 days. Various aspects of the test are considered in more detail in the following section.

Choice of test organisms and inoculum concentration

The test organisms used are the bacteria *Staphylococcus aureus*, *P. aeruginosa* and *E. coli* (which is used for testing all product types in the USP test but for oral products only in the PhEur test), together with

the yeasts/moulds *Candida albicans* and *Aspergillus brasiliensis* (plus the osmophilic *Zygosaccharomyces rouxii* in the PhEur test for oral syrups). The current PhEur recommends that the designated organisms be supplemented, where appropriate, by other strains or species that may represent likely contaminants to the preparation. A similar recommendation was contained in earlier versions of the USP preservative test but not in the current test (United States Pharmacopeial Convention, 2016).

One problem with adding other organisms (such as those isolated from the manufacturing environment) is that they are not universally available, and so a particular product could be tested at different manufacturing sites of the same company and pass in one location yet fail in another simply because the organisms used locally were not the same. The possibility of using resistant strains isolated from previous batches of spoilt product has been advocated, but this too may pose problems because organisms may rapidly lose their preservative resistance unless they are routinely grown on medium supplemented with the preservative in question.

The inoculum concentration of 10^5–10^6 microorganisms mL^{-1} or g^{-1} of the preparation under test has been criticized as being unrealistic because it is much higher than that which would be acceptable in a freshly manufactured product. It is adopted, however, in order for the 1000-fold fall (described as a 3-log reduction in the pharmacopoeia) in microbial concentration that would be required from an effective parenteral or ophthalmic preservative to be easily measured. The test organisms are added separately to different containers rather than as a mixed inoculum.

Inactivation of preservative

It is quite possible for a sufficient amount of the preservative to be contained in, and carried over with, the sample removed from the container to prevent or retard growth of colonies on the Petri dishes. If the inoculum level of the test organism initially is approximately 10^6 cells mL^{-1} or g^{-1} of product, the problem of carryover may not arise because a dilution factor of 10^3 or 10^4 would be required to achieve a countable number of colonies on a plate; at this dilution most preservatives would no longer be active. When a high proportion of the cells in the product have died, however, little or no such dilution is required, so preservative carryover is a real problem which may artificially depress the count even more.

To avoid this, preservative inhibitors or antagonists may be used. There are several of these, common examples being glycine for aldehydes, thioglycollate or cysteine for heavy metals, and mixtures of lecithin and polysorbate 80 with or without Lubrol W for quaternary ammonium compounds, chlorhexidine and parabens. The use of these and other inactivators has been tabulated by Gilmore et al. (2011).

An alternative method of removing residual preservative is to pass the sample of inoculated product through a bacteria-proof membrane so that surviving organisms are retained and washed on the surface of the membrane and the preservative is thus physically separated from them. After washing, the membrane is transferred to the surface of a suitable agar medium and colonies of microorganisms develop on it in the normal way. It is necessary to incorporate controls (validate the method) to demonstrate both that the inactivator really works and that it is not, itself, toxic. The former usually involves mixing the inactivator with the concentrations of preservative likely to be carried over, then inoculating this mixture and demonstrating no viability loss. Details of these validation procedures are described more fully in chapter <1227> of the USP (United States Pharmacopeial Convention, 2016).

One further control is a viable count of the inoculum performed by dilution in peptone water to check the actual number of cells introduced into the product. This is necessary because even a 'zero-time sample' of the product will contain cells that have been exposed to the preservative for a short period as it usually takes 15–45 seconds or more to mix the inoculum with the product and then remove the sample. Some of the cells may be killed even in such a short time, and so a viable count of the inoculum culture will reflect this.

Interpretation of results

The extent of microbial killing required at the various sampling times for a preservative to be considered acceptable for use in parenteral or ophthalmic products is greater than that required for a preservative to be used in topical products, which in turn exceeds that for an oral product preservative (Table 14.2).

In the case of the first two product categories, the PhEur specifies two alternative performance criteria, designated A and B. The A criterion express the recommended efficacy to be achieved, whereas the B criterion must be satisfied in justified cases where the A criterion cannot be attained, e.g. because of an increased risk of adverse reactions. The baseline used as the reference point to assess the extent of killing is the concentration of microorganisms expected to arise in the product after addition and mixing of the inoculum, as calculated from a viable count performed on the concentrated inoculum suspension prior to its addition to the product. The viable count of the time-zero samples removed from the inoculated product is not the baseline.

Table 14.2 Log reductions required in viable counts of microorganisms used in the *European Pharmacopoeia* (2017) preservative efficacy tests methods

Product type	Microorganism	Criterion	6 h	24 h	48 h	7 days	14 days	28 days
Parenteral and ophthalmic	Bacteria	A	2	3				NR
	Pseudomonas aeruginosa *Staphylococcus aureus* *Escherichia coli*[a]	B		1		3		NI
	Fungi	A				2		NI
	Aspergillus brasiliensis *Candida albicans*	B					1	NI
Topical	Bacteria	A			2	3		NI
		B					3	NI
	Fungi	A					2	NI
		B					1	NI
Oral and rectal	Bacteria						3	NI
	Fungi						1	NI

[a]In oral products only.

NI, No increase (see the text); *NR*, no recovery.

Disinfectant evaluation

A variety of tests have been described over many years for the assessment of disinfectant activity. Those developed during the early part of the 20th century, e.g. the Rideal–Walker and Chick–Martin tests, were primarily intended for testing phenolic disinfectants against pathogenic organisms such as *Salmonella typhi*. Such phenol coefficient tests are now outmoded because *S. typhi* is no longer endemic in the United Kingdom and phenolics are no longer preeminent; indeed, they now represent a minor fraction of the total biocides used for floor disinfection in aseptic dispensing areas in British hospital pharmacies (Murtough et al., 2000).

In the second half of the 20th century, several other testing procedures were described for use in the UK which reduced the sampling or other problems associated with the early phenol coefficient tests; these included the Berry and Bean method, the British Standard 3286 test for quaternary ammonium compounds and the Kelsey–Sykes test. Other countries adopted procedures that were similar in concept but which differed in experimental detail; these and other tests used in the UK, Europe and the USA are described by Reybrouck (2004) and more recently by Gilmore et al. (2011). At present there is no *internationally* applicable and officially recommended disinfectant testing procedure, although good uniformity exists in Europe as a result of the establishment by the European Committee for Standardization in 1990 of Technical Committee 216, which has a responsibility for chemical disinfectants and antiseptics. The European standard BS EN 1276 (British Standards Institution, 2009) was the first result of the work of Technical Committee 216; this deals with assessment of bactericidal activity of disinfectants on bacteria in aqueous suspension. Other procedures applicable to more specialized situations, e.g. disinfection of solid surfaces, are described in various European standards and have been reviewed by Hanlon (2010).

A confusing variety of methods for describing and categorizing test procedures are in use. Some schemes classify tests according to the organisms to be killed (bactericidal, fungicidal, virucidal, etc.), but classification based on test design is more common, for example:

- suspension tests;
- capacity tests which measure the extent to which the disinfectant can withstand repeated additions of test organisms;
- carrier tests, where the organism is loaded or dried onto a carrier; and
- in-use tests, which are intended to simulate actual conditions of use as closely as possible.

Most suspension tests of disinfectants have in common the addition of a defined concentration of the test organism to the disinfectant solution at a specified temperature, followed by assessment of viability in samples removed after suitable periods. However, there are four aspects of disinfectant testing that merit special note:

1. Because disinfectants are normally used in circumstances where there is a significant amount of organic 'dirt' present, modern testing procedures invariably attempt to take this into consideration. Thus, yeast, albumin or other material is added in known concentration to the disinfectant/microorganism mixture.

2. Regardless of the method by which the antimicrobial activity is assessed (see later), it is a fundamental principle of disinfectant testing, just as it is with preservative efficacy tests, that the antimicrobial activity of the disinfectant must be halted (also referred to as neutralized, inactivated or quenched) in the sample when it is removed from the disinfectant/microorganism mixture. Clearly, meaningful results cannot be obtained if it is impossible to distinguish what fraction of the microbial killing occurred during the timed period of exposure to the disinfectant from that arising due to carryover of disinfectant into the incubation step that follows exposure. Verification that the disinfectant inactivation method is effective and that any chemical neutralizers used are, themselves, nontoxic to the test organisms is an integral part of the test.

3. It is in viability assessment that there is a fundamental difference of approach between relatively recently developed tests (exemplified by BS EN 1276) and many of the tests that originated before the 1980s. The simplest method of viability assessment, which was employed in the Rideal–Walker and Kelsey–Sykes tests, for example, is to transfer the sample from the disinfectant/microorganism mixture to a known volume of neutralizing broth, incubate the broth and examine it for growth (manifest as turbidity). This procedure contains the inherent defect that any growth in the tubes of broth may result from the transfer

of very few surviving cells, or from many. Thus it is possible for the disinfectant to kill a high proportion of the inoculum within a short period yet fail to kill a small fraction of the cells, possibly mutants, which have atypically high resistance. In this case, there is the risk that the disinfectant may be dismissed as insufficiently active despite the fact that it achieved a rapid and extensive initial kill. For this reason, it has become common for disinfectant and preservative efficacy tests to be very similar in design, in that both employ viable counting methods to assess microorganism survival but the former use a sampling period of minutes or hours, whereas the latter use a 28-day period.

4. When viable counting is used to assess the survival of test organisms, the adoption of disinfection performance criteria based on a required reduction in the number of surviving organisms is a logical strategy, just as it is in preservative testing. Thus the so-called 5–5–5 testing principle has found much favour. Here, five test organisms are (separately) exposed for 5 minutes to the disinfectant, which is considered satisfactory if a 5-log reduction in viable numbers (a 10^5 fall in the number of viable cells mL^{-1}) is recorded in each case. This principle is adopted in BS EN 1276, although only four bacterial strains are recommended for routine use; there is, however, the option to supplement the standard organisms with others

more relevant to the intended use of the disinfectant in question.

Microbiological quality of pharmaceutical materials

Nonsterile products

Nonsterile pharmaceutical products obviously differ from sterile products in that they are permitted to contain some viable microorganisms, but the PhEur (European Pharmacopoeia Commission, 2017) specifies the maximum concentrations acceptable in different types of product and the species of organism that are not permitted at all (these characteristics are known as product bioburdens; see Table 14.3). Similar specifications are present in the USP and other pharmacopoeias.

The required microbiological quality of the manufactured medicine cannot be achieved by the application of an antimicrobial process (heating, radiation, etc.) as the final production step for two reasons: first, an approach that uses poor-quality raw materials and manufacturing procedures and then attempts to 'clean up' the product at the end is not acceptable to the licensing authorities; second, some products would not withstand such antimicrobial treatment, e.g. heating an emulsion may cause cracking or creaming. Thus the most reliable approach to ensure that the manufactured medicine complies with the

Table 14.3 *European Pharmacopoeia* (2017) specifications for the microbiological quality of major categories of pharmaceutical products

Route of administration	Total aerobic microbial count (cfu g^{-1} or cfu mL^{-1})	Total yeast and mould count (cfu g^{-1} or cfu mL^{-1})	Specified microorganisms (must be absent in 1 g or 1 mL)
Nonaqueous oral products	10^3	10^2	*Escherichia coli*
Aqueous oral products	10^2	10^1	*Escherichia coli*
Rectal products	10^3	10^2	
Products for use in the mouth, nose, and ears and on the skin	10^2	10^1	*Staphylococcus aureus* *Pseudomonas aeruginosa*
Vaginal products	10^2	10^1	*Staphylococcus aureus* *Pseudomonas aeruginosa* *Candida albicans*

Specifications also exist for transdermal patches, inhalations and certain oral products of animal, vegetable or mineral origin.
cfu, Colony-forming unit (defined in Chapter 13).

pharmacopoeial specification is to ensure that the raw materials are of good quality and that the manufacturing procedures conform to the standards laid down in the latest edition of *Rules and Guidance for Pharmaceutical Manufacturers and Distributors* (Medicines and Healthcare products Regulatory Agency, 2017).

Implicit in these standards is the principle that the extent of product contamination originating from the manufacturing environment and production personnel should be subject to regular monitoring and control.

Environmental monitoring

Environmental monitoring is normally taken to mean regular monitoring of the levels of microbial contamination of the atmosphere, of solid surfaces and, less frequently, of the personnel in the production areas. Water used to clean floors, benches and equipment (as distinct from water incorporated in the product) may be considered as part of environmental monitoring but will not be considered here as the procedures for counting microorganisms in water are described later in this chapter.

Atmospheric monitoring is most commonly undertaken by means of settle plates, which are simply Petri dishes containing medium suitable for the growth of bacteria and/or yeasts and moulds, e.g. tryptone soya agar, which are exposed to the atmosphere for periods of, typically, 1–4 hours. Microorganisms in the air may exist as single cells, e.g. mould spores, but more commonly they are attached to dust particles, so any organisms in the latter category (for which the culture medium is suitable) will grow into visible colonies during incubation after dust particles have settled on the agar surface. The colony counts recorded on the plates are obviously influenced by:

- the duration of exposure;
- the degree of air turbulence, which determines the volume of air passing over the plate; and
- the intrinsic level of atmospheric contamination (microorganisms per litre of air), which in turn is often a reflection of the number and activity level of the operating personnel because skin scales shed by the operators are usually the most potent source of atmospheric contaminants.

The disadvantage of settle plates is that it is not possible to relate colony counts directly to air volume.

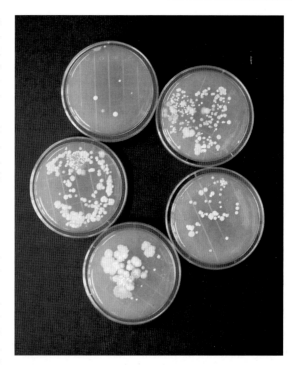

Fig. 14.8 • A selection of contact (e.g. RODAC™) plates used for sampling the following surfaces (from the *top left clockwise*): laminar flow cabinet; book cover; computer keyboard; tap handle; reagent bottle.

This limitation is overcome in active sampling methods, whereby a known volume of air is drawn over, or caused to impact on, the agar surface. These methods and the equipment available for active sampling have been reviewed by Johnson (2003).

Surface and equipment sampling is most frequently undertaken by swabbing or the use of contact plates (also known as RODAC™ – replicate organism detection and counting – plates; see Fig. 14.8). Swabbing a known area of bench, floor or equipment with a swab soaked in culture medium is convenient for irregular surfaces. The organisms on the swab may be counted after they have been dispersed by agitation into a fixed volume of suspending medium but it is not easy to quantify either the proportion of total organisms removed from the swabbed surface or the proportion dispersed in the diluent. This second limitation is overcome using contact plates, which are simply specially designed Petri dishes slightly overfilled with molten agar which, on setting of the molten agar, present a convex surface that projects above the rim of the plate. When the plate is inverted onto the surface to be sampled, microorganisms are transferred directly onto the agar.

Sampling of manufacturing personnel usually consists in sampling clothing, face masks or, more commonly, gloves. 'Finger dabs' is the phrase used to describe the process whereby an operator rolls the gloved surface of each finger over a suitable solid medium in a manner similar to that in which finger-prints are taken. Operator sampling by any means other than finger dabs is rare, particularly outside aseptic manufacturing areas.

Counting of microorganisms in pharmaceutical products

Most pharmaceutical raw materials are contaminated with microorganisms. The levels of contamination are often a reflection of the source of the raw material in question, with 'natural' products derived from vegetable or animal sources, or mined minerals such as kaolin and talc, being more heavily contaminated than synthetic materials whose microbial burden has been reduced by heat, extremes of pH or organic solvents during the course of manufacture. Determining the bioburden in these materials is often straight-forward, utilizing without modification the viable counting procedures described in Chapter 13. Occasionally the physical nature of the raw material makes this difficult or impossible, and this is often found to be the case with the finished manufactured medicine, where problems of dispersibility, sedimentation or viscosity cause complications. As a consequence, modifications to the standard viable counting procedures are necessary to reduce errors. Some of modifications and the circumstances that necessitate them are considered next.

Very low concentrations of microorganisms in aqueous solutions. The reliability of calculated viable cell concentrations becomes much reduced when they are based on colony counts much lower than approximately 10–15 per Petri dish. With use of a surface-spread method, it is rarely possible to place more than approximately 0.5 mL of liquid onto the agar surface in a standard Petri dish because it will not easily soak in. By a pour-plate method, 1 mL or more may be used but a point is reached where the volume of sample significantly dilutes the agar and nutrients. Thus, with a conventional plating technique, the lowest concentration conveniently detectable is of the order of 10–50 cells mL^{-1}. When the cell concentration is below this value, it is necessary to pass a known quantity of the liquid, typically 10 mL to 100 mL or even more, depending on the dosage form or specific product in question, through

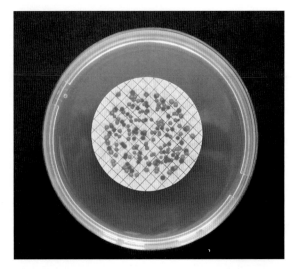

Fig. 14.9 • Membrane filter counting: colonies of the red pigmented bacterium *Serratia marcescens* growing on the surface of a cellulose nitrate filter membrane on agar in a Petri dish.

a filter membrane having a pore size sufficiently small to retain bacteria. The membrane is then placed with the organisms uppermost onto the agar surface in a Petri dish, which is incubated without inversion. As a result of diffusion of nutrients through the membrane, colonies grow on the surface in the normal way (Fig. 14.9). Diffusion may be assisted by the inclusion of a medium-soaked pad between the membrane and the agar. It is important to ensure that all the membrane is in contact with the pad or agar, otherwise elevated areas may become dry and no colonies will appear on them.

Insoluble solids. It is necessary to suspend an insoluble solid in a medium that will permit uniform dispersion and adequate wetting of the suspended material. Nutrient broth, peptone water or a buffered salt solution is frequently used, and a low concentration of a surfactant may be incorporated to promote wetting, e.g. polysorbate 80 (0.01% to 0.05%). Suspension in distilled water alone carries the risk of osmotic damage to sensitive cells, with a consequently low count; for this reason, it is best avoided. Having obtained the suspension, there are two options available depending on the nature and concentration of the suspended material.

The first is to remove a sample of the continuously mixed suspension, dilute it if necessary, and plate it in or on a suitable medium by a pour-plate or spread-plate method. If the concentration of suspended material is low, it may still be possible to see clearly the developing colonies. High concentrations may obscure the colonies and make counting impossible. The alternative is to dislodge the microbial cells from the solid to which they are attached, allow the solid to sediment out and then sample the supernatant. Methods of removal include vigorous manual shaking, the use of a vortex mixer or the use of equipment designed for the purpose, e.g. the Colworth 'stomacher', in which the aqueous suspension is placed in a sealed sterile bag which is repeatedly agitated by reciprocating paddles. The use of ultrasonics to dislodge the cells carries the risk of damage to, or lysis of, the cells themselves.

Assuming the suspended material has no antimicrobial activity, plating the 'whole suspension' is probably the easiest and most reliable method. The alternative strategy of sampling the supernatant involves the assumption that all the cells have been removed from the solid but this would have to be confirmed by control (validation) experiments in which a known quantity of similar organisms was artificially dried onto sterile samples of the material. The second method also relies on the solid sedimenting sufficiently rapidly for it to be separated from the bacteria in aqueous suspension above it. If all or part of the sample has a particle size similar to that of bacteria, yeasts or mould spores, i.e. approximately 1 μm to 5 μm, then a separation cannot easily be achieved.

Oils and hydrophobic ointments. These materials are usually not heavily contaminated because they are anhydrous and microorganisms will not multiply without water. Thus the microorganisms contained in oily products have usually arisen by contamination from the atmosphere, from equipment used for manufacture and from storage vessels. To perform a viable count, the oil sample must be emulsified or solubilized without the aid of excessive heat or any other agent that might kill the cells.

An oil-in-water emulsion must be produced using a suitable surfactant; nonionic emulsifiers generally have little antimicrobial activity. The proportion of surfactant to be used must be determined experimentally and validation experiments must be conducted to confirm that the surfactant is not toxic to the species that typically arise as contaminants of the sample in question; Millar (2000) has described the use of up to 5 g of polysorbate 80 added to a 10 g sample. Such an emulsion may be diluted in water or buffered salts solution if necessary, and aliquots may be placed on or in the agar medium in

the usual way. Alternatively, the oil may be dissolved in a sterile, nontoxic solvent and passed through a membrane filter. Isopropyl myristate, for example, is recommended in pharmacopoeial sterility testing procedures as a solvent for anhydrous materials but it may kill a significant fraction of the cells of some sensitive species, even during an exposure period of only a few minutes.

Creams and lotions. Oil-in-water emulsions do not usually represent a problem because they are miscible with water and thus are easily diluted. Water-in-oil creams, however, are not miscible and cannot be plated directly because bacteria may remain trapped in a water droplet suspended in a layer of oil on the agar surface. Such bacteria may not form colonies because the diffusion of nutrients through the oil would be inadequate. These creams are best diluted, dispersed in an aqueous medium and membrane filtered or converted to an oil-in-water type, and then counted by normal plating methods.

Dilution and emulsification of the cream in broth containing Lubrol W, polysorbate 80 or Triton X-100 is probably the best procedure, although the addition of approximately 0.1 g of the w/o emulsion sample to 25 g of isopropyl myristate followed by membrane filtration may be satisfactory.

Detection of specific hazardous organisms

In addition to placing limits on the maximum concentration of microorganisms that is acceptable in different materials, pharmacopoeias usually specify certain organisms that must not be present at all. In practice, this means that detection methods which are described in the pharmacopoeia must be applied to a known weight of material (typically 1 g to 10 g), and the sample passes the test if, on the culture plates, no organisms arise that conform to the standard textbook descriptions of those to be excluded. Typically, the pharmacopoeial methods involve preliminary stages using selective liquid culture media; these are designed to increase the concentration of the organism that is the subject of the test ('target' organism) and so render it more readily detectable. Commercially available identification kits or specific supplementary biochemical tests may also be used to confirm the identity of any isolates having the typical appearance of the target organisms. The PhEur used to recommend appropriate supplementary tests but these have been removed from the current edition, not because of a

Table 14.4 Media and procedures recommended in tests for specified microorganisms

Organism	Liquid enrichment medium (A) and solid (agar) medium (B) recommended in the *European Pharmacopoeia* (2017)	Appearance of colonies on solid (agar) medium	Typical supplementary tests[b]
Escherichia coli	A: MacConkey's broth B: MacConkey's agar	Pink colonies with precipitate of bile due to acid production	Indole production at 44 °C
Salmonella	A: Rappaport–Vassiliadis *Salmonella* enrichment broth B: XLD agar	Red colonies, sometimes with black centres	
Pseudomonas aeruginosa	A: casein soya bean digest broth[a] B: cetrimide agar	Colonies usually displaying a green or blue pigment	Positive oxidase test
Staphylococcus aureus	A: casein soya bean digest broth B: mannitol salt agar	Yellow colonies, possibly surrounded by a yellow zone in otherwise orange agar	Positive coagulase test
Clostridia	A: reinforced clostridial medium B: Columbia agar (incubated anaerobically)	White colonies	Rod-shaped cells with negative catalase reaction
Candida albicans	A: Sabouraud dextrose broth B: Sabouraud dextrose agar	Large, raised, white or off-white colonies	

[a]More commonly known as tryptone soya broth.
[b]Not part of *European Pharmacopoeia* (European Pharmacopoeia Commission, 2017) procedures.
XLD, Xylose–lysine–deoxycholate.

lack of reliability but because identification kits have become more common.

Both the PhEur (European Pharmacopoeia Commission, 2017) and the USP (US Pharmacopeial Convention, 2016) describe detection tests for *S. aureus*, *P. aeruginosa*, *E. coli*, salmonellae and *C. albicans*. In addition, the PhEur describes a test for clostridia, but this is unlikely to be applied to any material other than mined minerals, e.g. talc and bentonite, and to certain vaccines. The five organisms common to both pharmacopoeias are the subject of these tests primarily because of their potential to cause infections. However, they may also represent common contaminants of the products to which the tests are applied, or their presence may be indicative of the quality of the raw material or finished manufactured product. *E. coli*, for example, is a natural inhabitant of mammalian intestines and so its presence in a material such as gelatin (which originates in the slaughterhouse) would indicate unacceptable quality. The most likely source of *S. aureus* in a manufactured medicine is the production personnel, so if this origin were confirmed, it would indicate the need for higher manufacturing standards. In general, the tests are applied to pharmaceutical raw materials of 'natural' origin, e.g. carbohydrates, cellulose derivatives, gums and vegetable drugs. In addition, there is a requirement that products for use in the mouth, nose, or ears or on the skin should be free of both *P. aeruginosa* and *S. aureus* and vaginal products should also be free from *C. albicans*. Table 14.4 summarizes the PhEur (European Pharmacopoeia Commission, 2017) testing schemes for the five principal organisms of interest. These schemes are described in more detail elsewhere, together with photographs of the typical appearance of the organisms in question (Hodges, 2000).

Microbiological assays of B-group vitamins

Just as HPLC has become the favoured method of antibiotic assay, so too has it become the method of choice for assaying B-group vitamins. Turbidimetric assays are still occasionally used, however; for example, when insurmountable problems arise in resolving the many peaks that might arise in an HPLC chromatogram from a multivitamin product (which may contain 10 or more active ingredients plus excipients, all of which may cause assay interference).

Microbiological assays of B-group vitamins employ similar techniques to those used in turbidimetric assays of antibiotics (see earlier in this chapter). A culture medium is used which is suitable for the assay organism, except for the omission of the vitamin in question. The extent of bacterial growth in the medium is thus directly proportional to the amount of reference standard or test vitamin added. It is important to select an assay organism that has an absolute requirement for the substance in question and is unable to obtain it by metabolism of other medium components; species of *Lactobacillus* are often used for this purpose. 'Carryover' of the vitamin with the inoculum culture must be avoided because this results in some growth even when none of the test material has been added. Growth may be determined turbidimetrically or by acid production from sugars.

Sterile products

Sterile products must, by definition, be free of viable microorganisms, and it is important to understand that this is an absolute requirement. Thus, the presence of one single surviving microbial cell is sufficient to render the product nonsterile. There is not a level of survivors which is so small as to be regarded as negligible and therefore acceptable.

The principal component of microbiological quality assurance which has traditionally been applied to sterile products is, of course, the test for sterility itself. In essence, this is quite simple: a sample of the material to be tested is added to culture medium, which is incubated and then examined for signs of microbial growth. If growth occurs, the assumption is made that the contamination arose from the sample, which consequently fails the test. However, the limitations of this simplistic approach became more widely recognized in the second half of the 20th century, and there was an increasing awareness of the fact that contaminated products could pass the test and sterile ones apparently fail it (because of contamination introduced during the testing procedure itself). For these reasons the sterility test alone could no longer be relied on to provide an assurance of sterility, and that assurance is now derived from a strict adherence to high quality standards throughout the manufacturing process. These encompass:

- Adoption of the highest possible specifications for the microbiological quality of the raw materials. The rationale here is that sterilization processes are more likely to be effective when the levels of microorganisms to be killed or removed (bioburdens) are as low as possible to begin with. Procedures used to determine

bioburdens are described in Chapter 13 and earlier in this chapter.

- The rigorous application of environmental monitoring procedures (as described earlier in this chapter) during the course of manufacture, with more stringent limits for acceptable levels of microorganisms than those applicable during the manufacture of nonsterile products.

- Comprehensive validation procedures when sterilization processes are designed, together with regular in-process monitoring when those processes are in operation for product manufacture. Initial validation seeks to demonstrate that adequate sterilizing conditions are achieved throughout the load, and entails extensive testing with thermocouples, radiation dosimeters and biological indicators (see later) as appropriate.

The pharmacopoeias and regulatory authorities require a sterility assurance level for terminally sterilized products of 10^{-6} or better. This means that the probability of nonsterility in an item selected at random from a batch should be no more than 1 in 1 million. This sterility assurance level may be demonstrated in the case of some terminally sterilized products simply by reference to data derived from bioburdens, environmental monitoring and in-process monitoring of the sterilization procedure itself. In this case the sterility test may be unnecessary and omitted; the term 'parametric release' is used to describe the release of products for sale or use under these circumstances, although it should be emphasized that manufacturers must seek approval for parametric release from regulatory authorities; the decision is not made by the manufacturers themselves (Pharmaceutical Inspection Co-operation Scheme Secretariat, 2007).

Sterilization monitoring

Sterilization processes may be monitored physically, chemically or biologically (Denyer et al., 2011). Physical methods are exemplified by thermocouples, which are routinely incorporated at different locations within an autoclave load, whereas chemical indicators usually exhibit a colour change after exposure to a heat sterilization process. Biological indicators consist of preparations of spores of the *Bacillus* or *Geobacillus* species that exhibits the greatest degree of resistance to the sterilizing agent in question. The principle of their use is simply that if such spores are exposed to the sterilization process and fail to survive, it can be assumed that all other common organisms will also have been killed and the process is safe. Spores of *Geobacillus stearothermophilus* (often still indexed in the pharmaceutical literature under its former name of *Bacillus stearothermophilus*) are used to monitor autoclaves and gaseous hydrogen peroxide or peracetic acid sterilization processes, whereas *Bacillus atrophaeus* is the organism normally employed for dry heat, ethylene oxide and low-temperature steam–formaldehyde methods; *Bacillus pumilus* is used in radiation sterilization procedures.

Such biological indicators are regularly employed for validation of a sterilization process which is under development for a new product, or when a new autoclave is being commissioned; they are not normally used for routine monitoring during product manufacture. Spores possess the advantage that they are relatively easy to produce, purify and dry onto an inert carrier, which is frequently an absorbent paper strip or disc, or a plastic or metal support. Spore resistance to the sterilizing agent must be carefully controlled, and so rigorous standardization of production processes followed by observance of correct storage conditions and expiry dates is essential.

Tests for sterility

It is sufficient here to repeat that the test is really one for demonstrating the absence of gross contamination with readily grown microorganisms, and is not capable of affording a guarantee of sterility in any sample that passes the test.

The experimental details of these procedures are described in the PhEur (European Pharmacopoeia Commission, 2017). This section is therefore restricted to an account of the major features of the test and a more detailed consideration of those practical aspects that are important or problematical.

It is obviously important that materials to be tested for sterility are not subject to contamination from the operator or the environment during the course of the test. For this reason, it is essential that sterility tests are conducted in adequate laboratory facilities by competent and experienced personnel. Clearly, the consequences of recording an incorrect sterility result may be very severe. If a material which was *really* sterile were to fail the test, it would need to be resterilized or, more probably, discarded. This would have significant cost implications. If, on the other hand, a contaminated batch were to pass a test for sterility and be released for use, this would

obviously represent a significant health hazard. For these reasons, sterility testing procedures have improved significantly in recent years and failures are now viewed very seriously by the regulatory authorities. If a product does fail, it means either that the item in question is *really* contaminated, in which case the manufacturing procedures are seriously inadequate, or that the item is in fact sterile but the testing procedure is at fault. Either way, it is not possible to dismiss a failure lightly.

Sterility tests may be conducted in clean rooms or laminar flow cabinets which provide a grade A atmosphere as defined by the *Rules and Guidance for Pharmaceutical Manufacturers and Distributors* (Medicines and Healthcare products Regulatory Agency, 2017). However, it is becoming increasingly common for testing to be undertaken in an isolator that physically separates the operator from the test materials and so reduces the incidence of false-positive test results due to extraneous contamination introduced during the test itself. Such isolators are similar in principle to a glove box, and typically consist of a cabinet (supported on legs or a frame) that is sufficiently large for the operator, who is covered by a transparent hood of moulded flexible plastic forming the cabinet base, to sit or stand within it.

A sterility test may be conducted in two ways. The direct inoculation method involves the removal of samples from the product under test and their transfer to a range of culture media that might be expected to support the growth of contaminating organisms. After incubation, the media are examined for evidence of growth, which, if present, is taken to indicate that the product may not be sterile. It is not certain that the product is contaminated because the organisms responsible for the growth may have arisen from the operator or may have already been present in the media to which the samples were transferred, i.e. the media used for the test were not themselves sterile. Thus, in conducting a sterility test it is necessary to include controls that indicate the likelihood of the contaminants arising from these sources; these are discussed hereafter. The size and number of the samples to be taken are described in the PhEur (European Pharmacopoeia Commission, 2017).

It is necessary to inactivate any antimicrobial substances contained in the sample. These may be the active drug, e.g. an antibiotic, or a preservative in an eye drop or multidose injection. Suitable inactivators may be added to the liquid test media to neutralize any antimicrobial substances, but in the case of antibiotics particularly, no such specific inactivators are available (with the exception of β-lactamases, which hydrolyse penicillins and cephalosporins). This problem may be overcome using a membrane filtration technique. This alternative method of conducting sterility tests is obviously only applicable to aqueous or oily solutions that will pass through a membrane having a pore size sufficiently small to retain bacteria. The membrane, and hence the bacteria retained on it, is washed with isotonic salts solution, which should remove any last traces of antimicrobial substances. It is then placed in a suitable liquid culture medium. This method is certainly to be preferred to direct inoculation because there is a greater chance of effective neutralization of antimicrobial substances.

Solids may be dissolved in an appropriate solvent. This is almost invariably water because most other common solvents have antimicrobial activity. If no suitable solvent can be found, the broth dilution method is the only one available. If there is no specific inactivator available for antimicrobial substances that may be present in the solid, then their dilution to an ineffective concentration by use of a large volume of medium is the only course remaining.

The controls associated with a sterility test are particularly important because incomplete control of the test may lead to erroneous results. Failure to neutralize a preservative completely may lead to contaminants in the batch going undetected and subsequently initiating an infection when the product is introduced into the body.

The PhEur (European Pharmacopoeia Commission, 2017) recommends that four controls are incorporated. The so-called growth promotion test simply involves the addition of inocula with low counts (not more than 100 cells or spores per container) of suitable test organisms to the media used in the test to show that they do support the growth of the common contaminants for which they are intended. S aureus, Bacillus subtilis and P. aeruginosa are the three aerobic bacteria used, Clostridium sporogenes is the anaerobic bacterium used and C. albicans and A. brasiliensis are the fungi used. Organisms having particular nutritional requirements, such as blood, milk or serum, are not included, so they, in addition to the more obvious omissions such as viruses, cannot be detected in a routine sterility test because suitable culture conditions are not provided. On the other hand, it is impossible to design an all-purpose medium, and sterilization processes that kill the spore-forming bacteria and other common contaminants are likely

also to eradicate the more fastidious pathogens such as streptococci and Haemophilus species, which would be more readily detected on blood-containing media. This argument does not, however, cover the possibility of such pathogens entering the product, perhaps via defective seals or packaging, after the sterilization process itself and then going undetected in the sterility test.

The second control, termed the method suitability test, is intended to demonstrate that any preservative or antimicrobial substance has been effectively neutralized. This requires the addition of test organisms to containers of the various media as before but, in addition, samples of the material under test must also be added to give the same concentrations as those arising in the test itself. For the sterility test as a whole to be valid, growth must occur in each of the containers in these controls.

It is necessary also to incubate several tubes of the various media just as they are received by the operator. If the tubes are not opened but show signs of growth after incubation, this is a clear indication that the medium is itself contaminated. This should be an extremely rare occurrence but, in view of the small additional cost or effort, the inclusion of such a control is worthwhile.

A control to check the likelihood of contamination being introduced during the test should be included in the programme of regular monitoring of test facilities. The PhEur (European Pharmacopoeia Commission, 2017) recommends the use of 'negative controls', which may be used to check the adequacy of facilities and operator technique. These items, identical to the sample to be tested, are manipulated in exactly the same way as the test samples. If, after incubation, there are signs of microbial growth in the media containing these negative controls, the conclusion is drawn that the contamination arose during the testing process itself.

Some items present particular difficulties in sterility testing because of their shape or size, e.g. surgical dressings and medical devices. These problems are most conveniently overcome simply by testing the whole sample rather than attempting to withdraw a portion of it. So, for example, large clear plastic bags which have been radiation sterilized may be used to hold the entire medical device or complete roll or pack of dressings, which would then be totally immersed in culture medium. This method would only be valid if the culture medium gained access to the entire sample; otherwise the possibility exists, for example, of aerobic bacterial spores trapped within it failing to grow owing to insufficient diffusion of oxygen. This approach has the advantage of imposing a more rigorous test because a much larger sample is used. In the case of dressings, it may also reduce the risk of operator-induced contamination compared with the alternative approach, which would require the withdrawal of representative samples for testing from different areas of the roll or pack.

The final aspect of the test which is worthy of comment is the interpretation of the results. If there is evidence that any of the test samples are contaminated, the batch fails the test. If, however, there is convincing evidence that the test was invalid because the testing facility, procedure or media were inadequate, a single retest is permitted; this contrasts with earlier pharmacopoeial protocols, which under certain circumstances permitted two retests.

Endotoxin and pyrogen testing

This is an aspect of microbial contamination of medicines which is not usually considered part of microbiology but is discussed here because pyrogens are normally the products of microbial growth. A pyrogen is a material which when injected into a patient will cause a rise in body temperature (pyrexia). The lipopolysaccharides that constitute a major part of the cell wall of Gram-negative bacteria are called endotoxins, and it is these that are the most commonly encountered pyrogens (although any other substance that causes a rise in body temperature may be classified under the same heading). Bacterial cells may be pyrogenic even when they are dead and when they are fragmented, and so a solution or material that passes a test for sterility will not necessarily pass a pyrogen test. It follows from this that the more heavily contaminated with bacteria an aqueous injection becomes during manufacture, the more pyrogenic it is likely to be at the end of the process.

Two main procedures are used for the detection of pyrogens. The traditional method requires the administration of the sample to laboratory rabbits, whose body temperature is monitored for a period of time thereafter. The alternative procedure, which is now by far the most common, is to use the *Limulus* amoebocyte lysate test, in which the pyrogen-containing sample causes gel formation in the lysis product of amoebocytes of the giant horseshoe crab *Limulus polyphemus*. A detailed account of endotoxin testing is outside the scope of this chapter, but the review by Baines (2000) provides a comprehensive account of the practicalities of the method.

Please check your eBook at **https://studentconsult. inkling.com/** for self-assessment questions. See inside cover for registration details.

References

Baines, A., 2000. Endotoxin testing. In: Baird, R.M., Hodges, N.A., Denyer, S.P. (Eds.), Handbook of Microbiological Quality Assurance. Taylor and Francis, London.

British Standards Institution BS EN 1276, 2009. Chemical disinfectants and antiseptics. Quantitative suspension test for the evaluation of bactericidal activity of chemical disinfectants and antiseptics used in food, industrial, domestic and institutional areas. Test method and requirements (phase 2, step 1).

Denyer, S.P., Hodges, N.A., Talbot, C., 2011. Sterilization procedures and sterility assurance. In: Denyer, S.P., Hodges, N., Gorman, S.P., et al. (Eds.), Hugo and Russell's Pharmaceutical Microbiology, eighth ed. Wiley-Blackwell, Oxford.

European Pharmacopoeia Commission, 2017. European Pharmacopoeia, ninth ed. Council of Europe, Strasbourg.

Gilmore, B.F., Ceri, H., Gorman, S.P., 2011. Laboratory evaluation of antimicrobial agents. In: Denyer, S.P., Hodges, N., Gorman, S.P., et al. (Eds.), Hugo and Russell's Pharmaceutical Microbiology, eighth ed. Wiley-Blackwell, Oxford.

Hanlon, G., 2010. Disinfectant testing and the measurement of biocide effectiveness. In: Hodges, N.A., Hanlon, G.W. (Eds.), Industrial Pharmaceutical Microbiology: Standards and Controls. Euromed Communications, Haslemere.

Hewitt, W., Vincent, S., 1989. Theory and Application of Microbiological Assay. Academic Press, London.

Hodges, N.A., 2000. Pharmacopoeial methods for the detection of specified microorganisms. In: Baird, R.M., Hodges, N.A.Denyer, S.P. (Eds.), Handbook of Microbiological Quality Assurance. Taylor and Francis, London.

Johnson, S.M., 2003. Microbiological environmental monitoring. In: Hodges, N.A., Hanlon, G.W. (Eds.), Industrial Pharmaceutical Microbiology: Standards and Controls. Euromed Communications, Haslemere.

Medicines and Healthcare products Regulatory Agency, 2017. Rules and Guidance for Pharmaceutical Manufacturers and Distributors, tenth ed. Pharmaceutical Press, London.

Millar, R., 2000. Enumeration. In: Baird, R.M., Hodges, N.A. Denyer, S.P. (Eds.), Handbook of Microbiological Quality Assurance. Taylor and Francis, London.

Murtough, S.M., Hiom, S.J., Palmer, M., et al., 2000. A survey of disinfectant use in hospital pharmacy aseptic preparation areas. Pharm. J. 264, 446–448.

Pharmaceutical Inspection Co-operation Scheme Secretariat, 2007. Recommendation on Guidance for Parametric Release. http://www.gmp-compliance.org/guidemgr/files/PICS/PI%20005-3%20PARAMETRIC%20 RELEASE.PDF (Accessed 30 December 2016).

Reybrouck, G., 2004. Evaluation of the antibacterial and antifungal activity of disinfectants. In: Fraise, A.P, Lambert, P.A.Maillard, J.Y. (Eds.), Principles and Practice of Disinfection Preservation and Sterilization, fourth ed. Blackwell Science, Oxford.

United States Pharmacopeial Convention, 2016. United States Pharmacopeia, thirty-ninth ed. United States Pharmacopeial Convention, Rockville.

Wardlaw, A.C., 2000. Practical Statistics for Experimental Biologists, second ed. John Wiley & Sons, Chichester.

15

Action of physical and chemical agents on microorganisms

Geoffrey W. Hanlon   Norman A. Hodges

CHAPTER CONTENTS

KEY POINTS

- Although microorganisms are increasingly being used in a biotechnology role to manufacture medicines, it is still the case that the major pharmaceutical interest is in killing them, or at least controlling their growth. Consequently, a pharmacist or pharmaceutical scientist needs an understanding of the methods available to kill and remove living organisms from medicines.

- Microorganisms exposed to steam – the most commonly used method of product sterilization – normally die according to first-order kinetics. Parameters such as the *D* value and *Z* value describe, respectively, the microbial death rate at a given temperature and the effect of temperature change on that death rate.

- Steam causes microbial death by hydrolysis of nucleic acids and proteins; it is a far more effective sterilizing agent than dry heat at the same temperature, which kills cells by oxidation of macromolecules.

- Bacterial spores are much more resistant to heat than are vegetative bacteria, fungi or viruses.

- The measured heat resistance of a microorganism may be influenced substantially by the age of the cells, and by the pH, redox potential, water activity and chemical composition of the media in which they were grown and tested, so all of these factors need to be carefully controlled when heat resistance is measured.

- There is no such thing as an ideal biocide, and each class of compound has its advantages and disadvantages. Knowledge of the structure and physicochemical properties of biocides is required in order to make informed judgements on the appropriate use of these agents.

- Biocides may be used as disinfectants, antiseptics or preservatives depending on their activity and toxicity profile. These roles are quite different from each other, and so it is important to understand what is required of the biocide in a formulation.
- Biocides will interact with excipients within a formulation and also with the packaging components of the product. The choice of biocide for inclusion in a product must therefore form part of the original formulation process and not just be an add-on at the end.

Introduction

The subject of this chapter is of importance because pharmaceutical scientists have a responsibility for:

- the production of medicines which have as their prime function the destruction of microorganisms, e.g. antiseptic liquids and antibiotic formulations;
- the production of sterile pharmaceutical products containing no living microorganisms, e.g. injections and eye drops; and
- the production of a wide range of medicines which must be effectively protected against microbial spoilage.

Thus the major pharmaceutical interest in microorganisms is that of killing them, or at least preventing their growth. Consequently, it is necessary to have both an understanding of the physical processes, e.g. heating and ultraviolet or gamma radiation that are used to kill microorganisms, and knowledge of the more diverse subject of antimicrobial chemicals.

This background knowledge must include an understanding of the kinetics of cell inactivation, the calculation of parameters by which microbial destruction and growth inhibition are measured, and an appreciation of the factors that influence the efficiency of the physical and chemical processes used. These aspects, together with a synopsis of the major groups of antimicrobial chemicals, are the subject of this chapter.

Kinetics of cell inactivation

The death of a population of cells exposed to heat or ionizing radiation is often found to follow or approximate to first-order kinetics (see Chapter 7). In this sense, it is similar to bacterial growth during

Table 15.1 Death of *Bacillus megaterium* spores in pH 7.0 buffer at 95 °C

Time (min)	Viable cell concentration (mL^{-1})	Percentage of survivors	Log$_{10}$ percentage of survivors
0	2.50×10^6	100	2.000
5	5.20×10^5	20.8	1.318
10	1.23×10^5	4.92	0.692
15	1.95×10^4	0.78	−0.108
20	4.60×10^3	0.18	−0.745
25	1.21×10^3	0.048	−1.319
30	1.68×10^2	0.0067	−2.174

the logarithmic phase of the cycle, the graphs representing these processes being similar but of opposite slope. Assuming first-order kinetics (the exceptions will be considered later), an initial population of N_o cells per mL will, after a time t minutes, be reduced to N_t cells per mL, according to the following equations, in which k is the inactivation rate constant:

$$N_t = N_o e^{-kt}$$

(15.1)

$$\ln N_t = \ln N_o - kt$$

(15.2)

$$\log_{10} N_t = \log_{10} N_o \frac{-kt}{2.303}$$

(15.3)

Thus the data in Table 15.1 may be used to produce a plot of logarithm of cell concentration against exposure time (Fig. 15.1), where the intercept is log N_o and the slope is $-k/2.303$. This may be plotted with the logarithm of the percentage of survivors as the ordinate; thus the largest numerical value on this axis is 2.0 (100%). An important feature of Fig. 15.1 is the fact that there is no lower endpoint to the ordinate scale – it continues indefinitely. If the initial population was 1000 cells mL^{-1} the logarithmic value would be 3.0; at 100 cells mL^{-1} the value would be 2.0; at 10 cells mL^{-1} 1.0, and at 1 cell mL^{-1} zero. The next incremental point on the logarithmic scale would be −1, which corresponds to 0.1 cells mL^{-1}. It is clearly nonsense to talk of a fraction of a viable cell per mL but this value corresponds to one whole cell in 10 mL of liquid. The next point, −2.0,

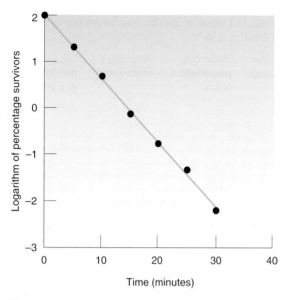

Fig. 15.1 • Heat inactivation of *Bacillus megaterium* spores at 95 °C.

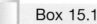

Box 15.1

Worked example

A batch of 1 mL ampoules contained 50 heat-resistant bacterial spores per millilitre before sterilization. These spores were known to die according to first-order kinetics when exposed to saturated steam at 121 °C; at this temperature they were found to have an inactivation rate constant of 1.6 min^{-1}. If they were exposed to the 'standard' steam sterilization cycle of 121 °C for 15 minutes, would the process achieve the required sterility assurance level of 10^{-6}?

Calculation:

Substituting $N_o = 50$ (so $\log_{10} N_o = 1.699$), $k = 1.6$ min^{-1} and $t = 15$ min in Eq. 15.3, we obtain

$$\log N = 1.699 - \frac{(1.6 \times 15)}{2.303}$$
$$\log N = 1.699 - 10.42$$
$$\log N = -8.72$$

Thus $N = 1.905 \times 10^{-9}$ surviving spores per millilitre after 15 minutes' exposure.

Because this value is much lower than the required sterility assurance level of 10^{-6}, the process should easily satisfy the pharmacopoeial requirement.

corresponds to one cell in 100 mL, and so on. Sterility is the complete absence of life, i.e. zero cells mL^{-1}, which has a log value of $-\infty$. *Guaranteed sterility* would therefore require an infinite exposure time.

Box 15.1 shows how Eq. 15.3 can be used to determine if a proposed sterilization process will satisfy the pharmacopoeial requirement that the probability of a nonsterile item in a batch should be no greater than 1 in 1 million (a sterility assurance level of 10^{-6}; see Chapter 17).

D value, or decimal reduction time

It is characteristic of first-order kinetics that the same percentage change in concentration occurs in successive time intervals. Thus in Fig. 15.1 it can be seen that the viable population falls to 10% of its initial value after 7.5 minutes; in the next 7.5-minute period, the population again falls to 10% of its value at the start of that period. This time period for a 90% reduction in count is related to the slope of the line and is one of the more useful parameters by which the death rate may be indicated. It is known as the decimal reduction time, or D value, and usually has a subscript showing the temperature in degrees Celsius at which it was measured, e.g. D_{121} or D_{134}. It is quite possible to indicate the rate of destruction by the inactivation rate constant calculated from the slope of the line, but the significance of this value cannot

be as readily appreciated during conversation as that of a D value, and so the former is rarely used.

If in the circumstances of the previous specimen calculation it was known that the D value for the spores in question was 1.44 minutes at 121 °C (which is the value corresponding to the inactivation rate constant used in the example), it is an easy calculation to say that in a 15-minute steam sterilization cycle the spore numbers would have fallen through 15/1.44 ($\sim$10.5) decimal reductions, so if there were only 50 spores per mL to start with, there would certainly be fewer than 5 × 10^{-9} per mL at the end. In other words, it is only necessary to divide the exposure time by the D value in order to appreciate how extensively the spore population is reduced. This is the basis of the inactivation factor described in Chapter 16.

Z value

When designing steam sterilization processes, it is necessary to know both the D value, which is a measure of the effectiveness of heat at any given temperature, and the extent to which a particular increase in temperature will reduce the D value, i.e.

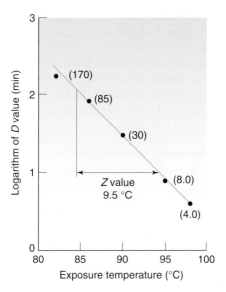

Fig. 15.2 • Relationship between logarithm of D value and exposure temperature for heated *Bacillus megaterium* spores. Individual D values are shown in parentheses.

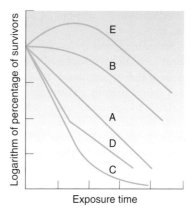

Fig. 15.3 • Alternative survivor plots for cells exposed to lethal agents.

it is necessary to have a measure of the effect of temperature change on death rate. One such measure is the Z value, which is defined as the number of degrees of temperature change required to achieve a 10-fold change in the D value, e.g. if the D value for *Geobacillus stearothermophilus* spores at 110 °C is 20 minutes and they have a Z value of 9 °C, this means that at 119 °C the D value would be 2.0 minutes and at 128 °C the D value would be 0.20 minutes. The relationship between D and Z values is shown in Fig. 15.2. The Z value is one of several parameters that relate change in temperature to change in death rate, and is the most commonly used and readily understood.

The activation energy obtained from an Arrhenius plot (see Chapter 7) or a temperature coefficient, a Q_{10} value (change in rate for a 10 °C change in temperature; see Chapter 14), does the same but is rarely used.

Alternative survivor plots

It was stated earlier that bacterial death often approximates to first-order kinetics, although exceptions do arise; some of the more common are illustrated in Fig. 15.3. The plot labelled A is that conforming to first-order kinetics, which has already been described. A shoulder on the curve, as in case B, is not uncommon, and various explanations have been offered. Cell aggregation or clumping may be responsible for such a shoulder, because it would be necessary to apply sufficient heat to kill all the cells in the clump, not merely the most sensitive, before a fall is observed in the number of colonies appearing on the agar. Under normal circumstances a single colony could arise both from one cell alone or, say, from 100 aggregated cells. In the latter case, if sufficient heat were applied to kill the 99 most sensitive cells in the clump, the colony count would be unaltered. Clumping is not the only explanation, because substantial shoulders may arise when using suspensions where the vast majority of cells exist individually.

Tailing of survivor curves, as in plot C, is often observed if the initial cell concentration is high. This has been attributed to the presence of mutants that are exceptionally resistant to the lethal agent. If the proportion of mutants is 1 in 10^6 cells and the initial concentration was only 10^5 cells mL^{-1} the mutant would not be detected, but an initial population of 10^9 cells mL^{-1} would permit easy detection if the inactivation plot were continued down to low levels of survivors. Again there are alternative explanations, one of the most common being that the cells dying during the early exposure period release chemicals which help to protect those that are still alive.

A sharp break in the line, as in plot D, usually indicates that there are two distinct populations of cells present which have markedly different resistances. Contamination of a cell suspension or culture is a possible explanation, or it may be that a mutant has arisen naturally and the culture conditions are such that it has a selective advantage and its numbers have increased until it is a substantial proportion of the population.

Plot E is uncommon and is usually only seen as a result of 'heat activation' of bacterial spores. This is a situation in which a significant proportion of a population of spores (usually a thermophile) remains dormant and fails to germinate and produce colonies under 'normal' conditions. If the suspension receives a heat stimulus or shock which is insufficient to kill the spores, some or all of those that would otherwise remain dormant become activated, germinate and thus produce a rise in the colony count.

First-order kinetics are less commonly observed when microorganisms are being killed by chemicals than when heat or ionizing radiation is the lethal agent. This is because the chemical must interact with a target molecule within the cell, and the concentration of both the chemical and the intracellular target might influence the death rate; this results in second-order kinetics. In practice, however, the antimicrobial chemical is often present in such a high concentration that the proportion of it that is 'used up' by interaction with the cell is negligible; this means its concentration is effectively constant, and pseudo-first-order kinetics result.

Antimicrobial effects of moist and dry heat

Moist heat (steam) and dry heat (hot air) both have the potential to kill microorganisms, but their efficiencies and their mechanisms of action differ. In autoclaves, dry saturated steam, i.e. 100% water vapour with no liquid water present, is used at temperatures between 121 °C and 135°C, at which it rapidly kills microorganisms. An advantage of the use of steam is that it possesses a large latent heat of vaporization, which it transfers to any object on which it condenses. It is essential to use dry saturated steam if maximal autoclaving efficiency is to be achieved. If the steam is wet, i.e. contains liquid water, penetration of vapour-phase steam into dressings may be retarded. If the steam is superheated, i.e. its temperature has been raised but the pressure remains constant, or the pressure has been lowered but the temperature remains constant, it contains less moisture and latent heat than dry saturated steam at the same temperature. In this case, the effect is similar to that of using a steam–air mixture at that temperature. The process by which steam kills cells is hydrolysis of essential proteins (enzymes) and nucleic acids. In contrast, dry heat causes cell death by oxidative processes, although again it is the proteins and nucleic acids that are the vulnerable targets. Dry heat is much less effective at killing microorganisms than steam at the same temperature. Exposure to 160 °C for not less than 2 hours (or an equivalent temperature–time combination) are recommended in the *European Pharmacopoeia* for sterilization by dry heat methods. The state of hydration of a cell is thus an important factor determining its resistance to heat.

Resistance of microorganisms to moist and dry heat

Numerous factors influence the observed heat resistance of microbial cells, and it is difficult to make comparisons between populations unless these factors are controlled. Not surprisingly, marked differences in resistance exist between different genera, species and strains, and between the spore and vegetative cell forms of the same organism. The resistance may be influenced, sometimes extensively, by the age of the cell, i.e. lag, exponential or stationary phase; its chemical composition, which in turn is influenced by the medium in which the cell is grown; and by the composition and pH of the fluid in which the cell is heated. It is difficult to obtain strictly comparable heat resistance data for grossly dissimilar organisms, but the values quoted in Table 15.2 indicate the relative order of heat resistance of the various microbial groups. Tabulation of D values at a designated temperature is perhaps the most convenient way of comparing resistance, but this is only suitable for first-order kinetics. Alternative methods of comparison include the time to achieve a particular percentage kill and the time required to achieve no survivors; the latter is, of course, dependent on the initial population level and is now rarely used.

The most heat-resistant infectious agents (as distinct from microbial cells) are prions, which are proteins rather than living cells and are the cause of spongiform encephalopathies, e.g. Creutzfeldt–Jakob disease (CJD) and bovine spongiform encephalopathy (BSE; or 'mad cow disease'). Prion proteins are so resistant to heat inactivation that an autoclave cycle of 134 °C to 138 °C for 18 minutes has been recommended for the decontamination of prion-contaminated materials, and the efficacy of even this extreme heat treatment has been questioned. The World Health Organization recommends that prion-contaminated surgical instruments be autoclaved at

Table 15.2 A 'league table' of heat resistances of different microorganisms and infectious agents

Organism or agent	Heat resistance (values are for fully hydrated organisms unless otherwise stated)
Prions	The most heat-resistant infectious agent. May survive steam sterilization at 134 °C to 138°C for 1 h
Bacterial spores (endospores)	Little or no inactivation at <80 °C. Some species survive boiling for several hours
Fungal spores	Ascospores of *Byssochlamys* species may survive at 88 °C for 60 min but most fungal spores are less resistant
Actinomycete spores	Spores of *Nocardia sebivorans* reported to survive for 10 min at 90 °C but most species are less resistant
Mycobacterium tuberculosis	May survive for 30 min at 100 °C in the dry state but when hydrated is killed by pasteurization (63 °C for 30 min or 72 °C for 15 s)
Yeasts	Ascospores and vegetative cells show little difference in resistance. Survival for 20 min at 60 °C is typical
Most nonsporing bacteria of pharmaceutical or medical importance	D_{60} of 1 min to 5 min is typical of staphylococci and many Gram-negative enteric organisms. Enterococci may be more resistant, and pneumococci may survive for 30 min at 110 °C when dry
Fungi and actinomycetes	Vegetative mycelia exhibit resistance similar to that of the nonsporing bacteria described above
Viruses	Rarely survive for >30 min at 55 °C to 60 °C except perhaps in blood or tissues, but papovaviruses and hepatitis viruses are more resistant
Protozoa and algae	Most are no more resistant than mammalian cells and survive for only a few hours at 40 °C to 45 °C. However, cysts of *Acanthamoeba* species are more resistant

121 °C for 1 hour in the presence of 1 M sodium hydroxide.

Bacterial endospores are invariably found to be the most heat-resistant *cell* type, and those of certain species may survive being in boiling water for many hours. The term 'endospore' refers to the spores produced by *Bacillus* and *Clostridium* species (and a few other genera that are unlikely to arise as pharmaceutical contaminants) and is not to be confused with the spores produced by other bacteria, such as actinomycetes, which do not develop within the vegetative cell. Most *Bacillus* and *Clostridium* species normally form spores which survive in water for 15–30 minutes at 80 °C without significant damage or loss of viability. Because endospores are more resistant than other cells, they have been the subject of a considerable amount of research in the food and pharmaceutical industries. Much of the earlier work was reviewed by Russell (1999), and more recently by Hancock (2013).

Mould spores and those of yeasts and actinomycetes usually exhibit a degree of moist heat resistance intermediate between that of endospores and vegetative cell forms; D values of the order of 30 minutes at 50 °C would be typical of such organisms, although some species may be substantially more resistant. Bacterial and yeast vegetative cells and mould mycelia all differ significantly in heat resistance: mycobacteria, which possess a high proportion of lipid in their cell wall, tend to be more resistant than others. Protozoa and algae are, by comparison, susceptible to heat, and when in the vegetative (uncysted) state they, like mammalian cells, rapidly die at temperatures much in excess of 40 °C. Information on the heat resistance of viruses is limited but the available data suggest that it may differ significantly between types. The majority of viruses are no more heat resistant than vegetative bacteria, but hepatitis viruses, particularly hepatitis B virus, is less susceptible, and exposure to 80 °C for 10 minutes or more is required for effective decontamination.

Resistance to dry heat by different groups of infectious agents and microorganisms usually follows a pattern similar to that in aqueous environments. Again, prions head the 'league table' by exhibiting extreme heat resistance, and endospores are substantially more resilient than other cell types, with those of *G. stearothermophilus* and *Bacillus atrophaeus* (formerly known as *Bacillus subtilis* var. *niger*) usually more resistant than other species. Exposure to 160

°C for at least 2 hours is required by the *European Pharmacopoeia* (European Pharmacopoeia Commission, 2017) to achieve an acceptable level of sterility assurance for materials sterilized by dry heat.

Cells of pneumococci have been reported to survive dry heat at 110 °C for 30 minutes but this represents exceptional resistance for vegetative cells, most of which may be expected to die after a few minutes heating at 100 °C or less.

Valid comparisons of dry heat resistance among dissimilar organisms are even less common than those for aqueous environments because there is the additional problem of distinguishing the effects of drying from those of heat. For many cells, desiccation is itself a potentially lethal process, even at room temperature, so experiments in which the moisture content of the cells is uncontrolled may produce results that are misleading or difficult to interpret. This is particularly so when the cells are heated under conditions where their moisture content is changing and they become progressively drier during the experiment.

Factors affecting heat resistance and its measurement

The major factors affecting heat resistance were listed in the previous section and will be considered in some detail here. The subject has been extensively studied, and again much of the experimental data and consequently many of the examples quoted in this section come from the field of spore research.

The measurement of heat resistance in fully hydrated cells, i.e. those suspended in aqueous solutions or exposed to dry saturated steam, does not normally represent a problem when it is conducted at temperatures less than 100 °C, but errors may occasionally arise when spore heat resistance is measured at higher temperatures. In these circumstances it is necessary to heat suspensions sealed in glass ampoules immersed in glycerol or oil baths, or to expose the spores to steam in a modified autoclave. Monitoring and control of heat-up and cool-down times become important, and failure to pay adequate attention to these aspects may lead to apparent differences in resistance, which may be simply due to factors such as variations in the thickness of glass in two batches of ampoules.

Species and strain differences

Variations in heat resistance between the species within a genus are very common, although it is difficult to identify from the published reports the precise magnitude of these differences because different species may require different growth media and incubation conditions, which, together with other factors, might influence the results. For example, one report described a 700-fold variation in spore heat resistance within 13 *Bacillus* species, but to produce the spore crops for testing, the authors necessarily had to use eight culture media, three incubation temperatures and six procedures for cleaning the spores. Differences between strains of a single species are, not surprisingly, more limited; D_{90} values ranging from 4.5 to 120 minutes have been reported for five strains of *Clostridium perfringens* spores.

Cell form

Vegetative cells of spore-forming species are considerably more heat sensitive than the spores themselves. Khoury et al. (1990) found that vegetative cells of a *B. subtilis* strain died at the same rate at 50 °C as the spores did at 90 °C. It is thus important to ensure that heat resistance data for *Bacillus* or *Clostridium* species are obtained from pure populations of either vegetative cells or spores but not a mixture of the two, otherwise the results are difficult to interpret.

The degree of heat resistance shown by vegetative cells may also be influenced by the stage of growth from which the cells were taken. It is normally found that stationary-phase cells are more heat resistant than those taken from the logarithmic phase of growth, although several exceptions have been reported.

Culture conditions

The conditions under which the cells are grown is another factor that can markedly affect heat resistance. Insufficient attention has been paid to this potential source of variation in a substantial part of the research conducted.

Factors such as growth temperature, medium pH and buffering capacity, oxygen availability and the concentrations of the culture medium components may all affect resistance.

Thermophilic organisms are generally more heat resistant than mesophilic organisms, which in turn tend to be more resistant than psychrophilic organisms. If a 'league table' of spore heat resistance were to be constructed, it is probable that *G. stearothermophilus*, *Bacillus coagulans* and *Clostridium thermosaccharolyticum* would head the list; all three have growth optima of 50 °C to 60 °C. Variable results have arisen when single species have been grown at a variety of temperatures. *Escherichia coli* and *Streptococcus faecalis* have both been the subject of conflicting reports on the influence of growth temperature on heat resistance, whereas Khoury et al. (1990) showed that for two different *B. subtilis* strains the heat resistance of both the vegetative cells and the spores was, in every case, directly proportional to the temperature at which the cells or spores were produced.

The effects of medium pH, buffering capacity, oxygen availability and the concentrations of the culture medium components are often complex and interrelated. An unsuitable pH, inadequate buffer or insufficient aeration may all limit the extent of growth, with the result that the cells that *do* grow each have available to them a higher concentration of nutrients than would be the case if a higher cell density had been achieved. The levels of intracellular storage materials and metal ions may therefore differ and so influence resistance to heat and other lethal agents. Cells existing in, or recently isolated from, their 'natural' environment, e.g. water, soil, dust or pharmaceutical raw materials, have often been reported to have a greater heat resistance than their progeny that have been repeatedly subcultured in the laboratory and then tested under similar conditions.

pH and composition of heating menstruum

It is frequently found that cells survive heating more readily when they are at neutrality (or their optimum pH for growth if this differs from neutrality). The combination of heat and an unfavourable pH may be additive or even synergistic in killing effects; for example, *G. stearothermophilus* spores survive better at 110 °C in dilute pH 7.0 phosphate buffer than at 85 °C in pH 4.0 acetate buffer. Differences in heat resistance may also result merely from the presence of the buffer, regardless of the pH it confers. Usually an apparent increase in resistance occurs when cells are heated in buffer rather than in water alone. A similar increase is often found to occur on the addition of other dissolved or suspended solids, particularly those of a colloidal or proteinaceous nature, e.g. milk, nutrient broth and serum.

Because dissolved solids can have such a marked effect on heat resistance, great care must be taken in attempts to use experimental data from simple solutions to predict the likely heat treatment required to kill the same cells in a complex formulated medicine or food material. An extreme case of protection of cells from a lethal agent is the occlusion of cells within crystals. When spores of *B. atrophaeus* were occluded within crystals of calcium carbonate, their resistances to inactivation were approximately 900 times and 9 times higher than for unoccluded spores when subjected to steam and dry heat respectively; an exposure period of 2.5 hours at 121 °C (moist heat) was required to eliminate survivors within the crystals. It is to minimize the risk of such situations arising that the *Rules and Guidance for Pharmaceutical Manufacturers and Distributors* (Medicines and Healthcare products Regulatory Agency, 2017) places such emphasis on hygiene and cleanliness in the manufacture of medicines.

The solute concentrations normally encountered in dilute buffer solutions used as suspending media for heat resistance experiments cause no significant reduction in the vapour pressure of the solution relative to that of pure water, i.e. they do not reduce the water activity, A_w, of the solution (which has a value of 1.0 for water). If high solute concentrations are used, or the cells are heated in a 'semidry' state, A_w is significantly lower and the resistance is increased, e.g. a 1000-fold increase in the D value has been reported for *Bacillus megaterium* spores when A_w was reduced from 1.0 to between 0.2 and 0.4.

Recovery of heat-treated cells

The recovery conditions available to cells after exposure to heat may influence the proportion of cells that produce colonies. A heat-damaged cell may require an incubation time longer than normal to achieve a colony of any given size, and the optimum incubation temperature may be several degrees lower. The composition of the medium may also affect the colony count, with a nutritionally rich medium giving a greater percentage survival than a 'standard' medium, whereas little or no difference can be detected between the two when unheated cells are used. Adsorbents such as charcoal and starch have been found to have beneficial effects in this context.

Ionizing radiation

Ionizing radiation can be divided into electromagnetic and particulate (corpuscular) types and is of sufficient energy to cause ejection of an electron from an atom or molecule in its path. Electromagnetic radiation includes γ-rays and X-rays, whereas particulate radiation includes α and β particles, positrons and neutrons.

Particulate radiation

The nuclear disintegration of radioactive elements results in the production of charged particles. α particles are heavy and positively charged, being equivalent to the nuclei of helium atoms. They travel relatively slowly in air, and although they cause a great deal of ionization along their paths, they have very little penetrating power, their range being just a few centimetres in air. α particles cannot penetrate skin but may cause damage when emitted by radionuclides inserted into the body. β particles are negatively charged and have the same mass as an electron. In air the penetrating power of these particles is a few metres but they will be stopped by a thin sheet of aluminium. β particles resulting from radioactive decay are therefore not sufficiently penetrative for use in sterilization processes, but the production of accelerated electrons from man-made machines (cathode rays) results in particles of great energy with enhanced penetrating power.

Electromagnetic radiation

γ radiation results when the nucleus still has too much energy even after the emission of α or β particles. This energy is dissipated in the form of very short wavelength radiation which, as it has no mass or charge, travels with the speed of light, penetrating even sheets of lead. Although travelling in a wave form, γ radiation behaves as if it is composed of discrete packets of energy called quanta (photons). A ^{60}Co source emits γ-rays with photons of 1.17 MeV and 1.33 MeV and the source has a half-life of 5.2 years. X-rays are generated when a heavy metal target is bombarded with fast electrons. They have properties similar to those of γ-rays despite originating from a shift in electron energy rather than from the nucleus.

Units of radioactivity

The unit of activity is the becquerel (Bq), which is equal to one nuclear transformation per second. This replaces the term *curie* (Ci); 3.7×10^{10} Bq = 1 Ci. The unit of absorbed dose according to the SI system is the gray (Gy), which is equal to one joule per kilogram. However, the old term 'rad' is still used occasionally and is equivalent to 100 ergs per gram of irradiated material (1 Gy = 100 rad).

The energy of radiation is measured in electronvolts (eV) or millions of electronvolts (MeV). An electronvolt is the energy acquired by an electron falling through a potential difference of one volt.

Effect of ionizing radiation on materials

Ionizing radiation is absorbed by materials in a variety of ways, depending on the energy of the incident photons:

1. *Photoelectric effect:* Low-energy radiation (<0.1 MeV) is absorbed by the atom of the material, resulting in the ejection or excitation of an electron.
2. *Compton effect:* Incident photons of medium energy 'collide' with atoms and a portion of the energy is absorbed with the ejection of an electron. The remaining energy impacts further atoms, and further electrons are emitted until all the energy is scattered.
3. *Pair production:* Radiation of very high energy is converted on impact into negatively charged electrons and positively charged particles called positrons. The positron has an extremely short life and quickly annihilates itself by colliding with an orbital electron.

The ionization caused by the primary radiation results in the formation of free radicals, excited atoms, etc., along a discrete track through the material. However, if secondary electrons contain sufficient energy, they may cause excitation and ionization of adjacent atoms, thereby effectively widening the track. Accelerated electrons used in electron-beam sterilizers are essentially equivalent to the secondary electrons arising from γ irradiation – they cause direct ionization of molecules within materials. The temperature rise during irradiation is very small, and even high-energy radiation resulting in pair production is accompanied by an increase of only approximately 2 °C, but nevertheless the chemical changes that occur in irradiated materials are very widespread. Of particular significance here are the deleterious changes that may occur in packaging materials at normal dosage levels. Such effects may include changes in tensile strength, colour, odour and gas formation of polymers. The materials most affected include acetal, fluorinated ethylene propylene, polytetrafluoroethylene and polyvinyl acetate. The total absorbed energy determines the extent of physical and chemical reactions that occur, and so damage is cumulative. For sterilization purposes, exposure times can be long, but the process is predictable and delivers a reproducible level of lethality.

The lethal effect of irradiation on microorganisms can occur in two ways:

1. *Direct effect*. In this case the ionizing radiation is directly responsible for the damage by causing a direct hit on a sensitive target molecule. It is generally accepted that cellular DNA is the principal target for inactivation, and that the ability to survive irradiation is attributable to the organism's ability to repair damaged DNA rather than to any intrinsic resistance of the structure. Further damage may be caused by free radicals produced within the cell but not directly associated with DNA. These radicals can diffuse to a sensitive site and react with it, causing damage.

2. *Indirect effect*. The passage of ionizing radiation through water causes ionization along and immediately next to the track and the formation of free radicals and peroxides. These peroxides and free radicals are highly reactive and destructive and are responsible for both the killing capability and the ability to modify the properties of polymers.

Some of the possible reactions are as follows:

$$radiation$$
$$H_2O \rightarrow H_2O^+ + e^-$$
$$H_2O^+ \rightarrow \cdot OH + H^+$$
$$e^- + H_2O \rightarrow OH^- + H\cdot$$
$$2H\cdot \rightarrow H_2$$
$$2\cdot OH \rightarrow H_2O_2$$

The presence of oxygen has a significant effect on the destructive properties of ionizing radiation owing to the formation of hydroperoxyl radicals:

$$H\cdot + O_2 \rightarrow \cdot HO_2$$

Peroxides and free radicals can act as both oxidizing and reducing agents according to the conditions.

Factors affecting the radiation resistance of microorganisms

Across the spectrum of microorganisms, viruses are the forms most resistant to the effects of radiation, followed by bacterial endospores, then Gram-positive cells and finally Gram-negative cells. Resistance to radiation is genetically determined, and a particularly resistant bacterium called *Deinococcus radiodurans* can withstand a radiation dose up to 5000 Gy, compared with *Escherichia coli*, which is killed by 800 Gy. For comparison, a dose of 5 Gy is lethal to humans. Fortunately, *D. radiodurans* does not have any clinical significance. It is worth noting that microbial products such as endotoxins will not be inactivated by normal doses of ionizing radiation. Consequently, it is important to ensure that initial bioburden levels are low.

Oxygen has already been mentioned as having a significant influence on the antimicrobial effects of radiation, as increased levels of hydroperoxyl radicals lead to marked increases in kill. Vegetative cells such as *E. coli* and *Pseudomonas aeruginosa* are 3 to 4 times more sensitive in the presence of oxygen than in its absence. The presence of moisture will also influence sensitivity, with dehydration causing an increase in resistance owing to an indirect effect on the formation and mobility of free radicals. Freezing increases radiation resistance owing to the reduction of mobility of free radicals in the menstruum, preventing them from diffusing to sites of action at the cell membrane. Above the freezing point there is very little effect of temperature.

A variety of organic materials provide a protective environment for microorganisms, and comparison of radiation resistance is greatly complicated by different complexities of the media used. Sulfhydryl (–SH) groups, such as may be found in amino acids and proteins, have a protective effect on microorganisms owing to their interaction with free radicals. In contrast, compounds that combine with –SH groups, such as halogenated acetates, tend to increase sensitivity. Some naturally occurring materials, particularly foods, may have a profound protective effect on contaminant bacteria. This is of concern to the food-processing industry.

Ultraviolet radiation

Although ultraviolet (UV) radiation covers a range of wavelengths from approximately 15 to 330 nm, its range of maximum bactericidal activity is much narrower (220–280 nm), with an optimum of approximately 265 nm. Whereas ionizing radiation causes electrons to be ejected from atoms in its path, UV radiation does not possess sufficient energy for this and merely causes the electrons to become excited.

It has much less penetrating power than ionizing radiation and tends to be used for the destruction of microorganisms in air, in water and on surfaces.

The bactericidal effect of UV light is due to the formation of linkages between adjacent pyrimidine bases in the DNA molecule to form dimers. These are usually thymine dimers, although other types have been identified. The presence of thymine dimers alters the structural integrity of the DNA chain, thereby hindering chromosome replication. Certain cells can repair damaged DNA in a variety of ways, enhancing their radiation resistance.

Exposure of UV-damaged cells to visible light (photoreactivation) enables a light-dependent photoreactivating enzyme to split the thymine dimers into monomers. A second mechanism is not light dependent and is called dark recovery. In this case, the thymine dimers are removed by a specific endonuclease enzyme that nicks the damaged DNA strand either side of the dimer. DNA polymerase then replaces the missing nucleotides and the ends are joined by a ligase enzyme.

Factors affecting resistance to UV light

As already mentioned, UV light has very little penetrating power, and anything that acts as a shield around the cells will afford a degree of protection. The formation of aggregates of cells will result in those cells at the centre of the aggregate surviving an otherwise lethal dose of radiation. Similarly, microorganisms suspended in water withstand considerably higher doses of radiation than in the dry state, owing to lack of penetration of the radiation. Suspension of bacteria in broth containing organic matter such as proteins increases the resistance of the cells still further. The stage of growth of the culture will affect the sensitivity of the cells, with maximum sensitivity being shown during the logarithmic phase.

Other factors shown to influence radiation resistance include pH, temperature and humidity, although the effect of the last parameter is still somewhat confused.

Gases

The use of gases as antimicrobial agents has been documented for centuries, although it is only recently that their mechanisms of action and factors affecting activity have been elucidated. A wide variety of gaseous agents has been used for their antimicrobial properties, and a few of the major ones will be considered here.

Ethylene oxide

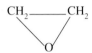

Ethylene oxide (C_2H_4O) is a gas at room temperature (with a boiling point at 10.7 °C) that readily permeates a variety of materials (plastics, cardboard, cloth, etc.) but not crystals. Its odour is reported as being rather pleasant, although the levels at which it is detected in the atmosphere (700 ppm) greatly exceed the 5 ppm maximum safety limit for humans. Toxicity problems include burns and blistering if the material comes into contact with the skin, whereas inhalation results in lachrymation, headache, dizziness and vomiting. Great care must be taken to ensure the removal of residual ethylene oxide from treated products (e.g. rubber gloves) to avoid the risk of skin reactions. Explosive mixtures are formed when ethylene oxide is mixed with air at any concentration above 3%, and this is especially dangerous if the gas mixture is confined. The addition of carbon dioxide or fluorinated hydrocarbons will eliminate this risk, and for sterilization purposes, gas mixtures of 10% ethylene oxide and 90% carbon dioxide are typically used.

Ethylene oxide is extremely effective at killing microorganisms, and its activity is related to its action as an alkylating agent. Reactive hydrogen atoms on hydroxyl, carboxyl, sulfhydryl and amino groups can all be replaced with hydroxyethyl groups, thereby interfering with a wide range of metabolic activities. Ethylene oxide inactivates the complete spectrum of microorganisms, including endospores and viruses. The difference in resistance between endospore-forming bacteria and vegetative cells is only of the order of 5 to 10 times, compared with several-thousand-fold differences with other physical and chemical processes. In addition, no microorganism of genetically determined high resistance has been found. Spores of *B. atrophaeus* are among the most resistant to the effect of ethylene oxide. The moist-heat-resistant spore former *G. stearothermophilus* and spores of *Clostridium sporogenes* are no more resistant than a number of vegetative organisms, such as *Staphylococcus aureus* and *Micrococcus luteus*.

Fungal spores exhibit the same order of resistance as vegetative cells.

Factors affecting the activity of ethylene oxide

The bactericidal activity of ethylene oxide is proportional to the partial pressure of the gas in the reaction chamber, the exposure time, the treatment temperature, and level and type of contamination. At room temperature, the time taken to reduce the initial concentration of cells by 90% can be very slow. For this reason, elevated temperatures of 50 °C to 60°C are recommended, and these result in greatly increased rates of kill. Concentrations of ethylene oxide between 500 mg L^{-1} and 1000 mg L^{-1} are usually used. Relative humidity (RH) has a most pronounced effect, as at very high humidities ethylene oxide may be hydrolysed to the much less active ethylene glycol. This is borne out by the observation that the gas is 10 times more active at 30% RH than at 97% RH. The optimum value for activity appears to be between 28% and 33% RH. Below 28% RH the alkylating action of ethylene oxide is inhibited by lack of water. The degree of dehydration of cells greatly influences activity, and it may not be possible to rehydrate very dry organisms simply by exposure to increased RH. The RH value chosen in practice is usually between 40% and 70%.

Microorganisms may be protected from the action of ethylene oxide by occlusion within crystalline material or when coated with organic matter or salts. *B. atrophaeus* spores dried from salt-water solutions are much more resistant to the gas than are suspensions dried from distilled water.

Biological indicators used to test the efficacy of ethylene oxide treatment employ spores of *B. subtilis* dried on to suitable carriers, such as pieces of aluminium foil.

Formaldehyde

Formaldehyde (HCHO) in its pure form is a gas at room temperature, with a boiling point of −19 °C but readily polymerizes at temperatures below 80 °C to form a white solid. The vapour, which is extremely irritating to the eyes, nose and throat, can be generated either from solid polymers such as paraformaldehyde or from a solution of 37% formaldehyde in water (formalin). Formalin usually contains approximately 10% methanol to prevent polymerization.

As with ethylene oxide, formaldehyde is a very reactive molecule, and there is only a small differential in resistance between bacterial spores and vegetative cells. Its bactericidal powers are superior to those of ethylene oxide (concentrations of 3 mg L^{-1} to 10 mg L^{-1} are effective) but it has weak penetrating power and is really only a surface bactericide. It is also more readily inactivated by organic matter. Adsorbed gas is very difficult to remove, and long airing times are required. Its mechanism of action is thought to involve the production of intramolecular cross-links between proteins, together with interactions with RNA and DNA. It acts as a mutagenic agent and an alkylating agent, reacting with carbonyl, thiol and hydroxyl groups. In order to be effective, the gas must dissolve in a film of moisture surrounding the bacteria. For this reason, relative humidities of the order of 75% are required. Formaldehyde used in conjunction with low-temperature steam is a very effective sterilization medium.

Peracetic acid

The toxic nature of ethylene oxide and formaldehyde has prompted the search for further gaseous sterilants. Peracetic acid has been widely used as an aqueous solution, but its use in the gas phase is more limited. It is a liquid at room temperature, requiring heat treatment to vaporize. Although it is highly active against bacteria (including mycobacteria and endospores), fungi and viruses, it is rather unstable and is damaging to certain materials such as metals and rubber.

Hydrogen peroxide

Hydrogen peroxide is similar to peracetic acid in that it is a solution at room temperature and must be heated to generate the gas phase. The main attraction of hydrogen peroxide as an antimicrobial agent is the fact that its decomposition products are oxygen and water. Most work on the antimicrobial properties of hydrogen peroxide has been carried out on aqueous solutions, where it has been shown to have a good range of activity, including against bacterial spores. The biocidal efficacy of the vapour phase is less than that in solution and is influenced by environmental conditions.

Chlorine dioxide

Chlorine dioxide is a gas at room temperature but is primarily used in aqueous solution, where it has good broad-spectrum activity. If it is to be employed in the gas phase, then it must be generated at the point of use, and in this form it is highly effective and relatively safe.

Propylene oxide

Propylene oxide is a liquid (boiling point 34 °C) at room temperature which requires heating to volatilize. It is inflammable between 2.1% and 21.5% by volume in air but this can be reduced if it is mixed with CO_2. Its mechanism of action is similar to that of ethylene oxide and involves the esterification of carbonyl, hydroxyl, amino and sulfhydryl groups present on protein molecules. It is, however, less effective than ethylene oxide in terms of its antimicrobial activity and its ability to penetrate materials. Whereas ethylene oxide breaks down to give ethylene glycol or ethylene chlorohydrin, both of which are toxic, propylene oxide breaks down to give propylene glycol, which is much less toxic.

Methyl bromide

Methyl bromide boils at 3.46 °C and so is a gas at room temperature. It is used as a disinfectant and a fumigant at a concentration of 3.5 mg L^{-1} with a relative humidity between 30% and 60%. It has inferior antimicrobial properties compared with the previous compounds but has good penetrating power.

Gas plasmas

A plasma is formed by application of energy to a gas or vapour under a vacuum. Natural examples are lightning and sunlight, but plasmas can also be generated under low energy such as in fluorescent strip lights. Within a plasma, positive and negative ions, electrons and neutral molecules collide to produce free radicals. The destructive power of these entities has already been described, and so plasmas can be used as biocidal agents in a variety of applications. This type of system can be produced at temperatures below 50 °C with use of vapours generated from hydrogen peroxide or peracetic acid. For more details on gas plasma sterilization the reader is referred to McDonnell (2013).

Antimicrobial effects of chemical agents

Chemical agents have been used since very early times to combat such effects of microbial proliferation

as spoilage of foods and materials, infection of wounds and decay of bodies. Thus, long before the role of microorganisms in disease and decay was recognized, salt and sugar were used in food preservation, a variety of oils and resins were applied to wounds and employed for embalming, and sulfur was burned to fumigate sick rooms.

The classic research work of Pasteur, which established microorganisms as causative agents of disease and spoilage, paved the way for the development and rational use of chemical agents in their control. There are different definitions to describe the antimicrobial use of chemical agents in different settings. Those agents used to destroy microorganisms on inanimate objects are described as *disinfectants*, whereas those used to treat living tissues, as in wound irrigation, cleansing of burns or eye washes, are called *antiseptics*. The term *preservative* describes those antimicrobial agents used to protect medicines, pharmaceutical formulations, cosmetics, foods and general materials against microbial spoilage. Other definitions have been introduced to give more precise limits of meaning: namely, *bactericide* and *fungicide* for chemical agents that kill bacteria and fungi respectively, and *bacteriostat* and *fungistat* for those that prevent the growth of a bacterial or fungal population. The validity of drawing a rigid demarcation line between those compounds that kill and those that inhibit growth without killing is doubtful. In many instances, concentration and time of contact are the critical factors. *Biocide* is a general term for antimicrobial chemicals but it excludes antibiotics and other agents used for systemic treatment of infections.

The mechanisms by which biocides exert their effects have been intensively investigated and the principal sites of their attack on microbial cells identified. These are the cell wall, the cytoplasmic membrane and the cytoplasm. Chemical agents may weaken the cell wall, thereby allowing the extrusion of cell contents, distortion of cell shape, filament formation or complete lysis. The cytoplasmic membrane, controlling as it does permeability and being a site of vital enzyme activity, is vulnerable to a wide range of substances that interfere with reactive groups or can disrupt its phospholipid layers. Chemical and electrical gradients exist across the cell membrane and these represent a proton-motive force which drives such essential processes as oxidative phosphorylation, adenosine triphosphate (ATP) synthesis and active transport; several agents act by reducing the proton-motive force. The cytoplasm, which is the site of genetic control and protein synthesis, presents a target for those chemical agents that disrupt ribosomes, react with nucleic acids or generally coagulate protoplasm.

Principal factors affecting activity

The factors most easily quantified are temperature and concentration. In general, an increase in temperature increases the rate of kill for a given concentration of the agent and inoculum size. The commonly used nomenclature is Q_{10} (temperature coefficient), which is the change in activity of the agent per 10 °C rise in temperature (e.g. Q_{10} for phenol is 4).

The effect of a change in concentration of a chemical agent on the rate of kill can be expressed as

$$\eta = \frac{\log t_2 - \log t_1}{\log C_1 - \log C_2}$$

(15.4)

where C_1 and C_2 represent the concentrations of the agent required to kill a standard inoculum in times t_1 and t_2. The concentration exponent η represents the slope of the line when log death time (t) is plotted against log concentration (C).

When $\eta > 1$, changes of concentration will have a pronounced effect. Thus, in the case of phenol, when $\eta = 6$, halving the concentration will decrease its activity by a factor of 2^6 (i.e. 64-fold), whereas for a mercurial compound, $\eta = 1$, and the same dilution will reduce its activity only twofold (2^1). Further details and tabulations of both temperature coefficients and concentration exponents may be found in Denyer & Wallhaeusser (1990).

Range of chemical agents

The broad categories of antibacterial chemical compounds have remained surprisingly constant over the years, with phenolics and hypochlorites constituting the major disinfectants, and quaternary ammonium compounds widely used as antiseptics. The compounds capable of being used as preservatives in preparations for oral, parenteral or ophthalmic administration are obviously strictly limited by toxicity requirements. As concerns regarding toxicity have intensified, the range of available preservatives has diminished: mercury-containing compounds, for example, are now

very little used for the preservation of parenteral and ophthalmic products. The high cost of research and testing coupled with the poor prospects for an adequate financial return militate against the introduction of new agents. For this reason, there is a tendency towards the use of existing preservatives in combination, with a view to achieving the benefits of synergy, a broader antimicrobial spectrum or reduced human toxicity resulting from the use of lower concentrations. Al-Adham et al. (2013) have described in detail the characteristics of commonly used biocides. Table 15.3 summarizes the properties and uses of the major groups of biocides.

Phenolics

A limited selection of phenolic compounds is shown in Fig. 15.4.

Various distillation fractions of coal tar yield phenolic compounds, including cresols, xylenols and phenol itself, all of which are toxic and caustic to skin and tissues. Disinfectant formulations traditionally described as 'black fluids' and 'white fluids' are prepared from higher-boiling coal tar fractions. The former make use of soaps to solubilize the tar fractions in the form of stable homogeneous solutions, whereas the latter are emulsions of the tar products and unstable on dilution.

Remarkable success has been achieved in modifying the phenol molecule by the introduction of chlorine and methyl groups, as in chlorocresol and chloroxylenol. This has the dual effect of eliminating toxic and corrosive properties while at the same time enhancing and prolonging antimicrobial activity. Thus, chlorocresol is used as a bactericide in injections and to preserve oil-in-water creams, whereas chloroxylenol is employed as a household and hospital antiseptic. Phenol may itself be rendered less caustic by dilution to 1% w/v or less for lotions and gargles, or by dissolving in glycerol for use as ear drops. Bisphenols, such as hexachlorophane and triclosan (Irgasan), share the low solubility and enhanced activity of the other phenol derivatives described, but have a substantive effect which makes them particularly useful as skin antiseptics. Formulated as creams, cleansing lotions or soaps, they have proved valuable in reducing postoperative infections and cross-infection. Again, toxicity concerns have emerged. Consequently, hexachlorophane, for example, is restricted in the UK both in respect of the concentrations that may be employed and the type of product in which it may be used.

Table 15.3 Properties and uses of the major groups of antimicrobial chemicals (biocides)

Chemical group	Examples	Mode(s) of action	Principal uses	Advantages	Disadvantages
Alcohols and phenols	Ethanol, 2-propanol, benzyl alcohol, chlorbutanol, phenylethyl alcohol, phenoxyethanol, phenol, chlorocresol, chloroxylenol	Membrane damage, protein denaturation, cell lysis	Ethanol and 2-propanol as skin antiseptics and disinfectants; other agents variously used as antiseptics, disinfectants and preservatives for injections, and some oral and topical products	Ethanol, 2-propanol and phenol are very water soluble and have good cleansing properties. Relatively low toxicity. Broad antimicrobial activity	Several alcohols are flammable. Activity much reduced on dilution, by organic matter and, for phenolics, by high pH. Phenolics absorbed by rubber and plastics. Little or no sporicidal activity at room temperature
Aldehydes	Formaldehyde, glutaraldehyde, o-phthalaldehyde	React with amino and other groups causing protein cross-linking and denaturation	Glutaraldehyde has limited use as a chemosterilant for surgical instruments, and formaldehyde has limited use as a gaseous sterilant	Little affected by organic matter. Broad antimicrobial spectrum including spores. Noncorrosive sterilants	Relatively high toxicity: may cause respiratory distress and dermatitis
Biguanides	Chlorhexidine	Membrane disruption and cytoplasmic coagulation at high concentration	Antiseptic	Relatively nontoxic. Good activity against Gram-positive bacteria	Less active against Gram-negative bacteria and fungi. Incompatible with many negatively charged materials
Halogens	Hypochlorites, iodine and iodophors	Interaction with thiol and amino groups causing enzyme and protein damage	Disinfectants	Broad antimicrobial spectrum, including spores	Chlorine liberated from hypochlorite is an irritant to skin, eyes and lungs. Hypochlorites are corrosive. Iodine stains
Organic acids	Benzoic acid, sorbic acid	Uncoupling agents that prevent the uptake of substrates requiring a proton-motive force to enter the cell	Preservatives in oral products	Sufficiently low toxicity for oral use	Activity much diminished with rising pH. Only useful for products with pH lower than approximately 5
Organic acid esters (parabens)	Methyl, ethyl, butyl, propyl and benzyl parabens and their salts	Exact mode of action uncertain. Thought to alter cell membrane properties causing intracellular leakage. May also inhibit transport of amino acids	Preservatives used principally in topical and oral products and in some injections	Relatively good activity against fungi. Activity little changed with rising pH. Relatively low toxicity	Poor water solubility and a tendency to partition into the oily phase of emulsions. Relatively weak activity against Gram-negative bacteria
Oxidizing agents	Hydrogen peroxide, peracetic acid	Oxidation of protein functional groups	Disinfectants and gas-phase sterilants for isolators and equipment	Broad antimicrobial spectrum, including spores	Peracetic acid has a pungent smell and is corrosive. Hydrogen peroxide is unstable
Quaternary ammonium compounds	Benzalkonium chloride, benzethonium chloride, cetrimide, cetylpyridinium chloride	Cell membrane damage and loss of essential chemicals from the cell. Cytoplasmic coagulation in high concentration	Disinfectants and antiseptics. Preservatives in ophthalmic, topical and some injectable products	Very water soluble and effective at neutral and alkaline pH. Good stability, noncorrosive and generally nonhazardous	Benzalkonium chloride causes skin and ophthalmic sensitization. Incompatible with many negatively charged materials

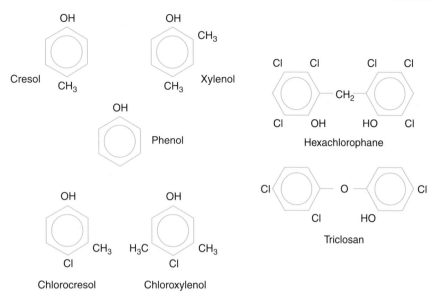

Fig. 15.4 • Chemical structures of a range of phenols.

Phenols are generally active against vegetative bacteria and fungi, are readily inactivated by dilution and organic matter and are most effective in acid conditions. Depending on the concentration, phenols may cause cell lysis at low concentrations or general coagulation of cell contents at higher concentrations.

Alcohols, aldehydes, acids and esters

Ethanol has long been used, usually as 'surgical spirit' for rapid cleansing of preoperative areas of skin before injection. It is most effective at concentrations of 60% to 70%. It is rapidly lethal to bacterial vegetative cells and fungi but has no activity against bacterial endospores and little effect on viruses. The effect of aromatic substitution is to produce a range of compounds which are less volatile and less rapidly active and find general use as preservatives, e.g. phenylethanol for eye drops and contact lens solutions, benzyl alcohol in injections and bronopol (2-bromo-2-nitropropane-1,3-diol) in shampoos and other toiletries. Phenoxyethanol, which has good activity against *P. aeruginosa*, has been used as an antiseptic. In general, the alcohols act by disrupting the bacterial cytoplasmic membrane and can also interfere with the functioning of specific enzyme systems contained within the membrane.

Formaldehyde and glutaraldehyde are both powerful disinfectants, denaturing protein and destroying vegetative cells and spores. Formaldehyde is used in sterilization procedures both as a gas and as a solution in ethanol. Glutaraldehyde solutions are also used to sterilize surgical instruments.

The organic acids sorbic acid and benzoic acid and their esters, because of their low toxicity, are well established as preservatives for food products and medicines (see Chapter 48). The exact mode of action of these agents on microorganisms is still uncertain but they have been shown to influence the pH gradient across the cell membrane. At higher concentrations, the parabens (esters of *p*-hydroxybenzoic acid) induce leakage of intracellular constituents.

Quaternary ammonium compounds

The chemical formula for quaternary ammonium compounds is shown in Fig. 15.5.

These cationic surface-active compounds are, as their name implies, derivatives of an ammonium halide in which the hydrogen atoms are substituted by at least one lipophilic group, a long-chain alkyl or aryl-alkyl radical containing 8 to 18 carbon atoms. In marked contrast to phenol and the cresols, these compounds are mild in use and active at such high dilutions as to be virtually nontoxic. Their surface-active properties make them powerful cleansing agents, a useful adjunct to their common use as skin antiseptics and preservatives in contact lens cleansing and soaking solutions. They are also safe for formulation into eye drops and injections, and are widely used in gynaecology and general surgery. Because they

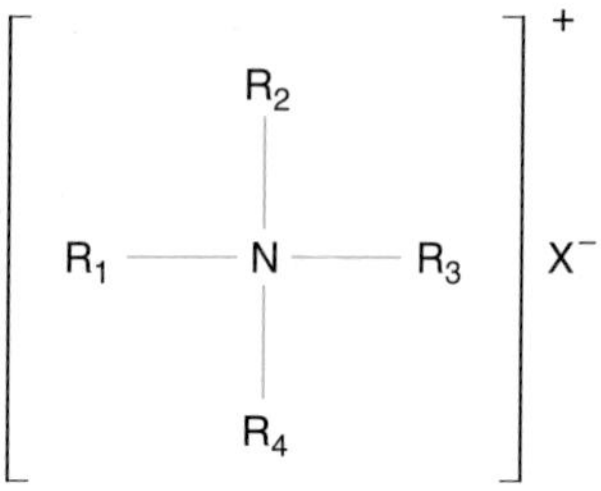

Cetrimide
$R_1R_2R_3$ — CH_3
R_4 — mainly $C_{14}H_{29}$
X — Br

Benzalkonium chloride
R_1R_2 — CH_3
R_3 — $C_6H_5CH_2$
R_4 — mainly $C_{13}H_{27}$
X — Cl

Fig. 15.5 • Chemical structure of cetrimide and benzalkonium chloride.

are active as cations, ambient pH is important, as is interference caused by anions. Thus alkaline conditions promote activity, and it is important that all traces of soap, which is anion active, are removed from the skin prior to treatment with a quaternary ammonium compound. Foreign organic matter and grease also cause inactivation.

One effect of the detergent properties of these compounds is to interfere with cell permeability such that susceptible bacteria (mainly Gram-positive bacteria) leak their contents and eventually undergo lysis. Gram-negative bacteria are less susceptible and, to widen the spectrum of activity to include these, mixtures of quaternary ammonium compounds with other antimicrobial agents such as phenoxyethanol or chlorhexidine are used.

Biguanides and amidines

Chlorhexidine (Fig. 15.6) is a widely used biocide which has activity against Gram-positive and Gram-negative bacteria but little activity against endospores or viruses. It is widely used in general surgery, both alone and in combination with cetrimide, and can

also be used as a preservative in eye drops. Polyhexamethylene biguanide (PHMB) is a polymeric biguanide used widely in the food, brewing and dairy industries. It has also found application as a disinfectant in contact lens cleaning solutions. The biguanides act on the cytoplasmic membrane, causing leakage of intracellular constituents.

The aromatic diamidines propamidine and dibromopropamidine are nontoxic antiseptics mainly active against Gram-positive bacteria and fungi. However, resistance to these agents can develop quickly during use.

Halogens and their compounds

Chlorine gas is a powerful disinfectant used in the municipal treatment of drinking water and in swimming baths. Solutions of chlorine in water may be made powerful enough for use as general household bleach, and disinfectant and dilute solutions are used for domestic hygiene. The high chemical reactivity of chlorine renders it lethal to bacteria, fungi and viruses, and to some extent spores. This activity is optimal at acid pH levels of approximately 5.0. Unionized hypochlorous acid (HOCl) is an extremely potent and widely used bactericidal agent that acts as a nonselective oxidant, reacting readily with a variety of cellular targets. Salt solutions subjected to electrolysis in an electrochemical cell yield a mixture of biocidal species, of which the predominant one is hypochlorous acid. This system is available commercially for use in endoscope washers.

Two traditional chlorine-containing pharmaceutical formulations, which are used much less frequently now, are Eusol (Edinburgh University solution of lime, also known as Chlorinated Lime and Boric Acid Solution BPC 1973) and Dakin's solution (Surgical Chlorinated Soda Solution BPC 1973), both of which are designed to provide slow release of chlorine.

An alternative method of obtaining more prolonged release of chlorine is by the use of organic chlorine compounds such as chloramine T (sodium p-toluenesulfonchloramide) and Halazone BPC 1973 (p-sulfondichloramide benzoic acid). These are used in pharmaceutical products much less frequently now

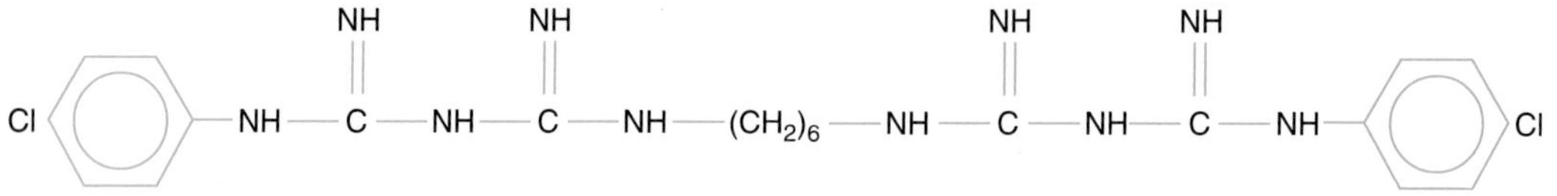

Fig. 15.6 • Chemical structure of chlorhexidine.

but have retained some application in the disinfection of water such as in whirlpool spas and in fish farms.

Iodine, which, like chlorine, is a highly reactive element, denatures cell proteins and essential enzymes by its powerful oxidative effects. Traditionally it has been used in alcoholic solutions such as Tincture of Iodine BP 1973 or complexed with potassium iodide to form an aqueous solution (Lugol's Iodine BP 1973). The latter product, although highly effective as a bactericide, probably fell out of favour because of the tendency to stain both the clothes and skin.

The staining and irritant properties of iodine have resulted in the development of iodophores, mixtures of iodine with surface-active agents, which hold the iodine in a micellar combination from which it is released slowly. Such a preparation is Betadine (polyvinylpyrrolidone–iodine formulated as 10% povidone–iodine), used as a nonstaining, nonirritant antiseptic.

Metals

Many metallic ions are toxic to essential enzyme systems, particularly those utilizing sulfhydryl (–SH) groups, but those used medically are restricted to mercury, silver and aluminium. The extreme toxicity of mercury has rendered its use obsolete apart from in organic combination. The organic compounds that still have a limited use in pharmacy are phenylmercuric nitrate (and acetate) as a bactericide in eye drops and injections, and thiomersal (sodium ethylmercurithiosalicylate) as a preservative in biological products and certain eye drops.

Silver, in the form of the nitrate, has been used to treat infections of the eyes, as have silver protein solutions. Aluminium foil has been used as a wound covering in the treatment of burns and venous ulcers. It has been shown to adsorb microorganisms and inhibit their growth.

The acridines

This group of compounds interferes specifically with nucleic acid function and has some ideal antiseptic properties. Aminacrine hydrochloride is nontoxic, nonirritant, nonstaining and active against Gram-positive and Gram-negative bacteria even in the presence of serum.

Please check your eBook at **https://studentconsult. inkling.com/** for self-assessment questions. See inside cover for registration details.

References

Al-Adham, I., Haddadin, R., Collier, P., 2013. Types of microbicidal and microbistatic agents. In: Fraise, A.P., Maillard, J.-Y., Sattar, S.A. (Eds.), Russell, Hugo and Ayliffe's Principles and Practice of Disinfection, Preservation and Sterilization, fifth ed. Wiley-Blackwell, Chichester.

Denyer, S.P., Wallhaeusser, K.H., 1990. Antimicrobial preservatives and their properties. In: Denyer, S.P., Baird, R. (Eds.), Guide to Microbiological Control in Pharmaceuticals. Ellis Horwood, Chichester.

European Pharmacopoeia Commission, 2017. European Pharmacopoeia, ninth ed. Council of Europe, Strasbourg.

Hancock, C.O., 2013. Heat sterilization. In: Fraise, A.P., Maillard, J.-Y., Sattar, S.A. (Eds.), Russell, Hugo and Ayliffe's Principles and Practice of Disinfection, Preservation and Sterilization, fifth ed. Wiley-Blackwell, Chichester.

Khoury, P.H., Qoronfleh, M.W., Streips, U.N., et al., 1990. Altered heat resistance in spores and vegetative cells of a mutant from Bacillus subtilis. Curr. Microbiol. 21, 249–253.

McDonnell, G., 2013. Gas plasma sterilization. In: Fraise, A.P., Maillard, J.-Y., Sattar, S.A. (Eds.), Russell, Hugo and Ayliffe's Principles and Practice of Disinfection, Preservation

and Sterilization, fifth ed. Wiley-Blackwell Chichester.

Medicines and Healthcare products Regulatory Agency, 2017. Rules and Guidance for Pharmaceutical Manufacturers and Distributors, tenth ed. Pharmaceutical Press, London.

Russell, A.D., 1999. Destruction of bacterial spores by thermal methods. In: Russell, A.D., Hugo, W.B., Ayliffe, G.A.J. (Eds.), Principles and Practice of Disinfection, Preservation and Sterilization, third ed. Blackwell Science, Oxford.

16

Principles of sterilization

Susannah E. Walsh   Jean-Yves Maillard

KEY POINTS

- A number of dosage forms, medical products and devices need to be free of microorganisms.
- Failure to achieve sterility and the lack of validation or documentation of a sterilization process have led to patient deaths.
- Pharmacopoeias usually recommend five processes for the sterilization of sterile dosage forms: steam (under pressure), dry heat, gaseous (ethylene oxide), ionizing radiation and filtration sterilization.
- The use of sterilization parameters allows the calculation of the efficacy of a given sterilization regimen for a given load/products and enables comparison of efficacy between processes.
- High-level disinfection is used for the 'sterilization' of certain medical devices.
- A number of new technologies, notably high-pressure and gas plasma sterilization, might offer appropriate alternatives to common sterilization processes.

Introduction

Previous chapters have described the types and properties of microorganisms (see Chapter 13) and the action of heat and chemical agents on them (see Chapter 15). This chapter will build on those fundamentals and describe the principles underlying the different methodologies available to achieve sterility. These will be described both for pharmaceutical preparations and for medical products and devices. This chapter will also describe the criteria used to measure sterility. The practicalities associated with the processes of sterilization are described in Chapter 17.

By definition, a sterile preparation is described as the absolute absence of viable microbial contaminants. In practice, this definition is not achievable as a preparation cannot be *guaranteed* to be sterile. This remark is discussed further in Chapter 17.

Certain pharmaceutical preparations, medical devices and items for which their use involves contact with broken skin, mucosal surfaces or internal organs, injection into the bloodstream and other sterile parts of the body are required to be sterile. These are frequently referred to in pharmacopoeias as sterile products or sterile dosage forms. Microbiological materials, such as soiled dressings and other contaminated items, also need to be sterilized before disposal or reuse.

Sterilization is the process by which a product is rendered sterile, i.e. by the destruction or removal of microorganisms. The majority of the processes recommended by pharmacopoeias (i.e. steam under pressure sterilization, dry heat sterilization, gaseous sterilization and ionizing radiation sterilization) are terminal sterilization processes for which the preparation is sterilized in its final container or packaging. For other multiple-component preparations that cannot be sterilized with such methods, filtration sterilization can be used. Finally, high-level disinfection is used for the 'sterilization' of medical devices.

Need for sterility

As mentioned in the introduction, certain pharmaceutical preparations, medical products and devices are required to be sterile (further information is given in Chapter 17, Table 17.1). Briefly, these include:

- injections – intravenous infusions, parenteral nutrition (PN) fluids, small-volume injections and small-volume oily injections;
- noninjectable sterile fluids – noninjectable water, urological irrigation solutions, peritoneal dialysis and haemodialysis solutions, nebulizer solutions;
- ophthalmic preparations – eye drops, lotions and ointments and some contact lens solutions;
- dressings;
- implants;
- absorbable haemostats;
- surgical ligatures and sutures (absorbable and nonabsorbable); and
- instruments and equipment – syringes, metal instruments, respirator parts, medical devices, endoscopes.

Failure to achieve sterility can result in serious consequences. In the best-case scenario, surviving microorganisms induce spoilage of the product (i.e. chemical and physical degradation) that might be identified before the preparation is used. The product (or batch of product) is then removed from use and destroyed. In the worst-case scenario, where microbial survival cannot be identified through deleterious effects on the product, infection (sometimes fatal) might result from the use of the contaminated preparation. There have been many reports in the literature of such incidents over the years. For example, in the Devonport incident (in 1971–1972), the death of five patients (from acute endotoxic shock) was traced to dextrose 5% infusion bottles 'sterilized' using a faulty autoclave. In 1996, in Romaira (Brazil), 35 newborn infants died of sepsis attributed to locally produced intravenous solutions (Centers for Disease Control and Prevention, 1998). In 2005 a contaminated heparin intravenous flush was responsible for infecting several patients in different states in the USA (Centers for Disease Control and Prevention, 2005). In these cases, inappropriate quality control procedures were implicated. These incidents emphasize that not only must an appropriate sterilization regimen be used but appropriate monitoring and control must also be performed. This requires an understanding of the principles of sterilizing processes and their control and validation.

Sterilization parameters

The inactivation kinetics of a pure culture of microorganisms exposed to a physical or chemical sterilization process is generally described by an exponential relationship between the number of organisms surviving and the extent of treatment (International Organization for Standardization, 2009), although variations from this are likely (Chapter 15 gives more details). Survivor curves have been used to generate inactivation data for specific sterilization processes using specific biological indicators (see Chapter 17). These data are important for the calculation of a number of sterilization parameters which help to establish a sterilizing regimen adapted to a specific preparation or product.

D value and Z value

One of the important concepts in sterilization is the D value (Fig. 16.1). This parameter is calculated as the time taken to achieve a 1-log (90%) reduction in the number of microorganisms. Another important concept is the Z value, which represents the increase in temperature for steam (under pressure) or dry heat sterilization, or the dose for radiation sterilization,

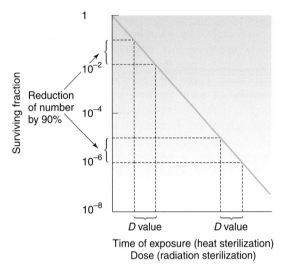

Fig. 16.1 • Calculation of the D value. Note that the D value remains the same although it is calculated with different surviving fractions.

required to produce a 1-log (90%) reduction in the D value for a particular microorganism. This parameter is used to compare the heat (or dose) resistance of different biological indicators following alterations in temperature or radiation. Chapter 15 provides more information on both these parameters.

Inactivation factor and most probable effective dose

The inactivation factor is the total reduction in the number of viable microorganisms brought about by a defined sterilization process. This parameter can be calculated from the D value but only if the destruction curve follows the linear logarithmic model. To overcome problems caused by variations from this model, a most probable effective dose can be used. This is the dose needed to achieve n decimal reductions in the number of microorganisms.

F value

The F value is a measure of the total lethality of a heat sterilization process for a given microorganism and is used to compare the lethality of different heat sterilization processes. A reference value (F_o) of *Geobacillus stearothermophilus* (formerly *Bacillus stearothermophilus*) spores at 121 °C is often used with a Z value of 10 °C. The total F_o of a process

includes the heating up and cooling down phases of the sterilization cycle.

For dry heat sterilization, the F value concept has some limited application. The F_H value is used and corresponds to the lethality of a dry heat process in terms of the equivalent number of minutes of exposure at 170 °C. A Z value of 20 °C is used for the calculation.

Principles of sterilization processes

Five main types of sterilization processes are usually recommended for pharmaceutical products (British Pharmacopoeia Commission, 2017). Among these, steam sterilization (sometimes referred to as steam under pressure sterilization or high-temperature steam sterilization) still represents the gold standard. Novel sterilization processes are being developed and have already been applied in the food industry. These are mentioned in the section entitled 'New technologies' later in this chapter.

Heat sterilization

Heat has been employed as a purifying agent since early historical times, and is now used worldwide in sterilization. Boiling is not a form of sterilization as higher temperatures are needed to ensure the destruction of all microorganisms.

Microorganisms vary in their response to heat. Species of bacterial spores are thought to be some of the most heat-resistant forms of life and can survive temperatures above 100 °C. Nonsporulating bacteria are destroyed at lower temperatures (50 °C to 60 °C) and vegetative forms of yeasts and moulds have a similar response. Cysts of amoebas (e.g. *Acanthamoeba polyphaga*) are less sensitive than their vegetative cells, which are inactivated at 55 °C to 60 °C. It is generally thought that viruses are less resistant than bacterial spores (McDonnell, 2007). The agents responsible for spongiform encephalopathies, the prions, are worth mentioning due to their infectious nature and high resistance to heat (current thermal sterilization procedures are not effective in inactivating prions; see Chapter 15).

Despite the widespread use of heat sterilization, the exact mechanisms and target sites involved are still uncertain. It is likely that several mechanisms and targets are implicated and those proposed include damage to the outer membrane (Gram-negative bacteria) and cytoplasmic membrane, RNA breakdown and coagulation, damage to DNA and denaturation of proteins, probably as a result of an oxidation process. For hydrated cells (steam sterilization), it is likely that the chemically lethal reactions occur more rapidly in the presence of water. The denaturation and coagulation of key enzymes and structural proteins probably result from a hydrolytic reaction.

The thermal death of bacterial cells and spores is usually thought to have first-order reaction kinetics. Although some controversy over this exists, the use of an exponential inactivation model for the kinetics of spores is unlikely to underestimate the heat required (Joslyn, 2001; McDonnell, 2007). One way to express the rate of death as a first-order reaction is

$$N_t = N_o e^{-kt}$$

$$(16.1)$$

This relationship is discussed further in Chapter 15.

Heat sterilization processes usually occur in three phases:

- the heating up phase, where the temperature within the chamber of the sterilizer is brought to the appropriate level;
- the holding phase – when the optimal temperature is reached, the holding time is maintained for the required duration (e.g. 15 minutes at 121°C); and
- the cooling down phase, where the chamber temperature is brought down before the preparation/product can be removed safely from the sterilizer.

Principles of steam sterilization

Steam sterilization relies on a combination of steam, temperature and pressure. Steam is used to deliver heat to the product to be sterilized. There are different types of steam, but only steam at the phase boundary (between water and steam) has the appropriate characteristics for maximum effectiveness (Fig. 16.2). Steam at the phase boundary between itself and its condensate has the same temperature as the boiling water that produced it but holds much more latent heat. This latent heat is available for transfer (without a decrease in temperature) when it condenses onto a cooler surface. This rapid transfer of latent heat is responsible for the rapid rise in temperature (to the sterilization temperature) of any

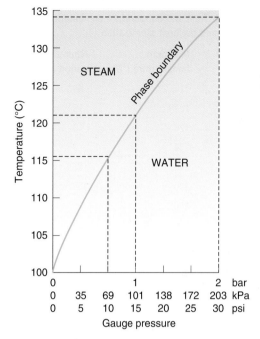

Fig. 16.2 • Saturated steam phase diagram for moist heat sterilization.

items it touches (Chapter 15 provides more information). The condensed water also aids the process by hydrating microorganisms and making them more sensitive. The condensation of steam contracts it to a very small volume that creates a pressure decrease into which more steam is drawn to reestablish the pressure. This aids the penetration of steam into porous items such as dressings. Wet saturated steam is less effective than dry saturated steam as not as much condensation is produced and the latent heat available is less (see Fig. 16.2). It can also saturate loads with free water and interfere with steam penetration. Superheated steam is another potential problem that must be limited (see Chapter 15). Although it is hotter than dry saturated steam, superheated steam is less efficient at releasing its heat to cooler objects, as it is only as efficient as hot air at the same temperature.

Principles of dry heat sterilization

Sterilization using dry heat is less efficient than sterilization using moist heat but is the preferred method for items that are thermostable but moisture sensitive or impermeable to steam (Sharp, 2000). This includes some metal devices, glassware, oils/oily injections and some powders (see Chapter 17,

Table 16.1 Time and temperature combinations used for moist and dry heat sterilization

Process	Minimum temperature (°C)	Minimum holding period (min)
Steam sterilization (autoclaving)	115	30
	121	15
	126	10
	134	3
Dry heat	140	180
	150	150
	160	120
	170	60
	180	30

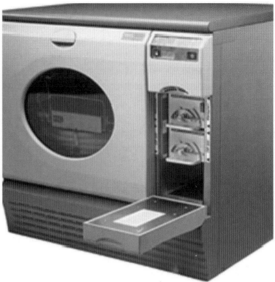

Fig. 16.3 • Endoscope washer from Steris Corporation.

Table 17.1). In addition, temperatures greater than 220°C are used for depyrogenation of glassware (in this case the process needs to demonstrate a 3-log reduction in the amount of heat-resistant endotoxin). The main advantage of dry heat sterilization over steam sterilization is its ability to penetrate items and kill microorganisms via oxidation. The process is generally slower and the holding times for dry heat sterilization are much longer than those needed for steam sterilization (Table 16.1).

Combination treatments

The amount of heat required for sterilization can be reduced by use of a combination treatment of heat plus a reduced pH (<4.5) or low water potential (A_w). Although some spores may survive the initial treatment, they then germinate and die, reducing the numbers of organisms present as time passes (a process called autosterilization). This technique has been used in the food industry with meat-based canned foods to avoid high-temperature sterilization. In addition, the combination of heat and hydrostatic pressure is thought to be synergistic. This is further discussed in the section entitled 'Ultrahigh pressure' later in this chapter.

In the pharmaceutical industry, another type of combination treatment involves low-temperature steam formaldehyde (LTSF). The steam is below atmospheric pressure (70°C to 80°C) and formaldehyde gas provides the sporicidal effect. Formaldehyde has been used to sterilize medical devices but care must be taken with its use as it is acutely toxic to humans and is also mutagenic and possibly

carcinogenic (Sharp, 2000). Some caution should be attached to the sterility assurance level (see Chapter 17) of the process, as it has been suggested that revival of spores after LTSF treatment is possible (McDonnell, 2007). Finally, the processing of thermolabile medical equipment such as endoscopes is conducted in automated washer disinfectors (Fig. 16.3). These make use of high-level disinfectants and slightly raised temperature. This is further discussed in the section entitled 'High-level disinfection' later in this chapter.

Alternative means for heat delivery and control

Systems for the delivery of heat via direct application of flame, heating using alternating electric currents and microwave energy have been developed and adopted in some parts of the world. The use of infrared radiation allows a rapid elevation of temperature. Advances in packaging have improved heat penetration and made it more uniform. These include flexible pouches, polypropylene rigid containers, thermoformed containers, tin-free steel and foil-plastic combinations.

Gaseous sterilization

When sterilization by heat is not possible, one alternative is to use a sterilizing gas. Not many gases are used in the pharmaceutical industry for sterilization, and it is important to note that some of these gases are also used for disinfection (as either a liquid or a gas) under different conditions. Pharmacopoeias usually recommend the use of ethylene oxide for gaseous sterilization of pharmaceutical preparations, although other chemicals are available, such as formaldehyde, hydrogen peroxide, chlorine dioxide, peracetic acid and ozone. The chemical biocides are generally divided, according to their mode of action, into alkylating and oxidizing agents.

Alkylating gases

Some alkylating gases can permeate through many polymeric materials and are therefore not limited to just surface applications.

Ethylene oxide is widely used in pharmaceutical manufacturing but less so in hospitals. It occurs in gaseous form at room temperature (boiling point 10.7°C) and penetrates narrow spaces well. Ethylene oxide has been shown to possess bactericidal, fungicidal, virucidal, sporicidal and protozoacidal properties (Dusseau et al., 2013).

The use of LTSF sterilization has been mentioned already. Formaldehyde is a surface sterilant only and cannot be used to sterilize occluded areas. Penetration into porous materials can be inhibited by the formation of polymers that cross-link, preventing further sterilant access (Chapter 15 provides more information).

Oxidizing gases

Oxidizing gases are relatively unstable, and their decomposition can lead to microenvironments within the load that are not exposed to the full concentration of the agent.

Hydrogen peroxide gas has been shown to be effective against spores at a range of temperatures. Its action is greatest when used at near-saturation levels on clean dry surfaces, and it does not leave a toxic residue (McDonnell, 2007). The vapour is usually obtained via evaporation of a heated stock solution. Water condensation on surfaces that are being sterilized can reduce local concentrations of hydrogen peroxide and hence its activity; decomposition by catalytic activity and absorption by cellulosic materials (e.g. paper) can also reduce its effectiveness. The combination of hydrogen peroxide with cold plasma, cupric or ferric ions, ozone or ultraviolet radiation has been shown to enhance activity (Dusseau et al., 2013).

Ozone has been demonstrated to be an effective sterilant, but the complex control of humidity required and corrosion problems have limited its applications, and it is not routinely used. Ozone as a disinfectant for water currently shows more promise, and commercial systems are available for several applications.

Chlorine dioxide is a broad-spectrum biocide with a sporicidal activity and is mainly used for the high-level disinfection of medical devices. Its applications are limited due to its effect on materials such as uncoated aluminium foil, uncoated copper, polycarbonate and polyurethane (McDonnell, 2007).

Peracetic acid exists as a liquid at room temperature and is used for high-level disinfection (discussed later). Vaporized peracetic acid can be used for the sterilization of surfaces and devices, although a long contact time is required. Peracetic acid can cause corrosion of certain metals and rubbers and has low penetrating power.

Vaporized oxidizing agents are often used in combination or with plasma. Formulations also contain excipients that reduce their negative impact, such as smell and corrosiveness.

Radiation sterilization

There are two main types of radiation: electromagnetic and particulate.

* electromagnetic radiation – γ-rays, X-rays, ultraviolet radiation (UV), infrared radiation (IR), microwave energy and visible light
* particulate radiation – α-particles, β-particles (high-speed electrons), neutrons and protons.

Of these, only γ-rays and high-speed electron beams are used for sterilization of pharmaceutical products, since other forms of radiation have not been shown to be effective as sterilants and/or are not suitable (McDonnell, 2007). Both γ-rays and β-particles are forms of ionizing radiation (Chapter 15 provides more information on the mode of action and resistance). One advantage of irradiation is that it does not cause a significant rise in temperature and hence has been called 'cold' sterilization. The main target site for radiation is DNA, but damage to other vital components such as RNA, enzymes and cell membranes is also involved. Single-stranded or double-stranded DNA breaks will inhibit DNA synthesis or cause errors in protein synthesis. Damage to the sugars and bases may also occur (McDonnell, 2007).

Ionizing radiation can be used to sterilize items that cannot be sterilized with heat (see Chapter 17, Table 17.1). This is not a process that is normally carried out in a standard pharmaceutical manufacturing facility; instead specialized plants are used (Sharp, 2000).

D values are used in radiation sterilization (see Fig. 16.1) and can be calculated from the formula

$$D = \text{radiation dose}/(\log N_0 - \log N)$$

(16.2)

where N_0 and N represent a 1-log difference in numbers.

As with heat sterilization, the dose–response curve to radiation can vary (shoulders and tailing off can occur) but in general the exponential model holds. The initial lag that causes a shoulder is thought to result from multiple targets being hit before death or from DNA repair taking place (see Chapter 17).

Despite having been shown to have activity against bacterial spores, viruses and vegetative cells, UV radiation is not used for sterilization of pharmaceutical products because of its low penetrative power and absorption by glass and plastics. It is used for disinfection of surfaces, including isolators and safety cabinets, and can be used as part of the treatment for drinking water (Lambert, 2013).

Filtration sterilization

Thermolabile solutions can be sterilized by filtration through filters that remove bacteria. Filtration sterilization is the complete removal of microorganisms within a specific size range from liquids or gases. It is a nonterminal sterilization process, and strict aseptic techniques need to be observed. Because of their small size, viruses are not removed by sterilization filtration and therefore, where possible, terminal sterilization processes should be preferred. Items that might be filter sterilized include heat-sensitive injections and ophthalmic solutions, biological products and air and other gases for supply to aseptic areas (Walsh & Denyer, 2013).

There are two main types of filtration mechanisms:

- Sieving, which makes use of synthetic membrane filters. This is an absolute mechanism since it ensures the exclusion of all particles above a defined size.
- Adsorption and trapping, which make use of depth filters. Depth filters have a high dirt-handling capacity and are often used as prefilters.

Generally, only membrane filters are thought to be suitable for the removal of microorganisms. The types used for pharmaceutical applications are usually made from cellulose esters or other polymers and are highly uniform with regular spaces or holes. When a liquid passes through the filter, all particles and microorganisms larger than the holes are retained. Membrane filters have the advantage of removing particles and microorganisms efficiently while retaining very little of the product in their holder or housing. However, they can become blocked quickly if the liquid being sterilized contains a lot of particles, and smaller particles can become trapped in the holes, causing a pressure differential (Levy, 2001). Because of this, prefilters are often used.

High-level disinfection

The term 'high-level' disinfection is often employed with chemical biocides that have demonstrated sporicidal activity. They are sometimes described as 'sterilants' or 'chemosterilants'. High-level disinfectants are usually considered to be highly reactive against macromolecules and are generally divided into two main groups of highly reactive biocides: alkylating and oxidizing agents (Table 16.2). Among the former, the aldehydes, notably formaldehyde (gas), glutaraldehyde and *ortho*-phthalaldehyde (OPA) are the most important. Oxidizing agents are composed of a wider family, such as peroxygen compounds (e.g. peracetic acid and hydrogen peroxide) chlorine dioxide and superoxidized water (McDonnell, 2007). Peracetic

Table 16.2 Sterilization and high-level disinfection using chemical biocides

Chemical agents	Use
Hydrogen peroxide	Gas plasma sterilization (endoscopes)
Peracetic acid	Endoscopes, pharmaceutical preparations
Chlorine dioxide	Gas-phase chlorine dioxide sterilization (medical equipment)
Glutaraldehyde	High-level disinfection (endoscopes)
o-Phthalaldehyde	High-level disinfection (endoscopes)
Formaldehyde	Gaseous sterilization (LTSF)
Ethylene oxide	Liquid and gaseous sterilization

LTSF, Low-temperature steam formaldehyde.

acid has also been used for the cold sterilization of some pharmaceutical preparations such as emulsions, hydrogels, ointments and powders.

Oxidizing agents have been shown to react extensively with macromolecules such as amino acids, peptides, proteins and lipids, notably through a reaction with sulfydryl (–SH) groups, sulphur bonds (S–S) and fatty acid double bonds (Finnegan et al., 2010); however, the mechanisms by which they are lethal to the bacterial cell have not been resolved, although there is evidence that the primary target site for oxidizing agents used at a high (in use) concentration is the bacterial nucleic acid. Oxidizing agents also lead to the formation of peroxyl radicals (fatty acids, lipids), hydroxyl radicals and other reactive species, although the role of these species in the lethality of these agents at a high concentration is subject to debate.

Alkylating agents have been shown to react with macromolecules through a reaction with amino, carboxyl, thiol, hydroxyl and imino groups and amide substituents. Their interactions with proteins and enzymes and their cross-linking ability are thought to be responsible for their mechanisms of bactericidal action. The lipophilicity of OPA is thought to be responsible for a better penetration of the aldehyde through the cell wall and for an increase in activity compared with glutaraldehyde (Fraud et al., 2003).

On occasion, the use of chemical biocides has been combined with elevated temperatures (e.g. LTSF as discussed earlier in this chapter). For the disinfection of medical devices such as endoscopes, high-level disinfectants are often used in automated washer disinfectors, which are designed for specific devices and ensure automation of the process, although a precleaning stage is often necessary before disinfection takes place.

New technologies

Although only five sterilization procedures are usually recommended in pharmacopoeias, there has been an interest in developing alternative methods to overcome the disadvantages of existing ones (see Chapter 17). Most of the progress has been made in the food area. These technologies include the use of ultrahigh pressure, high-intensity light pulses, ultrasonication and gas plasma, the last being the most promising for the sterilization of medical devices and products. The principles of these new sterilization processes, although they are not used for pharmaceutical preparations, are worth mentioning briefly.

Ultrahigh pressure

The principle of using high pressure is that vegetative microorganisms are inactivated at pressures above 100 MPa and bacterial spores are inactivated at pressures above 1200 MPa. The use of high-pressure processing for food preservation has been combined with the chemical effect of the preservative system, such as a low pH in certain foodstuffs (e.g. jams, fruit juices). The low pH ensures the prevention of outgrowth of bacterial spores. The advantage of this process is that the quality and taste of the products tend not to be affected by such a system. Indeed, high pressure tends to preferentially denature macromolecules rather than low molecular weight flavour and odour compounds (Yordanov & Angelova, 2010). The microbial cell offers multiple pressure-sensitive target sites (e.g. enzymes, membranes, genomic material), although bacterial spores are more resilient to high pressures. The combination of high pressure and elevated temperature has been shown to be synergistic, although the process varies depending on the combination and the type of spores.

The use of high pressure for the sterilization of pharmaceutical products has been considered and might offer an appropriate alternative to existing sterilization processes. High-pressure sterilization is an innocuous process that can be performed at a relatively low temperature. Another advantage of using high pressure is the rapid control of thermal processes. Indeed, the application of pressure raises the temperature but conversely the temperature decreases as the pressure is reduced. Hence rapid temperature changes following a rapid change in pressure can help in controlling a thermal process and reduce heat-induced damage to a product (Heinz & Knorr, 2001). However, detailed studies with pharmaceutical preparations and detailed process validation are needed for high pressure to be used for the sterilization of dosage forms (van Doorne, 2008).

High-intensity light pulses

The application of intense light, such as from a high-intensity laser, is known to inactivate microorganisms. This principle already has applications in the food industry and also in the medical area, notably in dentistry. Such processes have been shown to inactivate vegetative microorganisms and bacterial spores. In the food industry, broad-spectrum light with pulse durations from 10^{-6} to 10^{-1} seconds and with energy densities ranging from 0.1 J cm^{-2} to 50 J cm^{-2} is used. In dentistry, high-intensity light pulses (i.e. from a laser) have been combined with the use of antimicrobial dyes (e.g. toluidine blue) to achieve better inactivation of microorganisms in the treatment of root canal infections, and such a combination is also referred to as antimicrobial photodynamic treatment (Soukos & Goodson, 2011).

For pharmaceutical preparations, a potential application is the terminal sterilization of clear solutions such as water, saline, dextrose and ophthalmic products. The type of container is of prime importance since it must not hinder the transmission of light.

Ultrasonication

The use of sonication to inactivate microorganisms was first reported more than 30 years ago. The principle is based on cavitation through the material exposed, resulting in the formation and collapse of small bubbles. The ensuing shock waves associated with high temperatures and pressures can be sufficiently intense to disrupt the microbial cell; however, spores are highly resistant. A synergistic effect has been reported by combination of ultrasound and heat to a certain extent (O'Donnell et al., 2010). Such a combination has been reported to reduce the heat resistance of microorganisms.

Gas plasma

Gas plasma is generated with the application of a strong magnetic field to a gas-phase compound (e.g. hydrogen peroxide). This process creates a mixture of charged nuclei, free electrons and other reactive species such as free radicals that can then damage cellular components (e.g. membrane, nucleic acid), a mechanism of action similar to that of oxidizing agents. Plasma is generally considered the 'fourth' state of matter. This dry sterilization process is effective against vegetative microorganisms and also bacterial spores and has the advantage of being a nonthermal method (Moreau et al., 2008). The use of gas plasma offers an appropriate alternative to traditional sterilization processes and finds many applications for the sterilization of medical devices, but also in drug delivery with the treatment of biomaterials (Cheruthazhekatt et al., 2010; Fig. 16.4).

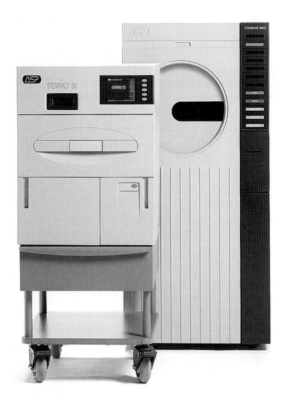

Fig. 16.4 • Gas plasma sterilizer from Advanced Sterilization Products.

Summary

Sterilization is an essential process for the manufacture of sterile dosage forms, and reprocessing medical devices and products. Several processes can be used to achieve appropriate sterilization for a given preparation or product/device. Each of these processes has advantages and disadvantages, although steam sterilization remains the reference standard. The advances in nonthermal sterilization and the coming new technologies, although mainly applied to the food industry to date, offer potentially valuable alternatives. The demonstration of sporicidal activity of a new technology, as well as its control and reproducibility, remains essential.

Common to all these processes is the need for the user to understand the technology, its activity and limitations, to follow the appropriate guidelines but also, importantly, to ensure the validation of the process. Failure to provide the appropriate documentation and to control a sterilization process adequately might result in failure of the process, with potentially fatal consequences.

It is important to note at this point that although terminal sterilization ensures the destruction of possible microbial contaminants, it needs to be operated alongside good manufacturing practice. Therefore suitable measures must be taken to ensure the microbiological quality of pharmaceutical preparations during manufacture but also during packaging, storage and distribution. These important aspects are discussed in more depth in Chapter 17.

Please check your eBook at **https://studentconsult. inkling.com/** for self-assessment questions. See inside cover for registration details.

References

British Pharmacopoeia Commission, 2017. British Pharmacopoeia. Appendix XVIII. Methods of sterilization (methods of preparation of sterile products). Stationery Office, London.

Centers for Disease Control and Prevention, 1998. Clinical sepsis and death in a newborn nursery associated with contaminated parenteral medications — Brazil, 1996. MMWR Morb. Mortal. Wkly. Rep. 47, 610–612.

Centers for Disease Control and Prevention, 2005. *Pseudomonas* bloodstream infections associated with a heparin/saline flush — Missouri, New York, Texas, and Michigan, 2004–2005. MMWR Morb. Mortal. Wkly. Rep. 54, 269–272.

Cheruthazhekatt, S., Cernak, M., Slavicek, P., et al., 2010. Gas plasmas and plasma modified materials in medicine. J. Appl. Biomed. 8, 55–66.

Dusseau, J.-Y., Duroselle, P., Freney, J., 2013. Gaseous sterilization. In: Fraise, P.A., Maillard, J.-Y.Sattar, S.A. (Eds.), Principles and Practice of Disinfection, Preservation and Sterilization, fifth ed. Blackwell Science, Oxford.

Finnegan, M., Denyer, S.P., McDonnell, G., et al., 2010. Mode of action of hydrogen peroxide and other oxidizing agents: differences between liquid and gas forms. J. Antimicrob. Chemother. 65, 2108–2115.

Fraud, S., Hann, A.C., Maillard, J.-Y., et al., 2003. Effects of ortho-phthalaldehyde, glutaraldehyde and chlorhexidine diacetate on *Mycobacterium chelonae* and *M. abscessus* strains with modified permeability. J. Antimicrob. Chemother. 51, 575–584.

Heinz, V., Knorr, D., 2001. Effects of high pressure on spores. In: Hendrickx, M.E.G., Knorr, D. (Eds.), Ultra High Pressure Treatments of Foods. Kluwer Academic/Plenum, New York.

International Organization for Standardization, 2009. ISO 14937:2009. Sterilization of health care products – general requirements for characterization of a sterilizing agent and the development, validation and routine control of a sterilization process for medical devices. International Organization for Standardization, Geneva.

Joslyn, L.J., 2001. Sterilization by heat. In: Block, S.S. (Ed.), Disinfection, Sterilization, and Preservation, fifth ed. Lippincott Williams & Wilkins, Philadelphia.

Lambert, P.A., 2013. Sterilization: radiation sterilization. In: Fraise, A.P., Maillard, J.-Y.Sattar, S.A. (Eds.), Russell, Hugo & Ayliffe's Principles and Practice of Disinfection, Preservation and Sterilization, fifth ed. Blackwell Science, Oxford.

Levy, R.V., 2001. Sterile filtration of liquids and gases. In: Block, S.S. (Ed.), Disinfection, Sterilization, and Preservation, fifth ed. Lippincott Williams & Wilkins, Philadelphia.

McDonnell, G., 2007. Antisepsis, Disinfection and Sterilization: Types, Action and Resistance. ASM Press, Washington, DC.

Moreau, M., Orange, N., Feuilloley, M.G.J., 2008. Non-thermal plasma technologies; new tools for bio-decontamination. Biotechnol. Adv. 26, 610–617.

O'Donnell, C.P., Tiwari, B.K., Bourke, P., et al., 2010. Effect of ultrasonic processing on food enzymes of industrial importance. Trends Food Sci. Technol. 21, 358–367.

Sharp, J., 2000. Quality in the Manufacture of Medicines and Other Healthcare Products. Pharmaceutical Press, London.

Soukos, N.S., Goodson, J.M., 2011. Photodynamic therapy in the control of oral biofilms. Periodontol. 2000 55, 143–166.

van Doorne, H., 2008. High-pressure treatment, a potential antimicrobial treatment for pharmaceutical preparations? A survey. PDA J. Pharm. Sci. Technol. 62, 273–291.

Walsh, S.E., Denyer, S.P., 2013. Sterilization: filtration sterilization. In: Fraise, A.P., Maillard, J.-Y.Sattar, S.A. (Eds.), Principles and Practice of Disinfection, Preservation and Sterilization, fifth ed. Blackwell Science, Oxford.

Yordanov, D.G., Angelova, G.V., 2010. High pressure processing for food preserving. Biotechnol. Biotechnol. Equip. 24, 1940–1945.

Bibliography

Block, S.S. (Ed.), 2001. Disinfection, Sterilization, and Preservation, fifth ed. Lippincott Williams & Wilkins, Philadelphia.

British Society for Gastroenterology Working Party, 1998. Cleaning and disinfection of equipment for gastrointestinal endoscopy. Gut 42, 585–593.

Fraise, A.P., Maillard, J.Y., Sattar, S.A. (Eds.), 2013. Principles and Practice of Disinfection, Preservation and Sterilization, fifth ed. Blackwell Science, Oxford.

17

Sterilization in practice

Jean-Yves Maillard   Susannah E. Walsh

CHAPTER CONTENTS

KEY POINTS

- Sterilization is essential to produce sterile dosage forms.
- Pharmacopoeias usually recognize four terminal sterilization processes – steam (under pressure), dry heat, gaseous (ethylene oxide) and ionizing radiation sterilization – and nonterminal sterilization by filtration.

- The choice of sterilization processes reflects the great diversity of pharmaceutical preparations, medical products and devices that are required to be sterile.
- A sterilization process is informed by a number of specific standard documents and guidelines, is tightly controlled and must be documented and validated.
- A clear understanding of the method, the product to be sterilized (including its packaging), the validation process and the overall documentation required is necessary to perform a successful sterilization.

Sterile products

Sterilization is an essential part of the processing of pharmaceutical dosage forms that are required to be sterile. By definition, a sterile product is completely free of viable microorganisms. In addition to the pharmaceutical products that need to be sterile, a number of medical devices that come into contact with sterile parts of the body or are reused in patients also need to be free of microorganisms (Table 17.1). The diversity of the items to be sterilized in terms of properties (e.g. heat sensitive or not), bulk, content and the number of items to be sterilized per load requires the use of distinct sterilization processes. The *British Pharmacopoeia* (British Pharmacopoeia Commission, 2017a), as an example, describes the use of five main sterilization processes to accommodate the range of products to be sterilized: steam, dry heat, gaseous, ionizing radiation and filtration sterilization. The first four methods are usually used

Table 17.1 Examples of sterile preparations and devices

Preparation/product/item	Typical volume	Typical container	Sterilization process
Injections			
Intravenous infusion, e.g. blood products	0.5 L	Plastic, glass	Steam Filtration (e.g. addition of additives)
Parenteral nutrition fluid	>3 L	Plastic, glass	Steam Filtration (e.g. addition of vitamins)
Small-volume injections, e.g. insulin, vaccines	1 mL to 50 mL	Plastic glass	Steam[a] Filtration
Small-volume oily injections		Glass	Dry heat
Noninjectable sterile fluids			
Noninjectable water, e.g. surgery, irrigation	0.5 L to 1 L	Plastic (polyethylene or polypropylene)	Steam
Urological irrigation solution	>3 L	Plastic (rigid)	Steam Filtration
Peritoneal dialysis and haemodialysis solutions	2.5 L	Plastic	Steam
Nebulizer solutions	Diluted in WFI	Plastic (polyethylene nebules)	Steam Filtration
Ophthalmic preparations			
Eye drops	0.3 mL to 0.5 mL	Plastic, glass	Steam[a] Filtration
Eye lotions	>0.1 L	Plastic, glass	Steam
Eye ointments	–	Plastic, aluminium	Dry heat Filtration
Contact lens solutions	Small	Plastic	Chemical disinfection
Dressings			
Chlorhexidine gauze dressing		Different wrapping[b]	Steam[c]
Polyurethane foam dressing			Dry heat
Elastic adhesive dressing			Ethylene oxide
Plastic wound dressings			Ionizing radiation Other effective method
Implants			
		Small, sterile cylinders of drug	Dry heat Chemical (0.02% phenyl mercuric nitrate, 12 h, 75 °C)
Absorbable haemostats			
Oxidized cellulose, human fibrin foam			Dry heat

Continued

Table 17.1 Examples of sterile preparations and devices—cont'd

Preparation/product/item	Typical volume	Typical container	Sterilization process
Surgical ligatures and sutures			
Sterilized surgical catgut			γ-radiation Chemical (96% ethanol + 0.002% phenyl mercuric nitrate + formaldehyde in ethanol 24 h before use; naphthalene or toluene at 160 °C for 2 h)
Nonabsorbable type			γ-radiation Steam
Instruments and equipment			
Syringes		Glass, plastic	Dry heat Steam γ-radiation Ethylene oxide
Metal instruments			Steam
Rubber gloves			γ-radiation Ethylene oxide
Respirator parts			Steam
Fragile heat-sensitive devices			Chemical disinfection

aDepends on the preparations (thermostable or thermolabile).
bDressings must be appropriately wrapped (aseptic handling) for their specific use.
cSterilization process depends on the stability of the dressing constituents (e.g. dressings containing waxes cannot be sterilized by moist heat) and the nature of their components.
WFI, Water for Injections.

to process products in their final containers (terminal sterilization). Regardless of the sterilization method used, it is important that the process itself is fully validated. A number of guidelines and European/international standard documents for specific product–sterilization method combinations exist and are followed by manufacturers and end users. Failure to control and/or document adequately a sterilization process can lead to serious incidents. This chapter aims to provide a brief overview of the recommended sterilization processes, their control and their validation.

Determination of sterilization protocols

Various technologies are available to achieve sterility of pharmaceutical preparations and medical devices (Table 17.2). Generally, sterilization of the product in its final container (terminal sterilization) is preferred. This implies that the container must not impinge on the optimum sterilization to be delivered and that the container and closure maintain the sterility of the product throughout its shelf life. The selected sterilization process must be suitable for its purpose, i.e. the sterilization of a given product, device and preparation, which means that the product and its container have to be rendered sterile and must not be damaged by the process.

The choice of an appropriate sterilization process depends on a number of factors (Table 17.3) related to the product to be sterilized, such as the type and composition of product and also the quantity to be sterilized. Additionally, the composition and the packaging of the product are significant factors that rule out some sterilization processes. For example, a heat-labile preparation would not be sterilized by heat sterilization, and a small oily injection would not be sterilized by steam sterilization (further

Table 17.2 Sterilization technologies (for pharmaceutical preparations and medical devices)

Type	Principle	Examples
Terminal sterilization		
Physical	Heat	Steam
		Dry heat
	Radiation	γ-radiation
		Accelerated electrons (particle radiation)
Chemical	Gaseous	Ethylene oxide
		Low-temperature steam formaldehyde
		Gas plasma
	Liquid	Glutaraldehyde, o-phthalaldehyde, formaldehyde, peracetic acid, hydrogen peroxide
Nonterminal sterilization		
Filtration	Aseptic procedure	

Box 17.1

Key points to achieve good manufacturing practice

- Qualified personnel with appropriate training
- Adequate premises
- Suitable production equipment, designed for easy cleaning and sterilization
- Adequate precautions to minimize the bioburden before sterilization (starting materials, etc.)
- Validated procedures for all critical production steps
- Environmental monitoring and in-process testing procedures

examples are given in Table 17.1). For specific types of products such as dressings, although moist heat sterilization is generally the method of choice, only certain types of autoclave, such as vacuum and pressure-pulsing autoclaves, are appropriate.

For any given preparation or product, it is difficult to predict the microbial bioburden prior to sterilization. It is assumed that the bioburden of pharmaceutical preparations will be minimal as the manufacturing process should adhere to good manufacturing practice (GMP) (Box 17.1). However, a sterilization process should be able to deal with a worst-case scenario. This is usually exemplified by the use of biological indicators (see the section entitled 'Process indicators' later in this chapter) such as bacterial spores, which are considered the most resistant microorganisms (with the exception of prions, the agents responsible for spongiform encephalopathies). This is usually the situation for official sterilization methods. Pharmacopoeial recommendations, as well as guideline documents, are derived from data generated from the use of biological indicators for a given sterilization process.

When a fully validated sterilization process has been conducted, the release of a batch of product can be based on process data obtained during sterilization rather than the results from sterility testing. Any change in the sterilization procedure (e.g. product

load, type of containers) requires revalidation to take place.

Resterilization of products/devices can cause their degradation (e.g. repeated irradiation or autoclaving) or may even cause them to become toxic (e.g. with ethylene oxide; Richards, 2004). Therefore, any proposed resterilization must be carefully investigated.

Recommended pharmacopoeial sterilization processes

Five main sterilization processes, which have different characteristics, are usually recommended by pharmacopoeias:

- steam (under pressure) sterilization (terminal);
- dry heat sterilization (terminal);
- ionizing radiation sterilization (terminal);
- gaseous (ethylene oxide) sterilization (terminal); and
- sterilization by filtration (nonterminal).

Although the use of other sterilization methods is not necessarily precluded, appropriate validation documentation for each product needs to be provided. More information can be found in Chapters 15 and 16, or in the relevant pharmacopoeia. At the time of writing, examples of these include the *European Pharmacopoeia* (European Pharmacopoeia Commission, 2017), the *United States Pharmacopeia* (US Pharmacopeial Convention, 2016) and the *British Pharmacopoeia* (British Pharmacopoeia Commission,

Table 17.3 Selection of a sterilization process

Type of product/preparation

Pharmaceutical preparations	Volume	Large, small injection
	Composition	Water, oil, powder
Medical devices	Size	Small, large, complex devices (e.g. endoscopes, respirator parts
	Composition	Plastic, glass, metal, porous (e.g. dressing)

Possible damage to the preparation/product

	Heat (heat-sensitive preparations)
	Radiation (water)
	Corrosiveness (oxidizing agents)

Possible damage to the product/container

	Water ballasting
	Moisture
	Glass breaking (on cooling)
	Change in composition (irradiation)
	Corrosiveness

Other considerations

Toxicity/safety	Gas sterilization (ethylene oxide, formaldehyde)
	Liquid sterilants: aldehydes
	Radiation sterilization: radioactive source
Level of bioburden	Expected heavy contamination
	Surgical instruments
Sterilization regimen	Local sterilization (portable autoclave)
	Large quantity of items to be sterilized
	Need for quarantine (desorption of toxic chemicals)
Cost of sterilization process	Equipment, e.g. autoclave, electron accelerator
	Facility, e.g. irradiation plant
	Running cost: gas, ^{60}Co
	Training of end users
Validation	Ease of validation; producing appropriate documentation
	Cost of audit
	Cost of validation

2017a) but it is always important to consult the most up-to-date texts and guidelines. The European Agency for the Evaluation of Medicinal Products publishes a decision tree for the selection of sterilization methods.

Steam (under pressure) sterilization

Steam sterilization is the most reliable, versatile and universally used form of sterilization and relies on the combination of steam, temperature and pressure. The typical cycle consists of a holding time of 15 minutes at a temperature of 121°C at 15 psi

(103 kPa) gauge pressure (Table 17.4). The aim is to deliver steam at the phase boundary (dry saturated steam; see Chapter 16, Fig. 16.2) to all areas of the load. This is achieved using steam and pressure (Table 17.5).

Steam under pressure is commonly used unless prohibited by lack of load penetration or heat and/or moisture damage. Steam can only kill microorganisms if it makes direct contact with them, so it is very important to avoid air pockets in the sterilizer during a sterilization process. In addition, air can reduce the partial pressure of the steam such that the temperature reached on surfaces will be less than

Table 17.4 Typical terminal sterilization cycles

Sterilization process	Temperature (°C)	Pressure (psig)	Relative humidity (%)	Holding time/dose	Concentration	Parametric release	Desorption
Heat							
Moist heat	121	15 (103 kPa)	–	15 min	–	Yes	No
	134	30 (207 kPa)	–	3 min	–	Yes	No
Dry heat	160	–	–	>2 h	–	Yes	No
Radiation							
γ-radiation	Room	–	–	25 kGy[a]	–	Yes	No
Particle radiation	Room	–	–	25 kGy	–	No	No
Gaseous	**Temp.**	**(°C)**	**Relative humidity (%)**	**Holding time**	**Conc.**	**Parametric release**	**Desorption**
Ethylene oxide[b]	40–50	–	40–80	30 min to 10 h	400 mg/L to 1000 mg/L	No	Yes[c]
LTSF[d]	70–80[e]	–	75–100	90 min	6 mg/L to 50 mg/L	No	Yes

[a]Standard dose. The time necessary to achieve this dose depends on the source. For γ-ray irradiation, the process can take up to 20 hours, whereas for high-energy electrons (particle radiation), only a few minutes may be required.
[b]Vacuum cycle; pretreatment of the load: preheating and humidification of the load. Pressurized cycle: always higher than atmospheric pressure; allows shorter contact time.
[c]Desorption could take up to 15 days; maximum threshold of ethylene oxide residues and evaluation documented in ISO 10993-7 (International Organization for Standardization, 2008).
[d]Values can differ slightly depending on the literature.
[e]Lower temperature of 55 °C to 56 °C can be used depending on the thermotolerance of the preparation.
LTSF, Low-temperature steam formaldehyde.

Table 17.5 Examples of temperature and pressure combinations used for steam sterilization

Temperature (°C)	Steam pressure	
	kPa	psig
115	69	10
121	103	15
126	138	20
134	207	30

Steam pressures are expressed in kilopascals (kPa) and pounds per square inch gauge (psig), the latter still finding continuing use.

that expected with the pressure used. Hence removal of air is an essential part of the process to ensure effective sterilization. To remove the air present when an autoclave is loaded, autoclaves are equipped with air removal/displacement systems (e.g. vacuum and displacement autoclaves). For porous loads, gravity displacement systems (downward-displacement autoclaves) are not adequate, and vacuum and pressure-pulsing autoclaves are preferred (McDonnell, 2007). Noncondensable gases must also be removed and monitored; these are atmospheric gases such as nitrogen and oxygen that form part of the initial atmosphere of the sterilizer. Other factors that affect the efficacy of steam sterilization are water content and steam purity. The optimal sterilization is obtained with saturated steam (as discussed in Chapter 16). Supersaturated steam (i.e. wetter steam) is associated with condensation and poor penetration. Superheated steam (i.e. drier steam) behaves like dry heat and is less efficient. Steam purity is determined by the quality of the water, which can be affected by a number of contaminants (e.g. pyrogens, amines, toxic metals, iron, chlorides) that can render the sterile product unsafe (e.g. toxicity caused by pyrogenic reactions, metallic poisoning) or damaged (e.g. discoloration of packaging, corrosion caused by iron and chlorides).

Steam under pressure is generated in autoclaves which can vary greatly in size and shape, ranging from portable bench-top units to industrial production facilities (Fig. 17.1). A cross-section through an autoclave is shown in Fig. 17.2.

Steam sterilization applications are informed/regulated by a number of European and international guidelines and standards providing information on sterilizer design and installation, quality of steam, requirement for pressure, development and validation and routine control, etc.

Dry heat sterilization

The most common dry heat sterilization method uses hot air ovens (Fig. 17.3). Other procedures, such as sterilizing tunnels using high-temperature filtered laminar air flow or infrared irradiation to achieve rapid heat transfer, are also available. Hot air ovens are usually heated electrically and often have heaters under a perforated bottom plate to provide convection currents (gravity convection type). Mechanical convection hot air ovens are equipped with a fan to assist air circulation and increase heat transfer by convection (Joslyn, 2001). Dry heat sterilization is less expensive than steam sterilization and is effective for the depyrogenation of containers/packaging (e.g. glassware). Overloading should be avoided, wrappings and other barriers minimized and the load positioned to allow optimal air circulation. Other problems include long heating up times (e.g. with large loads of instruments) and the charring or baking of organic

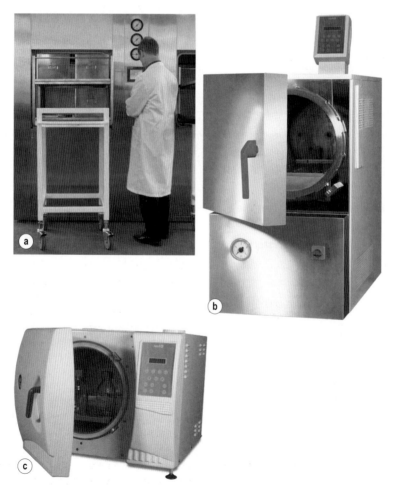

Fig. 17.1 • Examples of autoclaves. **(a)** Square section, **(b)** Swiftlock and **(c)** Swiftlock Compact autoclaves. Courtesy of Astell.

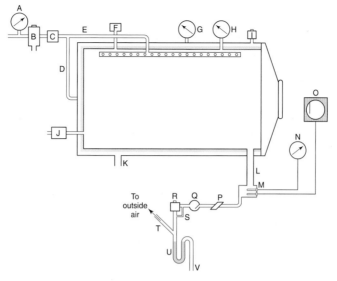

Fig. 17.2 • The features of a large steam sterilizer (for simplicity, the control valves have been omitted). *A,* Mains pressure gauge; *B,* separator; *C,* reducing valve; *D,* steam supply to jacket; *E,* steam supply to chambers; *F,* air filter; *G,* jacket pressure gauge; *H,* chamber pressure gauge; *I,* jacket air vent; *J,* vacuum pump; *K,* jacket discharge channel (detail not shown); *L,* chamber discharge channel; *M,* thermometer pocket; *N,* direct-reading thermometer; *O,* recording thermometer; *P,* strainer; *Q,* check valve; *R,* balanced-pressure thermostatic trap; *S,* bypass; *T,* vapour escape line; *U,* water seal; *V,* air-break.

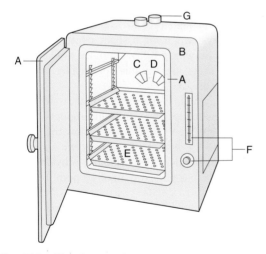

Fig. 17.3 • Hot air oven. *A,* Heat-resistant gasket; *B,* outer case containing glass-fibre insulation, and heaters in chamber wall; *C,* false wall; *D,* fan; *E,* perforated shelf; *F,* regulator; *G,* vents.

matter onto items. Dry heat sterilization cycles are generally longer than for moist heat sterilization, typically 2 hours at 160 °C (see Table 17.4). The process is thermostatically controlled and monitored using thermocouples.

Dry heat sterilization cannot be used for a number of products, such as rubber, plastics and other thermolabile items, or for aqueous solutions.

Integrated lethality in sterilization practice

All heat sterilization processes must include heating up and cooling down periods. These prolonged periods at a raised temperature may increase the degradation of the product. Integrated lethality attempts to examine the effects of heat on the inactivation process during these periods.

For steam sterilization, the F_o concept ('reference unit of lethality') is used. This takes into account the heating up and cooling down stages of the heating cycle and is expressed as the equivalent time in minutes at a temperature of 121 °C delivered by the process to the product in its final container with reference to microorganisms with a Z value of 10. Its calculation is complex, and further information can be found in the relevant pharmacopoeias. In practice, computer programs can be used to calculate the combined effect of whole processes, allowing a reduction in the total process time. It is important that

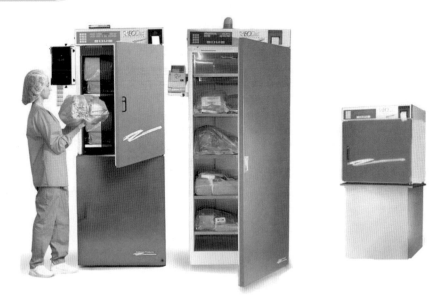

Fig. 17.4 • Examples of ethylene oxide sterilizers using slight negative pressure rather than the conventional vacuum system. These are suitable for smaller loads, e.g. hospital reprocessing loads, research and development work, short production runs and low-volume production. Courtesy of Andersen Caledonia.

the appropriate sterility assurance level is consistently achieved, and the routine use of biological indicators is recommended, although following process validation, parametric release might be preferred.

Gaseous sterilization

The gaseous sterilization method recommended by pharmacopoeias mainly employs ethylene oxide. It is usually used on a commercial scale for the sterilization of catheters, infusion giving sets, syringes, prostheses and some plastic containers and thermolabile powders (if humidity is not a problem; Sharp, 2000). The ethylene oxide sterilization cycle is complex since many factors need to be controlled over a long period (Table 17.4). The control of the temperature, concentration and relative humidity is critical. In addition, ethylene oxide is very flammable and can form explosive mixtures in air. It is therefore combined with an inert gas carrier (e.g. carbon dioxide or nitrogen). Ethylene oxide is also toxic, mutagenic and a possible human carcinogen. Gaseous sterilization using ethylene oxide is nevertheless a popular sterilization process, mainly because of the low temperature used during sterilization, but also because of the amount of information acquired on ethylene oxide sterilization processes over the years.

The sterilization procedure is usually carried out in a purpose-built, gas-tight stainless steel chamber which can withstand high pressures and a high vacuum. However, systems using a slight negative pressure rather than drawing a full vacuum are available (Fig. 17.4) and these are suitable for smaller, vacuum-sensitive loads.

Packaging should be permeable by air, water vapour and ethylene oxide. The sterilized products need to be quarantined after the process to allow the removal of gas. The *European Pharmacopoeia* and other international standards set limits for ethylene oxide residue levels (e.g. a maximum of 10 ppm for plastic syringes).

Low-temperature steam formaldehyde (LTSF, discussed in Chapter 16), although not included in this chapter's list of recommended methods, is used for the sterilization of certain preparations. As with ethylene oxide, its sterilization cycle is rather complex as several parameters have to be controlled (see Table 17.4).

Radiation sterilization

There are two types of radiation unit. The becquerel (Bq) measures the activity of a source of radiation (physical radiation). One Bq equates to a source that has one nuclear disintegration per second. The gray (Gy) measures the effect of radiation on living tissue. One Gy is equal to the transfer of 1 J of energy to 1 kg of living tissue. The gray has replaced the rad that quantified radiation absorbed dose. The electronvolt (eV) measures the energy of radiation and is usually expressed as millions of electronvolts (MeV).

The source of γ-rays for sterilization is usually cobalt-60. Caesium-137 can also be used but has less penetrating power. Cobalt-60 decays with the emission of two high-energy γ-rays (1.17 MeV and 1.33 MeV) and a lower-energy (0.318 MeV) β-particle. Gamma radiation is highly penetrative, causes negligible heating of the sterilized product at normal doses and induces no radioactivity in the final product.

Irradiation of a product can be carried out in batches but is more commonly a continuous process using a conveyor system. The products pass through the irradiation chamber and are irradiated from one or two sides. The source is shielded with concrete to protect the operators and the environment. The intensity of radiation decreases as it penetrates. For example, 100 mm of a product with a density of 1 g cm^{-3} would reduce the cobalt-60 intensity by 50%. A cobalt-60 source of 1×10^{16} Bq to 4×10^{16} Bq is used for industrial irradiation, and this provides a radiation dose in excess of 25 kGy. In most of Europe, 25 kGy is the standard dose (e.g. European Pharmacopoeia Commission, 2016). When not in use, the radioactive source is submerged in water for shielding and cooling.

Particle radiation sterilization uses β-particles that are accelerated to a high energy by application of high-voltage potentials (no radioactivity required). Their low energy means that beams from particle accelerators are less penetrating than γ-rays, with only 10 mm of a 1 g cm^{-3} material being penetrated per million electronvolts (MeV). However, an important advantage of particle radiation sterilization is that the source can be turned off and is directional (Lambert, 2013). The design of an accelerator can be customized to particular applications by including different energy and power requirements. The beam source is shielded with concrete and products are conveyed through the exposure area and irradiated. Another advantage is that shorter exposure times are required than those needed for γ-ray irradiation. High-energy beams with energies of 5 MeV to 10 MeV are used for sterilization, the accelerating field being generated using radiofrequency or microwave energy. Once it has been accelerated to the required energy, the beam of electrons is controlled by magnetic fields which can alter its size, shape or direction (McDonnell, 2007).

Radiation can affect a number of materials (e.g. polyethylene, silicone rubber, polypropylene, Teflon), aqueous solutions (e.g. through the process of water radiolysis), and packaging (discussed further in the 'Limitation of sterilization methods' section later in this chapter). Although radiation sterilization is considered a 'cold' process, intense radiation can cause an increase in temperature and as such possible overheating needs to be considered for a specific load.

Validation of radiation sterilization involves the use of *Bacillus pumilus* as a biological indicator and dosimetric analysis (discussed later in this chapter). The routine monitoring involves measurements to ensure that all products are receiving the required dose. The radiation sterilization procedure is highly regulated, and there are a number of European and international standards and guidelines available with information on requirements for the development, validation and routine control of the process (e.g. BS EN ISO 11137-1) and the dose required for sterilization (e.g. ISO 11137-2).

Filtration

Filtration is employed for nonterminal sterilization and has to be used under strict aseptic conditions. It is used for those preparations that cannot be sterilized by a terminal process or to which an agent (e.g. additive, heparin, vitamin) is added post-sterilization. Filtration is used to sterilize aqueous liquid, oils and organic solutions, and also air and other gases. Membrane filtration is an absolute process which ensures the exclusion of all particles larger than a defined size. Although many materials have been used to make filters, only a few are suitable for sterilization of pharmaceutical products.

Depth and surface filters are suitable for prefiltration of pharmaceutical products as they can retain large amounts of particles. Depth filters can be made of fibrous, granular or sintered material that is bonded into a maze of channels that trap particles throughout their depth. Surface filters are made of multiple layers of a substance such as glass or polymeric microfibres. Any particles that are larger than the spaces between the fibres are retained, and smaller particles may be trapped in the matrix (McDonnell, 2007). A membrane filter downstream is needed to retain any fibres shed from these filters, as well as small particles and microorganisms.

To sterilize a product, it is often necessary to combine several types of filtration (e.g. depth, surface and membrane filters) to achieve the removal of microorganisms. Depth and surface filtration are used to remove the majority of the particles by acting as prefilters. The final filtration step is accomplished using a membrane filter. This combined approach removes particles and microorganisms without the membrane filter being rapidly blocked up with large particles.

High-level disinfection

In addition to the processes previously described, high-level disinfectants (chemical biocides) have to be mentioned as they are used for the *chemosterilization* of medical devices, particularly high-risk items that come into contact with sterile parts of the body, such as surgical instruments, intrauterine devices and endoscopes (which are used for a wide range of diagnostic and therapeutic procedures) (Table 17.1).

Like the gaseous biocides, the activity of high-level liquid disinfectants depends on a number of factors (Maillard & McDonnell, 2012). Consequently, the training of the end user is of vital importance. Guidelines are often available from professional societies regarding the use of chemical biocides and specific devices; for example, the sterilization procedure and risk assessment for gastroscopes are published by the British Society of Gastroenterology (2014).

To ensure the efficacy of high-level disinfection, knowledge of the factors affecting efficacy, education of end users and compliance with manufacturers' instructions is essential (Maillard & McDonnell, 2012). The main advantage of using high-level disinfection is the low temperature used in processing medical devices. However, high-level disinfection might not give the same level of sterility assurance, and where possible, physical processing (e.g. steam sterilization) should be the method of choice.

The main disadvantages of high-level disinfection are exposure toxicity with regard to the end users, damage to materials and potential emerging microbial resistance; all high-level disinfectants are toxic at the concentration used. For example, there have been many reports of exposure toxicity from glutaraldehyde following endoscope reprocessing, and this has resulted in abandonment of the use of the dialdehyde in many countries. Damage to the materials following reprocessing can take the form of corrosion of metallic surfaces and increased rigidity of plastics. Problems associated with inappropriate high-level disinfection regimens, which resulted in microbial contamination, have been described since the 1990s. Reports have highlighted the potential for transmission of infection via medical devices and medical device reprocessors (Fisher et al., 2012; Deva et al., 2013; Verfaillie et al., 2015). It has been suggested that as many as 270 000 infections are transmitted by endoscopes each year (Lewis, 1999). These events are quite distinct from reports that microorganisms are becoming resistant to the in use concentrations of these disinfectants, including high-level ones (Maillard, 2010; Maillard et al., 2013).

Statistical considerations of sterility testing and sterility assurance level

The strict definition of sterility is the complete absence of viable microorganisms. In other words, after a successful sterilization process, the number of microbial survivors should be zero. This is an absolute definition which cannot be guaranteed, especially from a microbial point of view. To ensure the absence of viable microorganisms, one has to ensure all viable microorganisms can be detected and cultured. When one looks at microbial inactivation following, for example, exposure to heat or radiation, the inactivation usually follows first-order kinetics (see Chapters 15 and 16), although in practice microorganisms are inactivated at different rates, producing a deviation from linear inactivation. Thus assuring the complete elimination of microbial contaminants and thus sterility of the product cannot be *guaranteed* mathematically or practically.

Instead of our defining sterility in a strict microbiological sense, it is more appropriate to consider the likelihood of a preparation being free of microorganisms. This is best expressed as the probability of a product containing a surviving microorganism after a given sterilization process. Survival depends on the number and the type of microorganisms, soiling and the environmental conditions within the sterilizing equipment. The concept of a sterility assurance level (SAL) or microbial safety index provides a numerical value for the probability of survival of a single microorganism. The SAL is therefore the degree of

Box 17.2

Worked example

Consider steam sterilization. For an initial bioburden of 10^4 spores of *Geobacillus stearothermophilus*, an inactivation factor of 10^{10} will be required to achieve a sterility assurance level of 10^{-6}.

G. stearothermophilus has a *D* value of 1.5 for steam sterilization.

Thus according to Eq. 17.1, a 15-minute sterilization process (i.e. holding time) at 121 °C will be required to achieve an inactivation factor of 10^{10} (i.e. $10^{15/1.5}$).

The process will therefore reduce the level of microorganisms by 10 log cycles.

assurance for a sterilizing process to render a population of products sterile. For pharmaceutical preparations a SAL of 10^{-6} or better is required. This equates to not more than one viable microorganism per million items/units processed. Practically, the lethality of a sterilization process and in particular the number of log cycles required need to be calculated.

The inactivation factor, which measures the reduction in the number of microorganisms (of a known *D* value; see Chapters 15 and 16) brought about by a defined sterilization process, can be calculated as follows:

$$IF = 10^{t/D}$$

(17.1)

where IF is the inactivation factor, *t* is the contact time (for heat or gaseous process) or radiation dose (for ionizing radiation) and *D* is the *D* value appropriate to the process employed. An example calculation is shown in Box 17.2.

Calculation of the IF is based on one obtaining inactivation kinetics that follows a first-order process. In reality, this is not always the case. In the food industry, the calculation of the most probable effective dose (MPED) is preferred as it is independent of the slope of the survivor curve for the process. However, to establish an MPED that will achieve the required reduction in a number of microorganisms requires complex calculations.

Test for sterility of the product

Sterility testing assesses whether a sterilized pharmaceutical or medical product is free from viable microorganisms by incubating all or part of the product with a nutrient medium. Testing for sterility is a destructive process. For an item to be shown not to contain organisms, unfortunately it has to be destroyed. Due to the destructive nature of the test and the probabilities involved in sampling only a portion of a batch, it is only possible to say that no contaminating microorganisms have been found in the sample examined in the conditions of the test (British Pharmacopoeia Commission, 2017b). Thus the measurement of sterility relies on statistical probability. In other words, it is impossible to prove sterility since sampling may fail to select nonsterile containers, and culture techniques have limited sensitivity. In addition, not all types of microorganisms that might be present can be detected by conventional methods as not all microorganisms are affected by a sterilization process in the same way. It is possible that some may not be killed or removed. For example, a filter pore size of 0.22 μm is usually used for filtration sterilization, which means that smaller microorganisms such as viruses are allowed to pass through.

Detailed sampling and testing procedures are given in pharmacopoeias, and further details can be found in Chapter 14. For terminally sterilized products, biologically based and automatically documented physical proofs that show correct treatment during sterilization provide greater assurance than the sterility test. This method of assuring sterility is termed parametric release and is defined as the release of a sterile product based on process compliance with physical specifications. Parametric release is acceptable for all fully validated terminal sterilization processes recommended by the *European Pharmacopoeia*.

Validation of a sterilization process

The *British Pharmacopoeia* (British Pharmacopoeia Commission, 2017a) states:

The sterility of a product cannot be guaranteed by testing; it has to be assured by the application of a suitably validated production process. It is essential that the effect of the chosen sterilization procedure on the product (including its final container or package) is investigated to ensure effectiveness and the integrity of the product and that the procedure is validated before being applied in practice.

Clearly this statement points out that testing for sterility is not enough and a suitable production process should be appropriately validated. Any changes in the sterilization procedure (i.e. change in sterilization process, product packaging or load) require revalidation. For pharmaceutical preparations, good manufacturing practices (GMP) have to be observed for the entire manufacturing process, not just the sterilization procedure.

The process of validation requires that the appropriate documentation is obtained to show that a process is consistently complying with predetermined specifications. International organizations such as the International Organization for Standardization (http://www.iso.org) and the Food and Drug Administration in the USA (http://www.fda.gov) provide detailed documentation for the validation of sterilization of health care products or medical devices with various processes (e.g. steam, radiation and gaseous sterilization). For the validation of sterilization processes, two types of data are required: commissioning data and performance qualification data (Box 17.3). Commissioning data refer mainly to the installation and characteristics of the equipment, and the performance data ensure that the equipment will produce the required sterility assurance level. The performance qualification data can be divided into physical and biological performance data (Box 17.3).

Obtaining biological performance data is required for the validation and revalidation of the sterilization process for new preparations, new loads and new sterilization regimens and is usually not used routinely except when the sterilization conditions are not well defined (e.g. gaseous sterilization) or with nonstandard methods. The use of biological indicators (discussed in the next section) requires good knowledge of the inactivation kinetics (e.g. D value) for a given process. Performance qualification data must be reevaluated following a change to the preparation or product and its packaging, the loading pattern or the sterilization cycle.

Process indicators

For all methods of sterilization, it is essential that the equipment used works correctly. Routine tests

Box 17.3

Information required for the validation of a sterilization process

Commissioning data

- Evidence that the equipment has been installed in accordance with specifications
- Equipment is safe to use
- Equipment functions within predetermined limits

Performance qualification data

- Evidence that equipment will produce a product with an acceptable assurance of sterility
- Physical performance qualification – evidence that the specified sterilization conditions have been met throughout the sterilization cycle:
  - the tests performed depend on the sterilization process
  - data should be generated from the worst region in the sterilizer
  - the data generated should also show no detrimental effect on the product and its packaging
- Biological performance qualification – evidence that the specified sterilizing conditions deliver the required microbiological lethality to the preparation/product:
  - makes use of biological indicators
  - data are not required if the process is well defined (e.g. use of F value).

are carried out to demonstrate that all parts of the sterilizer have been correctly installed (installation qualification) and that they operate properly, with sterilizing conditions reaching every part of the load (operation qualification; McDonnell, 2007). The test methods used vary according to the sterilization method and may involve the use of physical indicators, chemical indicators and biological indicators.

Physical indicators measure parameters such as heat distribution (i.e. temperature) by thermocouples, pressure variation by gauges or transducers, gas concentration, steam purity, relative humidity by hygrometers or direct calorimetry, delivered dose and time exposure. Sensors must be maintained and calibrated regularly. They are usually the first indicators of a problem with a sterilization process. Sensors maintenance and calibration are essential to ensure the validity of parametric release (Berube et al., 2001).

Chemical indicators vary depending on the sterilization method but essentially they all change in physical or chemical nature in response to one or more

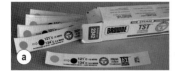
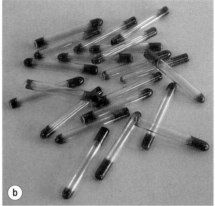
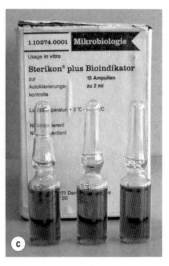

Fig. 17.5 • Examples of chemical and biological indicators. **(a)** Multiparameter (time, steam and temperature) indicators. **(b)** Sterilization control tubes. **(c)** *Geobacillus stearothermophilus/Bacillus stearothermophilus* biological indicators.

parameters. There are several types of chemical indicators (Fig. 17.5); temperature-specific indicators just show whether a specific temperature has been reached (single-variable indicators), whereas multiparameter/multivariable indicators can measure more than one variable at a time, e.g. heat and time or gas concentration and time, or time, steam and temperature.

Process indicators demonstrate that an indicator has gone through a process but they do not guarantee that sterilization was satisfactory. A common example is autoclave tape (single end-point indicator), which reflects the conditions inside the chamber environment but is not able to demonstrate that an item has been sterilized. Another example is a Temptube®, which is a glass tube containing a chemical with a specific melting point indicated by a colour change. More specific indicators, such as the 'Bowie–Dick tests', are used to monitor air removal from autoclaves. They must be used in the first cycle of the day as an equipment function test (McDonnell, 2007). The standardized test pack is placed in the centre of porous load sterilizers, and if the process is correct (i.e. air removal is appropriate), uniform colour change occurs across the test package (Fig. 17.6).

A common example of multivariable indicators is sterilization control tubes (e.g. Browne's tubes), which produce a colour change when the appropriate temperature and exposure time have been achieved.

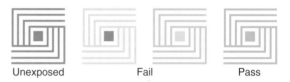

Unexposed   Fail   Pass

Fig. 17.6 • Bowie–Dick test pack used to monitor air removal from steam sterilizers; a uniform colour change indicates sufficient steam penetration.

Other chemical indicators are quantitative and indicate a combination of critical variables within a process. This is the case with dosimeters (e.g. Perspex®), which gradually change colour on exposure to radiation. The performance of chemical indicators can be altered by the storage conditions before and after use and by the method used.

Biological indicators consist of a carrier or package containing a standardized preparation of defined microorganisms of known resistance to a specific mode of sterilization (Berube et al., 2001; see Fig. 17.5). The carriers used are usually made of filter paper, a glass slide, stainless steel or a plastic tube. Some new versions incorporate ampoules containing a growth medium. The carrier is covered to prevent deterioration or contamination while still allowing entry of the sterilizing agent (British Pharmacopoeia Commission, 2017a). Different organisms are used for different processes (Table 17.6), but biological indicators usually consist of bacterial spores. In excess

Table 17.6 Organisms used as biological indicators for sterilization

Sterilization process	Spores used as a biological indicator
Dry heat	*Bacillus atrophaeus* ATCC 9372. NCIMB 8058 or CIP 77.18
Moist heat	*Geobacillus stearothermophilus* ATCC 7953. NCTC 10007. NCIMB 8157 or CIP 52.81
Ethylene oxide	*Bacillus atrophaeus* ATCC 9372. NCIMB 8058 or CIP 77.18
Radiation	*Bacillus pumilus* ATCC 27142. NCTC 10327. NCIMB 10692 or CIP 77.25
Filtration	*Pseudomonas diminuta* ATCC 19146. NCIMB 11091 or CIP 103020

of between 10^5 and 10^7 spores are used, the recommended number being dependent on the sterilization method being assessed. After exposure to the sterilization process, the indicators are removed aseptically and incubated in suitable media to detect the presence of surviving microorganisms. If no growth occurs, the sterilization process is said to have had sufficient lethality (Berube et al., 2001).

Testing filtration efficacy

Compared with other sterilization methods, the potential risk of failure is higher for filtration sterilization. This means that it may be advisable to add an extra prefiltration stage using a bacteria-retentive filter. Confidence in the filters used is of prime importance during filtration sterilization. Each batch of filters is tested to ensure that they meet the specifications for release of particulate materials, mechanical strength, chemical characteristics (e.g. oxidizable materials and leaching of materials) and filtration performance. The methods for testing filtration performance involve either a challenge test (which is destructive so cannot be conducted on every filter in a batch) or an integrity test (Walsh & Denyer, 2013).

The microbial challenge test is used to demonstrate that a filter is capable of retaining microorganisms. This is normally performed with a suspension of at least 10^7 colony-forming units (see Chapter 14) of *Pseudomonas diminuta* per square centimetre of active filter surface. *Pseudomonas diminuta*, also known

as *Brevundimonas diminuta*, is a small (0.2 μm to 0.9 μm) Gram-negative short rod that is a natural choice for this test because of its size and because it was originally isolated from contaminated filtered solutions (Levy, 2001). After filtration of a bacterial suspension prepared in tryptone soya broth, the filtrate is collected and incubated at 32 °C.

Integrity tests are used to verify the integrity of an assembled sterilizing filter before use and to confirm integrity after use. The tests used must be appropriate to the filter type and the stage of testing and may include bubble point tests, pressure hold tests and diffusion rate tests. The bubble point test is the oldest and one of the most widely used non-destructive tests. It measures the pressure (bubble-point pressure) needed to pass gas through the largest pore of a wetted filter. In practice, the pressure required to produce a steady stream of gas bubbles through a wetted filter is often used as the bubble point. The basis of the test relies on the holes through the filter resembling uniform capillaries passing from one side to another. If these capillaries become wet, then they will retain liquid via surface tension, and the force needed to expel the liquid with a gas is proportional to the diameter of the capillaries (pore diameter). The main limitations of this technique are that it is reliant on operator judgement and on the holes in the filter being perfect uniform capillaries (Walsh & Denyer, 2013).

Diffusion rate tests are especially useful for large-area filters. They measure the rate of flow of a gas as it diffuses through the water in a wetted filter. The pressure required to cause migration of the gas through the liquid in the pores can be compared with data specified by the filter's manufacturer to establish if the filter has defects (Levy, 2001).

Monitoring decontamination

The possibility of transmission of Creutzfeldt–Jakob disease (CJD) has increased the importance of protein removal from previously contaminated high-risk instruments. Visual inspection and ninhydrin or modified *o*-phthalaldehyde (OPA) methods may not be as sensitive as newer methods. Scanning electron microscopy (SEM) and energy-dispersive X-ray spectroscopy (EDX) analysis are not practical for health care professional use, so recent methods have concentrated on using fluorescent reagents coupled with digital imaging; for example, epifluorescence differential interference contrast microscopy (EFDIC)

Table 17.7 Limitations of sterilization processes

Sterilization processes	Limitations
Heat sterilization	
Steam	Heat; damage to preparation
	Vapour; damage to the container (wetting of final product, risk of contamination after sterilization)
	Pressure; air ballasting: damage to the container
Dry heat	Heat: damage to preparation
	Potentially longer exposure time needed
Gaseous sterilization	
Ethylene oxide	High toxicity: risk to the operator
	Decontamination required after the process
	Explosive: risk to the operator
	Slow process[a]
	Many factors to control
Formaldehyde	High toxicity: risk to the operator
	Damage to some materials (e.g. materials made from cellulose)
	Decontamination required after the process
	Slow process[a]
	Many factors to control
Radiation sterilization	
γ-radiation	Risk to the operator
	Water radiolysis: damage to the product
	Discolouration of some glasses and plastics (including PVC), destructive process may continue after sterilization has finished
	Liberation of gases (e.g. hydrogen chloride from PVC)
	Hardness and brittleness properties of metals may change
	Butyl and chlorinated rubber are degraded
	Changes in potency can occur
	High costs
Particle radiation	β-radiation: risk to the operator
	Water radiolysis: damage to the product
	Poor penetration of electrons exacerbated by density of product
	Significant product heating may occur at high doses
	High costs
Chemosterilants	
Glutaraldehyde and o-phthaladehyde	Toxicity: risk to the operator
	Activity: reports of microbial resistance
Peracetic acid	Corrosiveness: damage to the product/device
	Activity: reports of microbial resistance
Filtration sterilization	
	Not efficient for small particles (viruses, prions)
	Requires strict aseptic techniques
	Integrity of membrane filter
	Growth of microbial contaminants in depth filter
	Shedding of materials from depth filter

[a]Relative to moist heat sterilization.

and epifluorescence scanning (EFSCAN) (Baxter et al., 2014). Commercial products such as ProReveal® can produce a high level of confidence in the effectiveness of washer disinfector processes. More information can be found in ISO 15883-1.

Limitations of sterilization methods

Sterilization processes can involve some extreme conditions, such as high temperatures, high pressure, a vacuum and pressure pulsing, or the use of toxic substances, which can damage the product and/or its packaging. The alteration of a pharmaceutical preparation might lead to reduced therapeutic efficacy or patient acceptability, and damage to the container might lead to the poststerilization contamination of the product. There needs to be a balance between acceptable sterility assurance and acceptable damage to the product and container. Knowledge of the preparation and packaging design, and the choice and understanding of the sterilization technologies help in making the appropriate selection to achieve maximum microbial kill while decreasing the risk of product and packaging deterioration.

Nevertheless, each sterilization technology has its limitations (Table 17.7). Limitations associated with established and recommended procedures are usually linked to the nature of the process (e.g. heat, irradiation), whereas newer technologies tend to suffer from a lack of reproducibility.

Summary

The achievement of sterility is a complex process that requires proper documentation. Sterility in the microbiological sense cannot be guaranteed. Therefore the sterility of a product has to be assured by the application of an appropriate validation process. It is important that the sterilization methodology is compatible with the preparation or product, including its final container or packaging, and combines effectiveness and the absence of detrimental effects. Although not described in detail in this chapter, the choice of the container/packaging must allow the optimum sterilization to be applied and assure that sterility is maintained after the process. Sterilization occurs at the end of manufacturing but it does not replace or permit a relaxation of the principles of good manufacturing practice. In particular, the microbiological quality of ingredients for pharmaceutical preparations and the removal/reduction of bioburden must be monitored. Monitoring the critical parameters of the sterilization process will ensure that the predetermined conditions (during validation) are met. The lack of validation, or failure to follow a validated process, carries the risk of a nonsterile product, deterioration and possible infection.

Where possible, terminal sterilization is the method of choice. Processes that are fully validated allow the parametric release of the preparation/product and hence their rapid commercialization, since sterility testing, and the delay it incurs, might not be necessary.

A clear understanding of the method, the product to be sterilized (including its packaging), the validation process and the overall documentation required is therefore necessary to carry out a successful sterilization.

Please check your eBook at **https://studentconsult. inkling.com/** for self-assessment questions. See inside cover for registration details.

References

Baxter, H.C., Jones, A.C., Baxter, R.L., 2014. An overview of new technologies for the decontamination of surgical instruments and the quantification of protein residues. In: Walker, J.T. (Ed.), Decontamination in Hospitals and Healthcare. Woodhead Publishing, Cambridge.

Berube, R., Oxborrow, G.S., Gaustad, J.W., 2001. Sterility testing: validation of sterilization processes and sporicide testing. In: Block, S.S. (Ed.), Disinfection, Sterilization, and Preservation, fifth ed. Lippincott Williams & Wilkins, Philadelphia.

British Pharmacopoeia Commission, 2017a. British Pharmacopoeia. Appendix XVIII. Methods of sterilization (methods of preparation of sterile products). Stationery Office, London.

British Pharmacopoeia Commission, 2017b. British Pharmacopoeia. Appendix XVI A. Test for sterility. Stationery Office, London.

British Society for Gastroenterology, 2014. Guidance on Decontamination of Equipment for Gastrointestinal Endoscopy: 2014 Edition. The Report of a Working Party of the British Society of Gastroenterology Endoscopy Committee. British

Society for Gastroenterology, London.

Deva, A.K., Adams, W.P., Vickery, K., 2013. The role of bacterial biofilms in device-associated infection. Plast. Reconstr. Surg. 132, 1319–1328.

European Pharmacopoeia Commission, 2017. European Pharmacopoeia, ninth ed. Council of Europe, Strasbourg.

Fisher, C.W., Fiorello, A., Shaffer, D., et al., 2012. Aldehyde-resistant mycobacteria associated with the use of endoscope reprocessing systems. J. Hosp. Infect. 40, 880–882.

International Organization for Standardization, 2008. ISO 10993-7:2008. Biological Evaluation of Medical Devices – Part 7: Ethylene Oxide Sterilization Residuals. International Organization for Standardization, Geneva.

Joslyn, L.J., 2001. Sterilization by heat. In: Block, S.S. (Ed.), Disinfection, Sterilization, and Preservation, fifth ed. Lippincott Williams & Wilkins, Philadelphia.

Lambert, P.A., 2013. Radiation sterilization. In: Fraise, A.P., Maillard, J.-Y., Sattar, S.A. (Eds.),

Principles and Practice of Disinfection, Preservation and Sterilization, fifth ed. Blackwell Science, Oxford.

Levy, R.V., 2001. Sterile filtration of liquids and gases. In: Block, S.S. (Ed.), Disinfection, Sterilization, and Preservation, fifth ed. Lippincott Williams & Wilkins, Philadelphia.

Lewis, D.L., 1999. A sterilization standard for endoscopes and other difficult to clean medical devices. Practical Gastroenterology 23, 28–56.

Maillard, J.-Y., 2010. Emergence of bacterial resistance to microbicides and antibiotics. Microbiology Australia 31, 159–165.

Maillard, J.-Y., Bloomfield, S., Rosado Coelho, J., et al., 2013. Does microbicide use in consumer products promote antimicrobial resistance? A critical review and recommendations for a cohesive approach to risk assessment. Microb. Drug Resist. 19, 344–354.

Maillard, J.-Y., McDonnell, G., 2012. Use and abuse of disinfectants. In Pract. 34, 292–299.

McDonnell, G. (Ed.), 2007. Antisepsis, Disinfection and Sterilization: Types, Action and Resistance. ASM Press, Washington, DC.

Richards, R.M.E., 2004. Principles and methods of sterilization. In: Winfield, A.J., Richards, R.M.E. (Eds.), Pharmaceutical Practice. Churchill Livingstone, London.

Sharp, J., 2000. Quality in the Manufacture of Medicines and Other Healthcare Products. Pharmaceutical Press, London.

United States Pharmacopeial Convention, 2016. United States Pharmacopeia, thirty-ninth ed. United States Pharmacopeial Convention, Rockville.

Verfaillie, C.J., Bruno, M.J., Voor In 't Holt, A.F., et al., 2015. Withdrawal of a novel-design duodenoscope ends outbreak of a VIM-2-producing Pseudomonas aeruginosa. Endoscopy 47, 493–502.

Walsh, S.E., Denyer, S.P., 2013. Sterilization: filtration sterilization. In: Fraise, A.P., Maillard, J.-Y.Sattar, S.A. (Eds.), Principles and Practice of Disinfection, Preservation and Sterilization, fifth ed. Blackwell Science, Oxford.

Bibliography

Block, S.S. (Ed.), 2001. Disinfection, Sterilization, and Preservation, fifth ed. Lippincott Williams & Wilkins, Philadelphia.

Fraise, A.P., Maillard, J.-Y., Sattar, S.A. (Eds.), 2013. Principles and Practice of Disinfection, Preservation and Sterilization, fifth ed. Blackwell Science, Oxford.

International Organization for Standardization, 2006. ISO 15883-1:2006. Washer-Disinfectors Part 1: General Requirements, Terms and Definitions and Tests. International Organization for Standardization, Geneva.

Part 4: Biopharmaceutical principles of drug delivery

Introduction to biopharmaceutics

Marianne Ashford

CHAPTER CONTENTS

KEY POINTS

- Biopharmaceutics is the study of how the physicochemical properties of the drug, the dosage form and the route of administration affect the rate and extent of drug absorption.
- A dynamic equilibrium exists between the concentration of the drug in blood plasma and the concentration of the drug at the site of action.
- Pharmacokinetics is the study and characterization of the time course of drug absorption, distribution, metabolism and excretion (ADME) and it is determined by measuring a plasma profile.
- Pharmacodynamics is the relationship between the drug concentration at the site of action and the resulting effect.
- Bioavailability is the percentage of an administered dose of a drug that reaches the systemic circulation intact; it is therefore the ratio of the drug in the systemic circulation to that following an intravenous dose of the drug.
- The therapeutic window is the range of drug concentrations between the minimum effective concentration and the maximum safe concentration.

What is biopharmaceutics?

Biopharmaceutics can be defined as the study of how the physicochemical properties of drugs, dosage forms and routes of administration affect the rate and extent of drug absorption.

The relationship between the drug, its dosage form and the route by which it is administered governs how much of the drug enters the systemic circulation and at what rate. For a drug to be effective, a sufficient amount of it needs to reach its site(s) of action and stay there long enough to be able to exert its pharmacological effect. This is determined by the route of administration, the form in which the drug is administered and the rate at which it is delivered.

Background

Apart from the intravenous route, where a drug is introduced directly into the bloodstream, all other routes of administration, where the site of action is remote from the site of administration, involve the absorption of the drug into the blood. Once the drug reaches the blood, it partitions between the plasma and the red blood cells, the erythrocytes. Drug dissolved in the plasma partitions between the plasma proteins (mainly albumin) and the plasma water. It is the free or unbound drug in plasma water, and not the drug bound to the proteins, that passes out of the plasma through the capillary endothelium and to tissues and hence the site(s) of action.

A dynamic equilibrium normally exists between the concentration of the drug in the blood plasma and the concentration of the drug at its site(s) of action. This is termed *distribution*, the degree of which will depend largely on the physicochemical properties of the drug, in particular its lipophilicity. As it is frequently difficult to access the drug at its site(s) of action, its concentration in the plasma is often taken as a surrogate for the concentration at its site(s) of action. Even though the unbound drug in the plasma would give a better estimate of the concentration of the drug at its site(s) of action, this requires much more complex and sensitive assays than a measurement of the total concentration of the drug (i.e. the sum of the bound and unbound drug) within the blood plasma. Thus it is this total drug concentration within the plasma that is usually measured for clinical purposes and a calculation made to determine the free drug concentration. Plasma protein binding is therefore a critical parameter to consider when investigating the therapeutic effect of a drug molecule.

The concentration of the drug in blood plasma depends on numerous factors. These include the amount of an administered dose that is *absorbed* and reaches the systemic circulation, the extent of *distribution* of the drug between the systemic circulation and other tissues and fluids (which is usually a rapid and reversible process), and the rate of *elimination* of the drug from the body. The drug can either be enzymatically cleaved or biochemically transformed, in which case it is said to have been *metabolized*, or be *excreted* unchanged. The study and characterization of the time course of drug absorption, distribution, metabolism and excretion (ADME) is termed *pharmacokinetics*. In contrast, *pharmacodynamics* is the study of the biochemical and physiological effects of the drug on the body, or the relationship between drug concentration at the site of action and the resulting effect. The majority of drugs either mimic normal physiological or biochemical processes, or inhibit pathological processes. More simply, pharmacokinetics has also been defined as what the body does to the drug, whilst in contrast pharmacodynamics may be defined as what the drug does to the body. Pharmacokinetics can be used in the clinical setting to enhance the safe and effective therapeutic management of individual patients and is termed *clinical pharmacokinetics*. Increasingly pharmacodynamic markers are used to assess the success of therapy.

Fig. 18.1 illustrates some of the factors that can influence the concentration of the drug in the blood plasma and also at its site(s) of action. Biopharmaceutics is concerned with the first stage – getting the drug from its site of administration into the bloodstream or systemic circulation.

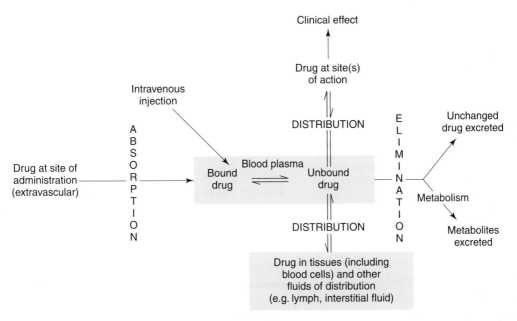

Fig. 18.1 • Drug absorption, distribution, metabolism and excretion. (ADME).

Concept of bioavailability

If a drug is given intravenously, it is administered directly into the blood and therefore we can be sure that all of the drug reaches the systemic circulation. The drug is therefore said to be 100% *bioavailable*. However, if a drug is given by another route, there is no guarantee that the whole dose will reach the systemic circulation intact. The amount of an administered dose of the drug that does reach the systemic circulation in the unchanged form is known as the *bioavailable dose*. The percentage of an administered dose of a particular drug that reaches the systemic circulation intact is known as the *bioavailability*.

Bioavailability is defined in the FDA's regulations as 'the rate and extent to which the active ingredient or active moiety is absorbed from a drug product and becomes available at the site of action'. Absolute bioavailability compares the bioavailability of the unchanged drug in the systemic circulation following a nonintravenous dose (e.g. oral, rectal, transdermal, sublingual, intramuscular, subcutaneous) with the bioavailability of the same drug following intravenous administration. The bioavailability exhibited by a drug is thus very important in determining whether a therapeutically effective concentration will be achieved at the site(s) of action.

In defining bioavailability in these terms, it is assumed that the administered drug is the therapeutically active form. This definition would not be valid in the case of prodrugs, whose therapeutic action normally depends on their being converted into a therapeutically active form prior to, or on reaching the systemic circulation. It should also be noted that, in the context of bioavailability, the term 'systemic circulation' refers primarily to venous blood (excluding the hepatic portal vein, which carries blood from the gastrointestinal tract to the liver in the absorption phase) and the arterial blood, which carries the blood to the tissues.

Therefore, for a drug which is administered orally to be 100% bioavailable, the entire dose must move from the dosage form to the systemic circulation. The drug must therefore:

- be completely released from the dosage form;
- be fully dissolved in the gastrointestinal fluids;
- be stable in solution in the gastrointestinal fluids;
- pass through the gastrointestinal barrier into the mesenteric circulation without being metabolized; and

- pass through the liver into the systemic circulation unchanged.

Anything which adversely affects either the release of the drug from the dosage form, its dissolution into the gastrointestinal fluids, its permeation through and stability in the gastrointestinal barrier or its stability in the hepatic portal circulation will influence the bioavailability exhibited by that drug from the dosage form in which it was administered.

Concept of biopharmaceutics

Many factors have been found to influence the rate and extent of absorption, and hence the time course of a drug in the plasma, and therefore at its site(s) of action. These include the foods eaten by the patient, the effect of the disease state on drug absorption, the age of the patient, the site(s) of absorption of the administered drug, the coadministration of other drugs, the physical and chemical properties of the administered drug, the type of dosage form, the composition and method of manufacture of the dosage form, the size of the dose and the frequency of administration.

Thus a given drug may exhibit differences in its bioavailability if it is administered:

- in the same type of dosage form by different routes of administration (e.g. an aqueous solution of a given drug administered by the oral and intramuscular routes);
- by the same routes of administration but in different types of dosage form (e.g. a tablet, a hard gelatin capsule and an aqueous suspension administered by the peroral route); or
- in the same type of dosage form by the same route of administration but with different formulations of the dosage form (e.g. different formulations of an oral aqueous suspension).

Variability in the bioavailability exhibited by a given drug from different formulations of the same type of dosage form, or from different types of dosage forms, or by different routes of administration, can cause the plasma concentration of the drug to be too high, and therefore cause side effects, or too low, and therefore the drug will be ineffective. Fig. 18.2 shows the plasma concentration–time curve following a single oral dose of a drug, indicating the parameters associated with a therapeutic effect. The therapeutic window is the drug concentrations which are above

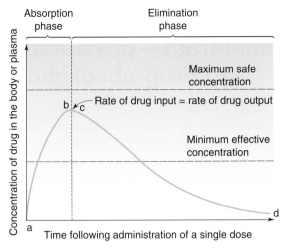

a–b rate of drug absorption > rate of drug elimination
c–d rate of drug elimination > rate of drug absorption

Fig. 18.2 • A typical blood plasma concentration–time curve obtained following the oral administration of a single dose of a drug in a tablet showing the therapeutic window of the drug.

the minimum effective concentration and below the maximum safe concentration.

Poor biopharmaceutical properties may result in:

- poor and variable bioavailability;
- difficulties in toxicological evaluation;
- difficulties with bioequivalence of formulations;
- multiple daily dosing;
- the requirement for a nonconventional delivery system;
- long and costly development times; and
- high cost of products.

Summary

Chapters 19 and 20 deal in more detail with the physiological factors, dosage form factors and intrinsic properties of drugs that influence the rate and extent of absorption for oral drugs. Chapter 21 looks at means of measuring the biopharmaceutical properties of compounds and assessing bioavailability.

A thorough understanding of the biopharmaceutical properties of a candidate drug is important both in the discovery setting, where potential drug candidates are being considered, and in the development setting, where it is important to anticipate formulation and manufacturing problems. The influence of variability and bioequivalence issues on clinical results must be studied to provide assurance to the regulatory authorities as to the robustness and quality of the drug substance and drug product.

Bibliography

Rowland, M., Tozer, T.N., 2010. Clinical Pharmacokinetics and Pharmacodynamics: Concepts and Applications. Lippincott Williams & Wilkins, Philadelphia.

Shargel, L., Yu, A.B.C., 2015. Applied Biopharmaceutics and Pharmacokinetics, seventh ed. McGraw-Hill Education, New York.

Spruill, W.J., Wade, W.E., DiPiro, J.T., et al., 2014. Concepts in Clinical Pharmacokinetics, sixth ed. American Society of Health System Pharmacists, Bethesda.

19

Gastrointestinal tract – physiology and drug absorption

Marianne Ashford

CHAPTER CONTENTS

KEY POINTS

- The gastrointestinal tract is complex, and many physiological factors affect absorption of drugs as they transit through the gastrointestinal tract.
- Physiological factors affecting absorption include the transit of dosage forms through the gastrointestinal tract, environmental factors, such as the pH, enzymes and food within the gastrointestinal tract, and disease states of the gastrointestinal tract.
- Barriers to drug absorption include environmental factors, such as pH and enzymes, the mucus and unstirred water layer, the gastrointestinal membrane and presystemic metabolism.
- Drugs are absorbed through the gastrointestinal membrane via transcellular, paracellular or active transport processes.

Introduction

The factors that influence the rate and extent of absorption depend on the route of administration. As stated in Chapter 18, the intravenous route offers direct access to the systemic circulation, and the total dose administered via this route is available in the plasma for distribution to other body tissues and the site(s) of action of the drug. Other routes will require an absorption step before the drug reaches the systemic circulation. The factors affecting this absorption will depend on the physiology of the administration site(s) and the membrane barriers present at the site or sites that the drug needs to cross to reach the systemic circulation. A summary of some of the properties of each route of administration is given in Chapter 1.

The gastrointestinal tract is discussed in detail in this chapter, and a detailed description of the physiology of some of the other more important routes of administration is given in the relevant chapters in Part 5. The oral route of delivery is by far the most popular, with approximately 50% of medicines being given by mouth, mainly because it is natural and convenient for the patient, and because it is relatively easy to

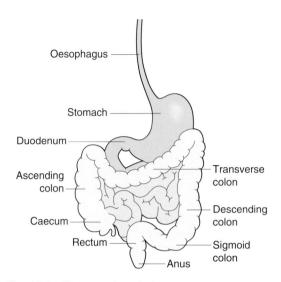

Fig. 19.1 • The gastrointestinal tract.

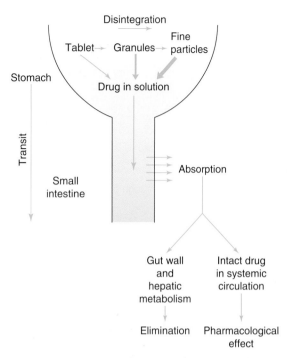

Fig. 19.2 • Steps involved before a pharmacological effect, after administration of a rapidly disintegrating tablet.

manufacture oral dosage forms. Oral dosage forms do not need to be sterilized, are compact and can be produced cheaply in large quantities by automated machines. This chapter and Chapter 20 will therefore be confined to discussing the biopharmaceutical factors (i.e. physiological, dosage form and drug factors) that influence oral drug absorption.

Physiological factors influencing oral drug absorption

The gastrointestinal tract is complex. Fig. 19.1 outlines some of the main structures involved in, and key physiological parameters that affect oral drug absorption. In order to gain an insight into the numerous factors that can potentially influence the rate and extent of drug absorption into the systemic circulation, a schematic illustration of the steps involved in the release and absorption of a drug from a tablet dosage form is presented in Fig. 19.2. It can be seen from this that the rate and extent of appearance of intact drug in the systemic circulation depend on a succession of kinetic processes.

The slowest step in this series, which is the rate-limiting step, controls the overall rate and extent of appearance of intact drug in the systemic circulation. The rate-limiting step will vary from drug to drug. For a drug which has a very poor aqueous solubility, the rate at which it dissolves in the gastrointestinal

fluids is often the slowest of all the steps, and the bioavailability of that drug is said to be *dissolution-rate limited*. In contrast, for a drug that has a high aqueous solubility, its dissolution will be rapid, and the rate at which the drug crosses the gastrointestinal membrane may be the rate-limiting step, termed *permeability limited*.

Other potential rate-limiting steps include the rate of drug release from the dosage form (this can be by design, in the case of controlled-release dosage forms), the rate at which the stomach empties the drug into the small intestine, the rate at which the drug is metabolized by enzymes in the intestinal mucosal cells during its passage through them into the mesenteric blood vessels, and the rate of metabolism of the drug during its initial passage through the liver, often termed the *'first-pass' effect*.

Physiology of the gastrointestinal tract

The gastrointestinal tract is a muscular tube, approximately 6 m in length with varying diameters. It stretches from the mouth to the anus and consists

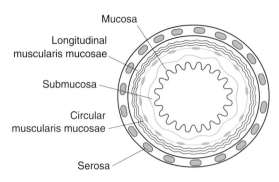

Fig. 19.3 • Cross-section through the gastrointestinal tract.

of four main anatomical areas; the oesophagus, the stomach, the small intestine and the large intestine, or colon. The luminal surface of the tube is not smooth but very rough, thereby increasing the surface area for absorption.

The wall of the gastrointestinal tract is essentially similar in structure along its length, consisting of four principal histological layers (Fig. 19.3):

1. The *serosa*, which is an outer layer of epithelium with supporting connective tissues which are continuous with the peritoneum.

2. The *muscularis externa*, which contains three layers of smooth muscle tissue, a thinner outer layer, which is longitudinal in orientation, and two inner layers, whose fibres are oriented in a circular pattern. Contractions of these muscles provide the forces for movement of gastrointestinal tract contents and physical breakdown of food.

3. The *submucosa*, which is a connective tissue layer containing some secretory tissue and which is richly supplied with blood and lymphatic vessels. A network of nerve cells, known as the submucous plexus, is also located in this layer.

4. The *mucosa*, which is essentially composed of three layers: the muscularis mucosae, which can alter the local conformation of the mucosa, a layer of connective tissue known as the lamina propria, and the epithelium.

The majority of the gastrointestinal epithelium is covered by a layer or layers of mucus. This is a viscoelastic translucent aqueous gel that is secreted throughout the gastrointestinal tract, acting as a protective layer and a mechanical barrier. Mucus is a constantly changing mix of many secretions and exfoliated epithelial cells. It has a large water

component (~95%). Its other primary components, which are responsible for its physical and functional properties, are large glycosylated proteins called mucins. Mucins consist of a protein backbone approximately 800 amino acids long and oligosaccharide side chains that are typically up to 18 residues in length.

The mucous layer ranges in thickness from 5 μm to 500 μm along the length of the gastrointestinal tract, with average values of approximately 80 μm.

Mucus is constantly being removed from the luminal surface of the gastrointestinal tract through abrasion and acidic and/or enzymatic breakdown, and it is continually replaced from beneath. The turnover time has been estimated at 4 to 5 hours, but this may well be an underestimate and is liable to vary along the length of the tract.

Oesophagus

The mouth is the point of entry for most drugs (so-called *peroral* – via the mouth – administration). At this point, contact with the oral mucosa is usually brief. Linking the oral cavity to the stomach is the oesophagus. The oesophagus is composed of a thick muscular layer approximately 250 mm long and 20 mm in diameter. It joins the stomach at the gastro-oesophageal junction, or cardiac orifice, as it is sometimes known.

The oesophagus, apart from the lowest 20 mm, which is similar to the gastric mucosa, contains a well-differentiated squamous epithelium of nonproliferative cells. Epithelial cell function is mainly protective; salivary glands in the mouth secrete mucins into the narrow lumen to lubricate food and protect the lower part of the oesophagus from gastric acid. The pH of the oesophageal lumen is usually between 5 and 6.

Materials are moved down the oesophagus by the act of swallowing. After swallowing, a single peristaltic wave of contraction, its amplitude linked to the size of the material being swallowed, passes down the length of the oesophagus at a rate of 20 mm s^{-1} to 60 m s^{-1}, speeding up as it progresses. When swallowing is repeated in quick succession, the subsequent swallows interrupt the initial peristaltic wave and only the final wave proceeds down the length of the oesophagus to the gastrointestinal junction, carrying material within the lumen with it. Secondary peristaltic waves occur involuntarily in response to any distension of the oesophagus and serve to move sticky lumps of material or refluxed material to the stomach. In the upright position, the transit of materials through the oesophagus is assisted by gravity. The oesophageal transit of dosage forms is extremely rapid, usually of the order of 10 to 14 seconds.

Stomach

The next part of the gastrointestinal tract to be encountered by both food and pharmaceuticals is the stomach. The two major functions of the stomach are:

- To act as a temporary reservoir for ingested food and to deliver it to the duodenum at a controlled rate.
- To reduce ingested solids to a uniform creamy consistency, known as chyme, by the action of acid and enzymatic digestion. This enables better contact of the ingested material with the mucous membrane of the intestines and thereby facilitates absorption.

Another, perhaps less obvious, function of the stomach is its protective role in reducing the risk of noxious agents reaching the intestine.

The stomach is the most dilated part of the gastrointestinal tract and is situated between the lower end of the oesophagus and the small intestine. Its opening to the duodenum is controlled by the pyloric sphincter. The stomach can be divided into four anatomical regions (Fig. 19.4): the fundus, the body, the antrum and the pylorus.

The stomach has a capacity of approximately 1.5 L, although under fasting conditions it usually contains no more than 50 mL of fluid, which is mostly gastric secretions. These include:

- Hydrochloric acid secreted by the parietal cells, which maintains the pH of the stomach between 1 and 3.5 in the fasted state.
- The hormone gastrin, which itself is a potent stimulator of gastric acid production and pepsinogen and is released by the G cells in the stomach. The release of gastrin is stimulated by peptides, amino acids and distension of the stomach and causes increased gastric motility.
- Pepsins, which are secreted by the chief cells in the form of its precursor pepsinogen. Pepsins are peptidases which break down proteins to peptides at low pH. Above pH 5, pepsin is denatured.
- Mucus, which is secreted by the surface mucosal cells and lines the gastric mucosa. In the stomach the mucus protects the gastric mucosa from autodigestion by the pepsin–acid combination.

Very little drug absorption occurs in the stomach owing to its small surface area compared to the small intestine. The rate of gastric emptying can be a controlling factor in the onset of drug absorption from the major absorptive site, the small intestine. Gastric emptying will be discussed later in this chapter.

Small intestine

The small intestine is the longest (4 m to 5 m) and most convoluted part of the gastrointestinal tract, extending from the pyloric sphincter of the stomach to the ileocaecal junction, where it joins the large intestine. It is approximately 25 mm to 30 mm in diameter. Its main functions are:

- *digestion* – the process of enzymatic digestion, which began in the stomach, is completed in the small intestine; and
- *absorption* – the small intestine is the region where most nutrients and other materials are absorbed.

The small intestine is divided into the duodenum, which is 200 mm to 300 mm in length, the jejunum, which is approximately 2 m in length, and the ileum, which is approximately 3 m in length.

The wall of the small intestine has a rich network of both blood and lymphatic vessels. The gastro-intestinal circulation is the largest systemic regional

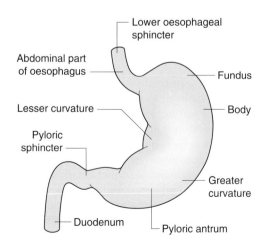

Fig. 19.4 • The anatomy of the stomach.

Lower oesophageal sphincter

Abdominal part of oesophagus

Fundus

Lesser curvature

Body

Pyloric sphincter

Greater curvature

Duodenum

Pyloric antrum

vasculature, and nearly one-third of the cardiac output flows through the gastrointestinal viscera. The blood vessels of the small intestine receive blood from the superior mesenteric artery via branched arterioles. The blood leaving the small intestine flows into the hepatic portal vein, which carries it via the liver to the systemic circulation. Drugs that are metabolized by the liver are degraded before they reach the systemic circulation; this is termed *hepatic presystemic clearance* or *first-pass metabolism*.

The wall of the small intestine also contains lacteals, which contain lymph and are part of the lymphatic system. The lymphatic system is important in the absorption of fats from the gastrointestinal tract. In the ileum there are areas of aggregated lymphoid tissue close to the epithelial surface which are known as Peyer's patches (named after the 17th-century Swiss anatomist Johann Peyer). These cells play a key role in the immune response as they transport macromolecules and are involved in antigen uptake.

The surface area of the small intestine is increased enormously, by approximately 600 times that of a simple cylinder, to approximately 200 m^2 in an adult, by several adaptations which make the small intestine such a good absorption site:

- *Folds of Kerckring* – these are submucosal folds which extend circularly most of the way around the intestine and are particularly well developed in the duodenum and jejunum. They are several millimetres in depth.
- *Villi* – these have been described as finger-like projections into the lumen (approximately 0.5 mm to 1.5 mm in length and 0.1 mm in diameter). They are well supplied with blood vessels. Each villus contains an arteriole, a venule and a blind-ending lymphatic vessel (lacteal). The structure of a villus is shown in Fig. 19.5.
- *Microvilli* – 600 to 1000 of these brush-like structures (~1 μm in length and 0.1 μm in width) cover each villus, providing the largest increase in surface area. These are covered by a fibrous substance known as glycocalyx.

The luminal pH of the small intestine increases to between 6 and 7.5. Sources of secretions that produce these pH values in the small intestine are:

- *Brunner's glands*. These are located in the duodenum and are responsible for the secretion of bicarbonate, which neutralizes the acid emptied from the stomach.

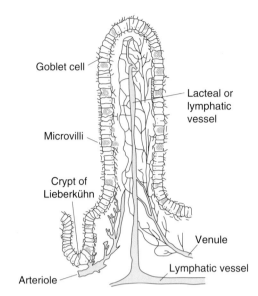

Fig. 19.5 • Structure of a villus.

- *Intestinal cells*. These are present throughout the small intestine and secrete mucus and enzymes. The enzymes, hydrolases and proteases, continue the digestive process.
- *Pancreatic secretions*. The pancreas is a large gland that secretes approximately 1 L to 2 L of pancreatic juice per day into the small intestine via a duct. The components of pancreatic juice are sodium bicarbonate and enzymes. The enzymes consist of proteases, principally trypsin, chymotrypsin and carboxypeptidases, which are secreted as inactive precursors or zymogens and are converted to their active forms in the lumen by the enzyme enterokinase. Lipase and amylase are both secreted in their active forms. The bicarbonate component is largely regulated by the pH of chyme delivered into the small intestine from the stomach.
- *Bile*. Bile is secreted by hepatocytes in the liver into bile canaliculi, concentrated in the gallbladder and hepatic biliary system by the removal of sodium ions, chloride ions and water, and delivered to the duodenum. Bile is a complex aqueous mixture of organic solutes (bile acids, phospholipids, particularly lecithin, cholesterol and bilirubin) and inorganic compounds (such as the plasma electrolytes sodium and potassium). Bile pigments, the most important of which is bilirubin, are excreted in the faeces but the bile acids are reabsorbed by

an active process in the terminal ileum. They are returned to the liver via the hepatic portal vein and, as they have a high hepatic clearance, are resecreted in the bile. This process is known as enterohepatic recirculation. The main functions of the bile are promoting the efficient absorption of dietary fat, such as fatty acids and cholesterol, by aiding its emulsification and micellar solubilization, and the provision of excretory pathways for degradation products.

Colon

The colon is the final major part of the gastrointestinal tract. It stretches from the ileocaecal junction to the anus and makes up approximately the last 1.5 m of the 6 m of the gastrointestinal tract. It is composed of the caecum (~85 mm in length), the ascending colon (~200 mm), the hepatic flexure, the transverse colon (usually longer than 450 mm), the splenic flexure, the descending colon (~300 mm), the sigmoid colon (~400 mm) and the rectum, as shown in Fig. 19.6. The ascending colon and the descending colon are relatively fixed, as they are attached via the flexures and the caecum. The transverse colon and the sigmoid colon are much more flexible.

The colon, unlike the small intestine, has no specialized villi. However, the microvilli of the absorptive epithelial cells, the presence of crypts and the irregularly folded mucosae serve to increase the surface area of the colon by 10 to –15 times that of a simple cylinder. The surface area nevertheless

remains approximately l/30 that of the small intestine.

The main functions of the colon are:

- The absorption of sodium ions, chloride ions and water from the lumen in exchange for bicarbonate and potassium ions. Thus the colon has a significant homeostatic role in the body.
- The storage and compaction of faeces.

The colon is permanently colonized by an extensive number (approximately 10^{12} per gram of contents) and variety of bacteria. This large bacterial mass is capable of several metabolic reactions, including hydrolysis of fatty acid esters and the reduction of inactive conjugated drugs to their active form. The bacteria rely on undigested polysaccharides in the diet and the carbohydrate components of secretions such as mucus for their carbon and energy sources. They degrade the polysaccharides to produce short-chain fatty acids (acetic, propionic and butyric acids), which lower the luminal pH, and the gases hydrogen, carbon dioxide and methane. Thus the pH of the caecum is approximately 6 to 6.5. This increases to approximately 7 to 7.5 towards the distal parts of the colon.

Recently there has been much interest in the exploitation of the enzymes produced by these bacteria with respect to targeted drug delivery to this region of the gastrointestinal tract.

Transit of pharmaceuticals in the gastrointestinal tract

As the oral route is the one by which the majority of pharmaceuticals are administered, it is important to know how these materials behave during their passage through the gastrointestinal tract. It is known that the small intestine is the major site of drug absorption, and thus the time a drug is present in this part of the gastrointestinal tract is extremely important. If sustained-release or controlled-release drug delivery systems are being designed, it is important to consider factors that will affect their behaviour and, in particular, their transit times through certain regions of the gastrointestinal tract.

In general, most dosage forms, when taken in an upright position, transit the oesophagus quickly, usually in less than 15 seconds. Transit through the oesophagus is dependent on both the dosage form and the posture.

Tablets/capsules taken in the supine (lying down) position, especially if taken without water, are liable

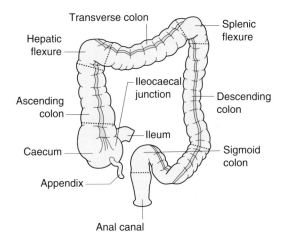

Fig. 19.6 • The anatomy of the colon.

Labels: Transverse colon, Splenic flexure, Hepatic flexure, Ileocaecal junction, Descending colon, Ascending colon, Ileum, Caecum, Sigmoid colon, Appendix, Anal canal

to lodge in the oesophagus. Adhesion to the oesophageal wall can occur as a result of partial dehydration at the site of contact and the formation of a gel between the formulation and the oesophagus. The chances of adhesion will depend on the shape, size and type of formulation. Transit of liquids, for example, has always been observed to be rapid, and in general faster than that of solids. A delay in reaching the stomach may well delay a drug's onset of action or cause damage or irritation to the oesophageal wall (e.g. potassium chloride tablets).

Gastric emptying

The time a dosage form takes to traverse the stomach is usually termed the *gastric residence time, gastric emptying time* or *gastric emptying rate*.

Gastric emptying of pharmaceuticals is highly variable and is dependent on the dosage form and the fed/fasted state of the stomach. Normal gastric residence times usually range between 5 minutes and 2 hours, although much longer times (>12 h) have been recorded, particularly for large single dosage units.

In the fasted state, the electrical activity in the stomach – the interdigestive myoelectric cycle or migrating myoelectric complex (MMC), as it is known – governs its activity and hence the transit of dosage forms. It is characterized by a repeating cycle of four phases. Phase I is a relatively inactive period of 40 to 60 minutes with only rare contractions occurring. Increasing numbers of contractions occur in phase II, which has a similar duration to phase I. Phase III is characterized by powerful peristaltic contractions which open the pylorus at the base and clear the stomach of any residual material. This is sometimes called the *housekeeper wave*. Phase IV is a short transitional period between the powerful activity of phase III and the inactivity of phase I.

The cycle repeats itself every 2 hours until a meal is ingested and the fed state or motility is initiated. In this state, two distinct patterns of activity have been observed. The proximal part of the stomach relaxes to receive food, and gradual contractions of this region move the contents distally. Peristalsis – contractions of the distal part of the stomach – serves to mix and break down food particles and move them towards the pyloric sphincter. The pyloric sphincter allows liquids and small food particles to empty while other material is retropulsed into the antrum of the stomach and is caught up by the next peristaltic wave for further size reduction before emptying.

Thus, in the fed state, liquids, pellets and disintegrated tablets will tend to empty with food, yet large sustained-release or controlled-release dosage forms can be retained in the stomach for long periods. In the fasted state the stomach is less discriminatory between dosage form types, with emptying appearing to be an exponential process and being related to the point in the MMC at which the formulation is ingested.

Many factors influence gastric emptying, as well as the type of dosage form and the presence of food. These include posture, the composition of the food and the effect of drugs and disease state. In general, food, particularly fatty foods, delays gastric emptying and hence the absorption of drugs. Therefore a drug is likely to reach the small intestine most rapidly if it is administered with water to a patient whose stomach is empty.

Small intestinal transit

There are two main types of intestinal movement – propulsive and mixing. The propulsive movements primarily determine the intestinal transit rate and hence the residence time of the drug or dosage form in the small intestine. As this is the main site of absorption in the gastrointestinal tract for most drugs, the small intestinal transit time (i.e. the time of transit between the stomach and the caecum) is an important factor with respect to drug bioavailability.

Small intestinal transit is normally considered to be between 3 and 4 hours, although both faster and slower transits have been measured. In contrast to the stomach, the small intestine does not discriminate between solids and liquids, and hence between dosage forms, or between the fed and the fasted state.

Small intestinal residence time is particularly important for:

- dosage forms that release their drug slowly (e.g. controlled-release, sustained-release or prolonged-release systems) as they pass along the length of the gastrointestinal tract;
- enteric-coated dosage forms which release drug only when they reach the small intestine;
- drugs that dissolve slowly in intestinal fluids;
- drugs that are absorbed by intestinal carrier-mediated transport systems; and
- drugs that are not absorbed well in the colon.

Colonic transit

The colonic transit of pharmaceuticals is prolonged and variable, and depends on the type of dosage form, diet, eating pattern, defecation pattern and frequency, and disease state.

Contractile activity in the colon can be divided into two main types:

- Propulsive contractions or mass movements that are associated with the aboral (away from the mouth) movement of contents.
- Segmental or haustral contractions that serve to mix the luminal contents and result in only small aboral movements. Segmental contractions are brought about by contraction of the circular muscle and predominate, whereas the propulsive contractions, which are due to contractions of the longitudinal muscle, occur only three to four times daily in normal individuals.

Colonic transit is thus characterized by short bursts of activity followed by long periods of stasis. Movement is mainly aboral (i.e. towards the anus). Motility and transit are highly influenced by defecation time; both the frequency of defecation and the likelihood of being included in a defecation event. Colonic transit times can range from 2 to 48 hours. In most individuals, total transit times (i.e. mouth to anus) are between 12 and 36 hours; however, they can range from several hours to several days.

Barriers to drug absorption

Fig. 19.7 shows some of the barriers to absorption that a drug may encounter once it is released from its dosage form and has dissolved in the gastrointestinal fluids. The drug needs to remain in solution, not become bound to food or other material within the gastrointestinal tract and not precipitate. It needs to be chemically stable so as to withstand the pH of the gastrointestinal tract and it must be resistant to enzymatic degradation in the lumen. The drug then needs to diffuse across the mucous layer without binding to it, across the unstirred water layer and subsequently across the gastrointestinal membrane, its main cellular barrier. After passing through this cellular barrier, the drug encounters the liver and all its metabolizing enzymes before it reaches the systemic circulation. Any of these barriers can prevent some or all of the drug reaching the systemic circulation and can therefore have a detrimental effect on its bioavailability.

Environment within the lumen

The environment within the lumen of the gastrointestinal tract has a major effect on the rate and extent of drug absorption.

Gastrointestinal pH

The pH of fluids varies considerably along the length of the gastrointestinal tract. Gastric fluid is highly

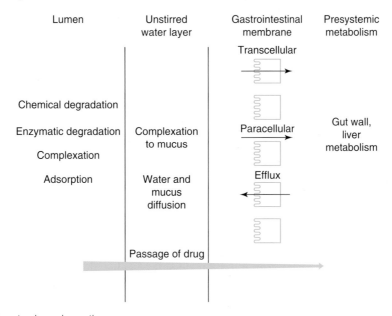

Fig. 19.7 • Barriers to drug absorption.

acidic, normally exhibiting a pH within the range from 1 to 3.5 in healthy people in the fasted state. Following the ingestion of a meal, the gastric juice is buffered to a less acidic pH that is dependent on meal composition. Typical gastric pH values following a meal are in the range from 3 to 7. Depending on the size of the meal, the gastric pH returns to the lower fasted-state values within 2 to 3 hours. Thus only a dosage form ingested with or soon after a meal will encounter these higher pH values. This may be an important consideration in terms of the chemical stability of a drug or in achieving drug dissolution or absorption.

Intestinal pH values are higher than gastric pH values owing to the neutralization of the gastric acid by bicarbonate ions secreted by the pancreas into the small intestine. There is a gradual rise in pH along the length of the small intestine from the duodenum to the ileum. Table 19.1 summarizes some of the literature values recorded for small intestinal pH in the fed and fasted states. The pH drops again in the colon as the bacterial enzymes, which are localized in the colonic region, break down undigested carbohydrates into short-chain fatty acids; this lowers the pH in the colon to approximately 6.5.

The gastrointestinal pH may influence the absorption of drugs in a variety of ways. If the drug is a weak electrolyte, the pH may influence the drug's chemical stability in the lumen, its rate and extent of dissolution or its absorption characteristics. Chemical degradation due to pH-dependent hydrolysis can occur in the gastrointestinal tract. The result of this instability is incomplete bioavailability, as only a fraction of the administered dose reaches the systemic circulation in the form of intact drug. The extent of

degradation of penicillin G (benzylpenicillin), the first of the penicillins, after oral administration depends on its residence time in the stomach and the gastric pH. This gastric instability has tended to preclude its oral use. The antibiotic erythromycin and proton pump inhibitors (e.g. omeprazole) degrade rapidly at acidic pH values and therefore have to be formulated as enteric-coated dosage forms to ensure good bioavailability (see Chapter 20). The effects of pH on the drug dissolution and absorption processes are also discussed in Chapter 20.

Luminal enzymes

The primary enzyme found in gastric juice is pepsin. Lipases, amylases and proteases are secreted from the pancreas into the small intestine in response to ingestion of food. These enzymes are responsible for most nutrient digestion. Pepsins and the proteases are responsible for the degradation of protein and peptide drugs in the lumen. Other drugs that resemble nutrients, such as nucleotides and fatty acids, may also be susceptible to enzymatic degradation. The lipases may also affect the release of drugs from fat/oil-containing dosage forms. Drugs that are esters can also be susceptible to hydrolysis in the lumen.

Bacteria, which are mainly localized within the colonic region of the gastrointestinal tract, secrete enzymes that are capable of a range of reactions. These enzymes have been utilized when designing drugs or dosage forms to target the colon. Sulfasalazine, for example, is a prodrug of 5-aminosalicylic acid linked via an azo bond to sulfapyridine. The sulfapyridine moiety makes the drug too large and hydrophilic to be absorbed in the upper gastrointestinal tract, and thus permits its transport intact to the colonic region. Here the bacterial enzymes reduce the azo bond in the molecule and release the active drug, 5-aminosalicylic acid, for local action in colonic diseases such as inflammatory bowel disease.

Influence of food in the gastrointestinal tract

The presence of food in the gastrointestinal tract can influence the rate and extent of absorption, either directly or indirectly via a range of mechanisms.

Complexation of drugs with components in the diet. Drugs are capable of binding to components within the diet. In general, this only becomes an

Table 19.1 pH in the small intestine in healthy humans in the fasted and fed states

Location	Fasted state pH	Fed state pH
Mid to distal part of duodenum	4.9	5.2
	6.1	5.4
	6.3	5.1
	6.4	
Jejunum	4.4–6.5	5.2–6.0
	6.6	6.2
Ileum	6.5	6.8–7.8
	6.8–8.0	6.8–8.0
	7.4	7.5

Data from Gray & Dressman (1996).

issue (with respect to bioavailability) where an irreversible or an insoluble complex is formed. In such cases the fraction of the administered dose that becomes complexed is unavailable for absorption. Tetracycline, for example, forms nonabsorbable complexes with calcium and iron, and thus patients are advised not to take products containing calcium or iron, such as milk, iron preparations or indigestion remedies, at the same time of day as the tetracycline. However, if the complex formed is water soluble and readily dissociates to liberate the 'free' drug, then there may be little effect on drug absorption.

Alteration of pH. In general, food tends to increase stomach pH by acting as a buffer. This is liable to decrease the rate of dissolution and subsequent absorption of a weakly basic drug and increase that of a weakly acidic one.

Alteration of gastric emptying. As already mentioned, some foods, particularly those containing a high proportion of fat, and some drugs tend to reduce gastric emptying and thus delay the onset of action of certain drugs. Food slows the rate of absorption, due to delayed gastric emptying, of the antiretroviral nucleoside analogues lamivudine and zidovudine; however, this is not considered to be clinically significant.

Stimulation of gastrointestinal secretions. Gastrointestinal secretions (e.g. pepsin) produced in response to food may result in the degradation of drugs that are susceptible to enzymatic metabolism and hence in a reduction in their bioavailability. The ingestion of food, particularly fats, stimulates the secretion of bile. Bile salts are surface-active agents and can increase the dissolution of poorly soluble drugs, thereby enhancing their absorption. However, bile salts have been shown to form insoluble and hence nonabsorbable complexes with some drugs such as neomycin, kanamycin and nystatin.

Competition between food components and drugs for specialized absorption mechanisms. In the case of those drugs that have a chemical structure similar to nutrients required by the body for which specialized absorption mechanisms exist, there is a possibility of competitive inhibition of drug absorption.

Increased viscosity of gastrointestinal tract contents. The presence of food in the gastrointestinal tract provides a viscous environment which may result in a reduction in the rate of drug dissolution. In addition, the rate of diffusion of a drug in solution from the lumen to the absorbing membrane lining the gastrointestinal tract may be reduced by an increase in viscosity. Both of these effects tend to decrease the bioavailability of a drug.

Food-induced changes in presystemic metabolism. Certain foods may increase the bioavailability of drugs that are susceptible to presystemic intestinal metabolism by interacting with the metabolic process. Grapefruit juice, for example, is capable of inhibiting the intestinal cytochrome P450 3A (CYP3A) family and thus, when taken with drugs that are susceptible to CYP3A metabolism, is likely to result in their increased bioavailability. Clinically relevant interactions exist between grapefruit juice and the antihistamine terfenadine, the immunosuppressant ciclosporin, the protease inhibitor saquinavir and the calcium channel blocker verapamil.

Food-induced changes in blood flow. Blood flow to the gastrointestinal tract and liver increases shortly after a meal, thereby increasing the rate at which drugs are presented to the liver. The metabolism of some drugs (e.g. propranolol) is sensitive to their rate of presentation to the liver; the faster the rate of presentation, the larger the fraction of drug that escapes first-pass metabolism. This is because the enzyme systems responsible for drug metabolism become saturated by the increased rate of presentation of the drug to the site of biotransformation. For this reason, the effects of food serve to increase the bioavailability of some drugs that are susceptible to first-pass metabolism.

It is evident that food can influence the absorption of many drugs from the gastrointestinal tract by a variety of mechanisms. Drug–food interactions are often classified into five categories: those that cause reduced, delayed, increased or accelerated absorption, and those on which food has no effect. The reader is referred to reviews by Varum et al. (2013) and Yasuji et al. (2012) for the effect of food on drug absorption and delivery.

Disease state and physiological disorders

Disease states and physiological disorders associated with the gastrointestinal tract are likely to influence the absorption and hence the bioavailability of orally administered drugs. Local diseases can cause alterations in gastric pH that can affect the stability, dissolution and/or absorption of the drug. Gastric surgery can cause drugs to exhibit differences in bioavailability from that in normal individuals. For example, partial or total gastrectomy results in drugs reaching the duodenum more rapidly than in normal individuals, and significant changes in fluid composition and volumes can significantly affect drug dissolution and therefore bioavailability. Patients with AIDS often have oversecretion of gastrin and thus low pH, which can adversely affect the dissolution and hence bioavailability of weakly basic drugs such as the antifungal drug ketoconazole. Lower pH values are often seen in disease states of the colon such as Crohn's disease and ulcerative colitis. In coeliac disease there is an increase in intestinal permeability due to a 'loosening' of the tight junctions.

Mucus and the unstirred water layer

Before drugs can permeate across the epithelial surface, the mucous layer and unstirred water layer need to be crossed. The mucus layer, whose thickness and turnover rates can vary along the length of the gastrointestinal tract, can hinder drug diffusion. The unstirred water layer or aqueous boundary layer is a more or less stagnant layer of water, mucus and glycocalyx adjacent to the intestinal wall. It is thought to be created by incomplete mixing of the luminal contents near the intestinal mucosal surface. This layer, which is approximately 30 µm to 100 µm in thickness, can provide a diffusion barrier to drugs. Some drugs are also capable of complexing with mucus, thereby reducing their availability for absorption.

Gastrointestinal membrane

Structure of the membrane

The gastrointestinal membrane separates the lumen of the stomach and intestines from the systemic circulation. It is the main cellular barrier to the absorption of drugs from the gastrointestinal tract. The membrane is complex in nature, being composed of lipids, proteins, lipoproteins and polysaccharides. It has a bilayer structure, as shown in Fig. 19.8. The barrier has the characteristics of a semipermeable membrane, allowing the rapid transit of some materials and impeding or preventing the passage of others. It

EXTRACELLULAR FLUID

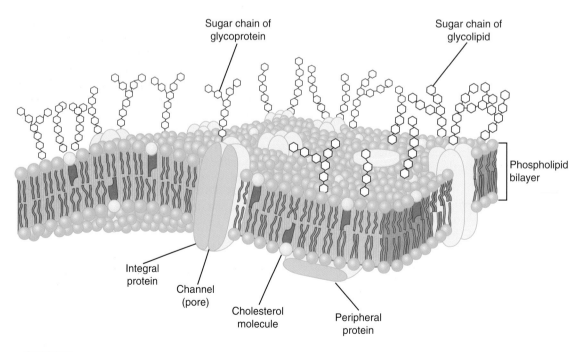

Sugar chain of glycoprotein

Sugar chain of glycolipid

Phospholipid bilayer

Integral protein

Channel (pore)

Cholesterol molecule

Peripheral protein

CYTOSOL

Fig. 19.8 • Structure of the gastrointestinal membrane.

is permeable to amino acids, sugars, fatty acids and other nutrients and is impermeable to plasma proteins. The membrane can be viewed as a semipermeable lipoidal sieve, which allows the passage of lipid-soluble molecules across it and the passage of water and small hydrophilic molecules through its numerous aqueous pores. In addition, there are a number of transporter proteins or membrane transporters that exist in the membrane and which, with the help of energy, transport materials back and forth across it.

Mechanisms of transport across the gastrointestinal membrane

There are two main mechanisms of drug transport across the gastrointestinal epithelium: transcellular (i.e. across the cells) and paracellular (i.e. between the cells). The transcellular pathway is further divided into simple passive diffusion, carrier-mediated or membrane transporter processes and transcytosis. These pathways are illustrated in Fig. 19.9.

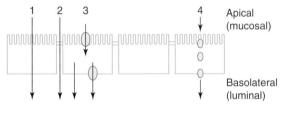

1 – Transcellular   3 – Carrier mediated
2 – Paracellular   4 – Transcytosis

Fig. 19.9 • Mechanisms of transport (absorptive).

Transcellular transport

Passive diffusion

This is the preferred route of transport for relatively small lipophilic molecules and thus many drugs. In this process, drug molecules pass across the lipoidal membrane via passive diffusion from a region of high concentration in the lumen to a region of lower concentration in the blood. This lower concentration is maintained primarily by blood flow. The rate of transport is determined by the physicochemical properties of the drug, the nature of the membrane and the concentration gradient of the drug across the membrane. The process initially involves the partitioning of the drug between the aqueous fluids within the gastrointestinal tract and the lipoidal-like membrane of the lining of the epithelium. The drug in solution in the membrane then diffuses across the epithelial cell(s) within the gastrointestinal barrier to blood in the capillary network in the lamina propria. On reaching the blood, the drug will be rapidly distributed, so maintaining a much lower concentration than that at the absorption site. If the cell membranes and fluid regions making up the gastrointestinal tract can be considered as a single membrane, then the stages involved in gastrointestinal absorption can be represented by the model shown in Fig. 19.10.

Passive diffusion of drugs across the gastrointestinal tract can often be described mathematically by Fick's first law of diffusion (see Chapter 2). When considered in the context of bioavailability, this indicates that the rate of diffusion across a membrane (dC/dt) is proportional to the difference in concentration on each side of that membrane. Therefore the rate of

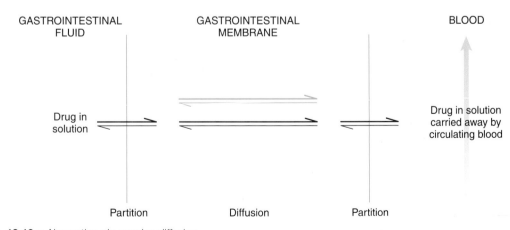

Fig. 19.10 • Absorption via passive diffusion.

appearance of drug in the blood at the absorption site is given by

$$dC/dt = k(C_g - C_b)$$

(19.1)

where dC/dt is the rate of appearance of drug in the blood at the site of absorption, k is the proportionality constant, C_g is the concentration of drug in solution in the gastrointestinal fluid at the absorption site and C_b is the concentration of drug in the blood at the site of absorption.

The proportionality constant k incorporates the diffusion coefficient of the drug in the gastrointestinal membrane (D), and the thickness (h) and surface area of the membrane (A):

$$k = \frac{DA}{h}$$

(19.2)

These equations indicate that the rate of gastro-intestinal absorption of a drug by passive diffusion depends on the surface area of the membrane that is available for drug absorption. Thus the small intestine, primarily the duodenum, is the major site of drug absorption, owing principally to the presence of villi and microvilli, which provide such a large surface area for absorption (discussed earlier in this chapter).

Eq. 19.1 also indicates that the rate of drug absorption depends on a large concentration gradient of drug existing across the gastrointestinal membrane. This concentration gradient is influenced by the apparent partition coefficients exhibited by the drug with respect to the gastrointestinal membrane–fluid interface and the gastrointestinal membrane–blood interface. It is important that the drug has sufficient affinity (solubility) for the membrane phase so that it can partition readily into the gastrointestinal membrane. In addition, after diffusing across the membrane, the drug should exhibit sufficient solubility in the blood such that it can partition readily out of the membrane phase into the blood.

On entering the blood in the capillary network in the lamina propria, the drug will be carried away from the site of absorption by the rapidly circulating gastrointestinal blood supply. It will then become diluted by distribution into a large volume of blood (i.e. the systemic circulation), by distribution into body tissues and other fluids, and by subsequent metabolism and excretion. In addition, the drug may bind to plasma proteins in the blood, which will

further lower the concentration of free (i.e. diffusible) drug in the blood. Consequently, the blood acts as a 'sink' for absorbed drug and ensures that the concentration of drug in the blood at the site of absorption is low in relation to that in the gastro-intestinal fluids at the site of absorption (i.e. $C_g \gg C_b$). The 'sink' conditions provided by the systemic circulation ensure that a large concentration gradient is maintained across the gastrointestinal membrane during the absorption process.

The passive absorption process is driven solely by the concentration gradient of the diffusible species of the drug that exists across the gastrointestinal tract. Thus Eqs 19.1 and 19.2 can be combined and written as

$$dC/dt = \frac{DAC_g}{h}$$

(19.3)

and because for a given membrane D, A and h can be regarded as constants, Eq. 19.3 becomes

$$dC/dt = kC_g$$

(19.4)

Eq. 19.4 is an expression for a first-order kinetics process (discussed in Chapter 7) and indicates that the rate of passive absorption will be proportional to the concentration of absorbable drug in solution in the gastrointestinal fluids at the site of absorption and therefore that the gastrointestinal absorption of most drugs follows first-order kinetics.

It has been assumed in this description that the drug exists solely as one single absorbable species. Many drugs, however, are weak electrolytes that exist in aqueous solution as two species: namely, the un-ionized species and the ionized species. Because it is the un-ionized form of a weak electrolyte drug that exhibits greater lipid solubility compared to than the corresponding ionized form, the gastrointestinal membrane is more permeable to the un-ionized species. Thus the rate of passive absorption of a weak electrolyte is related to the fraction of total drug that exists in the un-ionized form in solution in the gastrointestinal fluids at the site of absorption. This fraction is determined by the dissociation constant of the drug (i.e. its pK_a value) and by the pH of the aqueous environment, in accordance with the Henderson–Hasselbalch equations for weak acids and bases (discussed in Chapter 3). The gastrointestinal absorption of a weak electrolyte drug is enhanced

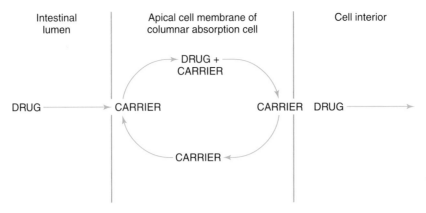

Fig. 19.11 • Active transport of a drug across a cell membrane.

when the pH at the site of absorption favours the formation of a large fraction of the drug in aqueous solution that is un-ionized. This forms the basis of the pH-partition hypothesis (see Chapter 20).

Membrane transporters

As already stated, the majority of drugs are absorbed across cells (i.e. transcellularly) by passive diffusion. However, certain compounds and many nutrients are absorbed transcellularly via membrane transporters.

A carrier or membrane transporter is responsible for binding a drug and transporting it across the membrane by a process illustrated in Fig. 19.11. Simplistically, carrier-mediated absorption is often explained by our assuming there is a shuttling process across the epithelial membrane. The drug molecule or ion forms a complex with the carrier/transporter in the surface of the apical cell membrane of the polarized enterocyte. The drug–carrier complex then moves across the membrane and liberates the drug on the other side of the membrane. The carrier (now free) returns to its initial position in the surface of the cell membrane adjacent to the gastrointestinal tract to await the arrival of another drug molecule or ion.

Membrane transport can be divided into *active transport* and *facilitated transport*. *Active transport* requires energy and is a process whereby materials can be transported against a concentration gradient across a cell membrane, i.e. transport can occur from a region of lower concentration to one of higher concentration. The energy arises either from the hydrolysis of ATP or from the transmembranous sodium gradient and/or electrical potential. *Facilitated transport* allows the passage of solutes (e.g. glucose,

amino acids, urea) across membranes down their electrochemical gradients and without energy expenditure. When substances are transported by facilitated transport, they are transported down the concentration gradient, but at a much faster rate than would be anticipated from the molecular size and polarity of the molecule. *Facilitated transport* differs from active transport in that it cannot transport a substance against a concentration gradient of that substance.

There are a large number of membrane transporters in the small intestine. More than 400 have been identified but only a few are thought to be involved in intestinal absorption. These can be present either on the apical membrane (brush border) or on the basolateral membrane of the enterocyte and can be classed as uptake or efflux transporters depending on the direction of transport. They have been classified into two main superfamilies; the solute carrier (SLC) family, members of which are the main uptake transporters, and the ATP-binding cassette (ABC) transporters, which are the main efflux transporters. These are illustrated schematically in Fig. 19.12. Uptake and efflux transporters, the gene that codes for them, their substrate specificity and examples of drug substrates are detailed in Tables 19.2 and 19.3.

Members of the SLC family of transporters are involved in the transport of many substrates, including amino acids, peptides, the nucleosides, sugars, bile acids, neurotransmitters and vitamins. Many nutrients are actively transported in this way. Each carrier system is generally concentrated in a specific segment of the gastrointestinal tract. The substance that is transported by that carrier will thus be absorbed preferentially in the location of highest carrier density. For example, the bile acid transporters are only found

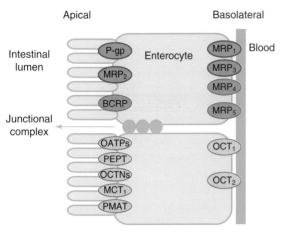

Fig. 19.12 • Major drug transporter proteins expressed at the intestinal epithelia, including intestinal uptake *(bottom)* and efflux *(top)* transporters. *BRCP,* Breast cancer resistance protein; *MCT,* monocarboxylate transporter; *MRP,* multidrug-resistance-associated protein; *OATPs,* organic anion transporting polypeptides; *OCT,* organic cation transporter; *OCTNs,* organic cation/carnitine transporters; *PEPT,* peptide transporter protein; *P-gp,* P-glycoprotein (multidrug resistance protein 1); *PMAT,* plasma membrane monoamine transporter.

in the lower part of the small intestine, the ileum. Each carrier/transporter has its own substrate specificity with respect to the chemical structure of the substance that it will transport. Some carriers/transporters have broader specificity than others. Thus if a drug structurally resembles a natural substance which is actively transported, then the drug is also likely to be transported by the same carrier mechanism.

The SLC superfamily includes many important transporters for drug absorption and drug disposition, such as proton-dependent oligopeptide transporters (e.g. peptide transporter proteins 1 PEPT1 and PEPT2), organic anion transporters (e.g. OAT), organic cation transporters (e.g. OCT), nucleoside transporters, plasma membrane monoamine transporter (PMAT) and the monocarboxylate transporters (MCT). The SLCO family is made up of the organic anion transporting polypeptides (e.g. OATP). These uptake transporters use a variety of porter mechanisms (i.e. uniporter, antiporter, symporter). Uniporters bind and transport only one type of substrate at a time. Symporters and antiporters are active transporters which can move more than one type of substrate at once, usually a drug molecule and a metal ion. Symporters (or cotransporters) transport ions and substrates simultaneously in the same direction, while antiporters (or counter transporters) simultaneously transport ions in one direction and substrates in the opposite direction. As the driving force for symporters and antiporters is voltage or ion gradients (usually sodium), they are also called ion-couple solute transporters; however, as the driving force for these transporters is voltage (H^+) or sodium, they can also be known as secondary active transporters. A number of substrates can usually bind to a transporter, and thus different drugs can compete for the same transporter. Thus the transporter can be inhibited, competitively, noncompetitively or uncompetitively. Competitive inhibition occurs when both the substrate and the inhibitor compete for the same binding site. Noncompetitive inhibition occurs when the inhibitor binds not to the transporter active site but to an allosteric site, which lowers the affinity of the transporter for the substrate due to changing the conformation of the transporter. Uncompetitive binding occurs when the inhibitor binds to the intermediate of the substrate–transporter complex to terminate the translocation step.

Many peptide-like drugs, such as the penicillins, cephalosporins, angiotensin-converting enzyme (ACE) inhibitors and renin inhibitors, rely on the peptide transporters for their efficient absorption. Nucleosides and their analogues for antiviral and anticancer drugs depend on the nucleoside transporters for their uptake. L-dopa (levodopa) and α-methyldopa are transported by the carrier-mediated process for amino acids. L-dopa has a much faster permeation rate than methyldopa, which has been attributed to the lower affinity of methyldopa for the amino acid carrier.

The most investigated transporters in the intestine are the ABC family of *efflux* transporters, P-glycoprotein (P-gp), multidrug-resistance-associated protein 2 (MRP 2) and breast cancer resistance protein (BCRP). These transporters are highly abundant at the apical (luminal) membrane of enterocytes, and many drugs, such as the statins, antibiotics, HIV protease inhibitors, immunosuppressants, anticancer drugs and cardiac drugs, have been shown to be substrates of these efflux transporters, and therefore their effective intestinal absorption is limited and there is a detrimental effect on bioavailability. Members of this ABC superfamily use ATP as an energy source, allowing them to pump substrates against a concentration gradient. Drugs can be simultaneously substrates and inhibitors of more than one efflux transporter, suggesting that ABC transporters exert a combined role in

Table 19.2 Drug uptake transporters and their substrates in the small intestine

Drug transporter	Gene family	Intestinal localization	Substrate specificity	Drug substrates
PEPT1	SLC15A	Apical	Dipeptides and tripeptides	Cephalosporins, penicillins, enalapril, renin inhibitors, thrombin inhibitors, bestatin
OCTN1	SLC22A	Apical	Carnitine and organic cations	Quinidine, verapamil
OCTN2	SLC22A	Apical	Carnitine and organic cations	Quinidine, verapamil, cephaloridine, imatinib, ipratropium, valproic acid, spironolactone
OCT1/OCT2	SLC22A	Basal	Low molecular weight organic cations	Metformin, acyclovir, zalcitabine, memantine, ranitidine
PMAT	SLC29	Apical	Organic cations	Serotonin, dopamine, adrenaline, noradrenaline, guanidine, histamine, metformin
OATP2B1	SLCO	Apical	Organic anions	Pravastatin, rosuvastatin, atorvastatin, pitavastatin, fexofenadine, mesalazine, glyburide, taurocholate, aliskiren
OATP1A2	SLCO	Apical	Organic anions	Bile salts, thyroid hormones, prostaglandin E_2, fexofenadine, opioid peptides, talinolol, celiprolol, atenolol, ciprofloxacin
MCT1	SLC16	Apical	Unbranched aliphatic and substituted monocarboxylates	Foscarnet, mevalonic acid, salicylic acid, carbenicillin indanyl sodium, phenethicillin, propicillin

Data from Estudante et al. (2013).
MCT1, monocarboxylate transporter 1; OATP1A2, organic anion transporter 1A2; OATP2B1, organic anion transporter 2B1; OCT1, organic cation transporter 1; OCT2, organic cation transporter 2; OCTN1, organic cation transporter 1; OCTN2, organic cation transporter 2; PEPT1, peptide transporter protein 1; PMAT, plasma membrane monoamine transporter.

detoxification in the intestine. In addition, drugs can either downregulate or induce these transporters, which can result in drug–drug interactions if other drugs are coadministered.

Unlike passive absorption, where the rate of absorption is directly proportional to the concentration of the absorbable species of the drug at the absorption site, active transport proceeds at a rate that is proportional to the drug concentration only at low concentrations. At higher concentrations, the carrier mechanism becomes saturated, and further increases in drug concentration will not increase the rate of absorption, i.e. the rate of absorption remains constant. Absorption rate–concentration relationships for active and passive processes are compared in Fig. 19.13.

Competition between two similar substances for the same transfer mechanism and the inhibition of absorption of one or both compounds and temperature dependence are characteristics of carrier-mediated

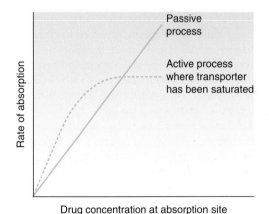

Fig. 19.13 • Relationship between rate of absorption and concentration at the absorption site for active and passive processes.

Table 19.3 Drug efflux transporters and their substrates in the small intestine

Drug transporter	Gene	Intestinal localization	Substrate specificity	Example drug substrates
MDR1/P-gp	*ABCB1*	Apical	Broad with preference for hydrophobic, amphipathic or cationic molecules	Steroid hormones, doxorubicin, daunorubicin, reserpine, vincristine, vinblastine, valinomycin, ciclosporin tacrolimus, tandutinib, aldosterone, hydrocortisone, dibucaine, talinolol, digoxin, ivermectin, paclitaxel, grepafloxacin, indinavir, nelfinavir, saquinavir, grepafloxacin, colchicine, darunavir, imatinib, methotrexate, mitoxantrone, prazosin, temocapril, SN-38
BCRP/MXR	*ABCG2*	Apical	Broad – acids and drug conjugates	Topotecan, irinotecan, SN-38, mitoxantrone, doxorubicin, daunorubicin, imatinib, gefitinib, tandutinib, prazosin, glyburide, dipyridamole, quercetin, temocapril, nitrofurantoin, zidovudine, lamivudine, efavirenz, ciprofloxacin, rifampicin, sulfasalazine, quercetin, methotrexate, gefitinib, rosuvastatin, atorvastatin, fluvastatin, simvastatin lactone
MRP1	*ABCC1*	Basal	Hydrophobic drugs, conjugates to glutathione, glucuronic acid or sulfate	Vinca alkaloids, anthracyclines, etoposide, teniposide, mitoxantrone, methotrexate
MRP2	*ABCC2*	Apical	Glutathione, glucuronide, sulfate and heavy metal conjugates, unconjugated organic anions	Vinblastine, irinotecan, SN-38, pravastatin, ceftriaxone, ampicillin, grepafloxacin, sulfasalazine, fexofenadine, lopinavir, fosinopril

Data from Estudante et al. (2013).
BCRP, breast cancer resistance protein; MDR1, multidrug resistance protein 1; MDR2, multidrug resistance protein 2; MRP1, multidrug-resistance-associated protein 1, MXR, mitoxantrone-resistance protein; P-gp, P-glycoprotein.

transport. Inhibition of absorption may also be observed with agents that interfere with cell metabolism. Some substances may be absorbed by simultaneous carrier-mediated and passive transport processes. The contribution of the carrier-mediated process to the overall absorption rate decreases with concentration, and at a sufficiently high concentration is negligible.

Membrane transporters play an important role in the pharmacokinetics, safety and efficacy of drugs. Transporters are the gatekeepers for cells and organelles, controlling uptake and efflux of crucial compounds such as sugars, amino acids, nucleotides, inorganic ions and drugs. For example, the P-glycoproteins were discovered because of their ability to cause multidrug resistance in tumour cells, preventing the intracellular accumulation of many cytotoxic cancer drugs by pumping the drugs back out of the tumours. Specific membrane transporters are expressed in the luminal and/or basolateral membranes of enterocytes, hepatocytes, renal tubular epithelial cells and other important barrier tissues, including the blood–brain barrier, blood–testis barrier and the placental barrier. Factors affecting membrane transporters in the intestine and the liver, which are the major organs a drug passes through before reaching the systemic circulation after an oral dose, will be important determinants of drug pharmacokinetics and bioavailability. Regulatory elements controlling protein levels, genetic polymorphisms leading to increased or reduced function, and coadministration with inhibitors are all important factors which will affect a transporter's ability to transport substrates.

Transcytosis

Transcytosis is a mechanism for transcellular transport in which a cell encloses extracellular material via an invagination of the cell membrane to form a vesicle (endocytosis), then moves the vesicle across the cell to eject the material through the opposite cell membrane by the reverse process (exocytosis). This is the process by which macromolecules, such as proteins or particles, are absorbed; it is not an important route for oral absorption of drugs that are in solution. Endocytosis can be further subdivided into four main processes: clathrin-mediated endocytosis, macropinocytosis, caveolin-mediated endocytosis and phagocytosis. Nanoparticles have been shown to be absorbed to a greater extent than microparticles, and there has been much debate whether this mechanism of uptake could be exploited further for peptide and protein drugs.

Transcytosis is also a means by which some viruses, bacteria and prion proteins can gain entry to the lymphatic system through absorption by enterocytes and specialized cells (M cells) in the gut-associated lymphoid tissue (GALT).

Paracellular pathway

The paracellular pathway differs from all the other absorption pathways as it is the transport of materials in the aqueous pores between the cells rather than across them. The cells are joined together via closely fitting tight junctions on their apical side. The intercellular spaces occupy only approximately 0.01% of the total surface area of the epithelium. The tightness of these junctions can differ considerably between different epithelia in the body. In general, absorptive epithelia, such as the epithelium of the small intestine, tend to be leakier than other epithelia. The paracellular pathway decreases in importance down the length of the gastrointestinal tract and as the number and size of the pores between the epithelial cells decrease.

The paracellular route of absorption is important for the transport of ions such as calcium ions and for the transport of sugars (e.g. mannitol), amino acids and peptides at concentrations above the capacity of their carriers. Small hydrophilic charged drugs (log $P < 0$) that do not distribute themselves into cell membranes cross the gastrointestinal epithelium via the paracellular pathway. The molecular mass cut-off for the paracellular route is usually considered to be 250 Da, although some larger drugs have been shown to be absorbed via this route. Drugs absorbed by the paracellular route include the H_2-antagonist cimetidine, the antidiarrheal loperamide, the β-blocker atenolol and the bisphosphonate tiludronate.

The paracellular pathway can be divided into convective ('solvent drag') and diffusive components. The convective component is the rate at which the compound is carried across the epithelium via the water flux.

In summary, drugs can be absorbed via passive diffusion, via membrane transporters or carrier-mediated pathways, paracellular transport or transcytosis. A drug can cross the intestinal epithelium via one pathway or a combination of pathways. The relative contribution of these pathways depends on the drug's location within the gastrointestinal tract, the formulation and the physicochemical properties of the drug, which are discussed in Chapter 20.

Presystemic metabolism

As well as having the ability to cross the gastrointestinal membrane by one of the routes described, drugs also need to be resistant to degradation and/or metabolism during this passage. All drugs that are absorbed from the stomach, small intestine and upper part of the colon pass into the hepatic portal system are exposed to the liver before reaching the systemic circulation. Therefore if the drug is going to be available to the systemic circulation, it must also be resistant to metabolism by the liver. Hence an oral dose of drug could be completely absorbed but incompletely available to the systemic circulation because of *first-pass* or *presystemic* metabolism by the gut wall and/or liver.

Gut wall metabolism

The gut walls contain a number of metabolizing enzymes that can degrade drugs before they reach the systemic circulation. For example, the major cytochrome P450 enzyme CYP3A, present in the liver and responsible for the hepatic metabolism of many drugs, is present in the intestinal mucosa, and intestinal metabolism may be important for substrates of this enzyme. This effect is also known as *first-pass metabolism by the intestine*. Cytochrome P450 levels tend to be higher in the intestine than in the colon.

Hepatic metabolism

The liver is the primary site of drug metabolism and thus acts as a final barrier for oral absorption. The first pass of absorbed drug through the liver may result in extensive metabolism of the drug, and a significant portion may never reach the systemic circulation, resulting in a low bioavailability of those drugs which are rapidly metabolized by the liver. The bioavailability of a susceptible drug may be reduced to such an extent as to render the gastrointestinal route of administration ineffective, or to necessitate an oral dose which is many times larger than the intravenous dose (e.g. propranolol). Although propranolol is well absorbed, only approximately 30% of an oral dose is available to the systemic circulation owing to the first-pass effect. The bioavailability of sustained-release propranolol is even less as the drug is presented via the hepatic portal vein more slowly than from an immediate-release dosage form, and the liver is therefore capable of extracting and metabolizing a larger portion. Other drugs which are susceptible to a large first-pass effect are the cholesterol-lowering agent atorvastatin, the anaesthetic lidocaine (lignocaine), the tricyclic antidepressant imipramine, diazepam and the analgesics pentazocine and morphine.

First-pass metabolism can be avoided by drug administration via the mouth (buccal or sublingual; see Chapter 30) or via the rectum (see Chapter 41).

The arrangement of the blood vessels in these regions means that absorbed drug does not pass through the liver first, before entering the systemic circulation.

Summary

There are many physiological factors that influence the rate and extent of drug absorption; these are initially dependent on the route of administration. For the oral route, the physiological and environmental factors of the gastrointestinal tract, the gastrointestinal membrane and presystemic metabolism can all influence drug bioavailability.

Please check your eBook at **https://studentconsult.inkling.com/** for self-assessment questions. See inside cover for registration details.

References

Estudante, M., Morais, J.G., Soveral, G., et al., 2013. Intestinal drug transporters: an overview. Adv. Drug Deliv. Rev. 65, 1340–1356.

Gray, V., Dressman, J., 1996. Change of pH requirements for simulated intestinal fluid TS. Pharmacopeial Forum 22, 1943–1945.

Varum, F.J.O., Hatton, G.B., Basit, A.W., 2013. Food, physiology and drug delivery. Int. J. Pharm. 457, 446–460.

Yasuji, T., Kondo, H., Sako, K., 2012. The effect of food on the oral bioavailability of drugs: a review of current developments and

pharmaceutical technologies for pharmacokinetic control. Ther. Deliv. 3, 81–90.

Bibliography

El-Kattan, A., Varma, M., 2012. Oral absorption, intestinal metabolism and human oral bioavailability. In: Paxton, J. (Ed.), Topics on Drug Metabolism. InTech, Rijeka.

Hu, M., Li, X. (Eds.), 2011. Bioavailability: Basic Principles, Advanced Concepts, and Applications. John Wiley & Sons, Hoboken.

McConnell, E.L., Fadda, H.M., Basit, A.W., 2008. Gut instincts: explorations in intestinal physiology and drug delivery. Int. J. Pharm. 34, 213–226.

Sugano, K., Kansy, M., Artursson, P., et al., 2010. Coexistence of passive and carrier-mediated processes in transport. Nat. Rev. Drug Discov. 9, 597–614.

Bioavailability – physicochemical and dosage form factors

20

Marianne Ashford

CHAPTER CONTENTS

KEY POINTS

- There are a number of factors influencing the bioavailability of a drug; these include the properties of the drug itself and the properties of the dosage form in which the drug is administered.
- Important drug properties are solubility and dissolution rate, and these can be influenced by the pH and environment in which a drug dissolves and the surface area of the drug.
- Lipid solubility and drug dissociation affect drug absorption.
- Drugs need to be in solution before they are absorbed.
- The type of dosage form and the choice of excipients within the dosage form affect the dissolution and hence the bioavailability of a drug.

Introduction

As discussed in Chapter 19, the rate and extent of drug absorption are influenced by the physiological factors associated with the structure and function of the gastrointestinal tract. This chapter discusses the physicochemical properties of the drug and dosage form factors that influence bioavailability. For a drug to be absorbed, it needs to be in solution and to be able to pass across the membrane. In the case of orally administered drugs, this is the gastrointestinal epithelium. The physicochemical properties of the drug that will influence its passage into solution and transfer across membranes include its dissolution rate, pK_a, lipid solubility, chemical stability and complexation potential.

Physicochemical factors influencing bioavailability

Dissolution and solubility

Solid drugs need to dissolve before they can be absorbed. The dissolution of drugs can be described by the Noyes–Whitney equation (Eqn 20.1). This equation, first proposed in 1897, describes the rate of diffusion of solute through boundary layers surrounding a dissolving spherical particle. When the dissolution process is diffusion controlled and involves no chemical reaction, then this equates to the rate of dissolution:

$$\mathrm{d}m/\mathrm{d}t = \frac{DA(C_s - C)}{h}$$

(20.1)

where $\mathrm{d}m/\mathrm{d}t$ is the rate of dissolution of the drug particles, D is the diffusion coefficient of the drug in solution in the gastrointestinal fluids, A is the effective surface area of the drug particles in contact with the gastrointestinal fluids, h is the thickness of the diffusion layer around each drug particle, C_s is the saturation solubility of the drug in solution in the diffusion layer and C is the concentration of the drug in the gastrointestinal fluids.

More details regarding the Noyes–Whitney equation and its limitations in describing the dissolution of drug particles are outlined in Chapter 2. The equation serves to illustrate and explain how various physicochemical and physiological factors can influence the rate of dissolution in the gastrointestinal tract. These are summarized in Table 20.1 and are discussed in more detail in the next section.

Fig. 20.1 illustrates the dissolution of a spherical drug particle in the gastrointestinal fluids.

Physiological factors affecting the dissolution rate of drugs

The environment of the gastrointestinal tract can affect the parameters of the Noyes–Whitney equation (Eqn 20.1) and hence the dissolution rate of a drug. For instance, the diffusion coefficient, D, of the drug in the gastrointestinal fluids may be decreased by the presence of substances that increase the viscosity of the fluids. Hence the presence of food in the

Table 20.1 Physicochemical and physiological factors affecting drug dissolution in the gastrointestinal tract

Factor	Physicochemical parameter	Physiological parameter
Effective surface area of drug	Particle size, wettability	Surfactants in gastric juice and bile. pH, buffer capacity, bile, food components
Solubility in diffusion layer	Hydrophilicity, crystal structure, melting point, salts, pK_a	pH, motility patterns
Concentration of drug in solution	Solubility of drug	Permeability, transit, gastrointestinal fluid composition and volume, coadministered fluids, gastrointestinal secretions
Diffusivity of drug	Molecular size	Viscosity of luminal contents
Boundary layer thickness		Motility patterns and flow rate

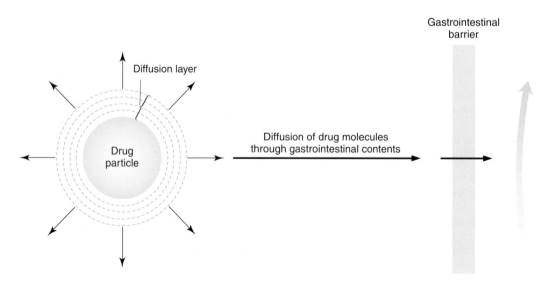

Fig. 20.1 • The dissolution of a drug particle in the gastrointestinal fluids.

gastrointestinal tract may cause a decrease in the drug dissolution rate by reducing the rate of diffusion of the drug molecules away from the diffusion layer surrounding each undissolved drug particle. Surfactants in gastric juice and bile salts will affect both the wettability of the drug, and hence its effective surface area, A, exposed to gastrointestinal fluids, and the solubility of the drug in the gastrointestinal fluids via micellization. The thickness of the diffusion layer, h, will be influenced by the degree of agitation experienced by each drug particle in the gastrointestinal tract. Hence an increase in gastric and/or intestinal motility may increase the dissolution rate of a sparingly soluble drug by decreasing the thickness of the diffusion layer around each drug particle.

The concentration of drug in solution in the bulk of the gastrointestinal fluids, C, will be influenced by such factors as the rate of removal of dissolved drug by absorption through the gastrointestinal tract and by the volume of fluid available for dissolution, which in turn will be dependent on the location of the drug in the gastrointestinal tract and the timing with respect to meal intake. In the stomach the volume of fluid will be influenced by the intake of fluid in the diet. According to the Noyes–Whitney equation, a low value of C will favour more rapid dissolution of the drug by virtue of increasing the value of the term $(C_s - C)$. In the case of drugs whose absorption is dissolution-rate limited, the value of C is normally kept very low by absorption of the drug. Hence dissolution occurs under sink conditions; that is, under conditions such that the value of $(C_s - C)$ approximates to C_s. Thus for the dissolution of a drug in the gastrointestinal tract under sink conditions, the Noyes–Whitney equation can be expressed as

$$dm/dt = \frac{DAC_s}{h}$$

(20.2)

Drug factors affecting the dissolution rate

Drug factors that can influence the dissolution rate are the particle size, the wettability, the solubility and the form of the drug (whether a salt or a free form).

Surface area and particle size

According to Eq. 20.1, an increase in the total surface area of the drug in contact with the gastrointestinal fluids will cause an increase in the dissolution rate.

Provided that each drug particle is intimately wetted by the gastrointestinal fluids, the effective surface area exhibited by the drug will be inversely related to the particle size of the drug. Hence the smaller the particle size, the greater the effective surface area exhibited by a given mass of drug and the higher the dissolution rate. Particle size reduction is thus likely to result in increased bioavailability, provided that the absorption of the drug is dissolution-rate limited.

One of the classic examples of particle size effects on the bioavailability of poorly soluble compounds is that of griseofulvin, where a reduction of particle size from about 10 μm (specific surface area of 0.4 m² g⁻¹) to 2.7 μm (specific surface area of 1.5 m² g⁻¹) was shown to produce approximately double the amount of drug absorbed in humans. Many poorly soluble, slowly dissolving drugs are routinely presented in micronized form to increase their surface area.

Examples of drugs where a reduction in particle size has been shown to increase the rate and extent of oral absorption and hence bioavailability are shown in Table 20.2. Such increases in bioavailability can

Table 20.2 Examples of drugs where a reduction in particle size has led to increases in bioavailability

Drug	Therapeutic class
Digoxin	Cardiac glycoside
Nitrofurantoin	Antibiotic
Medroxyprogesterone	Hormone
Danazol	Steroid
Tolbutamide	Antidiabetic
Aspirin	Analgesic
Sulfadiazine	Antibacterial
Naproxen	Nonsteroidal anti-inflammatory
Ibuprofen	Nonsteroidal anti-inflammatory
Phenacetin	Analgesic
Griseofulvin	Antifungal
Fenofibrate	Lipid-regulating agent
Aprepitant	Antiemetic
Rapamycin	Immunosuppressant
Lopinavir/ritonavir	HIV protease inhibitors

result in an increased incidence of side effects; thus for certain drugs it is important that the particle size is well controlled, and many pharmacopoeias state a requirement for particle size.

For some drugs, particularly those that are hydrophobic, micronization and other dry particle size reduction techniques can result in aggregation of the material. This will cause a consequent reduction in the effective surface area of the drug exposed to the gastrointestinal fluids and hence a reduction in its dissolution rate and bioavailability. Aspirin, phenacetin and phenobarbital are all prone to aggregation during particle size reduction. One approach that may overcome this problem is to micronize or mill the drug with a wetting agent or hydrophilic carrier. To overcome aggregation and to achieve particle sizes in the nanometre size range, wet milling in the presence of stabilizers has been used. The relative bioavailability of danazol has been increased by 400% by administering particles in the nanometre rather than the micrometre size range.

There are now several specialized drug delivery companies that can produce solid dosage forms with the drug stabilized in the nanometre size range to afford greater bioavailaility. Examples of commercialized products are the immunosuppressant Rapamune® (sirolimus), the antiemetic Emend® (aprepitant) and the lipid-regulating agent TriCor® (fenofibrate). Megace® ES is an orally administered nanosuspension of megestrol acetate for the treatment of appetite loss, severe malnutrition or unexplained significant weight loss in AIDS patients. It is a reformulation of the oral suspension using Nanocrystal® technology to increase the dissolution rate, absorption rate and bioavailability of the original formulation. The formulation is less viscous and allows a quarter of the volume to be dosed, thus aiding patient swallowing and adherence.

As well as by milling with wetting agents, the effective surface area of hydrophobic drugs can be increased by the addition of a wetting agent to the formulation. The presence of polysorbate 80 in a fine suspension of phenacetin (particle size less than 75 μm) greatly increased the rate and extent of absorption of the phenacetin in human volunteers compared with the same-size suspension without a wetting agent. Polysorbate 80 helps by increasing the wetting and solvent penetration of the particles and by minimizing aggregation of suspended particles, thereby maintaining a large effective surface area. Wettability effects are highly drug specific; however, wetting agents are routinely added to many formulations.

If an increase in the effective surface area of a drug does not increase its absorption rate, it is likely that the dissolution process is not rate limiting. For drugs such as penicillin G and erythromycin, which are unstable in gastric fluids, their chemical degradation will be minimized if they remain in the solid state. Thus particle size reduction would not only serve to increase their dissolution rate but would simultaneously increase chemical degradation and therefore reduce the amount of intact drug available for absorption.

Solubility in the diffusion layer, C_s

The dissolution rate of a drug under sink conditions, according to the Noyes–Whitney equation (Eqn 20.2), is directly proportional to its intrinsic solubility in the diffusion layer surrounding each dissolving drug particle, C_s. The aqueous solubility of a drug is dependent on the interactions between molecules within the crystal lattice, intermolecular interactions with the solution in which it is dissolving and the entropy changes associated with fusion and dissolution. In the case of drugs that are weak electrolytes, their aqueous solubility is dependent on pH (as discussed in Chapter 2). Hence in the case of an orally administered solid dosage form containing a weak electrolyte drug, the dissolution rate of the drug will be influenced by its solubility and the pH in the diffusion layer surrounding each dissolving drug particle. The pH in the diffusion layer – the microclimate pH – for a weak electrolyte will be affected by the pK_a and solubility of the dissolving drug, and the pK_a and solubility of the buffers in the bulk gastrointestinal fluids. Thus differences in dissolution rate will be expected in different regions of the gastrointestinal tract.

The solubility of weakly acidic drugs increases with pH, and so as a drug moves down the gastrointestinal tract from the stomach to the intestine, its solubility will increase. Conversely, the solubility of weak bases decreases with increasing pH, i.e. as the drug moves down the gastrointestinal tract. It is important therefore for poorly soluble weak bases to dissolve rapidly in the stomach, as the rate of dissolution in the small intestine will be much slower. The antifungal drug ketoconazole, a weak base, is particularly sensitive to gastric pH. Dosing ketoconazole 2 hours after the administration of the H_2-blocker cimetidine, which reduces gastric acid secretion, results in a significantly reduced rate and extent of absorption Similarly, in the case of the antiplatelet drug dipyrimidole, pretreatment with the H_2-blocker famotidine reduces the peak plasma concentration by a factor of up to 10.

Salts

The solubility of a weakly acidic drug in gastric fluid (pH 1–3.5) will be relatively low; however, it will be much greater in the higher pH environment of the intestine. The sodium salt of a weak acid will dissociate as follows:

$$DX \Leftrightarrow D + X$$

$$(20.3)$$

where D is the drug and X is the counterion. The concentration of the drug multiplied by the counterion concentration at any pH will give the solubility product K_{sp}, i.e.

$$K_{sp} = [D][X]$$

$$(20.4)$$

The pH solubility profile of a weak acid in the presence of counterions depends on the solubility product of the ionized drug and its counterions.

Many examples can be found of the effects of salts improving the rate and extent of absorption. The dissolution rate of the oral hypoglycaemic drug tolbutamide sodium in 0.1 M HCl is 5000 times faster than that of the free acid. Oral administration of a nondisintegrating disc of the more rapidly dissolving sodium salt of tolbutamide produces a very rapid decrease in blood glucose level (a consequence of the rapid rate of drug absorption), followed by a rapid recovery. In contrast, a nondisintegrating disc of the tolbutamide free acid produces a much slower rate of decrease in the blood glucose level (a consequence of the slower rate of drug absorption) that is maintained over a longer period of time. The barbiturates are often administered in the form of sodium salts to achieve a rapid onset of sedation and provide more predictable effects.

The nonsteroidal anti-inflammatory drug naproxen was originally marketed as the free acid for the treatment of rheumatoid arthritis and osteoarthritis. However, the sodium salt (naproxen sodium) is absorbed faster, owing to faster dissolution of the dosage from, and hence is more effective, and thus has now largely replaced the free form. Conversely, strongly acidic salt forms of weakly basic drugs (e.g. chlorpromazine hydrochloride) dissolve more rapidly in gastric and intestinal fluids than do the free bases (e.g. chlorpromazine). The presence of strongly acidic anions (e.g. Cl^- ions) in the diffusion layer around each drug particle ensures that the pH in that layer is lower than the bulk pH in either the gastric fluid or the intestinal fluid. This lower pH will increase the solubility of the drug in the diffusion layer.

The oral administration of a salt form of a weakly basic drug in a solid oral dosage form generally ensures that dissolution occurs in the gastric fluid before the drug passes into the small intestine, where pH conditions are unfavourable for dissolution. Thus the drug should be delivered to the major absorption site, the small intestine, in solution. If absorption is fast enough, precipitation of the dissolved drug is unlikely to significantly affect bioavailability. It is important to be aware that hydrochloride salts may experience a common-ion effect owing to the presence of chloride ions in the stomach (also discussed in Chapter 2). The in vitro dissolution of a sulfate salt of an HIV protease inhibitor analogue is significantly greater in hydrochloric acid than that of the hydrochloride salt. The bioavailability of the sulfate salt is more than three times greater than that of the hydrochloride salt. These observations are attributed to the common-ion effect of the hydrochloride.

The sodium salts of acidic drugs and the hydrochloride salts of basic drugs are by far the most common. However, many other salt forms are increasingly being employed (see Chapter 23). Some salts have a lower solubility and dissolution rate than the free form (e.g. aluminium salts of weak acids and pamoate salts of weak bases). In these cases, insoluble films of either aluminium hydroxide or pamoic acid are found to coat the dissolving solids when the salts are exposed to a basic or an acidic environment respectively. In general, poorly soluble salts delay absorption and may therefore be used to sustain the release of the drug. A poorly soluble salt form is generally used for suspension dosage forms.

Although salt forms are often selected to increase bioavailability, other factors such as chemical stability, hygroscopicity, manufacturability and crystallinity will all be considered during salt selection and may preclude the choice of a particular salt. The sodium salt of aspirin, sodium acetylsalicylate, is much more prone to hydrolysis than is aspirin, acetylsalicylic acid, itself. One way to overcome chemical instabilities or other undesirable features of salts is to form the salt in situ or to add basic/acidic excipients to the formulation of a weakly acidic or weakly basic drug. The presence of the basic excipients in the formulation of acidic drugs ensures that a relatively basic diffusion layer is formed around each dissolving particle. The inclusion of the basic ingredients aluminium dihydroxyaminoacetate and magnesium carbonate in aspirin tablets was found to increase their dissolution rate and bioavailability.

Crystal form

Polymorphism

Many drugs can exist in more than one crystalline form. This property is referred to as *polymorphism*, and each crystalline form is known as a polymorph (discussed further in Chapter 8). As discussed in Chapters 2 and 8, a metastable polymorph usually exhibits a greater dissolution rate than the corresponding stable polymorph. Consequently, the metastable polymorphic form of a poorly soluble drug may exhibit an increased bioavailability compared with the stable polymorphic form.

A classic example of the influence of polymorphism on drug bioavailability is provided by chloramphenicol palmitate. This drug exists in three crystalline forms designated A, B and C. At normal temperature and pressure, form A is the stable polymorph, form B is the metastable polymorph and form C is the unstable polymorph. Polymorph C is too unstable to be included in a dosage form, but polymorph B, the metastable form, is sufficiently stable. The plasma profiles of chloramphenicol from orally administered suspensions containing varying proportions of polymorphic forms A and B were investigated. The extent of absorption of chloramphenicol increased as the proportion of polymorphic form B of chloramphenicol palmitate was increased in each suspension. This was attributed to the more rapid in vivo rate of dissolution of the metastable polymorphic form, B, of chloramphenicol palmitate. Following dissolution, chloramphenicol palmitate is hydrolysed to give free chloramphenicol in solution, which is then absorbed. The stable polymorphic form, A, of chloramphenicol palmitate dissolves so slowly and consequently is hydrolysed so slowly to chloramphenicol in vivo that this polymorph is virtually ineffective. The importance of polymorphism for the gastrointestinal bioavailability of chloramphenicol palmitate is reflected by a limit being placed on the content of the inactive polymorphic form, A, in a chloramphenicol palmitate mixture.

Amorphous solids

In addition to different polymorphic crystalline forms, a drug may exist in an amorphous form (see Chapter 8). Because the amorphous form usually dissolves more rapidly than the corresponding crystalline form(s), the possibility exists that there will be significant differences in the bioavailabilities exhibited by the amorphous and crystalline forms of drugs that show dissolution-rate-limited bioavailability.

A classic example of the influence of amorphous versus crystalline forms of a drug on its gastrointestinal bioavailability is provided by the antibiotic novobiocin. The more soluble and rapidly dissolving amorphous form of novobiocin was readily absorbed following oral administration of an aqueous suspension. However, the less soluble and more slowly dissolving crystalline form was not absorbed to any significant extent. The crystalline form was thus therapeutically ineffective. A further important observation was made in the case of aqueous suspensions of novobiocin. The amorphous form slowly converts to the more thermodynamically stable crystalline form, with an accompanying loss of therapeutic effectiveness. Thus unless adequate precautions are taken to ensure the stability of the less stable, more therapeutically effective amorphous form of a drug in a dosage form, unacceptable variations in therapeutic effectiveness may occur.

Several delivery technologies for poorly soluble drugs rely on stabilizing the drug in its amorphous form to increase its dissolution and bioavailability. An example of this is Kaletra®, which is a combination tablet of the protease inhibitors lopinavir and ritonavir used for treatment of HIV infection, in combination with other antiretroviral drugs. These drugs are stabilized in their amorphous form by a polymer, copovidone, following melt extrusion of the drug with the polymer. The tablets provide a significant increase in bioavailability and variability such that two medium-sized tablets are equivalent to three large capsules of the old formulation.

Solvates

Another variation in the crystalline form of a drug can occur if the drug is able to associate with solvent molecules to produce crystalline forms known as solvates (discussed further in Chapter 8). When water is the solvent, the solvate formed is called a hydrate. Generally, the greater the solvation of the crystal, the lower is the solubility and dissolution rate in a solvent identical to the solvation molecules. As the solvated and nonsolvated forms usually exhibit differences in dissolution rates, they may also exhibit differences in bioavailability, particularly in the case of poorly soluble drugs that exhibit dissolution-rate-limited bioavailability.

An example is that of the antibiotic ampicillin. The faster dissolving anhydrous form of ampicillin is absorbed to a greater extent from both hard gelatin capsules and an aqueous suspension than is the more slowly dissolving trihydrate form. The anhydrous form of the hydrochloride salt of a protease inhibitor, an analogue of indinavir, has a much faster dissolution rate than the hydrated form in water. This is reflected in a significantly greater rate and extent of absorption and a more than doubling of the bioavailability of the anhydrous form.

Factors affecting the concentration of a drug in solution in the gastrointestinal fluids

The rate and extent of absorption of a drug depend on the effective concentration of that drug, i.e. the concentration of the drug in solution in the gastrointestinal fluids, which is in an absorbable form. Complexation, micellar solubilization, adsorption and chemical stability are the principal physicochemical properties that can influence the effective drug concentration in the gastrointestinal fluids.

Complexation. Complexation of a drug may occur within the dosage form and/or in the gastrointestinal fluids, and can be beneficial or detrimental to absorption.

Mucin, which is present in gastrointestinal fluids, forms complexes with some drugs. The antibiotic streptomycin binds to mucin, thereby reducing the available concentration of the drug for absorption. It is thought that this may contribute to its poor bioavailability. Another example of complexation is that between drugs and dietary components, as in the case of the tetracyclines, which is discussed in Chapter 19.

The bioavailability of some drugs can be reduced by the presence of some excipients within the dosage form. The presence of calcium (e.g. from the diluent dicalcium phosphate) in the dosage form of tetracycline reduces its bioavailability via the formation of a poorly soluble complex. Other examples of complexes that reduce drug bioavailability are those between amphetamine and sodium carboxymethylcellulose and between phenobarbital and polyethylene glycol 4000. Complexation between drugs and excipients probably occurs quite often in liquid dosage forms and may be beneficial to the physical stability of the dosage form.

Complexation is sometimes used to increase drug solubility, particularly of poorly water-soluble drugs. One class of complexing agents that is increasingly being employed is the cyclodextrin family (see Chapter 24). Cyclodextrins are enzymatically modified starches composed of glucopyranose units which form a ring of six (α-cyclodextrin), seven (β-cyclodextrin) or eight (γ-cyclodextrin) units. The outer surface of the ring is hydrophilic and the inner cavity is hydrophobic. Lipophilic molecules can fit into the ring to form soluble inclusion complexes. The ring of β-cyclodextrin is the correct size for the majority of drug molecules, and normally one drug molecule will associate with one cyclodextrin molecule to form reversible complexes, although other stoichiometries are possible. For example, the antifungal drug miconazole shows poor oral bioavailability owing to its poor solubility, but in the presence of cyclodextrin, the solubility and dissolution rate of miconazole are significantly enhanced (by up to 55-fold and 255-fold respectively). This enhancement of the dissolution rate resulted in a more than doubling of the oral bioavailability in a study in rats. There are numerous examples in the literature of drugs whose solubility, and hence bioavailability, have been increased by the use of cyclodextrins and their derivatives hydroxypropyl-β-cyclodextrin (HPβCD) and sulfobutyl ether β-cyclodextrin (SBEβCD): they include piroxicam, itraconazole, indometacin, pilocarpine, naproxen, hydrocortisone, diazepam and digitoxin. A number of products containing cyclodextrins as solubility enhancers are now available.

Micellar solubilization. Micellar solubilization can also increase the solubility of drugs in the gastrointestinal tract. The ability of bile salts to solubilize drugs depends mainly on the lipophilicity of the drug. Further information on solubilization and complex formation can be found in Chapter 5 and in Florence & Attwood (2016).

Adsorption. The concurrent administration of drugs and medicines containing solid adsorbents (e.g. antidiarrhoeal mixtures) may result in the adsorbents interfering with the absorption of drugs from the gastrointestinal tract. The adsorption of a drug onto solid adsorbents such as kaolin or charcoal may reduce its rate and/or extent of absorption owing to a decrease in the effective concentration of the drug in solution available for absorption. A consequence of the reduced concentration of free drug in solution at the site of absorption will be a reduction in the rate of drug absorption. Whether there is also a reduction in the extent of absorption will depend on whether the drug–adsorbent interaction is readily reversible. If the absorbed drug is not readily released from the solid adsorbent in order to replace the free drug that has been absorbed from the gastrointestinal tract, there will also be a reduction in the extent of absorption from the gastrointestinal tract.

An example of a drug–adsorbent interaction that gives a reduced extent of absorption is promazine–charcoal. The adsorbent properties of charcoal have been exploited as an antidote to overdoses of orally administered drugs.

Care also needs to be taken when insoluble excipients are included in dosage forms to ensure that the drug will not adsorb to them. Talc, which can be included in tablets as a glidant, is claimed to interfere with the absorption of cyanocobalamin by virtue of its ability to adsorb this vitamin.

Chemical stability of the drug in the gastrointestinal fluids. If the drug is unstable in the gastrointestinal fluids, the amount of drug that is available for absorption will be reduced, as will its bioavailability. Instability in gastrointestinal fluids is usually caused by acidic or enzymatic hydrolysis. When a drug is unstable in gastric fluid, its extent of degradation will be minimized (and hence its bioavailability increased) if it remains in the solid state in gastric fluid and dissolves only in intestinal fluid.

The concept of delaying the dissolution of a drug until it reaches the small intestine has been employed to increase the bioavailability of erythromycin in the gastrointestinal tract. Gastro-resistant coating of tablets containing the free base erythromycin has been used to protect the drug from gastric fluid. The gastro-resistant coating resists gastric fluid but is disrupted or dissolved at the less acid pH range of the small intestine (discussed later in this chapter and in Chapters 31 and 32). An alternative method of protecting a susceptible drug from gastric fluid, which has been employed for erythromycin, is the administration of chemical derivatives of the parent drug. These derivatives, or prodrugs, exhibit limited solubility (and hence minimal dissolution) in gastric fluid, but once in the small intestine liberate the parent drug to be absorbed. For instance, erythromycin stearate, after passing through the stomach undissolved, dissolves and dissociates in the intestinal fluid, yielding the free base erythromycin, which is absorbed.

The proton pump inhibitors omeprazole and esomeprazole are acid labile and are therefore formulated in a multiunit gastro-resistant coated pelleted system. Instability in gastrointestinal fluids is one of the reasons why many peptide-like drugs are poorly absorbed when delivered via the oral route.

Poorly soluble drugs

Poorly water-soluble drugs present a problem in terms of obtaining the satisfactory dissolution within the gastrointestinal tract that is necessary for good bioavailability. It is not only existing drugs that cause problems, and it is a challenge for medicinal chemists to ensure that new drugs are not only active pharmacologically but also have sufficient solubility to ensure fast enough dissolution at the site of administration, often the gastrointestinal tract. This is a particular problem for certain classes of drugs, such as the HIV protease inhibitors, many anti-infective drugs and anticancer drugs, where the targets are very lipophilic and thus designing potency and water solubility are challenging. Medicinal chemists are using approaches such as introducing ionizable groups, reducing melting points, changing polymorphs or introducing prodrugs to increase solubility.

Pharmaceutical scientists, as alluded to earlier in this chapter, are also applying a wide range of formulation approaches to increase the dissolution rate of poorly soluble drugs. These include formulating the drug in the nanometre size range, formulating the drug in a solid solution or dispersion or self-emulsifying drug delivery system, stabilizing the drug in the amorphous form or formulating the drug with cyclodextrins. Many drug delivery companies thrive on technologies designed to improve the delivery of poorly water-soluble drugs.

Drug absorption

Once the drug has successfully passed into solution, it is available for absorption. In Chapter 19, many physiological factors were described that influence drug absorption. Absorption, and hence the bioavailability of a drug once in solution, is also influenced by many drug factors, in particular the pK_a and hence the charge, lipid solubility, molecular weight, number of hydrogen bonds in the molecule and its chemical stability.

Drug dissociation and lipid solubility

The dissociation constant and lipid solubility of a drug and the pH at the absorption site often influence the absorption characteristics of a drug throughout the gastrointestinal tract. The interrelationship between the degree of ionization of a weak electrolyte drug (which is determined by its dissociation constant and the pH at the absorption site) and the extent of absorption is embodied in the pH-partition hypothesis of drug absorption, first proposed by Overton in 1899. Although it is an oversimplification of the complex process of absorption, the pH-partition hypothesis still provides a useful framework for understanding the transcellular passive route of absorption, which is that favoured by the majority of drugs.

pH-partition hypothesis of drug absorption

According to the pH-partition hypothesis, the gastrointestinal epithelium acts as a lipid barrier to drugs which are absorbed by passive diffusion, and those that are lipid soluble will pass across the barrier. As most drugs are weak electrolytes, the un-ionized form of weakly acidic or basic drugs (i.e. the lipid-soluble form) will pass across the gastrointestinal epithelium, whereas the gastrointestinal epithelium is impermeable to the ionized (i.e. poorly lipid-soluble) form of such drugs. Consequently, according to the pH-partition hypothesis, the absorption of a weak electrolyte will be determined chiefly by the extent to which the drug exists in its un-ionized form at the site of absorption.

The extent to which a weakly acidic or basic drug ionizes in solution in the gastrointestinal fluid may be calculated using the appropriate form of the Henderson–Hasselbalch equation (discussed further in Chapter 3). For a weakly acidic drug having a single ionizable group (e.g. aspirin, phenobarbital, ascorbic acid, i.e. vitamin C), the equation takes the form

$$\log \frac{[A^-]}{[HA]} = pH - pK_a$$

(20.5)

This is a slightly rearranged form of Eq. 3.16 where pK_a is the negative logarithm of the acid dissociation constant of the drug, [HA] and [A^-] are the respective concentrations of the un-ionized and ionized forms of the weakly acidic drug, which are in equilibrium and in solution in the gastrointestinal fluid, and pH refers to the pH of the environment of the ionized and un-ionized species (i.e. the gastrointestinal fluids).

For a weakly basic drug possessing a single ionizable group (e.g. chlorpromazine, erythromycin, morphine), the analogous equation is

$$\log \frac{[BH^+]}{[B]} = pK_a - pH$$

(20.6)

This is a slightly rearranged form of Eq. 3.19 where [BH^+] and [B] are the respective concentrations of the ionized and un-ionized forms of the weak basic drug, which are in equilibrium and in solution in the gastrointestinal fluids.

Therefore, according to these equations, a weakly acidic drug, pK_a 3.0, will be predominantly (98.4%) un-ionized in gastric fluid at pH 1.2 and almost totally (99.98%) ionized in intestinal fluid at pH 6.8, whereas a weakly basic drug, pK_a 5, will be almost entirely (99.98%) ionized at gastric pH of 1.2 and predominantly (98.4%) un-ionized at intestinal pH of 6.8. This means that, according to the pH-partition hypothesis, a weakly acidic drug is more likely to be absorbed from the stomach, where it is un-ionized, and a weakly basic drug is more likely to be absorbed from the intestine, where it is predominantly un-ionized. However, in practice, very little absorption occurs in the stomach and many other factors need to be taken into consideration.

Limitations of the pH-partition hypothesis

The extent to which a drug exists in its un-ionized form is not the only factor determining the rate and extent of absorption of a drug molecule from the gastrointestinal tract. Despite their high degree of ionization, weak acids are still quite well absorbed from the small intestine. In fact, the rate of intestinal absorption of a weak acid is often higher than its rate of absorption in the stomach, even though the drug is un-ionized in the stomach. The significantly larger surface area that is available for absorption in the small intestine more than compensates for the high degree of ionization of weakly acidic drugs at intestinal pH values. In addition, a longer small intestinal residence time and a microclimate pH (which exists at the surface of the intestinal mucosa and is lower than that of the luminal pH of the small intestine) are thought to aid the absorption of weak acids from the small intestine.

The mucosal unstirred layer is another recognized component of the gastrointestinal barrier to drug absorption that is not accounted for in the pH-partition hypothesis. During absorption, drug molecules must diffuse across this layer and then on through the lipid layer. Diffusion across this layer is liable to be a significant component of the total absorption process for those drugs that cross the lipid layer very quickly. Diffusion across this layer will also depend on the molecular weight of the drug.

A physiological factor that causes deviations from the pH-partition hypothesis is *convective flow* or *solvent drag.* The movement of water molecules into and out of the gastrointestinal tract will affect the rate of passage of small water-soluble molecules across the gastrointestinal barrier. Water movement occurs because of differences in osmotic pressure between blood and the luminal contents and because of differences in hydrostatic pressure between the lumen and the perivascular tissue. The absorption of water-soluble drugs will be increased if water flows from the lumen to the blood, provided that the drug and water are using the same route of absorption. This will have the greatest effect in the jejunum, where water movement is at its greatest. Water flow also affects the absorption of lipid-soluble drugs. It is thought that this is because the drug becomes more concentrated as water flows out of the intestine, thereby favouring a greater drug concentration gradient and increased absorption.

Lipid solubility

A number of drugs are poorly absorbed from the gastrointestinal tract despite their un-ionized forms predominating. For example, the barbiturates barbitone and thiopentone have similar dissociation constants – pK_a of 7.8 and 7.6 respectively – and therefore similar degrees of ionization at intestinal pH. However, thiopentone is absorbed much better than barbitone. The reason for this difference is that the absorption of drugs is also affected by the lipid solubility of the drug. Thiopentone, being more lipid soluble than barbitone, has a greater affinity for the gastrointestinal membrane and is thus far better absorbed.

An indication of the lipid solubility of a drug, and therefore whether that drug is liable to be transported across membranes, is given by its ability to partition between a lipid-like solvent and water or an aqueous buffer. This is known as the drug's *partition coefficient* and is a measure of its lipophilicity:

$$\text{partition coefficient} = \frac{\text{concentration of drug in organic phase}}{\text{concentration of drug in aqueous phase}}$$

(20.7)

The partition coefficient, P, is the ratio between the concentration of the drug in an organic phase that is not miscible with water and that in an aqueous phase at constant temperature. As this ratio normally spans several orders of magnitude, it is usually expressed as the logarithm, log P. The solvent that is usually selected to mimic the biological membrane, because of its many similar properties, is *n*-octanol.

The effective partition coefficient, taking into account the degree of ionization of the drug, is known as the *distribution coefficient*, and again is normally expressed as the logarithm (log D); it is given by the following equations for acids and bases:

For acids:

$$D = \frac{[HA]_{org}}{[HA]_{aq} + [A^-]_{aq}}$$

(20.8)

$$\log D = \log P - [1 + \text{antilog}(pH - pK_a)]$$

(20.9)

For bases:

$$D = \frac{[B]_{org}}{[B]_{aq} + [BH^+]_{aq}}$$

(20.10)

$$\log D = \log P - [1 + \text{antilog}(pK_a - pH)]$$

(20.11)

The lipophilicity of a drug is critical in the drug discovery process. Polar molecules, i.e. those that are poorly lipid soluble (log $P < 0$) and relatively large, such as gentamicin, ceftriaxone, heparin and streptokinase, are poorly absorbed after oral administration and therefore have to be given by injection. Smaller molecules that are poorly lipid soluble and hydrophilic in nature, such as the β-blocker atenolol, can be absorbed via the paracellular route. Lipid-soluble drugs with favourable partition coefficients (i.e. log $P > 0$) are usually absorbed after oral administration. Drugs which are very lipid soluble (log $P > 3$) tend to be well absorbed but are also more likely to be susceptible to metabolism and biliary clearance. Although there is no general rule that can be applied to *all* drug molecules, within a homologous series, such as the barbiturates or β-blockers, drug absorption usually increases as the lipophilicity rises.

Sometimes, if the structure of a compound cannot be modified to yield lipid solubility while maintaining pharmacological activity, medicinal chemists may investigate the possibility of making lipid-soluble prodrugs to increase absorption. A prodrug is a chemical modification, frequently an ester of an existing drug, which converts back to the parent compound as a result of metabolism by the body. A

Table 20.3 Prodrugs with increased lipid solubility and oral absorption

Prodrug	Active drug	Ester
Pivampicillin	Ampicillin	Pivaloyloxymethyl
Bacampicillin	Ampicillin	Carbonate
Carindacillin	Carbenicillin	Indanyl
Cefuroxime axetil	Cefuroxime	Acetylethyl
Enalapril	Enalaprilat	1-Carboxylic acid
Ibuterol	Terbutaline	Dibutyl
Valaciclovir	Aciclovir	L-Valyl (amino acid)
Fosamprenavir	Amprenavir	Phosphate

prodrug itself has no pharmacological activity. Examples of prodrugs which have been successfully used to increase the lipid solubility and hence absorption of their parent drugs are shown in Table 20.3.

Molecular size and hydrogen bonding

Two other drug properties that are important in permeability are the number of hydrogen bonds within the molecule and the molecular size.

For paracellular absorption, the molecular mass should ideally be less than 200 Da; however, there are examples where larger molecules (with molecular masses up to 400 Da) have been absorbed via this route. Shape is also an important factor for paracellular absorption.

In general, for transcellular passive diffusion, a molecular mass of less than 500 Da is preferable. Drugs with molecular masses greater than this are absorbed less efficiently. There are few examples of drugs with molecular masses greater than 700 Da being well absorbed.

Too many hydrogen bonds within a molecule are detrimental to its absorption. In general, no more than five hydrogen-bond donors and no more than 10 hydrogen-bond acceptors (the sum of the number of nitrogen and oxygen atoms in the molecule is often taken as a rough measure of the number of hydrogen-bond acceptors) should be present if the molecule is to be well absorbed. The large number of hydrogen bonds within peptides is one of the reasons why peptide drugs are poorly absorbed.

Summary

There are many properties of the drug itself that will influence its passage into solution in the gastrointestinal tract and across the gastrointestinal membrane, and hence its overall rate and extent of absorption.

Dosage form factors influencing bioavailability

Introduction

The rate and/or extent of absorption of a drug from the gastrointestinal tract has been shown to be influenced by many physiological factors and by many physicochemical properties associated with the drug itself. The bioavailability of a drug can also be influenced by factors associated with the formulation and production of the dosage form. Increasingly, many dosage forms are being designed to affect the release and absorption of drugs; for example, controlled-release systems (see Chapter 31) and delivery systems for poorly soluble drugs. This section summarizes how the type of dosage form and the excipients used in conventional oral dosage forms can affect the rate and extent of drug absorption.

Influence of the type of dosage form

The type of dosage form and its method of preparation or manufacture can influence bioavailability; that is, whether a particular drug administered in the form of a solution, a suspension or a solid dosage form can influence its rate and/or extent of absorption from the gastrointestinal tract. The type of oral dosage form will influence the number of possible intervening steps between administration and the appearance of dissolved drug in the gastrointestinal fluids, i.e. it will influence the release of the drug into solution in the gastrointestinal fluids (Fig. 20.2).

In general, drugs must be in solution in the gastrointestinal fluids before absorption can occur. Thus the greater the number of intervening steps, the greater will be the number of potential obstacles to absorption and the greater will be the likelihood of that type of dosage form reducing the bioavailability exhibited by the drug. Hence the bioavailability of a given drug tends to decrease in the following order of the types of dosage form: aqueous solutions > aqueous suspensions > solid dosage forms (e.g. hard capsules or tablets). Although this ranking is not universal, it does provide a useful guideline. In general,

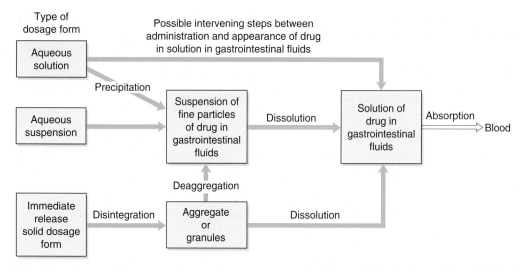

Fig. 20.2 • The influence of the dosage form on the appearance of a drug in solution in the gastrointestinal tract.

solutions and suspensions are the most suitable for administration of drugs intended to be rapidly absorbed. However, it should be noted that other factors (e.g. stability, patient acceptability) can also influence the type of dosage form in which a drug is administered via the gastrointestinal route.

Aqueous solutions

For drugs that are water soluble and chemically stable in aqueous solution, formulation as a solution normally eliminates the in vivo dissolution step and presents the drug in the most readily available form for absorption. However, dilution of an aqueous solution of a poorly water-soluble drug whose aqueous solubility had been increased by formulation techniques such as cosolvency, complex formation or solubilization can result in precipitation of the drug in the gastric fluids. Similarly, exposure of an aqueous solution of a salt of a weak acidic compound to gastric pH can also result in precipitation of the free acid form of the drug. In most cases the extremely fine nature of the resulting precipitate permits a more rapid rate of dissolution than if the drug had been administered in other types of oral dosage forms, such as an aqueous suspension, hard gelatin capsule or tablet. However, for some drugs this precipitation can have a major effect on bioavailability. For example, the same dose of an experimental drug was given to dogs in three different solution formulations: a polyethylene glycol solution and two different concentrations of hydroxypropyl-β-cyclodextrin. Bioavailabilities of 19%, 57% and 89%

were obtained for polyethylene glycol, the lower concentration of hydroxypropyl-β-cyclodextrin and the higher concentration of hydroxypropyl-β-cyclodextrin respectively. The difference in bioavailability of the three solutions was attributed to the difference in the rates of precipitation of the candidate drug from the three solutions on dilution. The experimental drug was observed to precipitate most quickly from the polyethylene glycol solution, and most slowly from the most concentrated hydroxypropyl-β-cyclodextrin solution.

Factors associated with the formulation of aqueous solutions that can influence drug bioavailability include:

- The chemical stability exhibited by the drug in aqueous solution and the gastrointestinal fluids.
- Complexation, i.e. the formation of a chemical complex between the drug and an excipient. The formation of such a complex can increase the aqueous solubility of the drug, which can increase bioavailability or increase the viscosity of the dosage form, which could have a detrimental effect on bioavailability.
- Solubilization, i.e. the incorporation of the drug into micelles to increase its aqueous solubility.
- The viscosity of a solution dosage form, particularly if a viscosity-enhancing agent has been included.

Information concerning the potential influence of each of these factors was given earlier in this chapter.

Further details concerning the formulation and uses of oral solution dosage forms are given in Chapter 24.

Aqueous suspensions

An aqueous suspension is a useful dosage form for administration of an insoluble or poorly water-soluble drug. Usually the absorption of a drug from this type of dosage form is dissolution-rate limited. The oral administration of an aqueous suspension results in a large total surface area of dispersed drug being immediately presented to the gastrointestinal fluids. This facilitates dissolution and hence absorption of the drug. In contrast to powder-filled hard gelatin capsule and tablet dosage forms, dissolution of all drug particles commences immediately on dilution of the suspension in the gastrointestinal fluids. A drug contained in a tablet or hard gelatin capsule may ultimately achieve the same state of dispersion in the gastrointestinal fluids but only after a delay. Thus a well-formulated, finely subdivided aqueous suspension is regarded as being an efficient oral drug delivery system, second only to a nonprecipitating solution-type dosage form.

Factors associated with the formulation of aqueous suspension dosage forms that can influence the bioavailabilities of drugs from the gastrointestinal tract include:

- the particle size and effective surface area of the dispersed drug;
- the crystal form of the drug;
- any resulting complexation, i.e. the formation of a nonabsorbable complex between the drug and an excipient such as the suspending agent;
- the inclusion of a surfactant as a wetting, flocculating or deflocculating agent; and
- the viscosity of the suspension.

Information concerning the potential influence of these factors on drug bioavailability was given earlier in this chapter. Further information concerning the formulation and uses of suspensions as dosage forms is given in Chapter 26.

Liquid-filled capsules

Liquids can be filled into capsules made from soft or hard gelatin or hydroxypropyl methylcellulose (HPMC). Both types combine the convenience of a unit dosage form with the potentially rapid drug absorption associated with aqueous solutions and suspensions. Drugs encapsulated in liquid-filled capsules for peroral administration are dissolved or dispersed in nontoxic, nonaqueous vehicles. Sometimes the vehicles have thermal properties such that capsules can be filled with them while they are hot, but they are solids at room temperature.

The release of the contents of capsules is affected by dissolution and breaking of the shell. Following release, a water-miscible vehicle disperses and/or dissolves readily in the gastrointestinal fluids, liberating the drug (depending on its aqueous solubility) as either a solution or a fine suspension, which is conducive to rapid absorption. In the case of capsules containing drugs in solution or suspension in water-immiscible vehicles, release of the contents will almost certainly be followed by dispersion in the gastrointestinal fluids. Dispersion is facilitated by emulsifiers included in the vehicle, and also by bile. Once dispersed, the drug may end up as an emulsion, a solution, a fine suspension or a nanoemulsion/microemulsion.

Well-formulated liquid-filled capsules are designed to improve the absorption of poorly soluble drugs and will ensure that no precipitation of drug occurs from the nanoemulsion or microemulsion formed in the gastrointestinal fluids. If the lipophilic vehicle is a digestible oil and the drug is highly soluble in the oil, it is possible that the drug will remain in solution in the dispersed oil phase and be absorbed (along with the oil) by fat absorption processes. For a drug that is less lipophilic or is dissolved in a nondigestible oil, absorption probably occurs following partitioning of the drug from the oily vehicle into the aqueous gastrointestinal fluids. In this case the rate of drug absorption appears to depend on the rate at which the drug partitions from the dispersed oil phase into the aqueous phase of the gastrointestinal tract. The increase in the interfacial area of contact resulting from dispersion of the oily vehicle in the gastrointestinal fluids will facilitate partitioning of the drug across the oil–aqueous interface. For drugs suspended in an oily vehicle, release may involve dissolution in the vehicle, diffusion to the oil–aqueous interface and partition across the interface.

Many poorly water-soluble drugs have been found to have greater bioavailabilities from liquid-filled capsule formulations. The cardiac glycoside digoxin, when formulated as a solution in a mixture of polyethylene glycol, ethanol and propylene glycol in a soft gelatin capsule, has been shown to be absorbed faster than from the standard commercial tablets.

More recently, far more complex capsule formulations have been investigated to increase the absorption of poorly soluble drugs. Ciclosporin is a large hydrophobic drug with poor gastro-intestinal permeability and solubility. It had low and variable oral bioavailability from its original liquid-filled soft gelatin capsule formulation (Sandimmune®) and was particularly sensitive to the presence of fat in the diet and bile acids. In its newer formulation (Neoral®), which is a complex mixture of hydrophilic and lipophilic phases, surfactants, cosurfactants and a cosolvent, it forms a nonprecipitating microemulsion on dilution with gastrointestinal fluids. It has a significantly increased bioavailability, with reduced variability, that is independent of the presence of food.

Many protease inhibitors (antiviral drugs) are peptidomimetic. They have high molecular weights and low aqueous solubility, are susceptible to degradation in the lumen and extensive hepatic metabolism, and consequently have poor bioavailability. Saquinavir has been reformulated from a powder-filled hard gelatin capsule (Invirase) to a complex soft gelatin capsule formulation (Fortovase). The latter shows a significant increase in bioavailability (3–4 times greater) over the standard hard gelatin capsule formulation and, as a consequence, a significantly greater viral load reduction.

Factors associated with the formulation of liquid-filled capsules that can influence the bioavailabilities of drugs from this type of dosage form include:

- the solubility of the drug in the vehicle (and gastrointestinal fluids);
- the particle size of the drug (if suspended in the vehicle);
- the nature of the vehicle, i.e. hydrophilic or lipophilic (and whether a lipophilic vehicle is a digestible or a nondigestible oil);
- the inclusion of a surfactant as a wetting/emulsifying agent in a lipophilic vehicle or as the vehicle itself;
- the inclusion of a suspending agent (viscosity-enhancing agent) in the vehicle; and
- the complexation, i.e. formation, of a nonabsorbable complex between the drug and any excipient.

More information on liquid-filled hard capsules and soft capsules can be found in Chapters 33 and 34 respectively.

Powder-filled capsules

Generally, the bioavailability of a drug from a well-formulated powder-filled hard gelatin or hydroxypropyl methylcellulose capsule dosage form will be similar to that from the same drug in a well-formulated compacted tablet. Provided the capsule shell dissolves rapidly in the gastrointestinal fluids and the encapsulated mass disperses rapidly and efficiently, a relatively large effective surface area of drug will be exposed to the gastrointestinal fluids, thereby facilitating dissolution. However, it is incorrect to assume that a drug formulated as a hard gelatin capsule is in a finely divided form surrounded by a water-soluble shell and that no bioavailability problems can occur. The overall rate of dissolution of drugs from capsules appears to be a complex function of the rates of different processes – such as the dissolution rate of the capsule shell, the rate of penetration of the gastrointestinal fluids into the encapsulated mass, the rate at which the mass disaggregates (i.e. disperses) in the gastrointestinal fluids and the rate of dissolution of the dispersed drug particles.

The inclusion of excipients (e.g. diluents, lubricants and surfactants) in a capsule formulation can have a significant effect on the rate of dissolution of drugs, particularly those that are poorly soluble and hydrophobic. Fig. 20.3 shows that a hydrophilic diluent (e.g. sorbitol, lactose) often serves to increase the rate of penetration of the aqueous gastrointestinal fluids into the contents of the capsule and to aid the dispersion and subsequent dissolution of the drug in these fluids. However, the diluent should exhibit no tendency to adsorb or complex with the drug as either can impair absorption from the gastrointestinal tract.

Both the formulation and the type and process conditions of the capsule-filling process can affect the packing density and liquid penetration into the capsule contents. In general, an increase in packing density (i.e. a decrease in porosity) of the encapsulated mass will result in a decrease in liquid penetration into the capsule mass and the dissolution rate, particularly if the drug is hydrophobic or if a hydrophilic drug is mixed with a hydrophobic lubricant such as magnesium stearate. If the encapsulated mass is tightly packed and the drug is hydrophobic, then a decrease in the dissolution rate would be expected unless a surfactant had been included to facilitate liquid penetration into the mass.

In summary, formulation factors that can influence the bioavailabilities of drugs from capsules include:

- the surface area and particle size of the drug (particularly the effective surface area exhibited by the drug in the gastrointestinal fluids);
- the use of the salt form of a drug in preference to the parent weak acid or weak base;

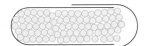

Hard gelatin capsule containing
only hydrophobic drug particles

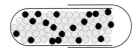

Hard gelatin capsule containing
hydrophobic drug particles (○)
and hydrophilic diluent particles (●)

In gastrointestinal fluids, hard gelatin capsule shell dissolves, thereby exposing contents to fluids

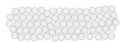

Contents remain as a capsule-shaped
plug. Hydrophobic nature of contents
impedes penetration of gastrointestinal
fluids

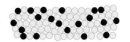

Particles of hydrophilic diluent
dissolve in gastrointestinal fluids,
leaving a porous mass of drug

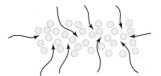

Gastrointestinal fluids can penetrate
porous mass

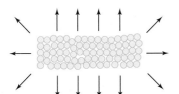

Dissolution of drug occurs only from
surface of plug-shaped mass. Relatively
low rate of dissolution

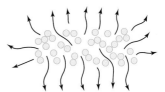

Effective surface area of drug and hence
dissolution rate is increased

Fig. 20.3 • Representation of how a hydrophilic diluent can increase the rate of dissolution of a poorly soluble,
hydrophobic drug from a hard gelatin capsule.

* the crystal form of the drug;
* the chemical stability of the drug (in the dosage form and in gastrointestinal fluids);
* the nature and quantity of the diluent, lubricant and wetting agent;
* drug–excipient interactions (e.g. adsorption, complexation);
* the type and conditions of the filling process;
* the packing density of the capsule contents;
* the composition and properties of the capsule shell (including gastro-resistant capsules); and
* interactions between the capsule shell and its contents.

More information on powder-filled hard capsules can be found in Chapter 33.

Tablets

Uncoated tablets

Tablets are the most widely used dosage form. When a drug is formulated as a compacted tablet, there is an enormous reduction in the effective surface area of the drug, owing to the compaction processes involved in tablet making. These processes necessitate the addition of excipients, which serve to return the surface area of the drug to its original precompacted state. Bioavailability problems can arise if a fine, well-dispersed suspension of drug particles in the gastrointestinal fluids is not generated following the administration of a tablet. Because the effective surface area of a poorly soluble drug is an important factor influencing its dissolution rate, it is especially important that tablets containing such drugs should disintegrate rapidly and completely in the gastrointestinal fluids if rapid release, dissolution and absorption are required. The overall rate of tablet disintegration is influenced by several interdependent factors, which include the concentration and type of drug, diluent, binder, disintegrant, lubricant and wetting agent, as well as the compaction pressure (discussed in Chapter 30).

The dissolution of a poorly soluble drug from an intact tablet is usually extremely limited because of the relatively small effective surface area of the drug exposed to the gastrointestinal fluids. Disintegration of the tablet into granules causes a relatively large increase in effective surface area of the drug, and the dissolution rate may be likened to that of a coarse, aggregated suspension. Further disintegration into small, primary drug particles produces a further large increase in the effective surface area and dissolution rate. The dissolution rate is probably comparable to that of a fine, well-dispersed suspension. Disintegration of a tablet into primary particles is thus important, as it ensures that a large effective surface area of a drug is generated so as to facilitate dissolution and subsequent absorption.

However, simply because a tablet disintegrates rapidly does not necessarily guarantee that the liberated primary drug particles will dissolve in the gastrointestinal fluids and that the rate and extent of absorption are adequate. In the case of poorly water-soluble drugs, the rate-controlling step is usually the overall rate of dissolution of the liberated drug particles in the gastrointestinal fluids. The overall dissolution rate and bioavailability of a poorly soluble drug from an uncoated conventional tablet are influenced by many factors associated with the formulation and manufacture of this type of dosage form. These include:

- the physicochemical properties of the liberated drug particles in the gastrointestinal fluids, e.g. wettability, effective surface area, crystal form, chemical stability;
- the nature and quantity of the diluent, binder, disintegrant, lubricant and any wetting agent;
- drug–excipient interactions (e.g. complexation);
- the size of the granules and their method of manufacture;
- the compaction pressure and speed of compaction used in tableting; and
- the conditions of storage and age of the tablet.

Because drug absorption and hence bioavailability are dependent on the drug being in the dissolved state, suitable dissolution characteristics can be an important property of a satisfactory tablet, particularly if it contains a poorly soluble drug. On this basis, specific in vitro dissolution test conditions and dissolution limits are included in many pharmacopoeias for tablets (and capsules) for certain drugs. That a particular drug product meets the requirements of a compendial dissolution standard provides greater assurance that the drug will be released satisfactorily from the formulated dosage form in vivo and be absorbed adequately (also discussed in Chapters 21 and 35).

More information on drug release from tablets can be found in Chapter 30.

Coated tablets

Tablet coatings may be used simply for aesthetic reasons, to improve the appearance of a tablet or to add a company identity, to mask an unpleasant taste or odour, to protect an ingredient from decomposition during storage or to protect health workers from the drug. Currently, the most common type of tablet coat is that created with a polymer film. However, several older preparations, such as tablets containing vitamins, ibuprofen and conjugated oestrogens, still have sugar coats.

The presence of a coating presents a physical barrier between the tablet core and the gastrointestinal fluids. Coated tablets therefore not only possess all the potential bioavailability problems associated with uncoated conventional tablets but are also subject to the additional potential problem of being surrounded by a physical barrier. In the case of a coated tablet which is intended to disintegrate/dissolve and release the drug rapidly into solution in the gastrointestinal fluids, the coating must dissolve or be disrupted before these processes can begin. The physicochemical nature and thickness of the coating can thus influence how quickly a drug is released from a tablet.

In the process of sugar coating, the tablet core is usually sealed with a thin continuous film of a poorly water-soluble polymer such as shellac or cellulose acetate phthalate. This sealing coat serves to protect the tablet core and its contents from the aqueous fluids used in the subsequent steps of the sugar-coating process. The presence of this water-impermeable sealing coat can potentially retard drug release from sugar-coated tablets. In view of this potential problem, annealing agents such as polyethylene glycols or calcium carbonate, which do not substantially reduce the water impermeability of the sealing coat during sugar coating but which dissolve readily in gastric fluid, may be added to the sealer coat to reduce the barrier effect and to aid rapid drug release.

The film coating of a tablet core by a thin film of a water-soluble polymer, such as hydroxypropyl methylcellulose, should have no significant effect on the rate of disintegration of the tablet core and subsequent drug dissolution, provided that the film coat dissolves rapidly and independently of the pH of the gastrointestinal fluids. However, if hydrophobic water-insoluble film-coating materials, such as ethylcellulose or certain acrylic resins, are used (see Chapter 32), the resulting film coat acts as a barrier which delays and/or reduces the rate of drug release. Thus these types of film-coating materials form barriers which can have a significant influence on drug absorption. Although the formation of such barriers would be disadvantageous in the case of film-coated tablets intended to provide rapid rates of drug absorption, the concept of barrier coating has been used (along with other techniques) to obtain more precise control over drug release than is possible with conventional uncoated tablets (see Chapters 31 and 32).

Gastro-resistant tablets

The use of barrier coating to control the site of release of an orally administered drug is well illustrated by gastro-resistant tablets (formerly known as enteric-coated tablets). A gastro-resistant coat is designed to resist the low pH of gastric fluids but to be disrupted or dissolve when the tablet enters the higher pH of the duodenum. Polymers such as cellulose acetate phthalate, hydroxypropyl methylcellulose phthalate, some copolymers of methacrylic acid and their esters and polyvinyl acetate phthalate can be used as gastro-resistant coatings. These materials do not dissolve in the gastric pH range but dissolve rapidly at the less acidic pH (about 5) associated with the small intestine. Gastro-resistant coatings should preferably begin to dissolve at pH 5 so as to ensure the availability of drugs which are absorbed primarily in the proximal region of the small intestine. Gastro-resistant coating thus provides a means of delaying the release of a drug until the dosage form reaches the small intestine. Such delayed release provides a means of protecting drugs which would otherwise be destroyed if they were released into gastric fluid. and hence can increase the oral bioavailability of such drugs. Gastro-resistant coating also protects the stomach against drugs which can cause nausea or mucosal irritation (e.g. aspirin, ibuprofen) if released at this site.

In addition to the protection offered by gastro-resistant coating, the delayed release of the drug also results in a significant delay in the onset of the therapeutic response of the drug. The onset of the therapeutic response is largely dependent on the residence time of the gastro-resistant tablet in the stomach. Gastric emptying of such tablets is an all-or-nothing process, i.e. the tablet is either in the stomach or in the duodenum. Consequently, the drug is either not being released or is being released. The residence time of an intact gastro-resistant tablet in the stomach can range from about 5 minutes to several hours (discussed further in Chapter 19). Hence there is considerable intrasubject and intersubject variation in the onset of therapeutic action exhibited by drugs administered as gastro-resistant tablets.

The formulation of a gastro-resistant product in the form of small individually coated granules or pellets (multiparticulates) contained in a rapidly dissolving capsule or a rapidly disintegrating tablet largely eliminates the dependency of this type of dosage form on the all-or-nothing gastric emptying process associated with intact (monolith) gastro-resistant tablets. Provided the coated granules or pellets are sufficiently small (around 1 mm in diameter), they will be able to exit from the stomach with liquids. Hence gastro-resistant granules and pellets exhibit a gradual but continual release from the stomach into the duodenum. This type of release also avoids the complete dose of the drug being released into the duodenum, as occurs with a gastro-resistant tablet. The intestinal mucosa is thus not exposed locally to a potentially toxic concentration of the drug.

Further information on coated tablets and multiparticulates is given in Chapter 32.

Influence of excipients for conventional dosage forms

Drugs are almost never administered alone but are rather administered in dosage forms that generally consist of a drug (or drugs) together with a varied number of other substances (*excipients*). Excipients are added to the formulation to facilitate the preparation, patient acceptability and functioning of the dosage form as a drug delivery system. Excipients include disintegrating agents, diluents, lubricants, suspending agents, emulsifying agents, flavouring agents, colouring agents, and chemical stabilizers.

Although historically excipients were considered to be inert in that they themselves should exert no therapeutic or biological action or modify the biological action of the drug present in the dosage form, they are now regarded as having the ability to influence the rate and/or extent of absorption of the drug. For instance, the potential influence of excipients on drug bioavailability has already been illustrated by the formation of poorly soluble, nonabsorbable drug–excipient complexes between tetracyclines and dicalcium phosphate, amphetamine and sodium carboxymethylcellulose, and phenobarbital and polyethylene glycol 4000.

Diluents

An important example of the influence that excipients employed as diluents can have on drug bioavailability is provided by the observed increase in the incidence of phenytoin intoxication which occurred in epileptic patients in Australia as a consequence of the diluent in sodium phenytoin capsules being changed. Many epileptic patients who had been previously stabilized with sodium phenytoin capsules containing calcium sulfate dihydrate as the diluent developed clinical features of phenytoin overdose when given sodium phenytoin capsules containing lactose as the diluent, even though the quantity of the drug in each capsule formulation was identical. The experimental data from this study are shown in Fig. 33.6. It was later shown that the excipient calcium sulfate dihydrate had been responsible for decreasing the gastrointestinal absorption of phenytoin, possibly because part of the administered dose of the drug formed a poorly absorbable calcium phenytoin complex. Hence although the size of the dose and the frequency of administration of the sodium phenytoin capsules containing calcium sulfate dihydrate gave therapeutic blood levels of phenytoin in epileptic patients, the efficiency of absorption of phenytoin had been lowered by the incorporation of this excipient in the hard gelatin capsules. Hence when the calcium sulfate dihydrate was replaced by lactose, without any alteration in the quantity of the drug in each capsule, or in the frequency of administration, an increased bioavailability of phenytoin was achieved. In many patients the higher plasma levels exceeded the maximum safe concentration for phenytoin and produced toxic side effects.

Surfactants

Surfactants are often used in dosage forms as emulsifying agents, solubilizing agents, suspension stabilizers or wetting agents. However, surfactants in general cannot be assumed to be 'inert' excipients as they have been shown to be capable of increasing, decreasing or exerting no effect on the transfer of drugs across biological membranes.

Surfactant monomers can potentially disrupt the integrity and function of a biological membrane. Such an effect would tend to enhance drug penetration and hence absorption across the gastrointestinal barrier, but may also result in toxic side effects. Inhibition of absorption may occur as a consequence of a drug being incorporated into surfactant micelles. If such surfactant micelles are not absorbed, which appears usually to be the case, then solubilization of a drug may result in a reduction of the concentration of 'free' drug in solution in the gastrointestinal fluids that is available for absorption. Inhibition of drug absorption in the presence of micellar concentrations of surfactant would be expected to occur in the case of drugs that are normally soluble in the gastrointestinal fluids, i.e. in the absence of surfactant. Conversely, in the case of poorly soluble drugs whose absorption is dissolution-rate limited, the increase in saturation solubility of the drug by solubilization in surfactant micelles could result in more rapid rates of dissolution and hence absorption.

The release of poorly soluble drugs from tablets and capsules may be increased by the inclusion of surfactants in their formulations. The ability of a surfactant to reduce the solid–liquid interfacial tension will permit the gastrointestinal fluids to wet the solid more effectively and thus enable it to come into more intimate contact with the solid dosage forms. This wetting effect may thus aid the penetration of gastrointestinal fluids into the mass of capsule contents that often remains when the hard gelatin shell has dissolved, and/or reduce the tendency of poorly soluble drug particles to aggregate in the gastrointestinal fluids. In each case the resulting increase in the total effective surface area of the drug in contact with the gastrointestinal fluids would tend to increase the dissolution and absorption rates of the drug. It is interesting to note that the enhanced gastrointestinal absorption of phenacetin in humans resulting from the addition of polysorbate 80 to an aqueous suspension of this drug was attributed to the surfactant preventing aggregation and thus increasing the effective surface area and dissolution rate of the drug particles in the gastrointestinal fluids.

The possible mechanisms by which surfactants can influence drug absorption are varied, and it is likely that only rarely will a single mechanism operate in isolation. In most cases the overall effect on drug absorption will probably involve a number of different actions of the surfactant (some of which will produce opposing effects on drug absorption), and the observed effect on drug absorption will depend on which of the different actions is the overriding one. The ability of a surfactant to influence drug absorption will also depend on the physicochemical characteristics and concentration of the surfactant, the nature of the drug and the type of biological membrane involved.

Lubricants

Both tablets and capsules require lubricants in their formulation to reduce friction between the powder and metal surfaces during their manufacture. Lubricants are often hydrophobic. Magnesium stearate is commonly included as a lubricant during tablet compaction and capsule-filling operations. Its hydrophobic nature often retards liquid penetration into capsule ingredients so after the shell has dissolved in the gastrointestinal fluids, a capsule-shaped plug frequently remains, especially when the contents have been formed into a consolidated plug by a machine (see Chapter 33). Similar reductions in the dissolution rate are observed when magnesium stearate is included in tablets. These effects can be overcome by the simultaneous addition of a wetting agent (i.e. a water-soluble surfactant) and the use of a hydrophilic diluent (e.g. stearic acid), or can be minimized by decrease of the magnesium stearate content of the formulation.

Disintegrants

Disintegrants are required to break up capsules, tablets and granules into primary powder particles in order to increase the surface area of the drug exposed to the gastrointestinal fluids. A tablet that fails to disintegrate or disintegrates slowly may result in incomplete absorption or a delay in the onset of action of the drug. The compaction force used in tablet manufacture can affect disintegration. In general, the higher the force, the longer the disintegration time. Even small changes in formulation may result in significant effects on dissolution and bioavailability. A classic example is that of tolbutamide where two formulations, the commercial product and the same formulation but containing half the amount of disintegrant, were administered to healthy volunteers. Both tablets disintegrated in vitro within 10 minutes,

meeting pharmacopoeial specifications, but the commercial tablet had a significantly greater bioavailability and hypoglycaemic response.

Viscosity-enhancing agents

Viscosity-enhancing agents are often employed in the formulation of liquid dosage forms for oral use in order to control properties such as palatability, ease of pouring and, in the case of suspensions, the rate of sedimentation of the dispersed particles. Viscosity-enhancing agents are often hydrophilic polymers.

There are a number of mechanisms by which a viscosity-enhancing agent may produce a change in the gastrointestinal absorption of a drug. Complex formation between a drug and a hydrophilic polymer could reduce the concentration of the drug in solution that is available for absorption. The administration of viscous solutions or suspensions may produce an increase in the viscosity of the gastrointestinal contents. In turn, this could lead to a decrease in the dissolution rate and/or a decrease in the rate of movement of drug molecules to the absorbing membrane.

Normally, a decrease in the rate of dissolution would not be applicable to solution dosage forms unless dilution of the administered solution in the gastrointestinal fluids caused precipitation of the drug.

In the case of suspensions containing drugs with bioavailabilities that are dissolution-rate dependent, an increase in viscosity could also lead to a decrease in the rate of dissolution of the drug in the gastrointestinal tract.

Summary

As well as physiological and drug factors, the dosage form can play a major role in influencing the rate and extent of absorption. Often this is by design. However, even with conventional dosage forms, it is important to consider whether changing the dosage form or excipients will affect the bioavailability of the drug. Some drugs will be more susceptible to changes in the rate and extent of absorption through dosage form changes than others; this will depend on the biopharmaceutical properties of the drug, which form the basis of Chapter 21.

Please check your eBook at **https://studentconsult. inkling.com/** for self-assessment questions. See inside cover for registration details.

Reference

Florence, A.T., Attwood, D., 2016. Physicochemical Principles of Pharmacy: In Manufacture, Formulation and Clinical Use, sixth ed. Pharmaceutical Press, London.

Bibliography

Buggins, T., Dickinson, P., Taylor, G., 2007. The effect of pharmaceutical excipients on drug disposition. Adv. Drug Deliv. Rev. 59, 1482–1503.

Elder, D.P., Holm, R., Lopez de Diego, H., 2013. Use of pharmaceutical salts and cocrystals to address the issue of poor solubility. Int. J. Pharm. 453, 80–100.

Taylor, L.S., Zhang, G.S., 2016. Physical chemistry of supersaturated solutions and implications for oral absorption. Adv. Drug Deliv. Rev. 101, 122–142.

Assessment of biopharmaceutical properties

21

Marianne Ashford

CHAPTER CONTENTS

KEY POINTS

- The measurable properties used to understand the biopharmaceutics of a product are the dissolution of a drug from its dosage form, its stability in physiological fluids, the drug's permeability across gastro-intestinal membrane and its metabolism by gastrointestinal enzymes.
- Various techniques ranging from in silico, to in vitro, to in vivo techniques in animals and humans can be used to calculate or measure the permeability of drugs. Bioavailability can be measured from comparison of the area under the curve of a plasma drug concentration versus time profile from a route of administration with the area under the curve of the same dose of the drug administered intravenously.
- The Biopharmaceutics Classification System classifies drugs into four classes according to their dose, their aqueous solubility over the gastrointestinal pH range and their permeability across the gastrointestinal mucosa.
- The Biopharmaceutical Drug Disposition Classification System is introduced.

Introduction

Biopharmaceutics is concerned with factors that influence the rate and extent of drug absorption. As discussed in Chapters 19 and 20, the factors that affect the release of a drug from its dosage form, its dissolution in physiological fluids, its stability within those fluids, its abililty to cross the relevant biological membranes and its presystemic metabolism will all influence its rate and extent of absorption (Fig. 21.1). Once the drug has been absorbed into the systemic circulation, its distribution within the body tissues (including to its site of action), its metabolism and its excretion are described by the *pharmacokinetics* of the compound (discussed in Chapter 18). This in turn influences the duration and magnitude of the therapeutic effect or the response of the compound, i.e. its *pharmacodynamics*.

The key biopharmaceutical properties that can be quantified and therefore give insight into the absorption of a drug are its:

- release from its dosage form into solution at the absorption site;

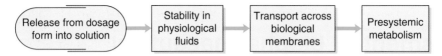

Fig. 21.1 • Key biopharmaceutical properties affecting drug absorption.

- stability in physiological fluids;
- permeability; and
- susceptibility to presystemic clearance.

As most drugs are delivered via the mouth, these properties will be discussed with respect to the peroral route. The bioavailability of a compound is an overall measure of its availability in the systemic circulation, and so the assessment of bioavailability will also be discussed. Other methods of assessing the performance of dosage forms in vivo will also be briefly mentioned.

The Biopharmaceutics Classification System (BCS), which classifies drugs according to dose and two of their key biopharmaceutical properties, solubility and permeability, is outlined, and the Biopharmaceutical Drug Disposition Classification System (BDDCS) is introduced.

Measurement of key biopharmaceutical properties

Release of a drug from its dosage form into solution

As discussed in Chapter 20 and Part 5, a dosage form is normally formulated to aid and/or control the release of a drug from it. For example, for an immediate-release tablet, the tablet needs to disintegrate to yield the primary drug particles. Furthermore, a suspension should not be so viscous that it impedes the diffusion of dissolving drug away from the solid particles.

The solubility of a drug across the gastrointestinal pH range will be one of the first indicators as to whether dissolution is liable to be rate limiting in the absorption process. Knowledge of the solubility across the gastrointestinal pH range can be determined by measuring the equilibrium solubility in suitable buffers or by using an acid or a base titration method.

Methods of measuring the dissolution rate of both a drug itself (intrinsic dissolution rate) and various dosage forms are discussed in Chapters 2 and 35, and in the chapters of Part 5.

The aim of dissolution testing is to find an in vitro characteristic of a potential formulation that reflects its in vivo performance. When designing a dissolution test to assess drug release from a biopharmaceutical perspective, it is important to mimic as closely as possible the conditions of the gastrointestinal tract. Clinical scientists increasingly want to rely on dissolution tests to establish in vitro–in vivo correlations between the release of the drug from the dosage form and its absorption. If this can be successfully achieved, it is possible that the dissolution test could replace some of the in vivo studies that need to be performed during product development and registration. Such correlations should have the benefits of reducing the use of animals to evaluate formulations and the size and number of costly clinical studies to assess bioavailability, as well as being used to allow formulation, process and site of manufacture changes.

An in vitro–in vivo correlation may be possible only for those drugs where dissolution is the rate-limiting step in the absorption process. Determining full dissolution profiles of such drugs in a number of different physiologically representative media will aid the understanding of the factors affecting the rate and extent of dissolution. The profiles can also be used to generate an in vitro–in vivo correlation. To achieve this, at least three batches that differ in their in vivo behaviour and their in vitro behaviour should be available. The differences in the in vivo profiles need to be mirrored by the formulations in vitro. Normally, the in vitro test conditions can be modified to correspond with the in vivo data to achieve a correlation. Very often, a well-designed in vitro dissolution test is found to be more sensitive and discriminating than an in vivo test. From a quality assurance perspective, a more discriminating dissolution method is preferred because the test will indicate possible changes in the product before the in vivo performance is affected.

In vitro dissolution testing of solid dosage forms is discussed fully in Chapter 35, to which the reader is referred for consideration of the apparatus available and suitable dissolution media to simulate as closely as possible gastric and intestinal fluids. This application of dissolution testing is discussed further here in the context of the assessment of biopharmaceutical properties.

A dilute hydrochloric acid based solution at pH 1.2 can simulate gastric fluid quite closely (but obviously not exactly), and phosphate-buffered solution at pH 6.8 can mimic intestinal fluid. However, dissolution media more closely representing physiological conditions may well provide more relevant conditions. A range of dissolution media that are widely accepted to mimic physiological parameters in gastric and intestinal fluids in the fed and fasted states are available. Each of these media takes into account not only the pH of the fluids in the different states but also their ionic composition, surface tension, buffer capacity and bile and lecithin contents. Details of simulated gastric and intestinal fluids for both the fed state and the fasted state are given in Tables 35.2 and 35.3.

The conditions within the stomach in the fed state are highly dependent on the composition of the meal eaten and are therefore difficult to simulate. In trying to produce an in vitro–in vivo correlation, it has been suggested that a more appropriate way of simulating the fed-state gastric fluids is to homogenize the meal to be used in clinical studies and then dilute it with water. Long-life milk has also been used to simulate gastric conditions in the fed state.

It has been proposed that the duration of the dissolution test should depend on the site of absorption of the drug and its timing of administration. Thus, when one is designing a dissolution test, some knowledge or prediction of the permeability properties of the drug is beneficial. If, for example, the drug is absorbed from the upper part of intestine and is likely to be dosed in the fasted state, the most appropriate dissolution conditions may be a short test (~5 min to 30 min) in a medium simulating gastric fluid in the fasted state. Alternatively, if it is advised that a drug should be administered with food and the drug is known to be well absorbed throughout the length of the gastrointestinal tract, a far longer dissolution test may be more appropriate. This could perhaps be several hours in duration with a range of media such as, initially, simulated gastric fluid to mimic the fed state, followed by simulated intestinal fluid to mimic both the fed state and the fasted state.

The volumes of fluid within, and the degree of agitation of, the stomach and intestines vary enormously, particularly between the fed state and the fasted state. Consequently, it is difficult to choose a representative volume and degree of agitation for an in vitro test. Guidance given to industry on the dissolution testing of immediate-release solid oral dosage forms suggests volumes of 500 mL, 900 mL or 1000 mL and gentle agitation conditions. Regulatory authorities will expect justification of a dissolution test to ensure that it will discriminate between a good formulation and a poor formulation, and thus see it as a critical quality test in submissions of applications for marketing authorizations.

Stability in physiological fluids

The stability of drugs in physiological fluids (in the case of orally administered drugs, the gastrointestinal fluids) depends on two factors:

- the chemical stability of the drug across the gastrointestinal pH range, i.e. the drug's pH stability profile between pH 1 and pH 8; and
- its susceptibility to enzymatic breakdown by the gastrointestinal fluids.

Means of assessing the chemical stability of a drug (alone and in its dosage form) are discussed in Chapters 47 and 49. The stability of a drug in gastrointestinal fluids can be assessed by simulated gastric and intestinal media or by obtaining gastrointestinal fluids from humans or animals. The latter provides a harsher assessment of gastrointestinal stability but is more akin to the in vivo setting. In general, the drug is incubated with either real or simulated fluid at 37 °C for 3 hours and the drug content is analysed. A loss of more than 5% of the drug indicates potential instability. Many of the permeability methods described in this chapter can be used to identify whether gastrointestinal stability is an issue for a particular drug.

For drugs that will still be in the gastrointestinal lumen when they reach the colonic region, resistance to the bacterial enzymes present in this part of the intestine needs to be considered. The bacterial enzymes are capable of a whole host of reactions. There may be a significant portion of a poorly soluble drug still in the gastrointestinal tract by the time it reaches the colon. If the drug is absorbed along the length of the gastrointestinal tract, and is susceptible to degradation or metabolism by the bacterial enzymes within the gastrointestinal tract, the drug's absorption and hence its bioavailability is liable to be reduced. Similarly, for sustained-release or controlled-release products that are designed to release their drug along the length of the gastrointestinal tract, the potential for degradation or metabolism by bacterial enzymes should be assessed. If a drug is metabolized to a metabolite which can be absorbed, the potential toxicity of this metabolite should be considered.

Permeability

There are a wealth of techniques available for either estimating or measuring the rate of permeation across membranes that are used to gain an assessment of oral absorption in humans. These range from computational (in silico) predictions to both physicochemical

methods and biological methods. The biological methods can be further subdivided into in vitro, in situ and in vivo methods. In general, the more complex the technique, the more information that can be gained and the more accurate is the assessment of oral absorption in humans. The range of techniques is summarized in Table 21.1. Some of the more widely used ones are discussed later in this chapter.

Partition coefficients

One of the first properties of a molecule that should be predicted or measured is its *partition coefficient*

Table 21.1 Some of the models available for predicting or measuring drug absorption

Model type	Model	Description
Computational/in silico	clog *P*	Commercial software that calculates the *n*-octanol–water partition coefficient on the basis of fragment analysis, known as the *Leo–Hansch method*
	mlog *P*	Method of calculating log *P*, known as the *Moriguchi method* (see the text)
Physicochemical	Partition coefficient	Measure of lipophilicity of a drug, usually measured between *n*-octanol and aqueous buffer via a shake-flask method
	Immobilized artificial membrane	Measures partition into more sophisticated lipidic phase on an HPLC column
Cell culture	Caco-2 monolayer	Measures transport across monolayers of differentiated human colon adenocarcinoma cells
	HT-29	Measures transport across a polarized cell monolayer with mucin-producing cells
Excised tissues	Cells	Measures uptake into cell suspensions, e.g. erythrocytes
	Freshly isolated cells	Measures uptake into enterocytes; however; the cells are difficult to prepare and are short-lived
	Membrane vesicles	Measures uptake into brush border membrane vesicles prepared from intestinal scrapings or isolated enterocytes
	Everted sacs	Measures uptake into intestinal segments/sacs
	Everted intestinal rings	Studies the kinetics of uptake into the intestinal mucosa
	Isolated sheets	Measures the transport across sheets of intestine
In situ studies	In situ perfusion	Measures drug disappearance from either closed or open loop perfusate of segments of intestine of anaesthetized animals
	Vascularly perfused intestine	Measures drug disappearance from perfusate and its appearance in blood
In vivo studies	Intestinal loop	Measures drug disappearance from perfusate of loop of intestine in awake animals
Human data	Loc-I-Gut	Measures drug disappearance from perfusate of human intestine
	High-frequency capsule	Noninvasive method; measures drug in systemic circulation
	InteliSite capsule	Noninvasive method; measures drug in systemic circulation
	Bioavailability	Deconvolution of pharmacokinetic data

HPLC, High-performance liquid chromatography.

between oil and a water phase (log *P*). This gives a measure of the lipophilicity of a molecule, which can be used to predict how well it will be able to cross a biological membrane. It is a very useful parameter for many reasons relating to formulation design and drug absorption, and is discussed in Chapters 2, 20 and 23. As discussed in Chapter 20, *n*-octanol is most commonly chosen as the solvent for the oil phase as it has properties similar to those of biological membranes, although other oil phases have been used (as considered in Chapter 23). One of the most common ways of measuring partition coefficients is to use the shake-flask method (Fig. 21.2). It relies on the equilibrium distribution of a drug between oil and an aqueous phase. Prior to the experiment, the aqueous phase should be saturated with the oil phase and vice versa. The experiment should be carried out at constant temperature. The drug should be added to the aqueous phase and the oil phase, which, in the case of *n*-octanol, as it is less dense than water, will sit on top of the water. The system is mixed and then left to reach equilibrium (usually at least 24 h). The two phases are separated and the concentration of the drug is measured in each phase and a partition coefficient is calculated. This technique is discussed further in the context of preformulation in Chapter 23.

If the aqueous phase is at a particular pH, the distribution coefficient at that pH is measured (log *D*); this then accounts for the ionization of the molecule at that pH. In the case of a weakly acidic or a weakly basic drug, the log *D* measured at an intestinal pH (e.g. 6.8) is liable to give a better prediction of the drug's ability to cross the lipid gastrointestinal membrane than its partition coefficient, log *P*, which does not take the degree of ionization into account.

As discussed in Chapter 20, within a homologous series, increasing lipophilicity (log *P* or log *D*) tends to result in greater absorption. A molecule is unlikely to cross a membrane (i.e. be absorbed via the transcellular passive route) if it has a log *P* less than 0.

Instead of our determining log *P* experimentally, computational methods can be used for its estimation; a number of software packages are available to do this. There is a reasonably good correlation between calculated and measured values. Log *P* can be estimated by breaking down the molecule into fragments and calculating the contribution of each fragment to the overall lipophilicity (often called the clog *P*). Another way of estimating log *P* is the Moriguchi method, which uses 13 parameters for hydrophobic and hydrophilic atoms, proximity effects, unsaturated bonds, intramolecular bonds, ring structures, amphoteric properties and several specific functionalities to obtain a value for the partition coefficient. This is often called mlog *P*. The advantages of these methods are in drug discovery, where an estimate of the lipophilicity of many molecules can be obtained before they are actually synthesized.

Another, more sophisticated physicochemical means of estimating how well a drug will partition into a lipophilic phase is by investigating how well the molecule can be retained on a high-performance liquid chromatography (HPLC) column. Such a column can be simply coated with *n*-octanol to mimic *n*-octanol–aqueous partition or, more elaborately, designed to mimic biological membranes. For example, the immobilized artificial membrane technique provides a measure of how well a solute (i.e. the drug) in the aqueous phase will partition into biological membranes (i.e. be retained on the column). Good correlations between these methods and biological in vitro methods of estimating transcellular passive drug absorption have been obtained.

Cell culture techniques

Cell culture techniques for measuring the intestinal absorption of molecules have been increasingly used in recent decades and are now a well-accepted model

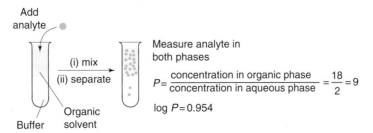

$$P = \frac{\text{concentration in organic phase}}{\text{concentration in aqueous phase}} = \frac{18}{2} = 9$$

log *P* = 0.954

Add analyte

(i) mix
(ii) separate

Measure analyte in both phases

Buffer   Organic solvent

Fig. 21.2 • The shake-flask method for determining the partition coefficient.

for absorption. The cell line that is most widely used is Caco-2.

Caco-2 cells are a human colon carcinoma cell line that was first proposed and characterized as a model for oral drug absorption by Hidalgo. In culture, Caco-2 cells spontaneously differentiate to form a monolayer of polarized enterocytes. These enterocytes resemble those in the small intestine, in that they possess microvilli and many of the transporter systems present in the small intestine; for example, those for sugars, amino acids, peptides and the P-glycoprotein efflux transporter. Adjacent Caco-2 cells adhere through tight junctions; however, the tightness of these junctions is more like that of those of the colon than that of those of the leakier small intestine.

There are many variations on growing Caco-2 monolayers and performing transport experiments with them. In general, the cells are grown on porous supports, usually for 15–21 days in a typical cell culture medium, Dulbecco's modified Eagle medium supplemented with 20% fetal bovine serum, 1% nonessential amino acids and 2 mM L-glutamine. The cells are grown at 37 °C in 10% carbon dioxide at a relative humidity of 95%. The culture medium is replaced at least twice each week. Transport experiments are performed by replacement of the culture medium with buffers, usually Hanks' balanced salt solution adjusted to pH 6.5 on the apical surface and Hanks balanced salt solution adjusted to pH 7.4 on the basolateral surface (Fig. 21.3).

After a short incubation period, usually approximately 30 minutes, when the cells are maintained at 37 °C in a shaking water bath, the buffers are replaced with fresh buffers, and a dilute solution of the drug is introduced to the apical chamber. At regular intervals, the concentration of the drug in the basolateral chamber is determined. The apparent permeability coefficient across cells can be calculated as follows:

$$P_{app} = dQ/dt(1/C_0 A)$$

(21.1)

where P_{app} is the apparent permeability coefficient (cm s^{-1}), dQ/dt is the rate of drug transport (µg s^{-1}), C_0 is the initial drug concentration in the donor chamber (mg mL^{-1}) and A is the surface area of the monolayer (cm^2).

To check that the monolayer has maintained its integrity throughout the transport process, a marker for paracellular absorption, such as mannitol, which is often radiolabelled for ease of assay, is added to the apical surface. If less than 2% of this crosses the monolayer in 1 hour, then the integrity of the monolayer has been maintained. Another way to check the integrity of the monolayer is by measuring the transepithelial resistance (TER).

To use the Caco-2 cells as an absorption model, a calibration curve needs to be generated. This is done for compounds for which the absorption in humans is known. Fig. 21.4 shows the general shape of the curve of the fraction absorbed in humans versus the apparent permeability coefficient in Caco-2 cells. As cells are biological systems, small changes in their source, their method of culture and the way in which the transport experiment is performed will affect the apparent permeability of a drug, such that this curve can shift significantly to the right or left, or alter in its gradient. Therefore, when carrying out Caco-2 experiments, it is important always to standardize the procedure within a particular laboratory and ensure that this procedure is regularly calibrated with a set of standard compounds.

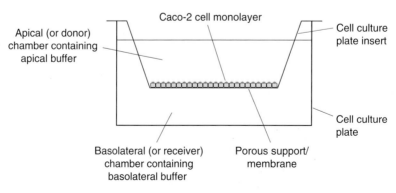

Fig. 21.3 • A Caco-2 cell culture system for determining apparent permeability.

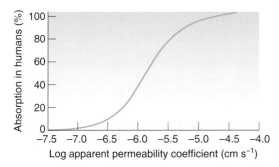

Fig. 21.4 • The relationship between the fraction absorbed in humans and the apparent permeability coefficient in Caco-2 cells.

Caco-2 monolayers can also be used to elucidate the mechanism of permeability. If the apparent permeability coefficient is found to increase linearly with increasing concentration of the drug (i.e. the transport is not saturated), is the same whether the drug transport is measured from the apical to basolateral direction or from the basolateral to apical direction, and is independent of pH, it can be concluded that the transport is a passive and not an active process. If the transport in the basolateral to apical direction is significantly greater than that in the apical to basolateral direction, then it is likely that the drug is actively effluxed from the cells by a countermembrane transporter, such as P-glycoprotein. If the transport of the drug is also inhibited by the presence of compounds that are known inhibitors of P-glycoprotein, this gives a further indication that the drug is susceptible to P-glycoprotein efflux.

To help elucidate whether other membrane transporters are involved in the absorption of a particular drug, further competitive inhibition studies can be performed with known inhibitors of the particular transporter. For example, the dipeptide glycosylsarcosine can be used to probe whether the dipeptide transporter is involved in the absorption of a particular drug.

To evaluate whether a compound is absorbed via the paracellular pathway or the transcellular pathway, the tight junctions can be artificially opened with compounds such as EDTA, which chelates calcium. Calcium is involved in keeping the junctions together. If the apparent permeability of a compound is not affected by the opening of these junctions, which can be assessed by use of a paracellular marker such as mannitol, one can assume the drug transport is via a transcellular pathway.

If the disappearance of the drug on the apical side of the membrane is not mirrored by its appearance on the basolateral side, and/or the mass balance at the end of the transport experiment does not account for 100% of the drug, there may be a problem with binding to the membrane porous support. This will need investigation, or the drug may have a stability issue. The drug could be susceptible to enzymes secreted by the cells and/or to degradation by hydrolytic enzymes as it passes through the cells, or it may be susceptible to metabolism by cytochrome P450 within the cell. Thus the Caco-2 cells are not only capable of evaluating the permeability of drugs but also have value in investigating whether two of the other potential barriers to absorption (namely, stability and presystemic metabolism) are likely to affect the overall rate and extent of absorption.

Caco-2 cells are very useful tools for understanding the mechanism of drug absorption and have furthered significantly our knowledge of the absorption of a variety of drugs. Other advantages of Caco-2 cells are that they are a nonanimal model, require only small amounts of compound for transport studies, can be used as a rapid screening tool to assess the permeability of large numbers of compounds in the discovery setting and can be used to evaluate the potential toxicity of compounds with regard to cells. The main disadvantages of Caco-2 monolayers as an absorption model are that, because of the tightness of the monolayer, they are more akin to the paracellular permeability of the colon rather than that of the small intestine and that they lack a mucous layer.

To further characterize permeability, a second cell line such as Madin–Darby canine kidney (MDCK) cells is often used. These cells are usually transfected with the *MDR1* gene, which codes for human P-glycoprotein, giving an MDR1-MDCK cell line which expresses human P-glycoprotein. This cell line is a useful model for the identification of P-glycoprotein substrates and inhibitors and their effect on permeability.

Further information on the use of Caco-2 monolayers as an absorption model can be obtained from Artusson et al. (1996) and Yang and Yu (2009).

Tissue techniques

A range of tissue techniques have been used as absorption models (see Table 21.1). Two of the more popular ones are the use of isolated sheets of intestinal

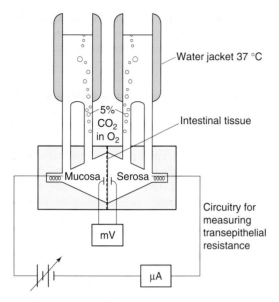

Fig. 21.5 • A diffusion chamber.

mucosa and the use of everted intestinal rings. These are discussed in more detail next.

Isolated sheets of intestinal mucosa are prepared by cutting the intestine into strips. The musculature is then removed and the sheet mounted and clamped in a diffusion chamber or an Ussing chamber filled with appropriate biological buffers (Fig. 21.5). The transepithelial resistance is measured across the tissue to check its integrity. The system is maintained at 37 °C and stirred so that the thickness of the unstirred water layer is controlled and oxygen provided to the tissue. The drug is added to the donor chamber and the amount accumulating in the receiver chamber is measured as a function of time. The permeability across the tissue can then be calculated.

Similarly to cell monolayers, the two sides of the tissue can be sampled independently, and thus fluxes from the mucosal to the serosal side and from the serosal to the mucosal side can be measured. Any pH dependence of transport can be determined by altering the pH of the buffers in the donor and/or receiver chambers. This system can also therefore be used to probe active transport.

One advantage of this technique over cell culture techniques is that permeability across different regions of the intestine can be assessed. It is particularly helpful to be able to compare permeabilities across intestinal and colonic tissue, especially when one is assessing whether a drug is suitable for a controlled-release delivery system. In addition, different animal

tissues that permit an assessment of permeability in different preclinical models can be used. The rat intestine is usually preferred for absorption studies as its permeability correlates well with that of human intestine. Human tissue and cell monolayers have also been used in this system.

Everted intestinal rings use whole intestinal segments rather than just sheets. The musculature is therefore intact. Intestinal segments are excised, again usually from rats. The segment is then tied at one end and carefully everted by placing it over a glass rod. It is cut into small sections or rings, and these rings are incubated in stirred oxygenated drug-containing buffer at 37 °C. After a set period of time, drug uptake is quenched by quickly rinsing the ring with ice-cold buffer and carefully drying it. The ring is then assayed for drug content, and the amount of drug taken up per gram of wet tissue over a specific period of time is calculated ($mol\ g^{-1}\ time^{-1}$). The advantage of the use of intestinal rings is that the test is relatively simple and quick to perform. A large number of rings can be prepared from each segment of intestine, which allows each animal to act as its own control. In addition, the conditions of the experiment can be manipulated and so provide insight into the mechanisms of absorption.

The disadvantages of this system are that it is biological and that care must be taken to maintain the viability of the tissue for the duration of the experiment. As the drug is taken up into the ring, the tissue needs to be digested and the drug extracted from it before it is assayed. This results in lengthy sample preparation and complicates the assay procedure. In addition, as this is an uptake method, no polarity of absorption can be assessed.

Both these absorption models can be calibrated with a standard set of compounds similar to the Caco-2 model. A similarly shaped curve for the percentage of drug absorbed in humans versus apparent permeability or uptake (moles per unit weight of tissue) for the isolated sheet and everted ring methods, respectively, is obtained.

Perfusion studies

Many variations of intestinal perfusion methods have been used as absorption models over the years. In general, because of its relative ease of use and similarity to the permeability of the human intestine, the rat model is preferred. In situ intestinal perfusion models have the advantage that the whole animal is

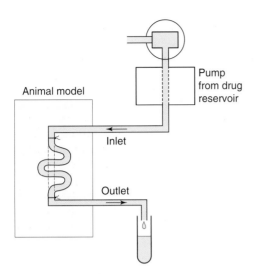

Fig. 21.6 • An in situ rat perfusion.

used, with the nerve, lymphatic and blood supplies intact. Therefore there should be no problem with tissue viability, and all the transport mechanisms present in a live animal should be functional.

The animal is anaesthetized and the intestine exposed. In the open loop method, a dilute solution of drug is pumped slowly through the intestine and the difference between the inlet and outlet drug concentrations is measured (Fig. 21.6). An absorption rate constant or effective permeability coefficient across the intestine can be calculated as follows:

$$P_{\mathrm{eff}} = Q\ln(C_i - C_0)/2\pi rl$$

$$(21.2)$$

where P_{eff} is the effective permeability coefficient (cm s^{-1}), Q is the flow rate (mL s^{-1}), C_i is the initial drug concentration, C_0 is the final drug concentration, r is the radius of the intestinal loop (cm) and, l is the length of intestinal loop (cm).

In the closed loop method, a dilute solution of drug is added to a section of the intestine and the intestine is closed. The intestine is then excised and the drug content is analysed immediately and after an appropriate time or time intervals, depending on the expected rate of absorption. Again, assuming there is a first-order rate process and hence an exponential loss of drug from the intestine, an absorption rate constant and effective permeability can be calculated. Like the intestinal ring method, the closed loop in situ perfusion model requires a lengthy digestion, extraction and assay procedure to analyse the drug remaining in the intestinal loop.

There is a lot of fluid moving in and out of the intestine, and so the drug concentrations in both these in situ perfusion methods need to be corrected for fluid flux. This is normally done by gravimetric means or by using a nonabsorbable marker to assess the effect of fluid flux on the drug concentration. As with other absorption models, correlations have been made with standard compounds where the fraction absorbed in humans is known (Fig. 21.4). In these models the 'absorption rate' is calculated by measuring the disappearance of the drug from the lumen and not its accumulation in the plasma. It is therefore important to check that the drug is not degraded in the lumen or intestinal wall as drug that has disappeared will be erroneously assumed to have been absorbed.

More sophisticated techniques are those involving vascular perfusion. In these techniques, either a pair of mesenteric vessels supplying an intestinal segment or the superior mesenteric artery and portal vein perfusing almost the entire intestine are cannulated. The intestinal lumen and sometimes the lymph duct are also cannulated for the collection of luminal fluid and lymph respectively. This model, although complicated, is very versatile as the drug can be administered into the luminal perfusate or the vascular perfusate. When the drug is administered to the intestinal lumen, drug absorption can be evaluated from both its disappearance from the lumen and its appearance in the portal vein. Using this method, both the rate and extent of absorption can be estimated, as can carrier-mediated transport processes. Collection of the lymph allows the contribution of lymphatic absorption for very lipophilic compounds to be assessed. One of the other advantages of this system is the ability to determine whether any intestinal metabolism occurs before or after absorption.

A further extension of this model is to follow the passage of drugs from the intestine through the liver, and several adaptations of rat intestinal–liver perfusion systems have been investigated. Such a combined system gives the added advantage of assessing the first-pass or presystemic metabolism through the liver, and determining the relative importance of the intestine and liver in presystemic metabolism.

The disadvantage of these perfusion systems is that as they become more complex, a larger number of animals are required to establish suitable perfusion conditions and the reproducibility of the technique. However, in general, as the complexity increases, so does the amount of information obtained.

Assessment of permeability in humans

Intestinal perfusion studies

Until relatively recently, the most common way to evaluate the absorption of drugs in humans was by performing bioavailability studies and deconvoluting the data available to calculate an absorption rate constant. This rate constant, however, is dependent on the release of the drug from the dosage form and is affected by intestinal transit and presystemic metabolism. Therefore very often it does not reflect the true intrinsic intestinal permeability of a drug.

Extensive studies have been carried out using a regional perfusion technique which has afforded greater insight into human permeability (Loc-I-Gut). The Loc-I-Gut is a multichannel tube system with a proximal and a distal balloon (Fig. 21.7). These balloons are 100 mm apart and allow a segment of intestine 100 mm long to be isolated and perfused. Once the proximal balloon passes the ligament of Treitz, both balloons are filled with air, thereby preventing mixing of the luminal contents in the segment of interest with other luminal contents. A nonabsorbable marker is used in the perfusion solution to check that the balloons work to occlude the region of interest. A tungsten weight is placed in front of the distal balloon to facilitate its passage down the gastrointestinal tract.

Drug absorption is calculated from the rate of disappearance of the drug from the perfused segment. This technique has afforded greater control in human intestinal perfusions, primarily because it isolates the luminal contents of interest, and has greatly facilitated the study of permeability mechanisms and the metabolism of drugs and nutrients in the human intestine.

Noninvasive approaches

There is concern that the invasive nature of perfusion techniques can affect the function of the gastro-intestinal tract, in particular the fluid content, owing to the intubation process altering the absorption and secretion balance. To overcome this problem, several engineering-based approaches have been developed to evaluate drug absorption in the gastrointestinal tract. These include the InteliSite®, Enterion and MAARS capsules.

The InteliSite capsule is a radiofrequency-activated, nondisintegrating delivery device. The capsule can be filled with either a liquid or a powder formulation, and the transit of the capsule is followed by γ-scintigraphy (see later in this chapter). Once the capsule reaches its desired release site, it is externally activated to open a series of windows to the drug reservoir within the capsule. The Enterion capsule is similar in that it contains a drug reservoir and γ-scintigraphy is used to locate the capsule in the gastrointestinal tract. However, its payload is released via an electromagnetic field triggering the actuation of a spring resulting in the instantaneous release of the formulation as a bolus. For both these systems, blood samples need to be taken to quantify drug absorption. The MAARS system is a magnetic active agent release system and thus relies on a magnetic impulse to disassemble the capsule and release the drug; this is a simpler system and can contain a large volume of drug. More sophisticated systems with cameras incorporated into capsules, such as the M2A capsule, are being developed to visualize the gastrointestinal tract. These can be used to help design better products.

Presystemic metabolism

Presystemic metabolism is the metabolism that occurs before the drug reaches the systemic circulation. Therefore, for an orally administered drug, this includes the metabolism that occurs in the gut wall and the liver. As discussed earlier, perfusion models that involve both the intestines and the liver allow an evaluation of the presystemic metabolism in both organs. In other models it is sometimes possible to design mass balance experiments that will assess whether presystemic intestinal metabolism is likely to occur.

Intestinal cell fractions, such as brush border membrane preparations that contain an abundance of hydrolytic enzymes, and homogenized preparations of segments of rat intestine can also be used to

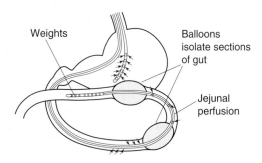

Fig. 21.7 • The Loc-I-Gut.

Weights

Balloons isolate sections of gut

Jejunal perfusion

determine intestinal presystemic metabolism. Drugs are incubated with either brush border membrane preparations or gut wall homogenate at 37 °C and the drug content is analysed.

Various liver preparations (e.g. subcellular fractions such as microsomes, isolated hepatocytes and liver slices) are used to determine hepatic metabolism in vitro. These are classified as phase I metabolism, which mainly involves oxidation but can be reduction or hydrolysis, and phase II metabolism, which follows phase I and involves conjugation reactions. Microsomes are prepared by high-speed centrifugation of liver homogenates, and are composed mainly of fragments of the endoplasmic reticulum. They lack cystolic enzymes and cofactors and are therefore suitable only to evaluate some of the metabolic processes (phase I metabolism) of which the liver is capable. Hepatocytes must be freshly and carefully prepared from livers and are viable for only a few hours. It is therefore difficult to obtain human hepatocytes. Hepatocytes are very useful for hepatic metabolism studies as it is possible to evaluate most of the metabolic reactions, i.e. both phase I and phase II metabolism. Whole liver slices again have the ability to evaluate both phase I and phase II metabolism. As liver slices are tissue slices rather than cell suspensions, and because they do not require enzymatic treatment in their preparation, they may give a higher degree of in vivo correlation than hepatocytes or microsomes.

Mechanistic physiologically based pharmacokinetic models

The concept of physiologically based pharmacokinetic (PBPK) modelling is to describe the concentration profile of a drug in various tissues over time, on the basis of the physicochemical characteristics of the drug, the site and means of administration and the physiological processes to which the drug is subjected. In PBPK modelling, the parameters determined from in vitro experiments are used in silico models to predict in vivo data.

The first commercial software describing the gastrointestinal tract in the context of a PBPK model was GastroPlus™, introduced in 1998, which used a series of mixing tanks to describe the movement of a drug from one region in the gastrointestinal tract to the next, with simple estimations of dissolution based on aqueous solubility, and absorption rate constants based on existing pharmacokinetic data.

This allowed an assessment of whether the absorption process or the solubility/dissolution would be the rate-limiting step for the drug's bioavailability. These models have been developed and become more sophisticated, and a number of other models, including Symcyp and PK-SIM®, are available, and several industries and academic groups have developed their own models. All of these programs strive to account for all relevant processes involved in the gastrointestinal absorption of drugs, including release from the dosage form, decomposition/complexation in the gastrointestinal tract, the various mechanisms of drug uptake and efflux and first-pass metabolism, whether this be in the gut wall or liver, and to describe the interplay of these factors in determining the rate and extent of drug absorption from the gastrointestinal tract and the resultant plasma profile.

These models are widely used in advance of information from the clinic to predict drug pharmacokinetics, and both the effect of physicochemical and dosage form factors such as the influence of salts and particle size on the predicted plasma profile and the effect of physiological factors such as gut lumen pH and bile salt concentrations, fasted–fed status, transit times and disease states (e.g. gastrectomy) on plasma concentrations. The PBPK models can be used to look at the impact of modified-release formulations, to design formulations for optimal exposure and to anticipate effects on bioequivalence. They can be modified iteratively as further in vitro or clinical information becomes available and can be used to inform the collection of additional data.

Assessment of bioavailability

Bioavailability is defined as the rate and extent to which the active ingredient or active moiety is absorbed from a drug product and becomes available at the site of action. The measurement of bioavailability therefore gives the net result of the effect of the release of a drug into solution in the physiological fluids at the site of absorption, its stability in those physiological fluids, its permeability and its presystemic metabolism on the rate and extent of drug absorption from the concentration–time profile of the drug in a suitable physiological fluid. The concentration–time profile also gives information on other pharmacokinetic parameters, such as the distribution and elimination of the drug. The most commonly used method of assessing the bioavailability of a drug involves the construction of a blood plasma concentration–time curve, but urine drug concentrations can also be used and are discussed later in this chapter.

Plasma concentration–time curves

When a single dose of a drug is administered orally to a patient, serial blood samples are withdrawn and the plasma is assayed for the drug concentration at specific time points after administration. This enables a plasma concentration–time curve to be constructed. Fig. 21.8 shows a typical plasma concentration–time curve following the oral administration of a tablet.

At zero time, when the drug is first administered, the concentration of the drug in the plasma will be zero. As the tablet passes into the stomach and/or intestine, it disintegrates, the drug dissolves and absorption occurs. Initially, the concentration of the drug in the plasma rises as the rate of absorption exceeds the rate at which the drug is being removed by distribution and elimination. The concentration continues to rise until a maximum (or peak) is attained. This represents the highest concentration of the drug achieved following the administration of a single dose, often termed C_{max} (or C_{pmax} in the specific case of maximum plasma concentration). It is reached when the rate of appearance of the drug in the plasma is equal to its rate of removal by distribution and elimination.

The ascending portion of the plasma concentration–time curve is sometimes called the *absorption phase*. Here the rate of absorption outweighs the rate of removal of the drug by distribution and elimination. Drug absorption does not usually stop abruptly at the time of peak concentration but may continue for some time into the descending portion of the curve. The early descending portion of the curve can thus reflect the net result of drug absorption, distribution, metabolism and excretion. In this phase the rate of drug removal from the blood exceeds the absorption rate, and therefore the concentration of the drug in the plasma declines.

Eventually drug absorption ceases when the bioavailable dose has been absorbed, and the concentration of the drug in the plasma is now controlled only by its rate of elimination by metabolism and/or excretion. This is sometimes called the *elimination phase* of the curve. It should be appreciated, however, that elimination of a drug begins as soon as it appears in the plasma.

Several parameters based on the plasma concentration–time curve that are important in bioavailability studies are shown in Fig. 21.9, and are discussed in the following paragraphs.

Minimum effective (or therapeutic) plasma concentration. It is generally assumed that some minimum concentration of drug in the plasma must be reached before the desired therapeutic or pharmacological effect is achieved. This is called the *minimum effective* (or *minimum therapeutic*) *plasma concentration*. Its value not only varies from drug to drug but also from individual to individual and with the type and severity of the disease state. In Fig. 21.9 the minimum effective concentration is indicated by the lower line.

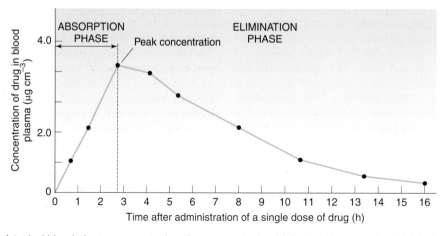

Fig. 21.8 • A typical blood plasma concentration–time curve obtained following the peroral administration of a single dose of a drug in a tablet.

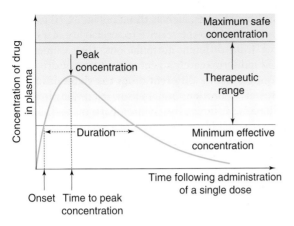

Fig. 21.9 • Relationship between the plasma concentration–time curve obtained following a single oral dose of a drug and parameters associated with the therapeutic or pharmacological response.

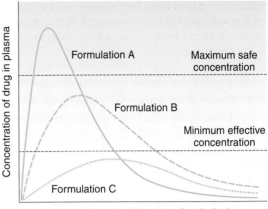

Fig. 21.10 • Plasma concentration–time curves for three different formulations of the same drug administered in equal single doses by the oral route.

Maximum safe concentration. The concentration of drug in the plasma above which side effects or toxic effects occur is known as the *maximum safe concentration*.

Therapeutic range or window. A range of plasma drug concentrations is also assumed to exist over which the desired response is obtained, yet toxic effects are avoided. This range is called the *therapeutic range* or *therapeutic window*. The intention in clinical practice is to maintain plasma drug concentrations within this range.

Onset. The *onset* may be defined as the time required to achieve the minimum effective plasma concentration following administration of the dosage form.

Duration. The *duration* of the therapeutic effect of the drug is the period during which the concentration of the drug in the plasma exceeds the minimum effective plasma concentration.

Peak concentration. The *peak concentration* represents the highest concentration of the drug achieved in the plasma, and is referred to as C_{max}.

Time to peak concentration. This is the time required to achieve the peak plasma concentration of the drug after the administration of a single dose. This parameter is related to the rate of absorption of the drug and can be used to assess that rate. It is often referred to as t_{max}.

Area under the plasma concentration–time curve. This is related to the total amount of drug absorbed into the systemic circulation following the administration of a single dose, and is often known as the area under the curve (AUC).

Use of plasma concentration–time curves in bioavailability studies

To illustrate the usefulness of plasma concentration–time curves in bioavailability studies for the assessment of the rate and extent of absorption, the administration of single equal doses of three different formulations, A, B and C, of the same drug to the same healthy individual by the same route of administration on three separate occasions can be considered. The assumption is made that sufficient time is allowed to elapse between the administration of each formulation such that the systemic circulation contained no residual concentration of the drug and no residual effects from any previous administrations. It is also assumed that the kinetics and pattern of distribution of the drug, its binding phenomena, the kinetics of elimination and the experimental conditions under which each plasma concentration–time profile is obtained are the same on each occasion. The plasma concentration–time profiles for the three formulations are shown in Fig. 21.10. The differences between the three curves are attributed solely to differences in the rate and/or extent of absorption of the drug from each formulation.

The three plasma profiles in Fig. 21.10 show that each of the three formulations (A, B and C) of the same dose of the same drug results in different peak plasma concentrations. The areas under the curves for formulations A and B are similar, indicating that the drug is absorbed to a similar extent from these two formulations. However, the absorption rate is different, with the drug being absorbed faster from formulation A than from formulation B. This means that formulation A shows a fast onset of therapeutic action, but as its peak plasma concentration exceeds the maximum safe concentration, it is likely that this formulation will result in toxic side effects. Formulation B, which has a slower rate of absorption than formulation A, shows a slower therapeutic onset than formulation A, but its peak plasma concentration lies within the therapeutic range. In addition, the duration of action of the therapeutic effect obtained with formulation B is longer than that obtained with formulation A. Hence formulation B appears to be superior to formulation A from a clinical viewpoint, in that its peak plasma concentration lies within the therapeutic range of the drug and the duration of the therapeutic effect is longer.

Formulation C gives a much smaller area under the plasma concentration–time curve, indicating that a lower proportion of the dose has been absorbed. This, together with the slower rate of absorption from formulation C (the time to peak concentration is longer than for formulations A and B), results in the peak plasma concentration not reaching the minimum effective concentration. Thus formulation C does not produce a therapeutic effect and consequently is clinically ineffective as a single dose.

This simple hypothetical example illustrates how differences in bioavailability exhibited by a given drug from different formulations can result in a patient being over medicated, undermedicated or correctly medicated.

It is important to realize that the study of bioavailability based on drug concentration measurements in the plasma (or urine or saliva) is complicated by the fact that such concentration–time curves are affected by factors other than the biopharmaceutical factors of the drug product itself. Some of the variables that can complicate the interpretation of bioavailability studies are:

- body weight;
- sex and age of the test participants;
- disease states;
- genetic differences in drug metabolism;
- distribution and excretion;
- food and water intake;
- concomitant administration of other drugs;
- stress; and
- time of administration of the drug.

As far as possible, studies should be designed to control these factors.

Although plots such as those in Fig. 21.10 can be used to compare the relative bioavailability of a given drug from different formulations, they cannot be used indiscriminately to compare different drugs. It is quite usual for different drugs to exhibit different rates of absorption, metabolism, excretion and distribution, different distribution patterns and differences in their plasma binding phenomena. All of these will influence the plasma concentration–time curve. Therefore it would be extremely difficult to attribute differences in the concentration–time curves obtained for different drugs presented in different formulations to differences in their bioavailabilities.

Cumulative urinary drug excretion curves

Measurement of the concentration of intact drug and/or its metabolite(s) in the urine can also be used to assess bioavailability.

When a suitable specific assay method is not available for the intact drug in the urine or the specific assay method available for the parent drug is not sufficiently sensitive, it may be necessary to assay the principal metabolite or intact drug plus its metabolite(s) in the urine to obtain an index of bioavailability. Measurements involving metabolite levels in the urine are valid only when the drug in question is not subject to metabolism prior to reaching the systemic circulation. If an orally administered drug is subject to intestinal metabolism or first-pass liver metabolism, then measurement of the principal metabolite or of intact drug plus metabolites in the urine would give an overestimate of the systemic availability of that drug. It should be remembered that the definition of bioavailability is in terms of the extent and the rate at which intact drug appears in the systemic circulation after the administration of a known dose.

The assessment of bioavailability by urinary excretion is based on the assumption that the appearance of the drug and/or its metabolites in the urine is a function of the rate and extent of absorption. This assumption is only valid when a drug and/or its metabolites are extensively excreted in the urine, and when the rate of urinary excretion is proportional to the concentration of the intact drug in the blood plasma. This proportionality does not hold if:

- the drug and/or its metabolites are excreted by an active transport process into the distal kidney tubule;

- the intact drug and/or its metabolites are weakly acidic or weakly basic (i.e. their rate of excretion is dependent on urine pH); or
- the excretion rate depends on the rate of urine flow.

The important parameters in urinary excretion studies are the cumulative amount of intact drug and/or metabolites excreted and the rate at which this excretion occurs. A cumulative urinary excretion curve is obtained by collecting urine samples (resulting from the total emptying of the bladder) at known intervals after a single dose of the drug has been administered. Urine samples must be collected until all the drug and/or its metabolites have been excreted (this is indicated by the cumulative urinary excretion curve becoming parallel to the abscissa) if a comparison of the extent of absorption of a given drug from different formulations or dosage forms is to be made. A typical cumulative urinary excretion curve and the corresponding plasma concentration–time curve obtained following the administration of a single dose of a given drug by the oral route to a study participant are shown in Fig. 21.11.

The initial segments (X–Y) of the curves reflect the *absorption phase* (i.e. where absorption is the dominant process), and the slope of this segment of the urinary excretion curve is related to the rate of absorption of the drug into the blood. The total amount of intact drug (and/or its metabolite(s))

excreted in the urine at point Z corresponds to the time at which the plasma concentration of intact drug is zero and essentially all the drug has been eliminated from the body. The total amount of drug excreted at point Z may be quite different from the total amount of drug administered (i.e. the dose) either because of incomplete absorption or because of the drug being eliminated by processes other than urinary excretion.

Use of urinary drug excretion curves in bioavailability studies

In order to illustrate how cumulative urinary excretion curves can be used to compare the bioavailabilities of a given drug from different formulations, let us consider the urinary excretion data obtained following the administration of single equal doses of the three different formulations, A, B and C, of the same drug to the same healthy individual by the same extravascular route on three different occasions. Assume that these give the same plasma concentration–time curves as shown in Fig. 21.10. The corresponding cumulative urinary excretion curves are shown in Fig. 21.12.

The cumulative urinary excretion curves show that the rate at which the drug appeared in the urine (i.e. the slope of the initial segment of each urinary excretion curve) from each formulation decreases in the order A > B > C. Because the slope of the initial segment of the urinary excretion curve is related to the rate of drug absorption, the cumulative urinary excretion curves indicate that the rates of absorption

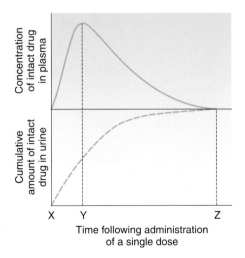

Fig. 21.11 • Corresponding plots showing the plasma concentration–time curve *(upper curve)* and the cumulative urinary excretion curve *(lower curve)* obtained following the administration of a single dose of a drug by the oral route.

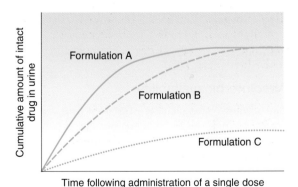

Fig. 21.12 • Cumulative urinary excretion curves corresponding to the plasma concentration–time curves shown in Fig. 21.10 for three different formulations of the same drug administered in equal single doses by the oral route.

of the drug from the three formulations decrease in the order A > B > C. The corresponding plasma concentration–time curves in Fig. 21.10 show that this is the case, i.e. peak concentration times (which are inversely related to the rate of drug absorption) for the three formulations increase in the order A < B < C. Although Fig. 21.12 shows that the rate of appearance of the drug in the urine from formulation A is faster than that from formulation B, the total amount of drug eventually excreted from these two formulations is the same, i.e. the cumulative urinary excretion curves for formulations A and B eventually meet and merge. As the total amount of intact drug excreted is assumed to be related to the total amount absorbed, the cumulative urinary excretion curves for formulations A and B indicate that the extent of drug absorption from these two formulations is the same. This is confirmed by the plasma concentration–time curves for formulations A and B in Fig. 21.10, which exhibit similar areas under their curves.

Thus both the plasma concentration–time curves and the corresponding cumulative urinary excretion curves for formulations A and B show that the extent of absorption from these formulations is equal, despite the drug being released at different rates from the respective formulations.

Consideration of the cumulative urinary excretion curve for formulation C shows not only that this formulation results in a slower rate of appearance of intact drug in the urine but also that the total amount of drug eventually excreted is much less than from the other two formulations. This is confirmed by the plasma concentration–time curve shown in Fig. 21.10 for formulation C.

Absolute and relative bioavailability

Absolute bioavailability

The absolute bioavailability of a given drug from a dosage form is the fraction (or percentage) of the administered dose which is absorbed intact into the systemic circulation. Absolute bioavailability may be calculated by comparison of the total amount of intact drug that reaches the systemic circulation after the administration of a known dose of the dosage form via a route of administration with the total amount that reaches the systemic circulation after the administration of an equivalent dose of the drug in the form of an intravenous bolus injection. An intravenous bolus injection is used as a reference to compare the systemic availability of the drug administered via different routes. This is because when a drug is delivered intravenously, the entire administered dose is introduced directly into the systemic circulation, i.e. it has no absorption barrier to cross, and is therefore considered to be totally bioavailable.

The absolute bioavailability of a given drug using plasma data may be calculated by comparing the total areas under the plasma concentration–time curves obtained following the administration of equivalent doses of the drug via any route of administration and following delivery via the intravenous route in the same individual on different occasions. Typical plasma concentration–time curves obtained by administering equivalent doses of the same drug by the intravenous route (bolus injection) and the gastrointestinal route are shown in Fig. 21.13.

For equivalent doses of administered drug,

$$\text{absolute bioavailability} = \frac{(AUC_T)_{abs}}{(AUC_T)_{iv}}$$

$$(21.3)$$

where $(AUC_T)_{abs}$ is the total area under the plasma concentration–time curve following the administration of a single dose via an absorption site and $(AUC_T)_{iv}$ is the total area under the plasma concentration–time curve following administration by rapid intravenous injection.

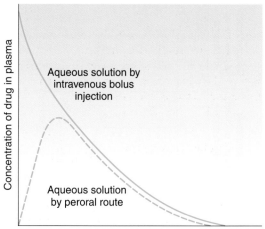

Fig. 21.13 • Typical plasma concentration–time curves obtained by administration of equivalent doses of the same drug by intravenous bolus injection and by the peroral route.

If different doses of the drug are administered by both routes, a correction for the sizes of the doses can be made as follows:

$$\text{absolute bioavailability} = \frac{(AUC_T)_{abs}/D_{abs}}{(AUC_T)_{iv}/D_{iv}}$$

(21.4)

where D_{abs} is the size of the single dose of drug administered via the absorption site and D_{iv} is the size of the dose of the drug administered as an intravenous bolus injection. Sometimes it is necessary to use different doses of drugs administered via different routes. Often the dose administered intravenously is lower to avoid toxic side effects and for ease of formulation. Care should be taken when different doses are used to calculate bioavailability data as sometimes the pharmacokinetics of a drug are nonlinear and different doses will then lead to an incorrect figure for the absolute bioavailability if it is calculated using a simple ratio, as in Eq. 21.4.

The absolute bioavailability based on urinary excretion data may be determined by comparing the total cumulative amounts of unchanged drug ultimately excreted in the urine following administration of the drug via an absorption site and the intravenous route (bolus injection) on different occasions to the same individual.

For equivalent doses of administered drug,

$$\text{absolute bioavailability} = \frac{(X_u)_{abs}}{(X_u)_{iv}}$$

(21.5)

where $(X_u)_{abs}$ and $(X_u)_{iv}$ are the total cumulative amounts of unchanged drug ultimately excreted in the urine following administration of equivalent single doses of the drug via an absorption site and as an intravenous bolus injection respectively.

If different doses of the drug are administered,

$$\text{absolute bioavailability} = \frac{(X_u)_{abs}/D_{abs}}{(X_u)_{iv}/D_{iv}}$$

(21.6)

The absolute bioavailability of a given drug from a particular type of dosage form may be expressed as a fraction or, more commonly, as a percentage.

Measurements of absolute bioavailability obtained by administration of a given drug in the form of a simple aqueous solution (which does not precipitate on contact with, or on dilution by, gastrointestinal fluids) by both the oral route and the intravenous route provide insight into the effects that factors associated with the oral route may have on bioavailability, e.g. presystemic metabolism by the intestine or liver, the formation of complexes between the drug and endogenous substances (e.g. mucin) at the site of absorption, and drug stability in the gastrointestinal fluids.

It should be noted that the value calculated for the absolute bioavailability will only be valid for the drug being examined if the kinetics of distribution and elimination are independent of the route and time of administration and the size of dose administered (if different doses are administered by the intravenous route and absorption site). If this is not the case, one cannot assume that the observed differences in the total areas under the plasma concentration–time curves or in the total cumulative amounts of unchanged drug ultimately excreted in the urine are due entirely to differences in bioavailability.

Relative bioavailability

In the case of drugs that cannot be administered by intravenous bolus injection, the relative (or comparative) bioavailability is determined rather than the absolute bioavailability. In this case the bioavailability of a given drug from a 'test' dosage form is compared with that of the same drug administered in a 'standard' dosage form. The latter is either an orally administered solution (from which the drug is known to be well absorbed) or an established commercial preparation of proven clinical effectiveness. Hence relative bioavailability is a measure of the fraction (or percentage) of a given drug that is absorbed intact into the systemic circulation from a dosage form relative to a recognized (i.e. clinically proven) standard dosage form of that drug.

The relative bioavailability of a given drug administered at equal doses of a test dosage form and a recognized standard dosage form, respectively, by the same route of administration to the same individual on different occasions may be calculated from the corresponding plasma concentration–time curves as follows:

$$\text{relative bioavailability} = \frac{(AUC_T)_{test}}{(AUC_T)_{standard}}$$

(21.7)

where $(AUC_T)_{test}$ and $(AUC_T)_{standard}$ are the total areas under the plasma concentration–time curves following the administration of a single dose of the test dosage form and of the standard dosage form respectively.

When different doses of the test and standard dosage forms are administered, a correction for the size of dose is made as follows:

$$\text{relative bioavilability} = \frac{(\text{AUC}_\text{T})_\text{test}/D_\text{test}}{(\text{AUC}_\text{T})_\text{standard}/D_\text{standard}}$$

(21.8)

where D_test and D_standard are the sizes of the single doses of the test and standard dosage forms respectively.

As for absolute bioavailability, relative bioavailability may be expressed as a fraction or as a percentage. Urinary excretion data may also be used to measure relative bioavailability as follows:

$$\text{relative bioavilability} = \frac{(X_\text{u})_\text{test}}{(X_\text{u})_\text{standard}}$$

(21.9)

where $(X_\text{u})_\text{test}$ and $(X_\text{u})_\text{standard}$ are the total cumulative amounts of unchanged drug ultimately excreted in the urine following the administration of single doses of the test dosage form and the standard dosage form respectively. If different doses of the test and standard dosage forms are administered on separate occasions, the total amounts of unchanged drug ultimately excreted in the urine per unit dose of the drug must be used in this equation.

It should be noted that measurements of relative and absolute bioavailability based on urinary excretion data may also be made in terms of either the total amount of the principal drug metabolite or the total amount of unchanged drug plus its metabolites ultimately excreted in the urine. However, the assessment of relative and absolute bioavailability in terms of urinary excretion data is based on the assumption that the total amount of unchanged drug (and/or its metabolites) ultimately excreted in the urine is a reflection of the total amount of intact drug entering the systemic circulation (as discussed for cumulative urinary excretion curves earlier).

Relative bioavailability measurements are often used to determine the effects of dosage form differences on the systemic bioavailability of a given drug. Numerous dosage form factors can influence the bioavailability of a drug. These include the type of dosage form (e.g. tablet, solution, suspension, hard gelatin capsule), differences in the formulation of

a particular type of dosage form, and manufacturing variables in the production of a particular type of dosage form. A more detailed account of the influence of these factors on bioavailability is given in Chapter 20.

Bioequivalence

Bioequivalence is the term used to describe the biological equivalence of two preparations of the same drug. If two products are said to be *bioequivalent*, they would be expected to have the same therapeutic effect. The US Food and Drug Administration (2016) defines *bioequivalence* as the absence of a significant difference in the rate and extent to which the active ingredient or active moiety in *pharmaceutical equivalents* or *pharmaceutical alternatives* (see later) becomes available at the site of drug action when administered at the same molar dose under similar conditions in an appropriately designed study. This relies on the fundamental assumption that when two products are equivalent in the rate and extent of absorption of the active drug into the plasma, the plasma concentration of the drug correlates with the concentration of the drug at the site of action (see Fig. 18.1), and therefore they will be therapeutically equivalent and can be used interchangeably.

This definition of bioequivalence contains two product types, *pharmaceutical equivalents* and *pharmaceutical alternatives*. *Pharmaceutical equivalents* means the drug products are in identical dosage forms that contain identical amounts of the identical active drug i.e. the same salt or ester of the drug. They do not necessarily contain the same excipients or inactive ingredients but the two products must meet the compendial or other applicable quality standards of identity, strength, purity and, if included, content uniformity, disintegration times, and/or dissolution rates. *Pharmaceutical alternatives* are drug products that contain the identical active drug, or its precursor, but not necessarily in the same amount or dosage form or as the same salt or ester. Each drug product should individually meet either the respective compendial quality standard or other applicable quality standard of identity, strength, quality, purity and, where included, content uniformity, disintegration times and/or dissolution rates.

The demonstration of bioequivalence is recognized by international consensus as the most appropriate method to prove therapeutic equivalence between two products that are pharmaceutical equivalents or pharmaceutical alternatives if the excipients in the product are inactive and therefore do not affect the safety and efficacy of the product.

In bioequivalence studies the plasma concentration–time profile of a test drug product is compared with that of a reference drug product. As it is unlikely that the plasma concentration–time (and/or urinary excretion) curves will be superimposable, predefined limits on pharmacokinetic parameters such as C_{max}, AUC and t_{max} which describe the rate and extent of absorption are set to demonstrate equivalent in vivo performance, i.e. similarity in terms of efficacy and safety and therefore bioequivalence (see later).

Regulatory requirements for bioequivalence

Studies to establish bioequivalence between two products are important for formulation or manufacturing changes that occur during the drug development process, for changes following registration of the product (postapproval changes) and for the introduction of new formulations and generic products. During development there are likely to be some changes in the formulation and/or the manufacturing process between early and late clinical trial formulations, differences between formulations used in clinical trials and formulations used in stability studies, differences between clinical trial formulations and marketed products, or different strengths of the same formulation. In these cases, the original product is likely to be the reference product and the new formulation is likely to be the test product. Postapproval changes to formulation components and composition, as well as to the manufacturing process and site also require demonstration of bioequivalence.

Demonstration of bioequivalence of a generic medicinal product is a fundamental concept for its approval via a simplified registration route (e.g. Abbreviated New Drug Application, ANDA). A generic medicinal product is a product which has the same qualitative and quantitative composition in active substances and the same pharmaceutical form as the reference medicinal product, and whose bioequivalence with the reference medicinal product has been demonstrated by appropriate bioavailability studies. The purpose of establishing bioequivalence is to demonstrate equivalence between the generic medicinal product and a reference medicinal product in order to allow bridging of preclinical tests and of clinical trials data, and therefore to avoid the need for further clinical efficacy or safety studies.

Pharmacokinetic studies to assess bioequivalence

Bioequivalence needs to be demonstrated between a test product and a reference product, and a number of methods can be used: pharmacokinetic methods, pharmacodynamics methods, in vitro methods and comparative clinical studies. Pharmacokinetic methods are by far the most common.

Determining bioequivalence via pharmacokinetic methods is essentially an extension of the concept of relative bioavailability. Determination of relative bioavailability involves comparing the total amount of a particular drug that is absorbed intact into the systemic circulation from a test product and from a recognized standard dosage form (the reference product). A common design for a bioequivalence study is a two-period two-sequence crossover study design which involves administration of the test and reference products on two occasions to volunteers, with each administration separated by a washout period. The washout period is chosen to ensure that the drug given in one treatment is entirely eliminated prior to administration of the next treatment. Just prior to administration, and for a suitable period afterwards, blood and/or urine samples are collected and assayed for the concentration of the drug substance and/or one or more metabolites to generate plasma/urine concentration–time curves for the two products. Pharmacokinetic measures, such as the AUC to assess extent of systemic exposure and C_{max} and t_{max} to assess the rate of systemic absorption, are generated. These metrics are calculated for each participant in the study, and the resulting values are compared statistically. The crossover design reduces variability caused by patient-specific factors, thereby increasing the ability to discern differences because of formulation.

The pharmacokinetic study to determine bioequivalence should be designed and standardized in such a way that the formulation effect can be distinguished from other effects, and to minimize interindividual and intraindividual variability. The participants should be healthy volunteers, if possible, with similar/defined age (usually 18–50 years) and weight range (within 10% of ideal body weight for height and body build). Healthy volunteers are likely to produce less pharmacokinetic variability than patients who may have confounding factors such as underlying and/or concomitant disease and concomitant medications that could affect the drug's pharmacokinetics. Male and female participants should be chosen so the sample is more representative, unless there is a reason to exclude one sex (e.g. for oral contraceptives that are intended to be used only in females). In some instances, for example when safety considerations preclude use of healthy individuals, it may be necessary to evaluate bioavailability and bioequivalence in patients for whom the drug product is intended. In this situation, sponsors and/or applicants should attempt to enrol patients whose disease process is stable during the study. The study is usually performed in fasted conditions after an overnight fast prior to dosing. Exercise, food, fluid and alcohol consumption are normally standardized or avoided during the study.

The number of participants included in the study will depend on the variability of the pharmacokinetic parameters to be evaluated (AUC, C_{max}, etc.). This should be determined from previous studies or a dedicated pilot study, the significance level desired ($\alpha = 0.05$) and the deviation from the reference product compatible with bioequivalence normally ±20%, but safety and efficacy considerations need to be taken into account in determining this. The minimum number of participants required is 12; however, in general, a bioequivalence study requires 18 to 24 participants to be statistically viable, but for a very variable drug a larger number will be required.

It is important that bioanalytical methods for measuring drug concentration in plasma (or urine) are accurate, precise, specific, sensitive and reproducible. Enough samples need to be taken at appropriate times, sufficient to fully characterize the plasma concentration–time profile and define the key pharmacokinetic parameters accurately; use of a pilot study can help in this design.

In determining bioequivalence following a single-dose study, C_{max} and AUC are analysed by analysis of variance (ANOVA). The data should be transformed prior to analysis with use of a logarithmic transformation and geometric means should be calculated. The assessment of bioequivalence is based on 90% confidence intervals for the ratio of the population geometric means (test/reference) for C_{max} and AUC. This method is equivalent to two one-sided tests with the null hypothesis of bioinequivalence at the 5% significance level. For these parameters the 90% confidence interval for the ratio of the test and reference products should be contained within the

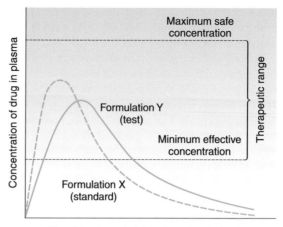

Fig. 21.14 • Plasma concentration–time curves for two chemically equivalent drug products administered in equal single doses by the oral route.

acceptance interval of 80.00% to 125.00%. A wider range may be acceptable on the basis of clinical justification.

The plasma concentration–time curves for two different products containing the same active drug following oral dosing are illustrated in Fig. 21.14. These formulations differ in terms of their rates of absorption (t_{max} and C_{max} are different); however, for both formulations the drug concentration is below the maximum safe concentration, so no big difference in tolerability would be expected and the two formulations are above the minimum effective concentration for a similar period so would be expected to perform similarly. To declare bioequivalence between these two formulations, however, the ratio of the geometric means of C_{max} and AUC for the test and reference products from a number of participants needs to be within predetermined statistical criteria (normally 80.00% to 125.00%).

In the case of drug products containing a drug which exhibits a narrow range between its minimum effective plasma concentration and its maximum safe plasma concentration (e.g. digoxin), the bioequivalence is critical, as in such cases small differences in the plasma concentration–time curves of chemically equivalent drug products may result in patients being overmedicated (i.e. exhibiting toxic responses) or undermedicated (i.e. experiencing therapeutic failure). These two therapeutically unsatisfactory conditions are illustrated in Fig. 21.15. Bioequivalence studies for products such as this, with narrow therapeutic windows, may well require tighter statistical limits.

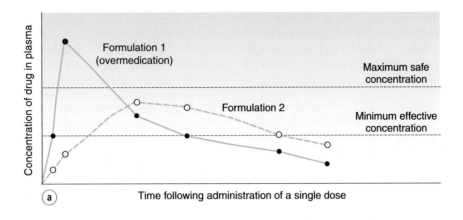

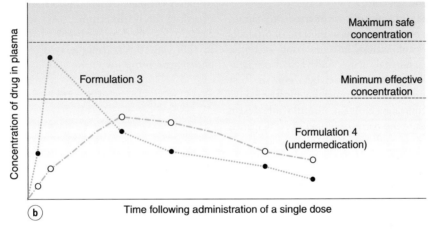

Fig. 21.15 • Plasma concentration–time curves for chemically equivalent drug products administered in equal single doses by the same extravascular route, showing potential consequences of bioinequivalence for a drug having a narrow therapeutic range, i.e. **(a)** overmedication and **(b)** undermedication.

Other methods of determining bioequivalence

It is possible to use in vitro methods to determine bioequivalence in some situations and waive the requirement for an in vivo bioequivalence study. This can usually be done to support minor changes to the formulation, process or scale during development, to compare different strengths of the formulation that have the same qualitative and quantitative composition and to justify minor changes in the formulation and manufacture after approval. The Biopharmaceutics Classification Scheme (see later) can be used to help justify the use of dissolution testing to determine bioequivalence. Normally, a representative number of dosage forms need to be tested (at least 12), and dissolution profiles of the product should be generated on all strengths using an appropriate dissolution method in three media (e.g. pH 1.2, 4.5 and 6.8) unless the dissolution of the product is not dependent on pH and strength. Further information on dissolution testing is available in Chapter 35.

Pharmacodynamics studies, i.e. measurement of a pathophysiological process over time, can be used to determine bioequivalence of two different products. This type of bioequivalence study is less common but can be undertaken where quantitative analysis in plasma or urine is not possible with a sufficient degree of accuracy and sensitivity, or where plasma concentration is not a surrogate for efficacy, e.g. topical formulations that do not have systemic exposure or targeted formulations that are designed to accumulate at the site of action. In addition, where claims of superiority of the product's effect are made, pharmacodynamics studies may be required. The pharmacodynamic parameters measured need to be relevant to the therapeutic effect and correlate with the efficacy of the drug and, potentially, safety. A pharmacodynamic effect dose–response curve is required so that it can be ensured that differences in formulation will be distinguished and no maximal effect of the response is likely to be seen during the study. The response needs to be measured quantitatively under double-blind conditions, repeatedly, so that the pharmacodynamic event can be accurately recorded (e.g. heart rate, key biomarkers, pupil diameter, blood pressure). As for pharmacokinetic studies the assay method needs to be precise, accurate, reproducible and specific.

Where no pharmacokinetic or pharmacodynamics parameters can be measured, as in the case of products intended for local action, not involving systemic absorption (e.g. dermal, ocular and vaginal preparations), comparative clinical tests between the test and the reference product must be performed to determine bioequivalence. Again, careful study design is needed to ensure the correct number of participants, clinical end points and potential safety end points are achieved. Acceptance criteria need to be determined on a case-by-case basis. There is likely to be greater variability with clinical studies than with pharmacokinetic studies.

Assessment of site of release in vivo

There are many benefits of being able to assess the fate of a dosage form in vivo, and the site and release pattern of the drug. Particularly for drugs that have poor oral bioavailability, or in the design and development of controlled-release or sustained-release delivery systems, the ability to follow the transit of the dosage form and the release of the drug from it is advantageous. Gamma scintigraphy is now used extensively and enables greater knowledge and understanding of the transit and fate of pharmaceuticals in the gastrointestinal tract to be gained.

Gamma (γ)-scintigraphy is a versatile, noninvasive and ethically acceptable technique that is capable of obtaining information both quantitatively and continuously. The technique involves the radiolabelling of a dosage form with a γ-emitting isotope of appropriate half-life and activity. Technetium-99m is often the isotope of choice for pharmaceutical studies because of its short half-life (6 h). The radiolabelled dosage

form is administered to an individual who is positioned in front of a γ-camera. γ-Radiation emitted from the isotope is focused by a collimator and detected by a scintillation crystal and its associated circuitry. The signals are assembled by computer software to form a two-dimensional image of the dosage form in the gastrointestinal tract. The anatomy of the gastrointestinal tract can be clearly seen from liquid dosage forms, and the site of disintegration of solid dosage forms can be identified. One can measure the release of the radiolabel from the dosage form by following the intensity of the radiation. By coadministration of a radiolabelled marker and a drug in the same dosage form, and simultaneous imaging and the taking of blood samples, the absorption site and release rate of a drug can be determined (e.g. with the InteliSite capsule described earlier in this chapter). When used in this way, the technique is often referred to as *pharmacoscintigraphy*.

Biopharmaceutics classification system

As a result of the plethora and variability of biopharmaceutical properties of existing and potential drugs, an attempt has been made to classify drugs into a small number of categories. The Biopharmaceutics Classification System (BCS) classifies drugs into four classes according to their dose, their aqueous solubility across the gastrointestinal pH range and their permeability across the gastrointestinal mucosa.

The scheme was originally proposed for the identification of immediate-release solid oral products for which in vivo bioequivalence tests may not be necessary. It is also useful to classify drugs and predict bioavailability issues that may arise during the various stages of the development process and is now used widely by many regulatory authorities.

The four classes are defined in terms of high and low aqueous solubility and high and low permeability:

- class I – high solubility/high permeability;
- class II – low solubility/high permeability;
- class III – high solubility/low permeability; and
- class IV – low solubility/low permeability.

A drug is considered to be highly soluble when the highest dose strength is soluble in 250 mL or less of an aqueous medium over the pH range from 1 to 8. The volume is derived from the minimum volume expected in the stomach when a dosage form is taken in the fasted state with a glass of water. If the volume of the aqueous medium needed to dissolve the drug in conditions ranging from pH 1 to pH 8 is greater than 250 mL, then the drug is considered to have low solubility. The classification therefore takes into account the dose of the drug as well as its solubility.

A drug is considered to be highly permeable when the extent of absorption in humans is expected to be greater than 90% of the administered dose. Permeability can be assessed with one of the methods discussed earlier in this chapter that has been calibrated with known standard compounds, or by pharmacokinetic studies.

Class I drugs. Class I drugs will dissolve rapidly when presented in immediate-release dosage forms, and are also rapidly transported across the gut wall. Therefore (unless they form insoluble complexes, are unstable in gastric fluids or undergo presystemic clearance) it is expected that such drugs will be rapidly absorbed and thus exhibit good bioavailability. The β-blockers propranolol and metoprolol are examples of class I drugs.

Class II drugs. In contrast, for drugs in class II, the dissolution rate is likely to be the rate-limiting step in oral absorption. For class II drugs it should therefore be possible to generate a strong correlation between in vitro dissolution and in vivo absorption (discussed earlier in this chapter). The nonsteroidal anti-inflammatory drug ketoprofen and the antiepileptic drug carbamazepine are examples of class II drugs. This class of drug should be amenable to formulation approaches to increase the dissolution rate and hence oral bioavailability.

Class III drugs. Class III drugs are those that dissolve rapidly but which are poorly permeable. The H_2-antagonist ranitidine and the β-blocker atenolol are examples. It is important that dosage forms containing class III drugs release them rapidly so as to maximize the amount of time these drugs, which are slow to permeate the gastrointestinal epithelium, are in contact with it.

Class IV drugs. Class IV drugs are those that are classed as poorly soluble and poorly permeable. These drugs are likely to have poor oral bioavailability, or the oral absorption may be so low that they cannot be given by the oral route. The diuretics hydrochlorothiazide and furosemide are examples of class IV drugs. Forming prodrugs of class IV compounds, the use of novel drug delivery technologies or finding an alternative route of delivery are approaches that have

to be adopted to significantly increase their absorption into the systemic circulation.

Biopharmaceutical drug disposition classification system

An extension of the BCS is the Biopharmaceutical Drug Disposition Classification System (BDDCS), which serves as a basis for predicting the importance of transporters in determining drug disposition, as well as in predicting drug–drug interactions. It was recognized that for drugs which exhibit high intestinal permeability (i.e. BCS classes I and II), the major route of elimination in humans is via metabolism, whilst drugs which exhibit low intestinal permeability rates (i.e. BCS classes III and IV) are primarily eliminated in humans as unchanged drug in the urine and bile. Although the two classification systems can be used to complement each other and both have the aim of speeding, simplifying and improving drug development, the purpose of the two classification systems is very different. The BCS is used to characterize drugs for which products of those drugs may be eligible for a biowaiver with regard to in vivo bioequivalence studies. The purpose of the BDDCS, however, is to predict drug disposition and potential drug–drug interactions in the intestine and the liver, and potentially the kidney and brain.

Summary

This chapter has discussed a range of approaches for assessing the biopharmaceutical properties of drugs that are intended for oral administration. Methods of measuring and interpreting bioavailability data were also described. The concepts of bioequivalence and the Biopharmaceutics Classification System of drugs were introduced.

It is imperative that the biopharmaceutical properties of drugs are fully understood, both in the selection of candidate drugs during the discovery process and in the design and development of efficacious immediate-release and controlled-release dosage forms.

Please check your eBook at **https://studentconsult. inkling.com/** for self-assessment questions. See inside cover for registration details.

References

Artusson, P., Palm, K., Luthman, K., 1996. Caco-2 monolayers in experimental and theoretical predictions of drug transport. Adv. Drug Deliv. Rev. 22, 67–84.

Food and Drug Administration, 2016. Code of Federal Regulations Title 21. Section 320.1. http://www.accessdata.fda.gov/scripts/cdrh/cfdocs/cfcfr/CFRSearch.cfm?fr=320.1.

Yang, Y., Yu, L.X., 2009. Oral drug absorption, evaluation and prediction. In: Qiu, Y., Chen, Y., Zhang, G.G.Z., et al. (Eds.), Developing Solid Oral Dosage Forms: Pharmaceutical Theory and Practice. Academic Press, London.

Bibliography

Benet, L.Z., 2013. The Role of BCS (Biopharmaceutics Classification System) and BDDCS (Biopharmaceutics Drug Disposition Classification System) in drug development. J. Pharm. Sci. 102, 34–42.

Bergström, C.A.S., Holm, R., Jørgensen, S.A., et al., 2014. Early pharmaceutical profiling to predict oral drug absorption: current status and unmet needs. Eur. J. Pharm. Sci. 57, 177–199.

Dickinson, P.A., Lee, W.W., Stott, P.W., et al., 2008. Clinical relevance of dissolution testing in quality by design. AAPS J. 10, 380–390.

Ehrhardt, C., Kim, K., 2008. Drug Absorption Studies: In Situ, In Vitro and In Silico Models. Springer, New York.

European Medicines Agency, 2010. Guideline on the Investigation of Bioequivalence. http://www.ema.europa.eu/docs/en_GB/document_library/Scientific_guideline/2010/01/WC500070039.pdf. (Accessed March 2016).

Food and Drug Administration, 2014. Guidance for Industry. Bioavailability and Bioequivalence Studies Submitted in NDAs/INDs – General Considerations. Draft Guidance. http://www.fda.gov/downloads/drugs/guidancecomplianceregulatoryinformation/guidances/ucm389370.pdf. (Accessed March 2016).

Kostewicz, E.S., Aarons, L., Bergstrand, M., et al., 2014. PBPK models for the prediction of in vivo performance of oral dosage forms. Eur. J. Pharm. Sci. 57, 300–321.

Kostewicz, E.S., Abrahamsoon, B., Brewster, M., et al., 2014. In vitro models for the prediction of in vivo performance of oral dosage forms. Eur. J. Pharm. Sci. 57, 342–366.

Lennernäs, K., 2014. Regional intestinal permeation: biopharmaceutics and drug development. Eur. J. Pharm. Sci. 57, 333–341.

Dosage regimens

22

Soraya Dhillon   Nkiruka Umaru   John H. Collett

CHAPTER CONTENTS

KEY POINTS

- Pharmacokinetics provides a mathematical basis to assess the time course of drugs in the body. It enables the following processes to be quantified: Absorption, Distribution, Metabolism and Excretion (ADME).

- The behaviour of drugs in the body can be characterized by one-compartment, two-compartment or multiple-compartment modelling. One-compartment pharmacokinetic modelling can be used in clinical pharmaceutical interpretation of drug levels, providing blood sampling is done after distribution.

- Most drugs show linear pharmacokinetic processes, where the rate of elimination is proportional to the plasma concentration.

- Some drugs such as phenytoin, high-dose theophylline or salicylates and alcohol show nonlinear drug handling, where increased or multiple doses of a medication can cause deviations from a linear pharmacokinetic profile and toxicity.

- The plasma–concentration time profile for a dosage form is influenced by the route of administration and the type of formulation.

- The time to reach steady-state plasma levels is independent of the route of administration or dosage formulation, but is determined by the drug's half-life.

- At the steady state, the plasma concentration fluctuates between a maximum and a minimum level within a dosing interval. Changing the dose and the dosing interval will impact the extent of the fluctuations, as well as the total concentration of the drug in the body. For drugs which have a narrow therapeutic range (e.g. theophylline), the dosage regimen should minimize the fluctuations. For drugs that have a wide therapeutic range, fluctuations may be less important and it is the total concentration of the drug that determines therapeutic response.

- Loading doses are required for drugs that have a long half-life and where an immediate clinical effect is required at a target drug concentration. Loading doses are dependent on the drug's volume of distribution.
- Understanding clinical pharmacokinetics is essential for effective medicines optimization.

Dosage regimens: influence on the plasma concentration-time profile of a drug in the body

The design of a dosage regimen determines the therapeutic benefit for patients. The principles of clinical pharmacokinetics are applied to design a dosage regimen for a patient that ensures the appropriate formulation of the drug is chosen for an appropriate route of administration. On the basis of the patient's drug handling parameters, which requires an understanding of absorption, distribution, metabolism and excretion (ADME), the appropriate dosage regimen for the medicine in a particular patient and condition will lead to effective medicines optimization. The pharmacist needs to ensure the appropriate regimen is prescribed to achieve optimal efficacy and minimal toxicity.

Clinical pharmacokinetics provides a basic understanding of the principles required to design a dosage regimen. Pharmacokinetics provides a mathematical basis to assess the time course of drugs and their concentrations in the body. It enables the following processes to be quantified:

- absorption;
- distribution;
- metabolism; and
- excretion.

It is these four pharmacokinetic processes, often referred to as ADME, that determine the drug concentration in the body following administration of a medicine (see also Chapter 18).

The influence that physiological factors, physicochemical properties of a drug, and dosage form factors can have in determining whether a therapeutically effective concentration of a drug is achieved in the plasma following oral administration of a *single* dose of the drug is discussed in Chapters 19 and 20.

Whilst a single dose of certain drugs (e.g. single-dose hypnotics, analgesics and antiemetics) may be used in some clinical situations, most medicines are given as a *multiple-dosage* regimen. For example, for the treatment of a respiratory tract infection, amoxicillin may be prescribed as one 500 mg capsule three times a day. The design of the regimen (i.e. formulation, route of administration, dose size and dosage frequency) is an important factor which influences what plasma concentration is achieved and maintained in the body over the prescribed course of drug treatment. Other factors to consider are patient choice and lifestyle, and thus the route of administration (the oral route is often preferred by patients) and the dosing interval (once, twice or three times a day) need to be suitable for a patient's life pattern. Moreover, the dosage form must be appropriate; for instance, a liquid may be preferable to a hard capsule for young and older patients or patients with swallowing difficulties.

Rates of ADME processes

To describe the processes of ADME, it is necessary to consider the rates of the various processes. In *zero-order* reactions the reaction proceeds at a constant rate and is independent of the concentration of a substance present in the body. An example is the elimination of alcohol. Drugs exhibiting this type of elimination will show accumulation of plasma levels of the drug, and hence nonlinear pharmacokinetics. In *first-order* reactions the reaction proceeds at a rate which is dependent on the concentration of a drug in the body. Most ADME processes follow first-order kinetics (see Chapter 7).

The majority of drugs used clinically at therapeutic dosages will exhibit first-order rate processes, i.e. the rate of elimination of most drugs will be first order. However, some drugs exhibit nonlinear rates of elimination (e.g., phenytoin and high-dose salicylates). First-order rate processes do not result in accumulation (i.e. as the amount of drug administered increases, the body is able to eliminate the drug accordingly). Hence if the dose is doubled, the steady-state plasma concentration is doubled. Whether a drug exhibits first-order or zero-order elimination is determined by its *Michaelis constant* (K_m). This parameter is the plasma concentration at which the elimination of the drug proceeds at half the maximum *metabolic capacity* (V_m). If normal therapeutic plasma levels of the drug exceed the drug's Michaelis constant, then the drug will exhibit nonlinear drug handling. For most drugs, the Michaelis constant is much higher than the levels achieved through normal therapeutic use.

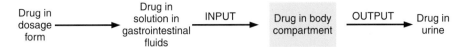

Fig. 22.1 • One-compartment open model of drug disposition for an orally administered drug.

One-compartment open model of drug disposition in the body

To understand how the design of a dosage regimen can influence the time course of a drug in the body, as measured by its plasma concentration–time profile, it is important to consider the complex pharmacokinetic processes of drug input (i.e. administration), output (i.e. elimination/metabolism) and distribution within the body. This can be described using the one-compartment open model of drug disposition, shown in Fig. 22.1.

Pharmacokinetic models are hypothetical constructs which describe the fate of a drug in a biological system following its administration. The purpose of modelling is to characterize the ADME profile for a drug to indicate how the drug is handled by the patient and to characterize basic parameters. These basic parameters describe the fate of the drug following administration and are used to optimize a dosage regimen. In a *one-compartment model* the drug is considered to be distributed instantly throughout the whole body following its release and absorption from the dosage form. Thus the body behaves as a single compartment in which absorbed drug is distributed so rapidly that a concentration equilibrium exists at any given time between the plasma, other body fluids and the tissues into which the drug has become distributed.

Rate of drug input versus rate of drug output

In a one-compartment open model the overall kinetic processes of drug input and drug output are described by first-order kinetics. Following administration of an oral dosage form, the process of drug input into the body compartment involves drug release from the dosage form and passage of the drug (absorption) across the cellular membranes, in this case the gastrointestinal barrier. The rate of drug input (absorption) at any given time is proportional to the concentration of the drug, which is assumed to be in an absorbable form, in solution in the gastrointestinal fluids at the site(s) of absorption, i.e. the effective concentration, C, of the drug at time, t.

Hence

$$\text{rate of drug input at time } t \propto C$$

(22.1)

and

$$\text{rate of drug input at time } t = -k_a C$$

(22.2)

where k_a is the apparent absorption rate constant.

The negative sign in Eq. 22.2 indicates that the effective concentration of the drug at the absorption site(s) decreases with time. The apparent absorption rate constant gives the proportion (or fraction) of the drug which enters the body compartment per unit time. Unlike the rate of drug input into the body compartment, the apparent absorption rate constant, k_a, is independent of the effective concentration of the drug at the absorption site(s). The rate of drug input will decrease gradually with time as the effective drug concentration at the site of absorption decreases (assumes first-order absorption). Other processes, such as chemical degradation and movement of the drug away from the absorption site(s), will also contribute to the gradual decrease in the drug concentration with time at the absorption site.

In the case of a one-compartment open model, the rate of drug output or elimination is a first-order process. Consequently, the magnitude of this parameter at any given time is dependent on the concentration of the drug in the body compartment at that time. Immediately following administration of the first dose of an oral dosage form, the rate of drug output from the body, i.e. elimination, will be low because a limited amount of drug has been absorbed into the body compartment. However, as absorption proceeds, initially at a higher rate than the rate of drug output, the net concentration of the drug in the body will increase with time. As the rate of drug output from the body compartment increases whilst the rate of drug input into the body compartment decreases with time, there will be a point at which the rate of drug input is equal to the rate of drug

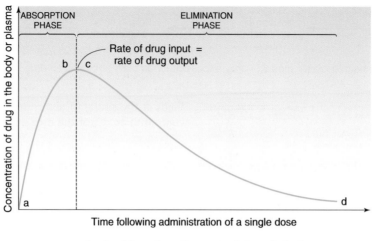

a–b rate of drug absorption > rate of drug elimination
c–d rate of drug elimination > rate of drug absorption

Fig. 22.2 • Plasma concentration–time course of a drug in the body following oral administration of a single dose of the drug which confers one-compartment open model characteristics on the body.

output, such that the net concentration of the drug in the body compartment will reach a peak value (C^{max}) and then begin to fall with time. At this stage the rate of drug output exceeds the rate of drug input.

These changes in the rates of drug input and output, relative to each other, with time are responsible for the characteristic shape of the concentration–time course of a drug in the body shown in Fig. 22.2 following oral administration of a single dose of a drug.

The shape of the curve is determined by the relationship between the rate of absorption and the rate of elimination. The greater the rate of drug input relative to the rate of drug output from the body compartment during the net absorption phase, the higher will be the peak concentration achieved in the body or plasma following oral administration of a single dose of the drug. This explains why increases in dose size and formulation changes in dosage forms, which produce increases in the effective concentration of a drug at the absorption site(s), result in higher peak plasma and body concentrations being obtained for a given drug. It should also be noted that any unexpected decrease in the rate of drug output relative to the rate of drug input, which may occur as the result of renal impairment or poor drug metabolism, is also likely to result in higher plasma and body concentrations of the drug than expected, and the possibility of the patient exhibiting toxic effects of the drug. The adjustment of dosage regimens in patients with severe renal impairment is considered

later. A summary of basic pharmacokinetic parameters is given in Box 22.1.

Elimination rate constant and biological half-life of a drug

In the case of a one-compartment open model, the rate of elimination or output of a drug from the body compartment follows first-order kinetics and is related to the concentration of the drug, C, remaining in the body compartment at time t by the following equation:

$$\text{rate of elimination at time } t = -k_e C$$

$$(22.3)$$

where k_e is the apparent elimination rate constant. The negative sign in Eq. 22.3 indicates that elimination is removing the drug *from* the body compartment.

The apparent elimination rate constant of a drug gives the proportion, or fraction, of that drug which is eliminated from the body per unit time. Its unit is in terms of reciprocal time. The apparent elimination rate constant of a given drug thus provides a quantitative index of the persistence of that drug in the body.

For example, the fraction of the drug remaining after time t is calculated from

$$C = C_0 e^{-kt}$$

$$(22.4)$$

Box 22.1

Basic pharmacokinetic parameters

The following describes various applications using the one-compartment open model system.

Elimination rate constant (k_e)

This is the basic parameter for drug elimination and can be used to estimate the amount of drug remaining or eliminated from the body per unit time.

Volume of distribution (V_d)

The volume of distribution (V_d) has no direct physiological meaning; it is not a 'real' volume and is usually referred to as the apparent volume of distribution. It is defined as *that volume of plasma in which the total amount of drug in the body would be required to be dissolved to reflect the drug concentration attained in plasma.*

The body is not a homogeneous unit even though a one-compartment model can be used to describe the plasma concentration–time profile of a number of drugs. It is important to realize that the concentration of the drug (C) in plasma is not necessarily the same as that in the liver, kidneys or other tissues.

V_d relates the total amount of drug in the body at any time to the corresponding plasma concentration. If the drug has a large V_d, this suggests the drug is highly distributed in tissues. On the other hand, if V_d is similar to the total plasma volume, this suggests the total amount of drug is poorly distributed and is mainly in the plasma.

Half-life ($t_{1/2}$)

The time required to reduce the plasma concentration to half of its initial value is defined as the *half-life ($t_{1/2}$)*.

This parameter is very useful to estimate how long it will take for plasma drug levels to be reduced to half the original concentration. This parameter can be used to estimate for how long use of a drug should be stopped if a patient has toxic drug levels, assuming the drug exhibits linear one-compartment pharmacokinetics.

Clearance (CL)

Drug clearance can be defined as the volume of plasma in the vascular compartment cleared of the drug per unit time by the processes of metabolism and excretion. Clearance is constant for all drugs that are eliminated by first-order kinetics. Drugs can be cleared by renal excretion or metabolism, or both. With respect to the kidney and liver, clearances are additive, i.e.

$$CL_{total} = CL_{renal} + CL_{nonrenal}$$

Mathematically, clearance is the product of the first-order elimination rate constant (k_e) and the apparent volume of distribution (V_d).

$$\text{Thus } CL_{total} = k_e \times V_d$$

The relationship with the half-life is

$$t_{1/2} = \frac{0.693 \times V_d}{CL}$$

If a drug has a clearance of 2 L h^{-1}, this tells us that 2 L of the volume of distribution is cleared of the drug per hour. If the concentration is 10 mg L^{-1}, then 20 mg of drug is cleared per hour.

Steady state

Most medicines are given as multiple doses, hence providing patients are given multiple doses before the preceding doses are eliminated, accumulation of the medicine will occur until a steady state is achieved. This occurs when the amount of drug administered (in a given period) is equal to the amount of drug eliminated in that same period. At the steady state, the plasma concentration of the drug (C_{ss}) at any time during any dosing interval and the peak and trough are similar. The time to reach steady-state concentrations is dependent on the half-life of the drug under consideration.

Bioavailability (F)

F is the fraction of an oral dose which reaches the systemic circulation, which following oral administration may be less than 100%. Thus when $F = 0.5$, then 50% of the drug is absorbed. Parenteral dosage forms (intramuscular and intravenous) assume a bioavailability of 100%, and so $F = 1$ and is therefore not considered, and is omitted from calculations. Absolute and relative bioavailabilities may be calculated (see Chapter 21).

Salt factor (S)

S is the fraction of the administered dose (which may be in the form of an ester or salt) which is the active drug. Aminophylline is the ethylenediamine salt of theophylline, and in this case S is 0.79. Thus 1 g of aminophylline is equivalent to 790 mg of theophylline.

Box 22.2

Calculation of the fractions of a drug eliminated from and remaining in the body with time

A patient receives a drug with an elimination rate constant of 0.08 h^{-1}. If the patient has a starting plasma concentration of the drug, C_0, of 20 mg L^{-1}, then at 4 hours the fraction remaining in the body (C) is equal to $C_0 e^{-kt}$

$$C = 20e^{-0.08 \times 4}$$

$C = 14.5$ mg L^{-1}, i.e. 72.6% of the drug is remaining and the fraction of the drug eliminated is

$$1 - e^{-kt} = 27.4\%$$

where C_0 is the starting concentration and e^{-kt} is the fraction of the drug remaining. The fraction eliminated is given by

$$1 - e^{-kt}$$

(22.5)

Application of these equations is shown in Box 22.2.

An alternative parameter used is the biological or elimination half-life of the drug, $t_{1/2}$. The biological half-life of a given drug is the time required for the body to eliminate 50% of the drug which it contained. Thus the larger the biological half-life exhibited by a drug, the slower will be its elimination from the body or plasma.

For a drug whose elimination follows first-order kinetics, the value of its biological half-life is independent of the concentration of the drug remaining in the body or plasma. Hence if a single dose of a drug with a biological half-life of 4 hours were administered orally, then after the peak plasma concentration had been reached, the plasma concentration of the drug would fall by 50% every 4 hours until the entire drug had been eliminated or a further dose was administered. The relationship between the numbers of half-lives elapsed and the percentage of the drug eliminated from the body following administration of a single dose is given in Table 22.1.

An appreciation of the relationship between the percentage of the drug eliminated from the body and the number of biological half-lives elapsed is useful when one is considering how much drug is eliminated from the body in the interval between

Table 22.1 Relationship between the amount of drug eliminated and the number of half-lives elapsed

Number of half-lives elapsed	Percentage of drug eliminated
0.5	29.3
1.0	50.0
2.0	75.0
3.0	87.5
3.3	90.0
4.0	94.0
4.3	95.0
5.0	97.0
6.0	98.4
6.6	99.0
7.0	99.2

Table 22.2 The biological half-life ranges for digoxin, theophylline, lithium and gentamicin in adult patients with uncompromised drug handling

Drug	Biological half-life (h)
Digoxin	36–51
Theophylline	6–8
Lithium	15–30
Gentamicin	2–3

successive doses in a multiple-dosage regimen. An understanding of this relationship can assist in determining an appropriate dosing interval. The biological half-life of a drug will differ from drug to drug. Biological half-lives for a number of drugs are given in Table 22.2.

There can also be significant interpatient variability influenced by disease state and lifestyle. For example, the drug theophylline has a half-life of 8.6 hours in healthy patients, yet in patients with heart failure or liver impairment it can be prolonged to 16 hours. For the same drug, in a patient who smokes will show a much shorter half-life; approximately 5 hours. For drugs such as lithium, gentamicin or digoxin, the half-life varies with age and renal function.

In the case of a drug whose elimination follows first-order kinetics, the biological half-life of the drug, $t_{1/2}$, is related to the apparent elimination rate constant, k_e, of that drug according to the following equation:

$$t_{1/2} = \frac{0.693}{k_e}$$

(22.6)

This equation indicates that the biological half-life of a drug will be influenced by any factor that influences the apparent elimination rate constant of the drug. This explains why factors such as genetic differences between individuals, age and certain diseases can affect the biological half-life exhibited by a given drug. The biological half-life of a drug is an important factor that influences the plasma concentration–time curve obtained following oral administration of a multiple-dosage regimen.

Concentration–time curve of a drug in the body following the oral administration of equal doses of a drug at fixed time intervals

In discussing how the design of multiple oral dosage regimens can influence the concentration–time course of a drug in the body, the following assumptions have been made.

- The drug exhibits the characteristics of a one-compartment open model.
- The values of the apparent absorption rate constant and the apparent elimination rate constant for a given drug do not change during the period for which the dosage regimen is administered to a patient.
- The fraction of each administered dose which is absorbed by the body compartment remains constant for a given drug.
- The aim of the dosage regimen is to maintain a concentration of the drug at the appropriate site(s) of action which is both clinically efficacious and safe for the desired duration of drug treatment.

If the time interval between each orally administered dose, i.e. dosing interval (τ), is longer than the time required for complete elimination of the previous dose, then the plasma concentration–time profile of the drug will exhibit a series of isolated single-dose profiles as shown in Fig. 22.3.

Consideration of the plasma concentration–time profile shown in Fig. 22.3 in relation to the minimum

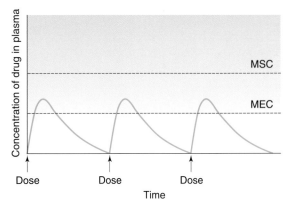

Fig. 22.3 • Plasma concentration–time curve following oral administration of equal doses of a drug at time intervals that allow complete elimination of the previous dose. *MEC*, minimum effective concentration of the drug in plasma; *MSC*, maximum safe concentration of the drug in plasma.

effective and maximum safe plasma concentrations for the drug reveals that this particular dosage regimen is unsatisfactory. The *therapeutic range* expresses the range of concentrations between which the drug will exhibit clinical efficacy and minimal toxicity. In this case the plasma concentration lies within the therapeutic range of the drug for only a relatively short time following the administration of each dose and the patient remains undermedicated for relatively long periods. If the dosing interval is reduced such that it is now shorter than the time required for complete elimination of the previous dose, then the resulting plasma concentration–time curve exhibits the characteristic profile shown in Fig. 22.4.

Fig. 22.4 shows that at the start of this multiple-dosage regimen, the maximum and minimum plasma concentrations of the drug observed during each dosing interval tend to increase with successive doses. This increase is a consequence of the time interval between successive doses being less than that required for complete elimination of the previous absorbed dose. Consequently, the total amount of the drug remaining in the body compartment at any time after a dose is equal to the sum of that remaining from all the previous doses. The accumulation of drug in the body and plasma with successively administered doses does not continue indefinitely. Providing drug elimination follows first-order kinetics, the rate of drug elimination will increase as the average concentration of the drug in the body (and plasma) rises. If the amount of drug supplied to the body compartment per unit dosing time interval remains constant, then a situation is eventually reached

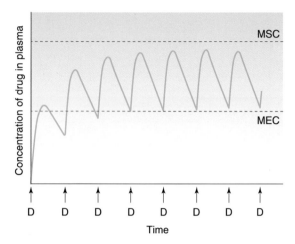

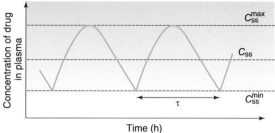

Fig. 22.5 • Fluctuation of drug concentration in the plasma at the steady state resulting from multiple oral administration of equal doses, D, of the drug at fixed time intervals, τ. C_{ss}^{max}, C_{ss}^{min} and C_{ss} represent the maximum, minimum and average plasma concentrations of the drug, respectively, achieved at the steady state.

Fig. 22.4 • Plasma concentration–time curve following oral administration of equal doses, D, of a drug every 4 hours. *MEC*, minimum effective concentration of the drug in plasma; *MSC*, maximum safe concentration of the drug in plasma.

when the overall rate of elimination of drug from the body in the dosing time interval becomes equal to the overall rate at which drug is being absorbed by the body compartment in the dosing time interval. The overall rate of elimination has effectively caught up with the overall rate of absorption of the drug by the body compartment in each dosing time interval. This is due to the elimination rate increasing as the residual concentration of the drug in the plasma rises (because elimination is first order here).

When the *overall* rate of drug supply equals the *overall* rate of drug output from the body compartment, a *steady state* is reached with respect to the *average* concentration of the drug remaining in the body in each dosing time interval. At the steady state, the amount of drug eliminated from the body in each dosing time interval is equal to the amount of drug that was absorbed by the body compartment following administration of the previous dose.

Fig. 22.5 shows that the amount of drug in the body, as measured by the plasma concentration of the drug, fluctuates between maximum and minimum values, which remain more or less constant from dose to dose. At the steady state, the average concentration of the drug in the plasma, C_{ss}, in successive dosing time intervals remains constant.

For a drug administered repeatedly in equal doses and at equal time intervals, the time required for the average plasma concentration to attain the corresponding steady-state value is a function only of the biological half-life of the drug and is independent of both the size of the dose administered and the dosing time interval. The time required for the average plasma concentration to reach 95% of the steady-state value corresponding to the particular multiple-dosage regimen is 4.3 times the biological half-life of the drug. The corresponding figure for 99% is 6.6 times. Therefore, depending on the magnitude of the biological half-life of the drug being administered, the time taken to attain steady-state plasma concentrations may range from a few hours to several days.

If we assume a patient is receiving repeated 100 mg doses of a drug and half the total amount is eliminated between doses, Table 22.3 shows the time required to reach a steady-state concentration in the body.

Table 22.3 Relationship between the dose, half-life and the amount of drug present in the body at the steady state

Repeated doses (mg)	Amount in the body (mg)	Amount eliminated (mg)	Number of half-lives
100	100	50	1
100	150	75	2
100	175	87.5	3
100	187.5	93.75	4
100	193.75	96.88	5
100	196.88	98.44	6
100	198.44	99.22	7
100	199.22[a]	99.61	8

[a]Beyond this dose, the amount of drug in the body will remain effectively constant.

In practice, the steady state is assumed to be reached after four to five half-lives. From a clinical viewpoint, the time required to reach the steady state is important because for a properly designed multiple-dosage regimen, the attainment of the steady state corresponds to the achievement and maintenance of maximal clinical effectiveness of the drug in the patient.

For some drugs, such as phenytoin, whose elimination is not described by first-order kinetics, the oral administration of equal doses at fixed time intervals may not result in the attainment of steady-state plasma levels of the drug. With repeated dosing, the average concentration of the drug in the body and plasma tends to continue to increase, rather than reaching a plateau. A glossary of pharmacokinetic equations is given in Table 22.4.

Important factors influencing steady-state plasma concentrations of a drug

Dose size and frequency of administration

The regimen must consider the plasma concentration profile at the steady state and in particular the fluctuations in C_{ss}^{max} and C_{ss}^{min}. A word here about symbols used for drug concentrations. In the case of drug levels measured at the steady state, 'ss' is often added to 'C' (i.e. C_{ss}). In the specific case of concentrations of a drug in blood plasma, an additional symbol denotes the maximum or minimum concentration at the steady state (e.g. C_{ss}^{max}, C_{ss}^{min}).

Only two factors can be adjusted for a given drug: namely, the size of the dose and the dosing interval. These are discussed in the following sections.

Size of dose

Fig. 22.6 shows the effects of changing the dose size on the concentration of the drug in the plasma following repetitive administration of oral doses at equal time intervals. As the size of the administered dose is increased, the corresponding maximum, minimum and average plasma drug levels (C_{ss}^{max}, C_{ss}^{min} and C_{ss} respectively) achieved at the steady state increase. An important factor to consider is the impact of the dose on the fluctuations in the plasma levels (i.e. they should be within the therapeutic range). The

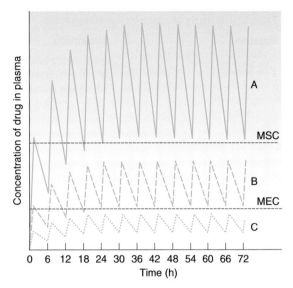

Fig. 22.6 • The effect of dose size on the plasma concentration–time curve obtained following oral administration of equal doses of a given drug at fixed intervals of time equal to the biological half-life of the drug. For curve A, each dose is 250 mg, for curve B, each dose is 100 mg and for curve C, each dose is 40 mg. *MEC*, minimum effective concentration of the drug in plasma; *MSC*, maximum safe concentration of the drug in plasma.

larger the dose administered, the larger the fluctuation between C_{ss}^{max} and C_{ss}^{min} during each dosing time interval. Large fluctuations between C_{ss}^{max} and C_{ss}^{min} may lead to toxicity if the maximum safe concentration is exceeded, or therapeutic failure may result if the minimum effective concentration is not achieved. This will impact clinically for drugs such as digoxin which have a narrow therapeutic range. Fig. 22.6 also illustrates that the time required to attain steady-state plasma concentrations of a drug is independent of the size of the administered dose.

Time interval between successive equal doses

Fig. 22.7 illustrates the effects of a constant dose administered at various dosing intervals. It is important to consider the relationship between the dosage interval and the half-life of the drug. If the dosage interval is less than the half-life, Fig. 22.7 shows that multiple administration results in higher steady-state plasma drug concentrations being obtained. The higher steady-state concentration is a consequence of the amount of the drug eliminated from the body in a dosing time interval equal to $0.5t_{1/2}$ being smaller

Table 22.4 Glossary of pharmacokinetic equations

Equation	Description	Practical use
$C_0 = \dfrac{S \times F \times D}{V_d}$	Initial plasma concentration at time zero following an intravenous bolus dose	To determine the maximum concentration following an intravenous bolus dose
$t_{1/2} = \dfrac{0.693}{k}$	Elimination half-life	Half-life can be used to: • determine the time to reach the steady state (e.g. four to five half-lives); and • determine when 50% of the measured serum concentration will fall by 50% (e.g. toxic drug levels for drugs with linear kinetics)
$CL = k \times V_d$	Clearance (CL) is the volume of plasma from which the drug is eliminated per unit time	Clearance can be used to determine how the patient is eliminating the drug. Clearance for drugs renally excreted is normally based on creatinine clearance and on the weight for drugs which are metabolized
$C = C_0 e^{-kt}$	*Single intravenous bolus injection.* Equation to describe the plasma concentration at any time (t) after a single intravenous bolus dose	C is the plasma concentration, and this equation can be used to: • determine the drug concentration at any time (t) following bolus administration; and • determine the change in drug concentration within a dosing interval at the steady state. This equation can also be rearranged to calculate the time taken for toxic drug levels to decay
$C = \dfrac{C_0 \times k_a}{(k_a - k)}(e^{-kt} - e^{-k_a t})$	*Single oral dose.* Equation to describe the plasma concentration at any time (t) after a single oral dose	C is the plasma concentration, and this equation can be used to determine the drug concentration at any time following a single oral dose. This can be applied to any dosage form where there is an absorption phase
$C_{ss} = C_0 \dfrac{e^{-kt}}{(1 - e^{-kt})}$	*Multiple intravenous bolus injections.* Equation to describe the concentration at any time (t) within a dosing interval	C_{ss} is the plasma concentration, and this equation can be used to determine the drug concentration at any time following multiple intravenous administrations
$C_{ss}^{max} = C_0 \dfrac{1}{(1 - e^{-kt})}$	*Multiple intravenous bolus injections.* Equation to describe the maximum drug concentration within a dosing interval	C_{ss}^{max} is the maximum concentration, and this equation can be used to determine the maximum (i.e. peak) drug concentration at the steady state
$C_{ss}^{min} = C_0 \dfrac{e^{-kt}}{(1 - e^{-kt})}$	*Multiple intravenous bolus injections.* Equation to describe the minimum drug concentration within a dosing interval	C_{ss}^{min} is the minimum drug concentration, and this equation can be used to determine the minimum (i.e. trough) drug concentration at the steady state
$C = \dfrac{D \times S(1 - e^{-kt})}{\tau \times CL}$	*Intravenous infusion before the steady state.* Equation to describe the concentration at any time (t) following the start of an intravenous infusion	C is the plasma concentration, and this equation can be used to determine the drug concentration at any time following the start of an intravenous infusion

Continued

Table 22.4 Glossary of pharmacokinetic equations—cont'd

Equation	Description	Practical use
$C_{ss} = \dfrac{D \times S}{\tau \times CL}$	*Intravenous infusion at the steady state.* Equation to describe the steady-state drug concentration	C_{ss} is the steady-state plasma concentration, and this equation can be used to determine the drug concentration at the steady state following the start of an intravenous infusion. The equation can be rearranged to calculate a starting dose (i.e. infusion rate) for a target concentration $R = D/\tau$
$C_{ss} = \dfrac{C_0 k_a}{(k_a - k)} \left(\dfrac{e^{-kt}}{(1 - e^{-kt})} - \dfrac{e^{-k_a t}}{(1 - e^{-k_a t})} \right)$	*Multiple oral dosing at the steady state.* Equation to describe the concentration at any time (t) within a dosing interval at the steady state	C_{ss} is the drug concentration at any time following multiple oral drug dosing. This equation can be used to determine the drug concentration at any time following multiple oral dosing (or following dosing by any route or for any dosage form where there is an absorption phase)
$t_{ss}^{max} = \dfrac{1}{(k_a - k)} \ln \left(\dfrac{k_a (1 - e^{-kt})}{k (1 - e^{-k_a t})} \right)$	Equation to calculate the time at which the maximum concentration occurs	t_{ss}^{max} is the time to achieve the maximum concentration and is determined by the absorption rate constant and the elimination rate constant
$C_{ss}^{max} = \dfrac{C_0 k_a}{(k_a - k)} \left(\dfrac{e^{-kt_{ss}^{max}}}{(1 - e^{-kt})} - \dfrac{e^{-k_a t_{ss}^{max}}}{(1 - e^{-k_a t})} \right)$	Equation to describe the maximum concentration within a dosing interval at the steady state	C_{ss}^{max} is the maximum concentration, and this equation can be used to determine the maximum (i.e. peak) drug concentration at the steady state following oral (or extravascular dosing)
$C_{ss}^{min} = \dfrac{C_0 k_a}{(k_a - k)} \left(\dfrac{e^{kt}}{(1 - e^{-kt})} - \dfrac{e^{-k_a t}}{(1 - e^{-k_a t})} \right)$	Equation to describe the minimum concentration within a dosing interval at the steady state	C_{ss}^{min} is the minimum concentration, and this equation can be used to determine the minimum (i.e. trough) drug concentration at the steady state following oral (or extravascular dosing)
$LD = \dfrac{V_d \times C}{S \times F}$	*Loading dose (LD).* Equation to calculate the loading dose at the initiation of therapy	LD is the loading dose (intravenous or oral), and this equation enables calculation of a suitable loading dose for a target drug concentration. The equation assumes the patient has not received this therapy previously
$LD = \dfrac{V_d \times (C_{desired} - C_{observed})}{S \times F}$	*Loading dose (LD).* Equation to calculate the loading dose for a patient who has already received the medication	LD is the loading dose (intravenous or oral), and this equation enables calculation of a suitable loading dose for a target drug concentration ($C_{desired}$). You need to estimate or measure the current concentration of the medicine in the plasma ($C_{observed}$). Population data can be used to estimate the drug concentration in the plasma for patients in whom this regimen has already been started
$C_{ss} = \dfrac{S \times F \times D}{CL \times \tau}$	Equation to describe the average steady-state concentration (C_{ss})	C_{ss} is the average plasma concentration at the steady state, and this equation can be used to determine the drug concentration at the steady state following oral, intravenous or other routes of administration. The equation can be rearranged to calculate the starting dose, i.e. D, for a given dosing interval (τ)
$t_{decay} = \dfrac{\ln C_1 - \ln C_2}{k}$	*Time for decay.* Equation to describe the decay/decline in toxic drug levels: linear pharmacokinetics	t_{decay} is the time taken for a toxic drug level to decay to a desired and safe drug concentration

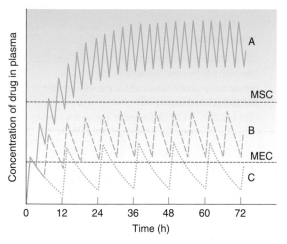

Fig. 22.7 • The effect of changing the dosing interval, t, on the plasma concentration–time curve obtained following multiple oral administration of equal-sized doses of a given drug. For curve A the dosing interval is 3 hours ($0.5t_{1/2}$), for curve B the dosing interval is 6 hours ($t_{1/2}$) and for curve C the dosing interval is 12 hours ($2t_{1/2}$). *MEC*, minimum effective concentration of the drug in plasma; *MSC*, maximum safe concentration of the drug in plasma.

than that which is eliminated when the dosing time interval is $t_{1/2}$.

Fig. 22.7 also shows the impact of the dosing interval if it is greater than the half-life of the drug, which results in lower steady-state plasma drug concentrations being obtained. This decrease is a consequence of a greater proportion of the drug being eliminated in a dosing time interval equal to $2t_{1/2}$ as compared with that which is eliminated when the dosing time interval is equal to $t_{1/2}$. The profile also shows greater fluctuation in C_{ss}^{max} and C_{ss}^{min}.

Summary of the effects of dose size and frequency of administration

Consideration of the effects of the administered dose size and the dosage time interval on the amount of a given drug in the body, as measured by the plasma concentration of the drug, following multiple oral administration of equal doses of the drug has revealed the following relationships:

- The magnitude of the fluctuations between the maximum and minimum steady-state amounts of the drug in the body is determined by the size of the dose administered or, more accurately, by the amount of drug absorbed following each dose administered.

- The magnitude of the fluctuations between the maximum and minimum steady-state plasma concentrations of a drug is an important consideration for any drug which has a narrow therapeutic range. The administration of smaller doses at more frequent intervals is a means of reducing the steady-state fluctuations without altering the average steady-state plasma concentration of the drug. For example, a 500 mg dose of a drug given every 12 hours will provide the same C_{ss} as a 250 mg dose of the same drug given every 6 hours, whilst the C_{ss}^{max} and C_{ss}^{min} fluctuation for the latter dose regimen will be decreased by a half.

- The average maximum and minimum amounts of a drug achieved in the body at the steady state are influenced by either the dose size or the dosage time interval in relation to the biological half-life of the drug, or both. The greater the dose size and the shorter the dosage time interval relative to the biological half-life of the drug, the greater are the average, maximum and minimum steady-state amounts of the drug in the body.

- For a given drug, the time taken to achieve the steady state is independent of the dose size and the dosage time interval.

- The maximum safe and minimum effective plasma drug concentrations (therapeutic range) are represented by the horizontal dashed lines in Figs 22.6 and 22.7. It is evident that the proper selection of the dose size and the dosage time interval is important with respect to achieving and maintaining steady-state plasma concentrations which lie within the therapeutic range of the particular drug being administered.

The characteristics of the drug concentration–time profile are determined by the selection of the dose size and the dosage time interval, which is crucial in ensuring that a multiple-dosage regimen provides steady-state concentrations of the drug in the body which are both clinically efficacious and safe, i.e. within the therapeutic range for that drug. Patient choice and social factors are also important to consider. For instance, most patients would prefer to take medication once or twice daily, rather than more frequently. Consequently, patient adherence to the prescribed regimen needs to be considered as well as the pharmacokinetic characteristics of the drug formulation.

Mathematical relationships which predict the values of the various steady-state parameters achieved in the body following repeated administration of doses at constant time intervals have been used to assist the design of clinically acceptable multiple-dosage regimens. A useful equation for predicting the average *concentration of a drug* (C_{ss}) achieved in the body at the steady state, following multiple oral administration of equal doses, D, at a fixed time interval, τ, is given by

$$D = \frac{C_{ss} \times CL \times \tau}{S \times F}$$

(22.7)

where F is the fraction of drug absorbed following administration of a dose, D, of the drug (thus $F \times D$ is the bioavailable dose of the drug), S is the salt factor, CL is the clearance and τ is the dosage interval. Eq. 22.7 can be rewritten in terms of the average steady-state plasma concentration of the drug as follows:

$$C_{ss} = \frac{S \times F \times D}{CL \times \tau}$$

(22.8)

If the average body amount or the average plasma concentration of a given drug at the steady state which gives a satisfactory therapeutic response in a patient is known, then Eq. 22.7 or Eq. 22.8 can be used to estimate, respectively, either the size of dose which should be administered at a preselected dosage time interval or the dosage time interval at which a preselected dose should be administered repeatedly. To illustrate a dosage regimen calculation, based on the average steady-slate plasma concentration of a drug, a worked example is shown in Box 22.3.

Mathematical equations which predict the maximum or minimum steady-state plasma concentrations of a drug achieved in the body following repeated administration of equal doses at fixed time intervals are also available for drugs whose time course in the body is described by the one-compartment open pharmacokinetic model.

Concept of loading doses

The time required for a given drug to reach 95% of the average steady-state plasma concentration is

---

Box 22.3

Calculation of a dosage regimen to achieve a desired steady-state plasma concentration

An antibiotic is to be administered repeatedly to a female patient weighing 50 kg. The antibiotic is available in the form of capsules each containing 250 mg of the drug. The fraction of the drug which is absorbed following oral administration of one 250 mg capsule is 0.9. The antibiotic has a biological half-life of 3 hours, and the patient has an apparent volume of distribution of 0.2 L per kilogram of body weight.

To estimate the dosing interval required for a multiple-dosage regimen to achieve a therapeutic average steady-state plasma concentration of 16 mg L^{-1}, the following approach can be used.

Use Eq. 22.8:

$$C_{ss} = \frac{S \times F \times D}{CL \times \tau}$$

where the average steady-state plasma concentration of the drug, C_{ss}, is 16 mg L^{-1}, the fraction of each administered dose absorbed, F, is 0.9, $S = 1$, the size of administered dose, D, is 250 mg, the elimination rate constant for the drug, k_e, is 0.23 h^{-1}, the apparent volume of distribution, V_d, is 0.2 L per kilogram of the patient's body weight, and the clearance, CL, is 2.31 L h^{-1}.

For a patient weighing 50 kg, $V_d = 0.2$ L kg^{-1} × 50 kg = 10 L

To calculate the dosing interval, τ, we have to substitute the aforementioned values into Eq. 22.7,

$$D = \frac{C_{ss} \times CL \times \tau}{S \times F}$$

after rearrangement to give

$$\tau = \frac{D \times S \times F}{CL \times C_{ss}}$$

$$\tau = \frac{250 \times 1 \times 0.9}{2.3 \times 16}$$

which gives approximately 6 hours.

Thus one 250 mg capsule should be administered every 6 hours to achieve the required average steady-state plasma concentration.

---

approximately 4.5 biological half-lives. Hence for a drug with a long half-life of 24 hours, it would take more than 4 days for the average drug concentration in the plasma to reach 95% of its steady-state value. For some drugs it is important to achieve plasma levels within the therapeutic range quickly for clinical efficacy, and it would be unacceptable to wait 4 days

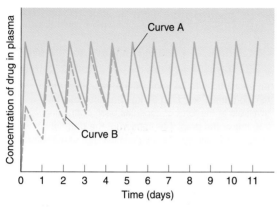

Fig. 22.8 • Representation of how the initial administration of a loading dose followed by equal maintenance doses at fixed time intervals ensures rapid attainment of steady-state plasma levels for a drug having a long biological half-life of 24 hours. Curve A represents the plasma concentration–time curve obtained following oral administration of a loading dose of 500 mg, followed by a maintenance dose of 250 mg every 24 hours. Curve B represents the plasma concentration–time curve obtained following oral administration of a 250 mg dose every 24 hours.

to achieve therapeutic levels. To reduce the time required for the onset of the full therapeutic effect of a drug, a large single dose of the drug may be administered initially in order to achieve a peak plasma concentration which lies within the therapeutic range of the drug and is approximately equal to the value of C_{ss}^{max} required. This initial dose is known as the *loading dose*. Thereafter, smaller, equal doses are administered at suitable fixed time intervals to maintain the plasma concentrations of the drug at the required maximum, minimum and average steady-state levels which provide the patient with the full therapeutic benefit of the drug.

Fig. 22.8 shows how rapidly therapeutic steady-state plasma concentrations of a drug are achieved when the dosage regimen consists of an initial loading dose followed by maintenance doses compared with a 'simple' multiple-dosage regimen of equal-sized doses administered at the same dosage intervals. Boxes 22.4 and 22.5 show the impact of giving a loading dose and the resulting plasma concentrations. The plasma concentration after the initial loading dose (LD) will fall, and the level will eventually fall below the therapeutic level; to maintain the steady-state level, the maintenance dose is given after the loading dose. This is illustrated for drugs with a long half-life and a short half-life.

Box 22.4

Loading dose and maintenance dose for a drug with a long biological half-life

A 70-year-old man requires oral digoxin therapy. Digoxin is an example of a drug with a long half-life. The half-life of this drug is 99 hours and hence a loading dose and a maintenance dose are required.

Parameters:

Weight: 68 kg
Volume of distribution (V_d): 7.2 L kg^{-1} = 490 L
Clearance (CL): 3.4 L h^{-1}
Elimination rate constant (k_e): 0.006939 h^{-1}
Half-life: 99 hours
Bioavailability (F): 0.65
Salt factor (S): 1
Target plasma level (C): therapeutic range from 1 microgram L^{-1} to 2 microgram L^{-1}

Loading dose (LD):

$$LD = \frac{V_d \times C}{S \times F}$$

(22.9)

$$LD = \frac{490 \times 1.5}{1 \times 0.65}$$

$$LD = 1130.8 \text{ microgram}$$

Consider the dosage forms available and give the patient a dose which enables an appropriate dose to be administered. Digoxin is available as 62.5 microgram, 125 microgram and 250 microgram tablet dosage forms. In practice the dose can be best given as 1 mg split into two 500 microgram doses. In clinical practice a higher single dose would cause nausea, and this patient would receive a 1 mg loading dose as 500 microgram in the morning and 500 microgram after 6 hours.

If no maintenance dose were administered, the target level of 1.5 microgram L^{-1} would decay to 1.26 microgram L^{-1} in 1 day and 1 microgram L^{-1} in 2 days.

Maintenance dose:

Use Eq. 22.7:

$$D = \frac{C_{ss} \times CL \times \tau}{S \times F}$$

$$D = \frac{1.5 \times 3.4 \times 24}{1 \times 0.65}$$

$$D = 188 \text{ microgram daily}$$

Hence the optimal dosage, based on available tablet strengths, will be 187.5 microgram daily and this patient would receive 187.5 microgram daily.

Box 22.5

Loading dose and maintenance dose for a drug with a short biological half-life

A 20-year-old woman requires theophylline for an acute asthma attack. Theophylline is an example of a drug with a short half-life. The half-life of this drug is 8 hours, and hence a loading dose and a maintenance dose, administered as aminophylline intravenous infusion, are required.

Parameters:

Patient weight: 50 kg

Volume of distribution (V_d): 0.5 L kg^{-1} = 25 L

Clearance (CL): 0.04 × weight = 2.0 L h^{-1}

Elimination rate constant (k_e): 0.08 h^{-1}

Half-life: 8.6 hours

Bioavailability (F): 1

Salt factor (S): 0.79

Target plasma level (C): therapeutic range from 10 mg L^{-1} to 20 mg L^{-1} (10 microgram mL^{-1} to 20 microgram mL^{-1})

Loading dose:

Use Eq. 22.9:

$$LD = \frac{V_d \times C}{S \times F}$$

Aim for C = 10 mg L^{-1}

$$LD = \frac{25 \times 10}{1 \times 0.79}$$

$$LD = 316\,mg$$

or

Aim for C = 15 mg L^{-1}

$$LD = \frac{25 \times 10}{1 \times 0.79}$$

$$LD = 474.7\,mg$$

Aminophylline infusion is available as a 25 mg mL^{-1} solution in a 10 mL ampoule. The easiest volume to use is two ampoules (20 mL), which is equivalent to 500 mg. As this patient has severe asthma, in clinical practice she would receive 500 mg as a loading dose.

If no maintenance dose was administered, the target level 10 microgram mL^{-1} would decay to 5 microgram mL^{-1} in 8.66 hours and 2.5 microgram mL^{-1} in 17 hours.

Maintenance infusion dose:

Use Eq. 22.7:

$$D = \frac{C_{ss} \times CL \times \tau}{S \times F}$$

$$D = \frac{10 \times 2 \times 1}{1 \times 0.79}$$

$$D = 25.32\,mg$$

This patient would receive an infusion dosage of 25 mg of aminophylline per hour.

Population data and basic pharmacokinetic parameters

To apply the principles of pharmacokinetics in practice, population data may be used. Population data are mean pharmacokinetic parameters, such as the apparent volume of distribution, which can be used to calculate predicted drug concentrations following a given dosage, or to calculate the dosage regimen, including loading and maintenance doses, required to achieve a particular drug concentration. Population data, i.e. basic pharmacokinetic parameters, can be found in standard reference sources or in original pharmacokinetic studies. It is important to identify the correct population data for the particular type of

patient. Interested readers are referred to the texts listed in the bibliography for further information and for examples of the use of such parameters.

Influence of changes in the apparent elimination rate constant of a drug: patients with renal impairment

Whilst the loading dose, maintenance dose and dosage time interval may be varied to design a clinically efficacious multiple-dosage regimen, one factor cannot normally be adjusted. That factor is the apparent elimination rate constant exhibited by the particular drug being administered. However, the elimination rate constant of a given drug does differ from patient to patient and is influenced by whether the patient has normal or impaired renal function.

Fig. 22.9 indicates the effects produced by changes in the apparent elimination rate constant on the plasma concentration–time curve obtained following multiple oral administration. Any reduction in the apparent elimination rate constant of a drug will produce a proportional increase in the biological half-life exhibited by that drug. This reduction, in turn, will result in a greater degree of accumulation of the drug in the body following multiple administrations before steady-state drug levels are achieved. The greater degree of drug accumulation is a consequence of a smaller proportion of the drug being eliminated from the body in each fixed dosage time interval when the biological half-life of the drug is increased.

Patients who develop severe renal impairment normally exhibit smaller apparent elimination rate constants and consequently longer biological half-lives for drugs which are eliminated substantially by renal excretion than do patients with normal renal function. For instance, the average apparent elimination rate constant for digoxin may be reduced from 0.021 h^{-1} in patients with normal renal function to 0.007 h^{-1} in patients with severe renal impairment. The average steady-state amount of the drug in the body is achieved and maintained when only the overall rate of drug supply equals the overall rate of elimination of the drug from the body in successive dosing intervals. Any reduction in the overall rate of elimination of a drug as a result of renal disease without a corresponding compensatory reduction in the overall rate of drug supply will result in increased steady-state amounts in the body. This effect may, in turn, lead to side effects and toxicity if the increased steady-state levels of the drug exceed the maximum safe concentration of the drug.

In order to illustrate this concept, consider that curves A and B in Fig. 22.9 correspond to the plasma concentration–time curves obtained for a given drug in patients with normal renal function and severe renal impairment respectively and that the upper and lower dashed lines represent the maximum safe and minimum effective plasma concentrations respectively. It is evident that administration of a drug according to a multiple-dosage regimen which produces therapeutic steady-state plasma levels of the drug in patients with normal renal function will result in plasma drug concentrations which exceed the maximum safe plasma concentration of the drug

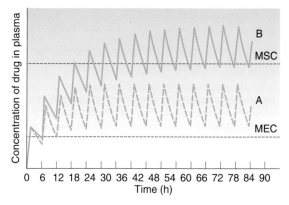

Fig. 22.9 • The effect of changing the biological half-life of a given drug on the plasma concentration–time curve exhibited by the drug following oral administration of one 250 mg dose every 6 hours. For curve A the biological half-life of the drug is 6 hours and for curve B the biological half-life of the drug is 12 hours. *MEC*, minimum effective concentration of the drug in plasma; *MSC*, maximum safe concentration of the drug in plasma.

in patients with severe renal impairment. Hence adjustment of multiple-dosage regimens in terms of dose size, frequency of administration or both is necessary if patients with renal disease are to avoid the possibility of overmedication. Further information is provided in the specialist pharmacokinetics texts in the bibliography.

Summary

This chapter has explained the interrelationship between the rate at which a drug enters the body and the rate at which it leaves. It has also discussed how, in turn, this balance influences the concentration of the drug in the blood plasma at any given time. It is clearly important for pharmacists and pharmaceutical scientists to understand these concepts so as to find ways of maintaining therapeutic drug levels appropriate to a particular disease state. This can be achieved by the careful design of the appropriate drug delivery system. The design and formulation of modified-release drug delivery systems extending drug release from a dosage form to prolong the therapeutic drug levels in the blood plasma are discussed fully in Chapter 31.

Please check your eBook at **https://studentconsult. inkling.com/** for self-assessment questions. See inside cover for registration details.

Bibliography

Dhillon, S., Kostrewski, A., 2006. Clinical Pharmacokinetics. Pharmaceutical Press, London.

Gibaldi, M., 1991. Biopharmaceutics and Clinical Pharmacokinetics, fourth ed. Lea & Febiger, Philadelphia.

Rowland, M., Tozer, T.N., 2010. Clinical Pharmacokinetics and Pharmacodynamics: Concepts and Applications, fourth ed. Lippincott Williams & Wilkins, Philadelphia.

Shargel, L., Yu, A.B.C., 2015. Applied Biopharmaceutics & Pharmacokinetics, seventh ed. McGraw-Hill, New York.

Winter, M., 2009. Basic Clinical Pharmacokinetics, fifth ed. Lippincott Williams & Wilkins, Philadelphia.

Part 5: Dosage form design and manufacture

Pharmaceutical preformulation

Simon Gaisford

CHAPTER CONTENTS

KEY POINTS

- Preformulation is the stage in drug and dosage form development before formulation proper.
- The aim of preformulation is to optimize the process of developing a drug candidate into a drug product.
- During preformulation, the physicochemical properties of drug candidates are determined.
- Solubility is usually the first parameter to be determined. In general, solubility greater than 10 mg mL^{-1} is optimal for oral delivery, whereas solubility less than 1 mg mL^{-1} may be problematic.
- Partition coefficients are determined between water and an organic (often n-octanol) phase. Partition coefficients are usually quoted as a log P value. Lipophilic compounds have a positive log P value; hydrophilic compounds have a negative log P value.
- Knowledge of solubility and partition coefficient allow a Biopharmaceutics Classification System (BCS) category to be assigned to the drug candidate, which gives an indication of the likely ease of formulation.
- Melting point and enthalpy of fusion are characteristic of the polymorphic form and allow calculation of ideal solubility.

- If the drug candidate has a pK_a, then its solubility will change with pH, and salt formation is possible.
- Salts enhance solubility by changing the pH on dissolution. Salt formation ideally requires a difference of 3 pK_a units between the free drug and the acid or base. Salts can also be used to enable isolation of the active substance, or to enhance stability or processability.
- Particle shape affects flow. Flow is assessed using a measure of compressibility (Carr's index or Hausner ratio) and angle of repose.
- Compaction requires good compression and cohesion properties.

The concept of preformulation

Formulation is the process of developing a drug candidate into a drug product. Initially, there may be a number of potential drug candidate molecules, each with a unique set of physicochemical properties and each showing activity towards a particular biological target. Ultimately, only one (at best) will be developed into a drug product. The decision to select a successful drug candidate to be developed does not depend on pharmacological efficacy alone. In practice, the physicochemical properties of the molecule affect how a material will be processed pharmaceutically, its stability, its interaction with excipients and how it will transfer to solution and, ultimately, will determine its bioavailability. It follows that characterizing the physicochemical properties of drug candidates early in the development process will provide the fundamental knowledge base upon which candidate selection, and ultimately dosage form design, can be made, reducing development time and costs.

It is an obvious point – but crucial to the task ahead – that usually nothing will be known about the physicochemical properties of a new drug candidate, and these facts must be ascertained by a combination of scientific consideration of the molecular structure and experimentation. At this stage of the development, the new drug candidate is often somewhat impure and in very short supply. Normal formulation studies have to be modified to deal with this scenario.

Physicochemical properties can be split into those that are *intrinsic* to the molecule and those that are *derived* from bulk behaviour (e.g. of the powder or crystals). Intrinsic properties are inherent to the molecule and so can only be altered by chemical modification, whereas derived properties are the result of intermolecular interactions and so can be affected by the solid-state form, physical shape and environment among other factors.

Determination of these properties for a new chemical entity is termed *preformulation* (literally the stage that must be undertaken before formulation proper can begin).

Assay development

No relevant physicochemical property can be measured without an assay, and so development of a suitable assay is the first step of preformulation. The first assay procedures should require minimal amounts of sample (since as little as 50 mg of each compound may actually exist). Ideally, experiments should allow determination of multiple parameters. For instance, a saturated solution prepared to determine aqueous solubility may subsequently be reused to determine a partition coefficient.

Note that at this stage the determination of *approximate* values is acceptable so as to make a 'go/no go' decision in respect of a particular drug candidate, and so assays do not need to be as rigorously validated as they do later in formulation development. Table 23.1 lists a range of properties to be measured

Table 23.1 Molecular properties and the assays used to determine them

Property	Assay	Requirement of sample
Solubility[a] Aqueous Nonaqueous	UV spectrophotometry	Chromophore
pK_a	UV spectrophotometry Potentiometric titration	Acid or basic group
P_w^0/log$P$	UV spectrophotometry TLC HPLC	Chromophore
Hygroscopicity	DVS TGA	No particular requirement
Stability Hydrolysis Photolysis Oxidation	HPLC, plus suitable storage conditions	No particular requirement

[a]Solubility will depend on the physical form.
DVS, dynamic vapour sorption; HPLC, high-performance liquid chromatography; TGA, thermogravimetric analysis; TLC, thin-layer chromatography; UV, ultraviolet.

Table 23.2 Macroscopic (bulk) properties and the techniques used to determine them

Derived property	Technique
Melting point	DSC or melting point apparatus
Enthalpy of fusion (and so ideal solubility)	DSC
Physical forms (polymorphs, pseudopolymorphs or amorphous)	DSC, XRPD, microscopy
Particle shape Size distribution Morphology Rugosity Habit	Microscopy Particle sizing BET (surface area)
Density Bulk Tapped True	Tapping densitometer
Flow	Angle of repose
Compressibility	Carr's index Hausner ratio
Excipient compatibility	HPLC, DSC

BET, Brunauer–Emmett–Teller; *DSC*, differential scanning calorimetry; *HPLC*, high-performance liquid chromatography; *XRPD*, X-ray powder diffraction.

during preformulation, in chronological order, and the assays that may be used to quantify them. These properties are a function of the molecular structure. Once these properties are known, further macroscopic (or bulk) properties of the drug candidate can be measured (Table 23.2). These properties result from intermolecular interactions. Note also that determination of the chemical structure is not required, as it is assumed the chemists preparing the candidate molecules will provide this information. Note also that solubility will be dependent on the physical form (polymorph, pseudopolymorph or amorphous).

The full characterization of a drug candidate (in the context of preformulation) should be possible with just ultraviolet (UV) spectrophotometry, high-performance liquid chromatography (HPLC), differential scanning calorimetry (DSC), dynamic vapour sorption (DVS) and X-ray powder diffraction (XRPD). This explains the popularity of these techniques in pharmaceutical development. Thin-layer chromatography (TLC) and thermogravimetric analysis (TGA) provide useful supporting data, but neither is essential during the early stages.

Solubility

Aqueous solubility is a critical attribute. No drug will reach its ultimate therapeutic target without first being in solution. Consequently, it is the first physicochemical parameter to be determined. It has been estimated that, historically, up to 40% of drug candidates have been abandoned because of poor aqueous solubility, and between 35% and 40% of compounds currently in development have an aqueous solubility less than 5 mg mL^{-1} at pH 7. The *United States Pharmacopeia* and the *European Pharmacopoeia* provide definitions of solubility based on concentration (see Chapter 2 and in particular Table 2.3).

Early determination of solubility gives a good indicator as to the ease of formulation of a drug candidate. Initial formulations, used for obtaining toxicity and bioavailability data in animal models, will need to be liquids for oral gavage or intravenous delivery, and a solubility greater than 1 mg mL^{-1} is usually acceptable. For the final product, assuming oral delivery in a solid form, solubility of the molecule greater than 10 mg mL^{-1} is preferable. If the solubility of the drug candidate is less than 1 mg mL^{-1}, then salt formation, if possible, is indicated. Where solubility cannot be manipulated through salt formation, then a novel dosage form will be required.

Dissolution is a phase transition and for it to progress, solid–solid bonds must be broken (effectively, the solid melts), while solvent–solvent bonds must be broken and replaced by solute–solvent bonds (the drug molecules become *solvated*) (see Chapter 2). With excess solid present, a position of equilibrium will be established between the solid and dissolved drug.

The concentration of the drug dissolved at this point is known as the *equilibrium solubility* (usually referred to simply as *solubility*), and the solution is *saturated*. If the drug has an ionizable group, then the equilibrium solubility of the un-ionized form is called the *intrinsic solubility* (S_o). This is important because ionizable drugs will dissociate to a greater or lesser extent, influenced by solution pH, and this will affect the observed solubility.

From a thermodynamic perspective, the energy input required to break the solid–solid bonds must equal the enthalpy of fusion (ΔH_f) required to melt the solid (because the same bonds are broken). Unlike melting, however, in the case of dissolution there is an additional enthalpy change because solvent–solvent bonds are broken and solute–solvent bonds are formed (shown diagrammatically in Fig. 2.2). The energy involved in this process is known as the enthalpy of mixing (ΔH_{mix}). The net enthalpy of dissolution (ΔH_{sol}) is thus the sum of the enthalpy of fusion and the enthalpy of mixing:

$$\Delta H_{sol} = \Delta H_f + \Delta H_{mix}$$

(23.1)

Knowledge of this relationship between solubility and bond energy can be used during preformulation to make predictions of solubility from thermal energy changes (e.g. during melting and other phase changes).

Thus dissolution in the presence of excess solid results in a position of equilibrium between the solid state and the dissolved state. The equilibrium constant (K_{sol}) for the overall process of dissolution can be represented as

$$K_{sol} = \frac{a_{aq}}{a_s}$$

(23.2)

where a_{aq} denotes the *activity* of the drug in solution and a_s denotes the activity of the drug in the solid phase. As the activity of a solid is defined as unity, and in dilute solution activity approximates to concentration (solubility in this case), then

$$K_{sol} = S_o = x_2$$

(23.3)

where S_o is again the intrinsic solubility, and x_2 denotes the saturated concentration of the drug in mole fraction units (x_1 being the mole fraction of the solvent).

It is possible to see from Eq. 23.1 that the crystal lattice energy might affect solubility. There will also be an effect of temperature on solubility, because the position of the equilibrium between the solid and dissolved drug will change. Both of these effects can be explored further through the concept of *ideal solubility*.

Ideal solubility

In the special case where the energy of the solute–solvent bond is equal to the energy of the solvent–solvent bond, solute–solvent bonds may form with no change in intermolecular energy (i.e. $\Delta H_{mix} = 0$), and dissolution is said to be *ideal*. Ideal dissolution (although unlikely in reality) leads to ideal solubility and is an interesting theoretical position because it

can be described in thermodynamic terms that allow calculation of the dependence of solubility on temperature.

From Eq. 23.1, if $\Delta H_{mix} = 0$, then ΔH_f is equal to ΔH_{sol}. Incidentally, because ΔH_f must be positive (i.e. endothermic), ΔH_{sol} must also be positive for ideal dissolution. For a process to occur spontaneously, the Gibbs free energy (ΔG) must be negative. The familiar thermodynamic relationship for dissolution is

$$\Delta G_{sol} = \Delta H_{sol} - T\Delta S_{sol}$$

(23.4)

where T is temperature. ΔG_{sol} is most likely to be negative when ΔH_{sol} is negative but, as noted previously, ΔH_{sol} is frequently positive for dissolution. This means that for dissolution to occur spontaneously, the driving force must be an increase in entropy.

Eq. 23.3 shows that solubility has the attributes of an equilibrium constant. This being so, it is possible to apply the van't Hoff equation (Eq. 23.9), yielding

$$\frac{d\ln x_2}{dT} = \frac{\Delta H_f}{RT^2}$$

(23.5)

Making the assumption that ΔH_f is independent of temperature, then integrating Eq. 23.5 from T_m to T results in

$$\ln x_2 = \frac{-\Delta H_f}{RT} + \frac{\Delta H_f}{RT_m}$$

(23.6)

where T_m is the melting temperature of the pure drug and T is the experimental temperature.

Eq. 23.6 is very useful in preformulation because it allows prediction of ideal solubility at a particular temperature if the melting temperature and enthalpy of fusion of the pure drug are known (an example of its application is shown in Box 23.1). This is why the melting point and enthalpy of fusion are the next physicochemical parameters to be determined during preformulation.

Determination of melting point and enthalpy of fusion using DSC

The energy changes discussed so far can be measured by differential scanning calorimetry (DSC). In DSC,

Box 23.1

Worked example

The melting temperature of aspirin is 137 °C and its enthalpy of fusion at the melting temperature is 29.80 kJ mol⁻¹. What is the ideal solubility of aspirin at 25 °C?

Applying Eq. 23.6, we obtain

$$\ln x_2 = \frac{-29800}{8.314 \times 298} + \frac{29800}{8.314 \times 410} = -3.286$$

$$x_2 = 0.037 \text{ (mole fraction)}$$

Table 23.3 Ideal (calculated) solubility for aspirin (at 25 °C, assuming a melting point of 137.23 °C and $\Delta H_f = 29.8$ kJ mol⁻¹) and paracetamol (at 30 °C, assuming a melting point of 170 °C and $\Delta H_f = 27.6$ kJ mol⁻¹) compared with experimentally determined solubilities in a range of solvents

Aspirin		Paracetamol	
Solvent	Solubility (mole fraction)	Solvent	Solubility (mole fraction)
Ideal (calculated)	0.037	Ideal (calculated)	0.031
Tetrahydrofuran	0.036	Diethylamine	0.389
Methanol	0.025	Methanol	0.073
Ethanol	0.023	Tetrahydrofuran	0.069
Acetone	0.018	Ethanol	0.066
Chloroform	0.015	1-Propanol	0.051
1-Propanol	0.011	Acetone	0.041
Acetonitrile	0.006	Acetonitrile	0.009
Water	0.00045	Water	0.002

the power required to heat a sample in accordance with a user-defined temperature programme is recorded, relative to an inert reference. The heating rate (β) can be linear or modulated by a mathematical function. When the sample melts, energy will be absorbed during the phase change and an endothermic peak will be seen (Fig. 23.1). The enthalpy of fusion is equal to the area under the melting endotherm, whilst the melting temperature may be determined either as an extrapolated onset (T_o) or the peak maximum (T_m).

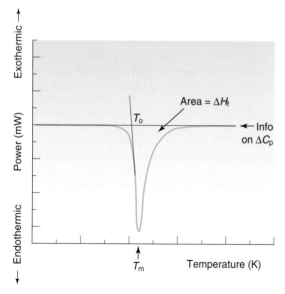

Fig. 23.1 • A typical differential scanning calorimetry (DSC) thermal curve for the melting of a solid. DSC data can be plotted with endothermic/exothermic peaks up or down because the data are the difference between the sample and the reference or the reference and the sample, depending on the instrument manufacturer. Note the direction indicated on the y-axis.

Invariably, real solutions do not show ideal behaviour because the assumptions made earlier that $\Delta H_{mix} = 0$ and that ΔH_f is independent of temperature are not always valid. A negative (exothermic) enthalpy of mixing increases solubility, whereas a positive (endothermic) enthalpy of mixing reduces solubility. Table 23.3 lists the experimentally measured solubilities for aspirin and paracetamol in a range of solvents. Note that solubility in water is by far the lowest among the solvents shown, while solubilities in tetrahydrofuran (THF) and methanol approach ideality in the case of aspirin, and exceed ideality in the case of paracetamol.

The reason that so many solvents, and water in particular, display such nonideal behaviour is because of significant intermolecular bonding resulting from their chemical structure and properties. The three primary chemical properties are the *dipole moment, dielectric constant* and capacity for forming *hydrogen bonds*.

A molecule has a dipole when there is a localized net positive charge in one part of the molecule and a localized net negative charge in another. Such molecules are said to be polar. Water is an example of a polar molecule. Drugs that have dipoles or dipolar character are generally more soluble in polar solvents.

Table 23.4 Dielectric constants of some common pharmaceutical solvents at 25 °C

Solvent	Dielectric constant (no unit, dimensionless)
Water	78.5
Glycerine	40.1
Methanol	31.5
Ethanol	24.3
Acetone	19.1
Benzyl alcohol	13.1
Phenol	9.7
Ether	4.3
Ethyl acetate	3.0

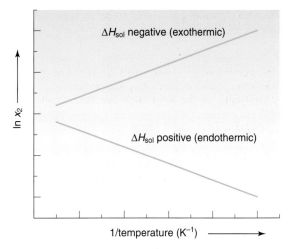

Fig. 23.2 • The change in solubility with temperature for drugs with endothermic and exothermic heats of solution.

Dielectric properties are related to the capacity of a molecule to store a charge and are quantified by a dielectric constant. Polar solvents may induce a dipole in a dissolved solute, which will increase solubility. The dielectric constants of a number of commonly used pharmaceutical solvents are given in Table 23.4. It can be seen that water has a high dielectric constant (78.5) relative to that of methanol (31.5) even though both are considered to be polar solvents.

Hydrogen bonding occurs when electronegative atoms (such as oxygen) come into close proximity to hydrogen atoms; electrons are pulled towards the electronegative atom, creating a reasonably strong force of interaction. A drug that has a functional group capable of forming a hydrogen bond with water (such as –OH, –NH or –SH) should have increased aqueous solubility.

Solubility as a function of temperature

Eq. 23.6 indicates that the heat of fusion should be determinable by experimentally measuring the solubility of a drug at a number of temperatures (as a plot of $\ln x_2$ versus $\frac{1}{T}$ should be linear and have a slope of $-\frac{\Delta H_f}{R}$). Because ΔH_f must be positive, Eq. 23.6 suggests that the solubility of a drug should increase with an increase in temperature. Generally, this agrees with everyday experience, but there are some drugs for which solubility decreases with

increasing temperature. This is because an assumption was made in the derivation of Eq. 23.6; namely, that ΔH_f is equal to ΔH_{sol}. However, as noted earlier and as demonstrated by the data in Table 23.3, ΔH_{mix} is frequently not zero. In cases where ΔH_{sol} is negative (i.e. the heat of solution is exothermic), solubility will decrease with increasing temperature. These effects are shown in Fig. 23.2.

Examples of data from three drug molecules plotted this way are given in Fig. 23.3. Although such plots are frequently found to be linear, the data are usually plotted over a very narrow temperature range and the heat of fusion so calculated is rarely ideal,

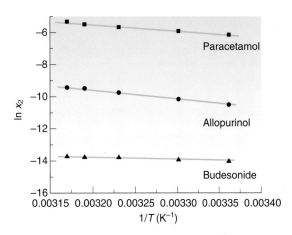

Fig. 23.3 • $\ln x_2$ versus $\frac{1}{T}$ for three drugs in water.

Solubility data from Mota et al., 2009.

although it can be considered to be an approximate heat of solution.

Solubility and physical form

If molecules in the solid state are able to align in different patterns (the phenomenon of polymorphism; see Chapter 8), then it is highly likely that the strength of the intermolecular bonds, and hence the crystal lattice energy, will vary. Two polymorphs of the same drug will thus have different melting temperatures and heats of fusion. Usually the stable polymorph has the higher melting point and greater heat of fusion and so, from Eq. 23.6, the lower solubility. Any metastable forms will, by definition, have lower melting points, lower enthalpies of fusion and so greater solubilities. The amorphous form, by virtue of not possessing a melting point, will have the greatest solubility. It is therefore clear that the solid-state structure of a new drug candidate should be determined during preformulation.

As discussed already, solubility is defined as the equilibrium between dissolved solute and the solid form. Thus if one prepares a saturated solution by dissolving a metastable form and the excess solid is removed by filtration, the solution will be supersaturated with respect to the stable form. Ultimately, the stable form will precipitate as the system reestablishes a position of equilibrium (Fig. 23.4). Formulating any

drug in a (solid) metastable form thus involves an element of risk, the risk being that the stable form will appear during storage or after dissolution. In either case, solubility will be reduced, with, potentially, a consequential reduction in bioavailability.

Measurement of intrinsic solubility

Initially, during preformulation, solubility should be determined in 0.1 M HCl, 0.1 M NaOH and water. These 'unsophisticated' choices are determined by the scarcity of material at this stage. Saturated solutions can be prepared by addition of an excess of solid to a small volume of solvent, agitating the mixture with time and then filtering.

UV spectrophotometry is the first-choice assay, for reasons of familiarity, cost, the small volume of solution needed and that the majority of drugs contain at least one functional group that absorbs in the UV region (190 nm to 390 nm). Table 23.5 lists the UV absorbance maxima for a series of common functional groups (called *chromophores*).

Excitation of the solute with the appropriate wavelength of light will reduce the amount of light passing through the solution. If the original light intensity is I_0 and the amount of light passing through the sample (the *transmitted light*) is I, then the amount of light absorbed will be a function of the concentration of the solute (C) and the depth of

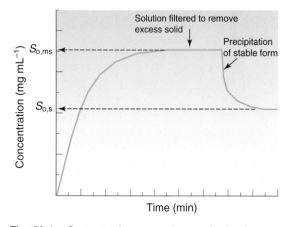

Fig. 23.4 • Concentration versus time profile for the dissolution of a metastable (ms) form of a drug. The system is in equilibrium until excess drug is removed by filtration, after which the solution is supersaturated with respect to the stable (s) form. Subsequently the stable form precipitates and a new position of equilibrium is reached.

Table 23.5 Ultraviolet absorbance maxima for a range of common functional groups

Chromophore	λ_{max} (nm)	Molar extinction (ε)
Benzene	184	46 700
Naphthalene	220	112 000
Anthracene	252	199 000
Pyridine	174	80 000
Quinoline	227	37 000
Ethylene	190	8000
Acetylide	175–180	6000
Ketone	195	1000
Nitroso	302	100
Amino	195	2800
Thiol	195	1400
Halide	208	300

From Wells (1988).

the solution through which the light is passing (the path length, l). This relationship is usually expressed as the Beer–Lambert equation:

$$\text{absorbance} = \log\left(\frac{I}{I_0}\right) = \varepsilon C l$$

(23.7)

where ε is a constant of proportionality called the molar extinction coefficient.

Higher values of ε mean greater UV absorbance by the solute. Values of ε for a range of functional groups are given in Table 23.5; it can be seen that groups containing large numbers of delocalized electrons, such as those containing benzene rings, have much greater ε values that groups containing simple carbon–carbon double bonds. The absorbance of a chromophore can be affected by the presence of an adjacent functional group if that group has unshared electrons (an *auxochrome*). A list of common auxochromes and their effects on the molar extinction coefficients of their parent benzene ring is given in Table 23.6.

Measurements of UV absorbance (thus solution concentration) should be recorded until the concentration remains constant and at a maximum. Care should be taken to ensure that the drug does not degrade during testing, if hydrolysis or photolysis are potential reaction pathways, and also that the temperature does not fluctuate. If the measured solubilities are the same in the three solvents, then the drug does not have an ionizable group. If solubility is highest in acid, then the molecule is a (weak) base, and if solubility is highest in alkali, then the molecule is a (weak) acid.

Solubility should be measured at a (small) number of temperatures:

4 °C	The reduced temperature minimizes the rate of hydrolysis (if applicable). Here, the density of water is at its greatest and thus presents the greatest challenge to solubility
25 °C	Standard room temperature
37 °C	Body temperature, and so an indication of solubility in vivo

Note that possession of solubility data as a function of temperature allows (approximate) determination of the heat of fusion from Eq. 23.6.

If the aim of the preformulation screen is to understand solubility in vivo, then solubility in biorelevant media should be determined. Assuming oral delivery, typical media would include simulated gastric fluid (SGF), fed-state simulated intestinal fluid (FeSSIF) and fasted-state simulated intestinal fluid (FaSSIF). The use of these fluids is discussed further in Chapters 21 and 35, and details of their composition are given in Tables 35.2 and 35.3. Biorelevant media tend to have higher ionic strengths, and hence the risk of salting out via the common-ion effect (see later) is greater.

Effect of impurities on intrinsic solubility

One potential consideration at this stage is the polymorphic form of the drug, which may initially be present in a metastable form. It is a good idea to use DSC or XRPD to determine the polymorphic form of the excess solid, filtered from the solubility experiments, to ensure there has been no form change to a stable polymorph, or that a hydrate has not formed (as both forms typically have lower solubilities).

Another issue for consideration at this stage is the chemical purity of the sample. If the drug is pure, then its phase-solubility diagram should appear as in Fig. 23.5. Initially, all drug added to the solvent dissolves, and the gradient of the line should be unity. When saturation is achieved, addition of further drug does not result in an increase in concentration, and the gradient becomes zero. However, new drug candidate material is rarely pure. When a single impurity is present, the phase-solubility diagram will appear as shown in Fig. 23.6. From the origin to

Table 23.6 The effect of auxochromes on the ultraviolet absorbance of the parent compound C_6H_5–R

Substituent	λ_{max} (nm)	Molar extinction (ε)
–H	203.5	7400
–CH$_3$	206.5	7000
–Cl	209.5	7400
–OH	210.5	6200
–OCH$_3$	217	6400
–CN	224	13000
–COO$^-$	224	8700
–CO$_2$H	230	11600
–NH$_2$	230	8600
–NHCOCH$_3$	238	10500
–COCH$_3$	245.5	9800
–NO$_2$	268.5	7800

From Wells (1988).

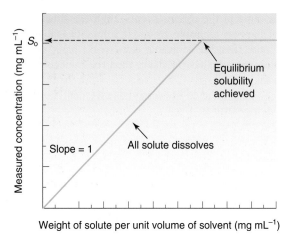

Fig. 23.5 • Phase-solubility diagram for a pure compound.

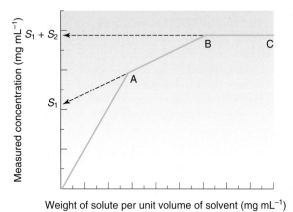

Fig. 23.6 • Phase-solubility diagram for a compound with one impurity.

point A, both components dissolve. At point A, the first compound has reached its solubility. The line AB represents the continued dissolution of the second compound. At point B, the second compound reaches its solubility and the gradient of the line BC is zero. The solubility of the first compound (S_1) can be determined by extrapolation of line AB to the y-axis. The solubility of the second compound (S_2) is the difference between the solubility at BC (= S_1 + S_2) and the y-intercept of the extrapolated line AB. The same principles apply if further impurities are present.

An alternative experiment is to prepare four solutions of the drug candidate with different phase ratios of drug to solvent (say, 3 mg, 6 mg, 12 mg and 24 mg of drug in 3 mL), measure the solubility of each and then extrapolate the data to a theoretical phase ratio of zero (Fig. 23.7). If the drug is pure,

then its solubility should be independent of the phase ratio. If the impurity acts to increase solubility (e.g., by self-association, complexation or solubilization), then the gradient of the plotted line will be positive, whereas if the impurity acts to suppress solubility (usually by the common-ion effect), then the gradient of the line will be negative. The point at zero phase ratio in Fig. 23.7 implies that the impurity concentration is zero, and thus the true solubility can be estimated.

The purity of a sample may also be checked with DSC because the presence of an impurity (even minor amounts) will lower and broaden the melting point of a material. Qualitatively, if the melting endotherm recorded by DSC is very broad, then the sample is likely to be impure (see Fig. 23.8).

If the melting point and heat of fusion of the pure drug are known, then the purity of an impure sample can be quantified by analysis of DSC data. Analysis requires determination of the fraction of sample melted as a function of temperature. This is easily achieved because integration of the peak area of melting gives the total heat of melting (Q). Partial integration of the melting endotherm to any particular temperature must therefore give a smaller heat (q). The fraction of material melted at any temperature (F_T) is then

$$F_T = \frac{q}{Q}$$

(23.8)

Changes in F_T as a function of temperature are easily measured. The van't Hoff equation (Eq. 23.9)

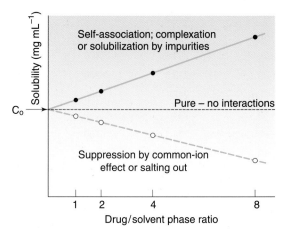

Fig. 23.7 • Effect of drug-to-solvent ratio when the drug is impure.

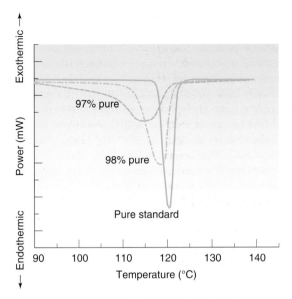

Fig. 23.8 • Differential scanning calorimetry thermal traces for benzoic acid of differing purity.

predicts that a plot of $\dfrac{1}{F_T}$ versus temperature should

be a straight line of slope $\dfrac{-RT_m^2x_2}{\Delta H}$, from which the

mole fraction of the impurity (x_2) can be calculated:

$$T = T_m \frac{-RT_m^2x_2}{\Delta H} \cdot \frac{1}{F_T}$$

(23.9)

Molecular dissociation

Approximately two-thirds of marketed drugs ionize between pH 2 and pH 12 (analysis of the 1999 World Drug Index by Manallack, 2007). Understanding acid and base behaviour is thus extremely important, not only because of the number of ionizable drugs available, but also because the solubility of an acidic or basic drug will be pH dependent (and because possession of an ionizable group opens up the possibility of solubility manipulation via salt formation). Determining the pK_a of a drug is the next step in preformulation characterization. This is particularly important with drugs intended for peroral administration as they will experience a range of pH environments, and it is important to know how their degree of ionization may change during passage along the gastrointestinal tract.

The principles of acid–base equilibria are discussed in Chapter 3, where the Henderson–Hasselbalch equations (Eqs 3.15 and 3.19) were derived for acid and base species.

The Henderson–Hasselbalch equations allow calculation of the extent of ionization of a drug as a function of pH, if the pK_a is known. When the pH is significantly below the pK_a (by at least 2 pH units), a weakly acidic drug will be completely un-ionized, and when the pH is significantly above the pK_a (by at least 2 pH units), a weakly acidic drug will be virtually fully ionized (and vice versa for a basic drug) (see Fig. 3.1).

The degree of ionization will affect solubility because ionized species are more freely soluble in water. Taking the acid-species Henderson–Hasselbalch equation as an example (i.e. Eq. 3.15), as $[A^-]$ represents the saturated concentration of ionized drug (S_i) and $[HA]$ represents the saturated concentration of un-ionized drug (i.e. the intrinsic solubility, S_o) the the equation may be re-written as

$$pK_a = pH + \log\frac{S_o}{S_i}$$

(23.10)

At any given pH, the observed total solubility (S_t) must be the sum of the solubilities of the un-ionized and ionized fractions, i.e.

$$S_t = S_o + S_i$$

(23.11)

Note that in this chapter the alternative symbol S (with appropriate subscript) is used for the specific concentration of the solution that corresponds to the saturated concentration or solubility. This is equally acceptable and is presented here, and later in the discussion of the intrinsic dissolution rate (IDR), as an alternative to annotation used elsewhere. This annotation is particularly useful when one is discussing various types of solubility, as here.

Rearranging Eq. 23.11 gives

$$S_i = S_t - S_o$$

(23.12)

Substituting this in Eq. 23.10 gives

$$pK_a = pH + \log\frac{S_o}{S_t - S_o}$$

(23.13)

Box 23.2

Worked example

What is the pK_a of chlordiazepoxide given the following solubility data? $S_o = 2$ mg mL^{-1}, at pH 4 $S_t =$ 14.6 mg mL^{-1} and at pH 6 $S_t = 2.13$ mg mL^{-1}.

For a weak acid,

$$pK_a = pH + \log\frac{S_t - S_o}{S_o}$$

At pH 4,

$$pK_a = 4 + \log\frac{14.6 - 2}{2} = 4.799$$

At pH 6,

$$pK_a = 6 + \log\frac{2.13 - 2}{2} = 4.813$$

The literature value is 4.8.

Or, in antilog form

$$S_t = S_o[1 + \text{antilog}(pH - pK_a)]$$

(23.14)

Eq. 23.14 allows calculation of the total solubility of an acidic drug as a function of pH. Total solubility will be equal to the intrinsic solubility at pH values below pK_a and will increase significantly at pH values above pK_a. In theory, Eq. 23.14 predicts an infinite increase in solubility when pH $\gg$ pK_a. In practice this is not attained, primarily because real systems exhibit nonideal behaviour. Nevertheless, Eq. 23.14 is a useful approximation over narrow, but useful, pH ranges.

A similar derivation can be made for weak bases following the same logic, resulting in

$$S_t = S_o[1 + \text{antilog}(pK_a - pH)]$$

(23.15)

Eq. 23.15 implies that, for weak bases, total solubility will be equal to the intrinsic solubility at pH values above pK_a and will increase significantly at pH values below pK_a.

An application of these equations is shown in Box 23.2.

Measurement of pK_a

Modern automated instrumentation is available that can determine pK_a values with very small amounts of drug (typically 10 mg to 20 mg). This is extremely useful in the context of preformulation, where material is scarce. Usually this instrumentation is based on a potentiometric pH titration. The drug is dissolved in water, forming either a weakly acidic or a weakly basic solution. Acid or base (as appropriate) is titrated and the solution pH recorded. A plot of volume of titrant solution added versus pH allows graphical determination of the pK_a, because when pH = pK_a, the compound is 50% ionized. This method has the significant advantage of not requiring an assay.

Alternative methods for determining pK_a include conductivity, potentiometry and spectroscopy. However, if the intrinsic solubility has been determined, measurement of solubility at a pH where the compound is partially ionized will allow calculation of pK_a from the Henderson–Hasselbalch equations.

Partitioning

No solute has complete affinity for either a hydrophilic or a lipophilic phase. In the context of preformulation, it is important to know early in the development stage how a molecule (or charged ion) will distribute itself between aqueous and fatty environments (e.g. between gut contents and lipid biological bilayers in the surrounding cell walls). When a solute is added to a mixture of two (immiscible) solvents, it will usually dissolve in both to some extent, and a position of equilibrium will be established between the concentrations (C) in the two solvents. In other words, the ratio of the concentrations will be constant and is given by

$$P_2^1 = \frac{C_1}{C_2}$$

(23.16)

where P is the *partition coefficient* and the superscript and subscript indicate the solvent phase. Note that it would be equally possible to define

$$P_1^2 = \frac{C_2}{C_1}$$

(23.17)

In a physiological environment, drugs partitions from an aqueous phase to numerous and complex lipophilic phases (typically various cell membranes; see also

Chapter 21). It would be difficult to develop an analytical method that allowed measurement of actual partitioning between such complex phases, and so a simple solvent model, commonly using n-octanol, is usually used instead. n-Octanol is taken to mimic the short-chain hydrocarbons that make up many biological lipid bilayers. A partition coefficient for the partitioning of a solute between water (w) and n-octanol (o) can be written as

$$P_w^o = \frac{C_o}{C_w}$$

(23.18)

Alternatively, the following could be defined:

$$P_o^w = \frac{C_w}{C_o}$$

(23.19)

By convention, P_w^o is the standard term.

When a drug is lipophilic (i.e. it has a high affinity for the octanol phase) the value of P_w^o will be greater than 1, and when the drug is hydrophilic the value of P_w^o will be less than 1. Because hydrophilic drugs will give very small P_w^o values, $\log P_w^o$ values are often quoted (abbreviated to log P), in which case hydrophilic drugs will have a negative value and lipophilic drugs a positive value.

Since only un-ionized solute can undergo partitioning (ionized species are too polar to dissolve in organic phases), the partition coefficient applies only if (1) the drug cannot ionize or (2) the pH of the aqueous phase is such that the drug is completely un-ionized. If the drug has partially ionized in the aqueous phase and partitioning is measured experimentally, then the parameter measured is the distribution coefficient, D:

$$D_w^o = \frac{C_o}{C_{w,ionized} + C_{w,un-ionized}}$$

(23.20)

The partition coefficient and the distribution coefficient are related by the fraction of solute un-ionized ($f_{un-ionized}$):

$$D_w^o = f_{un-ionized} P_w^o$$

(23.21)

Note also that partition coefficients may be defined between any organic phase and water. n-Octanol is

the most common choice, but it is by no means either the best choice or the only choice for the 'oil' phase, especially if partition coefficients are determined using chromatographic methods. However, many data exist for the n-octanol–water system, and its use continues.

Determination of log P

Log P values can be determined experimentally or can be calculated from the chemical structure of the drug candidate by means of group additivity functions. For the latter approach there are numerous computer models and simulation methods available; selection will reduce to personal choice and familiarity, and so these models will not be considered here. Rather, this text will focus on experimental determination. It is clear, however, that there is much value to be gained from comparison of calculated and experimentally determined log P values. The value of the calculation approach is greatest when one is selecting a lead candidate from a compound library when it would simply be neither possible nor practicable to measure the partitioning behaviour of the many thousands of compounds available.

Shake-flask method

Assuming that a UV assay is available, the shake-flask method is a quick, simple and near universally applicable way of determining the partition coefficient (see also Fig. 21.2). Prior to measurement, the solvents to be used should be mixed with each other and allowed to reach equilibrium. This is because each solvent has a small but significant solubility in the other (the solubility of n-octanol in water is 4.5×10^{-3} M; the solubility of water in n-octanol is 2.6 M).

The drug is dissolved in the aqueous phase to a known concentration. *Equal volumes* of aqueous drug solution and n-octanol are then mixed in a separating funnel. The mixture is shaken vigorously for some time (usually 30 min, to maximize the surface area of the two solvents in contact with each other) while the drug undergoes partition. The phases are allowed to separate (5 min) and then the concentration of the drug remaining in the aqueous phase is determined (Fig. 23.9). By difference, the concentration of the drug in the n-octanol phase is known:

$$C_{n\text{-octanol}} = C_{water,initial} - C_{water,final}$$

(23.22)

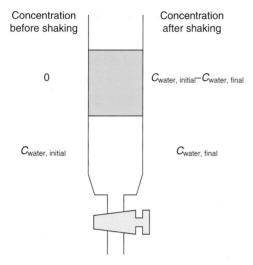

Concentration before shaking	Concentration after shaking
0	$C_{water,\ initial} - C_{water,\ final}$
$C_{water,\ initial}$	$C_{water,\ final}$

Fig. 23.9 • The shake-flask method for determination of the partition coefficient.

When the partition coefficient heavily favours distribution to the n-octanol phase, then a smaller volume of n-octanol can be used, as this will increase the concentration in the aqueous phase at equilibrium, reducing the error in the analytical determination of the concentration. The calculation for the partition coefficient needs to be corrected to account for the different volumes. For example, assuming a 1:9 n-octanol to water ratio, Eq. 23.18 becomes

$$P_w^o = \frac{10C_o}{C_w}$$

(23.23)

There are some drawbacks to the shake-flask method. One is that the volumes of solution are reasonably large, and another is that sufficient time must be allowed to ensure equilibrium partitioning is attained.

The use of n-octanol tends to reflect absorption from the gastrointestinal tract, which is why it is the default option; but n-octanol may not be the best organic phase. Hexane or heptane can be used as an alternative, although they will give different partition coefficient values from those obtained with n-octanol and are also considered to be less representative of biological membranes because they cannot form any hydrogen bonds with the solute. Where the aim of the experiment is to differentiate partitioning between members of a homologous series, the organic phase can be varied so as to maximize discrimination. n-Butanol tends to result in similar partition coefficients for a homologous series of solutes, whereas

heptane tends to exaggerate differences in solute lipophilicity. Solvents that are more polar than n-octanol are termed hypodiscriminating and those that are less polar than n-octanol are termed hyper-discriminating. Hyperdiscriminating solvents reflect more closely transport across the blood–brain barrier, whereas hypodiscriminating solvents give values consistent with buccal absorption. The discriminating powers of a range of common solvents, relative to n-octanol, are shown in Fig. 23.10.

Chromatographic methods

Separation of analytes by liquid chromatographic methods relies on interaction between the analytes (dissolved in a mobile phase) and a stationary (solid) phase. In normal-phase chromatography the stationary phase is polar and the mobile phase is nonpolar, and in reverse-phase chromatography the stationary phase is nonpolar and the mobile phase is polar. It follows that liquid chromatography may be used with single analytes to measure partitioning behaviour, as the extent of interaction must depend on the relative lipophilicity or hydrophilicity of the analyte. Typically, reverse-phase chromatography is used for partitioning experiments.

Reverse-phase TLC allows measurement of partition coefficients by comparing progression of a solute relative to progression of the solvent front (the ratio of the two being the resolution factor, R_f). The resolution factor achieved for each drug is converted to a TLC retention factor (R_m), which is proportional to log P:

$$R_m = \log\left(\frac{1}{R_f} - 1\right)$$

(23.24)

The stationary phase can be n-octanol but is more commonly silica impregnated with silicone oil. The mobile phase can, in principle, be water (or aqueous buffer), but unless the solute is reasonably hydrophilic, good resolution tends not to be achieved with water alone, and reasonably lipophilic compounds tend not to move from the 'starting line' at all (i.e. $R_f = 0$). Cosolvents (typically acetone, acetonitrile or methanol) can be added to the mobile phase to increase the migration of highly lipophilic compounds. The nearer the compound migrates to the solvent front, the higher the resolution factor (the maximum value attainable being 1). R_f can, in principle, range between 0 and 1 (corresponding to R_m values from $+\infty$ to $-\infty$, respectively) although in practice the measurable

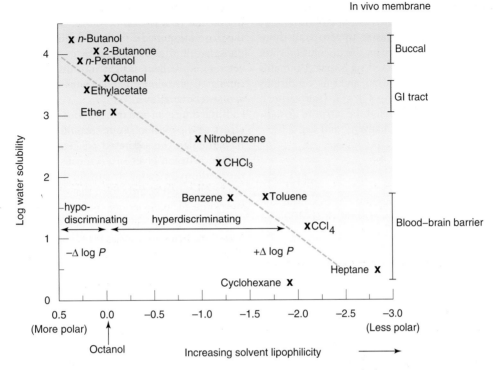

Fig. 23.10 • Discriminating power of various partitioning solvents. *GI*, gastrointestinal. From Wells, 1988.

range is approximately 0.03 to 0.97, corresponding to R_m values of 1.5 to −1.5, respectively.

Addition of a cosolvent can be used to modulate the value of R_f obtained, and the relationship is usually linear. This being so, it is possible to extrapolate to zero cosolvent and so calculate R_m in water.

Reverse-phase HPLC is an alternative, and widely used, technique for measurement of partition coefficients. The stationary phase comprises a nonpolar compound (typically a C_{18} hydrocarbon) chemically bound to an inert, solid support medium (such as silica). It is possible to use water saturated with *n*-octanol as the mobile phase, and a stationary phase covered in *n*-octanol, but the eluting power is not strong, for the same reason noted earlier for TLC, and so to measure an acceptable range of partition coefficients it is necessary to change the volume ratio of the mobile to stationary phase.

Because the hydrocarbon is bound to a solid substrate it cannot behave as a true liquid phase, and so conceptually it is not clear whether the interaction between the solute and the stationary phase constitutes surface adsorption or true phase partitioning. Although C_{18} hydrocarbons have been found to provide a better correlation to log *P* values, indicating that their greater reach from the solid surface of the support matrix means they behave more like a liquid phase, true partitioning is unlikely to occur.

Dissolution rate

Knowledge of solubility per se does not inform the dissolution rate since solubility is a position of equilibrium and not the speed at which it is attained. Thus high aqueous solubility does not necessarily mean that a compound will exhibit satisfactory absorption. Absorption can be assumed to be unimpeded if a drug candidate has an IDR (see the next section) greater than 1 mg cm^{-2} min^{-1}.

Intrinsic dissolution rate

One assumption in the use of the Noyes–Whitney equation (described in Chapter 2, Eqs 2.3 and 2.4) is that diffusion coefficient (D), the surface area of the dissolving solid (A) and the thickness of the stationary solvent layer surrounding the dissolving solid (h) remain constant. Assuming a constant stirring speed and that the solution does not increase in viscosity as the solid dissolves, this is appropriate for D and h but A must always change as the solid dissolves (see Fig. 2.5). Also, if a tablet disintegrates, for instance, then A would increase rapidly at the start of dissolution before decreasing to zero, and there will be a concomitant effect on the dissolution rate.

If the sample is constructed such that A remains constant throughout dissolution, and sink conditions are maintained so that $(S_t - C) \cong S_t$ (see earlier), then the measured rate is called the *intrinsic dissolution rate* (IDR) (see also Chapter 2 and Eq. 2.6):

$$IDR = KS_t$$

$$(23.25)$$

Wells (1988) suggested a method for measuring the IDR of a compound. A compact of the drug (300 mg) is prepared by compression (to 10 t load) in an infrared punch and die set (13 mm diameter, corresponding to a surface area on the flat face of 1.33 cm²). The metal surfaces of the punch and die should be prelubricated with a solution of stearic acid in chloroform (5% w/v). The compact is adhered to the holder of the rotating basket dissolution apparatus with use of low-melting paraffin wax. The compact is repeatedly dipped into the wax so that all sides are coated except the lower flat face (from which any residual wax should be removed with a scalpel blade). Dissolution is recorded while the disc is rotated (100 rpm) 20 mm from the bottom of a flat-bottomed dissolution vessel containing dissolution medium (1 L at 37 °C). The gradient of the dissolution line divided by the surface area of the compact gives the IDR.

IDR as a function of pH

Measurement of the IDR as a function of either pH or ionic strength can give good insight into the mechanism of drug release and the improvement in performance of salt forms, since, for weak acids, substitution of Eq. 23.14 into Eq. 23.25 yields

$$IDR = K(S_o[1 + \text{antilog}(pH - pK_a)])$$

$$(23.26)$$

and for weak bases substitution of Eq. 23.15 into Eq. 23.25 yields

$$IDR = K(S_o[1 + \text{antilog}(pK_a - pH)])$$

$$(23.27)$$

In either case, the measured IDR will clearly be affected either by the pH of the medium or by the pH of the microenvironment surrounding the solid

surface created by the dissolving salt. The effect of pH on the IDR is easily established by selection of the dissolution media. Standard media (0.1 M HCl, phosphate buffers, etc.) can be used or, in order to get a more realistic insight into dissolution in vivo, simulated gastrointestinal fluids (as discussed earlier) can also be employed.

If the drug is an acid or base, then the self-buffering effect as dissolution occurs should not be ignored. In particular, the saturated concentration of solute in the diffusion layer often means that the pH of the medium immediately surrounding the dissolving solid differs significantly from that of the bulk solvent and will lead to deviations from the ideal behaviour predicted by Eqs 23.26 and 23.27. A schematic representation of the buffering effect of salicylic acid is shown in Fig. 23.11.

IDR and the common-ion effect

The common-ion effect (discussed in Chapter 2) should not be ignored, especially for hydrochloride salts, as the chloride ion is often present in reasonably high concentrations in body fluids (0.1 M in gastric fluid and 0.13 M in intestinal fluid). For this reason, fed-state and fasted-state simulated intestinal fluids should contain 0.1 M Cl⁻ and 0.2 M Cl⁻ respectively.

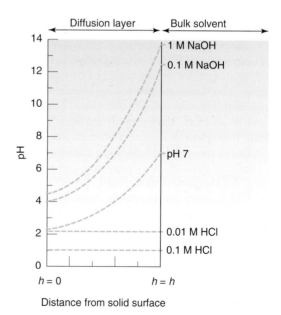

Fig. 23.11 • pH across the diffusion layer as a function of dissolution medium for salicylic acid. From Serajuddin & Jarowski, 1985.

Hence when the concentration of chloride in solution is high, the solubility advantage of choosing a hydrochloride salt is diminished. Li et al. (2005) demonstrated the effect of chloride concentration on the IDR of haloperidol salts and showed that dissolution of the hydrochloride salt was slower than that of either the phosphate salt or the mesylate salt.

Salt selection

If a drug candidate has poor aqueous solubility or is difficult to isolate or purify, but is a weak acid or base, then conversion to a salt form may be beneficial. A number of physicochemical properties may change on formation of a salt (Table 23.7). Any such changes may be beneficial or detrimental, and so a decision must be made early during preformulation as to which salt form (if any) is to be taken into development. This decision will not depend on solubility alone. The prevalence of salt forms of drugs in practice (estimated at approximately 50%) suggests that the benefits often outweigh the drawbacks. Salt selection should preferably be made before commencement of toxicity testing, because of the associated cost and potential time delay in development of switching to a different salt form. Each form is treated by regulatory authorities as a new entity.

Table 23.7 Possible advantages and disadvantages of salt formation

Advantages	Disadvantages
Enhanced solubility	Decreased percentage of active ingredient
Increased dissolution rate	Increased hygroscopicity
Higher melting point	Decreased chemical stability
Lower hygroscopicity	Increased number of polymorphs
Increased photostability	Reduced dissolution in gastric media
Better taste	No change in solubility in buffers
Higher bioavailability	Corrosiveness
Better processability	Possible disproportionation
Easier synthesis or purification	Additional manufacturing step
Potential for controlled release	Increased toxicity

Salt formation

A salt is formed when an acid reacts with a base, resulting in an ionic species held together by ionic bonds. In principle, any weak acid or base can form a salt, although in practice if the pK_a of the base is very low, the salt formed is unlikely to be stable at physiological pH values. Stephenson et al. (2011) noted that no marketed salt exists for a drug with a pK_a below 4.6. They suggested that 5 is a general value below which salt formation is unlikely to be effective. Because salts usually dissociate rapidly on dissolution in water, they are considered electrolytes. Sometimes a drug sounds from its name as if it is a salt but it may in fact be a single entity bound via covalent bonds, in which case electrolytic behaviour does not apply (e.g. fluticasone propionate).

Acids and bases can be classified as strong through to extremely weak, on the basis of their pK_a (Table 23.8). When strong acids react with strong bases, the reaction tends to go to completion, as both species will be fully ionized, and this is known as *neutralization*. For example,

$$HCl + NaOH \rightarrow NaCl + H_2O$$

(23.28)

In this instance the salt formed will precipitate once it is present at a concentration beyond its solubility. However, most drug candidates are either weak acids or bases, in which case their character is usually based on the Brønsted–Lowry definition: an acidic compound is a proton donor and a basic compound is a proton acceptor. The removal of a proton from an acid produces a *conjugate base* (A^-) and addition of a proton to an acceptor produces a *conjugate acid* (BH^+).

$$HA \rightleftharpoons H^+ + A^-$$

(23.29)

Table 23.8 Descriptions of acid and base strength

Description	pK_a	
	Acid	Base
Very strong	<0	>14
Strong	0–4.5	9.5–14
Weak	4.5–9.5	4.5–9.5
Very weak	9.5–14	0–4.5
Extremely weak	>14	<0

$$B + H \rightleftharpoons BH^+$$

(23.30)

Note that the Brønsted–Lowry definition requires acidic species to have an ionizable proton but does not require basic compounds to possess a hydroxyl group; simply that they can accept a proton (thus the theory does not consider KOH and the like to be a base but considers them to be a salt containing the basic OH^- moiety). In the case of a weak base (B) reacting with a strong acid, the conjugate acid and conjugate base may then form a salt:

$$B + HCl \rightleftharpoons BH^+ + Cl^- \rightleftharpoons BH^+Cl^-$$

(23.31)

When a salt dissolves in water, it will dissociate. Assuming dissolution of a basic salt, then the species in solution is the conjugate acid. The conjugate acid can donate its proton to water, reforming the free base:

$$BH^+ + H_2O \rightleftharpoons B + H_3O^+$$

(23.32)

All of the reasons for the change in solubility of salts are encompassed in Eq. 23.32. A basic salt contains the conjugate acid of the drug. On dissolution, the conjugate acid donates its proton to water and the free base is formed. The solute is thus the free base, but the pH of the solution in which it is dissolved has reduced because of the donated proton. Recall that the solubility of weak bases increases as the pH of the solution reduces. Thus dissolution of a basic salt increases solubility because there is a concomitant reduction in the pH of the solution.

The pH of a solution of a dissolved acid is given by

$$pH = \frac{1}{2}(pK_a - \log[acid])$$

(23.33)

and, because the acid species is BH^+, then

$$pH = \frac{1}{2}(pK_a - \log[BH^+])$$

(23.34)

A worked example is given in Box 23.3.

A similar situation occurs for the reaction of a weak acid with a strong base:

$$HA + NaOH \rightleftharpoons NaA + H_2O$$

(23.35)

Box 23.3

Worked example

What is the pH of a 0.2 M solution of ergotamine tartrate (pK_a 6.25)?

From Eq. 23.34,

$$pH = \frac{1}{2}(6.25 - \log 0.2) = 3.48$$

On dissolution of an acidic salt, the conjugate base is formed:

$$NaA \rightleftharpoons Na^+ + A^-$$

(23.36)

The conjugate base can then accept a proton from water, reforming the free acid and increasing the pH of the solution:

$$A^- + H_2O \rightleftharpoons AH + OH^-$$

(23.37)

The solute is thus the free acid, but the pH of the solution in which it is dissolved has increased because of the hydroxide ion generated. Recall again that the solubility of weak acids increases as the pH of the solution increases.

The pH of a solution of a base is given by

$$pH = \frac{1}{2}(pK_a + pK_w + \log[base])$$

(23.38)

and as A^- is a conjugate base,

$$pH = \frac{1}{2}(pK_a + pK_w + \log[A^-])$$

(23.39)

where pK_w reflects the ionization potential of water (and is 14 at 25 °C).

A worked example is given in Box 23.4.

Several consequences arise from this discussion. One is that salt formation might not best be achieved in aqueous solution, since dissolution of a salt in water generally results in formation of the free acid or base. For this reason, salts are often formed in organic solvents. Secondly, the increase in solubility of a salt over the corresponding free acid or base is a result only of the change in pH on dissolution. *The intrinsic solubility of the free acid or base does not change.* Thus if salts are dissolved in buffered solvents,

Box 23.4

Worked example

What is the pH of a 0.1 M solution of diclofenac sodium (pK_a 4.0)?
From Eq. 23.39,

$$pH = \frac{1}{2}(4.0 + 14 + \log 0.1) = 8.5$$

there will be no difference in the solubility profile of the salt relative to the corresponding free acid or base, because the buffer will act to neutralize any change in pH.

Selection of a salt-forming acid or base

For salt formation to occur there must be a sufficient difference in pK_a between the acid and the base

(the *reactivity potential*). For the transfer of a proton from an acid to a weak base, the pK_a of the acid must be less than that of the weak base and vice versa. As a general rule, a difference in pK_a (ΔpK_a) of 3 is indicated (although salt formation can sometimes occur with smaller differences; for instance, Wells (1988) notes that doxylamine succinate forms even though ΔpK_a is 0.2. The reason for this pK_a difference is to ensure both species are ionized in solution, thus increasing the chance of interaction. If ΔpK_a lies between 3 and 0, then knowledge of ΔpK_a per se is not predictive of whether salt formation will occur, and if ΔpK_a is less than 0, then co-crystal formation is the more likely outcome.

Thus selection of a salt-forming entity starts with knowledge of the pK_a of the entity and the pK_a of the drug. The pK_a values of some of the most common salt-forming acids and bases in water are given in Tables 23.9 and 23.10.

Ten of the most common anions and cations are shown in Table 23.11. For basic drugs the

Table 23.9 Values of pK_a for selected pharmaceutical acids

Acid	Anion	pK_a	Example
Hydrobromic	Hydrobromide	<−6.0	Galantamine
Hydrochloric	Hydrochloride	−6.0	Clindamycin
Sulfuric	Sulfate	−3.0, 1.92	Salbutamol
p-Toluenesulfonic	Tosilate	−1.34	Sorafenib
Methanesulfonic	Mesilate	−1.2	Benztropine
Naphthalene-2-sulfonic	Napsilate	0.17	Levopropoxyphene
Benzenesulfonic	Besilate	0.7	Amlodipine
Oxalic	Oxalate	1.27, 4.27	Escitalopram
Maleic	Maleate	1.92	Fluvoxamine
Phosphoric	Phosphate	1.96, 7.12, 12.32	Fludarabine
Pamoic	Pamoate	2.51, 3.1	Amitriptyline
Tartaric	Tartrate	3.02, 4.36	Metoprolol
Fumaric	Fumarate	3.03, 4.38	Formoterol
Citric	Citrate	3.13, 4,76, 6.40	Sildenafil
Hippuric	Hippurate	3.55	Methenamine
Benzoic	Benzoate	4.19	Emamectin
Succinic	Succinate	4.21, 5.64	Metoprolol
Acetic	Acetate	4.76	Megestrol
Carbonic	Carbonate	6.46, 10.3	Lithium

From Stahl & Wermuth (2011).

Table 23.10 Values of pK_a for selected pharmaceutical bases

Base	Cation	pK_a	Example
Potassium hydroxide	Potassium	~14	Benzylpenicillin
Sodium hydroxide	Sodium	~14	Diclofenac
Zinc hydroxide	Zinc	~14	Bacitracin
Calcium hydroxide	Calcium	12.6, 11.57	Fenoprofen
Magnesium hydroxide	Magnesium	11.4	Menbutone
Choline	Choline	>11	Theophylline
Lysine	Lysine	10.79, 9.18, 2.16	Ibuprofen
Benzathine	Benzathine	9.99, 9.39	Ampicillin
Piperazine	Piperazine	9.82, 5.58	Naproxen
Meglumine	Meglumine	9.5	Flunixin
Ammonia	Ammonium	9.27	Glycyrrhizic acid
Tromethamine	Trometamol	8.02	Lodoxamide
Aluminium hydroxide	Aluminium	>7	

From Stahl & Wermuth (2011).

Table 23.11 Frequency of pharmaceutical anions and cations of drugs (illustrated by data from the 2006 *United States Pharmacopeia* 29–*National Formulary* 24)

Anion	Frequency (%)	Cation	Frequency (%)
Hydrochloride	39.96	Sodium	62.79
Sulfate	10.58	Potassium	11.05
Acetate	6.70	Calcium	8.72
Phosphate	4.97	Aluminium	4.65
Chloride	4.54	Benzathine	2.33
Maleate	3.67	Meglumine	2.33
Citrate	3.02	Zinc	2.33
Mesilate	2.59	Magnesium	1.74
Succinate	2.38	Tromethamine	1.74
Nitrate	2.38	Lysine	1.16

hydrochloride salt is the most common form. In part this is because the pK_a of hydrochloric acid is so low it is very likely that it will form a salt with a weak base. Hydrochloride salts are also widely understood and form physiologically common ions and so are acceptable from a regulatory perspective. However, they do have some disadvantages, including the fact that the drop in pH on dissolution may be significant (which is not good for parenteral formulations). There are also risks of corrosion of the manufacturing plant and equipment, instability during storage (especially

if the salt is hygroscopic) and reduced dissolution and solubility in physiological fluids because of the common-ion effect.

Stahl and Wermuth (2011) organizes salt formers into three categories, which may be used as a guide to selection.

First-class salt formers are those that form physiologically ubiquitous ions or which occur as metabolites in biochemical pathways. These include hydrochloride and sodium salts and, as such, they are considered to be unrestricted in their use.

Second-class salt formers are those that are not naturally occurring but which have found common application and have not shown significant toxicological or tolerability issues (such as the sulfonic acids, e.g. mesilates).

Third-class salt formers are those that are used in special circumstances to solve a particular problem. They are not naturally occurring, nor are they in common use.

An additional factor to consider is that the salt formed should exist as a crystalline solid, to enable ease of isolation and purification. Amorphous salts are highly likely to cause problems in development and use and so should be avoided.

Salt screening

Once potential salt formers have been selected they must be combined with the free drug to see which of them preferentially form salts. As the potential number of permutations and combinations of salt formers and solvents is large, a convenient method for salt screening at the preformulation stage is to use a microwell plate approach. A small amount of drug (~0.5 mg) in solvent is dispensed into each well of a 96-well plate. To each well is added a solution of potential counterion. It is possible to construct the experiment in the well plates so that the effect of the solvent is examined in the x-direction and the effect of the counterion is examined in the y-direction. Solvents should be selected carefully. Commonly used solvents are listed in Table 23.12.

After an appropriate time, the presence in each well of salt crystals is checked with an optical device (e.g. a microscope or a nephelometer). If no crystals are seen, then the plate can be stored at a lower temperature. If the reduction in temperature does not cause precipitation, then as a last attempt the temperature can be increased to evaporate the solvent (although care must be taken in this case during subsequent analysis because the isolate may contain a simple mixture of the drug and the salt former, rather than the salt itself).

Once a potential salt has been identified, preparation can be undertaken with slightly larger sample masses (10 mg to 50 mg). XRPD may be used to get a preliminary idea of the polymorphic form, while melting points may be determined with a melting point apparatus, hot-stage microscopy (HSM) or DSC. Examination with HSM, if operated under cross-polarized filters, allows visual confirmation of

Table 23.12 Properties of some common solvents used for salt screening

Solvent	Boiling point (°C)	Dielectric constant (ε)
N,N-Dimethylformamide	153	37
Acetic acid	118	6.2
Water	100	78.4
1-Propanol	97	20.3
2-Propanol	83	19.9
Acetonitrile	82	37.5
2-Butanone	80	18.5
Ethanol	78	24.6
Ethyl acetate	77	6.0
n-Hexane	69	1.9
Isopropyl ether	68	3.9
Methanol	65	32.2
Acetone	57	20.7
Methylene chloride	40	8.9
Diethyl ether	35	4.3

melting and any other changes in physical form during heating, while analysis by DSC provides the heat of fusion in addition to the melting temperature (and so allows calculation of ideal solubility). Additional analyses by TGA and DVS will provide information on water content and hygroscopicity (see later). All of these experiments can be performed if approximately 50 mg of salt is available.

Solubility of salts

It is not a simple matter to predict the solubility of a salt. In particular, the common-ion effect cannot be ignored, especially when dissolution and solubility in biological media are considered. There are many empirical approaches in the literature for estimating the solubility of salts, but most require knowledge of the melting point of the salt, a value most reliably determined by preparing the salt and melting it (in which case the salt is available for solubility determination by experiment). This section will thus consider the underlying principle of solubility pH dependence, based on ionic equilibria, and assumes that solubility would be determined experimentally with the actual salt.

Solubility of basic salts

For a basic salt, at high pH the solubility will be equal to that of the un-ionized (or free) base (i.e. at its lowest) and at low pH the solubility will be that of the ionized base (i.e. at its highest). There will be a region between these extremes where the solubility will vary with pH, as shown in Fig. 3.1. The standard interpretation of a solubility profile of this form is based on the model of Kramer and Flynn (1972), who assumed that the overall profile is the sum of two solubility profiles (Fig. 23.12). In region 1 the dissolved solute is in equilibrium with solid salt, and in region 2 the dissolved solute is in equilibrium with solid free base. The point at which the two solubility profiles intersect is termed pH_{max}.

Data suggest that a basic salt will be most soluble in low-pH media (such as gastric fluid) but will become increasingly insoluble as the pH increases (as it would in intestinal fluids).

Solubility of acidic salts

A similar series of considerations can be made for salts of weak acids. In this case the free acid is the solid phase in equilibrium with the saturated solution below pH_{max} and the salt is the solid phase in equilibrium with the saturated solution above pH_{max}.

An acidic salt will be least soluble in low-pH media but will become increasingly soluble as the pH increases. Thus if an acidic salt is administered orally, its solubility will naturally increase as it progresses along the gastrointestinal tract. Indeed, a drug candidate's solubility in gastric fluid may be so low that it will naturally dissolve only lower in the gastrointestinal tract, which may be a formulation advantage.

The importance of pH_{max}

At pH_{max}, which in principle is a single point on the solubility profile, both the free acid/base and the salt coexist in the solid phase. For a basic salt (see Fig. 23.12), if the pH of a saturated solution containing excess solid free base is lowered below pH_{max}, then the solid will convert to the salt (although the pH will not drop below pH_{max} until enough acid has been added to convert all the free base to salt). Conversely, if the pH of a saturated solution containing excess solid salt is raised above pH_{max}, then the solid phase will convert to the free base. The opposite holds true for an acidic salt.

It should be apparent that pH_{max} is an important parameter and its value will change depending on the solubility of the salt form made. In particular:

- increasing pK_a by 1 unit (making the base stronger) will increase pH_{max} by 1 unit;
- increasing the solubility of the free base by an order of magnitude will increase pH_{max} by 1 unit; and
- increasing the solubility of the salt by an order of magnitude will decrease pH_{max} by 1 unit.

If a small amount of H^+ is added to the system at pH_{max}, then free base is converted to salt. Conversely, if alkali is added, salt is converted to free base. As the system is effectively acting as a buffer, the pH (and consequently the solubility) will not change until sufficient acid or alkali has been added to convert one solid phase completely to the other.

A similar analysis can be performed for an acidic salt. The value of pH_{max} can have a critical influence on the dissolution rate of salts, because the pH of the dissolution medium can cause conversion of a salt back to the free acid or base form.

Dissolution of salts

Salts have the potential to increase the dissolution rate because the saturated concentration in the boundary layer is much higher than that of the free acid or base

For acidic and basic drugs, solubility is pH dependent. Accordingly, the Noyes–Whitney model predicts that the dissolution rate must therefore also be pH

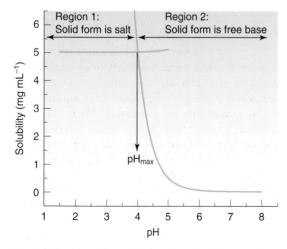

Fig. 23.12 • Solubility profile for a basic salt as a function of pH (pK_a 6.7).

dependent, with the solubility of the solute at the pH and ionic strength of the dissolution medium being the rate-controlling parameter. From the same argument, when the pH of the dissolution medium is approximately pH_{max}, the dissolution rates of the free acid or base and its salt should be the same (because their solubilities are roughly equal at this point). There are, however, numerous examples where this is not the case (e.g., doxycycline hydrochloride and doxycycline; sodium salicylate and salicylic acid; and haloperidol mesilate and haloperidol).

These differences suggest that the pH of the solution in which the solid is dissolving (i.e. the boundary layer) is materially different from that of the bulk solvent (and so the solubility of the dissolving species is different from that expected in the bulk solvent). The difference in pH between the boundary layer and bulk solvent arises because the boundary layer is a saturated solution and because dissolution of acids, bases or salts will result in a change in pH. When a solution (in this case the boundary layer) is saturated, the pH change is maximized. Nelson (1957) first noted this correlation during a study of the dissolution of various theophylline salts; salts with higher diffusion layer pH had greater in vitro dissolution rates and, importantly, faster in vivo absorption.

The pH of the boundary layer at the surface is termed the pH *microenvironment* (pH_{menv}) and is equal to the pH of a saturated solution of the dissolving solid in water. The Noyes–Whitney equation still governs the dissolution rate, but the solubility is not that of the solute in the dissolution medium but that in a medium of pH_{menv}. As the distance from the surface of the dissolving solid increases, the pH approaches that of the bulk medium (shown in Fig. 23.11).

Effect of salts on partitioning

Ionized species do not partition into organic solvents or nonpolar environments. Thus whilst solubility may be enhanced by formation of a salt, there is a considerable risk that partitioning will decrease (example data for partitioning of the sodium salt of ibuprofen are given in Table 23.13). There is thus a compromise to be reached between increasing solubility while maintaining bioavailability and it may well be the case that on this basis the most soluble salt is not taken forward for development.

Table 23.13 Log *P* and solubility data for ibuprofen sodium salt

pH	Solubility (mg mL^{-1})	log *P*	Un-ionization (%)
4	0.028	ND	73.81
5	0.156	3.28	21.98
6	1.0	2.42	2.74
7	340.51	0.92	0.28
8	299.04	0.63	0.03

From Sarveiya et al. (2004).
ND, no data.

Hygroscopicity

Hygroscopicity refers to the tendency of a substance to attract water from its immediate environment, either by absorption or by adsorption. An increase in water content usually results in a change in physicochemical properties. Typically, wet powders will become more cohesive and flowability is reduced. Water also acts to mediate many solid-state reactions, so an increase in water content can often increase the rate of chemical degradation of the active ingredient or interaction with any excipients. If the substance is amorphous, then absorption of water causes plasticization of the matrix (effectively the molecular mobility of the molecules is increased) and then major structural change. If the amorphous matrix is a freeze-dried powder, then absorption of water often causes structural collapse. At the extreme, absorption of water will cause amorphous materials to crystallize.

Salts, in particular, usually have a greater propensity to absorb water than the corresponding free acid or base, so the stability of salt forms with respect to environmental humidity must be assured. Some salts (e.g., potassium hydroxide or magnesium chloride) are so hygroscopic they will dissolve in the water they absorb, forming solutions. This process is called *deliquescence*. In any event, if water absorption is likely to cause a detrimental change in physicochemical properties, then appropriate steps must be taken to protect the drug candidate or drug product. Typically, this would involve selection of suitable packaging and advising the patient on correct storage.

From an analytical perspective, water uptake is usually determined through a change in mass (although chemical approaches, such as Karl Fischer titration, can also be used). TGA measures mass as a function of temperature, whilst DVS measures mass as a function of humidity at a constant temperature. TGA thus allows determination of water content *after* exposure of a sample to humidity, whilst DVS records the change in weight of a sample *during* exposure to humidity.

Physical form

The solid state is probably the most important state when one is considering development of a drug candidate into a drug product (discussed further in Chapter 8). Many solid-state (or physical) forms may be available, and each will have different physico-chemical properties (including solubility, dissolution rate, surface energy, crystal habit, strength, flowability and compressibility). In addition, physical forms are patentable, so knowing all of the available forms of a drug candidate is essential in terms of both optimizing final product performance and ensuring market exclusivity.

Polymorphism

When a compound can crystallize to more than one unit cell (i.e. the molecules in the unit cells are arranged in different patterns), it is said to be *polymorphic* (see Chapter 8). The form with the highest melting temperature (and by definition the lowest volume) is called the *stable* polymorphic form, and all other forms are *metastable*. Different polymorphs have different physicochemical properties, so it is important to select the best form for development. A defining characteristic of the stable form is that it is the only form that can be considered to be at a thermodynamic position of equilibrium (which means that over time all metastable forms will eventually convert to the stable form). It is tempting therefore to consider formulating only the stable polymorph of a drug, as this ensures there can be no change in polymorph on storage. The stable form might, however, have the worst processability (e.g., the stable form I of paracetamol has poor compressibility, whilst the metastable form II has good compressibility), or lowest bioavailability (e.g., the presence of the B form or the C form of chloramphenicol palmitate dramatically reduces bioavailability). Selection of polymorphic form is not necessarily straightforward, although if the stable polymorph shows acceptable

bioavailability, then it is of course the best option for development.

Polymorph screening

Polymorph screening at the preformulation stage is performed in much the same manner as described earlier for salt screening. Basic screening is achieved by crystallization of the drug candidate from a number of solvents or solvent mixtures of varying polarity. A small amount of the drug (approximately 0.5 mg) is added to each well of a 96-well plate. To each well is added a small volume of each solvent or solvent mixture. After an appropriate time, the presence in each well of crystals is checked with an optical device (e.g. a microscope or a nephelometer), with use of the strategies described previously for salt screening to facilitate crystallization.

XRPD provides structural data to identify and differentiate polymorphs. Fig. 23.13 shows the powder diffractograms for two polymorphs of sulfapyridine; it is immediately apparent that each has a unique set of intensity peaks and so the forms are qualitatively different. The 2θ angles for each peak provide a 'fingerprint' for each form, whilst the intensities of each peak can be used as the basis for a quantitative assay for each form.

DSC data differentiate polymorphs on the basis of their melting points and heats of fusion, thus providing thermodynamic information. This means DSC can identify which polymorph is stable and which polymorphs are metastable. In addition, the heat of fusion can be used to calculate ideal solubility.

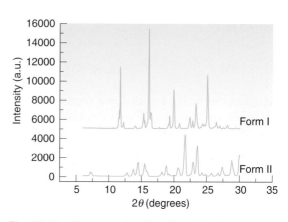

Fig. 23.13 • X-ray powder diffraction diffractograms for two polymorphs of sulfapyridine.

Assuming there is only one polymorph present in a sample, and that it is the stable form, heating the sample in the differential scanning calorimeter should result in a thermal curve showing only an endothermic melt, like that shown in Fig. 23.1. If the sample put into the differential scanning calorimeter initially is a metastable form, then an alternative thermal curve is likely (Fig. 23.14; top curve). Here three events are seen: an endotherm followed by an exotherm followed by an endotherm. To what phase transitions can these events be assigned? The low-temperature endotherm is easily assigned to melting of the metastable form. At a temperature immediately after the endotherm, the sample is thus molten, but because the form that melted was metastable, and so at least one higher melting point form is available, the liquid is *supercooled*. With time the liquid will crystallize to the next thermodynamically available solid form (in this case the stable polymorph). Crystallization is (usually) exothermic and so accounts for the exotherm on the DSC thermal curve. Finally, the stable form melts; the higher temperature endotherm. This pattern of transitions (endotherm–exotherm–endotherm) is a characteristic indicator of the presence of a metastable polymorph (indeed, if more than one metastable form is available, then an additional endotherm–exotherm sequence will be seen for each one). If the sample is cooled to room temperature and then reheated, often only the melting of the stable form is seen (Fig. 23.14; bottom curve). The combination of XRPD and DSC is very powerful and allows rapid assignment of polymorphic forms.

Amorphous materials

Several factors can make it difficult for molecules to orient themselves, in large numbers, into repeating arrays. One is if the molecular weight of the compound is very high (e.g. if the active ingredient is a derivatized polymer or a biological material). Another factor is if the solid phase is formed very rapidly (say, by quench-cooling or precipitation), wherein the molecules do not have sufficient time to align. It is also possible to disrupt a preexisting crystal structure with application of a localized force (e.g. by milling). In any of these cases the solid phase so produced cannot be characterized by a repeating unit cell arrangement, and the matrix is termed *amorphous* (see also Chapter 8).

Because amorphous materials have no lattice energy and are essentially unstable (over time they will convert to a crystalline form), they usually have appreciably higher solubilities and faster dissolution rates than their crystalline equivalents, and so offer an alternative to salt selection as a strategy to increase the bioavailability of poorly soluble compounds.

Confirmation that a material is amorphous can be achieved with XRPD. In this case, no specific peaks as a function of diffraction angle should be seen; rather, a broad diffraction pattern, known as a 'halo', is the defining characteristic, as shown in Fig. 23.15.

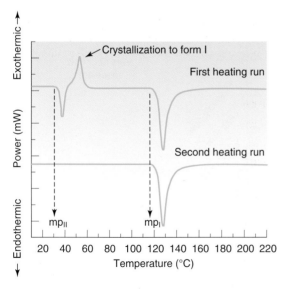

Fig. 23.14 • Differential scanning calorimetry thermal curves for a metastable polymorph on its first *(top)* and second *(bottom)* heating runs. *mp*, melting point.

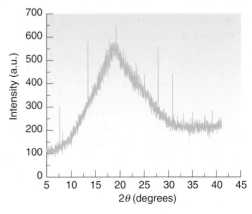

Fig. 23.15 • X-ray powder diffraction diffractogram for amorphous trehalose.

Powder properties

Manufacturing processes frequently involve the movement, blending, manipulation and compression of powders and so will be affected by powder properties. Powder properties that are affected by size and shape can be manipulated without changing the physical form by changing crystal habit.

Particle size and shape

Particle shape is most easily determined by visual inspection with a microscope (some typical particle shapes are shown in Fig. 23.16). Usually a light microscope will suffice, unless the material is a spray-dried or micronized powder, in which case scanning electron microscopy might be a better option. If the particles are not spherical but are irregularly shaped, it is difficult to define exactly which dimension should be used to define the particle size. Several semiempirical measures have been proposed, e.g. Feret's diameter and Martin's diameter (see Chapter 9, Fig. 9.3 and the associated text).

Powder flow

Powders must have good flow properties to fill tablet presses or capsule-filling machines and to ensure blend uniformity when mixed with excipients. This is discussed in Chapter 12.

Whilst poor powder flow will not hinder development of a dosage form, it may prove a major challenge for commercial manufacture, and so early assessment of powder flow allows time to resolve or reduce any problems. Assessment of powder flow is easy when large volumes of material are available, but during preformulation, methods must be used that require only small volumes of powder. The two most relevant methods of assessment at the preformulation stage involve the measurement of the angle of repose and measurement of bulk density. These measurements and their use in powder flow prediction are discussed in Chapter 12. The angle of repose (Tables 12.1 and 12.2), Carr's index (Eq. 12.13, Table 12.3) and the Hausner ratio (Eq. 12.12, Table 12.3) (the latter two are both calculated from measurements of bulk density) have proved to be the most useful parameters in predicting bulk properties when only a small amount of test material is available (Fig. 23.17).

Compaction properties

Compaction is a result of the compression and cohesion properties of a drug (see Chapter 30). These properties are usually very poor for most drug powders, but tablets are rarely made from the drug

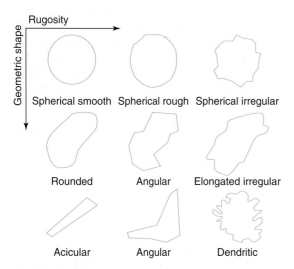

Fig. 23.16 • Some typical powder shapes.

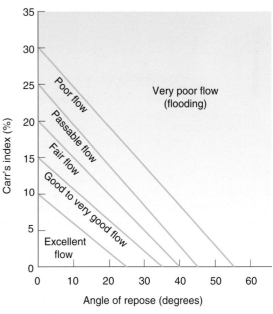

Fig. 23.17 • Relationship between Carr's index and angle of repose, and their correlation to powder flow characteristics.

alone. Excipients with good compaction properties are added. With low-dose drugs, the majority of the tablet comprises excipients and so the properties of the drug are less important. However, once the dose increases to more than 50 mg, the compaction characteristics of the drug will greatly influence the overall properties of the tablet.

Information on the compaction properties of a drug candidate is very useful at the preformulation stage. A material to be tableted should preferably have plastic properties (i.e. once deformed it should remain deformed), but brittleness is also a beneficial characteristic, because the creation of fresh surfaces during fragmentation facilitates bond formation. Water content may also be important as water frequently acts as a plasticizer, altering mechanical properties. A useful practical guide is that if a high-dose drug behaves plastically, the excipients should fragment. Otherwise the excipients should deform plastically.

It is possible to assess the mechanical properties of a drug candidate even when only a small amount of material is available. One method (requiring compaction of only three tablets) is to follow the scheme suggested by Wells (1988):

1. Accurately weigh three 500 mg aliquots of the drug and 5 mg (~1% w/w) magnesium stearate as a lubricant.
2. Blend two samples (A and B) with lubricant for 5 minutes and the third sample (C) for 30 minutes by tumble mixing.
3. Load sample A into a 13 mm infrared compact punch and die set and compress it quickly to 1 t, hold for 1 second and then release the pressure. Eject the compact and store it in a sealed container at room temperature overnight (to allow equilibration).
4. Repeat the process with sample B, but hold the load at 1 t for 30 seconds before releasing the pressure.
5. Compress sample C in precisely the same way as sample A.
6. After each compact has been stored, crush it diametrically in a tablet crushing apparatus and record the crushing force.

Table 23.14 Interpretation of the compression data, suggested by Wells (1988)

	Type of material	
	Plastic	**Fragmenting**
	Comparison of crushing force	
Compare strengths of compacts A and B	A < B	A = B
Compare strengths of compacts A and C	C < A	A = C
Overall	C < A < B	A = B = C

Interpretation of the results is given in Table 23.14. This simple test will yield a significant amount of information on the possible commercial tabletability of a drug candidate from very little material.

Summary

Preformulation studies have a significant part to play in anticipating formulation problems and identifying logical development paths for both liquid and solid dosage forms. The need for adequate drug solubility cannot be overemphasized. The availability of good solubility data should allow the selection of the most appropriate salt for development. DSC and XRPD data will define the physical form and indicate relative stability.

By comparing the physicochemical properties of each drug candidate within a therapeutic group, the preformulation scientist can assist the synthetic chemist to identify the optimum molecule, provide the biologist with suitable vehicles to elicit pharmacological response and advise the bulk chemist about the selection and production of the best salt with appropriate particle size and morphology for subsequent processing.

Please check your eBook at **https://studentconsult. inkling.com/** for self-assessment questions. See inside cover for registration details.

References

Kramer, S.F., Flynn, G.L., 1972. Solubility of organic hydrochlorides. J. Pharm. Sci. 61, 1896–1904.

Li, S., Doyle, P., Metz, S., et al., 2005. Effect of chloride ion on dissolution of different salt forms of haloperidol, a model basic drug. J. Pharm. Sci. 94, 2224–2231.

Manallack, D.T., 2007. The pK_a distribution of drugs: application to drug discovery. Perspect. Medicin. Chem. 1, 25–38.

Mota, F.L., Carneiro, A.P., Queimada, A.J., et al., 2009. Temperature and solvent effects in the solubility of some pharmaceutical compounds: measurements and modeling. Eur. J. Pharm. Sci. 37, 499–507.

Nelson, E., 1957. Solution rate of theophylline salts and effects from oral administration. J. Am. Pharm. Assoc. 46, 607–614.

Sarveiya, V., Templeton, J.F., Benson, H.A.E., 2004. Ion-pairs of ibuprofen: Increased membrane diffusion. J. Pharm. Pharmacol. 56, 717–724.

Serajuddin, A.T.M., Jarowski, C.I., 1985. Effect of diffusion layer pH and solubility on the dissolution rate of pharmaceutical acids and their sodium salts II: salicylic acid, theophylline and benzoic acid. J. Pharm. Sci. 74, 148–154.

Stahl, P.H., Wermuth, C.G. (Eds.), 2011. Handbook of Pharmaceutical Salts. Properties, Selection and Use, second ed. Wiley-VCH, Weinheim.

Stephenson, G.A., Aburub, A., Woods, T.A., 2011. Physical stability of weak bases in the solid-state. J. Pharm. Sci. 100, 1607–1617.

Wells, J.I., 1988. Pharmaceutical Preformulation. The Physicochemical Properties of Drug Substances. John Wiley & Sons, Chichester.

Bibliography

Biagi, G.L., Barbaro, A.M., Sapone, A., et al., 1994. Determination of lipophilicity by means of reversed-phase thin-layer chromatography: I. Basic aspects and relationship between slope and intercept of TLC equations. J. Chromatogr. A 662, 341–361.

Bird, A.E., Marshall, A.C., 1971. Reversed-phase thin layer chromatography and partition coefficients of penicillins. J. Chromatogr. A 63, 313–319.

Bogardus, J.B., Blackwood, R.K., 1979. Solubility of doxycycline in aqueous solution. J. Pharm. Sci. 68, 188–194.

Brittain, H.G., 2007. Strategy for the prediction and selection of drug substance salt forms. Pharm. Tech. 31, 78–88.

Brittain, H.G., 2008. Introduction and overview to the preformulation development of solid dosage forms. In: Adeyeye, M.C., Brittain, H.G. (Eds.), Preformulation in Solid Dosage Form Development. Informa Healthcare, New York.

Carr, R.L., 1965. Evaluating flow properties of solids. Chem. Eng. 72, 163–167.

Gaisford, S., Saunders, M., 2013. Essentials of Pharmaceutical Preformulation. Wiley-Blackwell, Oxford.

Govindarajan, R., Zinchuk, A., Hancock, B., et al., 2006. Ionization states in the microenvironment of solid dosage forms: effect of formulation variables and processing. Pharm. Res. 23, 2454–2468.

Rowe, R.C., Sheskey, P.J., Cook, W.G., et al., 2016. Handbook of Pharmaceutical Excipients, eighth ed. Pharmaceutical Press, London.

Valkó, K., 2004. Application of high-performance liquid chromatography based measurements of lipophilicity to model biological distribution. J. Chromatogr. A 1037, 299–310.

Weber, W.J. Jr., Chin, Y.-P., Rice, C.P., 1986. Determination of partition coefficients and aqueous solubilities by reverse phase chromatography—I. Theory and background. Water Res. 20, 1433–1442.

Zannou, E.A., Yatindra, Q.J., Joshi, M., et al., 2007. Stabilization of the maleate salt of a basic drug by adjustment of microenvironment pH in solid dosage form. Int. J. Pharm. 337, 210–218.

Solutions

24

Sudaxshina Murdan

KEY POINTS

- All the components in a solution are dispersed as molecules or ions.
- Pharmaceutical solutions contain the drug dissolved in a solvent system. The latter can be aqueous or oily. Water is the most common solvent.
- As the drug is already dissolved, it is immediately available for action or absorption.
- Solutions are given by many routes. The requirements of solutions are related to their route of administration.
- Solutions have many advantages (e.g. oral solutions are easy to swallow).
- Solutions also have some disadvantages (e.g. they are bulky and less stable than solid dosage forms).
- A variety of excipients may be included in solutions.

Introduction

This chapter concentrates on solution dosage forms and it is recommended that it be read in conjunction with Chapters 2 and 3, where the science of formation of solutions and their properties are discussed.

A solution, as defined in Chapter 2, is a homogeneous, molecular, mixture of two or more components. The simplest solution consists of two components, a solute dissolved in a solvent. The solute and the solvent could be in the solid, liquid or gaseous states of matter. Most commonly, pharmaceutical solutions are preparations in which the solid solutes, i.e. drug and excipients, are dissolved in a liquid solvent system. Water is the most common solvent, although organic solvents are used in combination with water or on their own. All the components of a solution are dispersed as molecules or ions, and the solution is optically clear. Solutions can be prepared by simple mixing of the solutes with the solvent system. In industry, solutions are prepared in large mixing vessels which are thermostatically controlled should a specific temperature be desired.

The solvent system

Aqueous solvents

The majority of pharmaceutical solutions are water-based. Water is the most commonly used solvent due to its many advantages, such as its lack of toxicity and low cost. Different types of 'water' have been defined in the pharmacopoeias, related to its purity. Those defined in the *European Pharmacopoeia* are

Table 24.1 Different types of water, as defined by the European Pharmacopoeia

Type of water	Use
Purified Water	Used for the preparation of medicines that do not have to be sterile and apyrogenic.
Highly Purified Water	Used for the preparation of medicines where water of high biological quality is needed, except where Water for Injections is required.
Water for Injections	Used for medicines for parenteral administration. Must be pyrogen-free.
Sterilized Water for Injections	Used for medicines for parenteral administration. Water has been sterilized by heat and is suitably packaged.

given as representative examples in Table 24.1. Other pharmacopoeias, such as the *United States Pharmacopeia*, have additional types, such as 'Bacteriostactic Water for Injection'.

Potable (drinking) water from a tap is not normally used for the manufacture of pharmaceutical solutions or for extemporaneous compounding, as it contains dissolved substances which could interfere with the formulation, (e.g. reduce drug solubility and stability). Potable water is therefore purified, for example, by distillation, ion exchange or reverse osmosis to produce 'Purified Water'. The latter is used for the preparation of nonparenteral solutions. For parenteral solutions, potable water is further purified to remove pyrogens (water-soluble, fever-producing compounds), thereby producing 'Water for Injections'. In certain instances, for example, in extemporaneous dispensing, potable water, freshly drawn from a mains supply and/or purified water, freshly boiled and cooled, can be used to prepare oral or external solutions that are not intended to be sterile.

On its own, water does not dissolve many drug compounds to a sufficient degree to enable the preparation of a pharmaceutical solution. Other water-miscible liquids with greater ability to dissolve drugs may therefore be added to water to enhance drug solubility. These liquids are called cosolvents. Commonly used examples include glycerol, propylene glycol, ethanol and polyethylene glycol. Cosolvents are generally less innocuous than water, and the concentration used in an aqueous solution is limited primarily by their toxicity, by drug solubility in the

formulation and finally cost. The mechanism of action of cosolvents is discussed in greater detail later in this chapter.

Nonaqueous solvents

Nonaqueous solvent systems are used when the drug is insufficiently soluble or stable in aqueous systems, or when a solution is intended for specific properties, such as sustained drug absorption. Nonaqueous solutions are, however, limited to certain delivery routes, such as intramuscular and topical, due to their unpalatability, toxicity, irritancy or immiscibility with physiological fluids. Although there are a huge number of organic liquids in which drugs can dissolve, the majority are toxic, and consequently only a few are used in pharmaceutical solutions. Examples of commonly used organic liquids are shown in Table 24.2. These liquids are used as cosolvents with water, as cosolvents with other organic liquids, or on their own.

The drug

The drug may be a small (low molecular weight) molecule such as aspirin, or a large biotherapeutic molecule, such as insulin or an antibody. As defined in Chapter 2, the drug is present in a solution as molecules or ions throughout the solvent. It is usual to ensure that the drug concentration in a pharmaceutical solution is well below its saturation solubility so as to avoid the possibility of the drug precipitating out of the solvent as a result of subsequent temperature changes during storage and use.

The excipients

Excipients – substances other than the drug or prodrug which are included in pharmaceutical solutions – are used for a number of reasons, such as to enhance product stability, bioavailability or patient acceptability, or to aid product manufacture and/or identification. Each excipient has a clear function in the product; thus the nature of an excipient used depends on the requirements of the pharmaceutical product. The excipient must be nontoxic, nonsensitizing and nonirritating, as well as compatible with all the other components of the formulation. The route of administration is important; many excipients are acceptable by certain, but not all, routes. For example, the preservative benzalkonium chloride is used in oral,

Table 24.2 Examples of nonaqueous solvents used in pharmaceutical solutions

Solvent	Use
Alcohols, including polyhydric ones (i.e. those containing more than one hydroxyl group per molecule)	*Ethanol* is the most common organic solvent used in pharmaceutical solutions. It is often used as a cosolvent in oral, topical and parenteral solutions. *Propylene glycol* ($CH_3CH(OH)CH_2OH$) contains two hydroxyl groups per molecule. It is often used as a cosolvent in oral, topical, parenteral and otic solutions. *Glycerol* contains three hydroxyl groups per molecule. It is widely used as a solvent or cosolvent with water in oral and parenteral solutions. *Low molecular weight polyethylene glycols* with the general formula $HOCH_2(CH_2CH_2O)nCH_2OH$. These are used as solvents or cosolvents with water or ethanol. Used in parenteral solutions.
Fixed vegetable oils	Fixed oils are expressed from the seeds, fruit or pit/stone/kernel of various plants. They are nonvolatile oils and are mainly triglycerides of fatty acids. Examples include olive oil, corn oil, sesame oil, arachis oil, almond oil, poppy seed oil, soya oil, cottonseed oil and castor oil. Historically, they have been used for intramuscular administration. They are used to a lesser extent now because of their irritancy and the possibility of allergic reactions to certain oils. They are being replaced by synthetic alternatives such as ethyl oleate.
Esters, such as ethyl oleate, benzyl benzoate and ethyl ethanoate	These are used as a vehicle in certain intramuscular injections.
Dimethyl sulfoxide	Used as a carrier for idoxuridine for topical application to the skin.
Glycofurol	Used as a cosolvent in parenteral solutions for intramuscular or intravenous injections.
Ethyl ether	Used as a cosolvent with ethanol in collodions.

Table 24.3 Traditional terms for different pharmaceutical solutions

Traditional term	Description
Aromatic waters	Saturated aqueous solutions of volatile oils or other aromatic or volatile substances.
Elixirs	Many oral solutions that contain alcohol as a cosolvent have traditionally been designated as elixirs. However, many other oral solutions containing significant amounts of alcohol are not designated as elixirs.
Spirits	Alcoholic or hydroalcoholic solutions of volatile substances. Some spirits are used as flavouring agents, others are medicinal.
Syrups	Oral aqueous solutions containing high concentrations of sucrose or other sugars. 'Syrup BP' is a solution of sucrose (66.7%) in purified water; it promotes dental decay and is unsuitable for diabetic patients. 'Sugar-free' syrups are obtained by replacing sucrose with hydrogenated glucose, mannitol, sorbitol, xylitol, etc.
Tinctures	Alcoholic or hydroalcoholic solutions prepared from vegetable materials or chemical substances. Because of the variability in the vegetable materials, drug concentration can vary.

but not nebulizer, solutions, as it causes bronchoconstriction. Like the drug, excipients may be small (e.g. sucrose) or large (e.g. hydroxypropyl methylcellulose) molecules.

Pharmaceutical solutions

Solutions are one of the oldest pharmaceutical formulations. They are administered by many different routes; they are often therefore classified by the intended route: for example, oral, otic (ear), and parenteral. Solutions are also classified by the nature of the formulation, or by the traditional name which relates to the solvent system used, such as syrups, elixirs, spirits and tinctures. The latter terms are described in Table 24.3. Whilst all pharmaceutical solutions must be stable, and acceptable to patients, other requirements of solutions administered by the different routes vary. For example, parenteral and ocular solutions must be sterile, oral solutions must be palatable, and solutions which come into contact with body fluids must be isotonic and at physiological pH, especially if large volumes are used. Multidose products often contain preservatives to ensure that the growth of any microorganisms that are accidentally introduced during product use is inhibited. The requirements of the different types of pharmaceutical solutions are detailed in Table 24.4. These requirements are achieved by the inclusion of a number of excipients, as detailed in Table 24.5.

Advantages of pharmaceutical solutions

Solutions have several advantages, and for many drugs, a solution is the only available dosage form. Advantages of solutions include:

- The drug is already dissolved in the solvent system; hence drug action can be rapid, allowing its use in emergencies (e.g. the use of adrenaline solution, as an injection, for the treatment of anaphylaxis).

Table 24.4 Requirements of pharmaceutical solutions with respect to their route of administration

Route of administration	Requirements of the solution
Oral	
Oral solutions are swallowed, in which case the drug may exert a local effect on the gastrointestinal tract or be absorbed into the blood and exert a systemic action.	Liquid oral solutions are aqueous formulations. To be acceptable to patients, these must be palatable. Flavouring, colouring and sweetening agents are therefore added to enhance their appearance and taste. Solution pH is usually 7.0, although a pH range of 2–9 can be tolerated. For convenience, the dose is usually in multiples of 5 mL, and the patient is given a 5 mL spoon with the solution. When smaller volumes are required, oral syringes are used. Viscosity should be appropriate for palatability and pourability. Solutions have a higher viscosity than water.
Oral cavity	
Mouthwashes and gargles are used to treat local infection and inflammation in the oral cavity. Gingival solutions are applied to the gingivae. These are not intended to be swallowed and the drug exerts a local effect in the mouth.	Solutions are aqueous formulations. They must be palatable and acceptable to patients. Flavouring, colouring and sweetening agents are often added. As far as possible, the pH should be around neutral.
Topical skin/nail/hair	
Solutions are applied to the skin for local and/or systemic effect. Solutions are also applied to the nails or hair for local effect.	The vehicle may be aqueous or nonaqueous, and different types of formulations are available. An *application* frequently contains parasiticides. A *lotion* is aqueous-based, and is intended for application without friction. A *liniment* is an alcoholic or oily solution (or emulsion) designed to be rubbed into the skin. *Paints* and *tinctures* are concentrated aqueous or alcoholic antimicrobial solutions. A *collodion* is a solution of a polymer, usually pyroxylin, in a volatile organic solvent system (a mixture of ethanol and ether). Following application to the skin, the solvents evaporate, leaving a polymeric film on the skin. *Nail solutions* are applied to the nail to treat nail diseases. All preparations must be acceptable to the patient. Formulations which are easy to transfer from the container and will spread easily and smoothly are preferred. The formulation must adhere to site of application, without being tacky or difficult to remove.

Continued

Table 24.4 Requirements of pharmaceutical solutions with respect to their route of administration—con'd

Route of administration	Requirements of the solution
Otic (ear, aural)	
Solutions are instilled in the outer ear to exert a local effect. They are used to remove ear wax or to deliver anti-infective, anti-inflammatory and analgesic drugs.	May be aqueous or nonaqueous solutions. Water, glycerol, propylene glycol and oils may be used as solvents. Nonaqueous vehicles are predominantly used when ear wax removal is desired as ear wax can dissolve in them. As the residence time in the ear is longer for viscous solutions, the viscosity of aqueous solutions is increased by the use of polymers. Propylene glycol and glycerol solutions are naturally viscous and these increase the residence time. Solutions do not need to be isotonic as they are external preparations.
Ocular	
Eye drops are used to treat local disorders of the eye, e.g. infection. Ocular solutions may also be used to treat intraocular disorders, such as glaucoma. *Eye lotions* are solutions for rinsing or bathing the eye, or for impregnating eye dressings.	Most ocular solutions are aqueous. They must be manufactured sterile as the product is to come in contact with tissues that are very sensitive to contamination. Once opened, a multidose ocular product should remain free from viable microorganisms during its period of use and must contain antimicrobial preservatives. Ideally the solution pH should be close to the physiological pH of tears (pH 7.4) or slightly more alkaline to reduce pH-induced lacrimation, irritation and discomfort. Physiological pH may not, however, be the optimum pH for drug solubility, absorption and stability, or for the function of other components of the solution; thus ocular solutions do not always have a pH of approximately 7.4. Fortunately, the eye can tolerate solutions with pH as low as 3.5 and as high as 9. Ideally, ocular solutions must be isotonic with the tears to minimize irritation and discomfort. Some deviation from isotonicity can be tolerated without marked discomfort when small volumes of solutions are administered, as the latter are rapidly diluted with tears. When large volumes are used (e.g. to wash the eyes), the solution must be approximately isotonic. Most products have a viscosity of 15 mPa s to 25 mPa s (for comparison, the viscosity of water is 1 mPa s). An increase in viscosity prolongs the solution's residence in the eye.
Nasal	
Nose drops and nasal sprays, used for local, e.g. decongestant, effect, or for systemic drug delivery.	*Nasal solutions* are aqueous formulations. Solution pH is in the normal pH range of nasal fluids (pH 5.5–6.5). Solutions are usually isotonic to nasal fluids. Solution viscosity is similar to that of nasal mucus (which is higher than that of water). Flavouring or sweetening agents are sometimes used to mask taste, as a small proportion of nasal solution may be swallowed following nasal administration. Multidose solutions require preservatives.
Pulmonary	
Inhaled solutions are administered by pressurized metered-dose inhalers or by nebulizers for local or systemic effect.	Solutions of drug and excipients dissolved in liquefied propellants, such as trifluoromonofluoroethane, are used in pressurized metered-dose inhalers. Solutions used in nebulizers are aqueous formulations. As relatively large volumes may be administered by nebulizers, the solutions must be isotonic and have a pH not lower than 3 and not higher than 10. Multidose preparations containing preservatives are available, although generally, sterile, single-unit doses without a preservative are used.
Rectal	
Solution enemas are usually administered for local or systemic drug action.	*Enemas* can be aqueous or oily solutions. *Micro enemas* have a volume of 1 mL to 20 mL, whereas macro enemas have volumes of 50 mL or more. *Macro enemas* should be warmed to body temperature before administration.

Continued

Table 24.4 Requirements of pharmaceutical solutions with respect to their route of administration—con'd

Route of administration	Requirements of the solution
Vaginal	
Vaginal solutions are administered for local effect, for irrigation or for diagnostic purposes.	*Vaginal solutions* are aqueous. Excipients to adjust the pH may be included.
Parenteral	
'Parenteral' refers to the injectable routes of administration. Drugs are most commonly injected into the veins (intravenous), into the muscles (intramuscular) and into (intradermal) and under (subcutaneous) the skin, although they can also be injected into arteries, joints, joint fluid areas, the spinal column, spinal fluid and the heart.	*Parenteral solutions* must be sterile and pyrogen-free. Preservatives, such as benzyl alcohol, are included under certain conditions such as in multidose products. Intravenous – the solution must be aqueous, as oil droplets can occlude the pulmonary microcirculation. Intramuscular and subcutaneous – the solution can be aqueous or nonaqueous. Ideally, a parenteral aqueous solution should have a pH close to physiological pH (which is 7.4) to avoid pain, phlebitis and tissue necrosis. A pH of 7.4 may not, however, be the optimum pH for drug solubility and product stability, and as a reasonably wide pH range can be tolerated, the pH of most licensed parenteral solutions is between 3 and 9. A wide pH range is tolerated as the administered solution is diluted on administration, most notably with the intravenous route. Parenteral solutions must be isotonic when large volumes are administered by intravenous infusion. When smaller volumes are used, a wider range of tonicity can be tolerated as dilution with body fluids occurs.

Table 24.5 Excipients used in pharmaceutical solutions

Excipients	Examples of excipients
Cosolvents	Ethanol, glycerol, propylene glycol. The concentration of ethanol should be limited as it exerts a pharmacological action following oral administration.
Flavouring agents	Used to mask the taste of drugs, many of which have a very unpleasant taste. Synthetic or naturally occurring flavourings such as vanilla, raspberry, orange oil, and lemon oil are used for oral solutions. Menthol is used in both oral and nasal solutions. Certain flavours appeal to certain patient populations and certain parts of the world; this must be borne in mind by the formulator. For example, fruit and bubble gum flavours are acceptable to children, whilst mint flavour is not.
Colouring agents	A colouring agent should correlate with the flavouring agent, e.g. green with mint flavour, red with cherry flavour. As for flavours, colour preference differs between cultures.
Sweeteners	Sucrose, sorbitol, mannitol, saccharin sodium, xylitol and high-fructose corn syrup are used to improve the palatability of oral solutions. Sweetened, but sugar-free, preparations containing aspartame are suitable for diabetic patients and are not cariogenic.
Antimicrobial preservatives	Used to preserve multidose preparations. Examples include benzalkonium chloride, benzyl alcohol, chlorobutanol, thimerosal and combinations of parabens (methyl, propyl, butyl).
Antioxidants	Sodium metabisulfite, sodium sulfite, sodium bisulfate, ascorbic acid, used to stabilize solutions.
Chelating agents	Disodium edetate, used to increase solution stability.
pH adjusters	Acids, e.g. citric acid, buffers. Alkalis, e.g. sodium hydroxide, buffers.
Isotonicity adjusters	Sodium chloride, potassium chloride, mannitol, dextrose, glycerol.
Viscosity enhancers	Hypromellose, hydroxyethylcellulose, poly(vinyl alcohol), povidone, dextran, carbomer 940.

- When drug absorption is required prior to drug action (e.g. following oral administration), the drug in a solution is already in a molecular form and thus available for absorption.
- Solutions provide dose uniformity, and specific volumes of the liquid solutions that can be measured accurately; this allows a range of different doses to be easily administered.
- Oral solutions are easily swallowed, and this is beneficial for patients for whom swallowing may be difficult (e.g. young children and older people).
- Solutions are generally easier to manufacture than other dosage forms.

Disadvantages of solutions

The disadvantages of solutions compared with other dosage forms include:

- Many drugs are inherently unstable, and instability is increased when a drug is present in solution (i.e. as molecules). The solution formulation is therefore not feasible for certain drugs. For other drugs, stability can be enhanced by optimization of the formulation (see later).
- Many drugs are poorly soluble in water. Their formulation as a solution is challenging (see later).
- Liquids are bulky and less easy for the patient to carry (e.g. the daily dose) than solid dosage forms. Liquids are also more expensive to transport, which increases the medicine's cost. The packaging of pharmaceutical solutions requires materials of higher quality (see Chapter 46).

Solution stability

A pharmaceutical solution must be stable for the duration of its shelf life (period of storage and use). That is, it must retain the same physical, chemical, microbiological, therapeutic and toxicological properties that it possessed at the time of its manufacture. The product's physical properties (e.g. colour, clarity, viscosity, odour, taste) and efficacy must not change, and there should be no significant increase in toxicity. The product should remain sterile or resistant to

microbial growth, and the drug's chemical nature and potency must not change.

However, many drug molecules undergo chemical reactions, such as, hydrolysis, oxidation, decarboxylation, epimerization, and dehydration, with hydrolysis, oxidation and reduction being the most common. Chemical reactions occur more readily at high temperature, at certain pH values, in the presence of UV light and of substances which can act as a catalyst, and in solutions where the drug is present as molecules. The resulting loss of drug molecules can reduce the efficacy of the formulation and increase the latter's toxicity if the products of the chemical changes are toxic. Pharmaceutical solutions are therefore formulated at the pH favouring drug stability, and often include excipients to enhance product stability. To reduce photooxidation, solutions are packaged in containers that do not allow light transmission. To reduce oxidation, antioxidants and/or metal chelators (as heavy metal ions catalyse oxidation) are used. Alternatively, oxygen can be excluded, by the purging of the solution with nitrogen and the creation of a nitrogen headspace within the container. To inhibit microbial growth during use, preservatives are used in multidose products. All the excipients used within a solution must be of suitable quality, nontoxic, compatible with the drug and with one another, and active at the solution pH. In addition, the excipient must remain in the solution throughout the shelf life of the product. That is, the concentration of the excipient must not decrease, which could happen, for example, if the excipient degraded or was adsorbed onto (or absorbed into) the container walls.

Further detailed information about drug and product stability can be found in Chapters 47, 48 and 49.

Enhancement of drug solubility

As mentioned already, water is the most commonly used vehicle in pharmaceutical solutions. Many drugs are water soluble, solubility being defined as the concentration of the drug in a solution when equilibrium exists between dissolved and undissolved drug. As described in Chapter 2, drug solubility in water depends on a number of factors, such as the drug's molecular structure, crystal structure, particle size and pK_a and the pH of the medium (if the drug is a weak acid/base or a salt).

Unfortunately, many drugs are not sufficiently soluble in water, and aqueous drug solubility must be increased by the inclusion of other solvents/chemicals. The nature of the solubility enhancer depends on the drug molecule and the route of administration, as well as the intended patient population. Certain enhancers may be safely administered via the oral route, but not parenterally due to their greater toxicity when administered parenterally. Others, e.g. ethanol, although widely used in medicines, should be avoided where possible in paediatric formulations. Different approaches to enhancing drug solubility are described in the following sections.

pH adjustment

Most existing drugs are either weak acids or weak bases. In solution, an equilibrium exists between the undissociated drug molecules and their ions. The equilibrium may be represented as

$$\text{weak acid: HA} \leftrightarrow H^+ + A^-$$

(24.1)

$$\text{weak base: B} + H^+ \leftrightarrow BH^+$$

(24.2)

Depending on the circumstances (discussed in Chapter 3), these equilibria will shift towards either the undissociated form or the dissociated form.

Since ions are more soluble in water than neutral molecules, changing the pH of the medium to increase ionization of the drug is a common technique for increasing drug solubility in an aqueous medium. Weakly acidic drugs are ionized when the pH of the solvent is increased. Conversely, lowering the pH favours ionization of weakly basic drugs. The pH required to achieve drug ionization can be calculated using the Henderson–Hasselbalch equations (see Chapter 3), and the pH can be adjusted using acids or alkalis, or by using buffers such as citrate, acetate, phosphate and carbonate buffers. Extremes of pH should be avoided however so that the solution is physiologically acceptable; the pH ranges tolerated for the different routes are shown in Table 24.4.

The selected pH should not adversely affect the stability of the drug and excipients. As mentioned already, the rate of chemical reactions which lead to degradation can be pH dependent. The pH for optimal drug solubility may not be the same as that for optimal stability. The pH can also be important for the optimal functioning of excipients. For example, the ionization

and subsequently the activity of a preservative may be influenced by the pH of the medium. Bioavailability of the drug should also not be compromised by a change in pH, un-ionized drug molecules being absorbed to a greater extent through biological membranes than their ionized counterparts. The pH of a pharmaceutical solution is thus a compromise between drug solubility, stability and bioavailability, the function of excipients, and physiological acceptability of the product.

Cosolvents

Cosolvents are often used to increase the water solubility of drugs which do not contain ionizable groups and whose solubility can thus not be increased by pH adjustment. The principle 'like dissolves like' was outlined in Chapter 2. That is, polar drugs generally dissolve in polar solvents and nonpolar drugs generally dissolve in nonpolar solvents. Thus nonpolar drugs are poorly soluble in water – a polar solvent. To increase the solubility of such drugs in water, the latter's polarity should be lowered. This can be achieved by addition of a third component such as a water-miscible organic liquid with a low polarity. Such a liquid, when used in this context, is called a cosolvent.

Most water-miscible organic liquids are toxic, and only a few are used as cosolvents in pharmaceutical solutions. Examples include glycerol, propylene glycol, ethanol and the low molecular weight polyethylene glycols. The solubility of nonpolar drugs in water can be increased by several orders of magnitude with cosolvents. Typically, a linear increase in cosolvent fraction results in logarithmic increases in drug solubility. The concentration of the cosolvent is, however, limited by its physiological acceptability. The cosolvent must be nontoxic at the concentrations used, and for the route of administration.

Complexation with cyclodextrins

Cyclodextrins (CDs) are nonreducing cyclic glucose-based oligosaccharides, comprising a variable number of D-glucose residues linked by α-(1,4) glycosidic linkages. The three most important CDs are α-CD, β-CD and γ-CD, which consist of six, seven and eight d-glucopyranosyl units respectively arranged in a ring. Three-dimensionally, CDs can be visualized as a hollow truncated cone (Fig. 24.1). The cavity in the cone has different diameters dependent on

pH affects stability
= speeds up reaction rate.

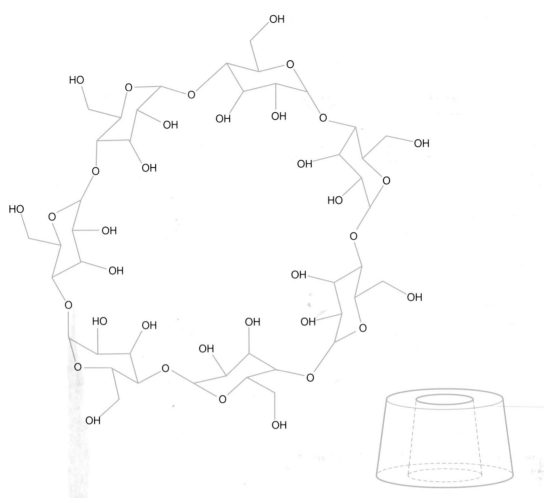

Figure 24.1 • The structure of a cyclodextrin molecule. The sketch shows both the chemical structure and the three-dimensional physical structure. The inside surface of the structure is hydrophobic and the exterior is hydrophilic.

the number of glucose units in the ring; α-CD has a cavity diameter of approximately 0.55 nm, β-CD has a cavity diameter of approximately 0.70 nm and γ-CD has a cavity diameter of approximately 0.90 nm, with cavity volumes of 0.10 mL g^{-1}, 0.14 mL g^{-1} and 0.20 mL g^{-1} respectively. The side rim depth is the same for all three (approximately 0.8 nm).

The interior cavity of CDs is apolar, whilst their exterior is hydrophilic. The representation in Fig. 24.1 needs careful interpretation as the –OH groups shown are actually attached to the top and bottom rims of the structure and not to either the inside or the outside walls. The hydrophobic nature of the inside surface arises from the location of the –O– and C–H bonds of the glucose molecules being oriented there.

The hydrophilic exterior results in CDs being soluble in water. Concurrently, the less polar interior can accommodate nonpolar drug molecules via noncovalent interactions, thereby allowing the nonpolar drug to be 'hidden', enabling it to be molecularly dispersed in water. Thus drug inclusion within CDs effectively increases the aqueous solubility. Each CD molecule can form inclusion complexes with one or more drug molecules. Drug–CD complexes can also self-associate, and the water-soluble structures formed can further solubilize the drug through noninclusion complexation.

On administration, for example orally, of a solution containing a drug–CD complex, the drug can be released from the CD molecule and the free drug can then be absorbed through the gastrointestinal tract.

Surfactants and micelles

As described in Chapter 5, surfactants (surface-active agents) and amphiphiles are molecules which have two distinct regions in their chemical structure. One region is hydrophilic and the other is hydrophobic. Because of this, such molecules tend to accumulate at the boundary between two phases, such as water–air or water–oil interfaces. They reduce the surface tension of liquids, and self-assemble to form micelles once the critical micellar concentration (CMC) is reached. Poorly water-soluble drugs can be solubilized in micelles to enhance their aqueous solubility. The location of the solubilizate (the drug which is solubilized within the micelles) depends on its nature: nonpolar solubilizates are located within the micelles' hydrophobic interior cores, solubilizates containing polar groups are oriented with the polar group at the micellar surface and slightly polar solubilizates partitions between the micelle surface and the core. Solubilizates may also be found in the palisade layer of nonionic surfactant micelles. The maximum amount of solubilizate which can be incorporated into a given system at a fixed concentration is known as the maximum additive concentration (MAC).

The aqueous solubility of a wide range of drugs has been increased by surfactants, especially for oral administration and parenteral administration. For example, solubilization of steroids with polysorbates has allowed their formulation in aqueous ophthalmic preparations, and solubilization of the water-insoluble vitamins A, D, E and K has enabled the preparation of aqueous injections. The surfactant chosen for a particular drug must solubilize the drug and be compatible with it and all the other components of the solution. For example, the surfactant should not adversely influence the drug's stability. The surfactant must also be nontoxic at the concentration used for the particular route of administration.

The different means of enhancing drug solubility are often used in combination, as one approach is often insufficient to achieve the target drug concentration in a pharmaceutical solution. For example, pH adjustment and cosolvents are often used in combination.

Please check your eBook at **https: studentconsult. inkling.com/** for self-assessment q tions. See inside cover for registration details.

Bibliography

British Pharmacopoeia Commission, 2017. British Pharmacopoeia. Stationery Office, London.

European Pharmacopoeia Commission, 2017. European Pharmacopoeia, ninth ed. Council of Europe, Strasbourg.

Florence, A.T., Attwood, D., 2016. Physicochemical Principles of Pharmacy: In Manufacture, Formulation and Clinical Use,

sixth ed. Pharmaceutical Press, London.

Jones, D., 2016. FASTtrack Pharmaceutics – Dosage Form and Design, second ed. Pharmaceutical Press, London.

Liu, R., 2008. Water-Insoluble Drug Formulation, second ed. CRC Press, Boca Raton.

Rowe, R.C., Sheskey, P.J., Cook, W.G., et al. (Eds.), 2016. Handbook of

Pharmaceutic. cipients, eighth ed. Pharmace Press, London.

Sweetman, S.C. , 2014. Martindale: Th omplete Drug Reference, thir ighth ed. Pharmaceutical ss, London.

United States Pha copeial Convention, 2(United States Pharmacopeia. Pharmacopeial Convention, Roc ille.

Clarification

25

Andrew M. Twitchell

KEY POINTS

- Clarification processes are widely used in the pharmaceutical industry in the preparation of drug substances and drug products.
- Clarification can be achieved using either filtration or centrifugation techniques.
- The main pharmaceutical uses of clarification are to remove unwanted solid particles from fluids or to separate a required solid from a fluid.
- Straining/sieving and impingement are the main mechanisms by which filtration occurs.
- The rate at which a filtration process occurs depends on the properties of the product being filtered and the design and operation of the filtration equipment.
- Darcy's equation combines the factors responsible for determining the filtration rate and shows how these factors may be manipulated to control the rate of filtration.
- Filters used for liquid products may be classified as gravity filters (e.g. simple laboratory filters), vacuum filters (e.g. the rotary vacuum filter) or pressure filters (e.g. cartridge filters).
- Centrifugal force can be used to enhance the separate of solids from liquids (e.g. perforated-basket centrifuges).

Introduction

Clarification is a term used to describe processes that involve the removal or separation of a solid from a fluid, or a fluid from another fluid. The term 'fluid' encompasses both liquids and gases. Clarification can be achieved by either filtration or centrifugation techniques, both of which are described in this chapter.

In pharmaceutical processing there are two main reasons for such processes:

- to remove unwanted solid particles from either a liquid product or air; and
- to collect the solid as the product itself (e.g. following crystallization).

Filtration

Types of filtration

Solid–fluid filtration

Solid–fluid filtration can be defined as the separation of an insoluble solid from a fluid by means of a porous medium that retains the solid but allows the fluid to pass. It is the most common type of filtration encountered during the manufacture of pharmaceutical products. Solid–fluid filtration may be further subdivided into two types: namely, solid–liquid filtration and solid–gas filtration.

Solid–liquid filtration. There are numerous applications of solid–liquid filtration in pharmaceutical processing, some of which are listed here:

- Improvement of the appearance of solutions, mouthwashes, etc., to give them a 'sparkle' or 'brightness'; this is often referred to as 'clarifying' a product.
- Removal of potential irritants (e.g. from eye drop preparations or solutions applied to mucous membranes).
- Production of water of appropriate quality for pharmaceutical production.
- Recovery of desired solid material from a suspension or slurry (e.g. to obtain a drug or excipient after a crystallization process).
- Certain operations, such as the extraction of vegetable drugs with a solvent, may yield a turbid product with a small quantity of fine suspended colloidal matter. This can be removed by filtration.
- Sterilization of liquid or semisolid products where processes involving heat (such as autoclaving) are not appropriate.
- Detection of microorganisms present in liquids. This can be achieved by analysis of a suitable filter on which the bacteria are retained. This method can also be used to assess the efficiency of preservatives.

Solid–gas filtration. There are two main applications of solid–gas filtration in pharmaceutical processing. One of particular importance in manufacturing is the removal of suspended solid material from air so as to supply air of the required standard for either processing equipment or manufacturing areas. This includes the provision of air for equipment such as fluidized-bed processors (see Chapters 28 and 29), film-coating machinery (see Chapter 32) and bottle-cleaning equipment so that product appearance and quality are maintained. The use of suitable filters also enables the particulate contamination of air in manufacturing areas to be maintained at an appropriate level for the product being manufactured; for example, air free from microorganisms can be supplied to areas where sterile products are being manufactured.

It is also often necessary to remove particulate matter generated during a manufacturing operation from the process air so as to prevent the material being vented to the atmosphere. Examples of this include filtering of exhaust air from fluidized-bed and coating processes.

Fluid–fluid filtration

Flavouring oils are sometimes added to liquid preparations in the form of a spirit (i.e. dissolved in alcohol). When these spirits are added to aqueous-based formulations, some of the oil may come out of solution, giving the product a degree of turbidity. Removal of the oil droplets by passing them through an appropriate filter (a liquid/liquid filtration process) is used to produce the desired product appearance.

Compressed air is used in a number of pharmaceutical processes, e.g. film-coating spray guns (see Chapter 32), bottle-cleaning equipment and fluid energy mills (see Chapter 10). Before use, the compressed air needs to be filtered to ensure that any entrained oil or water droplets are removed. This is an example of a fluid–gas filtration process.

Mechanisms of filtration

The mechanisms by which material may be retained by a filter medium (i.e. the surface on or in which material is deposited) are discussed in the following sections.

Straining/sieving

If the pores in the filter medium through which the fluid is flowing are smaller than the material that is required to be removed, the material will be retained. Filtration occurs on the surface of the filter in this case, and therefore the filter can be very thin (typically approximately 100 µm). Filter media of this type are referred to as membrane filters. Because filtration occurs on the surface there is a tendency for the filter to become blocked unless it is carefully designed (see later). Filters using the straining mechanism are used where the contaminant level is low or small volumes need to be filtered. Examples of the use of membrane filters include the removal of bacteria and fibres from parenteral preparations.

Impingement

As a flowing fluid approaches and passes an object (e.g. a filter fibre), the fluid flow pattern is disturbed,

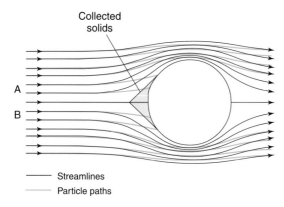

—— Streamlines
—— Particle paths

Fig. 25.1 • Filtration by impingement.

as shown in Fig. 25.1. Suspended solids may, however, have sufficient momentum such that they do not follow the fluid path but impinge on the filter fibre and are retained, owing to attractive forces between the particle and the fibre. Where the pores between filter fibres are larger than the material being removed, some particles may follow the fluid streamlines and miss the fibre, this being more likely if the particles are small (owing to their lower momentum) and as the distance from the centre of the fibre towards which they approach increases. To ensure the removal of all unwanted material, filter media that use the impingement mechanism must be sufficiently thick so that material not trapped by the first fibre in its path is removed by a subsequent one. These types of filter are therefore referred to as depth filters. The fluid should flow through the filter medium in a streamlined manner to ensure the filter works effectively, as turbulent flow may carry the particles past the fibres. Depth filters are the main type of filter used for removal of material from gases.

Attractive forces

Electrostatic and other surface forces may exert sufficient hold on the particles to attract and retain them on the filter medium (as occurs during the impingement mechanism).

Air can be freed from dust particles in an electrostatic precipitator by passing the air between highly charged surfaces, which attract the dust particles.

Autofiltration

Autofiltration is the term used to describe the situation when filtered material (termed the filter cake) acts as its own filter medium. This mechanism is used by the metafilter, which is discussed later in this chapter.

Factors affecting the rate of filtration

The filtration process chosen must not only remove the required 'contaminants' or product but must also do so at an acceptably fast rate to ensure that the manufacturing process can be performed economically. The laboratory Büchner funnel and flask (Fig. 25.2) is a convenient filter that can be used to illustrate the factors that influence the rate at which a product can be filtered. This filter is used for solid–liquid filtration processes, but the same basic principles are valid whatever filtration process is being evaluated.

The rate of filtration – volume of filtered material (V; m³) obtained in unit time (t; s) – depends on the following factors:

* The area available for filtration (A; m²), which in this case is the cross-sectional area of the funnel.
* The pressure difference (ΔP; Pa) across the filter bed (filter medium and any cake formed). With the Büchner funnel apparatus, this difference is due to the 'head' of unfiltered suspension and therefore it decreases as filtration proceeds and the level drops. It is the

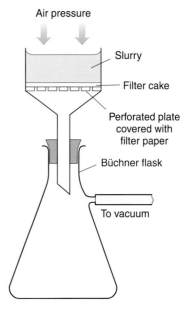

Fig. 25.2 • Büchner funnel and vacuum flask.

pressure difference across the filtration medium that is important, and this can be increased if the pressure in the collection flask is reduced to create a vacuum. The difference between atmospheric pressure and the lower pressure in the flask is added to the pressure due to the unfiltered product to give the total pressure difference.

- The viscosity of the fluid passing through the filter, i.e. the filtrate (μ; Pa s). A viscous fluid will filter more slowly than a mobile one owing to the greater resistance to movement offered by more viscous fluids (see Chapter 6).
- The thickness of the filter medium and any deposited cake (L; m). The cake will *increase* in thickness as filtration proceeds, so if it is not removed, the rate of filtration will fall.

Darcy's equation

The factors affecting the rate of filtration are combined in Darcy's equation:

$$\frac{V}{t} = \frac{KA\Delta P}{\mu L}$$

(25.1)

In this equation the driving force for this particular 'rate process' is the pressure difference across the filter, and the resistance to the process is a function of the properties of the filter bed, its thickness and the viscosity of the filtrate. The contribution to resistance to filtration from the filter medium is usually small compared with that of the filter cake, and can often be disregarded in calculations.

The proportionality constant K (m^2) expresses the permeability of the filter medium and cake and will increase as the porosity of the bed increases. It is clearly desirable that K should be large so as to maximize the filtration rate. If K is taken to represent the permeability of the cake, it can be shown that K is given by

$$K = \frac{e^2}{5(1-e)^2 S^2}$$

(25.2)

where e is the porosity of the cake and S is the surface area of the particles making up the cake. If the solid material is one that forms an impermeable cake, the filtration rate may be increased by adding a filter aid (discussed later), which aids the formation of open porous cakes.

Methods used to increase the filtration rate

Darcy's equation can be used to determine ways in which the filtration rate can be increased or controlled in practice. These are now discussed.

Increase the area available for filtration. The total volume of filtrate flowing through the filter will be directly proportional to the area of the filter, and hence the rate of filtration can be increased by using either larger filters or a number of small units in parallel. Both of these approaches will also distribute the cake over a larger area and thus decrease the value of L, thereby further increasing the filtration rate.

Increase the pressure difference across the filter cake. The simplest filters, e.g. a laboratory filter funnel, use the gravitational force of the liquid 'head' to provide the driving force for filtration. Often this driving force is too low for an acceptably fast filtration rate and there is a requirement to increase it. If a vacuum is 'pulled' on the far side of the filter medium (see Fig. 25.2), then the pressure difference can be increased up to atmospheric pressure, i.e. approximately 100 kPa, or 1 bar. In practice, however, it will be less, as liquids will boil in the collecting vessel if the pressure is reduced to too low a value. Despite the limited pressure difference generated, vacuum filtration is used in the laboratory, where there are safety advantages in using glassware, because if the glassware is damaged, it will implode rather than explode. One important industrial filter, the rotary vacuum filter, also uses a vacuum; this is described later in this chapter.

With industrial-scale liquid filtration, commonly used means of obtaining a high-pressure difference are either pumping the material to be filtered into the filter with a suitable pump or using a pressurized vessel to drive the liquid through the filter. Most industrial filters have a positive-pressure feed; the pressure used is limited only by the pump capacity and the ability of the filter to withstand the high-pressure stress. Pressures up to 1.5 MPa (15 bar) are commonly used.

Although increasing the ΔP value in the absence of any other changes will cause a proportional increase in the filtration rate, care needs to be taken to ensure that a phenomenon known as cake compression does not occur. Too high an applied pressure may cause the particles making up the cake to deform and therefore decrease the voidage (bed porosity). It can be seen from Eq. 25.2 that small decreases in the value of the porosity (e) lead to large decreases in cake permeability (K), and therefore in the filtration rate. The effect of decreasing K greatly outweighs any increase in the filtration rate arising from a thinner cake. There is also a danger of 'blinding' the filter medium at high pressures by forcing particles into it. This is most likely in the early stages before a continuous layer of cake has formed. As a general rule, filtration should start at moderate pressure, which can be increased as filtration proceeds and the cake thickness builds up.

Decrease the filtrate viscosity. The flow through a filter cake can be considered as the total flow through a large number of capillaries formed by the voids between the particles of the cake. The rate of flow through each capillary is governed by Poiseuille's law, which is a mathematical relationship that includes viscosity as a factor contributing to the resistance to flow. To increase the filtration rate, the viscosity of the filtrate can be reduced in most cases by heating of the formulation to be filtered. Many industrial filters (e.g. the metafilter) can be fitted with a steam jacket which can control temperature and hence viscosity. Care needs to be taken with this approach when one is filtering formulations containing volatile components, or if the components are thermolabile. In such cases, dilution of the formulation with water may be an alternative means of reducing the viscosity providing that the increase in the filtration rate exceeds the effect of increasing the total volume to be filtered.

Decrease the thickness of the filter cake. Darcy's equation (Eq. 25.1) shows that the filtration rate decreases as the cake increases in thickness. This effect is commonly observed when one is filtering formulations in the laboratory using filter paper in a funnel. In some cases, if the cake is allowed to build up, the process slows to an unacceptable rate, or may almost stop. In these situations, it may be necessary to remove the cake periodically or to maintain it at a constant thickness, as occurs, for example, with the rotary drum filter. As previously mentioned, the cake thickness can be kept lower by using a larger filter area.

Increase the permeability of the cake. One way of increasing the permeability of the cake is to include filter aids. A filter aid is a material that, when included in the formulation to be filtered, forms a cake of a more open, porous nature and thus increases the K value in Darcy's equation. In addition, it may reduce the compressibility of the cake and/or prevent the filtered material blocking the filter medium. Filter aids that are used include diatomite (a form of diatomaceous earth) and perlite (a type of naturally occurring volcanic glass), which has been used in the filtration of, for example, penicillin and streptomycin. The use of filter aids is obviously not appropriate if the filtered material is the intended end product.

Filtration equipment

The filtration equipment described in this chapter is that used for filtering liquids. Equipment for filtering gases (mainly air) is also available.

Equipment selection

Ideally the equipment chosen should allow a fast filtration rate to minimize production costs, be cheap to buy and use, be easily cleaned and resistant to corrosion, and be capable of filtering large volumes of product before the filter needs to be stripped down for cleaning or replacement.

There are a number of product-related factors that should be considered when one is selecting a filter for a particular process. These include:

- The chemical nature of the product. Interactions with the filter medium may lead to leaching of the filter components, degradation or swelling of the filter medium or adsorption of components of the filtered product onto the filter. All of these may influence the efficiency of the filtration process or the quality of the filtered product.
- The volume to be filtered and the filtration rate required. These dictate the size and type of equipment and the amount of time needed for the filtration process.
- The operating pressure needed. This is important in governing the filtration rate (Eq. 25.1) and influences whether a vacuum filter (where the pressure difference is limited to approximately 100 kPa) is appropriate. High operating pressures require that the equipment is of sufficient strength and that appropriate safe operating procedures are adopted.
- The amount of material to be removed. This will influence the choice of the filter, as a large 'load' may necessitate the use of prefilters or may require a filter where the cake can be continuously removed.

- The degree of filtration required. This will dictate the pore size of membrane filters or the filter grade to be used. If sterility is required, the equipment should itself be capable of being sterilized and care must be taken to ensure that contamination does not occur after the product has passed the filter.
- The product viscosity and filtration temperature. A high product viscosity may require elevated pressures to be used. The incoming formulation can be heated, or steam-heated jackets can be fitted to the equipment. Care should be taken to ensure the equipment seals, for example, can operate at elevated temperatures.

Industrial filtration equipment

Filters for liquid products may be classified by the method used to drive the filtrate through the filter medium. Filters can be organized into three classes: namely, gravity, vacuum and pressure filters.

Gravity filters

Filters that rely solely on gravity generate only low operating pressures and therefore their use on a large scale is limited. Gravity filters are, however, simple and cheap, and are frequently used in laboratory filtration, where volumes are small and a low filtration rate is relatively unimportant.

Vacuum filters

The rotary vacuum filter

In large-scale filtration, continuous operation is often desirable, and this may be difficult to achieve when it is necessary to filter slurries containing a high proportion of solids. The rotary vacuum filter is continuous in operation and has a system for removing the cake so that it can be run for long periods handling concentrated slurries. A rotary drum filter is shown in Fig. 25.3. It can be visualized as two concentric cylinders with the annular space between them divided into a number of septa by radial partitions. The outer cylinder is perforated and covered with a filter cloth. Each septum has a radial connection to a complicated rotating valve whose function is to perform the sequence of operations listed in Table 25.1.

The cylinder rotates slowly in the slurry, which is kept agitated, and a vacuum applied to the segments

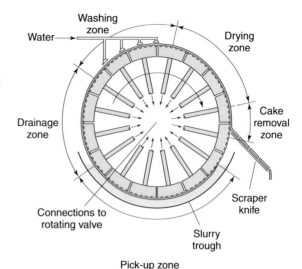

Fig. 25.3 • Rotary drum filter.

Table 25.1 Rotary vacuum filter operation

Zone	Position	Service	Connected to
Pick-up	Slurry trough	Vacuum	Filtrate receiver
Drainage	–	Vacuum	Filtrate receiver
Washing	Wash sprays	Vacuum	Wash water receiver
Drying	–	Vacuum	Wash water receiver
Cake removal	Scraper knife	Compressed air	Filter cake conveyor

In some cases, for example when the solid is the required product, the same receiver may be used for the filtrate and for wash water.

draws filtrate into the septa, depositing cake on the filter cloth. When the deposited cake leaves the slurry bath, the vacuum is maintained to draw air through the cake, thus aiding liquid removal. This is followed by washing and then further drainage in the drying zone. The cake is removed by the scraper blade aided by compressed air forced into the septa. It is the function of the rotary valve to direct these services into each septum when required.

Rotary filters can be up to 2 m in diameter and 3.5 m in length, with a filtration area of approximately 20 m². The drum rotates slowly, typically between 10 and 60 revolutions per hour. Cake compression rollers are often fitted to improve the efficiency of washing and draining if the cake on the drum becomes cracked. Difficult solids, which tend to block the

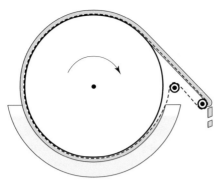

Fig. 25.4 • String discharge rotary drum filter.

filter cloth, necessitate a preliminary precoat of a filter aid to be deposited on the cloth prior to filtration of the slurry. During the actual filtration, the scraper knife is set to move slowly inwards, removing the blocked outer layer of the filter aid and exposing fresh surface.

If removal of the cake presents problems, a string discharge filter may be employed. This is useful for filtration of the fermentation liquor in the manufacture of antibiotics, when a felt-like cake of mould mycelia must be removed. The filter cloth in this case has a number of bands passing round the drum and over two additional small rollers, as shown in Fig. 25.4. In operation, the bands lift the cake off the filter medium. The cake is broken by the sharp bend over the rollers and collected, and the bands return to the drum.

The advantages of the industrial rotary vacuum filter can be summarized as follows:

* It is automatic and continuous in operation, so labour costs are low.
* The filter has a large capacity.
* Variation of the speed of rotation enables the cake thickness to be controlled, and for solids that form an impenetrable cake, the thickness may be limited to less than 5 mm. On the other hand, if the solids are coarse and form a porous cake, the thickness may be 100 mm or more.

The disadvantages of the rotary vacuum filter include the following:

* The rotary filter is a complex piece of equipment with many moving parts and is very expensive. In addition to the filter itself, ancillary equipment such as vacuum pumps, vacuum receivers and traps, slurry pumps and agitators are required.

* The cake tends to crack because of the air drawn through by the vacuum system, so washing and drying are not efficient.
* Because it is a vacuum filter, the pressure difference is limited to 100 kPa (1 bar). Yet some hot filtrates may boil because of the reduced pressure.
* The rotary filter is suitable only for straightforward slurries, being less satisfactory if the solids form an impermeable cake or will not separate cleanly from the cloth.

Small rotary vacuum filter units with a drum approximately 120 mm long and 75 mm in diameter are also available. These are simpler in construction than the larger industrial-type units as they do not have a cake-washing facility. They have disposable filter drums and can filter batches from approximately 100 L to 700 L at a rate of 1 L min^{-1} to 2 L min^{-1}.

The rotary filter is most suitable for continuous operation on large quantities of slurry, especially if the slurry contains considerable amounts of solids (i.e. in the range 15% to 30%).

Examples of pharmaceutical applications include the collection of calcium carbonate, magnesium carbonate and starch, and the separation of the mycelia from the fermentation liquor in the manufacture of antibiotics.

Pressure filters

Pressure filters feed the product to the filter at a pressure greater than that which would arise from gravity alone. This is the most common type of filter used in the processing of pharmaceutical products.

The metafilter. In its simplest form, the metafilter consists of a grooved drainage rod on which a series of metal rings are packed. These rings, usually made of stainless steel, are approximately 15 mm in inside diameter, 22 mm in outside diameter and 0.8 mm thick, with a number of semicircular projections on one surface (Fig. 25.5). The height of the projections and the shape of the section of the ring are such that when the rings are packed together and tightened on the drainage rod, channels are formed that taper from approximately 250 μm down to 25 μm. One or more of these packs is mounted in a vessel and the filter is operated by pumping in the slurry under pressure.

In this form the metafilter can be used for separating coarse particles, but for finer particles, a bed of a suitable material (such as a filter aid) is first built

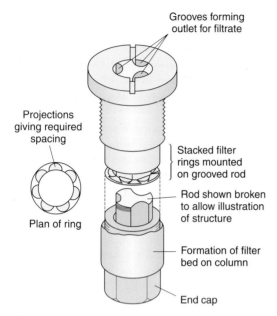

Grooves forming outlet for filtrate

Projections giving required spacing

Plan of ring

Stacked filter rings mounted on grooved rod

Rod shown broken to allow illustration of structure

Formation of filter bed on column

End cap

Fig. 25.5 • Metafilter. Construction of the filter element.

up over the rings by recirculation of a filter aid suspension. The pack of rings, therefore, serves essentially as a base on which the true filter medium is supported.

The advantages of the metafilter can be summarized as follows:

- It possesses considerable strength, and high pressures can be used with no danger of bursting the filter medium.
- As there is no filter medium as such, the running costs are low and it is very economical.
- The metafilter can be made from materials (such as stainless steel) that can provide excellent resistance to corrosion and avoid contamination of the product.
- By selection of a suitable grade of material to form the filter bed, it is possible to remove very fine particles. In fact, it is possible to sterilize a liquid with this filter.

The small surface area of the metafilter restricts the amount of solid that can be collected. This, together with the ability to separate very fine particles, means that the metafilter is used almost exclusively for clarification of liquids where the contaminant level is low. Furthermore, the strength of the metafilter permits the use of high pressures (up to 1.5 MPa, 15 bar), making the method suitable for viscous liquids.

Specific examples of pharmaceutical uses include the clarification of syrups, injection solutions and intermediates such as insulin liquors.

Cartridge filters. Cartridge filters are now commonly used in the preparation of pharmaceutical products, as they possess a very large filtration area in a small unit and are easy and relatively cheap to operate. In simple form, they consist of a cylindrical cartridge containing highly pleated material (e.g. polytetrafluoroethylene, cellulose acetate or nylon) or 'string-wound' material (i.e. wound like a ball of string). This cartridge then fits in a metal supporting cylinder and the product is pumped under pressure into one end of the cylinder surrounding the filter cartridge. The filtrate is forced through the filter cartridge from the periphery to the inner hollow core, from where it exits through the other end of the support cylinder. The filter cartridges are often disposable and are good for applications where there is a low contaminant level, e.g. during the filtration of liquid products as they are filled into bottles.

Cross-flow microfiltration. It is possible to form membrane filters within 'hollow fibres'. The membrane, which may consist of polysulfone, acrylonitrile or polyamide, is laid down within a fibre which forms a rigid porous outer support (Fig. 25.6). The lumen of each fibre is small, typically 1 μm to 2 μm. However, a large number of fibres can be contained in a surrounding shell to form a cartridge, which may have an effective filtration area greater than 2 m^2.

In use, the liquid to be treated is pumped through the cartridge in a circulatory system, so that it passes through many times. The filtrate, which in this technique is often called the 'permeate', flows radially through the membrane and porous support. The great advantage of this mode of operation is that the high fluid velocity and turbulence minimize blocking of the membranes. Fresh liquid enters the system from a reservoir as filtration proceeds. Because the fluid flow is across the surface, rather than at right angles, this technique is known as cross-flow microfiltration.

The method has been used for fractionation of biological products by first using a filter of pore size sufficient to let through all the molecules the same size as or smaller than those required, and then passing the permeate through a second filter that will retain the required molecules whilst allowing passage of smaller unwanted molecules. Blood plasma can be processed to remove alcohol and water and prepare concentrated purified albumin with this method. The

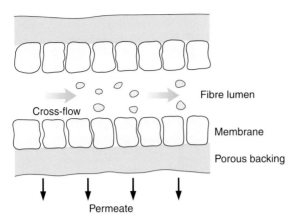

Fig. 25.6 • Cross-flow microfiltration through an individual fibre.

process has also been used for the recovery of antibiotics from fermentation media.

Centrifugation

Centrifugal force can be used either to provide the driving force (ΔP) for the filtration process (see Darcy's equation, Eq. 25.1) or to replace the gravitational force in sedimentation processes (refer to Stokes's law; see Chapters 5 and 6). Centrifuges are often used in the laboratory to separate solid material from a liquid, the solid typically forming a 'plug' at the bottom of the test tube at the end of the process.

Principles of centrifugation

If a particle (mass m; kg) spins in a centrifuge (radius r; m) at a velocity (v; m s^{-1}), then the centrifugal force (F; N) acting on the particle equals mv^2/r. The same particle experiences gravitational force (G; N) equal to $m \times g$ (where g is the gravitational constant).

The centrifugal effect (C) is the ratio of these two forces, so $C = F/G$, i.e. C indicates how many times greater F is than G. Therefore $C = v^2/gr$. If the rotational velocity is taken to be πdn, where n is the rotation speed (s^{-1}) and d is the diameter of rotation (m), then $C = 2.01dn^2$.

To increase the centrifugal effect, it is more efficient to increase the centrifuge speed than use a larger diameter at the same speed. Larger centrifuges generate greater pressures on the centrifuge wall for the same value of C, so are more costly to manufacture.

Industrial centrifuges

Two main types of centrifuge are used to achieve separation on an industrial scale: those using perforated baskets, which perform a filtration-type operation (like a spin-dryer), and those with a solid-walled vessel, where particles sediment towards the wall under the influence of the centrifugal force.

Perforated-basket centrifuges (centrifugal filters)

A diagram of a perforated-basket centrifuge is shown in Fig. 25.7. It consists of a stainless steel perforated basket (typically 1 m to 2 m in diameter) lined with a filter cloth. The basket rotates at a speed which is typically less than 25 s^{-1}, higher speeds tending to stress the basket excessively. The product enters centrally and is thrown outwards by centrifugal force and held against the filter cloth. The filtrate is forced through the cloth and removed via the liquid outlet; the solid material is retained on the cloth. The cake can be washed, if required, by the spraying of water into the centrifuge.

The centrifugal filter has been used for separation of crystalline materials from the preparation liquor (e.g. in the preparation of drug crystals) and for removal of precipitated proteins from, for example, insulin. It has the advantages of being compact and efficient, a 1 m diameter centrifuge being able to process approximately 200 kg in 10 minutes. It can also handle concentrated slurries, which might block other filters. The spinning action gives a product with a low moisture content (typically approximately 2% w/w), which saves energy during subsequent drying.

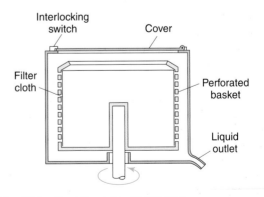

Fig. 25.7 • Centrifugal dewatering filter.

The centrifuge described here is operated batch-wise, but continuous centrifuges are available for large-scale work. These have a means for automatic discharge of the cake from a basket, which rotates around a horizontal axis, in contrast to the vertical axis. Most of the energy required to run a centrifuge is used to bring it up to the operating speed and little more is needed to maintain that speed. Continuous centrifuges are therefore cheaper to run but the initial cost is considerably higher.

Tubular-bowl centrifuges (centrifugal sedimenters)

These consist of a cylindrical 'bowl', typically approximately 100 mm in diameter and 1 m long, that rotates at a high speed, 300 s^{-1} to 1000 s^{-1}. The product enters at the bottom, and centrifugal force causes solids to be deposited on the wall as it passes up the bowl, the clear liquid overflowing from the top (Fig. 25.8). This type of centrifuge can also be adapted to separate immiscible liquids. The inlet rate needs to be controlled so that there is sufficient time for sedimentation to occur before the product leaves the bowl.

The uses of centrifugal sedimenters include:

- liquid–liquid separation, e.g. during antibiotic manufacture and purification of oils from natural sources (e.g. fish oils);
- the removal of very small particles;
- the removal of solids that are compressible or 'slimy' and which easily block filter media;
- the separation of blood plasma from whole blood (C of approximately 3000 is required);

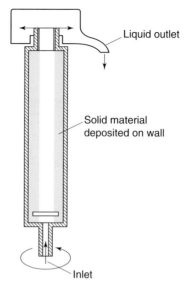

Fig. 25.8 • Tubular-bowl centrifuge.

- the separation of different particle size fractions; and
- examination of the stability of emulsions.

These centrifuges are compact, have a high separating efficiency and are good for separating 'difficult' solids. However, they have a limited capacity and are complicated to construct to achieve the required speed and minimize vibration.

Please check your eBook at **https://studentconsult. inkling.com/** for self-assessment questions. See inside cover for registration details.

Bibliography

Jornitz, M.W., Meltzer, T.H., 2008. Filtration and Purification in the Biopharmaceutical Industry. Informa Healthcare, London.

Perlmutter, B.A., 2015. Solid-Liquid Filtration. Butterworth-Heinemann, Oxford.

Sparks, T., Chase, G., 2015. Filters and Filtration Handbook. Butterworth-Heinemann, Oxford.

Suspensions

26

Susan A. Barker

CHAPTER CONTENTS

KEY POINTS

- Suspensions are dispersions of solid materials, generally the drug, in a liquid medium.
- All normal considerations that apply to pharmaceutical products, such as chemical stability and dose integrity, apply equally to pharmaceutical suspensions, but with the added issues of particulate behaviour.
- Formulators must have a working understanding of the electrical double layer and the Derjaguin–Landau–Verwey–Overbeek theory of particulate behaviour in a suspension.
- Many formulation excipients have the potential to affect particulate interaction and sedimentation behaviour. Therefore the formulation needs to be considered holistically and the effects of individual additives need to be studied.

Introduction

Suspensions are probably one of the most challenging pharmaceutical formulations that students and formulators are likely to encounter. Many of the issues relating to solution formulation development apply equally to suspension formulations, but there are several additional considerations relating to the solid component of the system and the interface between the solid and the liquid components. This chapter presents these issues and discusses them in context so that the reader will have a fundamental understanding of the science behind suspension formulation, as well as the more patient-focused aspects.

The most important consideration in suspension formulation development is the interaction between the solid particles and the liquid vehicle, so this aspect will be considered in detail first. Secondly, other considerations relating to the solid component will be discussed, and finally, aesthetic, patient-focused and practical matters will be reviewed.

Definition of a suspension

It is appropriate here to review the definition of a solution before we consider the definition of a suspension. Solutions are discussed in detail in Chapters 2, 3 and 24. They can be formed from various combinations of phases. However, in pharmacy, the word 'solution', without further description, is generally understood to refer to a liquid system. A solution is a one-phase system where at equilibrium all the ingredients are dispersed evenly at a molecular level. Solutions are therefore optically clear as there are no solid particles remaining to disperse the light. In the context of a pharmaceutical formulation, the drug (solute) is added as a solid to the vehicle (solvent, most commonly water) and dissolves completely to give the formulation (a solution). Other formulation components, such as preservatives, buffers and flavours, are added as required.

A pharmaceutical suspension is also a liquid system. However, in this case the solid material (usually the drug) does not dissolve in the vehicle to any appreciable extent but remains as solid particles which are distributed throughout the vehicle. Technically, the term *suspension* describes a dispersion of a solid material (the dispersed phase) in a liquid (the continuous phase) without reference to the particle size of the solid material. However, the particle size of the solid material can affect both its physical behaviour and its chemical behaviour, so a distinction is usually made between a *colloid* or *colloidal suspension* with a particle size range of up to approximately 1 μm (see Chapter 5) and a 'coarse dispersion' with larger particles. Unfortunately, pharmaceutical suspensions fall across the borderline between colloidal and coarse dispersions, with solid particles generally in the range of 0.1 to 10 μm. Suspensions are not optically clear and will appear cloudy unless the size of the particles is within the colloidal range.

In the ideal suspension, the particles of the solid material are monodisperse spheres and are evenly suspended in three dimensions throughout the vehicle and remain so even after prolonged periods. Here, every dose from the suspension will contain the same amount of drug and will give the same clinical effect to the patient; such reproducibility is absolutely vital for all formulations, but is difficult to achieve with suspensions.

Solid particle–liquid vehicle interactions

Solid particle–liquid vehicle interactions determine the behaviour of suspensions, and hence it is vital to have a working knowledge of them. Water is by far the most common vehicle used for pharmaceutical suspensions, owing to its lack of toxicity; hence it is the interaction between water and the particles which is important. The behaviour of an individual particle will be discussed first, then the interactions between multiple particles. These issues are discussed in Chapter 5 in the context of dispersed systems in general, and Chapter 4 discusses solid–liquid interfaces. The emphasis in this chapter is on pharmaceutical suspensions and the importance of particle charge and particle–particle interactions in successful suspension formulation.

The 'electrical double layer' theory

A solid material will not dissolve in a liquid vehicle unless it has some chemical similarity. Thus drugs which are hydrophobic will not dissolve very well in water. Many modern drugs have very low aqueous solubility, because they are designed to fit into hydrophobic biological receptors, so although they may be very efficient once they are at their site(s) of action, they present a real challenge to the formulator, and many may be developed as suspension formulations.

An apparently odd characteristic of such hydrophobic drugs is that once they have been dispersed as solid particles in an aqueous environment, they will acquire a charge. This is counterintuitive, as hydrophobic materials will generally repel water; if they could ionize, they would be expected to show a reasonable degree of aqueous solubility and would not remain as solid particles within the aqueous dispersion. However, the charge produced is not as a result of ionization of the drug, rather it is due to the ionization of water:

$$H_2O \leftrightarrow H^+ + OH^-$$

(26.1)

The liberated protons will then be solvated by intact water molecules to form hydronium ions (H_3O^+) and larger structures with more water molecules. One result of this is that they are generally less mobile than the hydroxide ions (OH^-) produced from the initial ionization reaction shown in Eq. 26.1. Some of the hydroxide ions will then collect on solid surfaces within the aqueous dispersion and give rise to an apparent negative charge on these surfaces. Overall, within the system, electrical neutrality must be maintained, so there will be a gradation of charge from a high negative charge on the surface of the particle down to no charge (overall neutrality) in the bulk vehicle. This gradation of charge occurs in two stages, giving rise to two 'layers' of charge surrounding the particle, hence the term *electrical double layer*.

Fig. 26.1 illustrates a single solid particle in water, showing a negatively charged surface arising from the OH^- ions. The innermost layer or 'halo' around the particle has a predominance of positively charged ions. The outer layer or *halo* also has a predominance of positively charged ions, but to a lesser extent than the inner layer. Finally, the bulk vehicle has no overall net charge. Charges in the inner layer are held tightly to the particle, and this layer is therefore known as the *fixed layer*, whereas charges within the outer layer are more mobile and can move away from the solid surface and hence this layer is denoted the 'diffuse layer'. The two layers, fixed and diffuse, are also known as the *Stern* and *Gouy–Chapman layers* respectively.

The rigidity with which the charges are held to the particle affects the intensity of the charge at any point between the charged surface and the bulk external liquid. Throughout the fixed layer, there is a linear decrease of overall charge from the particle surface (high) to the edge of the fixed layer (lower). From this point until the edge of the diffuse layer, i.e. the beginning of the bulk liquid, there is an exponential decrease of charge. This phenomenon is discussed in Chapter 5.

Factors affecting the electrical double layer

The addition of formulation excipients can change the behaviour of a solid particle in a suspension, by affecting either the fixed layer or the diffuse layer, or both. Materials which can ionize (e.g. sodium chloride) will increase the amount of mobile charges

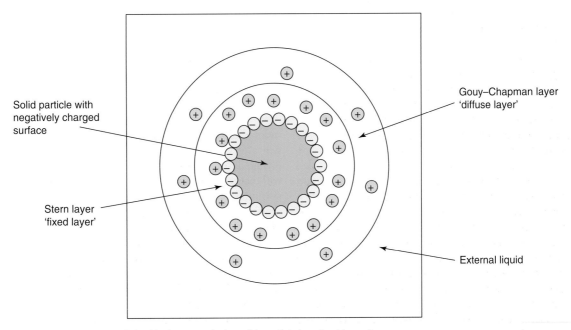

Solid particle with negatively charged surface

Stern layer 'fixed layer'

Gouy–Chapman layer 'diffuse layer'

External liquid

Fig. 26.1 • The electrical double layer: a single solid particle in a liquid medium.

(a) low concentrations of
added ionic materials ⊖

(b) high concentrations of
added ionic materials ⊖

(c) addition of
surfactants ●

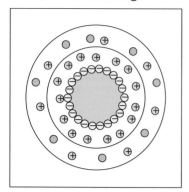
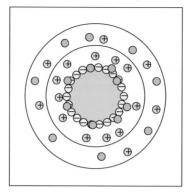
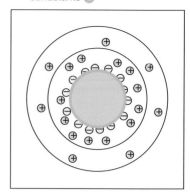

Fig. 26.2 • The location of added materials in the electrical double layer of a single solid particle in a liquid medium: **(a)** low concentrations of added ionic materials; **(b)** high concentrations of added ionic materials; **(c)** addition of surfactants.

available in the system. At low to medium concentrations (e.g. 0.01 M), such charges are generally located only within the diffuse layer, as shown in Fig. 26.2a, and therefore will not affect the surface potential ψ_o or the Stern potential ψ_δ (see Chapter 5 for explanations). The increase in the number of individual charges within the diffuse layer will result in easier neutralization of the remaining charge from the particle (ψ_δ) and hence will lead to a thinning of the diffuse layer. Mathematically, this is because the distance over which ψ_δ becomes ψ_δ/e, i.e. $1/\kappa$ (the 'Debye–Hückel length'; see Chapter 5), is smaller. It should be evident from the previous discussion that an increased concentration of the additional charges would be expected to lead to a greater reduction of $1/\kappa$. In fact, the relationship is a square root one, in that $1/\kappa$ is inversely proportional to the square root of the ionic strength of the medium. This is the same as saying that κ (the Debye–Hückel length parameter; see Chapter 5) is directly proportional to the square root of the ionic strength of the medium. Care must be taken, therefore, to consider the chemistry of dissolved ionic materials: the ionic strength of a calcium chloride ($CaCl_2$) solution is higher than that of a sodium chloride (NaCl) solution of the same molar concentration. The effects of these two solutions on the electrical double layer will consequently be different.

Higher concentrations of ionic materials (e.g. 0.1 M) will not just result in a greater effect on the diffuse layer, but some of the charges will migrate through it into the fixed layer and become adsorbed onto the surface of the particle itself, shown in Fig.

26.2b. In this case the charge on the particle surface will decrease, which will have the automatic effect of lowering the Stern potential and a secondary effect of reducing the zeta potential, as the charge reduction across the diffuse layer will begin at a different value.

Surfactants added to the system at concentrations below their critical micelle concentration (cmc) will localize on the surface of the particles, as shown in Fig. 26.2c. At concentrations above the cmc, surfactant micelles will be formed, with a central hydrophobic core into which the hydrophobic drug may dissolve (see Chapters 5 and 24). To avoid this, it is necessary to ensure that the surfactant concentration remains below the cmc. The addition of the surfactant to the surface of the particle will change the particulate charge, certainly in its magnitude but possibly also in its sign. The effects will be dependent on the chemistry of the surfactant itself, i.e. whether it is cationic, anionic or nonionic. Such charge modification will affect the fixed layer directly, rather than the diffuse layer, and a variation in the surface charge will naturally lead to an alteration of the Stern potential. As described earlier, this will then have a secondary effect on the zeta potential, as the charge decay across the diffuse layer will start from a different value. Ionic surfactants can also release ionic components into the medium (e.g. Na^+ ions from sodium lauryl sulfate), which will then have their own direct effects on the diffuse layer. The overall effect of addition of surfactants will need to be considered on a case-by-case basis, on the basis of their chemistry.

The Derjaguin–Landau–Verwey–Overbeek (DLVO) theory

Pharmaceutical suspensions are composed not of a single particle of drug suspended in a liquid medium but rather of multiple particles; this leads to multiple particulate interactions. These interactions can, to some extent, be thought of as the interactions of the diffuse layers around individual particles, and hence the electrical double layer provides the basis for understanding interparticulate interactions. The Derjaguin–Landau–Verwey–Overbeek (DLVO) theory describes these interactions.

The DLVO theory (Chapter 5 provides more detail) is concerned with predicting the stability of lyophobic ('solvent-hating') colloids and is relevant here because of the particle size of pharmaceutical suspensions. Essentially, it calculates the energies of attraction and repulsion between similar particles and predicts the overall energy of interaction. From this, deductions can be made as to the likely behaviour of the suspension, e.g. whether particles coalesce and settle, or remain evenly dispersed throughout the medium. This is arguably the most important question in pharmaceutical suspension formulation development, as a fundamental specification for such a formulation is dose reproducibility, which is most easily achieved with a system which remains well dispersed under all conditions.

To calculate the total energy of interaction, V_T, between two particles, the values of V_A and V_R are summed, as shown in Eq. 26.2:

$$V_T = V_A + V_R$$

(26.2)

V_R is the energy of electrical repulsion and by convention this carries a positive sign. V_A is the energy of van der Waals attractions and by convention is given a negative sign.

Fig. 26.3 shows the values of V_A, V_R and V_T for two similar particles suspended in a medium and interacting. Further detailed relationships involving V_A and V_R can be found in Chapter 5. It is important to note that the V_A and V_R curves shown in Fig. 26.3 are not mirror images of each other.

The easiest way to consider what happens when two particles interact is to remember that the V_T line gives the overall energy of interaction and that this will change depending on the distance between the two particles. There are three important zones, or values of V_T, in the DLVO diagram – the primary

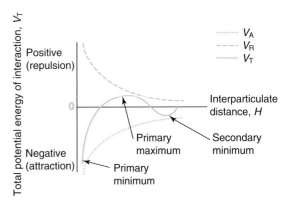

Fig. 26.3 • The energy of interaction between two similar particles, as described by the Derjaguin–Landau–Verwey–Overbeek theory.

minimum, the secondary minimum and the primary maximum – and the behaviour of the suspension will be dependent on which zone the particles are in. It must also be remembered that all particles will have some thermal energy and will show some movement, whether caused by Brownian motion, the effects of gravity or external agitation.

The primary minimum

The 'primary minimum' zone is described as a 'minimum' because the total energy is calculated to be below zero (remember that repulsive energy is described as positive and attractive energy as negative). It is described as 'primary' because it is the largest negative deviation from zero. Particles in the primary minimum zone show a higher energy of attraction than repulsion and are therefore likely to move closer together. Imagine two particles are just far enough apart that the energy of attraction balances out the energy of repulsion, so the overall energy of interaction is zero. Any movement of the particles which brings them closer together will result in an overall mathematical decrease in V_T, i.e. V_T is now attractive and the particles will continue to move closer together. As they do so, the strength of the overall attractive forces increases, moving the particles still closer together, resulting in a further increase in the attractive forces, and so on. The kinetic energy that the particles have (kT, where k is the Boltzmann constant and T the temperature in kelvins) is not high enough to overcome V_T, which at this point is overall attractive. Consequently the particles will eventually aggregate irreversibly. Particles will initially show 'flocculation', whereby the individual particles are loosely attracted to each other but still act

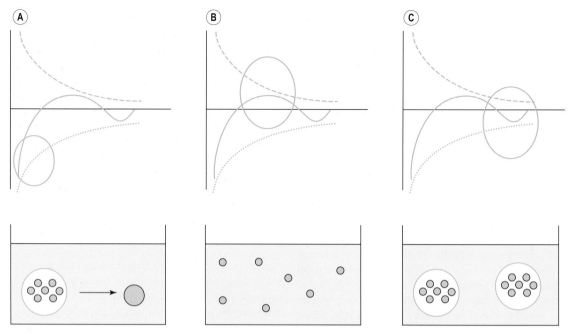

Fig. 26.4 • Flocculation and deflocculation consequences of the Derjaguin–Landau–Verwey–Overbeek theory for pharmaceutical suspensions The top panel of the diagrams indicates energy of interaction between two similar particles as a consequence of the DLVO theory. The ringed zones indicates particles in: **(a)** the primary minimum, **(b)** the primary maximum, **(c)** the secondary minimum. The lower panel shows the flocculation and deflocculation consequences at each zone.

independently; subsequently they will demonstrate 'coagulation', where particles will collide and form larger particles. Such behaviour is undesirable for pharmaceutical suspensions as it will have serious negative effects on the reproducibility of dosing from the system. These changes are illustrated in Fig. 26.4a.

The primary maximum

The naming of the 'primary maximum' zone follows the same conventions as for the primary minimum. The primary maximum zone is described as a 'maximum' because the total energy is calculated to be above zero (from the convention of repulsive energy being positive and attractive energy being negative). It is described as 'primary' because it is the largest positive deviation from zero. Particles in the primary maximum zone show a higher energy of repulsion than attraction and are therefore likely to remain separate or 'deflocculated'. This is illustrated in Fig. 26.4b. At first sight this would appear to be a good formulation strategy for pharmaceutical suspensions, as if the particles can be forced into the primary maximum zone, then they should remain independent and hence dosing would be expected to be reproducible. This is true when the kinetic energy

of the particles is less than V_T and they are, if anything, more likely to move away from each other, which will have the effect of decreasing the magnitude of V_T but maintaining an overall repulsive effect. However, if the kinetic energy of the particles is high enough (e.g. if the temperature is increased), then this can overcome the energy barrier imposed by V_T with the result that the particles can then move closer together. In this case, V_T will initially decrease but remain repulsive, so the particles will still exist as independent entities. However, the magnitude of the difference between V_T and the particles' kinetic energy is now greater and therefore they are likely to move even closer together. At some point the particles will be sufficiently close such that the overall energy of interaction becomes negative, i.e. it is now predominantly attractive, and the particles enter the primary minimum zone with the consequences described previously. In summary, therefore, formulating pharmaceutical suspensions so that the particles are in the primary maximum zone can be considered to be risky.

The secondary minimum

Fig. 26.4c shows the behaviour within the secondary minimum zone. As its name suggests, the 'secondary minimum' gives rise to an overall attractive energy of interaction between particles, but of a lower magnitude than that seen in the primary minimum. The particles here show an overall limited attraction to each other and behave as 'floccules', loose aggregates of individual particles. Depending on the kinetic energy of the particles, their behaviour will vary slightly. If the kinetic energy is less than V_T, then the particles will move closer together under the influence of V_T, but will not collide and coalesce as V_T is still relatively weak. As the particles move further together, the attractive forces will reach their highest point (although not as strong as in the primary minimum zone) then decrease and overall V_T becomes weakly repulsive, which will have the effect of forcing the particles apart. At this stage, V_T once again dominates over the kinetic energy and the particles will be attracted weakly to each other. In essence, the particles are maintained in their flocculated state (i.e. they still exist as individual particles but are loosely grouped together in floccules). If, however, the kinetic energy of the particles is greater than V_T, then the particles will be able to move further apart. As they do this, the overall V_T will become less attractive and ultimately will become, to all practical purposes, zero. In this case the particles will behave independently, will not flocculate and will not coalesce. In either case (kinetic energy greater than or less than V_T), coalescence and coagulation of particles are minimal, and hence this is usually the desired strategy for developing pharmaceutical suspensions.

Controlling particulate behaviour in suspensions

From the previous discussion, it can be seen that the behaviour of particles in suspension is complex, even when only two individual interacting particles are considered, the behaviour ultimately being dependent on the relative contribution of the repulsive and attractive energies at any separation distance. Examination of the equations that govern these two aspects (Eqns 5.24 and 5.25 respectively, repeated here for convenience) can give some clues as to which factors can be manipulated during suspension formulation to alter the behaviour of the particles and which factors cannot be altered:

$$V_R = 2\pi\varepsilon a\psi_0^2 \exp(-\kappa H)$$

(5.24)

$$V_A = -Aa/12H$$

(5.25)

A, the Hamaker constant (Eqn 5.25). This factor is constant for each combination of particle and medium. As the particulate material within a pharmaceutical suspension is the drug, the formulator has no opportunity to change the physicochemical nature of the particles. Although theoretically the medium may be altered, which will then change the Hamaker constant, most pharmaceutical suspensions, certainly those intended for oral drug delivery, are aqueous. Hence the two components in the suspension which contribute to the Hamaker constant (the drug and water) are fixed, and this factor is, in effect, not modifiable.

ε, the permittivity of the medium (Eqn 5.24). The permittivity of the medium is related to its polarity, so therefore varying the medium will have a direct effect on the repulsive energy between particles in the system. Water is the most common medium for pharmaceutical suspensions, and addition of dissolved solids, such as electrolytes, to water will have a relatively minor effect on its permittivity, compared with the effect of changing the medium from water to, for example, oil. Overall, therefore, for the purposes of pharmaceutical suspensions, the permittivity can be considered to be that of water and will have limited variability.

H, the distance between particles (Eqns 5.24 and 5.25). The distance between particles can be considered to be both a cause and an effect of the balance between the attractive and repulsive energies of the system, as discussed in the previous section: particles very far apart will have very limited interaction and particles close to each other will be attracted or repelled depending on exactly how far apart they are, and may move in response to the dominant V_T. Interparticulate distance is difficult to control directly. It will be partly dependent on the mobility of the particles, i.e. their kinetic energy, which itself is dependent on the ambient temperature. The range of temperatures to which a pharmaceutical product is exposed is quite small, from fridge temperature (~5 °C) to 40 °C during product testing, so reducing the temperature to reduce mobility is not really a viable option. The interparticulate distance is also dependent on the concentration of particles within the system, a higher concentration making it more likely that the particles will be physically located close to each other.

ψ_o, the surface potential (Eqn 5.24). The physicochemical nature of the particles is fixed, as the formulator must work with the drug that is required; therefore the fundamental surface potential of the particles in an aqueous medium will also be fixed. However, it is easy to modify the surface potential of the particles by causing materials to adsorb at their surface, such materials most commonly being surfactants below their cmc.

κ, the Debye–Hückel reciprocal length parameter (Eqn 5.24). The Debye–Hückel reciprocal length parameter is related to the distance over which the charge on the particle is reduced. It is dependent on the ionic strength of medium and can therefore be controlled easily by the addition of ionizable materials, such as sodium chloride.

a, the radius of the particle (Eqns 5.24 and 5.25). The radius of the particle (assuming sphericity) appears in both equations and so will affect both the attractive energy and the repulsive energy. It can be relatively easily controlled by the milling or micronization of larger particles to achieve a desired small particle size, or by crystal engineering techniques, intended to produce small particles directly from a solution. Assuming all other parameters in the two equations remain constant, variation in the particle size will have the same magnitude of effect on both V_A and V_R, and thereby V_T. For example, doubling the particle size will double all three calculated values, and halving the particle size will halve them. In all cases, the sign of the V_T, i.e. whether overall repulsive or attractive, will remain constant. Changing the particle size will have an effect, therefore, on the magnitudes of both the primary minimum and the primary maximum and, depending on the relative extent of the kinetic energy compared with V_T and the interparticulate distance, may lead to increased or lowered stability, following the arguments already presented.

Effects of additives

As indicated in the previous section, the addition of ionic or surfactant materials to a suspension formulation is likely to have an effect on the particulate behaviour, by changing the relative values of V_A and V_R. The effects can be rationalized by our considering the electrical double layer on individual particles and how this affects the interaction between particles. Addition of low to medium concentrations of ionizable materials will result in higher concentrations of the positively charged ion in the diffuse layer surrounding a particle (remember that the particle will carry a negative charge in the absence of any absorbed material on its surface), which will allow charge neutralization to occur over a shorter range, i.e. the diffuse layer becomes thinner.

The practical significance of this is that the secondary minimum will be deeper, i.e. it will have a larger magnitude. This in turn means that the energy barrier to escaping the secondary minimum is now higher and the particles will require a larger kinetic energy to do so. Hence more particles will be kept within this separation range. As described previously, the secondary minimum is generally considered to be desirable for pharmaceutical suspensions, as the particles will remain as loose floccules rather than becoming aggregated, and so it follows that addition of low to medium concentrations of ionic materials will be beneficial for pharmaceutical suspension formulations. However, the height of the energy barrier at the primary minimum will also be decreased, so if the particles have a high enough kinetic energy (e.g. from exposure to high temperatures or caused by vigorous shaking), then they could overcome this repulsive force and move closer together, finally entering the primary minimum and coalescing.

If the concentration of the ionic material is sufficiently high, then some of the counterion charges will penetrate to the particle surface and reduce the overall surface charge ψ_o and hence the Stern potential, ψ_δ, i.e. the charge at the edge of the fixed layer. Taken together with a high concentration of the added counterion charges in the diffuse layer, which will reduce the Debye–Hückel length, $1/\kappa$, very quickly, this will have the effect of reducing V_T to such an extent that V_A will dominate in the V_T calculation at all separation distances. Hence, the particles remain attracted to each other at all length scales and are more likely to aggregate and coalesce.

Adding surfactants to the suspension formulation at a level below their cmc will result in their adsorption on the particle surface. This will alter the surface charge (ψ_o), thereby changing the value of V_R, with a consequent effect on V_T. However, the size and magnitude of this effect will be dependent on the chemical characteristics of the surfactant and addition of surfactant may result in an increased or decreased chance of flocculation.

Particle movement in suspensions

There will always be some particle motion in a suspension formulation: very small particles will exhibit Brownian motion (Chapter 5), gravity will cause the particles to sediment and the suspension may be shaken by the patient or during transportation. This motion can therefore affect the interparticulate distance and by consequence the values of V_A, V_T and V_R, potentially affecting the flocculation status of the suspension. When considering the effects of movement, one must remember that deflocculated systems behave as individual small particles, whilst flocculated systems behave as individual large particles with a porous structure. Flocculated and deflocculated systems will show different particulate behaviour as a result.

Diffusion

Brownian motion (see Chapter 5) is the irregular movement of particles through the medium and is shown by particles with radius below approximately 1 µm to 2 µm. The result of Brownian motion is diffusion of the particles throughout the medium, from an area of high concentration to one of low concentration. Diffusion (see Chapter 3) will therefore result in an improved, more homogeneous distribution of the particles throughout the system. It can be described by the Stokes–Einstein diffusion equation (Eqn 3.30). From Eq. 3.30, it can be seen that reducing the particle size will increase the diffusion constant and, conversely, increasing the particle size will reduce it. There is an effective size range above which diffusion will be negligible, and for particles of radius greater than approximately 1 µm to 2 µm, diffusion can be ignored. As pharmaceutical suspensions may contain particles in the sub-micrometre range, diffusion may be an important contributor to particle movement. However, it is most likely to be observed with deflocculated systems, as these behave as independent particles, and less likely to be seen with flocculated systems. The latter behave as larger particles because of their agglomerated status, and they are therefore likely to be of a size above the effective cut-off for diffusional movement. Diffusion can be reduced by an increase in the viscosity of the medium, with a value of 5 mPa s effectively reducing diffusion to zero. For comparison, water at 20 °C has a viscosity of 1 mPa s, and a 2% w/v solution of low molecular weight hydroxypropyl methylcellulose has a viscosity of 5 mPa s at 20 °C.

Sedimentation

Sedimentation (also discussed in Chapters 5 and 6) is the downward movement of particles under gravity,

and is observed for particles with radii of approximately 0.5 µm or greater. The vast majority of pharmaceutical suspensions will contain particles in this size range, so sedimentation is a significant cause of particle motion. Sedimentation is described by Stokes's sedimentation equation (Eqn. 26.3), with the sedimentation velocity, v, predicting the speed of settling expected under particular conditions; higher values of v suggest greater likelihood of sedimentation. Here, the Stokes equation has been given in two equivalent forms, defined by the particle radius and diameter:

$$v = \frac{2a^2 g(\rho - \rho_\circ)}{9\eta} = \frac{d^2 g(\rho - \rho_\circ)}{18\eta}$$

$$(26.3)$$

where v is the sedimentation velocity, a and d are the particle radius and diameter respectively (the particle is assumed to be spherical), g is the acceleration due to gravity, ρ and $\rho_\circ$ are the densities of the particles and the medium respectively, and η is the viscosity of the medium.

In the context of suspension formulation, Eq. 26.3 shows that reducing the particle size will reduce the sedimentation rate, and conversely increasing the particle size will result in increased settling. Both flocculated and deflocculated systems will show sedimentation. Because of their relative sizes, flocculated systems will settle quickly, whereas deflocculated systems will settle more slowly. Increasing the viscosity of the medium will reduce sedimentation, as will reducing the difference in density between the medium and the particle.

Controlling particulate movement in suspensions

Diffusion and sedimentation of particles within the suspension formulation will have opposite, but not equal, effects, sedimentation leading to increased proximity of particles and diffusion leading to greater dispersion of particles within the system. Particulate movement is almost inevitable in a liquid suspension system, with the overall result of a variation in the separation distance between particles, which has a direct consequence for the energies of interaction between particles and hence their flocculation behaviour. Increasing the separation distance will initially move particles away from the primary maximum zone into the secondary minimum zone, changing the nature of the system from a deflocculated one to a flocculated one. Further outward movement will take the particles out of the secondary minimum zone and into an area of very little interaction, again changing the nature of the suspension, this time from a flocculated system to an effectively deflocculated system. Decreasing the separation distance between particles will initially move them from the secondary minimum zone, showing flocculated behaviour, to the primary maximum zone, showing deflocculated behaviour. Further inward movement will result in the particles entering the primary minimum zone, leading to irreversible coagulation. It must be remembered that gravity works only in one direction (downwards) and that the base of the container is immobile, so ultimately the first settling particle or floccule will reach a point at which its travel stops and it rests on the inside bottom surface of the container. The second and subsequent sedimenting particles or floccules, will then approach the first, fixed one from above. The combination of gravitational force on the sedimenting particles or floccules and mechanical forces exerted by the mass of the sedimenting particles or floccules on those below will overcome V_R, moving the particles into the primary minimum zone and resulting in irreversible coagulation.

Controlling the movement of particles within the suspension formulation is extremely important to maintain the desired flocculation status. Examination of Eqs 3.30 and 26.3, for diffusion and sedimentation respectively, will allow assessment of which factors can be manipulated and the likely results of such manipulation.

a, the radius of the particle. Manipulation of particle size is relatively easily accomplished mechanically or via manipulation of crystallization techniques. Reducing the particle size will increase diffusion and reduce sedimentation, with a larger effect on the sedimentation rate. Particle size reduction would generally be regarded as beneficial because of these effects. However, particle size is a key parameter governing particulate interactions as described by the DLVO theory and so manipulation of particle size will have a direct effect on V_T and flocculation behaviour. Particle size will also have an effect on the dissolution behaviour of the drug, which is discussed later.

ρ, the density of the particle. Particles are generally denser than the medium in which they are dispersed, and the greater the density difference, the faster the sedimentation rate. Reducing the particle density by changing crystallization methods is possible, but this will result in an increased particle size (if the total number of particles remains constant) or an increased number of particles (if the particle size remains constant), both of these leading to a change in the DLVO characteristics and flocculation behaviour of the system. So, although manipulation of the density of the particles seems an easy way of reducing the sedimentation rate, it has potential serious disadvantages. Diffusion is unaffected by particulate density.

ρ₀, the density of the medium. Reducing the density difference between the particles and the suspending medium will lead to a reduction in the sedimentation rate, which is beneficial for pharmaceutical suspensions. We can most easily achieve this by increasing the density of the medium. Although most pharmaceutical suspensions are based on water, addition of materials such as dextrose or some polymers will raise the density of the product sufficiently to reduce the observed sedimentation. It is best if these materials are nonionic, as ionic materials will lead to a change in the flocculation behaviour of the particles, via movement of the counterion into the diffuse layers surrounding the particles.

η, the viscosity of the medium. Raising the viscosity of the suspending medium will reduce diffusion of the particles, with a value of 5 mPa s effectively decreasing the diffusion to zero. An increased viscosity will also reduce the particulate sedimentation rate. Overall, an increased viscosity is beneficial for pharmaceutical suspensions. The viscosity of water is very low (1 mPa s at 20 °C) but it can be easily modified via additives such as polymers, for example hydroxypropyl methylcellulose or sodium carboxymethylcellulose. In the latter case, however, effects on the electrical double layer around the particles and hence flocculation behaviour are likely to be seen because of the mobile Na^+ ion.

T, temperature (in kelvins). Increasing the temperature will lead to an increase in the diffusion constant and hence greater particle mobility. Although not expressed explicitly in Eq. 26.3, the viscosity of a given substance will change with temperature, affecting both diffusion and sedimentation. In reality, however, the range of temperatures to which a suspension is exposed (or should be exposed) is limited but uncontrolled outside the place of manufacture, and temperature should not be used as a tool with which to control particulate behaviour. Repeated cyclical variations in temperature will lead to Ostwald ripening, a deleterious effect, which will be discussed later.

Measuring particle movement

It is not straightforward to measure diffusion in a suspension formulation, but bulk sedimentation is very easy to observe. A known volume of the suspension with the solid particles dispersed as optimally as possible is placed in a graduated cylinder and left to stand, allowing sedimentation to occur. At certain time intervals, the volume of sediment is measured and the sedimentation volume ratio, F, calculated, as shown in Eq. 26.4 (F is in the range of 0 to 1):

$$F = \frac{V_f}{V_o}$$

(26.4)

where F is the sedimentation volume, V_o is the initial volume of suspension before settling and V_f is the final volume of sediment. Fig. 26.5 illustrates this diagrammatically. The speed and extent of sedimentation can be observed visually and used to assess the behaviour of the formulation.

The sedimentation patterns of flocculated and deflocculated systems are different. In a flocculated system, the particles are arranged in loose aggregates or floccules, which behave as large, porous individual particles. These floccules will begin to sediment quickly, generally within a few minutes, leaving a clear supernatant, and sedimentation will reach a maximum within a few hours or days. The sediment formed is loose and fluffy and can be easily redispersed by shaking, as both the individual floccule and the bulk sediment formed have the solvent medium incorporated into it. A high volume of sediment is observed, with calculated values of the sedimentation volume ratio, F, being up to 0.6. Fig. 26.6 illustrates this, showing the initial condition, an 'intermediate' condition after a short period and the 'final' condition after a prolonged period.

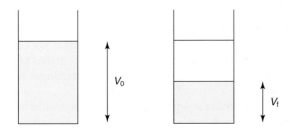

Fig. 26.5 • Calculation of the sedimentation volume ratio for a suspension. *Blue* indicates a suspension, *no colour* indicates an optically clear medium.

Deflocculated systems show a different pattern of sedimentation. As the particles behave independently, they will sediment slowly, reflecting their small size. Sedimentation takes some time, measured in days and weeks rather than minutes. In the initial stages of sedimentation, a small amount of compact sediment is observed at the base of the cylinder, with no, or limited, clear supernatant being observed. Subsequently, the volume of sediment and the volume of clear supernatant both increase. The sediment formed is dense and compacted, described as being 'caked'. Redispersion of the caked sediment is difficult, as little, if any, of the solvent medium can penetrate into it. A low final volume of sediment is observed, with calculated values of the sedimentation volume ratio, F, being as low as 0.1. Fig. 26.7 illustrates this, showing the initial condition, an 'intermediate' condition after a short period (although longer than for flocculated systems) and the 'final' condition after a prolonged period.

What is the desired sedimentation pattern?

The question then arises as to what sedimentation pattern is best for a pharmaceutical suspension. Two factors need to be considered: speed of sedimentation and reversibility. A slow sedimentation rate would be optimal, suggesting that a deflocculated system is more desirable; however, reversibility is key to ensuring that dosing from the suspension is reproducible, and so a flocculated system would be better in this respect. Overall, as in many formulation challenges, a balance between opposing factors must be struck. Formulators may choose to develop a deflocculated system with no or minimal sedimentation, which will require greater viscosity and density adjustments to maintain the initial dispersion of particles. If the suspension is too viscous, then it may be difficult to pour it from the container or to judge a dose accurately. A greater potential problem, though, is that, should changes to the particulate dispersion pattern occur, for example as a result of prolonged exposure to high temperatures, the particles may enter the primary minimum zone and irreversibly coagulate, resulting in catastrophic failure of the product. Alternatively, formulators may choose to develop a flocculated system with controlled slow sedimentation. This will require fewer viscosity and density adjustments than for a deflocculated system and will allow easy redispersion of particles on shaking. However, patients and health

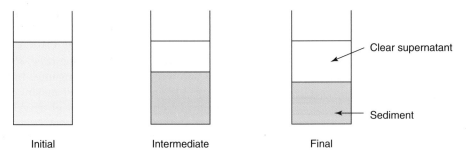

Fig. 26.6 • The sedimentation behaviour of a flocculated suspension. *Pale blue* indicates the initial suspension, *dark blue* indicates the resulting sediment and *no colour* indicates an optically clear medium.

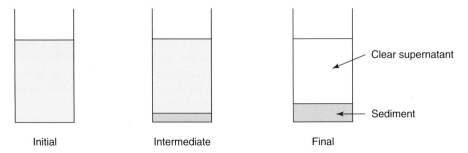

Fig. 26.7 • The sedimentation behaviour of a deflocculated suspension. *Pale blue* indicates the initial suspension, *dark blue* indicates the resulting sediment and *no colour* indicates an optically clear medium.

care providers will need to be educated as to the vital importance of shaking the product before dispensing a dose, and some people may find the separated product unexpected or unsightly.

Dispersibility issues – surface wetting

This chapter has focused on the interactions of particles with the suspending medium, but with an implicit assumption that there is a suitable initial dispersion of the particles in the medium. It is vital that this initial dispersion is homogeneous at the single-particle level to ensure that reproducible dosing is possible. However, pharmaceutical suspensions, by their very nature, involve the interaction of a nondissolving hydrophobic solid with water, and a homogeneous individual particulate dispersion is not, in most cases, simple to produce. A measurable surface tension will exist at the interface between the water and the solid, and the solid will not be easily wetted by the water (discussed in Chapter 4). To reduce this surface tension and obtain a more energetically favourable situation, the solid particles are likely to clump together. In this way the total particulate surface area in contact with the water is reduced; hence the total surface tension is reduced. The natural consequence is that the product is nonhomogeneous and inelegant, and reproducible dosing is not possible. A reduction in the surface tension between the particles and water is usually necessary to increase the contact between the solvent and solid, which will then promote even movement of the solvent across the particle surface and good dispersion of the particles throughout the medium. This is usually produced by the addition of a surfactant, below its cmc, to the medium.

Whether or not a given solid is likely to present dispersion problems can be assessed by examination of the contact angle made between the solid and a liquid when both are exposed to air. A compact of the solid is made and a drop of the liquid placed on its surface. The angle that the drop makes on the surface is then measured, as described in Chapter 4.

Generally, contact angle measurement should be used as a guide only, with values less than 90° indicating reasonable wetting would be expected and values greater than 90° suggesting that problems are likely to be observed during dispersion. Overinterpretation of very similar values of the contact angle should be avoided. Wettability can be increased by the use of a surfactant below its cmc, comparison of the contact angles in the presence and absence of the surfactant aiding the assessment of its effectiveness.

Dissolution issues

Drugs are formulated as suspensions for oral delivery because they show limited aqueous solubility related to their target dose, and hence an aqueous solution formulation is not feasible. However, for the drug to be absorbed orally, it must be dissolved within the gastrointestinal tract and so dissolution behaviour must be considered. The Noyes–Whitney equation (Eqn 2.3) governs the rate of dissolution of solid materials into a liquid medium. The Noyes–Whitney equation, dissolution and solubility are discussed in greater detail in Chapter 2.

It is clear from the Noyes–Whitney equation that increasing the surface area, whilst keeping the total quantity of drug the same, will increase the dissolution rate of the drug. This in turn is likely to promote oral bioavailability, as typically poorly water-soluble drugs show dissolution-rate-limited absorption. Surface area is related to particle size by

$$A = 4\pi a^2 = \pi d^2$$

(26.5)

where A is the surface area of the particles, and a and d are the particle radius and diameter respectively.

Reducing the particle size of the drug will therefore result in increased dissolution once a pharmaceutical suspension is taken orally by the patient. However, there are a number of cautions to be borne in mind at this point. Changing the particle size will affect the interparticulate interactions, as discussed earlier, and may alter the flocculation behaviour of suspensions. As the bioavailability is likely to be dependent on particle size, close control of the particle size and particle size distribution is required to maintain batch-to-batch uniformity and promote a consistent therapeutic response after ingestion.

Ostwald ripening

Even though the vast majority of the drug will be in the particulate state in a pharmaceutical suspension, there will always be a small amount in solution, dependent on its solubility. The equilibrium solubility of a solid in a liquid will change with temperature: raising the temperature will lead to an increase in the solubility, with a lowering of temperature resulting in a decrease in solubility. An unfortunate result of this temperature effect is *Ostwald ripening*, whereby small particles in suspension seem to disappear and large particles seem to grow after repeated temperature changes in both directions. This can be explained as follows. There will always be a range of particle sizes in the suspension, although this range should be as narrow as possible to maintain consistency, and the product will ideally be formulated to be stored at room temperature (approximately 25 °C). If the suspension is exposed to a higher temperature, e.g. by it being placed in direct sunlight or during transportation, then the equilibrium solubility of the drug in the dispersing medium will increase. Dissolution proceeds from the surface of the particles, so even though the instantaneous removal of an individual drug molecule from a small particle into solution will be the same as that from a large particle, there are fewer molecules on the surface of a small particle and hence the particle surface of a smaller particle appears to recede more quickly than that of a larger particle. The net result is that all particles are slightly smaller and there is more drug in solution. If the suspension is then placed in lower-temperature conditions, e.g. by storage in a refrigerator with a temperature of approximately 5 °C (usual range 2 °C to 8 °C), the equilibrium solubility of the drug will decrease to below the concentration now in solution (i.e. immediately after exposure to the higher temperatures) and the system is now supersaturated, which is energetically unfavoured. Some of the 'excess' drug will now precipitate out and will do so preferentially onto the larger particles, with their greater surface area, analogous to crystallization by seeding. At equilibrium of this stage, the smaller particles may have grown slightly but the larger particles will have grown more. Overall, therefore, after one hot and cold cycle, the particle size distribution has changed in that the smaller particles are smaller and the larger particles are larger. Repeated temperature cycling aggravates this situation, with the result that the smaller particles dissolve completely and larger particles grow, the whole process being known as *Ostwald ripening*. This is summarized in Fig. 26.8. A corresponding phenomenon occurs with droplets in emulsions (see Chapter 27).

Ostwald ripening is a problem for pharmaceutical suspensions, as the particle size and particle size

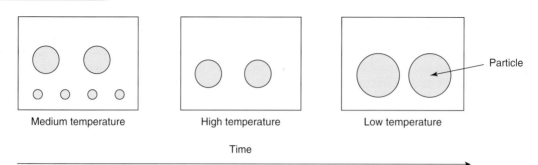

Fig. 26.8 • Ostwald ripening in suspensions.

distribution will change as a result. Consequent effects on the DLVO behaviour of the particles will alter the flocculation profile of the suspension and hence the sedimentation behaviour. The dissolution profile following oral administration will also change, leading to potential bioavailability issues and variability in clinical effect. As the temperature cycling is likely to happen outside the manufacturer's control (e.g. in the patient's home), it is difficult to control, and variable effects between batches or between containers from the same batch are to be expected. The formulator needs to be aware of this, and one relatively easy way of minimizing this is to ensure that the solubility profile of the drug in water is 'flat', i.e. over the temperature range that the product is likely to experience, the solubility changes only marginally.

General suspension formulation 1considerations

Pharmaceutically, suspensions are used in a wide range of applications, although oral dosing is the most common. The different routes of administration will present their own specific challenges. For example, a suspension prepared for nebulized inhalation therapy would need to be sterile, as would a suspension intended for ocular delivery. In both these cases, sterilization by filtration would be unsuitable, as the suspended particles would generally be too large to pass through the 0.22 μm filters commonly used for microbial sterilization. Similarly, autoclaving is unlikely to be suitable, as the high temperatures involved would affect the solubility of the drug and the physical structure of the suspension. Hence aseptic preparation would have to be used to manufacture sterile suspensions. In oral dosing, organoleptic considerations apply, necessitating the use of colours and flavours, which

are not relevant to the formulation of suspensions intended for topical application.

Solubility

The choice of developing a solution or a suspension formulation is ultimately made on the basis of the aqueous solubility of the drug. The dose of the drug required will be decided by the clinical profile of the drug and therefore cannot be varied. Similarly, the dosing volume is largely fixed: an oral product would have a dosing volume of 5 mL and an eye-drop formulation a dosing volume of 10 μL. Once the equilibrium solubility of the drug in water is known, a simple calculation will establish whether a solution is likely to be possible or not. However, the situation is slightly more complex. A drug in a solution formulation must be monomolecularly dispersed in the vehicle at manufacture, and remain so throughout the shelf life of the product. A solution formulation, therefore, should not be produced near its solubility limit, as variations downwards in temperature, e.g. by refrigerated storage, will decrease the equilibrium solubility and potentially lead to precipitation. A general recommendation for solution formulations is to use the equilibrium solubility at 5 °C for solubility calculations and apply a safety factor, so that the maximum concentration of the formulation is significantly less than the equilibrium solubility and the chances of precipitation are minimized.

If the solubility calculations indicate that a suspension formulation is required, then the solubility profile of the drug as a function of temperature needs to be established. A fundamental requirement for suspension formulations is that the drug is suspended in the medium initially and remains so throughout its shelf life. However, as discussed in previous sections, the drug needs to remain in the same dispersion state, i.e. degree of flocculation, throughout the shelf life of the product, not merely remain in suspension. Ostwald ripening must be avoided because of its potential deleterious consequences for product stability and clinical effect. An ideal solubility profile is flat (i.e. there is minimal change in the equilibrium solubility of the drug with temperature). Usually, the lower the aqueous solubility, the greater the chance of a flat profile being obtained. If the drug has some aqueous solubility, but not sufficient for a straightforward solution to be developed, then the solubility of the drug may need to be suppressed, so as to maintain the suspended nature of the drug. Solubility suppression may be achieved by the addition of an antisolvent. Antisolvents act in the opposite manner to cosolvents in that they reduce the aqueous solubility of the drug rather than enhance it, but they may be chemically the same as cosolvents (e.g. ethanol or polyethylene glycol). Variation of the pH of the medium may be appropriate if the drug is ionizable. Generally, pH manipulation is used to increase the solubility of drugs by causing the ionic species to form and allowing greater interaction with water, but the opposite intention can be used to find the pH of minimum solubility and use that for suspension formulation, assuming of course that the pH is acceptable for the intended route of administration. A weak acid will show low solubility in low-pH conditions, whereas a weak base will show low solubility in high-pH conditions. A prodrug such as an ester is also likely to show lower aqueous solubility than its counterpart 'real' drug, so is a potential formulation option. However, changes in the chemical structure of the drug will necessitate further expensive safety studies on the prodrug as well as the actual drug.

Formulation excipients

A range of formulation excipients may need to be added to the suspension formulation. In each case the potential effect of the excipient on the DLVO interaction of drug particles needs to be quantified and the formulation amended as necessary.

Flavours, sweeteners and colours

Products intended for oral dosing to children will generally require a colourant, sweetener and flavour to make them palatable (see Chapter 45). Although the intensity of the taste of a drug molecule will be less in a suspension formulation than in a solution formulation, it still needs to be considered. The topic of taste masking is outside the scope of this chapter, but as a general rule, children prefer sweet and fruity tastes, although bitter tastes (most drugs are bitter) are best masked by another bitter taste such as grapefruit. The effects of flavours and colours on the physical behaviour of the suspension are likely to be limited, because of the low concentrations used, especially for colours. Traditionally, sugar (sucrose) has been used to sweeten oral formulations, but the use of sugar is now severely restricted because of concerns over dental caries and potential interference with diabetic glucose control. Several sweeteners are available, all of which are much sweeter than sugar, and hence are used in much lower concentrations. All of the common sweeteners are ionizable: saccharin is commonly used as the sodium salt and acesulfame is provided as the potassium salt; hence the effect of the mobile ions on the electrical double layer needs to be considered. Another consideration applies to aspartame: its degradation products include phenylalanine, so it should not be ingested by patients with phenylketonuria, and hence it may be reasonable to avoid its use, depending on the patient population to be treated.

Antimicrobial preservatives

Any time water is present in a multidose or nonsterile suspension formulation, an antimicrobial preservative is required to prevent microbial contamination. A range of potential preservatives are available, including sorbic acid, benzoic acid, parabens, sucrose and benzalkonium chloride (see Chapter 48). Sucrose has a preservative action at concentrations greater than or equal to 67% w/v. It is unlikely to be used in commercial products because of its cariogenic potential but may be encountered in extemporaneous products, albeit more likely in solution formulations. Sucrose will not interfere with the DLVO behaviour of the system as it does not ionize, so will not be localized in the diffuse layer, and will not adsorb onto the particle surface. It will, however, affect the density and viscosity of the system, and so will have an effect on the sedimentation profile of the suspension. Benzalkonium chloride is typically used in aqueous eye-drop formulations at concentrations of approximately 0.01% w/w (approximately 0.3 mM). It is a cationic surfactant and will dissociate in aqueous solutions to produce Cl^- ions and a long-chain ionized surfactant moiety. Hence it is likely to affect both the surface potential of the solid drug by deposition of the benzalkonium part of the molecule and the diffuse layer surrounding the solid particle by production of mobile Cl⁻ anions. Benzalkonium chloride is not a 'pure' product, in that a range of molecules with differing hydrocarbon chain lengths will exist in each batch of 'benzalkonium chloride' (see Fig. 15.5), and thus interbatch variation in its effect on the flocculation behaviour of the suspension may be expected. Sorbic acid and benzoic acid are both weak acids used in oral formulations at approximately 0.2% w/v (approximately 15 mM). They are most effective as preservatives in the un-ionized state, in which state they will not interfere with the flocculation behaviour of the drug. However, they both show mid-range pK_a values (4.8 for sorbic acid and 4.2 for benzoic acid), so will be partially ionized in the pH conditions likely to be encountered in oral formulations. Some effect of charged moieties arising from this ionization is likely to be seen in the diffuse layer, and hence this will directly affect the flocculation behaviour of the suspension. Sorbic acid is commonly used as the potassium salt and benzoic acid is commonly used as the sodium salt. In this case, dissolution of the salt form into the aqueous vehicle will release the K^+ or Na^+ ions, which will directly affect the diffuse layer and hence flocculation. The parabens are a family of molecules based on p-hydroxybenzoic acid, with alkyl group esterification at the acid group. These are commonly used at a preservative concentration of approximately 0.2% w/v (approximately 10 mM). Parabens will not ionize at the pH conditions to be expected in a pharmaceutical product, so they are unlikely to interfere with the flocculation behaviour of the particles.

Buffers

A buffer is defined as a mixture of a weak acid or base and one of its salts and is designed to maintain the pH of an aqueous system within very narrow limits. Buffers may be used in suspension formulations if a particular pH is required because of the route of administration, or if the solubility of the drug is suppressed by it being formulated at a particular pH, as discussed earlier. Because of its ionic nature, a buffer system will contribute charges to the formulation, which will affect the flocculation behaviour of the suspension by virtue of their being associated with the diffuse layer surrounding the particle. The use of a buffer may also affect the ionization state of other components, such as preservatives, with subsequent effects on their efficacy and the concentration required.

Chemical stabilizers

A range of chemical stabilizers may be used to increase the chemical stability of the drug. These include antioxidants, such as ascorbic acid, used at concentrations of approximately 0.2% w/v (approximately 10 mM), and sodium metabisulfite, used at levels of approximately 0.1% w/v (approximately 5 mM), and chelators such as ethylenediaminetetraacetic acid (EDTA), commonly used as the disodium salt. As discussed earlier, if the additive ionizes to any appreciable extent, then it will potentially affect the stability of the product by interfering with the diffuse layer.

Density and viscosity modifiers/suspending agents

Increasing the density of the suspension formulation may help to reduce the sedimentation rate of the dispersed particles. This may be achieved by the addition of a sugar such as dextrose or sucrose, which would not be expected to change the flocculation behaviour other than by retarding sedimentation. Sugars in low concentration provide an energy source for microbial contamination (at much higher concentrations, sugar solutions are hypertonic, leading to lysis of bacterial cells, and so are self-preserving), so adequate antimicrobial preservation would be required. Additionally, most medicines are formulated, if at all possible, as sugar-free products, so this would not necessarily be a recommended formulation strategy.

Viscosity modifiers are also known as *suspending agents* as they will reduce the sedimentation of the particles and keep them suspended for longer. The viscosity of the system can be easily adjusted by the addition of polymeric materials or inorganic materials such as clays. The target viscosity for each preparation needs to be defined so as to maintain the particles in their suspended state for as long as possible, i.e. to retard sedimentation. However, this must be balanced against the ease of use of the product; whilst a very viscous suspension will show little, if any, sedimentation, it is unlikely to be patient-friendly. The product must be pourable from a bottle onto a spoon for oral use or dispensable through a nozzle if it is intended for ocular or nasal use.

Cellulosic materials are commonly used as viscosity enhancers in suspension formulations. Cellulose itself is a linear polymer of D-glucose, with individual glucose units being linked via β(1→4) glycosidic bonds; the number of repeating units may run into the thousands. Cellulose ethers are more often used, and these are obtained from native cellulose by chemical treatment with an appropriate reagent, replacing the hydrogen on the hydroxyl group of the glucose residue with an appropriate alkyl, hydroxyalkyl or carboxyalkyl group. There are three hydroxyl groups on each glucose residue in the cellulose chain, and the extent of conversion is measured by the degree of substitution. This can take values of anything up to 3, with noninteger numbers (e.g. 1.5) reflecting the fact that there will be an element of inhomogeneity along the cellulose backbone after reaction. Methyl ($-CH_3$) group substitution gives methylcellulose, which is water soluble, but ethyl ($-CH_2CH_3$) group substitution produces ethylcellulose, which is water insoluble. Substitution with a 2-hydroxypropyl ($-CH_2CH(OH)CH_3$) group produces hydroxypropyl cellulose, and mixed substitution of methyl and 2-hydroxypropyl groups results in hydroxypropyl methylcellulose. Carboxymethylcellulose is prepared from cellulose by the addition of carboxymethyl groups ($-CH_2COOH$) to the glucose residues. It is often used as its sodium salt, denoted sodium carboxymethylcellulose. All five cellulosic polymers mentioned (methylcellulose, hydroxypropyl cellulose, hydroxypropyl methylcellulose, carboxymethylcellulose and sodium carboxymethylcellulose) are water soluble and are available in a range of molecular weights and degrees of substitution, which leads to a range of solution viscosities being easily obtainable by manipulation of the chemical properties and concentrations of the polymers used. Generally speaking, the polymers will not interfere with the flocculation behaviour of the particles. However, the ionic nature of sodium carboxymethylcellulose will directly lead to the production of Na^+ ions in solution, which will migrate into the diffuse layer around the particles and affect their flocculation behaviour, so care should be taken with this excipient.

Alginic acid, a polymer derived from seaweed, can also be used to enhance the viscosity of the medium and reduce sedimentation. It comprises residues of β-d-mannuronic acid and α-l-guluronic acid joined via a (1→4) link; macroscopically, the polymer consists of linear blocks of one or other of the two individual components, with a third type of block showing an alternating structure of the two residue types. This structural variety is a consequence of its natural origin, different sources producing alginic acid with different blocking arrangements, and gives rise to differing properties in solution. Alginic acid is easily ionized and is commonly used as the sodium

salt, so in this case it will have a direct effect on flocculation behaviour. In the presence of divalent cations, such as calcium (Ca^{2+}), alginic acid will behave as a chelator, with one Ca^{2+} ion being bound to two ionized acid residues ($-COOH$), giving rise to an 'egg box' structure for the polymer and an increase in viscosity in the solution. In terms of suspension formulation, therefore, addition of alginic acid, either as the intact acid or as the sodium salt, will extract Ca^{2+} ions from the surroundings if they are present in the formulation. The effects of this will be both to change the flocculation behaviour of the particles and to increase the viscosity of the system.

Traditionally, clays and gums were used to thicken suspensions and to retard sedimentation. Clays are water-insoluble inorganic materials that, when dispersed in water, will absorb water into their structure rather than dissolve. A clay suspension shows some rheological structuring and will retard the sedimentation of other materials suspended with it, such as the drug in pharmaceutical suspensions. Ultimately, the clay will itself sediment as it is in suspension rather than in solution, as are the polymers already discussed. An example of a clay is bentonite, used in the *British Pharmacopoeia* (BP) formula for Calamine Lotion BP. Gum arabic is derived from the sap of *Acacia* trees and chemically is composed of a complex mixture of saccharides and glycoproteins. Once dissolved in water, gum arabic forms a reasonably viscous solution which can be used to retard sedimentation of suspended materials. Depending on the source, for example precisely which species of *Acacia*, the chemical composition will be different and hence the suspending capabilities will be variable. Tragacanth, sometimes known as gum tragacanth, is another complex polysaccharide mixture, derived from the sap of plants of the genus *Astragalus*. As with gum arabic, it is used to increase the viscosity of the suspending medium and to retard sedimentation of the drug particles. Clays and gums are natural materials and are subject to much greater batch-to-batch variation than synthetic or semisynthetic materials, and so have fallen out of favour as pharmaceutical excipients, where close control and predictability of physical and/or chemical behaviour is a prerequisite.

Wetting agents

Wetting agents are used to improve the flow of the liquid vehicle across the particle surface, which in turn increases the homogeneity of distribution of the drug particles throughout the formulation. They do this by reducing the interfacial tension between the solid particle and the liquid medium, as discussed earlier. Wetting agents are typically surfactants below their cmc. Above the cmc, micelles are formed with a hydrophobic core, and the hydrophobic drug will begin to dissolve into this region, thus affecting the structure of the system. Hence the level of the surfactant is kept below the cmc. Surfactants will localize on the surface of the particle, affecting the surface charge, ψ_o. The overall effect will be determined by the chemical nature of the surfactant and may be an increase or a decrease in the magnitude of the charge, but keeping the same sign (i.e. negative), or may even result in a change of sign (i.e. the particle effectively becomes positively charged). Each of these changes will have a direct effect on the Stern potential, ψ_δ, and an indirect effect on the thickness of the diffuse layer, resulting in alteration of the flocculation behaviour of the system. Additionally, ionic surfactants such as sodium lauryl sulfate will release mobile ions when dissolved and will have a separate effect on the diffuse layer.

Flocculation modifiers

In previous sections, the necessity of understanding particulate behaviour in suspension was stressed. The electrical double layer surrounding individual particles will have a significant effect on the DLVO behaviour of interacting particles (see Chapter 5), leading to flocculation or deflocculation depending on the relative extent of the attractive and repulsive energies at any separation distance. Materials which deposit onto the surface of the particle, such as surfactants, will affect the surface potential, ψ_o, leading to a secondary effect on the thickness of the diffuse layer by changing the Stern potential, ψ_δ. Materials which ionize in solution, such as preservatives and buffers, will lead to mobile charges being taken into the diffuse layer, resulting in a thinning of the diffuse layer and, generally, increased flocculation behaviour.

Excipients are added to pharmaceutical suspension formulations for various good scientific reasons, such as buffering, antimicrobial preservation and viscosity modification, as discussed earlier. However, their combined effects on the particulate behaviour must be understood and quantified. The last excipient to be added to the suspension formulation is the flocculation modifier, its function being to adjust the flocculation status of the particles to that which is intended. The quantity of flocculation modifier required must be determined last, once the levels

and effects of all other functional excipients have been established. It is no good, for example, to define the level of the flocculation modifier to give perfect flocculation behaviour and then add a buffer to the system, which will release mobile ions into the diffuse layer and change the flocculation status. Flocculation modifiers are ionic materials which ionize once in solution in the suspension medium. Typically, sodium chloride (NaCl) is used. The effect of the flocculation modifier on the flocculation behaviour of the particles is dependent on the ionic strength in solution, and therefore a multivalent salt (e.g. calcium chloride, $CaCl_2$) will have a greater effect than a monovalent salt (e.g. NaCl).

Colloid stabilizers

A colloid stabilizer is a material which will prevent or retard the coalescence of particles suspended in a medium and, as such, will encompass any material acting on the particle surface or in the diffuse layer. However, the term is usually understood to mean surfactants which are deposited on the particle surface, which were discussed earlier.

Stability considerations for suspensions

General chemical stability considerations apply to suspensions as much as to any other formulation. The drug must remain chemically stable over the intended shelf life of the product (and some time must be allowed as a 'margin of error' afterwards) and specifications will be in place for the maximum permitted levels of specified degradation products (these will be determined for each drug independently, on the basis of safety considerations). If the chemical degradation pathway of the drug is determined, then the appropriate chemical preservative(s) can be added to the suspension. Similarly, the effect of temperature on the chemical stability of the drug needs to be established, to assess whether any temperature restrictions are necessary during storage or transport.

However, physical stability is equally important for suspension formulations. Sedimentation should ideally be kept to a minimum, as discussed previously, and where sedimentation is permitted or unavoidable, easy redispersion of the sediment is necessary. The patient or carer should be able to redisperse the sediment by inversion and gentle shaking of the bottle only; the bottle should carry an appropriate instruction.

The redispersion pattern should be established, with testing at suitable time intervals and under various storage conditions, and used as a measure during shelf-life determinations. Visual assessment of sediment redispersion on shaking is useful but can provide only a general indication of whether there is a problem or not. A more quantitative approach involves assessment of the particle size distribution and drug content of representative samples taken from the top, middle and bottom of the container. Ideally, these should be consistent across depth and over time, meeting the preset product specifications.

Manufacturing considerations

Suspensions are more challenging to prepare than solution formulations. On both a dispensary scale and a factory scale, the most important part of the process is the initial dispersion stage, whereby the powdered drug is mixed with the carrier vehicle. If this is not performed adequately, then the particles are liable to cake. Poor initial dispersion will also lead to swift coagulation and sedimentation. Suspensions are bulky for manufacturers to produce. They require large quantities of pharmaceutical-grade water, necessitating in most cases a water processing plant to produce the water (on a dispensary scale, prepackaged Purified Water BP would be used). Packaging of the suspension into containers will require a stirred hopper to minimize settling during the packaging process, and the effect of shear at the dispensing nozzle on the suspension will need to be considered. A consideration with all products is cost. The drug is usually the most expensive item in the formulation, particularly for an investigative drug not yet licensed, and this will be no different for suspensions.

Summary

Suspensions are one of the most challenging pharmaceutical formulations that students and formulators are likely to meet. Successful suspension development is dependent on a basic understanding of the interactions between particles in the suspension and between particles and other formulation ingredients.

Please check your eBook at **https://studentconsult. inkling.com/** for self-assessment questions. See inside cover for registration details.

Bibliography

Kulshreshtha, K.A., Singh, O.N., Wall, G.M., 2009. Pharmaceutical Suspensions: From Formulation Development to Manufacturing. Springer, New York.

Nielloud, F., Marti-Mestres, G., 2000. Pharmaceutical Emulsions and Suspensions. Marcel Dekker, New York.

Rowe, R.C., Sheskey, P.J., Cook, W.G., et al., 2016. Handbook of Pharmaceutical Excipients, eighth ed. Pharmaceutical Press, London.

Schramm, L.L., 2014. Emulsions, Foams, Suspensions and Aerosols: Microscience and Applications, second ed. Wiley-VCH, Weinheim.

Emulsions and creams

Gillian M. Eccleston

CHAPTER CONTENTS

KEY POINTS

- Emulsions are dispersions of at least two immiscible (or partially miscible) liquids. Oil-in-water (o/w) emulsions contain oil droplets dispersed in water, and water-in-oil (w/o) emulsions contain water droplets dispersed in oil.
- Although emulsions may be formulated for virtually all the major routes of administration, most commercial products are for the intravenous route (o/w emulsions) or the topical route (o/w and w/o emulsions) of administration.
- Structured and semisolid emulsions for dermatological use (lotions and creams) are the largest class of emulsions used medically.
- Sterile intravenous o/w emulsions are used in parenteral nutrition as a source of calories and essential fatty acids, and as carriers for drugs of limited aqueous solubility, including diazepam, propofol and vitamin K.
- Emulsions are thermodynamically unstable and will attempt to return to separate oil and water phases (i.e. crack) by the processes of coalescence or Ostwald ripening (partially miscible oils) unless they are kinetically stabilized by the addition of emulsifiers.
- The choice of oil and emulsifier in pharmaceutical emulsions is severely limited by toxicity and/or irritancy. Synthetic ionic or

nonionic surfactants are used at low concentration in dermatological emulsions, whereas parenteral o/w emulsions contain mainly vegetable oils stabilized by lecithin.

- Emulsifiers impart kinetic stability to dilute emulsions by the formation of an interfacial film at the oil–water interface which increases droplet–droplet repulsion by the introduction of electrostatic repulsive forces (ionic emulsifiers) or hydration repulsive forces (nonionic emulsifiers). The interfacial film also provides a mechanical barrier to prevent coalescence if droplets collide.

- Mixtures of emulsifiers generally provide emulsions with greater stability than those achieved with individual emulsifiers as they form more rigid, close packed interfacial films.

- Mixtures of nonionic surfactants may be selected on the basis of the hydrophile–lipophile balance (HLB) system. Each oil has a required HLB. Blends of surfactants of high and low HLB with compositions calculated to give the required HLB are tested to find which blend forms the most stable emulsion. Stable emulsions will be many degrees below their phase inversion temperatures.

- Many emulsions contain mixed emulsifiers in excess of the quantity required to form an interfacial film. The excess emulsifier interacts with water either at the oil droplet interface or in the bulk continuous phase to form specific lamellar liquid crystalline phases (lecithin) or crystalline gel network phases (emulsifying wax).

- The gel network theory of emulsion stability established that the semisolid structure and the stability of o/w creams are dominated by the swelling properties of an α-crystalline gel network phase formed when the mixed emulsifier, in excess of the quantity required to form an interfacial film at the oil–water interface, interacts with continuous phase water. The gel networks immobilize droplets within their structure, thus preventing flocculation and coalescence.

- Aqueous creams are composed of four phases: dispersed oil phase stabilized by a mixed monomolecular film, α-crystalline gel phase composed of bilayers of surfactant and alcohol separated by layers of interlamellar fixed water, α-crystalline hydrates that show limited swelling in water, and bulk continuous phase free water.

Introduction

An emulsion is a dispersion of two immiscible (or partially miscible) liquids, one of which is distributed uniformly in the form of fine droplets (the dispersed phase) throughout the other (the continuous phase). The immiscible liquids are by convention described as 'oil' and 'water', as invariably one liquid is nonpolar (e.g. an oil, wax or lipid) and the other is polar (e.g. water or aqueous solution). For simplicity and consistency, the terms 'oil' and 'water' are used in this context throughout this chapter.

Oil-in-water (o/w) emulsions contain oil droplets dispersed in water, and water-in-oil (w/o) emulsions contain water droplets dispersed in oil (Fig. 27.1). Multiple emulsions can also be formed from oil and water by the reemulsification of an existing emulsion to form two dispersed phases. For example, multiple emulsions can be described as oil-in-water-in-oil (o/w/o) emulsions. These are o/w emulsions which are further dispersed in an oil continuum. Conversely water-in-oil-in-water (w/o/w) type multiple emulsions can be prepared by further emulsification of a w/o emulsion in water (Fig. 27.2).

Emulsion formation

When two *immiscible* liquids are placed together in a container, they will form distinct layers with a minimum area of contact (interfacial area) between

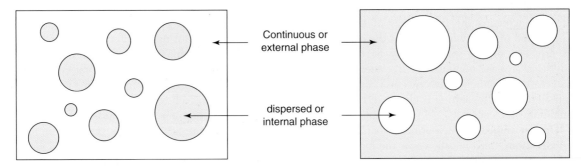

Continuous or external phase

dispersed or internal phase

Fig. 27.1 • An oil-in-water emulsion *(left)* and a water-in-oil emulsion *(right)*. The *shaded area* represents the oil.

447

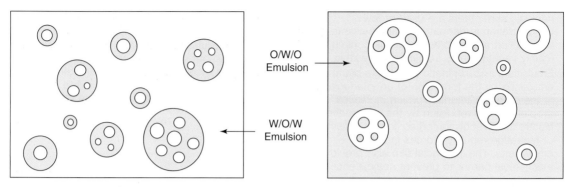

Fig. 27.2 • A multiple water-in-oil-in-water (w/o/w) emulsion and an oil-in-water-in oil (o/w/o) emulsion. The *shaded area* represents the oil.

the two liquids. In this state the surface free energy, G, is at a minimum. On mixing or mechanical agitation (i.e. input of energy), both liquids will form droplets of various sizes, thereby increasing the interfacial area between the liquids, with a corresponding increase in the surface free energy of the system. Emulsions are therefore thermodynamically unstable.

The increase in surface free energy ΔG brought about by the formation of droplets and the corresponding increase in surface area ΔA is given in Eq. 27.1:

$$\Delta G = \gamma \Delta A$$

(27.1)

where γ is the surface (or interfacial) tension.

In order to reduce this surface free energy, the droplets assume a spherical shape; this gives a minimum surface area per unit volume. On contact, droplets will coalesce (merge and recombine) in an attempt to reduce the total interfacial area (and thus the total surface energy, as indicated by Eqn 27.1).

Thus emulsification can be considered to be the result of two competing processes that occur simultaneously. The first process requires energy input to disrupt the bulk liquids and form fine droplets, thereby increasing the free energy of the system. The second process, which involves the coalescence of droplets, occurs spontaneously to reduce the interfacial area and minimize the free energy. If agitation ceases altogether, coalescence will continue until complete phase separation is obtained, the state of minimum free energy.

Droplet diameters vary enormously in pharmaceutical emulsions, but typically cover the range 0.1 μm (100 nm) to 25 μm. The visual appearance of an emulsion reflects the influence of droplet size on light scattering, and ranges from transparent or translucent for emulsions composed of small nanosized droplets (smaller than ~200 nm) to milky white and opaque for emulsions containing larger droplets.

Because emulsions are thermodynamically unstable, they will revert to separate oil and water continuous phases unless they are kinetically stabilized by the addition of emulsifying agents (see the sections entitled 'Emulsifying agents (emulsifiers)' and 'Emulsion stability').

Partially miscible liquids

When oil and water phases are partially miscible, droplet growth with eventual phase separation may occur by Ostwald ripening rather than coalescence. Ostwald ripening is an irreversible process which involves the growth of large droplets at the expense of smaller ones; it is considered later in this chapter in the section entitled 'Emulsion stability'. Ostwald ripening does not require any contact between droplets and is an important mechanism of instability in sub-micrometre pharmaceutical emulsions.

Emulsions in pharmacy

Emulsions can be formulated for virtually all the major routes of administration, although most commercial products are developed for the oral, parenteral and topical routes. Oral and intravenous emulsions are almost exclusively of the o/w type, whereas dermatological emulsions, and emulsions for subcutaneous or intramuscular injection may also be formulated as w/o emulsions.

Medicinal o/w emulsions for oral administration have a long tradition of use to deliver medicinal oils for the local treatment of constipation (e.g. mineral oil, castor oil) and as oral food supplements (e.g. fish liver oils and vegetable oils) in a more palatable and acceptable form. The unpleasant taste of the oil is masked by the aqueous phase and any odour is suppressed when it is administered as the internal phase of an o/w emulsion.

O/w emulsions containing vegetable oils are also used for the oral delivery of drugs and vitamins of low aqueous solubility. Intestinal absorption is generally enhanced when an oily solution of a drug is presented in the form of small sub-micrometre oil droplets, because of the larger interfacial area available for contact at the absorption site. Absorption is also generally faster and more complete than from suspension or tablet forms, because the drug in oral emulsions is already solubilized in the oil, thus eliminating the dissolution step prior to absorption.

Oral drug delivery using emulsions can be unpredictable because emulsions may become unstable in the low-pH environment of the stomach. Emulsion concentrates, described as self-emulsifying drug delivery systems, are available commercially to minimize instability. Self-emulsifying drug delivery systems (SEDDS) are composed of the drug, oil(s), surfactants and sometimes cosolvents. They are not themselves emulsions, but form an emulsion on mild agitation in the aqueous environment of the stomach.

Sterile intravenous lipid o/w emulsions are used clinically as a source of calories and essential fatty acids for debilitated patients. Such emulsions (e.g. Intralipid®) are also used as intravenous drug carriers for drugs of limited water solubility; marketed products are available for drugs such as diazepam (Diamuls®), propofol (Diprovan®) and vitamin K (Phytonadione®). The advantages of such intravenous emulsions over solution formulations (in which the drug is solubilized by various cosolvents, and/or surfactants and/or pH control) include a higher drug payload, lower toxicity, less pain on injection and protection of labile drugs by the oily environment.

Emulsions incorporating contrast agents (iodized oils, bromized perfluorocarbon oils) are used in diagnostic imaging, including X-ray examinations of body organs, computed tomography and magnetic resonance imaging.

W/o emulsions administered by the subcutaneous or intramuscular routes can be used to prolong the delivery of water-soluble antigens and thus provide a longer-lasting immunity. The antigen or drug must first diffuse from the aqueous droplets through the oily external phase before it reaches the tissues. Such emulsions are sometimes difficult to inject because of the high viscosity of the oily continuous phase. Multiple w/o/w emulsions, which are less viscous, have also been investigated for the prolonged release of drugs and vaccines incorporated in the innermost aqueous phase (see Chapter 36).

Dermatological emulsions are the largest class of emulsions used in pharmacy, and range in consistency from structured fluids (lotions, liniments) to semisolids (creams). Both o/w and w/o emulsions are extensively used as vehicles to deliver drugs to the skin, and for their therapeutic properties. Patient acceptance of such formulations is based on sensory attributes such as appearance, texture and 'skin feel'. W/o emulsions tend to be greasy, and although this conveys a greater feeling of richness, w/o emulsions do not mix well with aqueous wound exudates and are also sometimes difficult to wash off the skin. They do, however, hydrate the skin by occlusion, an important factor in drug permeation. In contrast, o/w lotions and creams readily mix with tissue exudates and are more easily removed by washing.

Dermatological emulsions (see Chapter 40) facilitate drug permeation into and through the skin by occlusion, by the incorporation of penetration-enhancing components and/or by evaporation on the skin surface. As most o/w creams are applied and rubbed onto the skin as a thin film, the drug delivery system is not the bulk emulsion but rather a dynamic evaporating film in which the dissolution environment and partitioning environment alter as the relative concentrations of the volatile ingredients change. Rapid evaporation may temporarily supersaturate the film, increasing thermodynamic activity and drug permeation.

Whilst dermatological emulsions and creams are two-phase systems, single-phase systems, including ointments and gels, are also available for topical application. These are described in Chapter 40.

Development of pharmaceutical emulsions

Although emulsions have many distinct advantages over other dosage forms, often increasing bioavailability and reducing side effects, there are relatively few commercial oral or parenteral emulsions available. This comparative lack of use is due to the fundamental problems of maintaining emulsion stability. Unstable emulsions are unsightly, give unpredictable drug-release profiles and may be toxic; for example, droplet size increases in parenteral emulsions may cause thrombosis following injection. However, there is currently a large increase in research into all aspects of emulsions, although as yet there are few new products. This resurgence of interest, which is mainly focused on lipid emulsions for local or intravenous delivery, combines nanoscience with the drive for cell-selective drug targeting and delivery.

Nanoemulsions

Nomenclature relating to nanoemulsions

It is necessary to spend a little time here considering the nomenclature of nanoemulsions as unfortunately there is some confusion in the literature, and definitions may vary.

Conventional emulsions (macroemulsions) and nanoemulsions. According to the convention for nanoscale materials, nanoemulsions are defined in the wider literature as *clear* or *transluscent* emulsions containing droplets of size typically smaller than approximately 200 nm (0.2 μm). In the pharmaceutical literature however, confusion arises because the term 'nanoemulsion' is sometimes used to include milky white emulsions containing droplets of up to 500 nm (0.5 μm) in diameter. In this chapter, milky white emulsions containing submicroscopic droplets smaller than 1 μm will be called colloidal, sub-micrometre emulsions, whilst the term 'nanoemulsion' will be reserved here for transparent emulsions containing droplets with diameters less than approximately 200 nm.

Microemulsions and nanoemulsions. The interchangeable use of the terms 'microemulsion' and 'nanoemulsion' is a more serious error that is becoming increasingly common in the pharmaceutical literature, causing confusion and inaccurate reporting. Although both microemulsions and nanoemulsions are clear and transparent, they are structurally quite different. Nanoemulsions are thermodynamically unstable dispersions of oil and water that contain individual small droplets less than 200 nm in diameter. In contrast, so-called microemulsions are *not emulsions*. They are thermodynamically stable, *single-phase* systems that form spontaneously and have a number of different microstructures depending on the nature and concentration of the components (see also Chapter 5).

Properties of nanoemulsions

Nanoemulsions are relatively stable physically, as the droplets do not collide as frequently as in ordinary emulsions and their small droplet sizes enable them to penetrate deep into the tissues through fine capillaries. Thus such emulsions are being investigated extensively as drug carriers and for their ability to target specific sites in the body, including the liver and the brain. The surface properties of emulsions can be modified by control of the charged nature of the interfacial film or by incorporation of homing devices into the film to target specific tissues and organs after injection.

Negatively charged droplets are cleared more rapidly from the blood than neutral or positively charged ones. Lipid emulsions modified with apolipoprotein E specifically target the parenchymal cells of the liver, and cationic emulsions complexed with plasmid DNA show promise in gene delivery.

Positively charged (cationic) nanoemulsions have also been shown to increase skin permeation of poorly soluble antifungal drugs and ceramides due to their interaction with the negatively charged skin epithelia cells. W/o nanoemulsion formulations are under investigation in cancer chemotherapy for prolongation of drug release after intramuscular or intratumoral injection, and as a means of enhancing the transport of anticancer agents via the lymphatic system.

Emulsion theory related to pharmaceutical emulsions and creams

The classical theories of emulsification for simple *two-phase* oil and water model emulsions based on droplet interactions and interfacial films are considered in Chapter 5. However, commercial pharmaceutical emulsions (even dilute mobile fluids for intravenous administration) are rarely such simple oil and water systems. They are more often complex multiphase emulsions containing phases (e.g. liquid crystalline) additional to oil and water. A unified theory of emulsification cannot be applied quantitatively to such multiphase emulsions, which range in consistency from mobile or structured fluids to soft or stiff semisolids.

Formulation of emulsions

When a formulator is formulating a pharmaceutical emulsion, the choice of oil, emulsifier and emulsion type (o/w, w/o or multiple emulsion) will depend on the route of administration and its ultimate clinical use. The formulator must optimize the processing conditions as these control droplet size distributions and rheological properties, which in turn influence emulsion stability and therapeutic response. The potential toxicity of all the excipients, their cost and possible chemical incompatibilities in the final formulation must also be identified. It is sometimes difficult to isolate these effects in practical emulsions as each is dependent on, and influenced by, the other. Thus ingredient selection is made often by trial and error and is dependent on the experience of the formulator.

Selection of the oil phase

The oil used in the preparation of pharmaceutical emulsions may be the medicament itself or it may function as a carrier for a lipid-soluble drug. The selection of the oil phase will depend on many factors, including the desired physical properties of the emulsion, the miscibility of the oil and aqueous phases, the solubility of the drug (if present) in the oil and the desired consistency of the final emulsion. Some oils, in particular unsaturated oils of vegetable origin, are liable to undergo auto-oxidation and become rancid, and so antioxidants or preservatives must be incorporated into the emulsion to inhibit this degradation process.

For externally applied emulsions, oils based on hydrocarbons are widely used. Liquid paraffin, either alone or combined with soft or hard paraffin, is used in numerous dermatological lotions and creams, both as a vehicle for the drug, and for the occlusive and sensory characteristics imparted when the emulsion is spread onto the skin. Turpentine oil, benzyl benzoate and various silicone oils are examples of other externally applied oils that are formulated as emulsions.

In oral emulsions, the most widely used medicinal oils are castor oil and liquid paraffin, which are nonbiodegradable and provide a local laxative effect in the gastrointestinal tract, fish liver oils (e.g. cod or halibut) that are high in vitamins A and D or various fixed oils of vegetable origin (e.g. arachis oil) as nutritional supplements. Vegetable oils are also used as drug carriers as they are readily absorbed in the gastrointestinal tract. The oil phase is rarely inert, as it may have an impact on bioavailability by its influence on gastric emptying time.

The choice of oil is severely limited in emulsions for parenteral administration, as many are inherently toxic. Although purified mineral oil is used in some w/o depot preparations for intramuscular injection, where its potential toxicity (e.g. abscess formation at the injection site) is balanced against its efficacy, it is too toxic to be incorporated into intravenous emulsions. A range of purified vegetable oils have been used, almost exclusively over many years in lipid emulsions for parenteral nutrition and as intravenous carriers for drugs of limited aqueous solubility.

The purified vegetable oils used in parenteral products comprise mixtures of long-chain triglycerides (LCTs) containing C_{12}–C_{18} saturated and unsaturated fatty acid moieties, mainly oleic, linoleic, palmitic and stearic acids. Although a large number of vegetable oils have been investigated as possible stable, nontoxic oils for use in lipid emulsions, most commercial products contain soya bean or safflower oils because of their high content of the essential fatty acid linoleic acid. Medium-chain triglycerides (MCTs), which contain shorter fatty acid moieties (approximately C_6–C_{10}) are obtained by the reesterification of fractionated coconut oil fatty acids (mainly capric and caprylic acids) with glycerol. These provide a more rapidly available source of energy, as well as enhancing the solubilizing capacity for lipid-soluble drugs, including ciclosporin.

Mixtures containing both long-chain and medium-chain triglycerides have been adopted in some commercial preparations (Table 27.1). Structured

Table 27.1 Selected commercial lipid emulsions for parenteral nutrition

Trade name	Oil phase	Emulsifier	Other components
Intralipid® (Fresenius Kabi)	Soya (10%, 20% and 30%)	Purified egg phospholipids (1.2%)	Glycerol (2.2%), phosphate (1.5 mmol)
Omegaven® (Fresenius Kabi)	Refined fish oils (10%)	Egg phosphatides (1.2%)	Glycerol (2.5%)
ClinOleic® 20% (Baxter)	Purified olive and soya (20%)	Egg phosphatides (1.2%)	Glycerol (2.25%)
Lipofundin MCT/LCT® (Braun)	1:1 soya and MCT (10% and 20%)	Egg lecithin (0.75% and 1.2%)	Glycerol (2.5%)

LCT, long-chain triglyceride; *MCT*, medium-chain triglyceride.

triglycerides, formed by modifying the oil enzymatically to produce 1,3-specific triglycerides with a mixture of long-chain and medium-chain fatty acids within the same molecule are under investigation as possible alternatives to physical mixtures of LCTs and MCTs.

Emulsified perfluorochemicals are also considered acceptable for intravenous use provided that they are excreted relatively quickly. A major problem in the formulation of the early perfluorocarbon emulsions as blood substitutes was that the oils that formed the most stable emulsions were not cleared rapidly from the body.

Selection of the emulsifying agent (emulsifier)

Emulsifiers are used to control emulsion stability during a shelf life that can vary from days for extemporaneously prepared emulsions to months or years for commercial preparations. In practice, combinations of emulsifiers rather than single agents are generally used. The choice of emulsifier depends on the type of emulsion to be prepared, emulsifier toxicity (or irritancy if applied to the skin) and potential cost and availability. The final clinical use of the emulsion is also an important consideration, as emulsifiers control the in vivo fate of emulsions by their influence on droplet size distribution, and the charge and surface properties of the individual droplets.

The functionality and types of emulsifying agent are of such importance for the properties of the emulsion that emulsifiers are considered in a separate section entitled 'Emulsifying agents (emulsifiers)'.

Other excipients

Preservatives

The aqueous continuous phase of an o/w emulsion can produce ideal conditions for the growth of bacteria and fungi. The potential sources of contamination may be from the water used, from the raw materials (especially if these are natural products), from the manufacturing and packaging equipment or introduced by the patient during use. Such contamination, which may constitute a health hazard, can also affect the physicochemical properties of the formulation, causing colour, odour or pH changes and even phase separation. W/o emulsions are less susceptible to such contamination because the aqueous phase is essentially enclosed and protected by the oil.

An ideal preservative should exhibit a wide spectrum of activity against bacteria and fungi; it should also be free from toxic, irritant or sensitizing activity (see Chapter 48). Large-volume injectable fat emulsions do not contain preservatives, and sterilization is achieved by autoclaving without a preservative. Phenoxyethanol, benzoic acid, and the p-hydroxybenzoates are used as preservatives in oral and topical emulsions. The preservative will partition between the oil and aqueous phases, with the oil phase acting as a reservoir. Aqueous pH is an additional factor to be considered, as a sufficient concentration of the un-ionized form must be present to ensure proper preservation. Compatibility problems can occur between emulsifiers and preservatives (e.g. polyoxyethylene nonionic surfactants emulsifiers and phenolic preservatives), destroying not only their microbial activity but also the emulsification properties of the surfactant.

Antioxidants and humectants

Antioxidants are added to some emulsions to prevent oxidative deterioration of the oil, emulsifier or the drug itself during storage. Such deterioration imparts an unpleasant, rancid odour and taste. Some oils are supplied containing suitable antioxidants. The antioxidants commonly used in pharmacy include butylated hydroxyanisole and butylated hydroxytoluene at concentrations up to 0.2%, and the alkyl gallates, which are effective at very low concentrations (0.001% to 0.1%). α-Tocopherol is added to some commercial lipid emulsions to prevent peroxidation of unsaturated fatty acids.

Humectants, such as propylene glycol, glycerol and sorbitol at concentrations up to 5%, are often added to dermatological preparations to reduce the evaporation of the water from the emulsion during storage and use. However, high concentrations may also remove moisture from the skin, causing dryness.

Emulsifying agents (emulsifiers)

Function of emulsifying agents

The function of an emulsifying agent (emulsifier) is to maintain the dispersion state of the emulsion for an extended period of time after the cessation of agitation, i.e. to impart kinetic stability to the emulsion. The dispersed droplets do not retain their initial character because the emulsion becomes thermodynamically stable (for the free energy is still high) but rather because the added emulsifiers inhibit or delay the processes of coalescence and Ostwald ripening (described later).

Emulsifiers generally impart time-dependent stability by the formation of a mechanical or electrostatic barrier at the droplet interface (an interfacial film) or in the external phase (a rheological barrier). The formation of interfacial films by adsorption of the emulsifier at the oil–water interface is discussed in Chapter 5.

The interfacial film may increase droplet–droplet repulsion by the introduction of electrostatic or steric repulsive forces to counteract the van der Waals forces of attraction. Electrostatic repulsions are important in o/w emulsions stabilized by ionic emulsifiers, whereas steric repulsive forces, which arise when hydrated polymer chains approach one another, dominate with nonionic emulsifiers and in w/o emulsions. The interfacial film may also provide a mechanical barrier to prevent droplet coalescence, particularly if it is close packed and elastic. Generally, mixtures of emulsifiers provide stronger interfacial films. Surfactant emulsifiers lower the interfacial tension between the oil and water. Although this facilitates the formation of droplets during emulsification and reduces the thermodynamic tendency for coalescence, interfacial tension reduction is not a major factor in maintaining long-term stability.

Interfacial films do not have the dominant role in maintaining stability in many practical emulsions in which the external phase is thickened by the emulsifier, i.e. in which the emulsifier significantly increases the viscosity of the continuous phase. In these, the structured continuous phase forms a rheological barrier which prevents the movement and hence the close approach of droplets. Emulsifiers that thicken the external phase but do not form an interfacial film are variously described as *auxiliary emulsifiers*, *co-emulsifiers* or *viscosity enhancers*. Many pharmaceutically important mixed emulsifiers, including lecithin and the emulsifying waxes, form interfacial films at low concentration and also structure the external phase at higher concentrations by the formation of additional lamellar liquid crystalline phases (with lecithins) or crystalline gel network phases (with emulsifying waxes).

Emulsion type

The type of emulsion that forms (whether o/w or w/o or multiple emulsion) and the droplet size distribution depend on a number of interrelated factors, including the method of preparation (energy input), the relative volumes of the oil and water phases and the chemical nature of the emulsifying agent. When oil and water are mixed vigorously in the absence of an emulsifier, droplets of both liquids are produced initially, with the more rapidly coalescing droplets forming the continuous phase. Generally this is the liquid present in the greater amount because the greater number of droplets formed increases the probability of droplet collision and subsequent coalescence. With the inclusion of an emulsifier, the type of emulsion that forms is no longer a function of phase volume alone, but also depends on the relative solubility of the emulsifier in the oil and water phases. In general, the phase in which the emulsifying agent is more soluble (or in the case of solids, more easily wetted by) will form the continuous phase. Thus hydrophilic surfactants and polymers promote o/w emulsions and lipophilic emulsifiers – with low hydrophile–lipophile balance (HLB; see the section entitled 'Emulsifier selection') – promote w/o systems.

Theoretically, the dispersed phase of an emulsion can occupy up to a maximum of 74% of the phase volume. Whilst such high internal phase o/w emulsions stabilized by suitable emulsifiers have been produced, it is more difficult to form w/o emulsions with greater than 50% dispersed phase because of the steric mechanisms involved in their stabilization. In practice, pharmaceutical emulsions usually contain 10% to 30% dispersed phase.

Classification of emulsifying agents

Emulsifying agents may be classified into two groups: (1) synthetic or semisynthetic surface-active agents and polymers and (2) naturally occurring materials and their derivatives. Examples of typical pharmaceutical emulsifying agents are shown in Tables 27.2 and 27.3.

Surface-active agents and polymers

Surface-active agents (surfactants for short) are further classified as ionic (i.e. anionic or cationic) or nonionic according to their characteristics on dissociation. Most are mixtures of long-chain homologues having

Table 27.2 Synthetic surface-active emulsifying agents

Class	Example	Structure	Emulsion type	Route of administration
Anionic				
Alkyl sulfates	Sodium lauryl sulfate	$C_{12}H_{25}OSO_3^-Na^+$	Oil in water	Topical
Monovalent salts of fatty acids	Sodium stearate	$C_{17}H_{35}COO^-Na^+$	Oil in water	Topical
Divalent salts of fatty acid	Calcium oleate	$(C_{17}H_{35}COO^-)_2Ca^{2+}$	Water in oil	Topical
Cationic				
Quaternary ammonium compounds	Cetrimide	$C_{16}H_{33}N^+(CH_3)_3$	Oil in water	Topical
Nonionic				
Alcohol polyethylene glycol ethers	Cetomacrogol 1000	$CH_3(CH_2)_n(OCH_2CH_2)_mOH$ $n = 15$ or 17; $m = 20–24$	Oil in water	Topical
Fatty acid polyethylene glycol esters	Polyethylene glycol 40 stearate	$CH_3(CH_2)_{16}CO(OCH_2CH_2)_{40}OH$	Oil in water	Topical
Sorbitan fatty acid esters	Sorbitan monooleate (Span 80)	See the text	Water in oil	Topical
Polyoxyethylene sorbitan fatty acid esters	Polyoxyethylene sorbitan monooleate (Tween 80)	See the text	Oil in water	Topical, parenteral
Polymeric				
Polyoxyethylene–polyoxypropylene block copolymers	Poloxomers (Pluronic F-68)	$OH(C_2H_4O)_a(C_3H_6O)_b(C_2H_4O)_a$	Oil in water	Parenteral
Fatty amphiphiles				
Fatty alcohols	Cetyl alcohol	$C_{16}H_{33}O^-H^+$	Water in oil	Topical
Fatty acids	Stearic acid	$C_{16}H_{33}COO^-H^+$	Water in oil	Topical
Monoglycerides	Glyceryl monostearate		Water in oil	Topical

Table 27.3 Emulsifying agents of natural origin

Class	Example	Emulsion type	Route of administration
Polysaccharide	Acacia	Oil in water	Oral
	Methylcellulose	Oil in water	Oral
Phospholipid	Purified lecithins	Oil in water	Oral, parenteral
Sterol	Wool fat	Water in oil	Topical
	Cholesterol and its esters	Water in oil	Topical
Finely divided solid	Bentonite	Oil in water and water in oil	Topical
	Aluminium hydroxide	Oil in water	Oral

hydrocarbon chain lengths between 12 and 18 carbon atoms with a hydrophilic head group. Their emulsifying power is influenced by batch variations in the homologue composition, with pure homologue surfactants proving to be very poor emulsifiers.

There are an enormous number of synthetic surfactants available commercially, and they form by far the largest group of emulsifiers studied in the general scientific literature. Unfortunately, the majority of the synthetic surfactants are toxic (many are haemolytic) and irritant to the skin and the mucous membranes of the gastrointestinal tract. In general, cationic surfactants are the most toxic and irritant and nonionic surfactants the least. Thus, for pharmaceutical emulsions, ionic synthetic surfactants are used only in external topical preparations, where they are present at relatively low concentration. Both ionic and nonionic surfactants are combined with fatty alcohols to produce anionic, cationic or nonionic emulsifying waxes, which are used to both stabilize and structure aqueous lotions and creams. A limited number of nonionic surfactants (e.g. the polysorbates, discussed later) are also used internally in oral and parenteral emulsions, although lecithin (a mixture of anionic and neutral phospholipids) is the main emulsifier in commercial lipid emulsions. The nonionic block copolymer poloxomer 188 (Pluronic® F68) has been used in perfluorochemical emulsions for intravenous infusion, although some patients are sensitive to this emulsifier.

Anionic surfactants

Anionic surfactants dissociate at high pH to form a long-chain anion with surface activity. Emulsifying properties are lost and emulsions are unstable in acid conditions and in the presence of cationic materials, such as cationic surfactants and polymers. Examples of anionic surfactants are described in the following paragraphs:

Alkyl sulfates. Sodium lauryl sulfate (sodium dodecyl sulfate) was until recently the most widely used surfactant in topical products. The commercial sulfate is actually a mixture containing predominantly the C_{12} homologue, but also contains some C_{14} and C_{16} homologues. Sodium lauryl sulfate alone is a weak emulsifier of the o/w type, but forms a powerful o/w blend when it is used in conjunction with cetostearyl alcohol.

Monovalent salts of fatty acids. Emulsifiers in this group consist mainly of the alkali salts of long-chain fatty acids, e.g. $C_{17}H_{35}COO^-X^+$, where X may be Na, K, NH_4 or triethanolamine (TEA). Alone, these 'soaps' promote rather unstable, mobile o/w emulsions, but when combined with fatty acids, they form powerful o/w emulsifying blends that stabilize a number of dermatological products.

In many formulations, the 'nascent soap' method of preparation is used, in which soap is formed in situ from the partial neutralization of a fatty acid (which may be a component of the oil phase) with the appropriate alkali. For example, in white liniment, ammonium oleate is formed in situ from the reaction between ammonia solution and oleic acid. TEA soaps, formed in situ by the partial neutralization of fatty acid (generally stearic acid) by TEA have a long history of use in the formulation of cosmetic and pharmaceutical o/w vanishing creams.

Divalent salts of fatty acids. Calcium salts of fatty acids containing two hydrocarbon chains form w/o emulsions because of their limited solubility in water. These are generally formed in situ by the interaction of calcium hydroxide with a fatty acid. In zinc cream, calcium oleate is formed in situ from the interaction between oleic acid and calcium hydroxide. This approach is also used in some formulations of oily calamine cream, in which oleic acid and some of the free fatty acid component of arachis oil are partially neutralized by calcium hydroxide to form a calcium oleate–oleic acid mixed emulsifier.

Cationic surfactants

Cationic surfactants dissociate at low pH to form a long-chain surface-active cation. Emulsions containing cationic surfactant as the emulsifier are unstable at high pH and in the presence of anionic materials, including anionic surfactants and polymers.

Quaternary ammonium compounds. These constitute an important group of cationic emulsifiers in dermatological preparations because they also have antimicrobial properties. Cetrimide (cetyltrimethylammonium bromide) is blended with cetostearyl alcohol to form cationic emulsifying wax, which is the mixed emulsifier used in cetrimide cream.

Nonionic surfactants

There are an enormous number of nonionic surfactants available commercially with different oil and water solubility producing either o/w emulsions or w/o emulsions. Nonionic surfactants are particularly useful as emulsifiers because they are less toxic and irritant than ionic surfactants, and therefore a limited number (e.g. polysorbate 80; Tween® 80) are used in parenteral and oral products. In addition, nonionic surfactants do not ionize to any extent and thus are more resistant than ionic surfactants to changes in pH and the presence of electrolytes and polyvalent ions. Most nonionic surfactants are based on:

- A hydrophobic moiety with 12–18 carbon atoms. The starting material may be a fatty acid or sorbitan.

- A hydrophilic moiety composed of an alcohol (–OH) and/or ethylene oxide groups linked to form long polyoxyethylene chains.

For each starting material the polyoxyethylene chain can be modified and water solubility increased by the systematic addition of ethylene oxide.

Polyoxyethylene glycol ethers (macrogols). These are a series of nonionic surfactant condensation products of fatty alcohols with hydrocarbon chain lengths from C_{12} to C_{18} and polyethylene glycol. They are used as both o/w emulsifiers and w/o emulsifiers as their oil and water solubility can be controlled by altering both the length of the hydrocarbon chain and the length of the polyoxyethylene (POE) chain. The most widely used emulsifier in this class is cetomacrogol 1000 (Table 27.2), which is used combined with cetostearyl alcohol to stabilize o/w lotions and creams, including Cetomacrogol Cream BP.

Sorbitan esters. The sorbitan esters are a series of surfactants, widely known as the Spans®, that are produced by the esterification of one or more of the hydroxyl groups of sorbitan with a fatty acid (hence the synonym *sorbitan fatty acid esters*). Various fatty acids are combined, resulting in a range of commercial products, e.g. sorbitan monolaurate (Span 20), sorbitan monopalmitate (Span 40), sorbitan monostearate (Span 60) and sorbitan monooleate (Span 80). The structure of sorbitan monooleate (Span 80) is shown below.

The series of sorbitan esters are hydrophobic and by themselves produce w/o emulsions.

Polyoxyethylene sorbitan esters (polysorbates). The polysorbates are more hydrophilic polyoxyethylene derivatives of the sorbitan esters (full name, polyoxyethylene sorbitan fatty acid esters). The following grades are used in pharmacy: polyethylene 20 sorbitan monolaurate (polysorbate 20), polyethylene 20 sorbitan monopalmitate (polysorbate 40), polyethylene 20 sorbitan monostearate (polysorbate 60) and polyethylene 20 sorbitan monooleate (polysorbate 80). These are marketed under the name Tween®. The 20 in the name refers to the number of POE groups in the molecule. The formula for polyoxyethylene 20 sorbitan monooleate (Tween 80) is shown below.

In this molecule, the subscripts w, x, y and z add up to 20. The group R is the fatty acid chain – in this case $-CH_2COOC_{17}H_{33}$.

An enormous range of polysorbate surfactants of differing oil and water solubilities are available from control of the fatty acid and the length of the polyethylene glycol chains in the molecule. Thus the polysorbates are able to stabilize both w/o and o/w emulsions, depending on their HLB value (see the section entitled 'Emulsifier selection'). Mixtures of sorbitan esters and their POE derivatives are used to form stable emulsions.

Fatty amphiphiles

Fatty alcohols and fatty acids. These are sometimes described in older texts as auxiliary emulsifiers. When used alone, they are weak w/o emulsifiers. However, in the presence of ionic or nonionic surfactants (e.g. when formulated as emulsifying waxes), they are very powerful o/w blends.

Glycerol monoesters. Glyceryl monostearate and glyceryl monooleate are the most common monoesters used in dermatological formulations. The amphiphilic glycerol monoesters, described as nonemulsifying grades in the various pharmacopoeias, are poor w/o emulsifiers. Self-emulsifying grades, which are similar to the emulsifying waxes, are produced either by the partial neutralization of some of the free fatty acid component of the monoester using alkali or by the addition of approximately 5% ionic or nonionic surfactant.

Most fatty amphiphiles are not pure homologues. For example, cetostearyl alcohol is a mixture of C_{16} cetyl alcohol (20% to 35%) and C_{18} stearyl alcohol (50% to 70%). Similarly, stearic acid is generally composed of approximately 55% palmitic acid (C_{16}) and 45% stearic acid (C_{18}) homologues. Such mixes show considerable intermanufacturer and interbatch variations. In creams, the homologue composition of the fatty amphiphile markedly influences structure and stability (see later in this chapter).

Polymeric surfactants

The poloxamers (also known as Pluronics®, e.g. poloxamer 188 is Pluronic® F68) are a series of neutral synthetic polyoxyethylene–polyoxypropylene block copolymers which are used either alone or as auxiliary emulsifiers with lecithin in small-volume parenteral injections. Poloxamer 188 is resistant to breakdown during autoclave sterilization, and its combination with lecithin may stabilize the emulsion by giving a more closely packed interfacial film.

Natural macromolecular materials

Many traditional emulsifying agents are derived from natural plant or animal sources and show considerable batch-to-batch variation in their composition which may result in variable emulsifying properties. Many are also susceptible to microbial contamination and degradation by oxidation or hydrolysis of components. In order to reduce such instabilities and extend product shelf life, purified and semisynthetic derivatives are generally used in commercial preparations.

Phospholipids

Purified lecithins are natural surfactants derived from egg yolk or soya bean oil. They are used extensively as o/w emulsifiers in parenteral and oral lipid emulsions (Table 27.3). Lecithins are composed of complex mixtures of neutral and negatively charged phospholipids, of which the major components are phosphatidylcholine and phosphatidylethanolamine (~90%) (which are uncharged at physiological pH), with smaller quantities of phosphatidylserine, phosphatidylglycerol and phosphatidic acid (which are negatively charged). The lecithins stabilize lipid emulsions by increasing the surface charge of the droplets, and by the formation of interfacial liquid crystalline phases. The emulsifying properties are related to the relative proportions of neutral and anionic lipids, which vary with the phospholipid source and degree of purification. Currently, egg-yolk lecithin is the emulsifier of choice (Table 27.1).

Hydrophilic colloids; polysaccharides

Polysaccharides, including gums, such as acacia and tragacanth, and alginate and cellulose derivatives are hydrophilic colloids that are predominantly used as emulsifying agents in oral preparations. They render an unpleasant feel to topical emulsions. They are susceptible to degradation, in particular by depolymerization. Polysaccharides provide a good growth medium for microorganisms, so preservation of emulsions containing them is essential. Whilst they do not lower interfacial tension, some polysaccharides, including acacia and purified and semisynthetic derivatives of methylcellulose, stabilize o/w emulsions by the formation of thick multilayered films which are highly resistant to film rupture. As an example, methylcellulose 20 is used at a concentration of 2% to stabilize Liquid Paraffin Oral Emulsion BP. Other polysaccharides form poor interfacial films and are relatively inefficient emulsifiers when used alone. They act mainly as viscosity modifiers as they increase the consistency of the external phase and thereby inhibit creaming and coalescence (see the section entitled 'Emulsion stability').

Steroidal emulsifiers

Examples of steroidal emulsifying agents derived from animal sources include wool fat (lanolin), wool alcohols (lanolin alcohols), beeswax and cholesterol. They are generally complex mixtures of cholesterol, long-chain alcohols and related sterols. Purified derivatives are still widely used in traditional dermatological emulsions, such as creams, as w/o emulsifiers, and for their emollient properties. They are prone to oxidation and hydrolysis, and antioxidants may need to be incorporated into the emulsion. Wool fat is used in combination with calcium oleate in oily calamine lotion, with beeswax in proflavine cream and with cetostearyl alcohol in zinc and ichthammol cream.

A large number of purified and chemically modified derivatives are available commercially that produce more stable w/o emulsions and retain desirable emollient properties. They are sometimes modified to produce o/w emulsions. For example, a series of nonionic water-soluble lanolin derivatives that promote the formation of o/w emulsions have been produced commercially by reacting lanolin with ethylene oxide.

Solid particles

Finely divided solid particles may stabilize emulsions if they are partially wetted by both the oil phase and the water phase and possess sufficient adhesion for one another to form a coherent interfacial film to give a mechanical barrier against droplet coalescence. If the particles are preferentially wetted by the aqueous phase, an o/w emulsion forms, whereas if the solid is preferentially wetted by oil, a w/o emulsion is produced. The particles must be orders of magnitude smaller than the droplets, and their effectiveness in stabilizing the emulsion will depend on particle size, shape and wettability, interparticle interactions and the emulsion medium. Emulsions stabilized by solid particles are sometimes described as Pickering emulsions or surfactant-free emulsions. Magnesium hydroxide is used as the emulsifier in liquid paraffin and magnesium hydroxide oral emulsion.

Solid particles may also act as viscosity modifiers. Clays, such as bentonite and aluminium magnesium silicate, are often incorporated into cosmetic creams. There is a resurgence in interest in Pickering emulsions, especially for the topical delivery of drugs, and a number of new types of hydrophobically modified colloidal silica particles are being investigated.

Emulsifier selection

The hydrophile-lipophile balance (HLB) method

As previously discussed, pharmaceutical emulsions generally contain mixtures of emulsifiers, as these form more stable emulsions. The HLB method provides a systematic method for selecting mixtures of emulsifying agents to produce physically stable emulsions. Although originally applied to nonionic surfactants, its use has now been extended to ionic surfactants.

Each surfactant is allocated an HLB number between 0 and 20 which expresses numerically the size and strength of the polar portion relative to the nonpolar portion of the molecule. Thus the higher the HLB number, the more hydrophilic or water soluble the surfactant, and the lower the HLB number, the more lipophilic or oil soluble the surfactant. The HLB values of ionic surfactants are much higher (up to 50) as they are based on ionization properties. Table 27.4 gives HLB values for commonly used surfactant emulsifiers. The theoretical concept of HLB values is discussed more fully in Chapter 5.

Determination of 'required HLB' value

The HLB value of the emulsifier blend giving the most stable emulsion is known as the 'required HLB value' for that oil phase. The HLB value required to most effectively form an emulsion for a range of individual oils, fats and waxes may be obtained from the literature. If a mixed emulsifier system is used in a formulation and the HLB values of the individual components in an oily mixture are known, the required HLB value can be calculated theoretically from the proportions of each component in the oil phase. Alternatively, if the required HLB value of the oil is not available, it can be found by experimentation. To perform such experiments, a series of emulsions

Table 27.4 Hydrophile–lipophile balance values for some pharmaceutical nonionic surfactants

Commercial name	Pharmacopoeia name	HLB value
Span 85	Sorbitan trioleate	1.8
Span 80	Sorbitan oleate	4.3
Span 60	Sorbitan monostearate	4.7
Span 20	Sorbitan monolaurate	8.6
Brij 98	Polyoxyethylene 10 stearyl ether	12
Tween 60	Polysorbate 60 (polyoxyethylene 20 sorbitan monostearate)	14.9
Tween 80	Polysorbate 80 (polyoxyethylene 20 sorbitan oleate)	15
Cetomacrogol 1000	Macrogol cetostearyl ether	15.7
Tween 20	Polysorbate 20 (polyoxyethylene 20 sorbitan monolaurate)	16.7
	Potassium oleate	20
	Sodium dodecyl sulfate (sodium lauryl sulfate)	40

HLB, hydrophile–lipophile balance.

Table 27.5 The 'required' hydrophile–lipophile balance values for oils and oil phase ingredients

Oil	Oil-in-water emulsion	Water-in-oil emulsion
Petrolatum	7–8	4
Liquid paraffin	10.5	4
Mineral oil, light	12	4
Castor oil	14	–
Lanolin, anhydrous	12	8
Beeswax	9	5
Cottonseed oil	6	–
Pine oil	16	–

using blends of a given pair of nonionic emulsifiers covering a range of HLB numbers is made. These HLB values can then be used to assess the suitability of other blends that may give a better emulsion.

The method of selection of emulsifying agents is based on the observation that different oils require emulsifying agents of different HLB numbers to produce close-packed interfacial films and stable emulsions. Thus individual oils are often given two 'required' HLB numbers – a high value to form o/w emulsions and a low one to form w/o emulsions (Table 27.5). A number of nonionic emulsifiers and their blends, chemically different but all with HLB values similar to the required HLB value of the oil, are then examined to find which emulsifying system forms the most stable emulsion. Assessments are based on physical properties, such as the droplet size distribution.

Calculation of ratio of emulsifier to produce a particular required HLB value

One of the most important aspects of the HLB system is that the HLB values are additive if the amount of each surfactant in a blend is taken into account. Thus blends of high and low HLB surfactants can be used to obtain the required HLB value of an oil. The HLB value of a mixture of surfactants consisting of fraction x of surfactant A and fraction $(1 - x)$ of surfactant B is assumed to be the algebraic mean of the two HLB numbers, i.e.

$$HLB_{mixture} = xHLB_A + (1 - x)HLB_B$$

$$(27.2)$$

An example calculation is shown in Box 27.1.

Limitations of the HLB method

Although the HLB system narrows the range of emulsifiers to select, and provides some sort of order to a seemingly endless choice of emulsifiers, it is limited by its strict relation to the molecular structure of individual surfactants. The system is insensitive to the affinity of the emulsifier components for the aqueous and oily phases. For example, when surfactants with widely different HLB numbers are mixed to give the optimum theoretical HLB value, unstable emulsions sometimes result because of the high solubility of the surfactants in the dispersed and continuous phases, which may change the balance of molecules at the interface, giving a weak interfacial film. In addition, the HLB method does not take into account the influence of additional components in the formulation or the profound influence of temperature changes on surfactant HLB.

Box 27.1

Worked example

A formulator is required to formulate an oil-in-water emulsion of the basic formula:

Liquid paraffin	50 g
Emulsifying agents (required HLB 10.5)	5 g
Water	to 100 g

To prepare this liquid paraffin-in-water emulsion, the nonionic emulsifier, or mixture of nonionic emulsifiers, should have the required HLB value of 10.5. This narrows the number of possible surfactants considerably. Although a single surfactant with this HLB value may be suitable, usually it is better to have a mixture of emulsifiers, one with a lower HLB value than required and the other with a higher HLB value than required. In this formulation, suitable emulsifiers are Tween 80 (with an HLB value of 15) and Span 80 (with an HLB value of 4.3).

To calculate the fraction x of Tween 80, Eq. 27.2 gives

$$10.5 = x \times 15 + (1 - x) \times 4.3$$
$$15x - 4.3x = 10.5 - 4.3, \text{ i.e. } 10.7x = 6.2$$
$$x = 0.58$$

Thus to match the required HLB of the oil, the fraction (or percentage = fraction × 100) of Tween 80 is 0.58 (58%) and that of Span 80 is 0.42 (42%). Thus 2.9 g (0.58 × 5) of Tween 80 and 2.1 g (0.42 × 5) of Span 80 are required for this formulation.

The HLB–phase inversion temperature system

This method extends the HLB method to include a characteristic property of the emulsion, the phase inversion temperature (PIT) of the system. If an o/w emulsion stabilized by a mixture of nonionic polyether surfactants is heated, phase inversion from an o/w emulsion to a w/o emulsion will occur at a specific temperature unique to the particular emulsion. Phase inversion can be seen visually.

Phase inversion is based on the fact that the stabilities of o/w emulsions containing nonionic surfactants are closely related to the degree of hydration of the interfacial films. O/w emulsions will form if the surfactant is predominantly hydrophilic, whereas w/o emulsions are produced when the lipophilic part of the molecule dominates.

As temperature increases, the HLB value of a nonionic surfactant will decrease as it becomes more hydrophobic. At the temperature at which its hydrophobic tendency just exceeds its hydrophilic tendency, the PIT, the emulsion will invert to form a w/o emulsion. Therefore, conditions which decrease the degree of hydration of the interfacial film (e.g. added salts or an increase in temperature) also decrease the stability of the emulsion. As a general rule, relatively stable o/w emulsions are obtained when the proposed storage temperatures are 20 °C to 60 °C below the PIT, because the interfacial films are then sufficiently hydrated.

Creams

Creams are white, semisolid preparations, often medicated, intended for external application to the skin and mucous membranes. Pharmaceutical and cosmetic creams are generally o/w emulsions (aqueous creams), although the term is also used occasionally to describe semisolid w/o emulsions (oily creams). In addition, other nonemulsion bases, such as the oil-free aqueous mixed emulsifier systems (described later), are referred to as creams as they are also white and semisolid. The aqueous continuous phase of an o/w cream may be structured (1) directly, by the addition of the appropriate amount of structuring agent (often described as a rheological modifier) such as clay particles or polymeric materials, and/or (2) indirectly by interactions between various emulsifier components and water to form lamellar gel network phases.

Table 27.6 Selection of commonly used fatty amphiphiles and surfactants

Fatty amphiphile	Surfactant
Cetostearyl alcohol	Cetomacrogol 1000
Commercial cetyl alcohol	Sodium lauryl sulfate
Commercial stearyl alcohol	Cetrimide
Triple-pressed stearic acid	Triethanolamine stearate
Glyceryl monostearate	Sodium stearate

Although the consistencies of some complex cream formulations are controlled by both mechanisms, the stability and rheological properties of most aqueous creams are due mainly to the presence of lamellar gel networks in the continuous phases.

Formulation of aqueous creams

In the preparation of o/w creams, sparingly soluble fatty amphiphiles combined with more water-soluble ionic or ionic surfactants are widely used (Table 27.6). The components of the emulsifier may be added separately during the preparation of the cream, or in the form of a preblended emulsifying wax (Table 27.7). Some emulsifier combinations contain the same components (e.g. fatty alcohols and ionic surfactants) as those investigated originally by Schulman and Cockbain in their classic work on interfacial films (discussed in Chapter 5). The properties of such films, although important, are not the main mechanisms in controlling shelf-life stability of practical o/w creams.

In creams, long-term stability is due to the formation of viscoelastic gel network phases which trap oil droplets, preventing their movement and interaction. However, it is emphasized that interfacial films are still important because even complex multiphase emulsions are sometimes fluid during their lifetime, so droplets are then free to interact. For example, the existence of a strong interfacial film is particularly important at the high temperatures of preparation before networks consolidate, and in nonionic creams in which networks consolidate only slowly on storage. During the emulsification process, surfactant emulsifiers reduce interfacial tension, making droplets easier to break up, and the interfacial film then reduces the tendency for freshly formed droplets to recombine.

Table 27.7 Typical emulsifying waxes and their component surfactants

Emulsifying wax	Components	Weight ratio of alcohol to surfactant	Molar ratio of alcohol to surfactant
Emulsifying Wax BP	Cetostearyl alcohol, sodium lauryl sulfate	9:1	~12:1
Cationic Emulsifying Wax BP	Cetostearyl alcohol, cetrimide	9:1	~12:1
Cetomacrogol Emulsifying Wax BP	Cetostearyl alcohol, cetomacrogol 1000	4:1	~20:1
Glyceryl Stearate SE (self-emulsifying)	Glyceryl monostearate, anionic soap	–	–

The gel network theory of emulsion stability

The gel network theory of emulsion stability gives a coherent explanation for the manner in which fatty amphiphiles and surfactant combined as mixed emulsifiers not only stabilize o/w lotions and creams but also control their consistencies between wide limits, from mobile lotions at low concentrations of emulsifying wax to soft or stiff semisolid creams at higher concentrations (self-bodying action). Although most early work was performed using long-chain alcohols, the same general principles apply whichever amphiphile or surfactant (ionic or nonionic) is used. The gel network theory established that the structure and stability of o/w creams are dominated by the swelling properties of an α-crystalline gel network phase formed when the mixed emulsifier, in excess of the quantity required to form an interfacial film at the oil–water interface, interacts with continuous phase water.

A valuable method of approach when developing the theory was to investigate the interaction of mixed emulsifiers and their components in water over the ranges of concentration and temperature relevant to the manufacture, storage and use of the emulsion. This protocol is now generally adopted to develop new formulations. Oil-free ternary systems, containing concentrations of mixed emulsifier similar to those used to stabilize emulsions, are useful *structural models* for the continuous phases of the corresponding emulsions.

Interaction of mixed emulsifiers in water

Fig. 27.3 illustrates the phases that form spontaneously when a fatty alcohol such as cetostearyl alcohol is dispersed in water alone, and when it is dispersed in the presence of small quantities of surfactant at low and high temperature. Other fatty amphiphiles show similar phase behaviour, although the terminology used to describe the polymorphs may differ.

Pure long-chain alcohols exist in three polymorphic forms. The high temperature α-form separates first from the melt and is stable over a narrow temperature range. At lower temperatures, the β-form and the γ-form can coexist. Transition temperatures are lowered and polymorphic temperature ranges extended with homologue admixtures such as cetostearyl alcohol, and in the presence of water. Thus at room temperature, cetostearyl alcohol may be in the α-form, whilst pure cetyl or stearyl alcohols may exist as β-crystalline and γ-crystalline polymorphs. Crystallization in the α-form is generally a prerequisite for the formation of the swollen crystalline and liquid crystalline phases described later.

In excess water, the α-crystals show limited swelling to form waxy crystalline hydrates (Fig. 27.3). However, in the presence of very small quantities of ionic or nonionic surfactant (molar ratios of alcohol to surfactant in the region of 10:1 to 30:1, which are the proportions present in commercial emulsifying waxes; see Table 27.7), the swelling in excess water increases spontaneously to give a viscoelastic, swollen α-crystalline gel phase. On heating, the gel phase transforms to lamellar liquid crystals at a specific temperature, the crystalline gel–liquid transition temperature. The liquid crystalline phase in which the hydrocarbon chains are in a dynamic disordered state is fluid as it does not swell as extensively as the low-temperature gel phase (Fig. 27.3).

With cetostearyl alcohol and other amphiphiles used in pharmaceutical emulsions, the gel–liquid crystalline transition temperature is approximately 40 °C to 50 °C, so although fluid liquid crystalline phases are present at the high temperatures of emulsion manufacture, when the emulsion cools they convert to a semisolid gel network phase composed of a swollen crystalline gel phase in equilibrium with hydrated

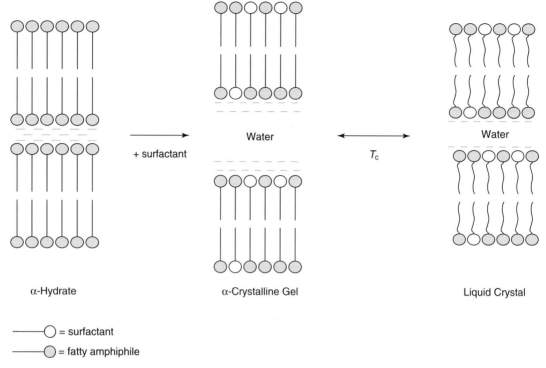

= surfactant

= fatty amphiphile

Fig. 27.3 • Illustration (not to scale) of the lamellar phases that form spontaneously at low and high temperatures when a fatty amphiphile and small quantities of ionic or nonionic surfactant are dispersed in water. T_c, gel–liquid crystalline phase transition temperature.

α-crystals and bulk free water. Many creams thicken at the transition temperature during the cooling process of manufacture, and this temperature is sometimes described as the 'setting temperature'.

Microstructure of creams

Fig. 27.4 shows a schematic diagram of a typical multiple-phase o/w cream. The emulsion is composed of four phases:

- dispersed oil phase stabilized by a mixed monomolecular film;
- α-crystalline gel phase composed of bilayers of surfactant and alcohol separated by layers of interlamellar fixed water;
- α-crystalline hydrates that show limited swelling in water; and
- bulk continuous phase free water.

This multicomponent continuous phase is viscoelastic, so the oil droplets are essentially immobilized in the structured continuous phase, preventing flocculation and coalescence.

Fig. 27.4 shows a general schematic representation. The overall consistency of the product (whether it is a structured liquid or a semisolid cream), its cosmetic appearance (shiny, pearly or matt), its rheological properties (fluid or semisolid) and its rheological stability on storage (thinning or thickening) are related to:

- the mechanisms and kinetics involved in the formation of the phases;
- the thickness of the interlamellar water layers;
- the proportion of the added water that is incorporated between the lamellae;
- the relative proportions of the three aqueous phases; and
- the stability of the three aqueous phases over a range of temperatures and batch variations of the components.

The gel network theory explains the manner in which formulation factors such as the nature of the fatty amphiphile and its homologue purity, the ionic or nonionic nature of the surfactant, the molar ratios of amphiphile to surfactant, and the total concentration of the mixed emulsifier will influence microstructure and properties.

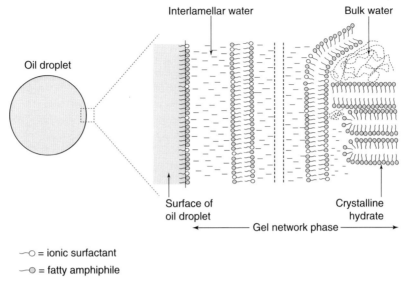

Fig. 27.4 • A typical oil-in-water cream showing the complex nature of the structured continuous phase. The interlamellar water thickness is not to scale.

Self-bodying action

The ability to control the consistency of o/w creams and the corresponding oil-free systems between wide limits by altering the mixed emulsifier concentration (self-bodying action) is related to the swelling ability of the lamellar gel network phase and its volume fraction. At low concentrations of mixed emulsifier, structured liquids form as the proportion of bulk (continuous phase) free water is relatively high. At higher concentrations of mixed emulsifier, the proportion of the swollen lamellar phase is increased, with a corresponding decrease in the amount of free bulk water, and emulsions become thicker or semisolid.

Fatty alcohol mixed emulsifiers

Ionic surfactants. Combinations of fatty alcohols and ionic surfactants exhibit a phenomenal swelling in the aqueous continuous phase of o/w emulsions, for the thickness of the water layers is more than 10 times the thickness of the hydrocarbon bilayers, as shown schematically in Fig. 27.5. The extensive swelling is electrostatic in nature. The surfactant molecules interpose among the fatty alcohol molecules, and electrical double layers arise from the dissociation and diffusion of counterions from the surfactant head groups at the surface of the bilayers into the surrounding water. Electrostatic repulsion between adjacent bilayers arises from the overlap of the electrical double layers, and is described by the Derjaguin–Landau–Verwey–Overbeek theory of colloid stability (see Chapter 5).

The addition of electrolytes, such as sodium chloride, to creams stabilized by ionic mixed emulsifiers reduces electrostatic swelling between the bilayers, thereby decreasing the gel network phase volume, with a corresponding increase in the quantity of bulk free water. Thus emulsions containing additional electrolyte are thinner, with lower apparent viscosities, than their electrolyte-free counterparts.

Nonionic polyoxyethylene surfactants. The fatty alcohols also swell in the presence of nonionic surfactants, although both the mechanism and the timescale are different from those for the ionic systems just described. With nonionic surfactants, the swelling of the α-crystals of fatty alcohol waxes is due to the hydration of the POE chains of the surfactant. These are oriented and extended into the interlamellar water, hydrated by this layer and stabilized by steric repulsions. With straight-chain POE surfactants, such as cetomacrogol 1000, containing a straight chain of 20–24 POE groups, the interlamellar thickness is approximately twice that of the extended chain length (Fig. 27.6).

Creams containing nonionic emulsifying waxes often show considerable structural changes on storage, sometimes changing from a milky liquid when first prepared to a semisolid on storage. Such changes are undesirable not only from a cosmetic point of view but also because variable bioavailability profiles may

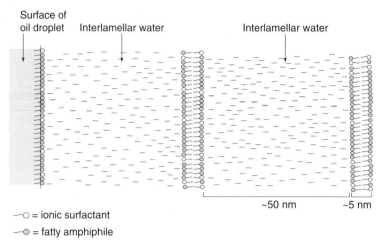

Fig. 27.5 • A multiphase oil-in-water cream stabilized by an ionic emulsifying wax to illustrate, to scale, the thickness of the interlamellar water layers.

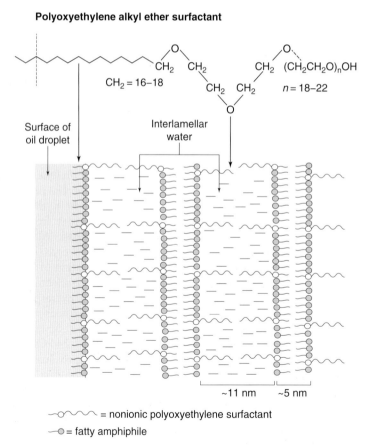

Fig. 27.6 • An oil-in-water cream stabilized by a fatty alcohol/nonionic (straight polyoxyethylene chain) surfactant emulsifying wax to illustrate, to scale, the thickness of the interlamellar water layers.

result. These changes can be explained by considering the relationship between temperature and hydration of POE chains. At the high temperature of preparation, the POE groups do not hydrate significantly. On cooling to below the transition temperature, the POE chains become increasingly soluble and bilayers form as the chains extend into and are hydrated by water. This means that the lamellar gel phase may only be partially formed after the cooling process, so the emulsion is thin immediately after preparation. On storage, the increased solubility of the POE chains allows additional gel phase to form, although this occurs very slowly because of the crystalline nature of the hydrocarbon chains. Thus emulsions thicken and gradually become semisolid on storage.

Fatty acid mixed emulsifiers

Fatty acids exhibit marked polymorphism, and also form lamellar gel network phases. Stearic acid is widely used as a component of 'vanishing' creams. Such creams are extensively used in cosmetics because they usually have an attractive pearlescent sheen, and appear to vanish during application, leaving a matt, nongreasy residue on the skin. Stearate creams are not traditional emulsions but are rather oil-free ternary systems composed of stearic acid, a stearate soap (i.e. an ionic surfactant) and water. The acid soap is formed in situ during the manufacture of the product from the partial neutralization (10% to 40%) of some of the fatty acid with alkali, traditionally triethanolamine, although sodium hydroxide and potassium hydroxide are also used in some formulations to produce potassium or sodium soaps. If an oil phase is included in the formulation, the stearic acid and its soap function as a mixed emulsifier to stabilize and control the consistency of the emulsion.

Stearate creams containing partially neutralized fatty acids show a more complicated phase behaviour than those prepared with alcohols, and they are extremely sensitive to mechanical disruption. Creams formed by the partial neutralization (35%) of stearic acid in situ by TEA contain a swollen lamellar gel phase with interlamellar water thickness ranging from 14 nm to 16 nm. This phase exists in equilibrium with crystals of stearic acid and bulk continuous phase water. The translucent nature of stearic acid crystals imparts a translucent sheen to the cream. In contrast, ordered swollen lamellar structures are not apparent in creams in which sodium hydroxide or potassium hydroxide is used to partially neutralize stearic acid. In these, the structure is a result of highly disordered interlinking bilayers of mixed emulsifier (twisted ribbons) holding vast amounts of water by capillary forces.

Self-emulsifying glyceryl monoesters

Glycerol monoesters are poor w/o emulsifiers. The self-emulsifying grades containing small quantities of either ionic or nonionic surfactant are essentially emulsifying waxes. When dispersed in water, the self-emulsifying grades form swollen lamellar gel network phases, and exhibit a self-bodying action in which mobile emulsions are obtained at low concentration and semisolid products are obtained at higher concentrations. In common with fatty acids, the network phases formed from self-emulsifying grades are very sensitive to mechanical disruption.

Molar ratio of fatty amphiphile to surfactant

For semisolid products structured by gel networks, a large excess of alcohol, in the region of at least 10–30 molecules of alcohol to one molecule of surfactant is essential. Commercial emulsifying waxes and those of the various pharmacopoeias contain such an excess of alcohol (Table 27.7). With higher surfactant concentrations, micellar phases rather than gel networks form. With excess alcohol, there is a broad range of molar ratios of alcohol to surfactant (from ~10:1 to 100:1) over which gel networks form. The ratio controls the relative proportions of the swollen gel, crystalline and water phases in the gel networks, and hence the appearance and rheological properties of the product. As the ratio of alcohol to surfactant increases, the proportion of crystals increases at the expense of swollen lamellar phase, and systems become progressively less structured and eventually fluid.

Source and batch variations of components

Source and batch variations of the components may cause undesirable changes in rheological behaviour, such as emulsion thinning or thickening during the shelf life. A thinner product may allow droplet interaction, leading to flocculation and coalescence on storage, whereas a thicker product may be cosmetically unacceptable.

Surfactants. The homologue composition of the hydrocarbon chains of the surfactant has little influence on the consistency of the product, owing to the low concentrations of surfactant chains in the bilayers. Batch variations of the POE chain length in nonionic surfactants can influence the consistency of the product, for there is a linear relationship between POE chain length, interlamellar water thickness and apparent viscosity. Batches with a higher proportion of long POE chains will produce thicker products, as more water is trapped between lamellae, and the opposite will occur with batches containing a higher proportion of shorter POE chains. Ionic impurities in charged surfactants may also cause minor variations in consistency by their influence in suppressing electrostatic swelling.

Fatty amphiphiles. In contrast, mixed homologue fatty alcohols and acids are essential for the formation of stable swollen gel network phases. Creams prepared from pure C_{16} or C_{18} alcohols, although initially semisolid, are rheologically unstable and break down on storage to form mobile crystalline fluids. This is because the gel network phase formed after a heating and cooling cycle of manufacture is unstable at low temperature. On storage, the swollen α-crystalline gel networks convert to nonswollen β-polymorphs and γ- polymorphs, and the system becomes fluid.

Similarly, pure homologue fatty acids do not form stable structured creams. Mixed homologue triple-pressed stearic acid, composed of approximately 45% stearic acid (C_{18}) and 55% palmitic acid (C_{16}) is generally used in cosmetic products.

Manufacture and processing of emulsions and creams

Fluid emulsions

When oil and water are mixed, energy in the form of agitation is necessary to produce the required droplet size distribution. Emulsifiers have an important role in the process of emulsification. Surfactant emulsifiers reduce interfacial tensions, making droplets easier to break up during mixing and reducing the tendency for them to recombine. Other emulsifiers, such as the polymeric macromolecules, alter the hydrodynamic forces generated during emulsification by their influence on rheological properties.

Emulsions are generally prepared experimentally on a small scale in the laboratory before their production is scaled up and they are manufactured in much larger quantities. Each scale of preparation involves similar generic steps. First, the emulsifying agents and other oil-soluble or water-soluble components are dissolved separately in the phase in which they are most soluble. When heat is required, for example to melt waxes in the oil phase during the preparation of lotions and creams, the oil phase and the water phase are heated separately to the same temperature (a few degrees above the highest melting point of the wax), and the elevated temperature is maintained as they are brought together and mixed. Prior heating of each phase to the same temperature before blending is important to avoid the formation of a granular or lumpy product by the premature solidification of the oil phase when it is mixed with the colder aqueous phase.

High temperature also has the advantage of reducing the consistency of the system, making it easier to mix. Generally, the dispersed phase is added to the external continuous phase with constant agitation to produce the required droplet size distribution. The emulsion is finally cooled (if necessary) to the storage temperature while mixing is continued. Volatile or heat-sensitive components are incorporated at the appropriate temperature as the emulsion cools.

A variation of this procedure is when o/w emulsions containing nonionic surfactant emulsifiers with PITs within the temperature range of normal processing (60 °C to 80 °C) are prepared by the phase inversion method. In this method, the external phase is added to the dispersed phase at temperatures above the PIT, temporarily forming a w/o emulsion. On cooling, the emulsion will revert to an o/w emulsion at a specific narrow temperature range, the PIT. Enormous forces are generated by phase inversion, and very fine nanosized droplets may be produced. This method is sometimes described as a low (applied) energy method as it utilizes the chemical energy of the system with minimal heat, rather than providing external energy from extreme agitation.

On an industrial scale, the oil and water phases are often heated separately in large tanks, and then combined by the pumping of each phase into the mixing vessel fitted with a suitable emulsification agitator, such as a mechanical mixer or homogenizer. Proprietary mixing vessels are available in a variety of sizes to accommodate a few hundred litres of emulsion in the initial scale-up, to several thousand litres for manufacture. The mixing vessel is usually made from stainless steel, jacketed so that heating or cooling can be applied, and sometimes fitted with baffles to modify circulation of the emulsion during mixing.

A wide range of agitation techniques are available for dispersing the internal phase into droplets. These include simple hand mixers, various stirrers and propeller or turbine mixers, homogenizers, microfluidizers, colloid mills and ultrasonic devices. Most disrupt droplets by shear forces in laminar flow, by inertial forces in turbulent flow or by cavitation during ultrasound agitation. Extensional flow, where there is a velocity gradient in the direction of flow, also has a very powerful droplet-breaking effect.

The choice of emulsification equipment for a particular emulsion depends on a number of inter-related factors, including:

- the volume of emulsion to be prepared, i.e. whether laboratory or production scale;
- the type of emulsifier used;
- the range of droplet sizes required; and
- the flow properties of the emulsion during the emulsification and cooling processes.

For the extemporaneous preparation of small quantities of a fluid emulsion, blending the oil and water phases in the presence of a suitable emulsifier in a mortar and pestle or by manual shaking or stirring is often sufficient to produce a coarse emulsion with droplets sizes in the region of 1 μm to 50 μm. Mechanical hand stirrers with the stirring rod held or placed directly into the system to be emulsified may also be used. Mechanical mixers, fitted with various impellers and paddles, are available in various sizes and with various motor speeds to prepare both small-scale and large-scale batches of emulsion.

When smaller droplets with narrower droplet size distributions are required, stronger agitation techniques are necessary. Nanoemulsion formulations that are unsuitable for preparation by the phase inversion method require extreme forces to overcome the large interfacial tension and form nanosized droplets. Parenteral emulsions also require a large input of energy to produce droplet sizes considerably smaller than 1 μm; thus lipid and perfluorochemical emulsions are usually prepared aseptically by homogenization at high temperature and pressure, or by microfluidization (see later).

Homogenizers are available for processing quantities of emulsions from a few millilitres in the laboratory up to several thousand litres for manufacture. Homogenizers function essentially by forcing the crude mixture of liquids through a small orifice under pressure. In some, the liquid impacts on a solid surface set at right angles to the direction of flow and, depending on the pressure applied, the intense extensional, shear and turbulent flow patterns develop to produce fine droplets smaller than 1 μm. Membrane homogenizers produce emulsions with uniform fine droplet sizes on a laboratory scale by forcing the internal phase to flow through specific glass membranes into the external phase under high external pressure.

Microfluidizers are also commonly used to prepare parenteral emulsions in both the laboratory and on scale-up. Separate oil and water phases are pumped into a chamber under high pressure, causing the liquids to accelerate at high velocity and interact with each other as they impinge on a hard surface. The shear and turbulent forces induced lead to the break-up of droplets to form an emulsion. Very small droplets are produced by recycling of the system a number of times through the microfluidizer.

Although both ultrasound and colloid mills also produce very small droplet sizes, their use is usually confined to laboratory-scale batches. Colloid mills generate considerable heat and so need extremely efficient cooling, which is expensive with large-scale batches. Ultrasound produces alternate regions of cavitation and compression in the emulsion, and very fine droplets form when the cavities collapse with extreme force. However, the energy density is highly localized, giving poorer reproducibility on a large scale.

Multiple emulsions

Multiple emulsions are generally prepared in two steps. In the first step a w/o or o/w emulsion (the primary emulsion) is prepared using a suitable emulsifier. The primary emulsion is then reemulsified during the second step to form a w/o/w or o/w/o multiple emulsion. The primary emulsion is prepared under high shear conditions to obtain small inner droplets, whilst the secondary emulsification step is performed at lower shear to avoid rupture of the internal droplets.

Creams

The processing and manufacture of commercial creams is more complex than for fluid emulsions because structure is formed in addition to droplet phases during their preparation. Scale-up, based on a previously developed laboratory procedure, is particularly challenging because of the difficulties in matching the exact laboratory conditions of preparation. Every type of emulsification equipment introduces energy into the system in a different way. On scale-up, energy input and hence emulsion microstructure can be affected by a change in the settings of a specific type of mixer when a larger volume is processed. Other relatively minor differences in processing such as the rate of the heating and cooling cycle, the order of adding the components and the extent of mixing may cause marked variations in the consistency and rheological profile of the resulting emulsions.

An essential approach to optimize processing conditions and obtain a reproducible cream is to identify the key structuring agents in the formulation, the mechanisms involved in forming the structure and the relationships between microstructure and processing variables. The knowledge gained can be used to optimize the manufacturing process to give a reproducible product using a minimum number of components. The processing conditions required to produce the swollen gel network phases when different types of emulsifying wax are incorporated can be identified using the gel network theory. For example, preparation techniques, in particular cooling rates and mixing, have a marked effect on the initial and final consistencies of creams prepared with fatty alcohol/nonionic POE surfactants. Shock cooling and limited mixing initially produces very mobile emulsions, which gel on storage. In contrast, slow cooling and increased mixing forms semisolid systems. These variations in rheological properties are related to the hydration of the POE groups and the mechanisms by which nonionic gel networks form, as discussed earlier in this chapter. To optimize the manufacture and minimize changes on storage (shelf-life stability) of such creams, slow cooling followed by vigorous agitation at temperatures just higher than the transition temperature are required.

Lamellar gel network phases formed in creams containing fatty acids are particularly sensitive to agitation. The ordered lamellar gel phases are metastable and convert to nonswollen crystals when mixed at high shear rates. The cream remains semisolid if mixing is discontinued at the transition temperature and the system is allowed to cool undisturbed. A more mobile system is formed if it is mixed below the transition temperature, and systems may need to 'rest' to allow the structure to rebuild.

Some complex commercial creams contain a number of different structuring agents within the same formulation, each of which needs different processing conditions to develop fully their structure. For example, rheological modifiers, such as clays, and natural and synthetic polymers, often have completely different processing requirements. Clays need to be processed under severe conditions of high temperatures and shear rates, with addition of electrolyte at the appropriate time, in order to ensure the structure is fully formed. Polymer hydration, on the other hand, often requires dispersion and wetting at a much lower temperature with much milder agitation to prevent polymer degradation and structure loss. Nonreproducible products with variable rheological profiles may result if the different sensitivities of each structuring mechanism to mixing, shear and temperature are not recognized and accommodated in the manufacturing process. In such cases, processing is optimized by identification of the optimum processing conditions for each individual structure beforehand, processing each structure off-line to ensure structure is fully formed before blending each fully developed structure together in a commercial mixing vessel.

Emulsion properties

Identification of emulsion type

It is important to confirm whether an emulsion is an o/w emulsion, a w/o emulsion or a multiple emulsion as this can significantly influence its application and properties. Generally, an emulsion exhibits the characteristics of its external (continuous) phase, and there are a number of simple tests based on this for distinguishing between o/w and w/o types of emulsion. The tests, some of which are described in the following paragraphs, essentially identify the continuous phase and do not identify a multiple emulsion. This can be resolved by microscopy.

Water or oil miscibility. An emulsion will only mix freely with a liquid that is miscible with its continuous phase. Thus a small quantity of water dropped onto the surface of an o/w emulsion will immediately mix with the external phase and disappear, whereas the water droplets will remain on the surface of a w/o emulsion. The reverse is true if a small quantity of oil is dropped onto the emulsion.

Filter paper test. The test involves putting a few drops of emulsion onto filter paper. If the droplet spreads rapidly into the filter paper, it is an o/w emulsion, as water (the external phase) tends to spread more rapidly throughout the filter paper than oil from a w/o emulsion.

Conductivity measurements. These are based on the principle that water conducts electricity better than oils. Thus, generally, o/w emulsions have a much higher electrical conductivity than w/o emulsions. A light source will glow when electrodes (connected in series to a battery and a suitable light source) are dipped into an o/w emulsion but not when they are placed in a w/o emulsion.

Dye solubility tests. These tests involve blending either a water-soluble dye or an oil-soluble dye with the emulsion. If a water-soluble dye is used, an o/w emulsion will be evenly coloured, whereas a w/o emulsion will be much paler. Microscopically, an o/w emulsion will appear as colourless droplets against a coloured background, whereas a w/o emulsion will appear as coloured droplets against a colourless background.

Droplet size distribution

It is important to control droplet sizes as they influence emulsion stability, biopharmaceutical properties, and clinical use. Droplet size distribution is related to the energy input during preparation, the viscosity difference between the phases and the characteristics of the emulsifier. Large droplets have a greater tendency to cream and coalesce, and a broad particle size distribution encourages an increase in droplet size by Ostwald ripening (see the section entitled 'Emulsion stability'). Thus the most physically stable pharmaceutical emulsions generally have small droplets and narrow size distributions. Ostwald ripening alone governs instability in nanoemulsions, as the very small droplets do not cream, flocculate or coalescence to any great extent (see the section entitled 'Emulsion stability').

For oral emulsions, gastrointestinal absorption increases as droplet sizes decreases. Whilst this is desirable with oral formulations of nutrient oils alone or with drugs dissolved in them, it may give adverse clinical effects with laxative oils that are used for a local effect and are toxic if absorbed. The clearance kinetics of parenteral emulsions is influenced by the droplet size distribution. Individual droplets should not exceed approximately 5 μm in diameter (the diameter of the smallest blood vessels) in intravenous emulsions because of the possibility of pulmonary embolism. Droplets smaller than 5 μm are rapidly cleared from the bloodstream by elements of the reticuloendothelial system, also known as the mononuclear phagocyte system (primarily by Kupffer cells of the liver). This natural targeting to the liver offers opportunities for the treatment of tropical diseases such as leishmaniasis and fungal infections

such as candidiasis. Drug delivery from dermatological preparations is also improved in lipid nanoemulsions.

Droplet charge provided by the emulsifier film influences the biological fate of the droplets as well as emulsion stability. For example, negatively charged droplets are cleared more rapidly from the blood than neutral or positively charged ones. Emulsions stabilized by nonionic POE surfactants circulate for longer in the blood and cationic emulsions are better for dermatological delivery.

Rheology

An emulsion should possess shear thinning rheological characteristics (see Chapter 6) appropriate to its intended use. For example, a dermatological cream must be thin enough to spread easily onto damaged skin without causing pain, but should rapidly regain structure so that it is thick enough to remain in place on the skin after application. The rheological properties of emulsions are influenced mainly by the phase volume ratio, the nature of the continuous phase, and, to a lesser extent, droplet size distributions. A variety of products ranging from mobile liquids to structured fluids and thick semisolids can be formulated by altering the dispersed phase volume and/or the nature and concentration of the emulsifiers.

For low internal phase volume emulsions, the consistency of the emulsion is similar to that of the continuous phase. Thus w/o emulsions are generally thicker than o/w emulsions. The consistencies of o/w systems are further increased by the addition of emulsifiers such as gums, clays, polymers and other thickening agents which impart plastic or pseudoplastic flow properties, often accompanied by thixotropy (see Chapter 6). At rest, the high apparent viscosity inhibits the movement of droplets, maintaining a physically stable emulsion. During use, higher shear rates are applied and apparent viscosities reduce (shear thinning), so the emulsion flows freely when injected or poured from a container.

Emulsifying waxes, used to stabilize structured lotions and semisolid creams, interact with water to form a viscoelastic continuous phase. Such emulsions are particularly difficult to characterize rheologically, because at rest solid properties dominate (hence the term *semisolid*), but on application of a force, structure is broken down *irreversibly* as systems thin and flow, producing very complex flow curves. Such flow curves, however, are sensitive to relatively small changes in consistency. Viscoelastic measurements are also useful in characterizing complex multiphase emulsions.

Emulsion stability

Definition of stability

A kinetically stable emulsion is one in which the dispersed droplets retain their initial character and remain uniformly dispersed throughout the continuous phase. In pharmaceutical emulsions, stability has a much wider definition as it is generally equated with a long shelf life. Thus in addition to kinetic stability, the emulsion must retain its original appearance, odour and consistency, and exhibit no microbial contamination.

Chemical instability

Ideally, all emulsion components should be chemically inert under the conditions of emulsification. Unfortunately, this is not always the case, so it is important to understand the chemical nature of all the emulsion components before a selection is made. Particular care has to be taken in the selection of pharmaceutical oils as they may be susceptible to oxidation by atmospheric oxygen or microbial contamination, developing an unpleasant odour and taste as they become rancid. Antioxidants and preservatives may be incorporated into the emulsion to minimize these effects. Polymeric emulsifiers may undergo depolymerization by hydrolysis or microbial degradation, with loss of emulsification power and consistency.

Interactions between the emulsifying agent and other components are of particular concern because emulsifying properties may be destroyed, causing the emulsion to break (see later). For example, POE nonionic emulsifiers form hydrogen bonds with phenolic preservatives, leading to poor preservation as well as loss of emulsifying power. Ionic emulsifying agents are usually incompatible with materials of the opposite charge. This occurs when cationic materials such as surfactants or drugs (e.g. cetrimide, neomycin sulfate) are added to a cream containing an anionic emulsifying agent such as sodium lauryl sulfate. The cream loses consistency on storage because lamellar structures in the continuous phase are destroyed by the resultant suppression of repulsive forces.

Physical instability

An emulsion without an emulsifier will quickly return to the original state of separate oil and water layers; that is, the emulsion will *break* or *crack*. In the presence of an emulsifier, this state is approached via four distinct processes, creaming, flocculation, coalescence and Ostwald ripening. Phase inversion, where a w/o emulsion inverts to an o/w emulsion or vice versa, is a special type of instability. The processes of instability are illustrated by the schematic representations in Fig. 27.7.

The destabilization processes are not independent and each may influence or be influenced by the others. In practice, they may proceed simultaneously or in any order. Coalescence and Ostwald ripening are the most serious types of instability, as they result in the formation of progressively larger droplets which will ultimately lead to phase separation. Creaming and flocculation, on the other hand, are subtler forms as they represent potential steps towards coalescence due to the close proximity of the droplets.

Creaming

Creaming is a process which occurs when the dispersed droplets separate under the influence of gravity to form a layer of more concentrated emulsion, the cream. Creaming occurs inevitably in any dilute emulsion containing relatively large droplets (~1 μm) if there is a density difference between the oil and water phases. Most oils are less dense than water, so that the oil droplets in an o/w emulsion rise to the surface to form an upper layer of cream, whereas water droplets sediment to form a lower layer in w/o emulsions. Although a creamed emulsion can be restored to its original state by gentle agitation, this is considered undesirable because the emulsion is inelegant and, more seriously, the patient may receive an inadequate dose if the emulsion is not agitated sufficiently before use.

The most effective way in practice to reduce creaming is to prepare emulsions with small droplet sizes, and to thicken the external phase by the addition of viscosity modifiers (see Stokes law, Chapters 5 and 6). Density adjustment to decrease the density difference between the two phases has received little attention.

Flocculation

Flocculation is a weak, reversible association between emulsion droplets which are separated by trapped continuous phase. Each cluster of droplets (floccule) behaves physically as a single kinetic unit, although every droplet in the floccule retains its individuality. Floccules can be redispersed by mild agitation, such

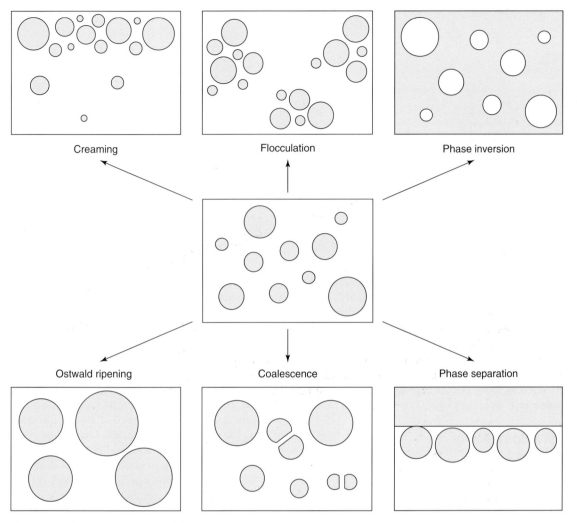

Fig. 27.7 • The processes of emulsion breakdown.

as shaking of the container. Flocculation is discussed in detail in Chapter 5 in terms of the attractive van der Waals forces pulling the droplets together and the repulsive forces tending to keep them apart. It occurs in the secondary minimum as illustrated in the schematic curve of the potential energy versus distance of separation plot (see Fig. 5.4) and is controlled by the properties of the emulsifier film, which modifies the repulsive forces between dispersed emulsion droplets. Thus the tendency for flocculation can be reduced by the use of a suitable emulsifier. Although the timescale between flocculation and coalescence can be extended almost indefinitely by the adsorbed emulsifier, flocculation is generally considered undesirable because floccules cream more

rapidly under the influence of gravity than individual emulsion droplets.

Coalescence

Coalescence describes the irreversible process in which dispersed phase droplets merge to form larger droplets. The process will continue until the emulsion breaks (cracks) and there is complete separation of the oil and water phases. Coalescence occurs when the emulsion droplets are able to overcome the repulsive energy barrier and approach the primary minimum (see Fig. 5.4). Once in this minimum, they are in very close proximity to each other, so stability against coalescence is determined essentially by the

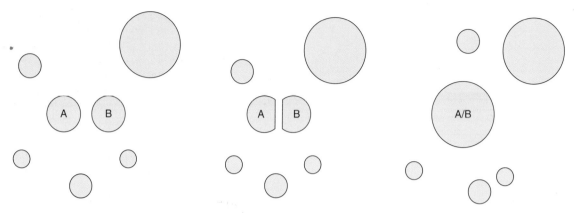

Fig. 27.8 • Flocculation and coalescence of dispersed droplets.

resistance of the interfacial film to rupture. Coalescence begins with the drainage of liquid films of continuous phase from between the oil droplets as they approach one another and become distorted, and ends with the rupture of the film (Fig. 27.8). Rigid close-packed elastic films formed by specific emulsifier mixtures and thick multilayered films provided by many polymers protect droplets against coalescence as they are highly resistant to film rupture.

Ostwald ripening

Ostwald ripening is an irreversible process which involves the growth of large droplets at the expense of smaller ones. Ostwald ripening occurs in emulsions containing small sub-micrometre droplets (smaller than ~600 nm), provided that the dispersed phase also has a significant solubility in the continuous phase. Ostwald ripening is a direct consequence of the Kelvin effect, which explains how the solubility of a partially miscible droplet increases markedly as its radius decreases. Thus small emulsion droplets have a higher solubility than larger droplets. In order to reach the state of equilibrium, the small droplets dissolve and their molecules diffuse through the continuous phase and redeposit onto larger droplets, which grow bigger (ripen), resulting in an overall increase in average droplet size. Ostwald ripening differs from coalescence in that it does not need any contact between the droplets.

Ostwald ripening, rather than coalescence, is the underlying mechanism of instability in many o/w fat emulsions and in perfluorocarbon emulsions. Although flocculation and coalescence are inhibited by the properties of surfactant interfacial films, Ostwald ripening may actually be enhanced if micelles are also present to further solubilize the oil. Ostwald ripening can be prevented by the addition of a small quantity of an immiscible second oil to the main partially miscible oil to reduce molecular diffusion of this major component. Fat emulsions containing local anaesthetics or local analgesics show enhanced stability in the presence of less soluble hydrophobic oils, and perfluorodecalin contrast media emulsions are more stable in the presence of small quantities of insoluble perfluorotributylamine. Ostwald ripening is also inhibited by the addition of the surfactant Pluronic F68®, which is strongly adsorbed at the o/w interface and does not form micelles in the continuous phase. Polymers that increase the viscosity of the emulsion external phase also inhibit Ostwald ripening as they slow down the molecular diffusion process.

Emulsion inversion

Emulsion inversion occurs occasionally in emulsions under specific conditions. A change in emulsifier solubility from water soluble at low temperature to oil soluble at high temperature (e.g. some nonionic surfactants) causes phase inversion at a specific temperature from an o/w emulsion to a w/o emulsion, and this phenomenon is used in the low-energy preparation of nanoemulsions. Emulsion inversion may also occur by specific interactions with other additives. For example, if a sodium salt is used to stabilize an o/w emulsion, the emulsion may invert to a w/o emulsion by the addition of divalent ions, such as Ca^{2+} ions, to form the calcium salt, which stabilizes a w/o emulsion.

Stabilization by use of mixed emulsifiers

It has already been indicated that pharmaceutical emulsions, whether they are dilute mobile systems for internal use or thick semisolid creams for application to the skin, contain mixtures of emulsifiers, as these form more stable emulsions. For example, mixtures of nonionic surfactants of high and low HLB generally form more stable emulsions than either surfactant alone. The lecithins used to stabilize oral and parenteral emulsions are natural mixtures of neutral and charged lipids. Mixtures of sparingly soluble fatty amphiphiles combined with more soluble ionic or nonionic surfactants are widely used in dermatological o/w lotions and creams, sometimes in the form of a preblended emulsifying wax.

Multiphase emulsions

Emulsifier concentration

In simple, dilute two-phase oil and water emulsions, the stabilizing effect of a mixed surfactant emulsifier at low concentration is generally attributed to its ability to form a close-packed mixed monolayer at the oil–water interface, which gives a mechanically strong condensed film. The interfacial film introduces repulsive forces (electrostatic or steric) to inhibit the close approach of droplets, and forms a mechanical barrier to coalescence if droplets do collide.

Most practical pharmaceutical emulsions, however, contain higher concentrations of a mixed emulsifier than are necessary to form a monomolecular film. The excess emulsifier interacts with water either at the oil droplet interface or in the bulk continuous phase to form specific lamellar liquid crystalline or crystalline gel network phases. Such emulsions that contain phases additional to oil and water are described as *multiphase emulsions* (not to be confused with the term *multiple emulsion*; see the section entitled 'Introduction'). Lamellar phases are particularly important in controlling the consistency and stability of aqueous lotions and creams stabilized by emulsifying waxes, and the stability of parenteral emulsions containing lecithin.

Lamellar liquid crystalline and gel phases

Lamellar phases are formed in o/w emulsions containing various synthetic and natural emulsifier mixtures under specific conditions. In such lamellar phases the surfactant molecules are arranged in bilayers separated by layers of water. The hydrocarbon chains of the bilayers can exist in a number of physical states, the most relevant to emulsions being the ordered α-crystalline gel state at low temperatures and the more disordered fluid liquid crystalline state at higher temperatures (Fig. 27.3).

α-Crystalline gel network phases. These phases dominate the rheological properties and stabilities of many structured o/w lotions and semisolid creams, and these vastly swollen phases were considered in detail earlier in this chapter. The viscoelastic gel network phases essentially stabilize emulsions kinetically by trapping the oil droplets, thus preventing their movement and consequent interaction.

Lamellar liquid crystalline phases. It has already been noted that the lecithins used to stabilize parenteral emulsions are complex mixtures of neutral lipids (amphiphiles) and small quantities of negatively charged lipids, i.e. the lecithins can be considered as natural emulsifying waxes. With commercial lecithins, the gel–liquid crystalline transition temperatures (which are influenced by the length and degree of saturation or branching of the hydrocarbon chains) are low, so swollen liquid crystalline phases (rather than crystalline gel network phases) stabilize parenteral emulsions (see Fig. 27.3). The liquid crystalline phases do not swell as extensively as crystalline gel network phases; thus parenteral emulsions are mobile liquids rather than semisolids.

Multilayers of viscous liquid crystals surround the oil droplets in oral and parenteral emulsions stabilized by lecithin which protect them from coalescence by two main mechanisms. Firstly, the multilayers reduce the van der Waals forces of attraction between oil droplets to a very low value, thereby reducing the tendency for collision, and secondly the high viscosity of the liquid crystalline arrays retards the film thinning process of coalescence if droplets do collide. The high viscosities of the liquid crystalline arrays may also protect the emulsion against Ostwald ripening by slowing down the molecular diffusion process.

Nanoemulsion stability

Although both emulsions and nanoemulsions are thermodynamically unstable, the kinetics of destabilization of nanoemulsions is extremely slow, so they are considered to possess a relatively high kinetic stability, sometimes lasting many years. The small droplet sizes of nanoemulsions confer stability against creaming and coalescence because the droplets do not collide as frequently as in an ordinary emulsion, so Ostwald ripening alone governs the destabilization process.

Stability testing

Only studies of an emulsion over its full shelf life will give an accurate picture of its stability. However, useful information can be obtained in a shorter period by use of accelerated stability testing programmes (see Chapter 49). This is accomplished by placement of an external stress on the emulsion and observation of the changes in one or more of its physical properties. The stresses most commonly used are freezing and thawing, elevated temperature, UV light sources and various mechanical stresses.

Evaluation of emulsion stability

Several techniques are used to evaluate the stability of the emulsion under one or more of the conditions just described. Instabilities of a chemical or physical nature are generally identified by changes in physical properties of the emulsion. The extent of instability is assessed by measuring the magnitude of the change with time. The techniques commonly used for fluid emulsions involve evaluating changes in appearance, droplet size distribution, droplet charge and rheological properties in real time, and under accelerated conditions of temperature or force (i.e. centrifugation). With structured and semisolid emulsions, phase changes on storage may cause changes in consistency which not only render the emulsion inelegant and difficult to use but can also influence drug delivery. For complex systems, additional methods to identify and evaluate structural changes on storage include thermal methods (differential scanning calorimetry, thermogravimetric analysis) and X-ray diffraction.

Appearance

An approximate estimation of physical stability can be made from a visible assessment of the extent of 'creaming' that occurs on storage. Centrifugation is sometimes employed as a means of speeding up this separation process, although the results may be misleading as the centrifugal forces may destroy floccules or structure in the emulsions, which would not occur under normal storage conditions.

Droplet size analysis

Coalescence and/or Ostwald ripening will cause increases in droplet sizes with time, and a number of direct and indirect techniques are available for measuring such changes. In emulsions containing droplets larger than 1 μm, optical microscopy is particularly useful because it provides a direct (and reassuring) measurement of individual droplet sizes. The tedium of counting droplets to obtain size distributions is reduced by the use of image analysis. Indirect methods generally involve laser light-scattering techniques (see Chapter 9) and are used extensively with emulsions containing sub-micrometre droplets. However, extreme caution should be exercised in interpreting data from such techniques. A major problem is that samples are often diluted before measurements are made (e.g. to reduce the turbidity for laser diffraction experiments), thus changing the phase volume ratio and characteristics of the original emulsion. In addition, flocculation can give an apparent increase in the droplet size distribution, and deflocculants added before measurements are made may also influence emulsion stability and droplet distribution.

Droplet charge, zeta potential

The zeta potential of emulsion droplets stabilized by a charged interfacial film (see Chapter 5) is particularly useful for assessing instability due to flocculation. It can be determined by observing the movement of droplets under the influence of an electric current (electrophoretic mobility measurements), often in conjunction with dynamic light scattering (photon correlation spectroscopy; see Chapter 9). This technique is particularly useful for assessing the stability of fat emulsions and other emulsions containing charged droplets, where the presence of additives may result in changes in the zeta potential and kinetic instability as droplet sizes increase. For example, decreased stability in fat emulsions after the addition of electrolytes or dextrose (which lowers the pH) can be correlated with a lowering of the zeta potential.

Rheological measurements

Rheological measurements are used extensively to evaluate emulsion stability over time (see Chapter 6). Changes in droplet size distributions, the degree of flocculation and creaming, or the phase behaviour of the emulsifiers usually alter the rheological properties. Generally multipoint cone and plate or concentric cylinder rheometers are used to plot the relationship between shear stress and shear rate between suitable limits, and to calculate the apparent viscosities at specific shear rates. Fluid emulsions generally exhibit shear thinning pseudoplastic or plastic behaviour, sometimes accompanied by thixotropy. Semisolid and structured emulsions give much more complex flow curves which are difficult to interpret, although attempts are made to correlate derived parameters, such as apparent viscosities and loop areas, with the qualitative term consistency. Despite difficulties in interpretation, such flow curves are very sensitive to minor changes in the emulsion. More fundamental viscoelastic (creep and oscillation) techniques where the emulsions are examined in their rheological ground states also enable instability on storage to be monitored. Rheological measurements performed above the phase transition temperature do not relate to the emulsion at rest.

Thermal techniques

Techniques such as differential thermal analysis and thermogravimetric analysis are particularly useful in investigating the phase behaviour of complex multiphase emulsions such as creams, and may be used to follow any phase changes that occur on storage.

X-ray diffraction

High- and low-angle X-ray diffraction experiments provide direct and accurate measurements of bilayer structure and interlamellar water spacing in creams. Such measurements, which were used extensively to develop the gel network theory, may also be used to investigate phase changes on storage, and to relate such changes to corresponding changes in rheological properties.

Please check your eBook at **https://studentconsult. inkling.com/** for self-assessment questions. See inside cover for registration details.

Bibliography

Anton, N., Vandamme, T.F., 2011. Nano-emulsions and micro-emulsions: clarifications of the critical differences. Pharm. Res. 28, 978–985.

Eccleston, G.M., 1997. The functions of mixed emulsifiers and emulsifying waxes in dermatological lotions and creams. Colloids and Surfaces 123, 169–182.

Eccleston, G.M., Behan-Martin, M.K., Jones, G., et al., 2000. Synchrotron X-ray Investigations into the lamellar gel phase formed in pharmaceutical creams prepared with cetrimide and fatty alcohols. Int. J. Pharm. 203, 127–139.

Eccleston, G.M., 2013. Emulsions and microemulsions. In: Swarbrick, J., Boylan, J.C. (Eds.), Encyclopaedia of Pharmaceutical Science and Technology, vol. 1, 4th ed. Informa Healthcare, New York.

Florence, A.T., Attwood, D., 2016. Physicochemical Principles of Pharmacy: In Manufacture, Formulation and Clinical Use, 6th ed. Pharmaceutical Press, London.

Jones, D., 2016. FASTtrack Pharmaceutics – Dosage Form and Design, 2nd ed. Pharmaceutical Press, London.

Rowe, R.C., Sheskey, P.J., Cook, W.G., et al., 2016. Handbook of Pharmaceutical Excipients, 8th ed. Pharmaceutical Press, London.

28

Powders, granules and granulation

Michael E. Aulton

CHAPTER CONTENTS

KEY POINTS

- Powders and granules are themselves dosage forms.
- Powders and granules can be filled into sachets and be administered as a dosage form. This is most commonly used for low-potency drugs.
- Powders can also be an intermediary for drugs normally administered as a solution or suspension in an aqueous vehicle. These are reconstituted just prior to use to avoid chemical degradation. Antibiotic powders for syrups and powders for injection are examples.
- Powders are also used for inhalation (pulmonary or nasal) and for external use (dusting powders).
- Granules are most commonly used as an intermediate in the manufacture of other dosage forms. Most pharmaceutical granules have a short lifetime before being incorporated into tablets (mainly) or hard capsule dosage forms.
- Powders are granulated for many reasons – to prevent segregation of the constituents of the powder mix, to improve the flow properties of the mix and to improve the compaction characteristics of the mix.
- There are many types of granulation process: dry granulation (roller compaction) and wet granulation (shear granulators, high-speed mixer granulators, fluidized-bed granulation, extrusion–spheronization and spray-drying). There is also water-free melt granulation for water-sensitive products.
- The mechanism of granule formation from powder particles will influence the structure of granules and therefore their properties.

Introduction to powders and granules

The scientific and technical aspects of powders and powder technology are discussed in Part 2. This chapter discusses the use of powders and granulated products in pharmaceutical dosage forms. Powders and granules are used as dosage forms in their own right, but by far the greatest use of granules in pharmaceutical manufacturing is as an intermediate during the manufacture of compressed tablets.

What is a powder?

A powder is generally considered to be composed of a collection of solid, loose, dry particles of the same or different chemical compositions having equivalent diameters less than approximately 1000 μm. When necessary, the term *primary powder particle* is used to distinguish individual power particles from bulk powder. The term 'powder', when used in the context of a dosage form, describes an administrable formulation in which drug powder has been mixed with other powdered excipients to produce a powdered final product. Two groups of powders are recognized by pharmacopoeias – *oral powders* and *topical powders*. The function of the added excipients depends on the intended use of the product. For example, colouring, flavouring, sweetening, and taste masking agents may be added to powders for oral use.

What is a granule?

Granules are preparations containing solid, dry aggregated groups of smaller powder particles, or individual larger particles that may have overall dimensions greater than 1000 μm.

The process of *granulation* is where dry primary powder particles (i.e. single, discrete powder particles) are processed to make them adhere to form larger multiparticulate entities called granules.

Pharmaceutical granules typically have a size range between 0.2 mm and 4.0 mm, depending on the subsequent use of the granules. In the majority of cases, when granules will be made as an intermediate product for tableting, they have a size range towards the lower end of this spectrum (typically 0.2 mm to 0.5 mm). When granules are prepared for use as a dosage form in their own right, they are usually larger (typically 1 mm to 4 mm).

Granules must have suitable mechanical properties. Those manufactured to be used as a dosage form must be sufficiently robust to withstand handling (packaging and transportation). Those intended to be compressed into tablets must also be robust and nonfriable but must also deform and bond during compression to ensure that a compact is formed.

Reasons for granulation

The reasons why granulation is often necessary are described in the following sections.

Prevention of segregation of the constituents of the powder mix

Segregation (or demixing, discussed in Chapter 11) occurs primarily due to differences in the size and/ or density of the components of the powder mix; the smaller particles and/or denser particles concentrate at the base of a container with the large particles and/or less dense ones above them. An ideal granulation will contain all the constituents of the mix in the correct proportion in each granule, and if this is achieved, segregation of individual ingredients will not occur (Fig. 28.1).

It is also important to control the particle size distribution of the granules because, although the individual components may not segregate, if there is a wide size distribution of the granules themselves, they may segregate. If this occurs in the hoppers of sachet-filling machines, capsule-filling machines or tableting machines, individual dose units having large weight variations will result. This is because these machines fill by volume rather than weight. If different regions in the hopper contain granules of different sizes (and hence different bulk density), a given volume from each region will contain a different weight of granules. This will lead to an unacceptable variability of the drug content within the batch of finished product even if the drug is evenly distributed, weight per weight, through individual granules.

Improvement of the flow properties of the mix

Many powders, because of their small size, irregular shape or surface characteristics, are cohesive and do not flow well. Poor powder flow will also often result in a wide weight variation within the final product due to, for example, variable fill of tablet dies. The resulting granules produced from irregular particles will be larger and more isodiametric, both factors contributing to improved flow properties (discussed more fully in Chapter 12).

Improvement of the compaction characteristics of the mix

Some primary powder particles are difficult to compact into tablets even if a readily compactable

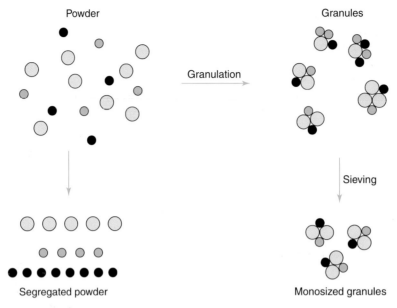

Fig. 28.1 • Illustration of how granulation can prevent powder segregation.

adhesive is included in the blend. Granules of the same formulation are often more easily compacted and produce stronger tablets. This is associated with the method employed to produce the granule and its resulting structure. Often solute migration (see Chapter 29) may occur during the post-wet granulation drying stage and this can result in the granules having a binder-rich outer layer. This in turn leads to direct binder–binder bonding, which assists the consolidation of weakly bonding materials.

Other reasons

The previous reasons are the primary reasons for the granulation of pharmaceutical products but there are other reasons which may necessitate the granulation of powdered material:

- The granulation of powdered toxic materials will reduce the hazard associated with the generation of toxic dust during handling. Suitable precautions must be taken to ensure that such dust is not a hazard during the granulation process itself (notably in the dry state, such as during the mixing of the dry ingredients and during drying of the granules). The granules produced should be nonfriable and have a suitable mechanical strength.
- Materials which are slightly hygroscopic may adhere and form a cake if stored as a powder.

Granulation may reduce this hazard as the granules will be able to absorb some moisture and yet retain their flowability because of their size.
- Granules, having a greater bulk denser than the parent powder mix, occupy less volume per unit weight. They are therefore more convenient for storage or shipment.

Powdered and granulated products as dosage forms

Powdered and granulated products are dispensed in many forms, which are discussed later. The advantages associated with this type of preparation as a dosage form are as follows:

1. Solid preparations are more chemically stable than liquid ones. The shelf life of powders for antibiotic syrups, for example, is 2–3 years, but once they are reconstituted with water it is only 1–2 weeks. The instability observed in liquid preparations is usually the primary reason for presenting some injections as powders to be reconstituted just prior to use.
2. Powders and granules are a convenient form in which to orally administer drugs with a high dose. The dose of Compound Magnesium

Trisilicate Oral Powder is 1 g to 5 g and, although it is feasible to manufacture tablets to supply this dose, it is often more acceptable to the patient to disperse powder or granules in water and swallow it as a draught.

3. Orally administered powders and granules of soluble medicaments have a faster dissolution rate than tablets or capsules, as these must first disintegrate before the drug dissolves. Drug release from such powdered or granulated preparations will therefore generally be faster than from the corresponding tablet or capsule.

The disadvantages of powdered and granulated dosage forms are as follows:

1. Bulk powders or granules (i.e. where doses are not predivided into individual aliquots) are far less convenient for the patient to carry than a small container of tablets or capsules, and are as inconvenient to self-administer as liquid preparations, such as mixtures. Modern packaging methods for divided preparations, such as heat-sealable laminated sachets (see Chapter 46), mean that individual doses can be carried conveniently by the patient.

2. The masking of unpleasant tastes may be a problem with this type of preparation. A method attempting taste masking involves formulating the powder into a pleasantly tasting or taste-masked effervescent product. However, the manufacture of tablets and capsules is a more appropriate option for low-dose products.

3. Bulk powders or bulk granules are not suitable for the administration of potent drugs with a low dose. This is because individual doses are extracted from the bulk with a 5 mL spoon. This method is subject to variation in spoon fill (e.g. 'level' or 'heaped' spoonful) and variation in the bulk density of different batches of the powder. It is therefore not an accurate method of measurement. Divided preparations have been used for more potent drugs, but tablets and capsules have replaced them for this purpose.

4. Powders and granules are not a suitable form for the administration of drugs that are inactivated in, or cause damage to, the stomach; these should be presented as gastro-resistant tablets, for example.

Powders and granules for oral administration

Oral powders

Oral powders are preparations consisting of solid, loose, dry particles of varying degrees of fine particle size. They contain one or more active substances, with or without excipients and, if necessary, approved colouring matter and flavouring. They are generally administered in or with water or another suitable liquid, or they may also be swallowed directly. They are presented as single-dose or multidose preparations in suitable containers.

Each dose of a single-dose powder is enclosed in an individual container (e.g. a sachet or a vial). Traditionally, single doses were wrapped in paper. This was unsatisfactory for most products, particularly if the ingredients were hygroscopic, volatile or deliquescent. Modern packaging materials of foil and plastic laminates have largely replaced such paper wrappings; they offer superior protective qualities and are amenable to use on high-speed packing machines. However, paper-wrapped powders continue to exist in some over-the-counter products.

Multidose oral powders are packed into a suitable bulk container, such as a wide-mouthed glass jar. They require the provision of a measuring device capable of delivering the quantity prescribed. Because of the difficulty in precisely measuring single doses from this type of preparation, the constituents are usually relatively nontoxic medicaments with a large dose. Relatively few proprietary examples exist, although many dietary/food supplements are packed in this way.

In the manufacture of oral powders, effort is made to ensure a suitable particle size is used with regard to the intended use. Additionally, during manufacture, packaging, storage and distribution of oral powders, suitable means must be taken to ensure microbial quality. All powders and granules should be stored in a dry place to prevent deterioration due to ingress of moisture. Even if hydrolytic decomposition of ingredients does not occur, the particles will adhere and cake, producing an inelegant, often unusable product.

Effervescent powders

Effervescent powders are presented as single-dose or multidose preparations and generally, in addition to the drug, contain acid substances and carbonates or hydrogen carbonates which react rapidly and effervesce when the patient adds the powder to water to produce a draught. Citric acid plus sodium bicarbonate is a common combination that releases carbon dioxide. The drug is quickly dissolved or dispersed in the water before administration.

It is preferred that effervescent powders are packed in individual dose units in airtight containers (laminated sachets are ideal; see Chapter 46). It is important to protect the powder from the ingress of moisture during manufacture and on subsequent storage to prevent the reaction occurring prematurely.

Granules

One disadvantage of powders is that, because of differences in particle size and density of the various ingredients, the ingredients may segregate (i.e. demix; see Chapter 11). This can take place either in the hoppers of packaging machines or on storage in the final bulk container. If this happens, the product will be nonuniform and the patient will not receive the same dose of the ingredients on each occasion. This can be minimized by efficient granulation of the mixed powders.

Granules are preparations consisting of solid, dry aggregates of powder particles sufficiently resistant to withstand handling. They are intended for oral administration. Some are swallowed as such, some are chewed and some are dissolved or dispersed in water or another suitable liquid before being administered.

Granules contain one or more active substances with or without excipients and, if necessary, suitable colouring and flavouring substances. They are mainly used for low-toxicity, high-dose drugs. Methylcellulose granules, for example, are used as a bulk-forming laxative and have a dosage of 1g to 4 g daily. Many proprietary preparations contain similar bulk-forming laxatives.

Granules are presented as single-dose or multidose preparations. Each dose of a multidose preparation is administered by means of a device suitable for measuring the quantity prescribed. For single-dose granules, each dose is enclosed in an individual package, (e.g. a sachet or a vial). If the preparation contains volatile ingredients or the contents have to be protected, they should be stored in an airtight container. For example, Methylcellulose granules should be kept in a wide-mouthed, airtight container.

Granules are subject to pharmacopoeial tests and standards that are very similar to those required for powders and include uniformity of dosage units, uniformity of content, uniformity of mass and uniformity of mass of delivered doses from multidose containers.

Like powders, granules should be stored in an airtight container.

There are several categories of orally administered granules:

- effervescent granules;
- coated granules;
- modified-release granules; and
- gastro-resistant granules.

Effervescent granules. Effervescent granules are uncoated granules generally containing, in addition to the drug, acid substances and carbonates or hydrogen carbonates which react rapidly in the presence of water to release carbon dioxide. Citric acid and sodium bicarbonate is a commonly used combination. Effervescent granules are intended to be dissolved or dispersed in water before administration. The effervescence and subsequent disintegration of the granules should be complete within 5 minutes, by which time the granule ingredients should be either dissolved or fully dispersed in the water. Effervescent granules should be stored in an airtight container.

Coated granules. Coated granules consist of granules coated with one or more layers of mixtures of various excipients. The substances used as coatings (generally polymers) are usually applied as a solution or suspension under conditions in which evaporation of the vehicle occurs leaving a film of coating (see Chapter 32). A suitable test should be performed to demonstrate the appropriate release of the active substance(s), for example one of the tests described in Chapter 35.

Modified-release granules. Modified-release granules are coated or uncoated granules that contain special excipients or which are prepared by special procedures, or both, designed to modify the rate, the place or the time at which the active substance or substances are released.

Modified-release granules may have prolonged-release or delayed-release properties. A suitable test must be performed to demonstrate the appropriate rate and extent of the release of the active substance(s) (as explained in Chapter 35).

Gastro-resistant granules. Gastro-resistant granules (previously referred to as enteric-coated granules) are delayed-release granules that are intended to resist the gastric fluid and to release the active substance(s) in the intestinal fluid. This is generally achieved by the covering of the granules with a gastro-resistant polymer (see Chapters 31 and 32). Again a suitable test should be performed to demonstrate the appropriate release of the active substance(s).

Powders for other routes of administration

Powders for inhalation

The use of dry-powder systems for pulmonary drug delivery is now extensive. This dosage form has developed into one of the most effective methods of delivering active ingredients to the lung for the treatment of asthma and chronic obstructive pulmonary disease. Its popularity is reflected in the number of commercial preparations available in a number of sophisticated and increasingly precise delivery devices. Pulmonary delivery is discussed fully in Chapter 37.

Nasal powders

Nasal powders are medicated powders intended for inhalation into the nasal cavity by means of a suitable device. Some potent drugs are presented in this way because they are rapidly absorbed when administered as a fine powder via the nose (see Chapter 38 for a detailed discussion of the nasal route of administration).

To enhance convenience and ensure that a uniform dose is delivered on each occasion, delivery devices have been developed. Sufficient drug for one dose may be presented in a hard gelatin capsule diluted with an inert, soluble diluent such as lactose. The capsule is placed in the body of the nasal delivery device and is broken when the device is assembled. The drug is inhaled, via the nose, by the patient as a fine powder. The size of the particles is such as to localize their deposition in the nasal cavity and is verified by adequate methods of particle size determination.

Powders for external use

Powders for cutaneous application (topical powders)

Powders for cutaneous application are preparations consisting of solid, loose, dry particles of varying degrees of fineness. They contain one or more active substances, with or without excipients and, if necessary, appropriate colouring matter.

Powders for cutaneous application are presented as single-dose powders or multidose powders. They should be free from grittiness (caused by the presence of some large primary powder particles). Powders specifically intended for use on large open wounds or on severely injured skin must be sterile.

Multidose powders for cutaneous application may be dispensed in sifter-top containers, in containers equipped with a mechanical spraying device or in pressurized containers.

In the manufacture of powders for cutaneous application, measures should be taken to ensure a suitable particle size is obtained (determined and controlled by sieving) with regard to the intended use. Additionally, suitable measures should be taken to ensure their microbial quality and if the label indicates that the preparation is sterile, the preparation must comply with a test for sterility.

Sterile powders used in cutaneous application must be prepared with materials and methods designed to ensure sterility and to avoid the introduction of contaminants and the growth of microorganisms.

The pharmacopoeial tests for topical powders are tests for fineness (by sieving), uniformity of dosage unit, uniformity of content and, where appropriate, sterility.

Dusting powders

Dusting powders are powders for cutaneous application which have a suitable fineness. An example is Talc Dusting Powder, which is a mix of 10% starch and 90% Purified Talc, where the particle size is controlled by size separation using, typically, a 250 μm sieve.

Dusting powders contain ingredients used for therapeutic, prophylactic or lubricant purposes and are intended for external use. Only sterile dusting powders should be applied to open wounds.

Dusting powders for lubricant purposes or superficial skin conditions need not be sterile but they should be free from pathogenic organisms. As minerals such as talc and kaolin may be contaminated at source with spores of organisms causing tetanus and gangrene, these should be sterilized before they are incorporated into a product. Talc Dusting Powder is a sterile cutaneous powder in which the talc is sterilized before incorporation with the starch, or the final product is subject to a suitable terminal sterilization procedure.

Dusting powders are normally dispensed in glass or metal containers with a perforated lid. The powder must flow well from such a container, so that it can be dusted over the affected area. The active ingredients must therefore be diluted with materials with reasonably good flow properties (e.g. purified talc or maize starch).

Hexachlorophene Dusting Powder contains an antibacterial agent, and Talc Dusting Powder is used as a lubricant to prevent chafing. Proprietary products are available, usually for the treatment of bacterial or fungal infections, e.g. Canesten® AF Powder (clotrimazole) is used as an antifungal agent.

Ear powders

Powders containing active ingredients can also be administered to the ear. Ear powders normally have to comply with the pharmaceutical requirements for powders for cutaneous application. They are supplied in containers fitted with a suitable device for application.

Preparations requiring further treatment at the time of dispensing

Some preparations for oral use are prepared from powders or granules to yield oral solutions or suspensions using a suitable vehicle. This may be performed at the dispensing stage or by the patient prior to administration. The vehicle for any preparations for oral use is chosen with regard to the nature of the active substance(s) and such that it provides organoleptic characteristics appropriate to the intended use of the preparation.

Several categories of preparations may be distinguished:

* powders and granules for oral solutions and suspensions;
* powders and granules for syrups;
* powders for oral drops; and
* powders for injection.

Powders and granules for solution or suspension

Powders and granules for the preparation of oral solutions or suspensions generally conform to the definitions in the normal pharmacopoeial standards for oral powders or granules as appropriate. They may contain excipients, in particular to facilitate dispersion or dissolution and to prevent caking. After dissolution or suspension, the resulting product should comply with the requirements for oral solutions or oral suspensions, as appropriate.

The label should explain the method of preparation of the solution or suspension from the powder or granules, and the conditions and the duration of storage after reconstitution.

Powders and granules for syrups

Syrups are aqueous preparations characterized by a sweet taste and a viscous consistency. They may contain sucrose at a concentration of at least 45%. The sweet taste can also be obtained by using other polyols or sweetening agents. Syrups usually contain aromatic or other flavouring agents.

All of the necessary ingredients for the syrup may be manufactured and stored in the dry powdered or granular state and then reconstituted (usually by the addition of water alone) at the time of dispensing or administration. After dissolution, the resulting syrup must comply with the normal pharmacopoeial requirements for syrups.

Antibiotic syrups. For patients who have difficulty taking capsules and tablets (e.g. young children), a liquid preparation of a drug offers a suitable alternative. Unfortunately, many antibiotics are physically or chemically unstable when formulated as a solution or suspension. The method used to overcome this instability problem is to manufacture the dry ingredients of the intended liquid preparation in a suitable container in the form of a powder or granules. When the product is dispensed, a given quantity of water is added to reconstitute the solution or suspension. This enables sufficient time for warehousing and distribution of the product and storage at the pharmacy without degradation. Once it is reconstituted, the patient must be warned of the short shelf life. A shelf life of 1–2 weeks for the reconstituted antibiotic syrup should not be a serious problem for the patient as the dosing would normally be completed by then. Amoxicillin Oral Suspension and Erythromycin Ethyl Succinate Oral Suspension are examples.

Powders for oral drops

Oral drops are solutions, emulsions or suspensions that are administered in small volumes, such as in drops, by the means of a suitable device. Powders for the preparation of oral drops would have to conform to the requirements of all other oral powders. They may contain excipients to facilitate dissolution or suspension in the prescribed liquid, or to prevent caking.

After dissolution or suspension, they comply with the specific pharmacopoeial requirements for prepre-pared oral drops. If the dose is measured in drops, the label should also state the number of drops per millilitre or per gram of preparation.

Powders for injection

Injections of medicaments that are unstable in aqueous solution must be made immediately prior to admin-istration. The ingredients are presented as sterile powders in ampoules or vials. Sufficient diluent (e.g. sterile Water for Injections) is added from a second container to produce the required drug concentration, and the injection is used immediately. The powder may contain suitable excipients in addition to the drug (e.g. sufficient additive to produce an isotonic solution when the injection is reconstituted).

Powders for injection are most often manufactured by a freeze-drying process (see Chapter 29). The sterilization of these 'lyophilized powders' is described in Chapter 17 and their use as parenteral products is discussed in more detail in Chapter 36.

The label for powders for injection should state (1) the amount of active ingredient contained in the sealed container, (2) the directions for preparing the injection or intravenous infusion from the powder and (3) that when dissolved or suspended, the preparation is intended for parenteral use.

Pharmacopoeial tests

The pharmacopoeial tests for assessing the quality of most powdered and granular dosage forms are very similar. The role of these tests is indicated by its title; details of procedures and standards can be found in the latest appropriate pharmacopeia.

Uniformity of dosage units. Single-dose oral powders should comply with a pharmacopoeial test for uniformity of dosage units or, where justified and authorized, with the tests for uniformity of content and/or uniformity of mass.

Uniformity of mass. Single-dose oral powders need to comply with a test for uniformity of mass of single-dose preparations. If the product complies with the uniformity of content test for all active substances, the test for uniformity of mass is not required.

Uniformity of content. In the case where the oral powder contains a particularly active drug, single-dose

oral powders must comply with a test for uniformity of content of active drug(s) in single-dose preparations. After each container has been shaken, it should be emptied as completely as possible; the test is per-formed on the individual contents. As an example, the *British Pharmacopoeia* defines an active substance as one where a single dose of powder or granules contains an amount of active substance less than 2 mg, or less than 2% of the total mass of the single-dose preparation.

Uniformity of mass of delivered doses from multidose containers. Oral powders and granules supplied in multidose containers must comply with this test.

Drug release. Where appropriate (e.g. coated granules, modified-release granules, gastro-resistant granules) the rate and extent of release of the active drug(s) must be quantified and compared with the required specification.

Sterility. When the label of the powder or granule product states that it is sterile, it must comply with the appropriate pharmacopoeial test for sterility.

Granules used as an intermediate in tablet manufacture

As indicated earlier in this chapter, by far the largest portion of pharmaceutical granules that are made will have a short lifetime before they are compacted into tablets (mainly) or filled into hard capsules. The methods of manufacture of granules are basically the same irrespective of the fate of the granules. However, in the context of manufacturing tablets, the mechani-cal properties of the granules and therefore the way in which they deform and bond are critical in the tableting process.

Pharmaceutical technology of granule production

Pharmaceutical granulation processes

Granulation methods can be divided into two types: *wet* methods, which use a liquid in the process, and *dry* methods, in which no liquid is used.

In a suitable formulation a number of different excipients will be needed in addition to the drug. The common types used are diluents, which are used to produce a unit dose weight of suitable size, and disintegrating agents, which are added to aid the break-up of the granule when it reaches a liquid medium (e.g. following ingestion by the patient). An adhesive (also known as a binder) in the form of a dry powder may also be added, particularly if dry granulation is employed. All ingredients will be mixed before granulation.

Dry granulation

In the dry methods of granulation, the primary powder particles are aggregated at high pressure. There are two main intermediate processes: either the production of a large tablet (known as a '*slug*') in a heavy-duty tableting press (a process known as *slugging*) or the squeezing of powder between two rollers to produce a sheet or flakes of material (*roller compaction*). In both cases the intermediate product is broken using a suitable milling technique to produce granular material which is usually sieved to separate the desired size fraction. The unused fine material may be reworked to avoid waste. This dry method may be used for drugs which do not compress well after wet granulation or those which are sensitive to moisture.

Wet granulation (involving wet massing)

Wet granulation involves the massing of a mix of dry *primary powder particles* using a *granulating fluid*. The granulating fluid contains a solvent that must be volatile, so that it can be removed by drying, and nontoxic. Typical suitable liquids include water, ethanol and 2-propanol either alone or in combination. The granulation liquid may be used alone or, more usually, as a solvent containing a dissolved *adhesive* (also referred to as a *binder* or *binding agent*), which is used to ensure particle adhesion once the granule is dry.

Water is commonly used for economic and ecological reasons. The disadvantages of water as a solvent are that it may adversely affect drug stability, causing hydrolysis of susceptible products, and it needs a longer drying time than organic solvents. This long drying time increases the duration of the process and again may affect chemical stability of the drug(s) because of the extended exposure to heat. The primary advantage of water is that it is nonflammable, which means that expensive safety precautions such as the use of flameproof equipment need not be taken. Organic solvents are used as an alternative to dry granulation when water-sensitive drugs are processed, or when a rapid drying time is required.

In the traditional wet granulation method, the wet mass is forced through a sieve to produce wet granules, which are then dried. A subsequent screening stage breaks agglomerates of granules and removes the fine material, which can be recycled. Variations of this traditional method are dependent on the equipment used, but the general principle of initial particle aggregation using a liquid remains in all of the processes.

An alternative to the traditional wet granulation process is melt granulation whereby thermosetting polymers are used to form the granules. This process is described later.

Effect of the granulation method on granule structure

The type and capacity of granulating mixers significantly influence the work input and time necessary to produce a cohesive mass, adequate liquid distribution and intragranular porosity of the granular mass. The method and conditions of granulation affect intragranular pore structure by changing the degree of packing within individual granules. It has been shown that precompacted granules, consisting of drug and binder particles, are held together by simple bonding formed during consolidation. Granules prepared by wet massing consist of intact drug particles held together in a sponge-like matrix of binder. Fluidized-bed granules are similar to granules prepared by the wet-massing process but possess greater porosity, and the granule surface is covered by a film of binding agent. With spray-dried systems, the granules consist of spherical particles composed of an outer shell with an inner core of particles or air. Thus the properties of the granule are influenced by the manufacturing process.

Granulation mechanisms

Particle bonding mechanisms

To form granules, bonds must be formed between powder particles so that they adhere, and these bonds must be sufficiently strong to prevent breakdown of the granule to powder in subsequent handling operations.

The five primary bonding mechanisms between particles are:

1. adhesion and cohesion forces in the immobile liquid films between individual primary powder particles;
2. interfacial forces in mobile liquid films within the granules;
3. the formation of solid bridges after solvent evaporation;
4. attractive forces between solid particles; and
5. mechanical interlocking.

Many different types of mechanism have been identified within these categories. The ones discussed next are those which are most relevant to pharmaceutical granulations.

Adhesion and cohesion forces in immobile films

If sufficient liquid is present in a powder to form a very thin, immobile layer, there will be an effective decrease in interparticulate distance and an increase in contact area between the particles. The bond strength between the particles will be increased because of this, as the van der Waals forces of attraction are proportional to the particle diameter and inversely proportional to the square of the distance of separation.

This situation will arise with adsorbed moisture and accounts for the cohesion of slightly damp powders. Although such films may be present as residual liquid after granules prepared by wet granulation have been dried, it is unlikely that they contribute significantly to the final granule strength. In dry granulation, however, the pressures used will increase the contact area between the adsorbed layers and decrease the interparticulate distance, and this will contribute to the final granule strength.

Thin, immobile layers may also be formed by highly viscous solutions of adhesives. The resulting bond strength will be greater than that produced by the mobile films discussed next. The use of starch mucilage in pharmaceutical granulations may produce this type of film.

Interfacial forces in mobile liquid films

During wet granulation, liquid is added to the powder mix and will be distributed as a film around and between the particles. Sufficient liquid is usually added to exceed that necessary for an immobile layer and this produces a mobile film. The three states of water distribution between particles are illustrated in Fig. 28.2.

At low moisture levels, termed the *pendular state*, the particles are held together by lens-shaped rings of liquid. These cause adhesion because of the surface tension forces of the liquid–air interface and the hydrostatic suction pressure in the liquid bridge. When all the air has been displaced from between the particles, the *capillary state* is reached, and the particles are held by capillary suction at the liquid–air interface, which is now only at the granule surface. The *funicular state* represents an intermediate stage between the pendular and capillary states. Moist granule tensile strength increases by approximately three times from the pendular state to the capillary state.

It may appear that the state of the powder bed is dependent upon the total moisture content of the wetted powders but the capillary state may also be reached by decreasing the separation of the particles. In the massing process during wet granulation, continued kneading/mixing of material originally in the pendular state will densify the wet mass, decreasing the pore volume occupied by air and eventually producing the funicular or capillary state without further liquid addition.

In addition to these three states, a further state, the droplet, is illustrated in Fig. 28.2. This will be important in the process of granulation by spray-drying

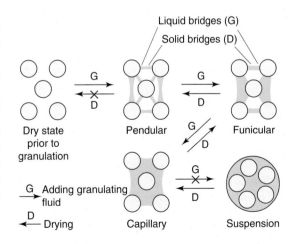

Fig. 28.2 • Water distribution between particles of a granule during formation and drying.

of a suspension. In this state the strength of the droplet is dependent upon the surface tension of the liquid used.

These wet bridges are only temporary structures in wet granulation because the moist granules will be dried. They are, however, a prerequisite for the formation of solid bridges formed by adhesives present in the liquid, or by materials which dissolve in the granulating liquid.

Solid bridges

These can be formed by:

- partial melting;
- hardening binders; or
- crystallization of dissolved substances.

Partial melting. Although not considered to be a predominant mechanism in pharmaceutical materials, it is possible that the pressures used in dry granulation methods may cause melting of low melting point materials where the particles touch and high pressures are developed. When the pressure is relieved, crystallization will occur, binding the particles together.

Hardening binders. This is the common mechanism in pharmaceutical wet granulations when an adhesive is included in the granulating solvent. The liquid will form liquid bridges, as discussed earlier, and the adhesive will harden or crystallize on drying to form solid bridges to bind the particles. Adhesives such as polyvinylpyrrolidone, the cellulose derivatives (such as carboxymethylcellulose) and pregelatinized starch function in this way.

Crystallization of dissolved substances. The solvent used to mass the powder during wet granulation may partially dissolve one of the powdered ingredients. When the granules are dried, crystallization of this material will occur and the dissolved substance then acts as a hardening binder. Any material soluble in the granulating liquid will function in this manner (e.g. lactose incorporated into powder blends granulated with water).

The size of the crystals produced in the bridge will be influenced by the rate of drying of the granules; the longer the drying time, the larger the particle size of the drug crystals. It is therefore important that the drug does not dissolve in the granulating liquid and recrystallize because it may adversely affect the dissolution rate of the drug if crystals larger than those of the drug starting material are produced.

Attractive forces between solid particles

In the absence of liquids and solid bridges formed by binding agents, there are two types of attractive force which can operate between particles in pharmaceutical systems.

Electrostatic forces may be of importance in causing powder cohesion and the initial formation of agglomerates (e.g. during mixing). In general, they do not contribute significantly to the final strength of the granule.

Van der Waals forces, however, are approximately four orders of magnitude stronger than electrostatic forces and contribute significantly to the strength of granules produced by dry granulation. The magnitude of these forces will increase as the distance between adjacent surfaces decreases, and in dry granulation this is achieved with use of pressure to force the particles together.

Mechanisms of granule formation

In the dry methods, adhesion of particles occurs because of applied pressure. A compact or sheet is produced which is larger than the granule size required and therefore the required size can be attained by milling and sieving.

In wet granulation methods, liquid added to dry powders has to be distributed throughout the powder by the mechanical agitation produced in the granulator. The particles adhere to each other because of liquid films, and further agitation and/or liquid addition causes more particles to adhere. The precise mechanism by which a dry powder is transformed into a bed of granules varies for each type of granulation equipment but the mechanism discussed in the following sections serves as a useful broad generalization of the process.

The proposed granulation mechanism can be divided into three stages: nucleation, transition and ball growth.

Nucleation

Granulation starts with particle–particle contact and adhesion due to liquid bridges. A number of particles will join to form the pendular state illustrated in Fig. 28.2. Further agitation densifies the pendular bodies to form the capillary state, and these bodies act as nuclei for further granule growth.

Transition

Nuclei can grow by two possible mechanisms: either single particles can be added to the nuclei by pendular bridges or two or more nuclei may combine. The combined nuclei will be reshaped by the agitation of the bed.

This stage is characterized by the presence of a large number of small granules with a fairly wide size distribution. Providing that the size distribution is not excessively large, this point represents a suitable end point for granules used in capsule and tablet manufacture as relatively small granules will produce a uniform tablet die or capsule fill. Larger granules may give rise to problems in small-diameter dies due to bridging across the die and uneven fill.

Ball growth

Further granule growth produces large, spherical granules, and the mean particle size of the granulating system will increase with time. If agitation is continued, granule coalescence will continue and produce an unusable, overmassed system, although this is dependent on the amount of liquid added and the properties of the material being granulated.

Although ball growth produces granules which may be too large for pharmaceutical purposes, some degree of ball growth will occur in planetary mixers and it is an essential feature of some spheronizing equipment.

The four possible mechanisms of ball growth are illustrated in Fig. 28.3.

Coalescence. Two or more granules join to form a larger granule.

Breakage. Granules break into fragments which adhere to other granules, forming a layer of material over the surviving granule.

Abrasion transfer. Agitation of the granule bed leads to attrition of material from granules. This abraded material adheres to other granules, increasing their size.

Layering. When a second batch of powder mix is added to a bed of granules, the powder will adhere to the granules, forming a layer over the surface and thus increasing the granule size. This mechanism is only of relevance to the production of layered granules using spheronizing equipment.

There will be some degree of overlap between these stages, and it will be very difficult to identify a given stage by inspection of the granulating system. For end-product uniformity, it is desirable to finish every

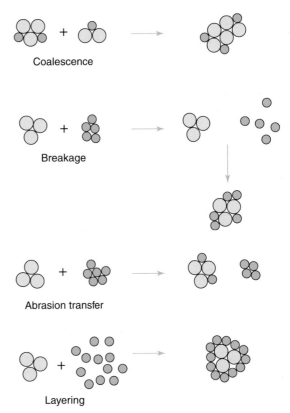

Fig. 28.3 • Mechanisms of ball growth during granulation.

batch of a formulation at the same stage, and this may be a major problem in pharmaceutical production.

Using the slower processes such as the planetary mixer, there is usually a sufficient length of time to stop the process before overmassing. With faster granulation equipment, the duration of granulation can only be used as a control parameter when the formulation is such that granule growth is slow and occurs at a fairly uniform rate. In many cases, however, the transition from a nongranulated to an overmassed system is very rapid and monitoring equipment is necessary to stop the granulation at a predetermined point. This is known as granulation end point control.

Pharmaceutical granulation equipment and processes

Wet granulators

Three main types of granulator are used in the pharmaceutical industry for wet granulation.

Shear granulators

The older shear granulators have largely disappeared and have been replaced by the much more efficient high-speed mixer/granulators. In the traditional shear (or planetary) granulation process, dry-powder blending usually has to be performed as a separate initial operation using different powder-mixing equipment. The older process suffered from a number of major disadvantages: its long duration, the need for several pieces of equipment and the high material losses which can be incurred because of the transfer stages between the different equipment. The process served the pharmaceutical industry well for many years but the advantages of modern mixer/granulators have proved too attractive for its continued use.

High-speed mixer/granulators

High-speed mixer/granulators (e.g. Diosna) are used extensively for pharmaceutical granulation. They were developed from traditional planetary mixers to speed up the process and to reduce the number of pieces of equipment and separate process steps required. The machines have a stainless steel mixing bowl containing a three-bladed main impeller which revolves in the horizontal plane and a three-bladed auxiliary chopper (or breaker blade) which revolves in either the vertical plane or the horizontal plane (Fig. 28.4). The main blade is designed to rotate at approximately 150–300 rpm and the high-speed chopper rotates at approximately 1500–3000 rpm.

The unmixed dry powders are placed in the bowl and mixed by the rotating impeller for a few minutes. Granulating liquid is then added via a port in the lid of the granulator while the impeller is turning. The granulating fluid is mixed into the powders by the impeller. The chopper is usually switched on when the moist mass is formed as its function is to break up the wet mass to produce a bed of granular material. Once a satisfactory granule has been produced, the granular product is discharged, passing through a wire mesh, which breaks up any large aggregates, into the bowl of a fluidized-bed dryer.

Like most modern process equipment, high-speed mixer/granulators are available in a wide range of sizes. These are often designed to have similar geometric and powder movement characteristics in an attempt to minimize scale-up problems when a product moves from development to production. Bowl volumes between 1 L and 1250 L are available. The weight of powder that each holds will depend on its bulk density and the optimum fill capacity (working volume) of each bowl. Bowls are manufactured from high-quality polished stainless steel.

The advantage of the process is that powder blending, wet massing and granulation are all performed in a few minutes in the same piece of equipment. The process needs to be controlled with care as the granulation progresses so rapidly that a usable granule can be transformed very quickly into an unusable, overmassed system. Thus it is often necessary to use a suitable monitoring system to

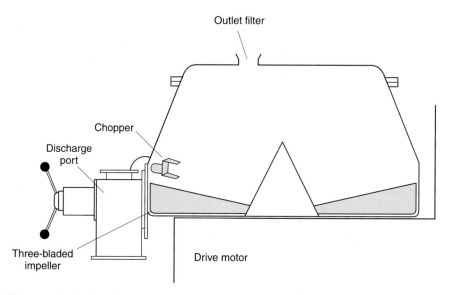

Fig. 28.4 • High-speed mixer/granulator.

indicate the end of the granulation process (i.e. when a granule of the desired properties has been attained). The process is also sensitive to variations in raw materials, but this may be minimized by using a suitable granulation end point monitor.

A variation of the Diosna type of design is the GEA UltimaGral mixer (GEA Collette, Vanguard) (Fig. 28.5). This is based on the bowl and overhead drive of the planetary mixer but the single paddle of a planetary mixer is replaced with two mixing shafts. One of these carries three blade arms which rotate in the horizontal plane at the base of the bowl and the second carries smaller blades which act as the chopper and rotate rapidly in the upper regions of the granulating mass. Thus the operating principle is similar to that of the Diosna type already described.

This design is available in sizes ranging from 10 L to 200 L volume (capable of processing approximately 3 kg to 80 kg batches respectively). The main mixing blade rotates at 450–600 rpm in the 10 L model and at 150–200 rpm in the 200 L model. This rotational speed variation is to attempt to maintain the same linear velocity of movement of the blades, as this helps scale-up. In all models the high-speed chopper rotates at 1500–3000 rpm.

An attractive feature of high-speed granulators is that the product is usually granular and a separate step to granulate the wet mass is avoided (the granules being produced by the action of the high-speed chopper). Occasionally this is not fully satisfactory, and the moist mass then has to be transferred to a granulator such as an oscillating granulator (Fig. 28.6). The rotor bars of the granulator oscillate at an adjustable rate between 60 and 100 rpm and force the moist mass through the sieve screen, the size of which determines the granule size. The mass should be sufficiently moist to form discrete granules when sieved. If excess liquid is added at the wet massing stage, strings of material will be formed, and if the mix is too dry, the mass will be sieved to a powder, and granules will not be formed.

Granulators of this type can also deal with the size reduction of dry material. They are available in a range of sizes capable of dealing with 300 kg to 500 kg of wet mass per hour or 700 kg to 1200 kg of dry mass per hour.

Fluidized-bed granulators

Fluidized-bed granulators (e.g. Aeromatic-Fielder, Glatt, Vanguard) have a design and operation similar to those of fluidized-bed dryers (i.e. the powder particles are fluidized in a stream of air), but in addition granulation fluid is sprayed from a nozzle onto the bed of powders (Fig. 28.7).

Heated and filtered air is blown or sucked through the bed of unmixed powders to fluidize the particles and mix the powders; fluidization is a very efficient mixing process. Granulating fluid is pumped from a reservoir through a spray nozzle or multiple nozzles positioned over the bed of particles. A variety of spray nozzles are available to cope with a wide range of products. The granulating fluid causes the primary powder particles to adhere when the droplets and powders collide. Escape of material from the granulation chamber is prevented by exhaust filters, which are periodically agitated to reintroduce the collected material into the fluidized bed. Sufficient liquid is sprayed to produce granules of the required size, at which point the spray is turned off – but the fluidizing air continues to be provided. The wet granulates are then dried in the heated fluidizing air stream.

Commercial apparatus ranges from laboratory models that, by changing the bowl, have a volume between 0.2 L and 2 L, giving a capacity of a few grams up to approximately 1 kg, to production

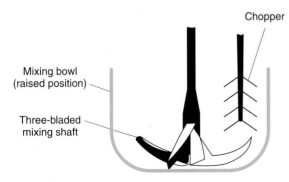

Fig. 28.5 • GEA Gral (Collette-type) of granulator: mixing shafts and bowl.

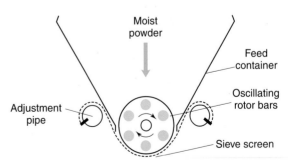

Fig. 28.6 • Oscillating granulator.

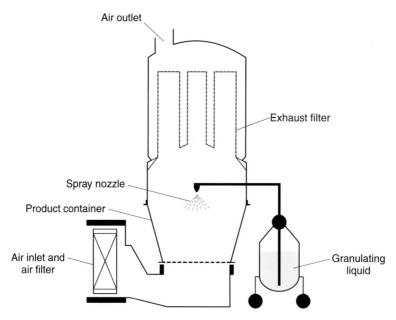

Fig. 28.7 • Fluidized-bed granulator.

machines. A wide range is available to cope with the wide variety of production volumes encountered in the pharmaceutical industry. They can be obtained in sizes suitable for batches between 5 kg and a massive 1550 kg, these calculations being based on an optimum 70% bowl fill and a powder/granule bulk density of 0.5 kg L^{-1}.

Advantages of fluidized-bed granulation. Fluidized-bed granulation has many advantages over conventional wet massing. All the granulation processes, which normally need separate equipment in the conventional method, are performed in one unit, saving labour costs, transfer losses and time. Another advantage is that automation of the process can be achieved once the conditions affecting the granulation have been optimized and validated.

Disadvantages of fluidized-bed granulation. On the downside, the equipment is initially expensive, and optimization of process (and product) parameters affecting granulation needs extensive development work, not only during initial formulation work but also during scale-up from development to production scale. Similar development work for the traditional process is not as extensive as that for high-speed granulators.

This long and very product specific development process has proved to be a serious problem with fluidized-bed granulation in the pharmaceutical industry. Numerous apparatus, process and product

parameters affect the quality of the final granule; these are listed in Table 28.1. The extent of this list, coupled with the fact that each formulation presents its own individual development problems, has led to fluidized-bed granulation not fulfilling its full potential in pharmaceutical production. This is exacerbated by the reality that most pharmaceutical companies have a wide range of products made at relatively small batch size, unlike other industries (fertilizer, herbicide, foodstuff), where fluidized-bed granulation is used successfully and extensively. Intelligent computer control of the whole process is available but requires careful setting up to cope with the sensitivity to small changes in formulation and process variables.

Spray-dryers

These differ from the method just discussed in that a dry, granular product is made from a solution or a suspension rather than from dry primary powder particles. The solution or suspension may be of the drug alone, a single excipient or a complete formulation.

The process of spray-drying is discussed more fully in Chapter 29. The resultant granules are free-flowing hollow spheres, and the distribution of the binder in such granules (at the periphery following solute migration during drying) results in good compaction properties.

Table 28.1 Apparatus, process and product variables influencing fluidized-bed granulation

Apparatus parameters	Process parameters	Product parameters
Air distribution place	Bed load	Type of binder
Shape of granulator body	Fluidizing air flow rate	Quantity of binder
Nozzle height	Fluidizing air temperature	Binder solvent
Positive or negative pressure operation	Fluidizing air humidity Atomization 　Nozzle type 　Spray angle 　Spraying regime 　Liquid flow rate 　Atomizing air flow rate 　Atomizing air pressure 　Droplet size	Concentration of granulating solution Temperature of granulating solution Starting materials 　Fluidization 　Powder hydrophobicity

This process can be used to make tablet granules, although it is probably economically justified for this purpose only when suitable granules cannot be produced by the other methods. Spray-drying can convert hard elastic materials into more ductile materials. Spray-dried lactose is the classic example, and its advantages over α-lactose monohydrate crystals when compacted are discussed in Chapter 30.

The primary advantages of the process are the short drying time and the minimal exposure of the product to heat because of the short residence time in the drying chamber. This means that little deterioration of heat-sensitive materials occurs, and it may be the only process suitable for this type of product.

Spheronizers/pelletizers

For some applications it may be desirable to have a dense, spherical pellet of the type difficult to produce with the equipment described in the previous sections. Such pellets are used for controlled drug release products following coating with a suitable polymer coat and the filling of hard capsules. Capsule filling with a mixture of coated and noncoated drug-containing pellets would give some degree of programmed drug release after the capsule shell dissolves.

A commonly used process involves the separate processes of wet massing, followed by extrusion of this wet mass into rod-shaped granules and subsequent spheronization of these granules. Because this process is used so frequently to produce modified-release multiparticulates, this process will be discussed in some detail.

Extrusion–spheronization

Extrusion–spheronization is a multistep process used to make uniformly sized spherical particles. It is primarily used as a method to produce multiparticulates for controlled drug release applications. The major advantage over other methods of producing drug-loaded spheres or pellets is the ability to incorporate high levels of active ingredients without producing excessively large particles (i.e. minimal excipients are necessary).

The main steps of the process are:

- *dry mixing of ingredients* to achieve a homogeneous powder dispersion;
- *wet massing* to produce a sufficiently plastic wet mass;
- *extrusion* to form rod-shaped particles of uniform diameter;
- *spheronization* to round off these rods into spherical particles;
- *drying* to achieve the desired final moisture content; and
- *screening* (optional) to achieve the desired narrow size distribution.

Applications of extrusion–spheronization

The potential applications are many but relate mainly to controlled drug release and improved processing.

Controlled drug release. Both immediate-release and controlled-release pellets can be formed. In turn, these pellets can either be filled into hard capsule shells or compacted with suitable excipients into tablets to form dosage forms. Pellets can contain two or more ingredients in the same individual unit or incompatible ingredients can be manufactured in separate pellets.

Pellets can be coated in subbatches to give, say, rapid-release, intermediate-release and prolonged-release pellets in the same capsule shell. Dense multiparticulates disperse evenly within the gastrointestinal tract and have less variable gastric emptying and intestinal transit times than single units, such as coated monolithic tablets.

Processing. The process of extrusion–spheronization can be used to increase the bulk density, improve flow properties and reduce the problems of dust usually encountered with low-density, finely divided active and excipient powders.

Extrusion–spheronization is a more labour-intensive process than other forms of granulation and therefore should be considered only when other methods of granulation are either not satisfactory for that particular formulation or are inappropriate (i.e. when spheres are required).

Desirable properties of pellets

Uncoated pellets have:

- uniform spherical shape;
- uniform size;
- good flow properties;
- reproducible packing (into hard capsules);
- high strength;
- low friability;
- low dust;
- smooth surface; and
- ease of coating.

Once coated, they:

- maintain all of the above properties; and
- have the desired drug release characteristics.

Process

Dry mixing of ingredients. This uses normal powder mixing equipment.

Wet massing. This stage also uses normal equipment and processes as used in wet granulation. There are two major differences in the granulation step compared with granulation for compaction:

- the amount of granulation fluid; and
- the importance of achieving a uniform dispersion of fluid.

The amount of fluid needed to achieve spheres of uniform size and sphericity is likely to be greater than that for a similar tablet granulation. Poor liquid dispersion will produce a poor-quality product.

Extrusion. Extrusion produces rod-shaped particles of uniform diameter from the wet mass. The wet mass is forced through dies and shaped into small cylindrical particles with uniform diameter. The extruded particles break at similar lengths under their own weight. Thus the extrudate must have enough plasticity to deform but not so much that the extruded particles adhere to other particles when collected or rolled in the spheronizer.

There are many designs of extruder but generally they can be divided into three classes, on the basis of their feed mechanism:

- screw-feed extruders (axial or endplate, dome and radial);
- gravity-feed extruders (cylinder roll, gear roll, radial); and
- piston-feed extruders (ram).

The first two categories (shown in Fig. 28.8) are used for both development and production but the latter is used only for experimental development work as it is easy to add instrumentation.

The primary extrusion process variables are:

- the feed rate of the wet mass;
- the diameter of the die;

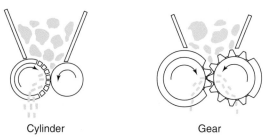

Screw-feed extruders

Axial   Radial

Gravity-feed extruders

Cylinder   Gear

Fig. 28.8 • Production extruders.

- the length of the die; and
- the water content of the wet mass.

The properties of the extrudate, and thus the resulting spheres, are very dependent on the plasticity and cohesiveness of the wet mass. In general, an extrudable wet mass needs to be wetter than that appropriate for conventional granulation by wet massing.

Spheronization. The function of the fourth step in the process (i.e. spheronization) is to round off the rods produced by extrusion into spherical particles.

This process is performed in a relatively simple piece of apparatus (Fig. 28.9). The working part consists of a bowl with fixed side walls, with a rapidly rotating bottom plate or disc. The rounding of the extrudate into spheres is dependent on frictional forces generated by particle–particle and particle–equipment collisions.

The bottom disc has a grooved surface to increase the strength of these forces. Two geometric patterns are generally used:

- a cross-hatched pattern with grooves running at right angles to one another; and
- a radial pattern with grooves running radially from the centre of the disc.

The transition from rods to spheres during spheronization occurs in various stages. These are best described by examination of the diagrams in Fig. 28.10.

If the moistened mass is too dry, spheres will not be formed; the rods will transform only as far as dumbbells.

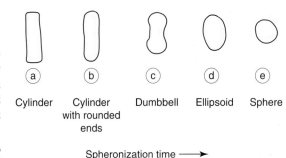

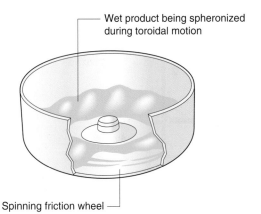

Fig. 28.9 • A spheronizer showing the characteristic toroidal (rope-like) movement of the forming pellets in the spheronizer bowl during operation.

Spheronization time ⟶

Fig. 28.10 • A spheronization mechanism, showing the transition from cylindrical particles *(a)* into cylindrical particles with rounded edges *(b)*, then dumbbells *(c)*, to ellipsoids *(d)* and finally spheres *(e)*.

Drying. A drying stage is required to achieve the desired moisture content. Drying is often the final step in the process. Drying of the pellets can be accomplished in any dryer that can be used for conventional wet granulations, including tray dryers and fluidized-bed dryers. Both are used successfully for extrusion–spheronization. If solute migration (see Chapter 29) occurs during drying of the wet spheres, this may result in:

- an increased initial rate of dissolution;
- stronger pellets; and
- modified surfaces which might reduce the adhesion of any added film coats.

Screening (optional). Screening may be necessary to achieve the desired narrow size distribution. Normal sieves are used. If all the previous stages are performed efficiently and with careful development of process and formulation conditions, this step may not be necessary.

Formulation variables

The composition of the wet mass is critical in determining the properties of the particles produced. During the granulation step, a wet mass is produced which must be plastic, deform when extruded and break off to form uniformly sized cylindrical particles which are easily deformed into spherical particles. Thus the process has a complex set of requirements that are strongly influenced by the ingredients of the pellet formulation.

Summary

Extrusion–spheronization is a versatile process capable of producing spherical granules having very useful properties. Because it is more labour-intensive than more common wet massing techniques, its use should be limited to those applications where a sphere is required and other granulation techniques are unsuitable.

The most common application of the process is to produce spherical pellets for controlled drug release.

Care must be taken to understand the required properties of the pellets and the manner in which the process and formulation influence the ability to achieve the required properties.

Rotorgranulation

This process allows the direct manufacture of spheres suitable for controlled-release solid dosage forms from a dry powder in one process. The powder mix is added to the bowl and wetted with granulating liquid from a spray or multiple sprays (Fig. 28.11). The base plate rotates at high speed and centrifugal force keeps the moist mass at the edges of the rotor. Here the velocity difference between the rotor and the static walls, combined with the upward flow of air around the rotor plate, causes the mass to move in a toroidal motion, resulting in the formation of discrete spherical pellets. This is a motion almost identical to that occurring in spheronizers, as shown in Fig. 28.10. The resulting spheres (actually, of course, wet granules) are dried by the heated inlet air from the air chamber.

With this technique, it is possible to continue the process and coat the pellets by subsequently spraying coating solution onto the rotating dried pellets. Additionally, layered pellets can be produced by using uncoated pellets as nuclei in a second granulation with a powder mix of a second ingredient or ingredients.

Rotorgranulators (e.g. Freund, Vanguard) are manufactured in size ranges between 45 L and 450 L capacity. Again, the corresponding fill weights will depend on the bulk density of the formulation and the optimum operating capacity of each bowl. This range requires corresponding bowl and rotor disc diameters between 300 mm and 1400 mm. Discs with different surface roughness patterns are available to cope with a wide range of materials. They also come with an adjustable air gap around the plate to assist in the manipulation of the resulting granule size. Powder charging and discharging are made easy, and there is precise liquid feeding. Intelligent computer control of the whole process is available.

Melt granulation

Introduction

Melt granulation is a size enlargement process in which a thermosetting material (*hot-melt binder*) is used to bind the primary powder particles into granules. It is a water-free alternative to wet granulation. The binder/granulating agent is a semisolid or solid hydrophilic polymer or a hydrophobic wax. There are two variants to the technique:

- The hot-melt binder is added as a solid powder to the drug–excipient powder mix at room

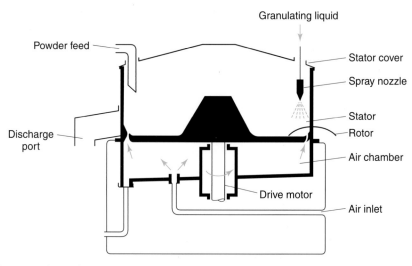

Fig. 28.11 • Rotorgranulator.

temperature and mixed while the temperature of the mix is raised to above the melting point of the binder (ideally at the low end of the range from 50 °C and 90 °C)

- The hot-melt binder is heated and melted then sprayed onto the powder in a fluidized-bed granulator or high-speed mixer granulator.

In either case, liquid bridges are formed by the molten binder, and powder agglomeration (i.e. granulation) occurs. The mechanism of granulation is analogous to that of wet granulation described earlier. The initial particle–particle bonds are formed by the surface tension of a liquid (this time the molten hot-melt binder). On subsequent cooling, the molten binder solidifies, forming solid bridges that permanently bind the particles together.

Hot-melt binders

Hot-melt binders can be either hydrophilic/water soluble or hydrophobic/water insoluble. The most commonly used hydrophilic water-soluble binders are the polyethylene glycols (PEGs). PEG is the ideal hot-melt binder for granules intended for immediate-release products. Grades between PEG 2000 and PEG 6000 can be used, with PEG 3000 being well suited (melting point 48 °C to 54 °C).

Hydrophobic water-insoluble binders are particularly useful in producing controlled-release dosage forms. Many different hydrophobic waxes have been found to be suitable. These include carnauba wax, hydrogenated castor oil, hydrogenated cottonseed oil, stearic acid and a wide variety of fatty acid derivatives (glyceryl behenate, glyceryl monostearate, glyceryl trilaurate, glyceryl trimyristate, glyceryl tripalmitate, glyceryl tristearate, hexadecyl palmitate, octadecyl stearate and sorbitan monostearate). Most of these are miscible when molten and can be used in combination.

Hot-melt processes

The heating procedure can be performed in a mixing vessel that is jacketed with hot water. In some formulations, the temperature rise can be generated by friction alone during agitation/mixing. High-speed mixers can sometimes generate a sufficient temperature rise in an acceptable processing time. Experimentation has shown that 60 °C can be achieved in as little as 10 minutes and that this can be reduced to 5 minutes with additional jacket heating.

There is also a variant of the standard extrusion–spheronization process in which low melting point waxes and heating are used in the extrusion process. Spheronization and cooling are performed simultaneously. This is *hot-melt extrusion–spheronization*.

The main factors influencing the efficiency of the hot-melt granulation process are the amount and melting point of the binder, its viscosity when molten, the impellor rotation speed, the massing time and the temperature achieved.

The amount of binder needed varies widely. Indeed, manipulation of the amount, and the creation of mixtures, of hydrophobic hot-melt binders can be part of the formulation development when one is designing modified-release products and adjusting the drug release versus time profile. For immediate-release systems, PEG 3000 of 25% to 30% by weight has been found to be a good starting point.

Following cooling of the melt granulation granules or pellets to room temperature, they follow the same fate as other granules, i.e. following an optional size reduction and screening procedure, they are either used in their own right as a dosage form, filled into hard capsule shells or they are compacted into tablets together with other excipients.

Advantages and limitations

The advantages of hot-melt granulation compared with aqueous wet granulation is that the use of water is avoided and so damage to hydrolytic drug molecules is minimized. Melt granulation also avoids the use of organic solvents that are sometimes used as an alternative in such cases. However, thermal degradation can still be a problem. A limitation in the use of melt granulation for immediate-release products is that at the moment there is little alternative to the use of PEGs.

Dry granulators

Dry granulation converts primary powder particles into granules using the application of pressure without the intermediate use of a liquid. It therefore avoids heat–temperature combinations which may degrade the product.

Two pieces of equipment are necessary for dry granulation: first, a machine for compressing the dry powders into compacts or flakes and second, a mill for breaking up these intermediate products into granules.

Slugging

The dry powders can be compacted using a conventional tablet machine or, more usually, a large heavy-duty rotary press can be used. This process is often known as *slugging*, the compacts made in the process (typically 25 mm diameter by approximately 10 mm to 15 mm thick) being termed *slugs*. A hammer mill is suitable for breaking the slugs. This is an old process that is being replaced by the more modern, and better, roller compaction process. Many pharmaceutical tableting materials suffer from a property known as *work hardening*, which results in poor recompaction of these already compacted granules.

Roller compaction

Roller compaction is an alternative, gentler method, the powder mix being squeezed between two counter-rotating rollers to form a compressed sheet (Fig. 28.12). The roller rotation speeds can be adjusted to allow variation of the compression time as the material passes between the rollers. Additionally,

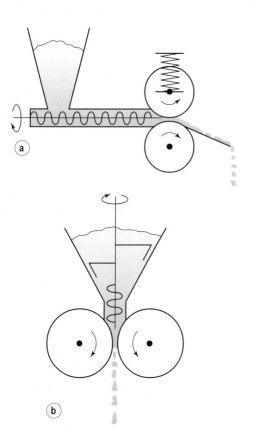

Fig. 28.12 • Roller compaction: **(a)** Alexanderwerk and **(b)** Protec types.

roller pressure can be adjusted and is maintained constant during a run by means of a hydraulic control system to yield granules of constant crushing strength. Even rollers with different surface grooves are available if a particular product is troublesome.

The sheet so formed is normally weak and brittle and breaks immediately into flakes that can be somewhat similar to cornflakes in their geometry. These flakes need gentler treatment to break them into granules. An oscillating granulator of the type shown in Fig. 28.6 can be used with care, but often the conversion of these flakes to granules can be achieved by screening alone. Separation of fines (small powder particles) formed during the size reduction stage is often necessary. With suitable documentation, these may be recycled.

Advantages of the roller compaction process

- The process is economical as it dispenses with the intermediate stages of wet massing and drying, and thus the associated energy and other processing costs.
- It can cope with a wide range of materials, particle size, bulk density and flowability. However, experience has shown that not all materials respond to roller compaction as they do not possess suitable deformation or cohesion properties.
- There are relatively low investment costs compared with alternative granulation processes using multiple, and more expensive, equipment.
- The process is easily scaled up.
- The product has uniform properties with respect to its mechanical strength.
- Additionally, the gentle 'squeeze' of roller compactors leaves the resulting granules capable of further compaction into tablets without the work-hardening problems encountered with slugging.

Again, as for most modern pharmaceutical process machinery, a wide range of sizes is available capable of operating with a wide range of throughputs and compaction forces (e.g. Alexanderwerk, Powtec). In the case of roller compactors, this range is enormous, being available for throughputs between 10 kg h^{-1} and 2000 kg h^{-1} and compaction forces between 16 kN and 64 kN per centimetre of roller length. This is achieved by the choice of machines with roller diameters of between 100 mm and 450 mm and roller lengths of 30 mm to 115 mm. This allows a wide range of active pharmaceutical ingredients (i.e. drugs) and excipients to be processed (or coprocessed) and enables easy scale-up from a few hundred grams in development to very large scale production of a successful product.

The Protec or Hutt type (Fig. 28.12b) has a vertical screw feeder in the hopper which produces an even flow of the material. Because of its design, it also has a precompacting and deaerating effect on the powder charge. The speed of the screw, and that of the rollers, can be adjusted to control the process.

Please check your eBook at **https://studentconsult. inkling.com/** for self-assessment questions. See inside cover for registration details.

Bibliography

Alvarez, L., Concheiro, A., Gomez-Amoza, J.L., et al., 2002. Effect of microcrystalline cellulose grade and process variables on pellets prepared by extrusion-spheronization. Drug Dev. Ind. Pharm. 28, 451–456.

Baert, L., 1992. Correlation of extrusion forces, raw materials and sphere characteristics. J. Pharm. Pharmacol. 44, 676–678.

Erkoboni, D.F., 2003. Extrusion/spheronization. In: Ghebre-Sellassie, I., Martin, C. (Eds.), Pharmaceutical Extrusion Technology. Marcel Dekker, New York.

Farag Badawy, S.I., 2000. Effect of process parameters on compressibility of granulation manufactured in a higher-shear mixer. Int. J. Pharm. 198, 51–61.

Faure, A., Grimsey, I.M., Rowe, R.C., et al., 1999. Applicability of a scale-up methodology for the wet granulation process in Collette Gral high shear mixer granulators. Eur. J. Pharm. Sci. 8, 85–93.

Florence, A.T., Siepmann, J. (Eds.), 2009. Modern Pharmaceutics, vol. 1 and 2, fifth ed. Informa, New York.

Gandhi, R., Kaul, C.L., Panchagnula, R., 1999. Extrusion and spheronization in the development of oral controlled-release dosage forms. Pharm. Sci. Technol. Today 2, 160–181.

Ghebre-Sellassie, I., Martin, C. (Eds.), 2003. Pharmaceutical Extrusion Technology. Marcel Dekker, New York.

Hapgood, K.P., Litster, J.D., 2010. Wet granulation processes. In: am Ende, D.J. (Ed.), Chemical Engineering in the Pharmaceutical Industry: R&D to Manufacture. John Wiley & Sons (in conjunction with AIChE), Hoboken.

Keleb, E.I., Vermeire, A., Vervaet, C., et al., 2004. Extrusion granulation and high shear granulation of lactose and highly dosed drugs: a comparative study. Drug Dev. Ind. Pharm. 30, 679–691.

Landin, M., York, P., Cliff, M.J., et al., 1999. Scale up of a pharmaceutical granulation in planetary mixers. Pharm. Dev. Technol. 4, 145–150.

Law, M.F., Deasy, P.B., McLaughlin, J.P., et al., 1997. Comparison of two commercial brands of microcrystalline cellulose for extrusion-spheronization. J. Microencapsul. 14, 713–723.

Lodaya, M., Mollan, M., Ghebre-Sellassie, I., 2003. Twin-screw wet granulation. In: Ghebre-Sellassie, I., Martin, C. (Eds.), Pharmaceutical Extrusion Technology. Marcel Dekker, New York.

Maejima, T., Kubo, M., Osawa, T., et al., 1998. Application of tumbling melt granulation (TMG) method to prepare controlled-release fine granules. Chem. Pharm. Bull. 46, 534–536.

Nürnberg, E., Wunderlich, J., 1999. Manufacturing pellets by extrusion and spheronization (part I). Pharm. Technol. Eur. 11 (2), 41–47.

Nürnberg, E., Wunderlich, J., 1999. Manufacturing pellets by extrusion and spheronization (part II). Pharm. Technol. Eur. 11 (3), 30–34.

Ogawa, S., Kamijima, T., Miyanoto, Y., et al., 1994. A new attempt to solve the scale-up problem for granulation using response surface methodology. J. Pharm. Sci. 83, 439–443.

Parikh, D.M., 2009. Handbook of Pharmaceutical Granulation Technology, third ed. Marcel Dekker, New York.

Rubino, O.R., 1999. Fluid-bed technology: overview and criteria for process selection. Pharm. Technol. 6, 104–113.

Schenck, L., Troup, G.M., Lowinger, M., et al., 2010. Achieving hot melt extrusion. In: am Ende, D.J. (Ed.),
Chemical Engineering in the Pharmaceutical Industry: R&D to Manufacture. John Wiley & Sons (in conjunction with AIChE), Hoboken.

Shah, R.D., Kabadi, M., Pope, D.G., et al., 1995. Physico-mechanical characterization of the extrusion-spheronization process. Part II: rheological determinants for successful extrusion and spheronization. Pharm. Res. 12, 496–507.

Sprockel, O.L., Stamato, H.J., 2010. Design and scale up of dry granulation processes. In: am Ende, D.J. (Ed.), Chemical Engineering in the Pharmaceutical Industry: R&D to Manufacture. John Wiley & Sons (in conjunction with AIChE), Hoboken.

Thoma, K., Ziegler, I., 1998. Investigations on the influence of the type of extruder for pelletization by extrusion-spheronization. I. Extrusion behavior of formulations. Drug Dev. Ind. Pharm. 24, 401–411.

Thoma, K., Ziegler, I., 1998. Investigations on the influence of the type of extruder for pelletization by extrusion-spheronization. II. Sphere characteristics. Drug Dev. Ind. Pharm. 24, 413–422.

Troy, D.B. (Ed.), 2006. Remington: The Science and Practice of Pharmacy, twenty-first ed. Lippincott Williams & Wilkins, Baltimore.

Vilhelmsen, T., Kristensen, J., Schaefer, T., 2004. Melt pelletization with polyethylene glycol in a rotary processor. Int. J. Pharm. 275, 141–153.

Wørts, O., 1998. Wet granulation – fluidized bed and high shear techniques compared. Pharm. Technol. Eur. 10, 27–30.

Zhang, F., McGinty, J.M., 1999. Properties of sustained-release tablets prepared by hot-melt extrusion. Pharm. Dev. Technol. 4, 241–250.

29

Drying

Michael E. Aulton   Satyanarayana Somavarapu

CHAPTER CONTENTS

KEY POINTS

- Drying is important at many stages of pharmaceutical manufacture to remove solvent (usually water) that could act as a vector for chemical and microbiological deterioration of the drug or product.
- The most common form of drying is heat-induced evaporation of the solvent. Great care must be taken (by controlling temperature and time) to minimize any thermal degradation during drying.
- Some fraction of the solvent is very easy to remove (known as *free moisture*) and the remainder is much more difficult or occasionally impossible to remove from a solid (*bound moisture*).
- Many different types of drying processes and equipment exist as there are numerous mechanisms by which moisture is lost from a wet product or intermediary.
- The selection of the best drying method for a product is a key decision.
- The phenomenon of solute migration during drying should be minimized.

Introduction

Drying is an important operation in primary pharmaceutical manufacture (i.e. the synthesis of active pharmaceutical ingredients or excipients) because it is often the last stage of manufacturing before packaging. It is important that the residual moisture, say from a final crystallization step, is rendered low enough to prevent product deterioration during storage and ensure free-flowing properties during use. It is equally important (and probably encountered more frequently) in secondary (dosage form) manufacture following the common operation of wet granulation (see Chapter 28) during the preparation of granules before tablet compaction. Hence stability (see Chapters 47 and 49), flow properties (see Chapter 12) and compactability (see Chapter 30) are all influenced by residual moisture.

This chapter is concerned with drying to the 'dry' solid state, starting with either a wet solid or a solution or suspension. The former is usually achieved by exposure of the wet solid to moving, relatively dry air. Elevated air temperatures to accelerate the process are common. The latter is possible with equipment such as the spray-dryer (see later in this chapter), which is capable of producing a dry product from a solution or suspension in one operation.

Most pharmaceutical materials are not completely free from moisture (i.e. they are not bone dry) but contain some residual water, the amount of which may vary with the temperature and humidity of the ambient air to which they are exposed. This is discussed in more detail in this chapter.

For the purpose of this chapter, drying is defined as the removal of all or most of the liquid associated with a wet pharmaceutical product. All drying processes of relevance to pharmaceutical manufacturing involve evaporation or sublimation of the liquid phase and the removal of the subsequent vapour. The process must provide the latent heat for these processes without a significant temperature rise. Naturally, the latter will enhance the potential of thermal degradation of the product. In most cases the 'liquid' will be water, but more volatile organic solvents, such as 2-propanol, may also need to be removed in a drying process. The physical principles of aqueous or organic solvent drying are similar, regardless of the nature of the liquid, though volatile solvents are normally recovered by condensation rather than being vented into the atmosphere. This is for environmental and economic reasons. In addition, the toxicity and flammability of organic solvents pose additional safety and process considerations.

Drying of wet solids

Fundamental properties and interrelationships

An understanding of the drying of wet solids requires some preliminary explanation of a number of important terms. To avoid confusion and repetition, these terms are defined and explained in the context of water (the most commonly used pharmaceutical solvent) but the explanations and concepts are equally applicable to other relevant liquids (e.g. ethanol, 2-propanol).

Moisture content of wet solids

The moisture content of a wet solid is expressed as kilograms of moisture associated with 1 kg of the moisture-free, or bone-dry, solid. Thus a moisture content of 0.4 means that 0.4 kg of water is present per kilogram of the bone-dry solid that will remain after complete drying. It is sometimes calculated as a percentage moisture content; thus this example would be quoted as 40% moisture content.

Total moisture content

Total moisture content is the total amount of liquid associated with a wet solid. Some of this water can be easily removed by the simple evaporative processes used by most pharmaceutical dryers and some cannot. The amount of easily removable water (*unbound water*) is known as the *free moisture content*, and the moisture content of the water that is more difficult to remove in practice (*bound water*) is the *equilibrium moisture content*. Thus the total moisture content of a solid is equal to its bound and unbound moisture content or, put another way, its free moisture content plus its equilibrium moisture content.

Unbound water. The unbound water associated with a wet solid exists as a liquid and it exerts its full vapour pressure. It can be removed readily by evaporation. During a drying process this unbound water is readily lost, but the resulting solid will not be completely free from water molecules as it remains in contact with atmospheric air, which inevitably contains some dissolved water. Consequently, the resulting solid is often known as *air dry*.

Equilibrium moisture content

As mentioned already, evaporative drying processes will not remove all the possible moisture present in a wet product because the drying solid equilibrates with the moisture that is naturally present in air. The moisture content of a solid under steady-state ambient conditions is termed the *equilibrium moisture content*. Its value will change with the temperature and humidity of the air, and with the nature of the solid (see later in this chapter).

Bound water. Part of the moisture present in a wet solid may be adsorbed on surfaces of the solid or may be absorbed within its structure to such an extent that it is prevented from developing its full vapour pressure and therefore from being easily removed by evaporation. Such moisture is described as *bound water* and is more difficult to remove than unbound water. Adsorbed water is attached to the surface of the solid as individual water molecules, which may form a monolayer (or bilayer) on the solid surface. Absorbed bound water exists as a liquid but is trapped in capillaries within the solid by surface tension.

Moisture content of air

An added complication to the drying process is that the drying air also contains moisture. Many pharmaceutical plants have air-conditioning systems to reduce the humidity of the incoming process air, but removing water from air is a very expensive process and therefore not all the water will be removed. The moisture content of air is expressed as kilograms of water per kilogram of bone-dry (water-free) air.

The moisture content of air is altered not only by changes in its temperature alone but also by changes in the amount of moisture taken up by the air. The moisture content of air should be carefully distinguished from the relative humidity.

Relative humidity of air

Ambient air is a simple solution of water in a mixture of gases and as such follows the rules of most solutions – such as increased water solubility with increasing temperature, a maximum solubility at a particular temperature (saturation) and precipitation of the solute on cooling (condensation, rain!). Incidentally, this is exactly why rain is sometimes called precipitation.

At a given temperature, air is capable of 'taking up' (i.e. dissolving) water vapour until it is saturated (at 100% relative humidity). Lower relative humidities can be quantified in terms of *percentage relative humidity*, which is given by

$$\frac{\text{vapour pressure of water vapour in air}}{\substack{\text{vapour pressure of water vapour in the} \\ \text{air saturated at the same temperature}}} \times 100$$

$$(29.1)$$

This is approximately equal to the percentage saturation, which is

$$\frac{\substack{\text{mass of water vapour present} \\ \text{per kilogram of dry air}}}{\substack{\text{mass of water vapour required to saturate} \\ 1\,\text{kg of dry air at the same temperature}}} \times 100$$

$$(29.2)$$

Percentage saturation is the more fundamental measure but the expression 'relative humidity' is most commonly used. The two differ only very slightly in practice and only because water vapour does not behave exactly like an ideal gas.

These relationships show that the relative humidity of air is dependent not only on the amount of moisture in the air but also on its temperature. This is because the amount of water required to saturate air is itself dependent on temperature. As mentioned before, in ambient air, water is in solution in the air gases, and in this case its solubility increases with increasing temperature. If the temperature of the air is raised whilst its moisture content remains constant, the air will theoretically be capable of taking up more moisture and therefore its *relative* humidity falls. A reexamination of Eqs 29.1 and 29.2 will show this.

It is important to understand the difference between moisture content and relative humidity of air. This is important in many contexts (powder properties, granulation, drying, compaction, storage conditions) but these terms are often confused.

An additional complication to be taken into account is that *during* a drying process both the temperature and the moisture content of the drying air (and therefore its relative humidity) could change significantly. This arises from two separate factors:

- Uptake into the drying air of water vapour that has evaporated from the drying solid. If evaporation is high and vapour removal inefficient, the drying efficiency will rapidly fall.
- The cooling of the supply air (and consequently the product) as the air transfers latent heat to the wet solid. This phenomenon is known as *evaporative cooling*. If the cooling is excessive, the temperature of the air may fall to a value known as the *dew point*. Here the solubility of water in the cooler air is reduced to such a point that the saturated solubility is exceeded and liquid water will condense and be deposited.

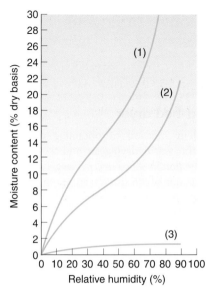

Fig. 29.1 • Typical equilibrium moisture contents at 20 °C for starch-based materials *(1)*, textiles and fibrous materials *(2)* and inorganic substances *(3)*, such as kaolin.

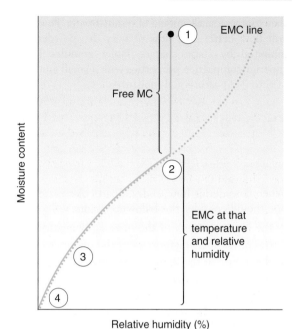

Fig. 29.2 • Loss of water from a drying solid. The wet solid before drying is at position 1. It can lose water by evaporation to position 2, its equilibrium moisture content (EMC) at that relative humidity. The only way the solid can lose more water is to reduce the relative humidity of the atmosphere, to position 3 with silica gel or to position 4 with phosphorus pentoxide. *MC*, moisture content.

Relationship between equilibrium moisture content, relative humidity and the nature of the solid

The equilibrium moisture content of a solid exposed to moist air varies with the relative humidity and with the nature of the solid; Fig. 29.1 shows some typical plots. If we assume that the atmospheric conditions are of the order of 20 °C and 70% to 75% relative humidity, a mineral such as kaolin will contain approximately 1% bound moisture, whilst a starch-based product may have as much as 30% or more.

Loss of water from wet solids

As explained already, unbound water is easily lost by evaporation until the equilibrium moisture content of the solid is reached. This is shown in Fig. 29.2. Once the solid reaches its equilibrium moisture content, extension of the time of drying will not change the moisture content as an equilibrium situation has been reached. The only way to reduce the moisture content of the solid shown in Fig. 29.2 is to reduce the relative humidity of the ambient air. This can be achieved on a large scale with an air-conditioning system. On a laboratory scale, desiccators are used. Silica gel (a common laboratory and packaging desiccant) does not directly take water from a solid; instead it acts by removing the water from the air, thereby reducing its relative humidity to approximately 5% to 10%. This in turn causes the equilibrium to move along the drying curve in Fig. 29.2 to the left, thus reducing the moisture content of the solids. Phosphorus pentoxide works in an identical manner but it has an even greater affinity for the water in the storage air.

If dried materials are exposed to humid ambient conditions, they will quickly regain moisture from the atmosphere as this relationship is an equilibrium. Fig. 29.1 shows this. Thus it is unnecessary to 'overdry' a product, and there is no advantage in drying a product to a moisture content lower than that which the material will have under the normal conditions of use.

If low residual moisture content is necessary because of a hydrolytic instability in the material, the dried product must be efficiently sealed during or immediately after the drying process to prevent ingress of moisture. It is also worth noting that some solid pharmaceutical materials perform better when they contain a small amount of residual water. Powders will flow better; the flow of very dry powders is inhibited by static charge. Tablet granules have superior compaction properties with a small amount (1% to 2 %) of residual moisture.

Types of drying method

Choice of drying method

When considering how to dry a particular material, one should consider the following points:

- the heat sensitivity of the material being dried;
- the physical characteristics of the material;
- the nature of the liquid to be removed;
- the scale of the operation;
- the necessity for asepsis; and
- the available sources of heat (steam, electrical).

The general principles for efficient drying can be summarized as:

- large surface area for heat transfer;
- efficient heat transfer per unit area (to provide sufficient latent heat of vaporization or heat of sublimation in the case of freeze-drying);
- efficient mass transfer of evaporated water through any surrounding boundary layers, i.e. sufficient turbulence to minimize boundary layer thickness; and
- efficient vapour removal, i.e. low relative humidity air moving at adequate velocity.

Dryers in the pharmaceutical industry

The types and variety of drying equipment have reduced in recent years as pharmaceutical companies strive for standardization and globalization of manufacturing. An additional trend is the manufacture of 'mini' versions of manufacturing equipment to be used in formulation and process development. The use of the miniaturized production equipment (processing just a few hundred grams) minimizes later problems that arise with scale-up to manufacturing batches (typically a few hundred kilograms).

A variety of pharmaceutical dryers are still used, and it is convenient to categorize these according to the heat transfer method that they use, i.e. convection, conduction or radiation.

Convective drying of wet solids

Dynamic convective dryers

Fluidized-bed dryer

An excellent method of obtaining good contact between the warm drying air and wet particles is found in the *fluidized-bed dryer*. The general principles of the technique of *fluidization* are summarized before its application to drying is discussed.

Consider the situation in which particulate matter is contained in a vessel, the base of which is perforated, enabling a fluid to pass through the bed of solids from below. The fluid can be a liquid or gas, but air will be assumed for the purposes of this description, as it is directly relevant to pharmaceutical drying processes.

If the air velocity through the bed is increased gradually and the pressure drop through the bed is measured, a graph of the operation shows several distinct regions, as indicated in Fig. 29.3. At first, when the air velocity is low, in the region from A to B, air flow occurs between the particles without causing disturbance, but as the velocity is increased a point, C, is reached when the pressure drop has attained a value where the frictional drag on the particle is equal to the force of gravity on the particle. Rearrangement of the particles occurs to offer least resistance, D, and eventually they are suspended in the air and move about. The pressure drop through the bed decreases slightly because of the greater porosity at D. Further increase in the air velocity causes the particles to separate and move freely, and the bed becomes *fully fluidized*, in the region from D to E. Any additional increase in velocity separates the particles further (i.e. the bed expands) without

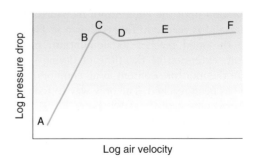

Fig. 29.3 • Effect of air velocity on pressure drop through a fluidized bed.

an appreciable change in the pressure drop. In the region from E to F, fluidization is irregular, much of the air flowing through in bubbles; the term *boiling bed* is used to describe this. At a very high air flow rate, F, the air velocity is sufficient to entrain the solid particles and transport them out of the top of the bed in a process known as *pneumatic transport*.

The important factor is that fluidization produces conditions of great turbulence, the particles mixing with good contact between air and particles. Hence if hot air is used, the turbulent conditions lead to high heat and mass transfer rates, and the fluidized-bed technique therefore offers a means of rapid drying.

The fluidized-bed dryer makes use of this process of fluidization to increase the efficiency of heat transfer and vapour removal compared with the older static tray dryers that it replaced. A reason for this is the more efficient transfer of the required latent heat of evaporation from the air to the drying solid. The rate of heat transfer (dH/dt) in convective drying may be written as

$$dH/dt = h_c A \Delta T$$

(29.3)

where h_c is the heat transfer coefficient for convective heat transfer, A is the surface area available for heat transfer and ΔT is the difference in temperature between the drying air and the solid to be dried. The heat transfer coefficient is high in a fluidized bed as the vigorous motion of the particles reduces the thickness of the boundary layer. Also, the process fluidizes individual powder particles or granules, and thus the surface area available for drying is maximized to the total surface area of the powder bed. An equivalent to Eq. 29.3 shows that the rate of mass transfer (in this case vapour removal in the opposite direction) is similarly increased.

Heat and mass transfer are therefore relatively efficient in a fluidized-bed dryer, and the process, even for a large manufacturing batch, takes between approximately 20 and 40 minutes.

The arrangement of a typical fluidized-bed dryer is shown in Fig. 29.4. Sizes are available with capacities ranging from approximately 400 g to 1200 kg. Commercially available fluidized-bed dryers are designed and manufactured so that the various dryers throughout the range have similar geometric and hydrodynamic features to aid scale-up from laboratory experiments to product manufacturing.

Advantages of fluidized-bed drying

1. Efficient heat and mass transfer gives high drying rates, so drying times are short. Apart

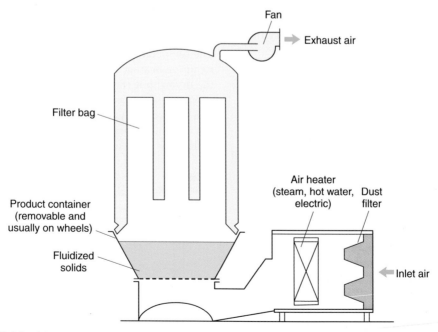

Fig. 29.4 • Fluidized-bed dryer.

from obvious economic advantages, the heat challenge to thermolabile materials is minimized.

2. The fluidized state of the bed ensures that drying occurs from the surface of all the individual particles. Hence most of the drying will occur at a constant rate.

3. The temperature of a fluidized bed is uniform throughout (as a result of the turbulence) and can be controlled precisely.

4. The turbulence in a fluidized bed causes some attrition of the surface of the granule. This produces a more spherical free-flowing product.

5. The free movement of individual particles reduces the risk of soluble materials migrating during drying (see later in this chapter).

6. Keeping the granules separate during drying also reduces the problems of aggregation and reduces the need for a sieving stage after drying.

7. The fluidization containers can be mobile, making handling and movement around the production area simple, thus reducing labour costs.

8. Short drying times mean that the unit achieves a high product output from a small floor space.

Disadvantages of fluidized-bed drying

1. The turbulence of the fluidized state may result in excessive attrition of some materials, with damage to some granules and the production of too much dust.

2. Fine particles may become entrained in the fluidizing air and must be collected by bag filters, with care to avoid segregation and loss of fines.

3. The vigorous movement of particles in hot dry air can lead to the generation of charges of static electricity, and suitable precautions must be taken. A mixture of air with a fine dust of organic materials such as starch and lactose can explode violently if ignited by sparking caused by static charges. The danger is increased if the fluidized material contains a volatile solvent. Adequate electrical earthing is essential and, naturally, is fitted as standard on all modern dryers.

Conductive drying of wet solids

In this process the wet solid is in thermal contact with a hot surface, and the bulk of heat transfer occurs by conduction.

Vacuum oven

This equipment is a good example of a conduction dryer, though it is not used as extensively as it was formerly. The vacuum oven (Fig. 29.5) consists of a jacketed vessel sufficiently strong in construction to withstand a vacuum within the oven and possibly steam pressure in the jacket. In addition, the supports for the shelves form part of the jacket, giving a larger area for heat transfer by conduction. The oven should be closed by a door that can be locked tightly to give an airtight seal. The oven is connected to a vacuum pump through a condenser and liquid receiver, although if the liquid to be removed is water and the pump is of the ejector type that can handle water vapour, the pump can be connected directly to the oven.

Operating pressure can be as low as 0.03 bar to 0.06 bar, at which water boils at 25 °C to 35 °C. Some ovens may be large (e.g. approximately 1.5 m³ and with 20 shelves).

The main advantage of a vacuum oven is that drying occurs at a low temperature, and because there is little air present, there is minimal risk of oxidation. The temperature of the drying solid can rise to the steam or heating water temperature at the end of the drying, but this is not usually harmful.

Vacuum ovens are rarely used nowadays for production but are still worthy of mention as they may be the only method available to dry particularly thermolabile or oxygen-sensitive materials. Additionally,

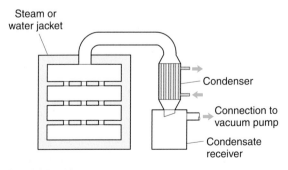

Fig. 29.5 • Vacuum oven.

small-scale vacuum ovens are frequently found in development laboratories, where they are commonly used for the drying of small development samples, particularly when the heat stability of the drug or formulation is uncertain.

Radiation drying of wet solids

Radiant heat transmission

Heat transmission by radiation differs from heat transfer by conduction or convection in that no transfer medium (solid, liquid or gaseous) needs be present. Heat energy in the form of radiation can cross empty space or travel through the atmosphere virtually without loss. If it falls on a body capable of absorbing it, then it appears as heat, although a proportion may be reflected or transmitted.

Use of microwave radiation

Use of microwave radiation in the wavelength range from 10 mm to 1 m has been found to be an efficient heating and drying method. Microwave dryers are used in the pharmaceutical industry.

Generation and action of microwaves

Microwaves are produced by an electronic device known as a magnetron. Microwave energy can be reflected down a rectangular duct (termed a waveguide) or simply beamed through a transparent polypropylene window into the drying chamber. To avoid interference with radio and television, the magnetron is permitted to operate only at certain frequencies, which are normally 960 MHz and 2450 MHz.

The penetration of microwaves into the wet product is so good that heat is generated uniformly within the solid.

When microwaves fall on substances of suitable electronic structure (i.e. small polar molecules, such as water), the electrons in the molecule attempt to resonate in sympathy with the radiation. The resulting molecular 'friction' generates heat. The large molecules of the solids do not resonate as well as, say, water molecules, so further heating may be avoided once the water is removed. This is indicated clearly by the 'loss factors' listed in Table 29.1. The loss factor is the ratio of the microwave energy absorbed by individual molecules to the microwave energy

Table 29.1 Microwave energy loss factors for some pharmaceutical solvents and excipients

Material	Loss factor
Methanol	13.6
Ethanol	8.6
Water	6.1
2-Propanol	2.9
Acetone	1.25
Maize starch	0.41
Magnesium carbonate	0.08
Lactose	0.02

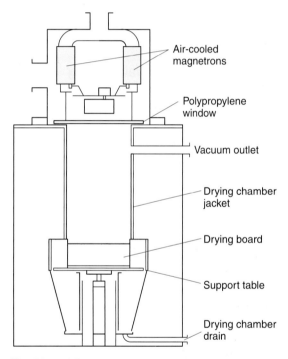

Fig. 29.6 • Microwave dryer. Courtesy of T.K. Fielder.

provided. Thus the higher the value, the greater is the absorption of microwave energy. Table 29.1 lists values for some common solvents and excipients. Clearly, the absorption of the microwave energy is far greater for small polar molecules than for larger and less polar molecules.

Microwave dryers for granulates

Fig. 29.6 shows a sketch of a microwave dryer used for drying granules. It is designed to operate under a slight vacuum. That, in itself, is not essential for the use of microwaves but the air flow through the chamber facilitates the continuous removal of evaporated solvent. The radiation is generated by multiple magnetrons each producing 0.75 kW at 2450 MHz. The radiation passes through the polypropylene window into the drying chamber, where it is absorbed by the liquid in the wet granules contained on a tray. The heat generated in the mass drives off the moisture.

The evolved vapour is drawn away in the air flow as it is formed. When drying is nearly complete, the radiation field intensity within the chamber will rise because the dry solids do not absorb as readily as water. This rise is detected, and the magnetrons are progressively turned down automatically to give an accurate control of the final moisture content and minimize the danger of overheating.

Advantages of microwave drying

The following advantages are claimed for microwave drying:

1. It provides rapid drying at fairly low temperatures.
2. The thermal efficiency is high as the dryer casing and the air remain cool. Most of the microwave energy is absorbed by the liquid in the wet material.
3. The bed is stationary, avoiding problems of dust and attrition.
4. Solute migration is reduced as there is uniform heating of the wet mass.
5. Equipment is highly efficient and refined. All the requirements of product and operator safety have been incorporated into machines without detracting from good manufacturing practice considerations.
6. Granulation end point detection is possible by measurement of the residual microwave energy (as this rises sharply within the dryer when there is little solvent left to evaporate).

Disadvantages of microwave drying

1. The batch size of commercial production microwave dryers is smaller than the batch sizes available for fluidized-bed drying.
2. Care must be taken to shield operators from the microwave radiation, which can cause damage to organs such as the eyes and testes.

This is ensured by fail-safe devices preventing generation of microwaves until the drying chamber is sealed.

Drying of solutions and suspensions

The objective of the dryers used for drying of solutions and suspensions is to generate a large surface area in the liquid for heat and mass transfer and to provide an effective means of collecting the dry solid. The most useful type disperses the liquid as a spray of small droplets – the spray-dryer.

Spray-drying

Spray-drying is a technique that converts a liquid into a dry powder and involves rapidly spraying the liquid or slurry into a hot drying medium. This method of drying is used widely in various industries to produce dry particles with desired properties. Pharmaceutically, spray-drying can be useful for engineering particles for characteristics such as size, morphology, water content and bulk density. The spray-dryer provides a large surface area for heat and mass transfer by atomizing the liquid feed into small droplets. These are sprayed into a stream of circulating hot air such that each liquid droplet dries and solidifies to an individual particle. In spray-drying technology, particle formation and drying occur in one continuous process.

There are many forms of spray-dryer (e.g. GEA, Niro, Buchi), and Fig. 29.7 presents a typical design in which the drying chamber resembles a cyclone. This ensures good circulation of air, facilitates heat transfer and mass transfer and encourages the separation of dried particles from the moving air by the centrifugal action.

The process of spray-drying involves the following fundamental steps:

1. atomization;
2. droplet drying and particle formation; and
3. particle collection.

Atomization

Atomization is the most critical step in spray-drying processes. Atomization is the process of converting fluid into a fine spray comprising high surface area droplets. The particle size of the final dry powder is

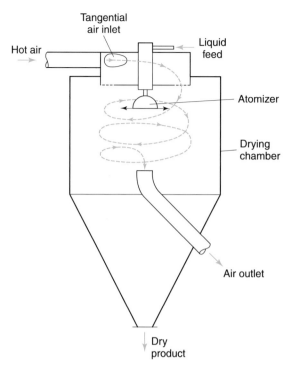

Fig. 29.7 • Spray-dryer.

primarily controlled by the initial feed droplet size. A wide variety of atomizers are available based on pressure, centrifugal, electrostatic and ultrasound techniques.

Pressure nozzle atomization. In this type of atomization, a spray is created by the forcing of the liquid through an orifice. The required pressure is supplied by the spray-dryer feed pump, with spray pressure having an influence on droplet size. Pressure nozzle atomization allows the narrowest range final product size distribution.

Two-fluid nozzle atomization. In two-fluid nozzle atomization (Fig. 29.8) the source of atomization energy is compressed gas, with a spray created by a high-speed gas steam (either air or nitrogen) blasting the liquid into droplets. In this context, the two fluids are the liquid product and the atomizing gas. A variety of twin-fluid designs exist, and these can generally handle feed rates between 30 L h^{-1} and 80 L h^{-1}. They can be positioned either to spray their droplets co-currently into the air stream from the top of the dryer or to spray their droplets from the base of the dryer in what is known as the 'fountain mode'. The two-fluid nozzles produce a narrow droplet size range, with the mean size being affected by the

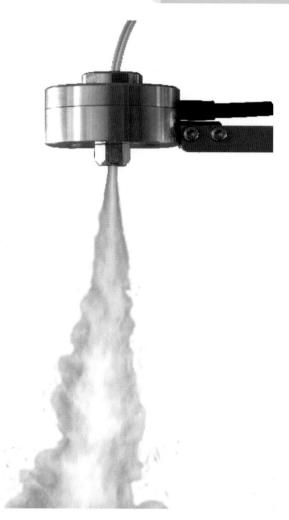

Fig. 29.8 • Two-fluid nozzle atomization. Courtesy of Buchi.

nozzle position. In general, a nozzle used co-currently will produce smaller droplets than one used in fountain mode. Rotary atomizers produce droplets in the mid range.

To illustrate this, data from one experiment performed under similar conditions for each mode and atomizer showed that the mean droplet size from a co-current two-fluid nozzle was 2 μm, from a rotary atomizer 50 μm and from a two-fluid nozzle used in fountain mode 100 μm. Two-fluid nozzles may not be useful for production of large particles. Two-fluid nozzle atomization is the least energy efficient method.

Centrifugal atomization. This is achieved by the use of rotary types of atomizer, one form of which is shown in Fig. 29.9. Liquid is fed onto the disc,

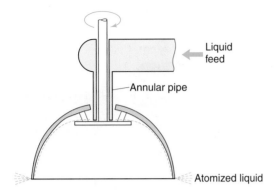

Fig. 29.9 • Rotary atomizer.

which is rotated at high speed (10 000–30 000 rpm). A liquid film is formed that spreads from the small disc to a larger, inverted hemispherical bowl. The film becomes thinner and is dispersed from the edge of the bowl in a fine spray of uniform droplet size. The rotary atomizer has the advantage of being equally effective with either solutions or suspensions of solids and can operate efficiently at various feed rates. This type of atomization is not suitable for highly viscous solutions.

Ultrasonic nozzles. The liquid feed is converted into a fine mist by high-frequency sound vibrations. Piezoelectric transducers convert electrical input into mechanical energy, which creates capillary waves in a liquid film. Droplet size is influenced by the frequency of vibration, viscosity of the feed, and surface tension. The range of frequencies used for ultrasonic nozzles is from 20 kHz to 180 kHz, with the smallest droplet size produced with the highest frequency.

Droplet drying and particle formation

Drying air enters the drying chamber via the gas dispenser. Drying chambers generally have a height-to-diameter ratio of approximately 5:1. The atomized droplets of the feed encounter hot air that can be flowing in co-current, countercurrent or a mixed mode in relation to the droplets. In the pharmaceutical industry, co-current mode is the most suitable method of supplying hot air.

The air enters the chamber tangentially and rotates the drying droplets around the chamber to increase their residence time and therefore the time available for drying. For pharmaceutical purposes, it is usual to filter the incoming air and to heat it indirectly by means of a heat exchanger. The rate of drying of atomized droplets is extremely fast because of the very large total surface area of the droplets, which facilitates fast evaporation of the solvent. The time taken to dry the particles in spray-drying is within the range of milliseconds to a few seconds.

A range of sizes of spray-dryers are available, from a laboratory model with a volume of 100 mL to 200 mL (capable of producing just a few grams of experimental material from aqueous or organic solution), through a pilot-scale model with a chamber diameter of 800 mm and a height of 3 m (capable of evaporating 7 kg of water per hour), to production-scale models that may have a chamber diameter of 3.5 m and be 6 m high (or even larger) with an evaporative capacity of approximately 50 kg to 100 kg water per hour. Larger spray-dryers, with a capacity of up to 4000 kg h^{-1}, are used in other industries, notably in food production. Typically, modern spray-dryers have a 60° cone at the base of the hollow cylinder.

Collection of dried product

Most of the dried particles separate from the drying gas at the bottom of the spray-dryer chamber. The separation of fine particles from the air is achieved by use of a special separation device, such as a cyclone or bag filter. The spray-drying process can be an open or closed system. In an *open system* the drying gas is air. In an open cycle the gas is not recirculated but enters the atmosphere. Open system spray-drying is cost-effective but may not be suitable for pharmaceuticals sensitive to oxygen. In a *closed system*, nitrogen is used as the drying gas. It is recycled, with the evaporated solvents being recollected.

Spray-dried product

Spray-dried product is easily recognizable, being uniform in appearance. The particles have a characteristic shape, in the form of hollow spheres sometimes with a small hole. This shape arises from the drying process because the droplet enters the hot air stream and dries from the outside to form an outer crust with liquid still in the centre. The internal liquid then vaporizes and the internal vapour escapes by blowing a hole in the sphere. Fig. 29.10 shows the mechanism of formation of the spherical product.

Nano spray-dryer

Spray-drying generally produces particles having sizes in the micrometre range. It is difficult to produce nano-sized particles with conventional spray-drying

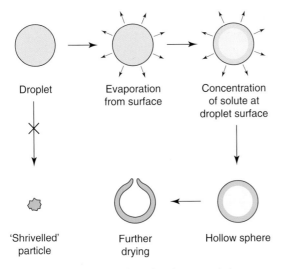

Fig. 29.10 • Formation of product in spray-drying.

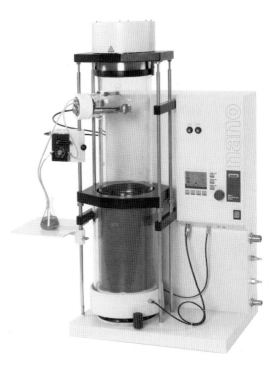

Fig. 29.11 • Nano spray-dryer. Courtesy of Buchi.

methods. This limitation is due to the design of the atomizers and powder collection systems used in conventional spray-drying systems. In a nano spray-dryer (Fig. 29.11) the fine droplets are generated by a vibrating mesh technology. A nano spray-dryer can produce particles of 300 nm, but as large as 5 μm if desired, with a uniform size distribution. An electrostatic precipitator is a novel element that allows collection of the extremely fine particles produced.

Advantages of the spray-drying process

1. There are millions of small droplets which give a large surface area for heat and mass transfer such that evaporation is very rapid. The actual drying time of a droplet is only a fraction of a second, and the overall time in the dryer is only a few seconds.
2. Because evaporation is very rapid, the droplets do not attain a high temperature. Most of the heat is used as latent heat of vaporization and the temperature of the particles is kept low by evaporative cooling.
3. Provided that a suitable atomizer is used and well controlled, the resulting powder will have a uniform and controllable particle size.
4. Labour costs are low, and the process yields a dry, free-flowing powder from a dilute solution, in a single operation with no handling.
5. It can be used as a continuous process if required.

6. The resulting product has many beneficial properties for pharmaceutical applications. These are discussed in the section entitled 'Pharmaceutical applications of spray-drying'.

Disadvantages of the spray-drying process

1. The equipment is very bulky and, with the ancillary equipment, is expensive.
2. The overall thermal efficiency is rather low as the air must still be hot enough when it leaves the dryer to avoid condensation of moisture. In addition, large volumes of heated air pass through the chamber without contacting a particle and thus not contributing directly to the drying process.

Pharmaceutical applications of spray-drying

Direct compressibility. Spray-drying can be useful for the manufacture of granule-sized particles that can be directly compressed. This avoids the need for any further granulation steps during tablet preparation.

This property results from the good flow properties, which, in turn, result from the size and spherical shape of the particles. The resulting hollow spheres are easily crushed and, particularly when binders and other excipients are co-sprayed with the drug, give a strongly bonding material. There are many directly compressible excipients produced by spray-drying. Spray-dried lactose is one example that is commonly used as an excipient in tablets.

Enhancement of the bioavailability of poorly water-soluble drugs. Crystalline drugs may exhibit poor bioavailability after oral administration, due to poor dissolution and solubility properties. One method to enhance the dissolution rate of such drugs is to convert them into the amorphous form by spray-drying. Co-spraying of insoluble drugs with a suitable excipient is a suitable method for producing 'amorphous solid dispersions'. These formulations will have a higher dissolution rate and enhanced bioavailability.

Modified release and taste masking. Spray-drying is a single-step process that can be applied to produce modified-release formulations by the co-spraying of a suitable excipient(s) and drug. Coating is also possible for taste-masking applications. By use of biodegradable polymers along with the drug, it is possible to engineer particles with the desired drug-release properties.

Dry powders for inhalation. Spray-drying is capable of producing spherical particles in the respirable range of approximately 1 μm to 5 μm for delivery of drugs to the lungs from dry powder inhalers (see Chapter 37). Spray-drying is considered an attractive alternative to milling (micronization), which is the established method of producing particles in this size range, as there is tighter control of particle size, particles dissolve more rapidly, porous particles having small aerodynamic diameters can be produced and the product has minimal exposure to heat. These advantages were exploited in Exubera®, the first (but no longer marketed) inhaled insulin product, which comprised spray-dried particles containing insulin, with a mean aerodynamic size of approximately 3 μm. Spray-drying is used to produce spherical tobramycin particles, permitting the efficient delivery of a high dose of the antibiotic from the Tobi® Podhaler.

Aseptic production with spray-drying. It is possible to operate spray-dryers aseptically with heated filtered air to dry products such as serum hydrolysate. In 2015 the US Food and Drug Administration approved the first aseptically spray-dried

fibrin sealant, which has application in controlling bleeding during surgery.

Fluidized spray-dryer

Two technologies, fluidized-bed drying and spray-drying, are combined in fluidized spray-drying. This process is useful mainly for the production of agglomerated powders. A development of the spray-dryer is the fluidized spray-dryer (GEA, Niro). This has a small fluidized bed mounted in the base of the cone at the point where the product is collected. The moving air created in the fluidized bed overcomes any cohesion of spray-dried particles after they fall into the collection chamber. This allows spheres with a higher moisture content to be handled and also ones to be made from stickier and more cohesive substances than were previously possible to process.

Freeze-drying (lyophilization)

In recent years, freeze-drying (also called lyophilization) has become an increasingly important process in the pharmaceutical and biotechnology industries. In the past, freeze-drying was mainly used for stabilization of labile products such as antibiotics, but more recently it has been applied in the production of various drug delivery systems. Freeze-drying is the process of choice in the pharmaceutical industry to stabilize and extend the shelf life of both small molecular therapeutics and biopharmaceuticals.

Freeze-drying is used to dry extremely heat-sensitive materials, and can allow drying, without excessive damage, of proteins, blood products, hormones, vaccines and even microorganisms, which retain a small but significant viability.

In freeze-drying the initial liquid solution or suspension is frozen, the pressure above the frozen state is reduced and the water is removed by sublimation. Thus an overall liquid-to-vapour transition occurs, as with all the previous dryers discussed, but here all three states of matter are involved: liquid to solid, then solid to vapour.

The phase diagram for water

The theory and practice of freeze-drying are based on an understanding and application of the phase diagram for the water system.

The phase diagram for the water system (Fig. 29.12) consists of three separate areas. Each area

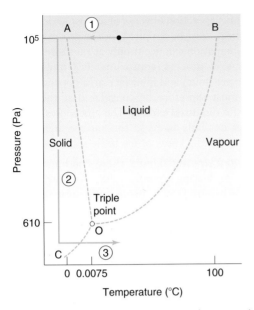

Fig. 29.12 • The phase diagram for water (not to scale) with the freeze-drying process superimposed.

represents a single phase of water – vapour, liquid or solid. Two phases can coexist along a line under the conditions of temperature and pressure defined by any point on the line. The point O is the one unique point where all three phases can coexist and is known as the *triple point*. Its coordinates for pure water are a pressure of 610 Pa (as a comparison, atmospheric pressure is approximately 10^5 Pa) and a temperature of 0.0075 °C.

The lines on the phase diagram represent the interphase equilibrium lines which show:

- The boiling point of water as it is lowered by reduction of the external pressure above the water (the line from B to O in Fig. 29.12).
- The variation of the melting point of ice on reduction of the external pressure above it. There is a very slight rise in the melting point (the line from A to O in Fig. 29.12).
- The reduction of the vapour pressure exerted by ice as the temperature is reduced (the line from C to O in Fig. 29.12).

On heating ice at *atmospheric* pressure, it will melt when the temperature rises to 0°C, i.e. at this temperature the ice will change to liquid water. Continued heating at atmospheric pressure will raise the temperature of the water to 100°C. If heating is continued, the liquid water will be converted into water vapour at 100°C.

If, however, solid ice is maintained at a pressure below the triple point, then on heating, the ice will sublime and pass directly to water vapour without an intermediary liquid phase. This sublimation, and therefore drying, will occur only at a temperature below that of the triple point. Thus it will only happen if the pressure is prevented from rising above the triple-point pressure during the process. To ensure that this is so, the vapour evolved must be removed as quickly as it is formed.

Application of the phase diagram for water to freeze-drying

The process of freeze-drying is superimposed on the phase diagram for water in Fig. 29.12. In its basic form, freeze-drying comprises three steps:

1. freezing the solution;
2. reducing the atmospheric pressure above the ice to below that of the triple point of the product; and
3. adding heat to the system to raise the temperature above the sublimation curve (the line from C to O in Fig. 29.12) and to provide the latent heat of sublimation.

These are discussed in detail next.

Stages of the freeze-drying process

Freezing stage

The freezing step is critical in the freeze-drying process. Freezing determines the morphology of the frozen material, which has an influence on the final freeze-dried product. The freezing process involves nucleation, crystallization of freeze concentrate, and freeze separation in eutectic products or amorphous products. The freezing protocol influences the pore size distribution and pore connectivity of the dried solid. The morphology of ice crystals in the frozen material strongly influences primary and secondary drying (see later).

The liquid material is frozen before the application of a vacuum so as to avoid frothing. The depression of the freezing point caused by the presence of dissolved solutes means that the solution must be cooled to well below the normal freezing temperature for pure water, and it is usual to work in the range from –10°C to –30°C, typically below –18°C. The presence of dissolved solutes will shift the pure-water phase diagram. Because the subsequent stage of sublimation is slow, several methods are used at this stage to produce a larger frozen surface to speed up that later stage.

Shell freezing. This is used for fairly large volumes, such as blood products. The bottles are rotated slowly and almost horizontally in a refrigerated bath. The liquid freezes in a thin shell around the inner circumference of the bottle. Freezing is slow and large ice crystals form, which is a drawback of this method as they may damage blood cells and reduce the viability of microbial cultures.

In vertical spin freezing, the bottles are spun individually in a vertical position so that centrifugal force produces a circumferential layer of solution, which is cooled by a blast of cold air. The solution supercools and freezes rapidly, with the formation of small ice crystals.

Centrifugal evaporative freezing. This is a similar method where the solution is spun in small containers within a centrifuge. This prevents foaming when the vacuum is applied. The vacuum causes boiling at room temperature, and this removes so much latent heat that the solution cools quickly and 'snap' freezes. Approximately 20% of the water is removed before freeze-drying, and there is no need for separate refrigeration. Ampoules are usually frozen in this way, a number being spun in an angled position (approximately 30° to the horizontal) in a special centrifuge head so that the liquid is thrown outwards and freezes as a wedge with a larger surface area.

Vacuum application stage

The containers and the frozen material must be connected to a source of a vacuum sufficient to reduce the pressure below the triple point and remove the large volumes of low-pressure vapour formed during drying. Again, an excess vacuum is normal in practice to ensure that the product in question is below the triple point of the formulation.

Commonly, a number of bottles or vials are attached to individual outlets of a manifold which is connected to a vacuum.

Sublimation stage

Heat of sublimation must be supplied. It may be thought that, as the process occurs at a low temperature, the additional heat needed to sublime the ice would be small. In fact, the latent heat of sublimation of ice is 2900 kJ kg^{-1}, appreciably larger than the latent

heat of evaporation of water at atmospheric pressure. This heat must be supplied for the process to occur.

Sublimation can occur only at the frozen surface. It is a slow process (approximately 1 mm thickness of ice per hour) and is surface area dependent. This step must therefore be considered at the freezing stage (as discussed earlier). The procedures discussed earlier not only increase the surface area but also reduce the thickness of ice to be sublimed.

Primary drying. Under these conditions the ice sublimes, leaving a porous solid which still contains approximately 0.5% moisture after primary drying. Further reduction can be effected by secondary drying. During the primary drying, the latent heat of sublimation must be provided and the vapour removed.

Heat transfer. Heat transfer is critical; insufficient heat input prolongs the process, which is already slow, and excess heat will cause melting.

Small ampoules may be left on the centrifuge head or may be placed on a manifold; in either case, heat gained from the atmosphere is sufficient. Large volumes (e.g. bottles of blood) are placed in individually heated cylinders or are connected to a manifold when heat can be taken from the surrounding environment. This heat must be replaced by some form of external heat source.

It is important to appreciate that, although a significant amount of heat is required, there should be no significant increase in temperature. The added heat should be sufficient to provide the latent heat of sublimation only and little sensible heat. Thus, in all cases, heat transfer must be controlled because only approximately 5 W m^{-2} K^{-1} is needed, and overheating may lead to thermal damage.

Vapour removal. The vapour formed must be removed continually to prevent the pressure within the container rising above the triple-point pressure and thus preventing sublimation. To reduce the pressure sufficiently, it is necessary to use efficient vacuum pumps, usually two-stage rotary pumps on the small scale and ejector pumps on the large scale. On the small scale, vapour is absorbed by a desiccant such as phosphorus pentoxide, or is cooled in a small condenser with solid carbon dioxide. Mechanically refrigerated condensers are used on the large scale.

For vapour flow to occur, the vapour pressure at the condenser must be less than that at the frozen surface, and a low condenser temperature is necessary. On a large scale, vapour is commonly removed by pumping, but the pumps must be of large capacity and must not be affected by moisture. The extent

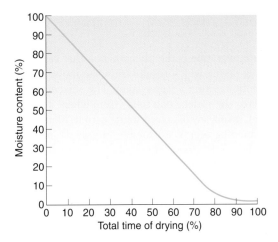

Fig. 29.13 • Sublimation drying: rate of drying curve.

of the necessary pumping capacity will be realized from the fact that, under the pressure conditions used during primary drying, 1 g of ice will form 1000 L of water vapour. Ejector pumps are most satisfactory for this purpose.

Rate of drying. The rate of drying in freeze-drying is very slow. The drying rate curve illustrated in Fig. 29.13 shows a shape similar to that of a normal drying curve, the drying being at constant rate for most of the time.

Computer control enables the drying cycle to be monitored. There is an optimum vapour pressure for a maximum sublimation rate, and the heat input and other variables are adjusted to maintain this value. Continuous freeze-drying is possible in modern equipment where the vacuum chamber is fitted with a belt conveyor and vacuum locks. Despite these advances, the overall drying rate is still slow.

Secondary drying

The removal of the final amounts of residual moisture at the end of primary drying is performed by the raising of the temperature of the solid to as high as 50°C or 60°C. This high temperature is permissible for many materials because the small amount of moisture remaining at the end of primary drying is not sufficient to cause spoilage.

Packaging

Attention must be paid to packaging freeze-dried products to ensure protection from moisture during storage. Containers should be closed without contacting the ambient atmosphere, if possible. Ampoules,

for example, are sealed on the manifold while still under a vacuum. Otherwise, the closing must be performed under controlled atmospheric conditions. The dry product often needs to be sterile.

Spray–freeze-drying

This is a novel concept combining two drying technologies in one system, consisting of elements of both freeze-drying and spray-drying. Spray–freeze-drying (SFD) involves spraying the liquid feed into a cryogenic medium instead of into a drying chamber; the atomized droplets are frozen and water is removed by sublimation. The SFD process thus involves atomization, followed by the steps encountered in conventional freeze-drying, i.e. freezing, primary drying and secondary drying. In SFD the therapeutic agent is exposed to lower temperatures than in spray-drying. SFD has application in the drying of biopharmaceuticals, preventing protein aggregation during drying because of the formation of glassy water. SFD gives a higher product yield compared with spray-drying and is useful in the production of porous particles which are suitable for dry powder formulations.

Advantages of freeze-drying

Freeze-drying, as a result of the character of the process, has certain special advantages:

1. Drying occurs at very low temperatures, so enzyme action is inhibited and chemical decomposition, particularly hydrolysis, is minimized.
2. As it is a frozen solution or suspension that sublimes, the final dry product is a porous solid occupying the same volume as the original solution. Thus the product is light and porous.
3. The porous form of the product gives rapid dissolution of the freeze-dried product.
4. There is no concentration of the solution before drying. Hence salts do not concentrate in the wet state and denature proteins, as occurs with other drying methods.
5. As the process occurs under a high vacuum, there is little contact with air, and oxidation is minimized.

Disadvantages of freeze-drying

There are two main disadvantages of freeze-drying:

1. The porosity, easy dissolution and complete dryness of the product results in it being very

hygroscopic. Unless the product is dried in the final container and the container is sealed in situ, packaging requires special consideration.

2. The process is very slow and uses complicated equipment that is very expensive. It is not a general method of drying, but should be limited to certain types of valuable products that, because of their heat sensitivity, cannot be dried by any other means.

Pharmaceutical applications of freeze-drying

Freeze-drying is used for those products which cannot be dried satisfactorily by any other heat method. These include biological products; for example, some antibiotics, blood products, vaccines (such as BCG, yellow fever, smallpox), enzyme preparations (such as hyaluronidase) and microbiological cultures. The latter enable specific microbiological species and strains to be stored for long periods. They have a viability of approximately 10% on reconstitution.

Freeze-dried tablets. One of the recent developments in tablet technology is the use of freeze-drying to prepare fast-dissolving tablets, which have gained a deal of popularity. Various pharmaceutical companies use freeze-drying technologies to prepared fast-dissolving tablets (e.g. Zydis®, Lyoc® and Quicksolv®). Freeze-dried tablets have a very high porosity that allows rapid dissolution of the tablet in just saliva, and hence these are termed *orodispersible*, *orally disintegrating* or *orally dissolving* tablets.

Freeze-dried wafers can also be useful for delivery of drugs through the buccal route and have huge potential in wound healing.

Stabilization of novel drug delivery systems. Novel drug delivery systems, such as liposomes, microparticles and nanoparticles, enhance the therapeutic potential of many drugs (see Chapter 44). One of the drawbacks with these systems is maintenance of physical and chemical stability in the liquid state. Consequently, freeze-drying is a very useful method to stabilize liposomes and other drug carrier systems, producing a stable powder, which can be reconstituted with an appropriate vehicle before administration. Excipients with cryoprotectant/lyoprotectant properties (such as trehalose, sucrose and mannitol) may need to be included in such preparations to protect the product against morphological changes resulting from freezing and subsequent removal of water.

Solute migration during drying

Solute migration is the phenomenon that can occur during drying which results from the movement of a solution within a wet system. The solvent moves towards the surface of a solid (from where it evaporates), taking any dissolved solute with it. Many drugs and binding agents are soluble in granulating fluid, and during the drying of granulates these solutes can move towards the surface of the drying bed or granule and be deposited there when the solvent evaporates. Solute migration during drying can lead to localized variability in the concentration of soluble drugs and excipients within the dried product.

Migration associated with drying granules can be of two types: intergranular migration (between granules) and intragranular migration (within individual granules).

Intergranular migration

Intergranular migration, where the solutes move from granule to granule, may result in gross maldistribution of the active drug. It can occur during the drying of static beds of granules (e.g. tray drying) because the solvent and accompanying solute(s) move from granule to granule towards the top surface of the bed, where evaporation occurs. When the granules are compressed, the tablets may have a deficiency or an excess of the drug. For example, experimentation found that only 12% of tablets made from a tray-dried warfarin granulate were within the *United States Pharmacopeia* limits for drug content.

Intragranular migration

Drying methods based on fluidization and vacuum tumbling keep the granules separate during drying and so prevent the intergranular migration that may occur in fixed beds. However, intragranular migration, where the solutes move towards the periphery of each granule, may occur.

Consequences of solute migration

Solute migration of either type can result in a number of problems and occasional benefits.

Loss of active drug

The periphery of each granule may become enriched, with the interior suffering depletion. This will be of

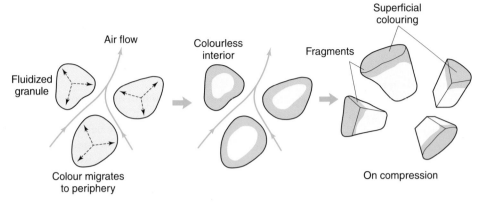

Fig. 29.14 • Mottling caused by intragranular solute migration.

no consequence unless the enriched outer layer is abraded and lost, as may happen during fluidized-bed drying when the fine drug-rich dust will be eluted in the air and carried to the filter bag or lost. The granules suffer a net loss of drug and as a result will be below specification with respect to the quantity of active ingredient.

Mottling of coloured tablets

Coloured tablets can be made by addition of soluble colour during wet granulation. Intragranular migration of the colour may give rise to dry granules with a highly coloured outer zone and a colourless interior (Fig. 29.14). During compaction, granule fracture occurs and the colourless interior is exposed. The eye then sees the coloured fragments against a colourless background and the tablets appear mottled.

Migration may be reduced by use of the insoluble aluminium 'lake' of the colouring material (in which the soluble dye is adsorbed strongly onto insoluble alumina particles) in preference to the soluble dye itself. Studies have indicated that the production of small granules, which do not fracture so readily, is preferable to the production of larger ones if mottling is troublesome.

Migration of soluble binders

Intragranular migration may deposit a soluble binder at the periphery of the granules and so confer on them a 'hoop stress' resistance, making the granules harder and more resistant to abrasion. This migration can aid the bonding process during tablet compaction as a result of binder–binder (rather than drug–drug or drug–excipient) contact and is therefore sometimes beneficial.

Many other factors, such as granule formulation, the drying method and the moisture content, affect solute migration.

Influence of formulation factors on solute migration

Nature of the substrate

The principles governing solute migration are similar to those of thin-layer chromatography. Thus if the granule substrate has an affinity for the solute, then migration will be impeded. Luckily, many of the common tablet excipients possess this affinity. The presence of absorbent materials, such as starch and microcrystalline cellulose, will minimize tablet solute migration.

The use of water-insoluble aluminium lakes (pigments) reduces mottling compared with the use of water-soluble dyes. This effect has also been seen with film-coat colours (see Chapter 32).

Viscosity of granulating fluid

The popular granulating fluids are solutions of polymers whose viscosity is appreciably greater than that of water alone. This viscosity impedes the movement of moisture by increasing the fluid friction. Increasing the concentration and therefore the viscosity of polyvinylpyrrolidone solutions has been shown to slow the migration of drugs in fixed beds of wet granules. Solutions of methylcellulose with comparable viscosities gave similar migration rates, showing that the effect is due to viscosity alone and not to any specific action of either of the binders.

Influence of process factors on solute migration

Drying method

Intergranular migration in fixed beds of granules will occur whenever a particular method of drying creates a temperature gradient. This results in greater evaporation from the hotter zones.

In slow convective drying (e.g. during static tray drying), the maximum concentration of solute that has migrated will normally occur in the surface of the drying bed because the process of drying is slow enough to maintain a capillary flow of solvent/solute to the surface over a long period.

Drying by microwave radiation results in uniform heating that in turn minimizes solute migration.

Drying methods which keep the granules in motion will abolish the problem of intergranular migration, but intragranular migration can still occur. This is marked in fluidized granules.

Initial moisture content

The initial moisture content of the granule will also influence the extent of migration. The greater the moisture content, the greater will be the moisture movement before the pendular state is reached, at which point migration cannot continue as there is no longer a continuous layer of mobile liquid water within the wet solid (see Fig. 28.2).

Some practical means of minimizing solute migration

The following measures can be taken to minimize migration:

- Use the minimum quantity of granulating fluid and ensure that it is well distributed. High-speed mixer/granulators give better moisture distribution than earlier equipment, and granules prepared in this way show less migration.
- Prepare the smallest granules that will flow easily and are generally satisfactory if mottling is troublesome.
- Avoid tray drying unless there is no alternative.
- If tray drying is unavoidable, then the dry granules should be remixed before compression. This will ensure that a random mix of enriched and depleted granules will be fed to the tablet machines. This remixing will be more effective if the granules are small as there will be a greater number of granules per die fill.
- If intragranular migration is likely to be troublesome, consider vacuum or microwave drying as an alternative to fluidized-bed drying.

Please check your eBook at **https://studentconsult. inkling.com/** for self-assessment questions. See inside cover for registration details.

Bibliography

Allen, L.V. (Ed.), 2012. Remington: The Science and Practice of Pharmacy, twenty second ed. Pharmaceutical Press, London.

Broadhead, J., Rouan, S.K., Hau, I., et al., 1994. The effect of process and formulation variables on the properties of spray-dried beta-galactosidase. J. Pharm. Pharmacol. 46 (6), 458–467.

Florence, A.T., Siepmann, J. (Eds.), 2009. Modern Pharmaceutics, vol. 1 and 2, fifth ed. Informa, New York.

Franks, F., Auffret, T., 2008. Freeze Drying of Pharmaceuticals and Biopharmaceuticals: Principles and Practice. RSC Publishing, London.

Koganti, V., Luthra, S., Pikal, M.J., 2010. The freeze-drying process: the use of mathematical modeling in process design, understanding, and scale-up. In: am Ende, D.J. (Ed.), Chemical Engineering in the Pharmaceutical Industry: R&D to Manufacture. John Wiley & Sons (in conjunction with AIChE), Hoboken.

Masters, K., 1991. Spray Drying Handbook, fifth ed. Longman Scientific and Technical, Harlow.

Travers, D.N., 1983. Problems with solute migration. Manuf. Chem. Aerosol News 53 (3), 67–71.

Tsotsas, E., Mujumbar, A.S., 2011. Modern Drying Technology, vol. 3. Wiley-VCH, Weinheim.

Walters, R.H., Bhatnagar, B., Tchessalov, S., et al., 2014. Next generation drying technologies for pharmaceutical applications. J. Pharm. Sci. 103, 2673–2695.

Wan, L.S., Heng, P.W., Chia, C.G., 1991. Preparation of coated particles using a spray drying process with an aqueous system. Int. J. Pharm. 77, 183–191.

Wendel, S., Çelik, M., 1997. An overview of spray-drying applications. Pharm. Tech. 10, 124–144.

30

Tablets and compaction

Göran Alderborn Göran Frenning

KEY POINTS

- Tablets of different types represent collectively the predominant type of dosage form.
- Tablets are used for oral administration for both systemic and local drug treatment.
- Several categories of tablets exist that are used in different ways, e.g. swallowed whole or retained in the mouth during the release of the drug.

517

- Tablets are normally formed by powder compression, i.e. the forcing of particles into close proximity to each other by the application of mechanical force.
- Besides the active ingredient, tablets normally contain a series of excipients that are included to control biopharmaceutical and other quality attributes, as well as to aid the manufacturing of the tablet.
- The release of the active pharmaceutical ingredient is a key product attribute and can be controlled by the formulation to achieve immediate release, delayed release or prolonged release of the drug.
- In the manufacturing of tablets, a series of unit operations are normally used, including mixing and granulation of active ingredient(s) and excipients.
- In the manufacturing of tablets, a number of technical problems can arise, such as high weight and dose variation, low mechanical strength, capping of the tablets, adhesion and high friction.
- The success of a tableting operation is related to the properties of the powder intended to be formed into tablets, and also to the design and conditions of the press and the tooling.
- Important tests of quality attributes of tablets include tablet disintegration and dissolution, tablet friability and tablet fracture resistance.

Introduction

The oral route is the most common way of administering drugs, and among the oral dosage forms, tablets of various kinds are the most common type of solid dosage form in contemporary use. The term 'tablet' (from Latin *tabuletta*) is associated with the appearance of the dosage form, i.e. tablets are small disc-like or cylindrical specimens. The Latin name of the dosage form 'tablet' in the *European Pharmacopoeia* (European Pharmacopoeia Commission, 2016) is *compressi*, which reflects the fact that the dominating process of tablet fabrication is powder compression in a confined space. Alternative preparation procedures are also in use, such as mouldings, freeze-drying and 3D printing. Tablet-like preparations prepared by freeze-drying are sometimes referred to as oral lyophilizates. Moulding (i.e. the shaping and hardening of a semisolid mixture of active substances and excipients), 3D printing, which creates tablets layer-by-layer using computer-aided design, and freeze-drying will not be further described in this chapter.

The idea of forming a solid dosage form by powder compression is not new. In 1843 the first patent for a hand-operated device used to form a tablet was granted. The use of tablets as dosage forms became of interest to the growing pharmaceutical industry, but within pharmacies the pill (a dosage form for oral administration formed by hand into spherical particles approximately 4 mm to 6 mm in diameter) remained the most popular solid dosage form for a long time.

A tablet consists of one or more drugs (active pharmaceutical ingredients), as well as a series of other substances (excipients), used in the formulation of a complete preparation. In the *European Pharmacopoeia* (European Pharmacopoeia Commission, 2016), tablets are defined as 'solid preparations each containing a single dose of one or more active substances. They are obtained by compressing uniform volumes of particles or by another suitable manufacturing technique, such as extrusion, moulding or freeze-drying (lyophilization). Tablets are intended for oral administration. Some are swallowed whole, some after being chewed, some are dissolved or dispersed in water before being administered and some are retained in the mouth where the active substance is liberated.'

Thus a variety of tablets exist, and the types of excipients and also the way in which they are incorporated in the tablet vary. Other dosage forms can be prepared in a similar way but are administered by other routes, such as suppositories.

Tablets are used mainly for systemic drug delivery but may also be used for local drug action. For systemic use the drug must be released from the tablet (i.e. normally it dissolves in the fluids of the mouth, stomach or intestine) and thereafter the drug is absorbed into the systemic circulation, by which it reaches its site of action. Alternatively, tablets can be formulated for local delivery of drugs in the mouth or gastrointestinal tract, or can be used to increase temporarily the pH of the stomach.

Tablets are popular for several reasons:

- The oral route is a convenient and safe way of drug administration.
- Compared with liquid dosage forms, tablets (and other solid dosage forms) have general advantages in terms of the chemical, physical and microbiological stability of the dosage form.
- The preparation procedure enables accurate dosing of the drug.
- Tablets are convenient to handle and can be prepared in a versatile way with respect to their use and the delivery of the drug.

- Tablets can be mass-produced relatively cheaply, with robust and quality-controlled production procedures giving an elegant preparation of consistent quality.

The main disadvantage of tablets as a dosage form is the problem of poor bioavailability of drugs because of unfavourable drug properties, e.g. poor solubility, poor absorption properties and instability in the gastrointestinal tract. In addition, some drugs may cause local irritant effects or otherwise cause harm to the gastrointestinal mucosa.

Quality attributes of tablets

Like all dosage forms, tablets should fulfil a number of product quality attributes regarding chemical, physical and biological characteristics. Quality issues relating to the final product are worth considering early in the development process (and thus early in this chapter) as they give an indication of the goal to be achieved during the development and manufacture of tablets.

The quality attributes that a tablet must possess can be summarized as follows:

1. The tablet should include the correct dose of the drug.
2. The appearance of the tablet should be elegant, and its weight, size and appearance should be consistent.
3. The drug should be released from the tablet in a controlled and reproducible way.
4. The tablet should be biocompatible, i.e. not include excipients, contaminants and microorganisms that could harm patients.
5. The tablet should be of sufficient mechanical strength to withstand fracture and erosion during handling at all stages of its lifetime.
6. The tablet should be chemically, physically and microbiologically stable during the lifetime of the product.
7. The tablet should be formulated into a product acceptable to the patient.
8. The tablet should be packaged in a safe manner.

In order to quantify these quality attributes, tests and specifications must be defined. Some tests and specifications are given in pharmacopoeias, such as dose content, dose uniformity, tablet disintegration, the release of the drug in terms of drug dissolution, and the microbial quality of the preparation. Another important quality attribute of tablets is their resistance to attrition and fracture.

Tablet manufacturing

Stages in tablet formation

The dominating technique of forming tablets (although alternative procedures are in use), as indicated in the definition of tablets in the *European Pharmacopoeia* (European Pharmacopoeia Commission, 2016), is by powder compression, i.e. forcing particles into close proximity to each other by confined compression. This enables the particles to cohere into a porous, solid specimen of defined geometry. The compression occurs in a die by the action of two punches, one lower and one upper, by which the compressive force is applied. *Powder compression* is defined as the reduction in volume of a powder owing to the application of a force. Because of the increased proximity of particle surfaces accomplished during compression, bonds are formed between particles which provide coherence to the powder, i.e. a compact is formed. *Compaction* is defined as the formation of a solid specimen of defined geometry by powder compression.

The process of tableting can be divided into three stages (sometimes known as the *compaction cycle*) (Fig. 30.1).

Die filling

This is normally accomplished by gravitational flow of the powder from a hopper via the die table into the die (although presses based on centrifugal die filling are also used). The die is closed at its lower end by the lower punch.

Tablet formation

The upper punch descends and enters the die, and the powder is compressed until a tablet is formed. During the compression phase the lower punch can be stationary or can move upwards in the die. After the maximum applied force has been reached, the upper punch leaves the powder, i.e. the decompression phase.

Tablet ejection

During this phase the lower punch rises until its tip reaches the level of the top of the die. The tablet is

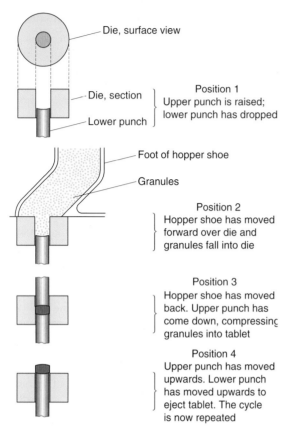

Die, surface view

Die, section
Lower punch

Position 1
Upper punch is raised;
lower punch has dropped

Foot of hopper shoe

Granules

Position 2
Hopper shoe has moved
forward over die and
granules fall into die

Position 3
Hopper shoe has moved
back. Upper punch has
come down, compressing
granules into tablet

Position 4
Upper punch has moved
upwards. Lower punch
has moved upwards to
eject tablet. The cycle
is now repeated

Fig. 30.1 • The sequence of events involved in the formation of tablets.

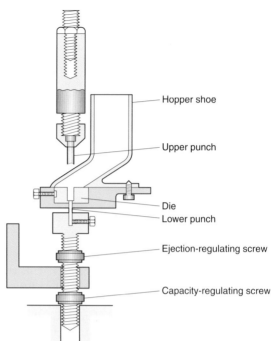

Hopper shoe

Upper punch

Die
Lower punch

Ejection-regulating screw

Capacity-regulating screw

Fig. 30.2 • A single-punch tablet press.

subsequently removed from the die table by a pushing device.

Tablet presses

There are two types of press in common use for tablet production: the single-punch press and the rotary press. In addition, hydraulic presses are used in research and development work for the initial evaluation of the tableting properties of powders and prediction of the effect of scale-up on the properties of the formed tablets (scale-up refers to the change to a larger apparatus for performing a certain operation on a larger scale).

Single-punch press (eccentric press)

A single-punch press possesses one die and one pair of punches (Fig. 30.2), i.e. a set of tableting tools. The powder is held in a hopper, which is connected to a hopper shoe located at the die table. The hopper

shoe moves to and fro over the die, by either a rotational or a translational movement. When the hopper shoe is located over the die, the powder is fed into the die by gravitational powder flow. The amount of powder with which the die is filled is controlled by the position of the lower punch. When the hopper shoe is located beside the die, the upper punch descends and the powder is compressed. The lower punch is stationary during compression, and the pressure is thus applied by the upper punch and controlled by the upper punch displacement. After ejection, the tablet is pushed away by the hopper shoe as it moves back to the die for the next tablet.

The output of tablets from a single-punch press is up to approximately 200 tablets per minute. A single-punch press thus has its primary use in the production of small batches of tablets, such as during formulation development and during the production of tablets for clinical trials.

Rotary press

The rotary press (also referred to as a multistation press) was developed to increase the output of tablets. The primary use of this machine is thus during scale-up in the latter part of the formulation work and during large-scale production. Outputs greater than

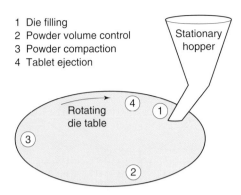

1 Die filling
2 Powder volume control
3 Powder compaction
4 Tablet ejection

Stationary hopper

Rotating die table

Fig. 30.3 • The events involved in the formation of tablets with a rotary press.

10 000 tablets per minute can be achieved by rotary presses.

A rotary press operates with a number of dies and sets of punches, which can range from three for small rotary presses to about 60 for large presses. The dies are mounted in a circle in the die table, and both the die table and the punches rotate together during operation of the machine, so that one die is always associated with one pair of punches (Figs 30.3 and 30.4). The vertical movement of the punches is controlled by tracks that pass over cams and rollers used to control the volume of powder fed into the die and the pressure applied during compression.

The powder is held in a hopper, whose lower opening is located just above the die table. The powder flows by gravity onto the die table and is fed into the die by a feed frame. The reproducibility of the die feeding can be improved by a rotating device, referred to as a force-feeding device. During powder compression both punches operate by vertical movement. After tablet ejection, the tablet is knocked away as the die passes the feed frame.

Computerized presses

For computerized presses the movement of the punches can be controlled and varied considerably. Thus tablets can be prepared under controlled conditions with respect to the loading pattern and loading rate. Possible applications are the investigation of the sensitivity of a drug to such variations, or to mimic the loading pattern of production presses to predict scale-up problems. Because of this latter application, this type of press is also referred to as a 'compaction simulator'.

Instrumentation of tablet presses

Significant research on the process of tablet preparation was initiated in the 1950s and 1960s, i.e. about 100 years after the introduction of tablets as a dosage form. An important step in the development of such fundamental research was the introduction of instrumented tablet machines. By this instrumentation, the forces involved in the compaction process, i.e. the press forces from the upper and lower punches, and the force transmitted to the die, as well as the displacement of the upper and lower punches during the compression and decompression phases, could be recorded.

Instrumented presses are used in research, in development and in the production of tablets. In research and development, instrumented machines are used to provide fundamental information on the mechanical and compaction properties of powders that should be used in tablet formulations. With this application, the work is normally done by instrumented single-punch presses or instrumented hydraulic presses (compaction simulators). The two main applications for an instrumented press in research and development are:

1. To prepare tablets under defined conditions, e.g. in terms of applied force during compaction. These tablets are thereafter characterized by different procedures, such as imaging, surface area and tensile strength analysis.

2. To describe and analyse the compression properties of materials by studying punch forces and punch displacements during the compression and decompression phases. A series of different procedures exists, involving, for example, the assessment of deformation behaviour of particles during compression and friction properties during ejection. Some of these are described later.

In production, instrumented production machines, i.e. rotary presses, are used to control the tableting operation and to ensure that tablets of consistent quality are produced. Normally, only force signals are used on production machines, and the variation in force signal during compression is monitored as it reflects variations in tablet weight.

The force transducers commonly used in the instrumentation of tablet machines are of two types. The most common type is called a *strain gauge*, which consists of wires through which an electric current is passed. The strain gauge is bonded to a punch or punch holder. During powder compression, a force

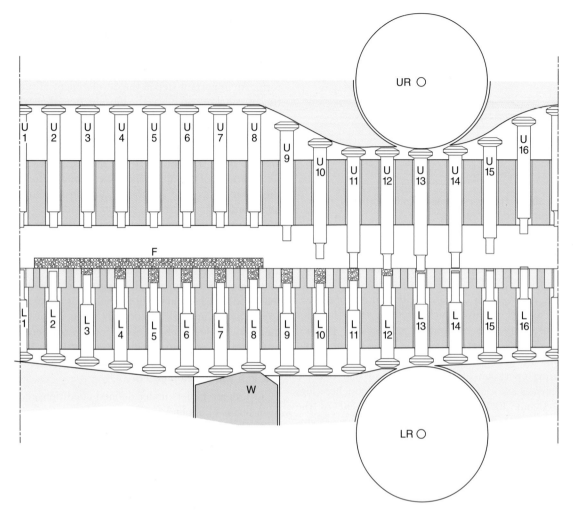

Fig. 30.4 • Punch tracks of a rotary tablet press. U1 to U8, upper punches in raised position; L1, lower punch at top position, tablet ejected; L2 to L7, lower punches dropping to lowest position and filling die with granules to an overfill at L7; L8, lower punch raised to expel excess granules giving correct volume; U9 to U12, upper punches lowering to enter die at U12; L13 and U13, upper and lower punches pass between rollers and granules are compacted to a tablet; U14 to U16, upper punch rising to top position; L14 to L16, lower punch rising to eject tablet. *F*, feed frame with granules; *LR*, lower roller; *UR*, upper roller; *W*, powder volume adjuster.

is applied to the punches and they will temporarily deform. The magnitude of this deformation is dependent on the elastic modulus of the punches and the force applied. When the punch is deformed, the wire of the strain gauge is also deformed and the electrical resistance of the strain gauge will change. This change in electrical resistance can be recorded and calibrated in terms of a force signal. Another, less common type of force transducer uses piezoelectric crystals. These are devices which emit an electrical charge when loaded, the magnitude of which is proportional to the applied force.

Displacement transducers measure the distance which the punches travel during the compression and decompression processes. The most common type of displacement transducer delivers an analogue signal. It consists of a rod and some inductive elements mounted in a tube. When the rod moves within the tube, a signal is obtained which directly reflects the position of the rod. The movable rod is connected to the punch so that they move in parallel, i.e. the signal from the displacement transducer reflects the position of the punch. Digital displacement transducers are also used in instrumented tablet machines.

Such transducers are based on differences in signal level depending on the position of an indicator.

Displacement transducers are necessarily mounted some distance from the punch tip. There is therefore a difference in the position given by the transducer and the real position of the punch tip owing to deformation of the punch along the distance between its tip and the connection point of the transducer. This deviation must be determined by a calibration procedure, e.g. by compressing the punch tips against each other, and a correction for this error must be made before the displacement data can be used.

The signals from the force and displacement transducers are normally amplified and sampled into a computer. After conversion into digital form, the signals are transformed into physically relevant units (e.g. newtons, pascals, millimetres) and organized as a function of time. To obtain reliable data, the calibration of the signals, the resolution of the measuring systems and the reproducibility of the values must be carefully considered.

Tablet tooling

Tablets are formed in a variety of shapes. The most common tablet shapes are circular, oval and oblong, but tablets may also have other shapes, such as triangular or quadratic. From a side view, tablets may be flat or convex and with or without bevelled edges. Tablets may also bear break marks or symbols and other markings. Break marks (or break lines) are used to facilitate breaking of tablets in a controlled way to ensure reproducible doses. Markings are used to facilitate identification of a preparation and are of two types: embossed and debossed. Debossed markings are indented into the tablet and embossed markings are raised on the tablet surface. The size, shape and appearance of a tablet formed by powder compaction are controlled by the set of tools and by tooling design; a large variation in tablet size, shape and appearance can thus be obtained.

Punches and dies for rotary presses are designed in a standardized way, and standard configurations and terms are in use. The terminology used in describing the punches includes head, neck, barrel, stem and tip and that used in describing the die includes face, chamfer and bore. The tools are normally fabricated in steel, and different steels may be used. Because of the high forces applied to the powder bed, tools may be damaged and under normal use they become worn. The toughness, wear resistance and corrosiveness differ between different types of steels, and the choice of steel grade depends on factors such as the tooling configuration, the formulation to be compacted and the cost. In addition, the surface of punches and dies may be coated with a thin layer of another metal, such as chrome, to modify its surface properties, such as hardness and corrosiveness.

Punches and dies are precision tools and they should thus be handled and stored with care. Manufacturing problems may be related to the quality of the compression tooling. Tooling inspection programmes should thus be used in the development and production of tablets.

Technical problems during tableting

A number of technical problems can arise during the tableting procedure, amongst which the most important are:

- high weight and dose variation of the tablets;
- low mechanical strength of the tablets;
- capping and lamination of the tablets;
- adhesion or sticking of powder material to punch tips; and
- high friction during tablet ejection.

Such problems are related to the properties of the powder intended to be formed into tablets and also to the design and conditions of the press and the tooling. They should therefore be avoided by ensuring that the powder possesses adequate technical properties and also by the use of a suitable, well-conditioned tablet press, e.g. in terms of the use of forced-feed devices and polished and smooth dies and punches.

Important technical properties of a powder that must be controlled to ensure the success of a tableting operation are:

- homogeneity and segregation tendency;
- flowability;
- compression properties and compactability; and
- friction and adhesion properties.

The technical properties of the powder are controlled by the ingredients of the formulation (i.e. the drug and excipients) and by the way in which the ingredients are combined into a powder during precompaction processing. The precompaction processing often consists of a series of unit operations in sequence. The starting point is normally the drug in a pure, most often crystalline form. The unit operations used during the subsequent precompaction treatment are

523

mainly particle size reduction, powder mixing, particle size enlargement and powder drying. For further details of these procedures see Chapters 10, 11, 28 and 29 respectively. Granulation of a fine powder is a common means used to preserve the fineness of the drug within larger particles that are suitable for tableting (see later), and granulation procedures are traditionally in common use in preparing a powder for tableting. To save time and energy, precompaction processing without a particle size enlargement operation is chosen if possible. This procedure is called *tablet production by direct compression* or *direct compaction*.

Tablet production via granulation

Rationale for granulating powders before tableting

Because both granulation and tableting involve the formation of aggregates, tablet production by granulation is based on the combination of two size-enlargement processes in sequence. The main rationales for granulating the powder (drug and filler mixture) before tableting are to:

- increase the bulk density of the powder mixture and thus ensure that the required volume of powder can be filled into the die;
- improve the flowability of the powder to ensure that tablets with a low and acceptable tablet weight variation can be prepared;
- improve mixing homogeneity and reduce segregation by mixing small particles which subsequently adhere to each other;
- improve the compactability of the powder by adding a solution binder, which is effectively distributed on the particle surfaces;
- ensure a homogeneous colour in a tablet by adding the colour in a manner that ensures its effective distribution over the particle surfaces; and
- affect the dissolution process for hydrophobic, poorly soluble particles by using a fine particulate drug which is thoroughly mixed with a hydrophilic filler and a hydrophilic binder.

Before granulation, the drug might be processed separately so as to obtain a suitable quality in terms of solid-state and particulate properties, such as by spray-drying and milling. Normally, the drug exists in dry particulate form before granulation. However, it might be suspended or dissolved in a liquid and be added to the filler as a part of the agglomeration liquid.

Different procedures may be used for granulation, amongst which the most important are the use of convective mixers, fluidized-bed dryers, spray-dryers and compaction machines. Chapter 28 discusses granulation in some detail, but the process is summarized here in the context of tableting.

Granulation by convective mixing

Agitation of a powder by convection in the presence of a liquid, followed by drying, is the main procedure for the preparation of pharmaceutical granules. This is often considered to be the most effective means in terms of production time and cost to prepare good-quality granules. The process is often referred to as *wet granulation*.

The ingredients to be granulated in a convective mixer are first dry-mixed. The objective is to achieve a good homogeneity. As the components are often cohesive powders, a convective mixer operating at high intensity is normally used (a high-shear mixer). The mixture often consists of the drug and a filler. A disintegrant may also be included (i.e. an intragranular disintegrant) but it is also common to add the disintegrant to the dry granulation (i.e. an extragranular disintegrant).

The drugs to be used in tablet formulations may have hydrophobic surfaces and thus are not wetted easily by water. In order to facilitate water-based wet granulation of such powders, a surface-active agent may be added to the granulation liquid used during wet massing of the powder. Improved wetting may promote a more uniform liquid distribution and better granule growth during wet granulation.

After wet mixing, the wet mass is dried in a separate dryer (usually a fluidized-bed dryer; see Chapter 29). Because granulation in a convective mixer is not a very well controlled operation, large granules (>1 mm) are often formed which must be broken down into smaller units. This is normally done by milling in a hammer mill or by pressing the granulation through a screen in an oscillating granulator. Granules ranging in size from approximately 100 μm to 800 μm are thus obtained.

The prepared granules are finally dry-mixed with the other ingredients, for example in a double-cone mixer, before tableting. Common excipients added in this final mixing operation are disintegrants, lubricants, glidants and colourants. Fig. 30.5 summarizes the sequence of unit operations used in the

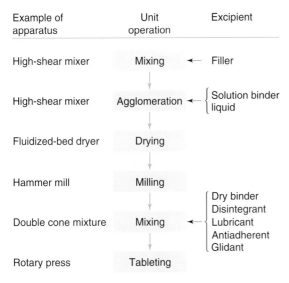

Fig. 30.5 • Overview of the sequence of unit operations used in the production of tablets with precompaction treatment by granulation.

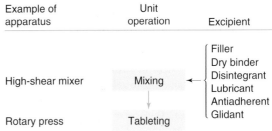

Fig. 30.6 • Overview of the sequence of unit operations used in the production of tablets by direct compaction.

production of tablets with precompaction treatment by granulation.

Alternative granulation procedures

A series of alternative granulation procedures may be preferable in certain situations. Granulation in a fluidized-bed apparatus is less common than the use of convective mixers as it is considered to be more time-consuming. However, granules of high quality in terms of homogeneity, flowability and compactability can be prepared by this operation.

By spray-drying a suspension of drug particles in a liquid, which can contain a dissolved binder, relatively small spherical granules with uniform size can be prepared. The process is of limited use, except for the preparation of fillers or diluents for direct compaction. The granules can show good compactability, and this presents the possibility of granulating a drug suspension without a separate drying step for the drug substance.

The formation of granules by compacting the powder into large compacts which are subsequently comminuted into smaller granules is an alternative approach to granulation. The approach can be used as a means of avoiding exposure of the powder to moisture and heat and is also referred to as *dry granulation*. In addition, for powders of very low bulk density, compaction can be an effective means to increase markedly their bulk density. The formation

of the compacts can be accomplished by powder compression in a die (slugging), giving relatively large tablet-like compacts, or by powder compression between rotating rollers (roller compaction), giving weak compacts with a flake or ribbon-like appearance. Roller compaction is a suitable operation for continuous granulation.

Tablet production by direct compaction

An obvious way to reduce the production time and hence cost is to minimize the number of operations involved in the pretreatment of the powder mixture before tableting. Tablet production by direct compaction can be reduced to only two operations in sequence: powder mixing and tableting (Fig. 30.6). The advantage with direct compaction is primarily a reduced production cost. However, in a direct compactable formulation, specially designed fillers and dry binders are normally required, which are usually more expensive than the traditional ones. They may also require a larger number of quality tests before processing. As heat and water are not involved, product stability can be improved. Finally, drug dissolution might be faster from a tablet prepared by direct compaction owing to fast tablet disintegration into primary drug particles.

The disadvantages of direct compaction are mainly technological. In order to handle a powder of acceptable flowability and bulk density, relatively large particles must be used which may be difficult to mix to a high homogeneity and may be prone to segregation. Moreover, a powder consisting mainly of a drug will be difficult to form into tablets if the drug itself has poor compactability. Finally, a uniform colouring of tablets can be difficult to achieve with a colourant in dry particulate form.

Direct compaction may be considered in two common formulation cases; firstly, relatively soluble drugs which can be processed as coarse particles (to ensure good flowability) and secondly, relatively potent drugs which are present in a few milligrams in each tablet and can be mixed with relatively coarse excipient particles (in this latter case the flow and compaction properties of the formulation are mainly controlled by the excipients).

Tablet excipients

In addition to the active ingredient(s), a series of excipients are normally included in a tablet; their role is to ensure that the tableting operation can run satisfactorily and that tablets of specified quality are prepared. Depending on the intended main function, the excipients to be used in tablets are subcategorized into different groups. However, one excipient can affect the properties of a powder or the tablet in a number of ways, and many substances used in tablet formulations can thus be described as multifunctional. The functions of the most common types of excipients used in tablets are described in the following sections. Examples of substances used as excipients in tablets are given in Table 30.1.

Filler (or diluent)

In order to form tablets of a size suitable for handling, a lower limit in terms of powder volume and weight is required. Tablets normally weigh at least 50 mg. Therefore a low dose of a potent drug requires the incorporation of a substance into the formulation to increase the bulk volume of the powder and hence the size of the tablet. This excipient, known as the *filler* or the *diluent*, is not necessary if the dose of the drug per tablet is high.

The ideal filler should fulfil a series of requirements, such as:

- be chemically inert;
- be nonhygroscopic;
- be biocompatible;
- possess good biopharmaceutical properties (e.g. water soluble or hydrophilic);
- possess good technical properties (such as compactability and dilution capacity);
- have an acceptable taste; and
- be cheap.

Table 30.1 Examples of substances used as excipients in tablet formulation

Type of excipient	Example of substances
Filler	Lactose Sucrose Glucose Mannitol Sorbitol Dicalcium phosphate dihydrate Calcium carbonate Cellulose
Disintegrant	Starch Cellulose Cross-linked polyvinylpyrrolidone Sodium starch glycolate Sodium carboxymethylcellulose
Solution binder	Gelatin Polyvinylpyrrolidone Cellulose derivative (e.g. hydroxypropyl methylcellulose) Polyethylene glycol Sucrose Starch
Dry binder	Cellulose Methylcellulose Polyvinylpyrrolidone Polyethylene glycol
Glidant	Silica Magnesium stearate Talc
Lubricant	Magnesium stearate Stearic acid Polyethylene glycol Sodium lauryl sulfate Sodium stearyl fumarate Liquid paraffin
Antiadherent	Magnesium stearate Talc Starch Cellulose

As all these requirements cannot be fulfilled by a single substance, different substances have been used as fillers in tablets, mainly carbohydrates but also some inorganic salts.

Lactose is the most common filler in tablets. It possesses a series of good filler properties, e.g. dissolves readily in water, has a pleasant taste, is nonhygroscopic, is fairly nonreactive and has good compactability. Its main limitation is that some people are lactose intolerant.

Lactose exists in both crystalline and amorphous forms. Crystalline lactose is formed by precipitation and, depending on the crystallization conditions, α-monohydrate or β-lactose (an anhydrous form) can be formed. By thermal treatment of the monohydrate form, crystalline α-anhydrous particles can be prepared. Depending on the crystallization conditions and the use of subsequent size reduction by milling, lactose of different particle sizes is obtained.

Amorphous lactose can be prepared by the spray-drying of a lactose solution (giving nearly completely amorphous particles) or a suspension of crystalline lactose particles in a lactose solution (giving aggregates of crystalline and amorphous lactose). Amorphous lactose dissolves more rapidly than crystalline lactose and has better compactability. Its main use is therefore in the production of tablets by direct compaction. Amorphous lactose is, however, hygroscopic and physically unstable, i.e. it will spontaneously crystallize if the crystallization conditions are met as a result of elevated temperature or high relative humidity (see Chapter 8 for more details).

Other sugars or sugar alcohols, such as glucose, sucrose, sorbitol and mannitol, have been used as alternative fillers to lactose, primarily in lozenges or chewable tablets, because of their pleasant taste. Mannitol has a negative heat of solution and imparts a cooling sensation when sucked or chewed.

Apart from the sugars, perhaps the most widely used fillers are powdered celluloses of different types. Celluloses are biocompatible, are chemically inert and have good tablet-forming and disintegrating properties. They are therefore also used as dry binders and disintegrants in tablets. They are compatible with many drugs but, owing to their hygroscopicity, may be incompatible with drugs prone to chemical degradation in the solid state.

The most common type of cellulose powder used in tablet formulation is microcrystalline cellulose. The name indicates that the particles have both crystalline and amorphous regions, depending on the relative position of the cellulose chains within the solid. The degree of crystallinity may differ depending on the source of the cellulose and the preparation procedure. The degree of crystallinity will affect the physical and technical properties of the particles, e.g. in terms of hygroscopicity and powder compactability.

Microcrystalline cellulose is prepared by hydrolysis of cellulose followed by spray-drying. The particles thus formed are aggregates of smaller cellulose fibres. Depending on the preparation conditions, aggregates of different particle size can be prepared which have different flowabilities.

A final important example of a common filler is an inorganic substance, dicalcium phosphate dihydrate. This is insoluble in water and nonhygroscopic, but is hydrophilic, i.e. easily wetted by water. The substance can be obtained in both a fine particulate form, mainly used in granulation, and an aggregated form. The latter possesses good flowability and is used in tablet production by direct compaction. Dicalcium phosphate dihydrate is slightly alkaline and may thus be incompatible with drugs sensitive to alkaline conditions.

Matrix former

In order to affect or control the release of the drug from the tablet, i.e. to speed up or to slow down its release rate, the drug may be dispersed or embedded in a matrix formed by an excipient or a combination of excipients. This type of excipient may thus be referred to as a matrix former. An alternative term is *base*, a term used in the *European Pharmacopoeia* (European Pharmacopoeia Commission, 2016) and defined there as 'the carrier, composed of one or more excipients, for the active substance(s) in semisolid and solid preparations'.

The matrix former is often a polymer or a lipid and may constitute a significant fraction of the total tablet weight. When the objective is to increase drug dissolution, the matrix former can be a water-soluble substance or a lipid, and the drug is dissolved or suspended as fine particles in the matrix. An example of a water-soluble matrix former is polyethylene glycol (PEG). When the objective is to prolong the drug release, the matrix former can be either an insoluble substance (a polymer or a lipid) or a substance that forms a gel in contact with water. The drug is normally dispersed in particulate form in the matrix (for more details, see later). A common gel-forming substance in tablets is hydroxypropyl methylcellulose (HPMC). Matrix formers are discussed in more detail in Chapter 31.

Disintegrant

A disintegrant is included in the formulation to ensure that the tablet, when in contact with a liquid, breaks up into small fragments, which promotes rapid drug dissolution. Ideally, the tablet should break up into individual drug particles so as to produce the largest possible effective surface area during dissolution.

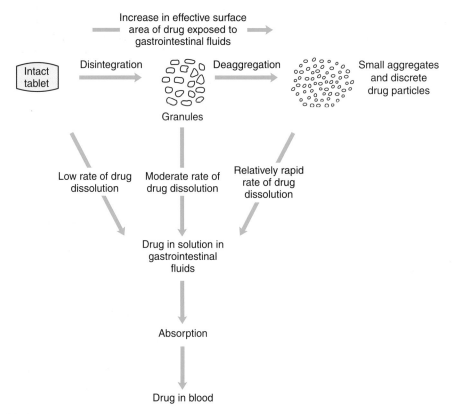

Fig. 30.7 • Mechanistic representation of the drug release process from a tablet by disintegration and dissolution. Adapted from Wells & Rubinstein, 1976.

The disintegration process for a tablet occurs in two steps. First, the liquid wets the solid and penetrates the pores of the tablet. Thereafter, the tablet breaks up into smaller fragments. The actual fragmentation of the tablet can also occur in steps, i.e. the tablet disintegrates into drug–excipient aggregates that subsequently deaggregate into smaller aggregates and discrete particles. Deaggregation into drug particles will set up conditions for the fastest possible dissolution of the drug. A scheme for the release of the drug from a disintegrating tablet is shown in Fig. 30.7.

The first step of the disintegration scheme described in Fig. 30.7, i.e. tablet disintegration, is an important step for the rate of drug release for the type of tablets referred to as disintegrating or conventional tablets (see later). The second step, granule disintegration or deaggregation, may result in the formation of smaller aggregates or, if driven to an ideal end point, discrete drug particles. The end point of the second step will probably depend on a series

of factors, such as the relative solubility and particle size of the drug and excipient particles of the granule. For example, in a situation where the drug particles are of low or very low solubility and are combined with a hydrophilic filler and binder of high solubility, the excipients may dissolve quickly, resulting in a dispersion of fine drug particles.

It should be pointed out that the term 'discrete drug particles' used in Fig. 30.7 should not be understood as meaning particles equivalent to the original drug particles. During formation of a tablet, the original drug particles may fracture, and the resultant size distribution of the drug particles may thus not necessarily equate to that of the original particles. Furthermore, the drug particles may also deform plastically during compression, which in addition may change their shape and appearance (see also later).

Several mechanisms of action of disintegrants have been suggested, such as swelling of particles, exothermic wetting reaction, particle repulsion and particle deformation recovery. However, as two main processes are involved in the disintegration event, the disintegrants to be used in plain tablets are classified here into two types:

1. *Disintegrants that facilitate water uptake.* These disintegrants act by facilitating the transport of liquids into the pores of the tablet, with the consequence that the tablet may break up into fragments. One obvious type of substance that can promote liquid penetration is surface-active agents. Such substances are used to make the drug particle surfaces more hydrophilic and thus promote the wetting of the solid and the penetration of the liquid into the pores of the tablet. It has also been suggested that other substances can promote liquid penetration, using capillary forces to suck water into the pores of the tablet. The additional presence of a surface-active agent may also facilitate penetration of water into the pore system of the aggregates formed during tablet disintegration and thus improve the deaggregation process of the aggregates too. Such a deaggregation and wetting process may ideally produce a fine dispersion of discrete wetted drug particles that will increase the surface area available for drug dissolution and thus the rate of dissolution.

2. *Disintegrants that will rupture the tablet.* Rupturing of tablets can be caused by swelling of the disintegrant particles during sorption of water. However, it has also been suggested that nonswelling disintegrants can break the tablet, and different mechanisms have been suggested. One such mechanism concerns a repulsion of particles in contact with water and another concerns the recovery of deformed particles to their original shape in contact with water, i.e. particles which have been deformed during compaction.

The disintegrant most traditionally used in conventional tablets is starch, among which potato, maize and corn starches are commonly used. The typical concentration range of starch in a tablet formulation is up to 10%. Starch particles swell in contact with water, and this swelling can subsequently disrupt the tablet. However, it has also been suggested that starch particles may facilitate disintegration by particle–particle repulsion.

The most common and effective disintegrants act via a swelling mechanism, and a series of effective swelling disintegrants have been developed which can swell dramatically during water uptake and thus quickly and effectively break the tablet. These are normally modified starch or modified cellulose. High-swelling disintegrants are included in the formulation at relatively low concentrations, typically 1% to 5% by weight.

Disintegrants can be mixed with other ingredients before granulation and can thus be incorporated within the granules (intragranular addition). It is also common for the disintegrant to be mixed with the dry granules before the complete powder mix is compacted (extragranular addition). The latter procedure will contribute to an effective disintegration of the tablet into smaller fragments.

A third group of disintegrants function by producing gas, normally carbon dioxide, when in contact with water. Such disintegrants are used in effervescent tablets and normally not in tablets that should be swallowed as a solid. The liberation of carbon dioxide is obtained by the decomposition of bicarbonate or carbonate salts in contact with acidic water. The acidic pH is accomplished by the incorporation of a weak acid in the formulation, such as citric acid or tartaric acid.

Dissolution enhancer

For drugs of low aqueous solubility, the dissolution rate of the drug may be the rate-limiting step in the overall drug release and absorption processes. Agents other than matrix formers may therefore sometimes be found in the composition of a tablet with the role to speed up the drug dissolution process by temporarily increasing the solubility of the drug during drug dissolution. An important example of a dissolution enhancer is the incorporation into the formulation of a substance that forms a salt with the drug during dissolution, e.g. increasing the dissolution rate of aspirin by using magnesium oxide in the formulation.

Another example of a dissolution-enhancing agent is a surfactant. As discussed already, a surfactant may facilitate wetting of hydrophobic drug particles and increase the surface area available for drug dissolution. A surfactant may also increase the rate of dissolution of poorly soluble drugs through a solubilization process. This may be conceptually described in terms of the formation of micelles in vivo followed by the dissolution of the drug into the micelles, increasing the apparent drug solubility. Sodium lauryl sulfate and polysorbates (polyoxyethylene sorbitan fatty acid esters) are examples of surfactants that may be used as such a dissolution-enhancing agent.

Absorption enhancer

For drugs with poor absorption properties, the absorption can be affected (see Chapter 20) by using substances in the formulation that affect the permeability of the intestinal cell membrane, and thus increase the rate at which the drug passes though the intestinal membrane. An additive that modulates the permeability of the intestine is often referred to as an *absorption enhancer*.

Binder

A *binder* (also sometimes called an *adhesive*) is added to a drug–filler mixture to ensure that granules and tablets can be formed with the required mechanical strength. Binders can be added to a powder in different ways:

- As a dry powder which is mixed with the other ingredients before wet agglomeration. During the agglomeration procedure, the binder might thus dissolve partly or completely in the agglomeration liquid.
- As a solution which is used as an agglomeration liquid during wet agglomeration. The binder is often referred to here as a *solution binder*.
- As a dry powder which is mixed with the other ingredients before compaction (slugging or tableting). The binder is often referred to here as a *dry binder*.

Both solution binders and dry binders are included in the formulation at relatively low concentrations, typically 2% to 10% by weight. Starch, sucrose and gelatin are common traditional solution binders. Polymers such as polyvinylpyrrolidone and cellulose derivatives (in particular hydroxypropyl methylcellulose), with improved adhesive properties, are more commonly used binders today. Microcrystalline cellulose and cross-linked polyvinylpyrrolidone are important examples of dry binders.

Solution binders are generally considered the most effective, and their use is therefore the most common way of incorporating a binder into granules; the granules thus formed are often referred to as binder–substrate granules. It is not uncommon, however, for a dry binder to be added to the binder–substrate

granules before tableting to further improve the compactability of the granulation.

Glidant

The role of the glidant is to improve the flowability of the powder. Glidants are used in formulations for direct compaction but are often also added to granules before tableting to ensure that sufficient flowability of the tablet mass is achieved for high production speeds.

Traditionally, talc has been used as a glidant in tablet formulations, in concentrations of approximately 1% to 2% by weight. Today, the most commonly used glidant is probably colloidal silica, added in very low proportions (approximately 0.2% by weight). Because the silica particles are very small, they adhere to the particle surfaces of the other ingredients (i.e. an ordered or structured mixture is formed; see Chapter 11) and improve flow by reducing interparticulate friction. Magnesium stearate, normally used as a lubricant, can also promote powder flow at low concentrations (< 1% by weight).

Lubricant

The function of the lubricant is to ensure that tablet formation and ejection can occur with low friction between the solid and the die wall. High friction during tableting can cause a series of problems, including inadequate tablet quality (capping or even fragmentation of tablets during ejection and vertical scratches on tablet edges), and may even stop production. Lubricants are thus included in almost all tablet formulations.

Lubrication is achieved mainly by two mechanisms: *fluid lubrication* and *boundary lubrication* (Fig. 30.8). In fluid lubrication a layer of fluid is located between and separates the moving surfaces of the solids from each other and thus reduces the friction. Fluid lubricants are seldom used in tablet formulations. However, liquid paraffin has been used, for instance in formulations for effervescent tablets.

Boundary lubrication is considered a surface phenomenon, as here the sliding surfaces are separated by only a very thin film of lubricant. The nature of the solid surfaces will therefore affect friction. In boundary lubrication the friction coefficient and wear of the solids are higher than with fluid lubrication. All substances that can affect the interaction between sliding surfaces can be described as boundary lubricants, including adsorbed gases. The lubricants used in tablet formulations acting by boundary lubrication are fine particulate solids.

A number of mechanisms have been discussed for these boundary lubricants, including that lubricants are substances that have a low resistance to shearing. The most effective of the boundary lubricants are stearic acid or stearic acid salts, such as magnesium

stearate. Magnesium stearate has become the most widely used lubricant owing to its superior lubrication properties. The stearic acid salts are normally used at low concentrations (< 1% by weight).

Besides reducing friction, lubricants may cause undesirable changes in the properties of the tablet. The presence of a lubricant in a powder is thought to interfere in a deleterious way with the bonding between the particles during compaction, thus reducing tablet strength (Fig. 30.9). Because many lubricants are hydrophobic, tablet disintegration and dissolution are often retarded by the addition of a lubricant. These negative effects are strongly related to the amount of lubricant present, and a minimum amount is normally used in a formulation, i.e. concentrations of 1% or below. In addition, the way in which the lubricant is mixed with the other ingredients should also be considered. It can, for example, be important if the excipients are added sequentially to a granulation rather than simultaneously. The total mixing time and the mixing intensity are also important in this context.

The commonly observed retardation of disintegration and dissolution of tablets is related to the hydrophobic character of the most commonly used lubricants. In order to avoid these negative effects, more hydrophilic substances have been suggested as alternatives to the hydrophobic lubricants.

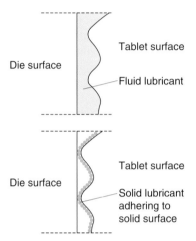

Fig. 30.8 • Illustration of lubrication mechanisms by fluid and boundary lubrication.

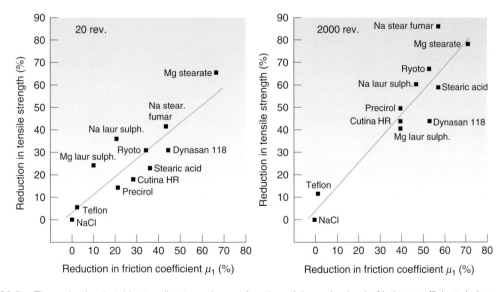

Fig. 30.9 • The reduction in tablet tensile strength as a function of the reduction in friction coefficient during tableting of a sodium chloride powder mixed with 0.1% by weight of a series of lubricants admixed at two different mixing intensities. *Mg laur sulph.*, magnesium lauryl sulfate; *Mg stearate*, magnesium stearate; *Na laur sulph.*, sodium lauryl sulfate; *Na stear fumar*, sodium stearyl fumarate. Adapted from Hölzer & Sjögren, 1981, with permission.

Surface-active agents and polyethylene glycol are examples. A combination of hydrophobic and hydrophilic substances might also be used.

The lubricant's effect on friction and on the changes in tablet properties is related to the tendency of lubricants to adhere to the surface of drugs and fillers during dry mixing. Lubricants are often fine particulate substances, which are thus prone to adhere to larger particles. In addition, studies on the mixing behaviour of magnesium stearate have indicated that this substance has the ability to form a film which can cover a fraction of the surface area of the drug or filler particles (the substrate particles). This film can be described as being continuous rather than particulate. A number of factors have been suggested to affect the development of such a lubricant film during mixing and hence also affect friction and changes in tablet properties, such as the shape and surface roughness of the substrate particles; the surface area of the lubricant particles; mixing time and intensity; and the type and size of the mixer.

Concerning the tablet-strength-reducing effect of a lubricant, apart from the degree of surface coverage of the lubricant film obtained during mixing, the compression behaviour of the substrate particles will also be important. Drugs and fillers can thus be evaluated in terms of their lubricant sensitivity, i.e. the reduction in the strength of a tablet due to the addition of a lubricant compared with the strength of a tablet formed from a powder without a lubricant. An important property for this lubricant sensitivity seems to be the degree of fragmentation the substrate particles undergo during compression (see later). It is thus assumed that, during compression, particle surfaces which are not covered with a lubricant film are formed during particle fragmentation and that these clean surfaces will bond differently from the lubricant-covered particle surfaces.

To explain the effect of lubricant film formation on the tensile strength of tablets, a coherent matrix model has been developed. This suggests that when a continuous matrix of lubricant-covered particle surfaces exists in a tablet, along which a fracture plane can be formed, the strength of the tablet is considerably lower than that of tablets formed from unlubricated powder. However, if the mixing and compression processes do not result in such a coherent lubricant matrix within the tablet (e.g. because of irregular substrate particles or particle fragmentation), the lubricant sensitivity appears to be lower.

Antiadherent

The function of an antiadherent is to reduce adhesion between the powder and the punch faces and thus prevent particles sticking to the punches. Many powders are prone to adhere to the punches, a phenomenon (known in the pharmaceutical industry as *sticking or picking*) which is affected by the moisture content of the powder. Such adherence is especially prone to happen if the tablet punches have markings or symbols. Adherence can lead to a build-up of a thin layer of powder on the punches, which in turn will lead to an uneven and matt tablet surface with unclear markings or symbols.

Many lubricants, such as magnesium stearate, also have antiadherent properties. However, other substances with limited ability to reduce friction can also act as antiadherents, such as talc and starch.

Sorbent

Sorbents are substances that are capable of sorbing some quantities of fluids in an apparently dry state. Thus oils or oil–drug solutions can be incorporated into a powder mixture which is granulated and compacted into tablets. Microcrystalline cellulose and silica are examples of sorbing substances used in tablets.

Flavour

Flavouring agents are incorporated into a formulation to give the tablet a more pleasant taste or to mask an unpleasant one. The latter can also be achieved by the coating of the tablet or the drug particles.

Flavouring agents are often thermolabile and so cannot be added before an operation involving heat. They are often mixed with the granules as an alcohol solution.

Colourant

Colourants are added to tablets to aid identification and patient adherence. Colouring is often accomplished during coating (see Chapter 32 for further information) but a colourant can also be included in the formulation before compaction. In the latter case, the colourant can be added as an insoluble powder or dissolved in the granulation liquid. The latter procedure may lead to a colour variation in the tablet caused by migration of the soluble dye during the drying stage (see Chapter 29 for more information on the phenomenon of solute migration).

Tablet types

Classification of tablets

Several categories of tablets may be distinguished, and the denomination and definitions of different types of tablets can be found in pharmacopoeias. The tablet dosage forms described in the *European Pharmacopoeia* (European Pharmacopoeia Commission, 2017) appear in the monographs for tablets and for oromucosal preparations (the monograph on oromucosal preparations includes some types of tablets, i.e. compressed lozenges, sublingual tablets and buccal tablets that are intended for administration by the oral cavity and/or the throat to obtain a local or systemic effect).

A common means of classifying tablets is based on the pattern of drug release from the tablets. The following categories are often used in this context: immediate release, prolonged release, pulsatile release and delayed release. The latter three types are also referred to as modified-release tablets.

For immediate-release tablets, the drug is intended to be released rapidly after administration, or the tablet is dissolved in liquid before intake and thus administered as a solution. Immediate-release tablets are the most common type of tablet and include disintegrating, chewable, effervescent, sublingual and buccal tablets.

Modified-release tablets should normally be swallowed intact. The formulation and thus also the type of excipients used in such tablets might be quite different from those of immediate-release tablets. The term *prolonged-release tablet* is used to indicate that the drug is released slowly at a nearly constant rate. If the rate of release is constant during a substantial period, a zero-order type of release is obtained, i.e. $M = kt$ (where M is the cumulative amount of drug released and t is the release time). This is sometimes described as an ideal type of prolonged-release preparation.

A pulsatile release is another means to increase the period of drug absorption after a single administration and is accomplished by releasing the drug in two or more pulses.

For delayed-release tablets the drug is liberated from the tablet some time after administration. After

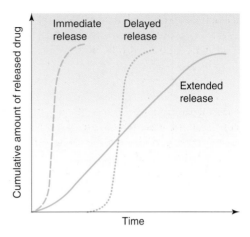

Fig. 30.10 • The cumulative amount of drug released from immediate-release, extended-release (prolonged-release) and delayed-release tablets.

this period has elapsed, the release is normally rapid. The most common type of delayed-release tablet is a *gastro-resistant* (also known as *enteric-coated*) tablet, for which the drug is released in the upper part of the small intestine after the preparation has passed the stomach. However, a delayed drug release can also be combined with a prolonged drug release, e.g. for local treatment in the lower part of the intestine or in the colon.

The type of release obtained from immediate-release, prolonged-release and delayed-release tablets is illustrated in Fig. 30.10. In the following sections, the most common types of tablets are described.

Disintegrating tablets

The most common type of tablet is intended to be swallowed and to release the drug a relatively short time thereafter by disintegration and dissolution, i.e. the goal of the formulation is fast and complete drug release in vivo. Such tablets are often referred to as conventional or plain tablets. A disintegrating tablet includes normally at least the following types of excipients: filler (if the dose of the drug is low), disintegrant, binder, glidant, lubricant and antiadherent.

As discussed earlier, the drug is released from a disintegrating tablet in a sequence of processes, including tablet disintegration, drug dissolution and drug absorption (Fig. 30.7). All these processes will affect, and can be rate-limiting steps for, the drug bioavailability. The rate of the processes is affected

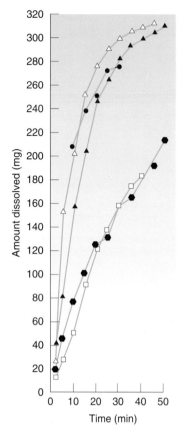

Fig. 30.11 • The dissolution rate of salicylic acid, as assessed by an in vitro dissolution method based on agitated baskets, from tablets formed from mixtures of salicylic acid (325 mg) and a series of different types of starches as disintegrant: potato starch *(squares)*, arrowroot starch *(hexagons)*, rice starch *(closed triangles)*, corn starch *(circles)*, compressible starch *(open triangles)*. Adapted from Underwood & Cadwallader, 1972.

by both formulation factors and production conditions.

The disintegration time of the tablet is a function of the composition and manufacturing conditions and may thus depend on several factors. Regarding composition, the choice of disintegrant (Fig. 30.11) is of obvious importance but other excipients, such as the type of filler and lubricant, can also be of significant importance for tablet disintegration.

Tablet disintegration may also be affected by production conditions during manufacture. Important examples that may affect the tablet disintegration time are the design of the granulation procedure (which will affect the physical properties of the granules), the mixing conditions during the addition of lubricants and antiadherents, the applied punch force during tableting and the punch force–time relationship. It has been reported that an increased compaction pressure can either increase or decrease the disintegration time, or give complex relationships with maximum or minimum disintegration times.

In many cases the drug dissolution rate is the rate-limiting step in the drug release process, especially for drugs that are poorly soluble in water but that are readily absorbed in the intestine (i.e. typically class II drugs in the Biopharmaceutics Classification System (BCS); see Chapter 21). Because many drugs have very poor solubility, the problem of the rate of drug dissolution is often a critical issue during the development of an immediate-release tablet. The most common means to achieve an acceptable drug dissolution rate for poorly soluble compounds are:

• control of apparent solubility of the drug;
• control of the surface area exposed to the dissolution medium; and
• addition of drug-dissolution-enhancing agents.

The apparent solubility can be increased by changing the solid-state form of the drug, such as a polymorph, using a salt of the drug or using amorphous particles. The surface area of a solid is inversely proportional to particle size, and particle size reduction is an obvious means to increase the drug dissolution rate. However, a reduced particle size will make a powder more cohesive. A reduction in drug particle size might produce aggregates of particles which are difficult to break up, with the consequence that the drug dissolution rate is not related to the surface area of the primary drug particles. It is thus important to ensure that the tablet is formulated in such a way that it will disintegrate and that the aggregates so formed break up into small drug particles so that a large surface area of the drug is exposed to the dissolution medium. The preparation and use of small particles, i.e. down to the sub-micrometre range (nanosized particles), and the use of drug dissolution enhancers and matrix formers in tablet compositions of poorly soluble drugs are important issues in the formulation of disintegrating, immediate-release tablets.

For drugs with poor absorption properties, the absorption can be affected (see Chapter 20) by modifying the drug's lipophilicity, e.g. by esterification of the drug, as well as by adding absorption enhancers.

Single disintegrating tablets can also be prepared in the form of multilayers, i.e. the tablet consists of concentric or parallel layers adhered to each other. Multilayer tablets are prepared by repeated compression of powders and are made primarily to separate incompatible drugs from each other, i.e. incompatible drugs can be incorporated into the same tablet. Although intimate contact exists at the surface between the layers, the reaction between the incompatible drugs is limited. The use of parallel-layered tablets where the layers are differently coloured is an approach to preparing easily identifiable tablets.

Another variation of the disintegrating tablet is coated tablets which are intended to disintegrate and release the drug quickly (in contrast to coated tablets intended for modified release). The rationale for using coated tablets and detailed descriptions of the procedures used for tablet coating are given in Chapter 32.

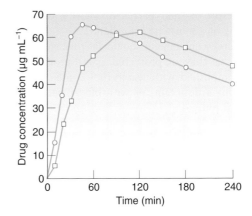

Fig. 30.12 • Concentration of salicylates in plasma after administration of acetylsalicylic acid tablets (1 g). *Circles*, effervescent tablet; *squares*, conventional tablet. Adapted from Ekenved et al., 1975, with permission.

Chewable tablets

Chewable tablets are chewed and thus are mechanically disintegrated in the mouth. The drug is, however, normally not dissolved in the mouth but swallowed and dissolves in the stomach or intestine. Thus chewable tablets are used primarily to accomplish a quick and complete disintegration of the tablet – and hence obtain a rapid drug effect – or to facilitate the administration of the tablet. A common example of the former is antacid tablets. In the latter case, the elderly and young children in particular have difficulty swallowing tablets and so a chewable tablet is an attractive form of medication. Vitamin tablets are important examples. Another general advantage of a chewable tablet is that this type of medication can be taken when water is not available.

Chewable tablets are similar in composition to conventional tablets except that a disintegrant is normally not included in the composition. Flavouring and colouring agents are common, and sorbitol and mannitol are common examples of fillers.

Effervescent tablets

Effervescent tablets are dropped into a glass of water before administration, during which carbon dioxide is liberated. This facilitates tablet disintegration and drug dissolution; the dissolution of the tablet should be complete within a few minutes. As mentioned earlier, the effervescent carbon dioxide is created by a reaction in water between a carbonate or bicarbonate and a weak acid such as citric acid or tartaric acid.

Effervescent tablets are used to obtain rapid drug action, for example for analgesic drugs (Fig. 30.12), or to facilitate the intake of the drug, for example for vitamins.

The amount of sodium bicarbonate in an effervescent tablet is often quite high (approximately 1 g). After dissolution of such a tablet, a buffered water solution will be obtained which normally temporarily increases the pH of the stomach. The result is a rapid emptying of the stomach, and the residence time of the drug in the stomach will thus be short. As drugs are absorbed in the small intestine rather than in the stomach, effervescent tablets can thus exhibit fast drug absorption, which can be advantageous, for example, for analgesic drugs. Another aspect of the short drug residence time in the stomach is that drug-induced gastric irritation can be avoided, e.g. for aspirin tablets, as the absorption of aspirin in the stomach can cause irritation.

Effervescent tablets also often include a flavour and a colourant. A water-soluble lubricant is preferable so as to avoid a film of a hydrophobic lubricant on the surface of the water after tablet dissolution. A binder is normally not included in the composition.

Effervescent tablets are prepared by both direct compaction and compaction via granulation. In the latter case, traditional wet granulation is seldom used; instead, granules are formed by the fusion of particles as a result of their partial dissolution during wet massing of a moistened powder.

Effervescent tablets should be packaged in such a way that they are protected against moisture. This is accomplished with waterproof containers, often including a desiccant, or with blister packs or aluminium foil.

Compressed lozenges

Compressed lozenges are tablets that dissolve slowly in the mouth and so release the drug dissolved in the saliva. Lozenges are used for systemic drug uptake or for local medication in the mouth or throat, e.g. with local anaesthetic, antiseptic and antibiotic drugs. The latter type of tablets can thus be described as slow-release tablets for local drug treatment.

Disintegrants are not used in the formulation, but otherwise such tablets are similar in composition to conventional tablets. In addition, lozenges are often coloured and include a flavour. The choice of filler and binder is of particular importance in the formulation of lozenges, as these excipients should contribute to a pleasant taste or feeling during tablet dissolution. The filler and binder should therefore be water soluble and have a good taste. Common examples of fillers are glucose, sorbitol and mannitol. A common binder in lozenges is gelatin.

Lozenges are normally prepared by compaction at high applied pressures to obtain a tablet of high mechanical strength and low porosity which can dissolve slowly in the mouth.

Sublingual tablets and buccal tablets

Sublingual tablets and buccal tablets are used for drug release in the mouth followed by systemic uptake of the drug. A rapid systemic drug effect can thus be obtained without first-pass liver metabolism. Sublingual tablets are placed under the tongue and buccal tablets are placed in the side of the cheek or high up between the inside of the upper lip and gum.

Sublingual and buccal tablets are often small and porous, the latter facilitating fast disintegration and drug release. Other designs, comprising high molecular weight hydrophilic polymers and/or gums, adhere in place by forming a gel. They remain in position, releasing the drug, for 1–2 hours (e.g. prochlorperazine maleate for nausea).

Prolonged-release and pulsatile-release tablets

Classification

In recent years there has been great interest in the development and use of tablets which should be swallowed and thereafter slowly release the drug in the gastrointestinal tract for approximately 12–24 hours. Such tablets are denominated in various ways, such as slow-release tablets, extended-release tablets, sustained-release tablets and prolonged-release tablets. They are often also referred to as controlled-release preparations. This latter term is somewhat misleading, as all tablets, irrespective of their formulation and use, should release the drug in a controlled and reproducible way. The nomenclature for prolonged-release preparations is subject to some debate, and no worldwide acceptable system exists. The reader is referred to Chapter 31 for further discussion of this subject.

After release from the tablet, the drug should normally be absorbed into the systemic circulation. The aim is normally to increase the time during which a therapeutic drug concentration in the blood is maintained. However, the aim can also be to increase the release time for drugs that can cause local irritation in the stomach or intestine if they are released quickly. Potassium chloride and iron salts are examples of the latter. In addition, drugs for local treatment of diseases in the large intestine are sometimes formulated as prolonged-release tablets.

A prolonged-release preparation can also be categorized as a single-unit or a multiple-unit dosage form. In the first case the drug dose is incorporated into a single release unit and in the latter case is divided into a large number of small release units. A multiple-unit dosage form is often considered to give a more reproducible drug action.

There are a series of rationales behind the increased interest in administering drugs orally for systemic uptake in the form of prolonged-release tablets. However, the drug must fulfil certain criteria to render itself suitable for sustained-release medication, otherwise another type of tablet is a more feasible option. These rationales and criteria, as well as the pharmacokinetic aspects of prolonged-release drug administration, are described in Chapters 22 and 31. In Chapter 31 the formulation principles used to achieve prolonged drug release are described.

Prolonged-release tablets are often categorized according to the mechanism of drug release. The following are the most common means used to achieve a slow, controlled release of the drug from tablets:

- drug transport control by diffusion;
- dissolution control;
- erosion control;
- drug transport control by convective flow (accomplished by, for example, osmotic pumping); and
- ion exchange control.

Diffusion-controlled release systems

In diffusion-controlled prolonged-release systems, the transport by diffusion of dissolved drugs in pores filled with gastric or intestinal juice or in a solid (normally polymer) phase is the release-controlling process. Depending on the part of the release unit in which the drug diffusion occurs, diffusion-controlled release systems are divided into matrix systems (also referred to as monolithic systems) and reservoir systems. The release unit can be a tablet or a nearly spherical particle approximately 1 mm in diameter (a granule or a millisphere). In both cases the release unit should stay more or less intact during the course of the release process. In matrix systems, diffusion occurs in pores located within the bulk of the release unit, and in reservoir systems, diffusion occurs in a thin water-insoluble film or membrane, often approximately 5 μm to 20 μm thick, which surrounds the release unit. Diffusion through the membrane can occur in pores filled with fluid or in the solid phase that forms the membrane.

Drug is released from a diffusion-controlled release unit in two steps:

1. The liquid that surrounds the dosage form penetrates the release unit and dissolves the drug. A concentration gradient of dissolved drug is thus established between the interior and the exterior of the release unit.
2. The dissolved drug will diffuse in the pores of the release unit or the surrounding membrane and thus be released or, alternatively, the dissolved drug will partition into the membrane surrounding the dose unit and diffuse in the membrane.

A dissolution step is thus normally involved in the release process but the diffusion step is the rate-controlling step. The rate at which diffusion will occur depends on three variables: the concentration gradient over the diffusion distance; the area and distance over which diffusion occurs; and the diffusion

coefficient of the drug in the diffusion medium. Some of these variables are used to modulate the release rate in the formulation.

Reservoir systems. In a reservoir system the diffusion occurs in a thin film surrounding the release unit (Fig. 30.13). This film is normally formed from a high molecular weight polymer. The diffusion distance will be constant during the course of the release and, as long as a constant drug concentration gradient is maintained, the release rate will be constant, i.e. a zero-order release ($M = kt$).

One possible process for the release of the drug from a reservoir system involves partition of the drug dissolved inside the release unit to the solid membrane, followed by transport by diffusion of the drug within the membrane. Finally, the drug will partition to the solution surrounding the release unit. The driving force for the release is the concentration gradient of dissolved drug over the membrane. The release rate (M/t) can be described in a simplified way by the following equation, which also summarizes the formulation factors by which the release rate can be controlled:

$$\frac{M}{t} = \frac{CAKD}{l}$$

(30.1)

where C is the solubility of the drug in the liquid, A and l are the area and thickness of the membrane, D is the diffusion coefficient of the drug in the membrane, and K is the partition coefficient for the drug between the membrane and the liquid at equilibrium.

In practice, the membrane surrounding the release unit often includes a water-soluble component. This can be small particles of a soluble substance, such as sucrose, or a water-soluble polymer, such as a water-soluble cellulose derivative (e.g. hydroxypropyl methylcellulose). In the latter case the polymer is used together with a water-insoluble polymer as the

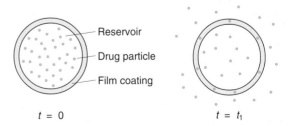

Fig. 30.13 • Illustration of the mechanism of drug release from a diffusion-based reservoir tablet. *t*, time.

film-forming materials that constitute the coating. In such a membrane the water-soluble component will dissolve and form pores filled with liquid in which the drug can thereafter diffuse. The area and length of these pores will thus constitute the diffusion area and distance. These factors can be estimated from the porosity of the membrane (ε) and the tortuosity (τ) of the pores (tortuosity refers to the ratio between the actual transport distance in the pores between two positions and the transport distance in a solution). The release rate can thus be described in a simplified way as follows:

$$\frac{M}{t} = \frac{CA\varepsilon D}{l\tau}$$

(30.2)

The membrane porosity and pore tortuosity can be affected by the addition of water-soluble components to the membrane.

For oral preparations the film surrounding the release units is normally based on high molecular weight, water-insoluble polymers, such as certain cellulose derivatives (e.g. ethylcellulose) and acrylates. The film often also includes a plasticizer. In the case of drug release through liquid-filled pores, a small amount of a water-soluble compound is also added, as described earlier. Reservoir systems today are normally designed as multiple-unit systems rather than single units.

Matrix systems. In a matrix system the drug is dispersed as solid particles within a matrix formed of a water-insoluble polymer, such as poly(vinyl chloride) (Fig. 30.14) or in a matrix forming a gel in contact with water (see later). Initially, drug particles located at the surface of the release unit will be dissolved and the drug will be released rapidly. Thereafter, drug particles at successively increasing distances from the surface of the release unit will be dissolved and released by diffusion in liquid-filled pores of the matrix or in the gel to the exterior of the release unit. Thus the diffusion distance of dissolved drug will increase as the release process proceeds. The drug release in terms of the cumulative amount of drug (M) released from a matrix can often be approximated to be proportional to the square root of time, i.e. $M = kt^{1/2}$.

The main formulation factors by which the release rate from a matrix system can be controlled are the amount of drug in the matrix, the porosity of the release unit, the length of the pores in the release unit (dependent on the size of the release unit and the pore tortuosity) and the solubility of the drug (which regulates the concentration gradient). The characteristics of the pore system can be affected by, for example, the addition of soluble excipients and by the compaction pressure during tableting.

Matrix systems are traditionally designed as single-unit systems, normally tablets, prepared by tableting. However, alternative preparation procedures are also used, especially for release units that are smaller than tablets. Examples of such techniques are extrusion, spray congealing and casting.

Dissolution-controlled release systems

In dissolution-controlled prolonged-release systems, the rate of dissolution of the drug or another ingredient in the gastrointestinal juices is the release-controlling process. It is obvious that a sparingly water-soluble drug can form a preparation of a dissolution-controlled prolonged-release type. Reduced drug solubility can be accomplished by preparing poorly soluble salts or derivatives of the drug. An alternative means of achieving prolonged release based on the dissolution-control principle is to incorporate

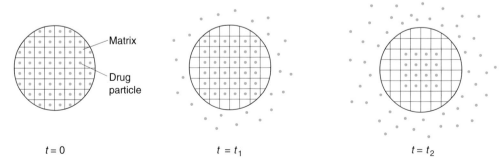

$t = 0$　　　　　　　　　$t = t_1$　　　　　　　　　$t = t_2$

Fig. 30.14 • Illustration of the mechanism of drug release from a diffusion-based matrix tablet. t, time.

the drug in a slowly dissolving carrier or by covering drug particles with a slowly dissolving coating. In the latter case, the release of the drug from such units occurs in two steps:

1. The liquid that surrounds the release unit dissolves the coating (rate-limiting dissolution step).
2. The solid drug is exposed to the liquid and subsequently dissolves.

In order to obtain an extended release based on dissolution of a coating, the tablet is formulated to release the drug in a series of consecutive pulses, i.e. a pulsatile release. This can be accomplished by dividing the drug dose into a number of smaller release units, often nearly spherical granules approximately 1 mm in diameter, which are coated in such a way that the dissolution time of the coatings will differ (Fig. 30.15). A variation in dissolution time of the coating can be accomplished by variation of its thickness or its solubility. Release units with different release times will be mixed and formed into a disintegrating tablet.

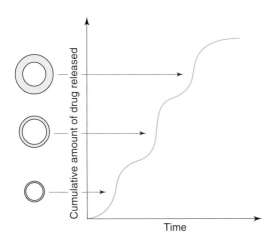

Fig. 30.15 • The cumulative amount of drug released from a dissolution-based (due to differences in coating thickness) pulsatile-release preparation.

Delayed-release tablets are normally formulated as dissolution-controlled preparations. In the case of gastro-resistant tablets, the dissolution is inhibited until the preparation reaches the higher pH of the small intestine, where the drug is released in a relatively short time.

Erosion-controlled release systems

In erosion-controlled prolonged-release systems, the rate of drug release is controlled by the erosion of the matrix in which the drug is dispersed. The matrix is normally formed by a tableting operation, and the system can thus be described as a single-unit system. The erosion in its simplest form can be described as a continuous liberation of matrix material (both drug and excipient) from the surface of the tablet, i.e. surface erosion. The consequence will be a continuous reduction in tablet weight during the course of the release process (Fig. 30.16). Drug release from an erosion system can thus be described in two steps:

1. Matrix material, in which the drug is dissolved or dispersed, is liberated from the surface of the tablet.
2. The drug is subsequently exposed to the gastrointestinal fluids and mixed with (if the drug is dissolved in the matrix) or dissolved in (if the drug is suspended in the matrix) the fluid.

The release rate of a drug from an eroding system can often approximate to zero order for a significant part of the total release time.

The eroding matrix can be formed from different substances. One example is lipids or waxes, in which the drug is dispersed. Another example is polymers that gel when in contact with water (e.g. hydroxyethyl cellulose). The gel will subsequently erode and release the drug dissolved or dispersed in the gel. However, as discussed earlier, a prolonged-release tablet based on a gel-forming matrix may also be classified as a diffusion-controlled release system. Diffusion may be the dominating release mechanism in some cases.

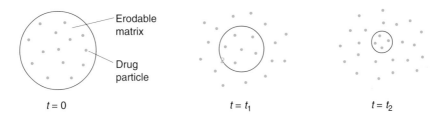

Fig. 30.16 • Illustration of the mechanism of drug release from an erosion tablet.

Osmosis-controlled release systems

In osmosis-controlled prolonged-release systems, the flow of liquid into the release unit, driven by a difference in osmotic pressure between the inside and the outside of the release unit, is used as the release-controlling process. Osmosis can be defined as the flow of a solvent from a compartment with a low concentration of solute to a compartment with a high concentration. The two compartments are separated by a semipermeable membrane, which allows flow of solvent but not of solute.

In the simplest type of osmosis-controlled drug release, the following sequence of steps is involved in the release process:

1. osmotic transport of liquid into the release unit;
2. dissolution of the drug within the release unit; and
3. convective transport of a saturated drug solution by pumping of the solution through a single orifice or through pores in the semipermeable membrane.

The pumping of the drug solution can be accomplished in different ways. One example is a tablet which includes an expansion layer, i.e. a layer of a substance that swells in contact with water, the expansion of which will press the drug solution out of the release unit. Alternatively, the increased volume of fluid inside the release unit will increase the internal pressure and the drug solution will thus be pumped out.

If the flow rate of incoming liquid to the release unit is the rate-controlling process, the drug release rate can be described as

$$\frac{M}{t} = \frac{CV}{t}$$

$$(30.3)$$

where V is the volume of incoming liquid. The flow rate of incoming liquid under steady-state conditions is a zero-order process, and the release rate of the drug will therefore also be a zero-order process. The water flow is not affected by the flow and pH of the dissolution medium. However, the water flow rate and hence the drug release rate can be affected by a number of formulation factors, such as the osmotic pressure of the drug solution within the release unit, the drug solubility, and the permeability and mechanical properties of the membrane.

Osmosis-controlled release systems can be designed as single-unit or multiple-unit tablets. In the first case, the drug solution can be forced out from the

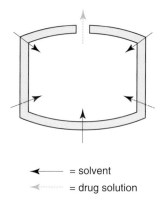

= solvent

= drug solution

Fig. 30.17 • Illustration of the mechanism of drug release from an osmosis-controlled release system designed as a single-unit tablet with a single release orifice.

tablet through a single orifice (Fig. 30.17) formed in the membrane by it being bored with a laser beam. Alternatively, the drug solution can flow through a number of pores formed during the uptake of water. Such pores can be formed by the dissolution of water-soluble substances present in the membrane, or by straining of the membrane owing to the increased internal pressure in the release unit. In the case of multiple-unit release tablets, the transport occurs in the pores formed.

Tablet testing

Test methods

In tablet formulation development and during the manufacture of tablets, a number of procedures are used to assess the quality of the tablets. Some test methods are described in pharmacopoeias, and these tests are traditionally concerned with the content and the in vitro release of the active ingredient. Test methods not described in pharmacopoeias are sometimes referred to as noncompendial and concern a variety of quality attributes that need to be evaluated, such as the porosity of tablets. Some of the tests used in the quality evaluation of tablets are briefly described in the following sections.

Uniformity of content of active ingredient

A fundamental quality attribute for all pharmaceutical preparations is the requirement for a constant dose

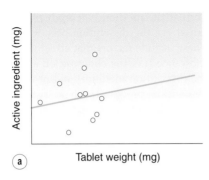

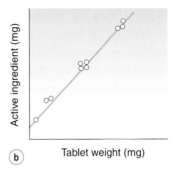

Fig. 30.18 • Correlation between the amount of active ingredient and tablet weight for **(a)** a low-dose tablet (drug content 23% of tablet weight) and **(b)** a high-dose tablet (drug content 90% of tablet weight). Adapted from Airth et al. 1967, with permission.

of drug between individual tablets. In practice, small variations between individual preparations are accepted, and the limits for this variation appear as standards in pharmacopoeias. Traditionally, uniformity of dose or dose variation between tablets is tested in two separate tests: uniformity of weight (mass) and uniformity of active ingredient.

The test for uniformity of weight is performed by collecting a sample of tablets from a batch and determining their individual weights. The average weight of the tablets is then calculated. The sample complies with the standard if the individual weights do not deviate from the mean by more than is permitted in terms of percentage.

If the drug substance forms the greater part of the tablet mass, any weight variation obviously indicates a variation in the content of active ingredient. Compliance with the standard thus helps to ensure that uniformity of dosage is achieved. However, in the case of potent drugs which are administered in low doses, the excipients form the greater part of the tablet weight and the correlation between tablet weight and amount of active ingredient can be poor (Fig. 30.18). Thus the test for weight variation must be combined with a test for variation in content of the drug substance. Nevertheless, the test for uniformity of weight is a simple way to assess variation in drug dose, which makes the test useful as a quality control procedure during tablet production.

The test for uniformity of drug content is performed by collecting a sample of tablets followed by determination of the amount of drug in each tablet. The average drug content is calculated, and the content of the individual tablets should fall within specified limits.

Disintegration

As discussed already, the process of drug release from tablets often includes a step in which the tablet disintegrates into smaller fragments. To assess this, disintegration test methods have been developed, and examples of these can be found in pharmacopoeias.

The test is performed by agitation of a given number of tablets in an aqueous medium at a defined temperature, and the time to reach the end point of the test is recorded. The preparation complies with the test if the time to reach this end point is below a given limit. The end point of the test is the point at which all visible parts of the tablets have been eliminated from a set of tubes in which the tablets have been held during agitation. The tubes are closed at the lower end by a screen, and the tablet fragments formed during the disintegration are eliminated from the tubes by passing the screen openings, i.e. disintegration is considered to be achieved when no tablet fragments remain on the screen (fragments of coating may, however, remain).

A disintegration instrument (Fig. 30.19) normally consists of six chambers, i.e. tubes open at the upper end and closed by a screen at the lower end. Before disintegration testing, one tablet is placed in each tube and usually a plastic disc is placed over the tablet. The tubes are placed in a water bath and raised and lowered at a constant frequency in the water in such a way that at the highest position of the tubes the screen (and thus the tablet held down by the plastic disc) remains below the surface of the water.

Tests for disintegration do not normally seek to establish a correlation with in vivo behaviour. Thus

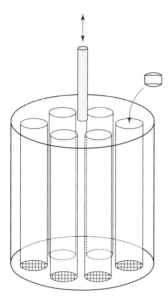

Fig. 30.19 • A disintegration instrument for the testing of tablet disintegration time.

compliance with the specification is not a guarantee of an acceptable release and uptake of the drug in vivo and hence an acceptable clinical effect. However, it is reasonable to assume that a preparation which fails to comply with the test is unlikely to be efficacious. Disintegration tests are, however, useful for assessing the potential effect of formulation and process variables on the biopharmaceutical properties of the tablet, and as a control procedure to evaluate the quality reproducibility of the tablet during production.

Dissolution

Dissolution testing is the most important way to study, under in vitro conditions, the release of a drug from a solid dosage form, and is thus an important tool to assess factors that affect the bioavailability of a drug from a solid preparation. During a dissolution test, the cumulative amount of drug that passes into solution is measured as a function of time. The test thus evaluates the overall rate of all the processes involved in the release of the drug into a bioavailable form. The reasons for and the procedures to enable the dissolution testing of solid dosage forms are discussed in detail in Chapter 35 but will be covered here briefly in the context of this chapter.

Dissolution is accomplished by locating the tablet in a chamber containing a flowing dissolution medium.

So that the method is reproducible, all factors that can affect the dissolution process are standardized. These include factors that affect the solubility of the substance (i.e. the composition and temperature of the dissolution medium) and others that affect the dissolution process (such as the concentration of dissolved substance in and the flow conditions of the fluid in the dissolution chamber).

A number of compendial and noncompendial methods exist for dissolution testing which can be applied to both drug substances and formulated preparations. With respect to preparations, the main test methods are based on forced convection of the dissolution medium and can be classified into two groups: stirred-vessel methods and continuous-flow methods.

The composition of the dissolution medium might vary between different test situations. Pure water or water mixed with acids or bases to adjust the pH is frequently used. In addition, liquids showing a closer resemblance to physiological conditions may also be used. These are often referred to as simulated gastric or intestinal fluids or biorelevant fluids (see Chapter 35). Other dissolution media might be used, such as solvent mixtures, if the water solubility of the drug is very low. Finally, dissolution studies may be carried out in water–ethanol solutions to assess the potential effect of intake of alcoholic drinks at a time close to the administration of a tablet.

Stirred-vessel methods

The most important stirred-vessel methods are the rotating-basket method (Fig. 30.20) and the paddle method (Fig. 30.21). Details of these can be found in monographs in the European or US pharmacopoeias, and are further discussed in Chapter 35. Both use the same type of vessel, which is filled with a dissolution medium of controlled volume and temperature. In the paddle method, the tablet is placed in the vessel and the dissolution medium is agitated by a rotating paddle. In the rotating-basket method, the tablet is placed in a small basket formed from a screen. This is then immersed in the dissolution medium and rotated at a given speed.

Continuous-flow methods

In the continuous-flow method (e.g. *United States Pharmacopeia* Apparatus 4; see Chapter 35), the preparation is held within a flow cell, through which the dissolution medium is pumped at a

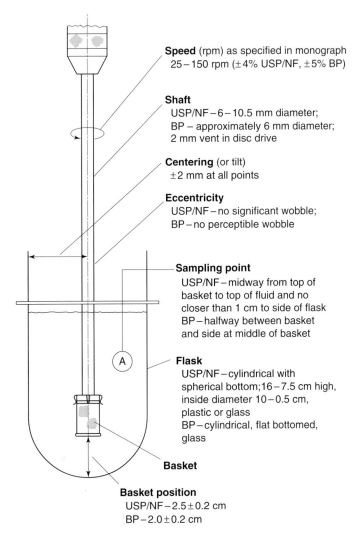

Speed (rpm) as specified in monograph
25–150 rpm (±4% USP/NF, ±5% BP)

Shaft
USP/NF–6–10.5 mm diameter;
BP – approximately 6 mm diameter;
2 mm vent in disc drive

Centering (or tilt)
±2 mm at all points

Eccentricity
USP/NF–no significant wobble;
BP–no perceptible wobble

Sampling point
USP/NF–midway from top of
basket to top of fluid and no
closer than 1 cm to side of flask
BP–halfway between basket
and side at middle of basket

Flask
USP/NF–cylindrical with
spherical bottom;16–7.5 cm high,
inside diameter 10–0.5 cm,
plastic or glass
BP–cylindrical, flat bottomed,
glass

Basket

Basket position
USP/NF–2.5±0.2 cm
BP–2.0±0.2 cm

Fig. 30.20 • A dissolution instrument based on the rotating-basket method for the testing of tablet dissolution rate. *BP, British Pharmacopoeia*; *NF, National Formulary*; *USP, United States Pharmacopeia*. From Banakar, 1992, with permission.

controlled rate from a large reservoir. The liquid which has passed the flow cell is collected for analysis of drug content. The continuous-flow cell method may have advantages over stirred-vessel methods, e.g. it maintains sink conditions throughout the experiment and avoids floating of the preparation.

The amount of drug dissolved is normally analysed more or less continuously as the concentration in the vessel as a function of time. However, sometimes a single measurement can be performed if required in the pharmacopoeial or product specification, i.e. the amount of drug dissolved at a certain time point is determined.

Mechanical strength

The mechanical strength of a tablet is associated with the resistance of the solid specimen to fracturing and attrition. An acceptable tablet must remain intact during handling at all stages, i.e. during production, packaging, warehousing, distribution, dispensing and administration by the patient. Thus an integral part of the formulation and production of tablets is the determination of their mechanical strength. Such testing is carried out to:

• assess the importance of formulation and
  production variables for the resistance of a

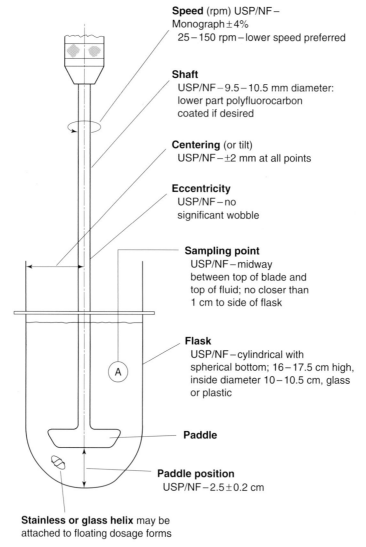

Speed (rpm) USP/NF–
Monograph±4%
25–150 rpm–lower speed preferred

Shaft
USP/NF–9.5–10.5 mm diameter:
lower part polyfluorocarbon
coated if desired

Centering (or tilt)
USP/NF–±2 mm at all points

Eccentricity
USP/NF–no
significant wobble

Sampling point
USP/NF–midway
between top of blade and
top of fluid; no closer than
1 cm to side of flask

Flask
USP/NF–cylindrical with
spherical bottom; 16–17.5 cm high,
inside diameter 10–10.5 cm, glass
or plastic

Paddle

Paddle position
USP/NF–2.5±0.2 cm

Stainless or glass helix may be
attached to floating dosage forms

Fig. 30.21 • A dissolution instrument based on the rotating paddle method for the testing of tablet dissolution rate. *NF, National Formulary; USP, United States Pharmacopeia.* From Banakar, 1992, with permission.

tablet to fracturing and attrition during formulation work, process design and scaling up;

- control the quality of tablets during production (in-process and batch control); and
- characterize the fundamental mechanical properties of materials used in tablet formulation.

A number of methods are available for measuring mechanical strength, and they give different results. In addition, the hardness of a tablet is sometimes measured by indentation testing. The hardness of a specimen is associated with its resistance to local permanent deformation and is thus not a measure of the resistance of the tablet to fracturing.

The most commonly used methods for strength testing can be subcategorized into two main groups: attrition resistance methods (friability tests) and fracture resistance methods.

Attrition resistance methods

The idea behind attrition resistance methods is to mimic the kind of forces to which a tablet is subjected during handling between its production and its administration. These are also referred to as friability tests; a friable tablet is one that is liable to erode mechanically during handling. During handling, tablets are subjected to stresses from collisions and tablets sliding towards one another and other solid surfaces, which can result in the removal of particles or particle clusters from the tablet surface. The result will be a progressive reduction in tablet weight and a change in its appearance. Such attrition can occur even though the stresses are not high enough to break or fracture the tablet into smaller pieces. Thus an important property of a tablet is its ability to resist attrition so as to ensure that the correct amount of drug is administered and that the appearance of the tablet does not change during handling. Another application of a friability method is to detect incipient capping, as tablets with no visible defects can cap or laminate when stressed by an attrition method.

The most common experimental procedure for determining attrition resistance involves the rotation of tablets in a cylinder, followed by the determination of weight loss after a given number of rotations. Another approach is to shake tablets intensively in a jar of dimensions similar to those of a pack-jar. Normally, weight loss of less than 1% during a friability test is required. In addition, the tablets should not show capping or cracking during such testing.

Fracture resistance methods

Analysis of the fracture resistance of tablets involves the application of a load on the tablet and the determination of the force needed to fracture or break the specimen along its diameter or another axis.

In order to obtain a controlled loading during the test, care must be taken to ensure that the load is applied under defined and reproducible conditions in terms of the type of load applied (compression, pulling, twisting, etc.) and the loading rate.

For compressive loading of tablets, the test is simple and reproducible under controlled conditions, and the diametral compression test therefore has broad use during formulation development and tablet production. In such compression testing the tablet is placed against a platen (a flat metal plate) and the load is applied along its diameter by a movable platen. The tablet fails ideally along its diameter, i.e. parallel to the compression load, in a single fracture into two pieces of similar size (Fig. 30.22) and the fracture force is recorded. This mode of failure is actually a tensile failure even though it is accomplished here

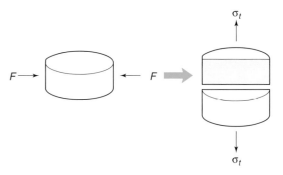

Fig. 30.22 • The tensile failure of a tablet during diametral compression.

by compressive loading. The force needed to fracture the tablet by diametral compression is often somewhat unfortunately referred to as the crushing strength of the tablet. The term 'hardness' is also used in the literature to denote the failure force, which is in this context incorrect as hardness is a deformation property of a solid.

The force needed to fracture a tablet depends on the tablet's dimensions. An ideal test, however, should allow comparison between tablets of different sizes or even shapes. This can be accomplished by assessing the strength of the tablet, i.e. the force needed to fracture the tablet per unit fracture area. A strength test requires that the fracture mode (i.e. the method by which the crack is formed) can be controlled and that the stress state along the fracture plane can be estimated. The simplest and most common tensile strength test is the indirect diametral compression test described previously. For a cylindrical flat-faced tablet, the tensile strength (σ_T) can be calculated by Eq. 30.4, provided that the tablet fails in a tensile fracture mode characterized by a single linear fracture across the diameter of the cylindrical specimen:

$$\sigma_T = \frac{2F}{\pi Dh}$$

(30.4)

where F is the force needed to fracture the tablet and D and h are the diameter and the height of the cylindrical flat-faced tablet respectively.

In practice, failure characteristics more complicated than tensile failure are often obtained during diametral compression (Fig. 30.23), which will prevent the strict application of the calculation procedure. It should be pointed out that the tensile strength of

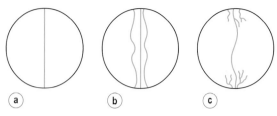

Fig. 30.23 • Examples of different types of failure induced by diametral compression. **(a)** Simple tensile failure. **(b)** Triple cleft failure. **(c)** Failure due to shear at platen edges. Adapted from Davies & Newton, 1996, with permission.

convex-faced tablets can also be calculated by use of other equations.

Alternative procedures to measure the tensile strength of a tablet include breaking the tablet in a bending test or directly pulling the tablet apart until it fractures. The latter may be used to detect weaknesses in the compact in the axial direction, which is an indication of capping or lamination tendencies in the tablet.

Fundamental aspects of the compression of powders

Mechanisms of compression of particles

The compressibility of a powder is defined as its propensity, when held within a confined space, to reduce in volume when subjected to a load. The compression of a powder bed is normally described as a sequence of processes. Initially, the particles in the die are rearranged, resulting in a more closely packed structure and reduced porosity. At a certain load the reduced space and the increased interparticulate friction will prevent any further interparticulate movement. The subsequent reduction of the tablet volume is therefore associated with changes in the dimensions of the particles.

Particles, either all or some, can change their shape temporarily by elastic deformation and permanently by plastic deformation (Fig. 30.24). Particles can also fracture into a number of smaller, discrete particles, i.e. particle fragmentation. The particle fragments can then find new positions, which will further decrease the volume of the powder bed. When the applied pressure is further increased, the smaller particles formed could again undergo deformation. Thus a single particle may undergo this cycle of events

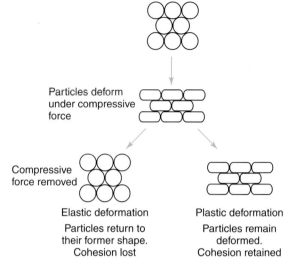

Fig. 30.24 • Particle deformation, elastic and plastic, during compression. Adapted from Armstrong, 1982, with permission.

several times during one compression. As a consequence of compression, particle surfaces are brought close to each other and particle–particle bonds can be formed.

Elastic and plastic deformations of particles are time-independent processes, i.e. the degree of deformation is related to the applied stress and not the time of loading. However, deformation can also be time dependent, i.e. the degree of deformation is related to the applied stress and the time of loading. This deformation behaviour is referred to as viscoelastic and viscous deformation of a material. The consequence is that the compression behaviour of a material might depend on the loading conditions during the formation of a tablet in terms of the punch displacement–time relationship. Many pharmaceutical substances seem to have a viscous character, i.e. are strain-rate sensitive, and the properties of the tablet are thus dependent on the punch displacement–time relationship for the compression process.

Elastic deformation can be described as a strain of the particle due to a small movement of the cluster of molecules or ions that forms the particle, e.g. a crystal lattice or a cluster of disordered molecules. Plastic deformation is considered to occur by the sliding of molecules along slip planes within the particles. For real crystals, such slip planes are formed at defects in the crystal lattice, especially dislocations.

The majority of powders handled in pharmaceutical production consist not of nonporous primary particles but rather of granules, i.e. porous secondary particles formed from small dense primary particles. For granules, a larger number of processes are involved in their compression. These can be classified into two groups:

- physical changes in the granules, i.e. the secondary particles; and
- physical changes in the primary particles from which the granules are formed.

The latter concern changes in the dimensions of the primary particles due to elastic and plastic deformation and fragmentation. Such processes may be significant for the strength of tablets. It is, for example, common for a capping-prone substance, when compacted as dense particles, to also be prone to cap or laminate during compaction in the form of granules, such as substrate–binder granules. However, in terms of the evolution of the tablet structure, the physical changes in the granules that occur during compression are of primary importance.

At low compression forces the reduction in volume of the bed of granules can occur by a rearrangement within the die. However, granules are normally fairly coarse, which means that they spontaneously form a powder bed of relatively low voidage (i.e. the porosity of the intergranular spaces). Therefore this initial rearrangement phase is probably of limited importance with respect to the total change in bed volume of the mass. With increased loading, a further reduction in bed volume therefore requires changes in the structure of the granules. The granules can deform, both elastically and permanently, but also densify, i.e. reduce their intragranular porosity. By these processes, granules can still be described as coherent units but their shape and porosity will change.

Granules can also be broken down into smaller units by two different mechanisms:

- Primary particles might be removed from the surface of granules when they slide against each other or against the die wall. This can be described as erosion or attrition, rather than fracturing. This mechanism occurs primarily for granules with a rough surface texture.
- Granules can fracture into a number of smaller ones, i.e. granule fragmentation.

Studies on the compression properties of granules formed from pharmaceutical substances have indicated that granules are not prone to fracture into smaller units during compression over the normal range of applied pressures. Thus permanent deformation and

Table 30.2 Dominating compression mechanisms for dense particles and granules (porous particles)

Dense particles	Granules
Repositioning of particles	Repositioning of granules
Particle deformation 　Elastic 　Plastic 　Viscous/viscoelastic	Granule deformation (is permanent, i.e. plastic) Granule densification Granule fragmentation/attrition
Particle fragmentation	Deformation of primary particles

densification dominate the compression event although cracking and attrition may occur in parallel, especially for irregular, rough granules.

The dominating compression mechanisms for dense particles and granules are summarized in Table 30.2. The relative occurrence of fragmentation and deformation of solid particles during compression is related to the fundamental mechanical characteristics of the substance, such as its elasticity and plasticity. For granules, both the mechanical properties of the primary particles from which the granules are formed and the physical structure of the granules, such as their porosity and shape, will affect the relative occurrence of each compression mechanism.

Evaluation of compression behaviour

Procedures

The procedures used in research and development work to evaluate the compression behaviour of particles and the mechanisms of compression involved in the volume reduction process are of two types:

- characterization of ejected tablets; and
- characterization of the compression and decompression events.

Concerning the characterization of ejected tablets, the most important procedures used are inspection and the determination of the pore structure of the tablet, in terms of the mean pore size, pore size distribution and specific surface area. A less common approach is to calculate ratios between the mechanical strengths of tablets measured in different directions.

Concerning characterization of the compression and decompression events, the procedures are based on relationships between parameters that can be

Table 30.3 Parameters used in procedures to describe compression and decompression events

Upper punch force/pressure versus compression time[a]
Lower punch force/pressure versus compression time[b]
Upper punch force/pressure versus lower punch force/pressure
Upper punch force versus die wall force
Punch force versus punch displacement (mainly upper punch)
Tablet relative volume versus upper punch pressure/force
Tablet porosity versus upper punch pressure/force

[a]Used both during ordinary compression and also as prolonged loading after maximum applied force/pressure has been reached (referred to as stress relaxation measurements).
[b]Used primarily to describe the ejection phase.

derived from the compaction process (Table 30.3). Some of the most common approaches used in this context are described in the following sections.

Inspection of tablets

The inspection of tablets, e.g. by scanning electron microscopy and by profilometry, is an important means of studying changes in the physical properties of particles during compression. Such changes include fragmentation into smaller particles, permanent shape changes due to deformation and the formation of cracks within the particles. Such inspection will also give information about the relative positions of particles within the tablet and hence the interparticulate pore structure. The fracture path during strength testing, i.e. failure around or across the particles, can also be estimated from inspection of the tablet fracture surface.

In addition to the inspection of intact tablets, studies of the fragmentation of particles during compression can be performed by analysing the size and size distribution of particles obtained by deaggregation of a tablet. Such deaggregation can occur spontaneously by disintegration of the tablet in a liquid or can be created mechanically. Studies on such deaggregated tablets have indicated that powder compression can effectively reduce the size of particles and result in a wider particle size distribution of the cohered particles within a tablet.

Pore structure and specific surface area of tablets

One of the most important ways to study the evolution of tablet structure during compression is to measure some characteristic of the pore structure of the tablet. Information on the pore size distribution can be obtained by use of mercury intrusion measurements and by gas adsorption–desorption. However, the most common way to evaluate the pore system of a tablet has been to measure the surface area of the tablet by air permeability or gas adsorption. The former has also been used to derive an indication of the mean pore size in a tablet.

Surface area measurements have been used as a means to assess fragmentation during compaction by measuring the specific surface area of a particulate solid before and after compaction, or by measuring changes in tablet surface area with compaction pressure.

The slope of the relationship between tablet surface area and applied pressure is an indication of the degree of fragmentation that occurs during compression and can be used to classify materials with respect to their fragmentation propensity (Fig. 30.25). It should be pointed out that the calculation of tablet surface area from air permeability measurements may give erroneous values as a result of the assumptions made in the derivation of the calculation procedure. In spite of this, the method has been shown to give useful data in terms of describing the fragmentation propensity of a substance.

The relationship between tablet surface area and applied pressure is, however, strongly dependent on the original surface area of the powder, i.e. the tablet surface area increases more markedly with applied pressure when the original particle size was smaller. Attempts have been made in the literature to derive an expression similar to those describing the size reduction of particles during milling (see Chapter 10), by which a measure of the propensity of particles to fragment independent of the original powder surface area can be calculated.

It is generally assumed that a change in the size of a particle affects the mechanics of particle deformation, i.e. how a particle responds to an applied load. Such a size-related change in the mechanics of particles can, for example, be attributed to a reduced probability of the presence of flaws in the crystal structure at which a catastrophic failure is initiated. It seems possible, therefore, that at a limiting particle size, fragmentation might cease. Examples of such transitions from a brittle to a plastic behaviour have been reported, and the particle size at which this transition takes place is referred to as the critical particle size. This critical size has been suggested to differ markedly between different substances.

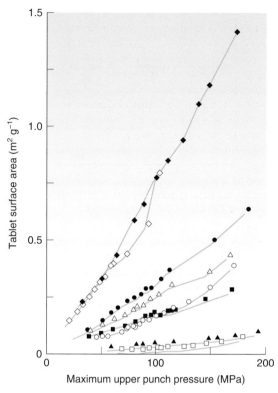

Fig. 30.25 • The tablet surface area, measured by air permeametry, as a function of compaction pressure for a series of pharmaceutical substances: sodium chloride *(open squares)*, sodium bicarbonate *(closed triangles)*, saccharose *(open circles)*, sodium citrate *(closed squares)*, ascorbic acid *(open triangles)*, lactose *(closed circles)*, paracetamol *(open diamonds)*, Emcompress *(closed diamonds)*. Adapted from Alderborn et al., 1985.

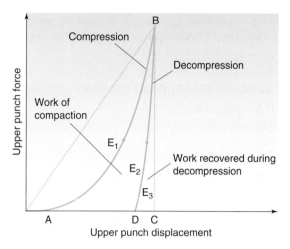

Fig. 30.26 • The relationship between upper punch force and upper punch displacement during compression and decompression of a powder. Adapted from Ragnarsson, 1996.

Force–displacement profiles

The relationship between upper punch force and upper punch displacement during compression, often referred to as the force–displacement profile, has been used as a means to derive information on the compression behaviour of a powder and to make predictions on its tablet-forming ability. The area under a force–displacement curve represents the work or energy involved in the compression process. Different procedures have been used to analyse the curves.

One approach is based on the division of the force–displacement curve into different regions (denoted E_1, E_2 and E_3 in Fig. 30.26). It has been suggested that the areas of E_1 and E_3 should be as small as possible for a powder to perform well in a tableting operation and give tablets of high mechanical strength. An alternative approach is based on mathematical analysis of the force–displacement curve from the compression phase, e.g. in terms of a hyperbolic function.

Force–displacement curves have some use in pharmaceutical development as an indicator of the tablet-forming ability of powders, including the assessment of the elastic properties of materials from the decompression curve. They can also be used as a means to monitor the compression behaviour of a substance so as to document and evaluate reproducibility between batches.

Force–displacement measurements have also been used in fundamental studies on the energy changes during compaction of powders, i.e. a thermodynamic analysis of the process of compact formation. The energy applied to the powder can be calculated from the area under the force–displacement curve. This compaction energy is used to overcome friction between particles, to deform particles both permanently and reversibly and to create new particle surfaces by fragmentation. The thermal energy released during compaction can be assessed by calorimetry, i.e. the die is constructed as a calorimeter. The heat released during compression is the result of particle deformation, i.e. energy is consumed during deformation and thereafter partly released when the deformation is completed, and the result of the formation of interparticulate bonds.

Data have been reported indicating that the net effect of a compaction process is exothermic, i.e. more thermal energy is released during compaction than is applied to the powder in terms of mechanical energy. The main explanation for this is released bonding energy in the form of heat due to the formation of bonds between particles.

Tablet volume–applied pressure profiles

In both engineering and pharmaceutical sciences, the relationship between volume and applied pressure during compression is the main approach to deriving a mathematical representation of the compression process. A large number of tablet volume–applied pressure relationships exist. In addition to tablet volume and applied pressure parameters, such expressions include some constants which are often defined in physical terms. However, only for a few equations has the physical significance of the constants been generally accepted. Among these, the most recognized expression in pharmaceutical science is the tablet porosity–applied pressure function according to Heckel (see Duberg & Nyström, 1986).

Heckel equation

Tablet porosity can be measured either on an ejected tablet or on a powder column under load, i.e. in a die. The latter approach is more common as it can be performed rapidly with a limited amount of powder. A problem might be that the compression time is different at each pressure, which could affect the profile for materials having pronounced time-dependent compression behaviour.

The compression of a powder can be described in terms of a first-order reaction where the pores are the reactant and the densification is the product. On the basis of this assumption, the following expression was derived:

$$\ln\left(\frac{1}{\varepsilon}\right) = KP + A$$

(30.5)

where ε is the tablet porosity, P is the applied pressure, A is a constant suggested to reflect particle rearrangement and fragmentation and K is the slope of the linear part of the relationship, which is suggested to reflect the deformation of particles during compression. The reciprocal of the slope value K is often calculated and considered to represent the yield stress or yield pressure (P_y) for the particles, i.e.

$$\ln\left(\frac{1}{\varepsilon}\right) = \frac{P}{P_y} + A$$

(30.6)

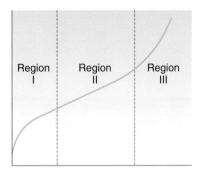

Region I   Region II   Region III

Fig. 30.27 • A typical example of a Heckel profile indicating the three regions of powder compression. Adapted from Sun & Grant, 2001, with permission.

The yield stress is defined as the stress at which plastic deformation of a particle is initiated. To be able to use the Heckel yield pressure to compare different substances, it is important to standardize the experimental conditions, such as tablet dimensions and speed of compaction.

Fig. 30.27 shows a typical Heckel profile. The profile often shows an initial curvature (region I) which is associated with particle fragmentation and repositioning. Thereafter, the relationship is often linear over a substantial range of applied pressures (region II) and thus obeys the expression. The linear part is considered to reflect a situation where particle deformation controls the compression process, and from the gradient of this linear part, the yield pressure can be calculated. Finally, the profile again deviates from the linear relationship (region III), and this curvature is considered to reflect elastic deformation of the whole tablet.

Strain rate sensitivity

Another proposed use of yield pressures from Heckel profiles is to assess the time-dependent deformation properties of particles during compression by comparing yield pressure values derived under compression at different punch velocities. A term denoted the *strain rate sensitivity* (SRS) has been proposed (Roberts & Rowe, 1985) as a characteristic of the time dependency of a powder:

$$SRS = \frac{P_y' - P_y''}{P_y''}$$

(30.7)

where P_y' is the yield pressure derived at a high punch velocity and P_y'' is that derived at a low punch velocity.

P_y' is normally higher than P_y'' and the SRS is thus a positive value.

The discussion on the use of Heckel profiles to derive a measure of the compression yield pressure is applicable to the compression of powders consisting of solid particles. It should be emphasized that the interpretation of $1/K$ in terms of a mean yield stress for the particles is under debate. Nevertheless, support has been presented that such an interpretation is valid for solid (nonporous) particles. For porous particles, i.e. granules and pellets, the Heckel procedure is inadequate for the derivation of a measure of deformability or granule strength. The problem of applying the Heckel approach to the compression of porous particles is related to the need to assess the porosity of the reactant pore system. The pore space of interest in relation to the Heckel equation is intergranular and the problem of quantifying this was discussed earlier in this chapter.

Kawakita equation

A promising means of assessing the compression mechanics of granules is to calculate a compression shear strength from the Kawakita equation. This was derived from the assumption that, during powder compression in a confined space, the system is in equilibrium at all stages, so the product of a pressure term and a volume term is constant. The equation can be written in the following linear form:

$$\frac{P}{C} = \frac{P}{a} + \frac{1}{ab}$$

(30.8)

where P is applied pressure, C is the degree of volume reduction and a and b are constants. The degree of volume reduction relates the initial height of the powder column (h_o) to the height of the powder column (the compact) at an applied pressure P (h) as follows:

$$C = \frac{h_o - h}{h_o}$$

(30.9)

This equation has been applied primarily to powders of solid particles. However, it has been suggested (Adams et al., 1994) that the compression parameter $1/b$ corresponds to the compression strength of granules. The procedure thus represents a possible means to characterize the mechanical property of granules from a compression experiment.

Powder and particle scale modelling

It is often of interest to see how tablet properties, such as the porosity, vary between different locations within a tablet. In a modelling context, such questions are generally addressed by use of models of a continuum type, in which the particulate nature of the powder is disregarded. Continuum models require material-specific equations (referred to as constitutive equations) that delineate how the powder behaves when subjected to external stresses. These are combined with generic balance equations (such as the balance of mass and momentum; the latter being analogous to Newton's equations) to form a system of equations that are typically solved numerically by the finite element method (FEM). As a result of the multifaceted behaviour of powders, the material-specific constitutive equations tend to be rather complex and generally require quite extensive experimental calibration before use. Most often, models have been adopted from the field of soil mechanics and, in particular, a model referred to as the Drucker–Prager cap (DPC) model is in widespread use (Han et al., 2008). Once a calibrated model is in place, continuum modelling is very powerful and can readily be used to investigate various aspects of powder compression. One example is provided in Fig. 30.28, in which experimental and numerical density distributions within convex tablets are compared. Because individual particles are not resolved, continuum models tend to be efficient in the sense that they do not require extensive computational powder (often a PC is sufficient).

For a more fundamental understanding, there is a need to relate the mechanical properties of the individual particles to the behaviour of the powder when it is subjected to load. To this end, particle dynamics simulations are commonly used, not only for confined compression but also to study various aspects of powder flow. In particle dynamics simulations, all particles and their mutual interactions are taken into account. In this manner, detailed information about phenomena that occur at the particulate scale can be obtained. The most commonly used method, referred to as the discrete element method (DEM), allows particles to overlap slightly, and the contact forces are considered to be functions of the particle overlaps. Moreover, multiple contacts on individual particles are considered to be independent. These assumptions are adequate for most dynamic processes but can result in inaccurate determinations of contact forces during confined compression, when

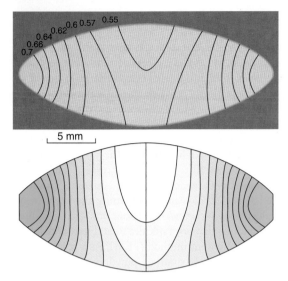

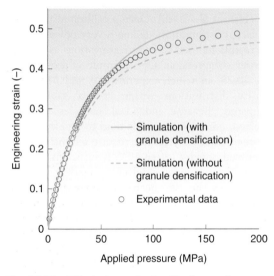

Fig. 30.28 • Density gradients of a tablet, assessed by experiment *(top)* and by modelling *(bottom)* for tablets with high tablet to die wall friction. From Sinka et al., 2003, with permission.

Fig. 30.29 • Effect of granule densification on the overall compression profile as obtained from discrete element method simulations. From Persson & Frenning, 2015, with permission.

individual particles deform considerably. For this reason, more elaborate models that take contact dependence and spatial confinement into account have started to appear in the literature. Confined compression of initially porous granules formed from microcrystalline cellulose has been studied with a model of this type. As shown in Fig. 30.29, granule

densification appears to have a significant effect on the overall compression profile, although a residual porosity remains in the granules. These observations are consistent with experimental results.

Evaluation of die wall friction during compression

Friction is a serious problem during tableting. Consequently, a series of procedures have been developed with the aim of assessing the friction between the powder or tablet and the die wall during compression and ejection, which can be used during tablet formulation to evaluate lubricants and formulations. These methods are based mainly on the use of force signals during powder compression or tablet ejection. The type of compression situation most commonly used in this context is a single-punch press with a movable upper punch and a stationary lower punch. In such a rig the force is applied by the upper punch and transmitted axially to the lower punch and also laterally to the die. The ejection of the tablet involves the application of an ejection force by the lower punch. Typical force profiles during compression in a single-punch press with a stationary lower punch are given in Fig. 30.30.

When the descending upper punch establishes contact with the powder bed in the die, the force increases with compression time. The applied force rises to a maximum value and thereafter decreases during the decompression phase to zero. Parallel with the force trace from the upper punch, force traces from the lower punch and the die will be obtained.

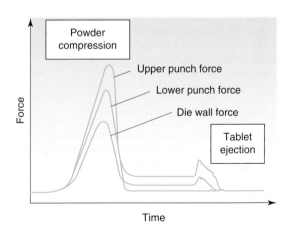

Fig. 30.30 • Force–time signals (from punches and die) during uniaxial powder compression.

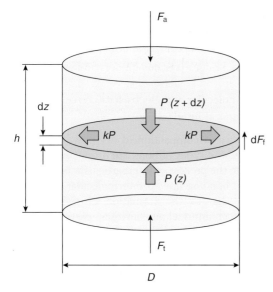

Fig. 30.31 • Illustration of the Janssen analysis of force transmission during uniaxial powder compression in a cylindrical die.

These can be described as transmitted forces, and the force values are thus generally lower than the applied force. The force transmitted from the upper punch to the lower punch is considered to depend on a number of factors, including the friction between the powder and the die wall.

A simplified but useful model for stress transmission through powder beds dates back to work performed by Janssen in 1895 and uses an approximate method that is called the method of differential slices (Nedermann, 1992). Consider a powder bed of cylindrical shape with diameter D and height h as illustrated in Fig. 30.31. The powder deforms under the influence of an applied force F_a exerted by a mobile upper punch and transmits a force F_t to a stationary lower punch. Focusing on a differential slice of thickness dz, one may express the difference in force between the upper and lower faces of the slice as the product of the cross-sectional area ($\pi D^2/4$) and the change in axial pressure P (i.e. the pressure that acts on planes parallel to the punch surfaces), as seen on the left-hand side of Eq. 30.10. The difference in force is balanced by friction between the tablet and the die (indicated by dF_f in Fig. 30.31). An approximation commonly made is to consider the radial pressure (i.e. the pressure that acts on the die wall) to be proportional to the axial pressure; hence the radial pressure is written as kP, where k is a constant (often referred to as the Janssen

constant). The lateral surface area of the differential slice equals the product of the circumference πD and the height dz. Multiplying the radial pressure and the lateral surface area, one obtains the normal force on the lateral surface area of the differential slice. On multiplication by the friction coefficient μ, the friction force is finally obtained, as indicated on the right-hand-side of Eq. 30.10:

$$\frac{\pi D^2}{4} \times [P(z+dz) - P(z)] = \mu \times \pi D dz \times kP(z)$$

(30.10)

Dividing this by $\pi D^2 dz/4$ and letting dz tend to zero, one obtains the following differential equation:

$$\frac{dP}{dz} - \frac{4\mu k}{D} P = 0$$

(30.11)

The solution can be expressed as

$$P(z) = P_0 e^{4\mu kz/D}$$

(30.12)

where P_0 is the pressure at zero height, i.e. the pressure at the lower punch. For a tablet of height h, the ratio between the transmitted and applied forces is obtained as

$$R = \frac{F_t}{F_a} = \frac{P_0}{P_h} = e^{-4\mu kh/D}$$

(30.13)

This analysis thus suggests that the force transmission ratio $R = F_t/F_a$ decreases exponentially with increasing friction coefficient and increasing ratio between the tablet height and the tablet diameter. Moreover, the total friction force can be determined as the difference between the applied and the transmitted forces:

$$F_f = F_a - F_t = F_a(1 - e^{-4\mu kh/D})$$

(30.14)

Both the difference between the applied and the transmitted force (i.e. the total friction force F_f, see Eq. 30.14) and the ratio between the applied and the transmitted force (i.e. the force transmission ratio R; see Eq. 30.13) are used as measures of die wall friction during compression. For a well-lubricated powder, the force transmission corresponds to $R > 0.9$.

After the upper punch has lost contact with the tablet and its force has consequently decreased to zero, the tablet will be positioned in the die in contact with the lower punch and the die wall. In this situation the tablet will apply a force to both the lower punch and the die wall. The magnitude of these forces is dependent on the mechanical character of the particles formed into the tablet and also on the friction conditions at the interface between the tablet and the die wall.

The ejection of the tablet will result in an increased force signal from the lower punch, referred to as the ejection force. This is a function of the lateral die wall force and also of the friction condition at the interface between the tablet and the die wall. The maximum ejection force is thus also used as a measure of friction between the tablet and the die wall. One approach to assess friction during ejection is to calculate the dimensionless friction coefficient (μ) as the ratio between the ejection force (F_e) and the die wall force (F_w) at the beginning of the ejection phase, i.e.

$$\mu = \frac{F_e}{F_w}$$

(30.15)

To summarize, the following procedures are mainly used to derive measures of friction between the powder or tablet and the die wall from force signals during tableting in a single-punch press:

- force difference between the upper and the lower punch;
- force ratio between the lower and the upper punch;
- maximum ejection force; and
- friction coefficient during ejection.

Fundamental aspects of the compaction of powders

Bonding in tablets

The transformation of a powder into a tablet is fundamentally an interparticulate bonding process, i.e. the increased strength of the assembly of particles is the result of the formation of bonds between them. The nature of these bonds is traditionally subdivided into five types, known as the *Rumpf classification*:

1. solid bridges;
2. bonding by liquids (capillary and surface tension forces);
3. binder bridges (viscous binders and adsorption layers);
4. intermolecular and electrostatic forces; and
5. mechanical interlocking.

In the case of compaction of dry powders, two of the suggested types of bond are often considered to dominate the process of interparticulate bond formation, i.e. bonding due to intermolecular forces and bonding due to the formation of solid bridges. Mechanical interlocking between particles is also considered as a possible but less significant bond type in tablets.

Bonding by intermolecular forces is sometimes also known as *adsorption bonding*, i.e. the bonds are formed when two solid surfaces are brought into intimate contact and subsequently adsorb to each other. Among the intermolecular forces, dispersion forces are considered to represent the most important bonding mechanism. These forces operate in a vacuum and in a gaseous or liquid environment at separation distances between the surfaces of approximately 10 nm to 100 nm.

The formation of solid bridges, also referred to as the *diffusion theory of bonding*, occurs when two solids are mixed at their interface and accordingly form a continuous solid phase. Such a mixing process requires that molecules in the solid state are movable, at least temporarily, during compression. An increased molecular mobility can occur because of melting or as a result of a glass–rubber transition of an amorphous solid phase.

Mechanical interlocking is the term used to describe a situation where strength is provided by interparticulate hooking. This phenomenon usually requires that the particles have an atypical shape, such as needle-shaped, or highly irregular and rough particles.

For tablets with porosity in the range from 5% to 30%, it is normally assumed that bonding by adsorption is the dominant bond type between particles. In tablets formed from amorphous substances or from substances with low melting points, it is possible that solid bridges can be formed across the particle–particle interface. It is also reasonable that if tablets of very low porosity, i.e. close to zero, are formed, particles can fuse together to a significant degree.

Often granules, i.e. secondary particles formed by the agglomeration of primary particles, are handled in a tableting operation. When granules are compacted, bonds will be formed between adjacent granule surfaces. For granules that do not include a binder, the fusion of adjacent surfaces during compaction is probably not a significant bonding mechanism. Thus intermolecular bonding forces acting between intergranular surfaces in intimate contact will probably be the dominant bond type in such tablets.

Granules often include a binder. When such binder–substrate granules are compacted, it is reasonable to assume that the binder also plays an important role in the formation of intergranular bonds. The binder may fuse together locally and form binder bridges between granule surfaces which cause the granules to cohere. Such bridges may be the result of a softening or melting of binder layers during the compression phase. However, different types of adsorption bonds may be active between granule surfaces. These may be subdivided into three types: binder–binder, binder–substrate and substrate–substrate bonds.

For adsorption bonds between granules in a tablet, the location of the failure during fracturing of the tablet can vary. Fractures occurring predominantly through binder bridges between substrate particles, as well as predominantly at the interface between the binder and the substrate particle, may occur. The location of the failure has been attributed to the relative strength of the cohesive (binder bridge) and adhesive (binder–substrate interface) forces acting within the granules, which can be affected by, for example, the surface geometry of the substrate particles.

The main bond types in tablets formed from dense particles (interparticulate bonds) and from granules (intergranular bonds) are summarized in Table 30.4.

Compactability of powders and the strength of tablets

The compactability of a powder refers to its propensity to form a coherent tablet and thus is a critical powder property in successful tableting operations. The ability of a powder to cohere is understood in this context in a broad sense, i.e. a powder with high compactability forms tablets with high resistance towards fracturing and without tendencies to cap or laminate (Fig. 30.32). In practice, the most common way to assess powder compactability is to study the effect of compaction pressure on the strength of the resulting

Table 30.4 Predominant bond types in tablets formed from dense particles (interparticulate bonds) and from granules (intergranular bonds)

Interparticulate bonds	Intergranular bonds
Adsorption bonds (intermolecular forces)	Adsorption bonds of three types: binder–binder binder–substrate substrate–substrate
Solid bridges	Solid binder bridges

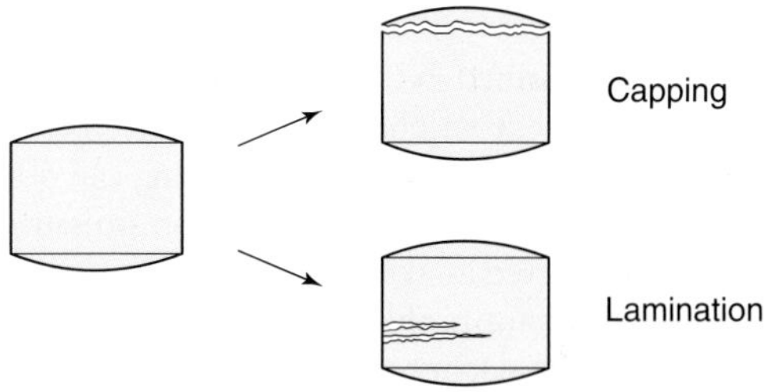

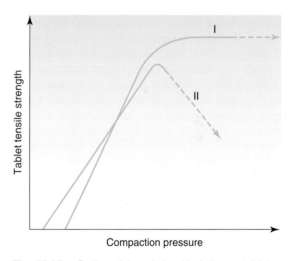

Fig. 30.32 • Illustration of tablet defects referred to as capping and lamination.

Fig. 30.33 • Outline of the relationship between tablet tensile strength and compaction pressure for tablets showing no lamination (I) and for tablets showing lamination or capping (II).

tablet, as assessed by the force needed to fracture the formed tablet while it is loaded diametrically, or the tensile strength of the tablet. Such relationships are often nearly linear (Fig. 30.33) above a lower pressure threshold needed to form a tablet, and up to a pressure corresponding to a tablet of low porosity. At low porosities the relationship between tablet strength and compaction pressure will often level out. This relationship can thus be described simply in terms of a three-region relationship characterized by lower and upper tablet strength thresholds and an intermediate region in which the tablet strength is pressure dependent in an almost linear way.

Compactability profiles are sometimes also described by sigmoidal curves that can be divided principally into the three regions already described. At low pressures the tensile strength of tablets increases as a power function with applied pressure, followed by a nearly linear region that finally levels off.

If cracks are formed in the tablet during tableting, e.g. during the ejection phase, this will often affect the assessed strength. Cracking and capping can often be induced at relatively high compaction pressures. This may be reflected as a drop in the tablet strength–compaction pressure profile.

A series of approaches to quantitatively describe or to model the compactability profile of a powder can be found in the literature. Some modelling approaches aim at describing the microstructure of a tablet in terms of an interparticulate bond structure and are based on the view that bond formation during compaction is significant for the development of coherence, i.e. it is postulated that the tensile strength of a tablet has some proportionality to the interparticulate bonds that act over the fracture area. Such models can thus be described as bond summation approaches and implicit is that all bonds are separated simultaneously during strength assessment. Because this is not consistent with the real mode of failure of a solid, the models are not fundamental approaches to understanding the strength of a tablet (see later).

Examples of equations describing compactability profiles have been given by Leuenberger (1982) and Alderborn (2003). In both cases the bond structure is modelled and related to an end point representing the maximum tensile strength (T_{max}) that can be obtained for tablets of a specific powder. Leuenberger's approach is based on the concept of effective numbers of interparticulate bonds in a cross-section of the tablet. It is assumed that over a cross-section of a tablet, a number of bonding and nonbonding sites exist. The number depends on the applied pressure during compression (P) and the tablet relative density (ρ, which is equivalent to 1 minus the tablet porosity, ε). In the derivation of the expression, the term *compression susceptibility* (γ) was introduced, which described the compressibility of the powder

and has the dimension of reciprocal pressure. The equation takes the following form:

$$T = T_{max}(1 - e^{\gamma P \rho})$$

(30.16)

The compactability profile as described by the expression stems from the origin of the tensile strength–compaction pressure axes; the tensile strength will initially increase with compaction pressure and finally level off (see the previous discussion of compactability profiles).

Alternatives to tablet strength–compaction pressure relationships for representing the compactability of powders are also used, such as the relationship between tablet strength and tablet porosity and the relationship between tablet strength and the work done by the punches during tablet formation.

Compaction is fundamentally a bonding process, i.e. strength is provided by bonds formed at the interparticulate junctions or contact sites during the compression process. Studies on the structure of fractured tablets indicate that a tablet generally fails by the breakage of interparticulate bonds, i.e. an interparticulate fracture process. However, especially for tablets of low porosity, the tablet can also fracture by breakage of the particles that form the tablet, i.e. a combination of an interparticulate and an intraparticulate fracture process. In general terms it seems, though, that the interparticulate contacts in a tablet represent the preferred failure path during fracturing. This conclusion is applicable to both tablets formed from solid particles and tablets formed from porous secondary particles (granules and pellets). Consequently, factors that affect the microstructure at the interparticulate junctions have been considered significant for the compactability of a powder.

Our understanding of the mechanical strength of a solid is based on the resistance of a solid body to fracture while loaded. It might seem reasonable that the sum of the bonding forces that cohere the molecules forming the solid will represent the strength of that solid. However, solids fail by a process of crack propagation, i.e. the fracture is initiated at a certain point within the solid and is thereafter propagated across a plane, thereby causing the solid to break. The consequence in terms of the strength of the solid is that the sum of the bonding forces acting over the fracture surface will be higher than the stress required to initiate failure. It is known, for example, that for crystalline solids the theoretical strength due to the summation of intermolecular bonds is much higher than the measured strength of the solid.

To understand the strength of solids, the process of fracture has attracted considerable interest in different scientific areas. In this context, important factors associated with the fracturing process and the strength of a specimen are the size of the flaw at which the crack is initiated and the resistance of the solid to fracturing. The latter property can be described by the critical stress intensity factor, which is an indication of the stress needed to propagate a crack. Another fracture mechanics parameter, which is related to the critical stress intensity factor, is the strain energy release rate, which is a measure of the energy released during crack propagation.

The tensile strength of the solid (T) is considered to be proportional to the ratio between the critical stress intensity factor (K_{Ic}) and the square root of the flaw size (c):

$$T \propto \frac{K_{Ic}}{\sqrt{c}}$$

(30.17)

The critical stress intensity factor varies with tablet porosity. It has therefore been suggested that for compacts, such as tablets, factors such as the size of the particles within the tablet and the surface energy of the material will affect the critical stress intensity factor (Kendall, 1988). These factors are also considered to control the interparticulate bond structure in a tablet.

Procedures to determine the critical stress intensity factor for a particulate solid have been described. Such procedures normally involve the formation of a beam-shaped compact in which a notch is formed. When the compact is loaded, the fracture is initiated at the notch. The force needed to fracture the compact is determined and the critical stress intensity factor is calculated. In order to assess a material characteristic, compacts of a series of porosities are formed and the series of values for the critical stress intensity factor subsequently determined are plotted as a function of the compact porosity (Fig. 30.34). The relationship may sometimes be extrapolated to zero porosity, and the value thus derived is sometimes considered a fundamental material characteristic.

In addition to the evaluation of compactability profiles and fracture mechanics studies, indices and expressions have been derived within pharmaceutical

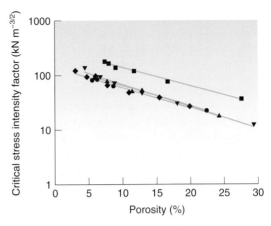

Fig. 30.34 • A log–linear relationship between the critical stress intensity factor and the compact porosity for beams formed from polyethylene glycols of different molecular weight. Adapted from Al-Nasassrah et al., 1998.

science which can be described as indicators of the compactability of a powder. There are several applications of such indicators during pharmaceutical development, such as:

- the evaluation of the compactability of small amounts of particles;
- the selection of drug candidates during preformulation on the basis of technical performance;
- the detection of batch variations of drugs and excipients; and
- the selection of excipients and the evaluation of the compactability of formulations.

The indices of tableting performance derived by Hiestand (Hiestand, 1996) are examples of such indicators which have found industrial use. Hiestand derived three indices of tableting performance, among which the *bonding index* (BI) and the *brittle fracture index* (BFI) are suggested to reflect the compactability of the powder. These indices are dimensionless ratios between mechanical properties of compacts formed at some porosity. The BI is proposed to reflect the ability of particles to form a tablet of high tensile strength, whereas the BFI is proposed to reflect the ability of a tablet to resist fracturing and lamination during handling. These indices are defined as follows:

$$BI = \frac{T}{H}$$

(30.18)

and

$$BFI = \frac{1}{2}\left(\frac{T}{T_0} - 1\right)$$

(30.19)

where T is the tensile strength of a normal compact, T_0 is the tensile strength of a compact with a small hole and H is the hardness of the compact.

Postcompaction tablet strength changes

The compactability of a powder is normally understood in terms of the ability of particles to cohere during the compression process and hence to form a porous specimen of defined shape. However, the mechanical strength of tablets can change, increase or decrease, during storage without the application of any external mechanical force. The underlying mechanisms for such changes are often a complex function of the combination of the ingredients in the tablet and the storage conditions, such as relative humidity and temperature.

During storage at a fairly high relative humidity, tablets can be softer and their tensile strength can be reduced. With increased relative humidity, the state of water adsorbed at the solid surface can change from an adsorbed gas to a liquid, i.e. water condenses in the tablet pores. Furthermore, if the solid material is freely soluble in water, it can dissolve. Both the presence of condensed water in the pores and the dissolution of a substance in the condensed water can drastically decrease tablet strength and eventually lead to the collapse of the whole tablet. However, the dissolution of a freely soluble substance in condensed pore water can also result in an increase in tablet strength if the water is allowed to evaporate owing to a change in temperature or relative humidity. The result of this evaporation can be crystallization of solid material, with the subsequent formation of solid bridges between particles in the tablet and increased tablet strength.

In addition to the mechanisms involving the presence of condensed pore water, several other mechanisms have been proposed to cause an increase in tablet strength during storage at a relative humidity at which condensation of water is unlikely to occur. One such mechanism is a continuing viscous deformation of particles after the compaction process has been completed. This phenomenon is referred to as *stress relaxation* of tablets. The increase in tablet strength can be significant with no, or minor, detectable changes in its physical structure. However, viscous deformation of small parts of particles might change the microstructure of the tablet in terms of the relative orientation of particle surfaces and the geometry of the interparticle voids and thus affect the resistance to fracturing of a tablet. A characteristic feature for stress relaxation changes is that the tablet strength changes occur for a limited time in connection with the compaction phase. An increase in tablet strength during storage may also be related to a polymorphic transformation, i.e. a change in the crystal structure of the particles.

Relationships between material properties and tablet strength

Factors of importance for powder compactability

A number of empirical studies exist in the pharmaceutical literature with the aim of mapping factors that affect the structure of a tablet and its mechanical strength, i.e. tensile strength, resistance to attrition and capping tendencies. These factors can be classified into three groups: material and formulation factors; processing factors (choice of tablet machine and operation conditions); and environmental factors (e.g. relative humidity).

Of special importance from a formulation perspective are the physical and mechanical properties of the particles used in the formulation, and how these particles are combined in granulation and mixing steps. Relationships for powders consisting of one component, two components, such as a filler and a lubricant or a dry binder, or several components have been discussed in this context.

Compaction of solid particles

As discussed already, it is often assumed that the evolution of the interparticulate structure of a tablet, in terms of bonds between particles and the pores between the particles, will be significant for the mechanical strength of the tablet. Thus the material-related factors that control the evolution of the microstructure of the tablet have been discussed as important factors for the compactability of a powder. In this context, the compression behaviour and the original dimensions of the particles have received special interest.

As already mentioned, the degree of fragmentation and permanent deformation that particles undergo during compression are significant for tablet structure and strength. It has been suggested that both fragmentation and deformation are strength-producing compression mechanisms. The significance of particle fragmentation has been considered to be related to the formation of small particles which constitute the tablet, with the consequence that a large number of contact sites between particles at which bonds can be formed will be developed and the voids between the particles will be reduced in size. The significance of permanent deformation has been explained in terms of an effect on the area of contact of the interparticulate contact sites, with a subsequent increased bonding force. The relative importance of these mechanisms for the bonding between particles in a tablet and the resistance of a tablet to fracturing has not, however, been fully clarified. Elastic deformation, which is recoverable, is considered as a disruptive rather than a bond-forming mechanism. Poor compactability, in terms of low tablet strength and capping/lamination, has been attributed to elastic properties of the solid. A summary of advantages and disadvantages of the different particle compression mechanisms for the ability of the particles to form tablets is given in Table 30.5.

It is sometimes considered that one of the most important properties of particles for the mechanical strength of a tablet is their size before compaction. A number of empirical relationships between particle dimensions before compaction and the mechanical strength of the resultant tablet can thus be found in the literature. As a rule, it is normally assumed that a smaller original particle size increases tablet strength. However, it is also suggested that the effect of original particle size is in relative terms limited for powder compactability, with the possible exception of very small (i.e. micronized) particles. Reported data show, however, that different and sometimes complex relationships between particle size and tablet strength can be obtained, with maximum or minimum tablet strengths. Complex relationships might be associated with a change in the shape, structure (such as the formation of aggregates) or degree of disorder of the particles with particle size. It seems also that increased compaction pressure stresses the relationship between the original particle size and tablet strength in absolute terms.

Some studies have specifically reported on the effect of original particle shape on tablet strength. The results indicate that for particles that fragment to a limited degree during compression, increased particle irregularity increased their compactability. However, for particles that fragmented markedly during compression, the original shape of the particles did not affect tablet strength. Moreover, an increased compaction pressure increased the absolute difference in strength of compacts of different original particle shape. Thus the shape characteristics of particles that fragment markedly during compression seem not to affect the microstructure and the tensile strength of

Table 30.5 Advantages and disadvantages of the different compression mechanisms in relation to the tablet-forming ability of the powder

Compression mechanism	Advantages	Disadvantages	Others
Fragmentation	No effect of particle shape Low sensitivity to additives Strain-rate insensitive	May cause fracturing of tablets (e.g. capping)	Bond-forming ability (and tablet strength) dependent on degree of particle fragmentation
Plastic deformation	Resistant to fracturing of tablets (e.g. capping) Strain-rate insensitive	Sensitive to additives and variations in original particle shape	Bond-forming ability (and tablet strength) dependent on degree of particle deformation
Elastic deformation	–	May cause fracturing of tablets (e.g. capping)	–
Time-dependent deformation	–	Strain-rate sensitive Prone to change tablet strength after compaction because of stress relaxation	–

tablets, but the converse applies for particles that showed limited fragmentation.

Compaction of granules

The rationale for granulating a powder mixture before tableting was discussed earlier in the chapter, one reason being to ensure good tableting behaviour, including compactability. When granules are compacted, the mechanical characteristics of the primary particles and the properties of other excipients will affect the tableting behaviour of the powder. For example, it is a common experience that capping-prone material will show capping tendencies in the granulated form of the substance also. However, the design of the granulation process, such as the method of granulation, will control the physical properties of the granules formed, e.g. in terms of granule size, shape, porosity and strength, which subsequently will affect the evolution in the microstructure of the tablets during compaction. It has, for example, been shown (Fig. 30.35) that tablets formed from granules prepared by roller compaction exhibit a tensile strength that depends on the compaction force used during the dry granulation process. Thus the evolution of the intergranular tablet microstructure during compression, as well as the evolution of tablet strength, is related to the following two factors:

- the composition of the granules (e.g. choice of filler and binder); and
- the physical properties of the granules (e.g. size, porosity and mechanical strength).

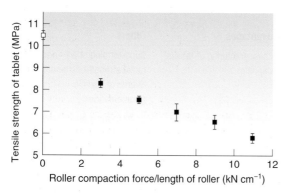

Fig. 30.35 • Tensile strength of tablets formed by compaction of a cellulose powder *(open square)* and of cellulose granules formed by roller compaction at different roller-compaction forces *(closed squares)*.
Adapted from Herting & Kleinebudde, 2008.

During compression of granules, the granules tend to keep their integrity, and the formed tablet can in physical terms be described as granules bonded together. When subjected to a load, tablets formed from granules often fail because of breakage of these bonds. Hence the bonding force of the intergranular bonds and the structure of the intergranular pores will be significant for the tensile strength of the tablets.

In terms of the physical properties of granules, their porosity and compression shear strength are significant properties that influence compactability that can be modulated by the granulation process and by the composition. In general terms, increased porosity and decreased compression shear strength will increase the compactability of the granules. As discussed earlier, pharmaceutical granules seem to fragment to only a limited degree during compression. The importance of these granule properties for compactability has thus been discussed in terms of a sequential relationship between the original physical character of the granules, the degree of deformation they undergo during compression and the area of contact and the geometry of the intergranular pores of the formed tablet. The formation of large intergranular areas of contact and a closed pore system promote a high tablet strength.

Traditionally, the most important means of controlling the compactability of granules has been to add a binder to the powder to be granulated. This is normally done by adding the binder in a dissolved form, thereby creating binder–substrate granules. An increased amount of binder can correspond to an increased compactability, but this is not a general rule. The importance of the presence of a binder for the compactability of such granules can be explained in two ways. First, it has been suggested that intergranular bonds that involve binder-coated granule surfaces can be described as comparatively strong, i.e. difficult to break. Second, binders are often comparatively deformable substances, which can reduce the compression shear strength of the whole granule and thus facilitate the deformation of the granules during compression. An increased degree of granule deformation is sometimes proposed to increase the compactability of the granules. Thus the binder might have a double role in the compactability of granules, i.e. to increase granule deformation and increase bond strength. Except for the presence of a binder in the granules, the combination of fillers in terms of the hardness and dimensions of the particles can affect the compression shear strength

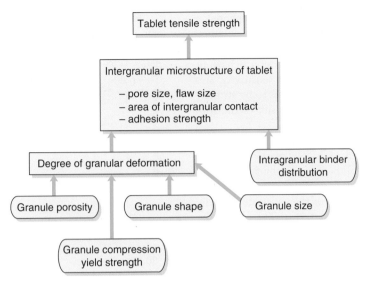

Fig. 30.36 • Overview of physical granule properties of importance for the compactability of granules.

and hence the deformation properties of the granules during compression.

In the preparation of binder–substrate granules, the intention is normally to spread out the binder homogeneously within the granules, i.e. all substrate particles are more or less covered with a layer of binder. However, it is possible that the binder will be concentrated at different regions within the granules, e.g. because of solute migration during drying. The question of the importance of a relatively homogeneous distribution versus a peripheral localization of the binder, i.e. concentration at the granule surface, has been addressed in the literature. It has been argued that a peripheral localization of the binder in the granules before compression should be advantageous, as the binder can thereby be used most effectively for the formation of intergranular bonds. However, the opposite has also been suggested, i.e. a homogeneous binder distribution is advantageous for the compactability of granules. This observation was explained by the assumption that, owing to extensive deformation and some attrition of granules during compression, new extragranular surfaces will be formed originating from the interior of the granule. When the binder is distributed homogeneously, such compression-formed surfaces will show a high capacity for bonding.

Fig. 30.36 gives an overview of the physical granule properties that may affect the compression behaviour and compactability of granules.

Compaction of binary mixtures

Most of the fundamental work on powder compaction has been carried out on one-component powders. It is, however, of obvious interest to derive knowledge that enables the prediction of the tableting behaviour of mixtures of powders from information on the behaviour of the individual components. In this context, powder mixtures of two components, i.e. binary mixtures, have often been the system of choice in pharmaceutical studies. Binary mixtures can be of two types: simple physical mixtures, i.e. nearly randomized mixtures of particles, and interactive (ordered) mixtures. Most of the studies in this context are empirical, although models for the compaction of binary powder mixtures have been derived.

For simple binary mixtures, the importance of the relative proportions of the ingredients has been studied in relation to the compactability of, or compression parameters for, the respective single component. The mixture can show a linear dependence of the properties of the single powders, but deviations from such a simple linear relationship, both positively and negatively, have also been reported. Such nonlinear behaviour has been explained in terms of differences between the components in their mechanical and adhesive properties.

Interactive mixtures, especially their compactability after the admixture of lubricants and dry binders, have been studied. The tablet-strength-reducing effect of a lubricant mixed with solid particles depends on the surface coverage of the lubricant film obtained during mixing, on the compaction properties of the lubricant per se and on the compression behaviour of the substrate particles. Lubricant sensitivity, also referred to as dilution capacity, seems to be strongly related to the fragmentation propensity of the substrate particles, as discussed earlier.

Concerning the tablet-strength-increasing effect of a dry binder mixed with solid particles, similar factors seem to control the compactability of the dry binder mixture as for the lubricant mixture, i.e. the degree of surface coverage of the substrate particle, the binding capacity and deformability of the dry binder and the fragmentation propensity of the substrate particles (Fig. 30.37).

The dilution capacity of interactive mixtures between granules and lubricants or dry binders seems to be related to the degree of deformation the granules undergo during compression, i.e. a high degree of deformation will give a lower sensitivity to a lubricant but also a less positive effect of a dry binder.

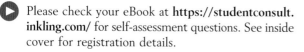 Please check your eBook at **https://studentconsult. inkling.com/** for self-assessment questions. See inside cover for registration details.

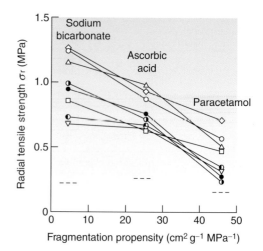

Fig. 30.37 • The tensile strength of tablets formed from three substrate substances of different fragmentation propensities in binary mixtures with some fine-particulate dry binders, i.e. microcrystalline cellulose (circles), methylcellulose (triangles) and polyvinylpyrrolidone (squares and diamonds) of different particle size. The *dashed lines* represent the tensile strength of tablets formed from the single substrate substances. Adapted from Nyström & Glazer, 1985.

References

Adams, M.J., Mullier, M.A., Seville, J.P.K., 1994. Agglomerate strength measurement using a uniaxial confined compression test. Powder Technol. 78, 5–13.

Airth, J.M., Bray, D.F., Radecka, C., 1967. Variability of uniformity of weight test as an indicator of the amount of active ingredient in tablets. J. Pharm. Sci. 56, 233–235.

Alderborn, G., 2003. A novel approach to derive a compression parameter indicating effective particle deformability. Pharm. Dev. Technol. 8, 367–377.

Alderborn, G., Pasanen, K., Nyström, C., 1985. Studies on direct compression of tablets. XI. Characterization of particle fragmentation during compaction by permeametry measurements of tablets. Int. J. Pharm. 23, 79–86.

Al-Nasassrah, M.A., Podczeck, F., Newton, J.M., 1998. The effect of an increase in chain length on the mechanical properties of polyethylene glycols. Eur. J. Pharm. Biopharm. 46, 31–38.

Armstrong, N.A., 1982. Causes of tablet compression problems. Manufacturing Chemist October, 62.

Banakar, U.V., 1992. Pharmaceutical Dissolution Testing. Marcel Dekker, New York.

Davies, P.N., Newton, J.M., 1996. Mechanical strength. In: Alderborn, G., Nyström, C. (Eds.), Pharmaceutical Powder Compaction Technology. Marcel Dekker, New York.

Duberg, M., Nyström, C., 1986. Studies on direct compression of tablets. XVII. Porosity-pressure curves for the characterization of volume reduction mechanisms in powder compression. Powder Technol. 46, 67–75.

Ekenved, G., Elofsson, R., Sölvell, L., 1975. Bioavailability studies on a buffered acetylsalicylic acid preparation. Acta Pharm. Suec. 12, 323–332.

European Pharmacopoeia Commission, 2017. European Pharmacopoeia, ninth ed. Council of Europe, Strasbourg.

Han, L.H., Elliott, J.A., Bentham, A.C., et al., 2008. A modified Drucker-Prager cap model for die compaction simulation of pharmaceutical powders. Int. J. Solids Struct. 45, 3088–3106.

Herting, M.G., Kleinebudde, P., 2008. Studies on the reduction of tensile strength of tablets after roll compaction/dry granulation. Eur. J. Pharm. Biopharm. 70, 372–379.

Hiestand, E.N., 1996. Rationale for and the measurement of tableting indices. In: Alderborn, G., Nyström, C. (Eds.), Pharmaceutical Powder Compaction Technology. Marcel Dekker, New York.

Hölzer, A.H., Sjögren, J., 1981. Evaluation of some lubricants by the comparison of friction coefficients and tablet properties. Acta Pharm. Suec. 18, 139–148.

Kendall, K., 1988. Agglomerate strength. Powder Metallurgy 31, 28–31.

Leuenberger, H., 1982. The compressibility and compactability of powder systems. Int. J. Pharm. 12, 41–55.

Nedermann, R., 1992. Statics and Kinematics of Granular Materials. Cambridge University Press, Cambridge.

Nyström, C., Glazer, M., 1985. Studies on direct compression of tablets. XIII. The effect of some dry binders on the tablet strength of compounds

with different fragmentation propensity. Int. J. Pharm. 23, 255–263.

Persson, A.-S., Frenning, G., 2015. An experimental evaluation of discrete element simulations of confined powder compression using an extended truncated-sphere model. Powder Technol. 284, 257–264.

Ragnarsson, G., 1996. Force-displacement and network measurements. In: Alderborn, G., Nyström, C. (Eds.), Pharmaceutical Powder Compaction Technology. Marcel Dekker, New York.

Roberts, R., Rowe, R., 1985. The effect of punch velocity on the compaction of a variety of materials. J. Pharm. Pharmacol. 37, 377–384.

Sinka, I.C., Cunningham, J.C., Zavaliangos, A., 2003. The effect of wall friction in the compaction of pharmaceutical tablets with curved faces: a validation study of the Drucker–Prager cap model. Powder Technol. 133, 33–43.

Sun, C., Grant, D.J.W., 2001. Influence of elastic deformation of particles on Heckel analysis. Pharm Dev Technol 6, 193–200.

Underwood, T.W., Cadwallader, D.E., 1972. Influence of various starches on dissolution rate of salicylic acid from tablets. J. Pharm. Sci. 61, 239.

Wells, J.I., Rubinstein, M.H., 1976. Importance of generated surface area in tablet performance. Pharm. J. 217, 629–631.

Bibliography

Alderborn, G., Nyström, C. (Eds.), 1996. Pharmaceutical Powder Compaction Technology. Marcel Dekker, New York.

Augsburger, L.L., Hoag, S.W., 2008. Pharmaceutical Dosage Forms: Tablets, vol. 1–3, 3rd ed. Informa Healthcare, New York.

Chulia, D., Deleuil, M., Pourcelot, Y., 1991. Powder Technology and

Pharmaceutical Processes. Elsevier, Amsterdam.

Frenning, G., 2010. Compression mechanics of granule beds: a combined finite/discrete element study. Chem. Eng. Sci. 65, 2464–2471.

Levin, M., 2002. Pharmaceutical Process Scale-up. Marcel Dekker, New York.

Podczeck, F., 1998. Particle-Particle Adhesion in Pharmaceutical Powder Handling. Imperial College Press, London.

Salman, A.D., Hounslow, M.J., Seville, J.P.K., 2007. Granulation. Handbook of Powder Technology, vol. 11. Elsevier, Amsterdam.

Sandell, E., 1993. Industrial Aspects of Pharmaceutics. Swedish Pharmaceutical Press, Stockholm.

31

Modified-release oral drug delivery

Emma L. McConnell   Abdul W. Basit

CHAPTER CONTENTS

KEY POINTS

- Modified-release drug delivery aims to deliver drugs at specific rates, times or physiological sites.
- Modified release can refer to extended, sustained, controlled, delayed or gastro-resistant release.
- Modified release can be employed to achieve once-daily dosing, to reduce side effects, to have long-acting medicines or to target a site in the gastrointestinal tract, e.g. the colon.
- Extended release can be achieved by using matrix polymer tablets, polymer-coated pellets or osmotic-based systems.
- Gastroretention is a type of extended release which aims to keep the drug in the upper gastrointestinal tract (stomach and upper part of the small intestine).
- Gastro-resistant coatings (pH controlled) protect a drug from the acidic environment of stomach and can be used for delivery to the small intestine or colon.
- Drugs can be targeted to the colon by using bacterial enzymes to initiate drug release.

Modified-release oral drug delivery

Administration of medicines by the oral route can seem like the most straightforward option for patients. It is the most commonly used route, with more than 70% of all medicines being delivered in this way. Oral medicines are easy to administer, improve patient adherence and are cheaper than some of the alternatives (e.g. injections). Most medicines administered by the oral route provide what is known as 'immediate-release' drug delivery or 'conventional' drug delivery. A common example is the use of paracetamol (acetaminophen) for a headache; the tablet or capsule disintegrates quickly in the stomach fluids, releasing the drug to provide rapid onset of effect, following dissolution and absorption in the gastrointestinal tract. However, there are some situations in which this rapid onset is not desirable, and a modification of the drug release pattern (or profile) is necessary to slow it down or make the drug's effects last longer (e.g. for 24 h). These more advanced oral drug delivery formulations are often referred to as oral modified-release drug delivery systems.

Modified-release drug delivery refers to the manipulation or modification of drug release from a dosage form (e.g. tablet, pellet, capsule) with the

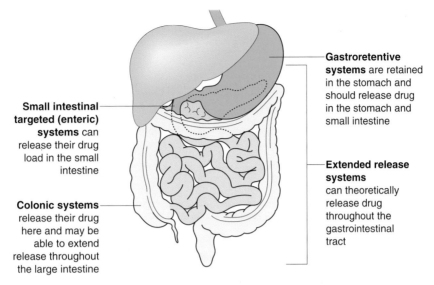

Gastroretentive systems are retained in the stomach and should release drug in the stomach and small intestine

Small intestinal targeted (enteric) systems can release their drug load in the small intestine

Extended release systems can theoretically release drug throughout the gastrointestinal tract

Colonic systems release their drug here and may be able to extend release throughout the large intestine

Fig. 31.1 • The site of release for various oral modified-release drug delivery systems.

specific aim of delivering active pharmaceutical ingredients (API) at:

1. desired rates;

2. predefined time points; or

3. specific sites in the gastrointestinal tract.

Modified-release drug delivery is a broad term which covers a variety of different approaches. These will be dealt with in further detail throughout this chapter. Briefly, the different types are:

- *Delayed-release dosage forms*: These release the drug at a time later than immediately after administration (i.e. there is a lag time between a patient taking a medicine, and the drug being detected in the blood). *Site-specific targeting* is a type of delayed release which aims to target specific regions of the gastrointestinal tract, e.g. the small intestine or colon.
- *Gastro-resistant dosage forms*: These are designed to have a type of delayed release mechanism which enables the drug to be released when a certain environmental pH is met. A common example of this type of dosage form ensures that the drug is not released in the acid of the stomach but in the higher-pH environment of the small intestine. Such products may also be known as enteric dosage forms.
- *Extended-release dosage forms*: These allow a reduction in dosing frequency compared with when the drug is present in an immediate-release dosage form (i.e. the drug plasma levels are sustained for longer periods). These are also known as *prolonged-release* or *sustained-release* dosage forms and are also referred to as *controlled-release* dosage forms. Extended-release systems which are retained in the stomach are known as *gastroretentive systems*.

The site of release of each of these systems is shown in Fig. 31.1.

The concept of modified-release dosage forms has been around since the late 1800s when the idea of protecting the stomach from irritant drugs triggered a search for gastro-resistant materials. As knowledge of the gastrointestinal tract increased (pH, bacteria, transit times), the success and scope of the dosage forms targeted to the gastrointestinal tract improved. In the last decade there has been a huge increase in the number of patents filed for modified-release dosage forms (Fig. 31.2), highlighting the intense interest of the pharmaceutical industry in exploiting the benefits of these technologies to improve product performance.

What modified-release drug delivery means for the patient

Keeping the drug in the therapeutic range. Modified release is often used to improve therapeutic outcomes for a patient relative to an immediate-release medication. For example, a drug which is

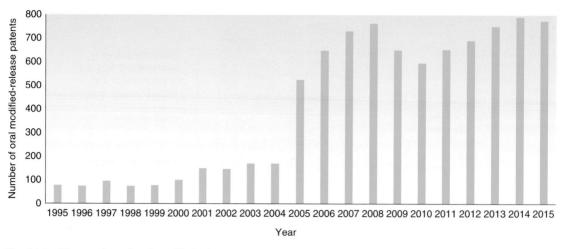

Fig. 31.2 • The number of oral modified-release patents granted from 1995 to 2015.

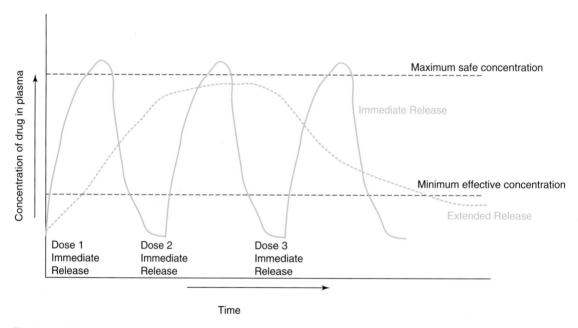

Fig. 31.3 • Theoretical plasma (blood) profiles of immediate-release and extended-release formulations. The immediate-release dosage form requires three doses to keep the drug levels effective over the period shown, and the maximum concentration (C_{max}) exceeds the maximum safe concentration in this example. The extended-release profile *(dotted line)* represents one dose of a sustained-release dosage form over the same period. The latter reduces C_{max} and extends the time that an effective concentration is maintained.

rapidly absorbed and eliminated can have a steep plasma profile in an immediate-release formulation. An extended-release formulation can keep the drug at therapeutic levels for longer (Fig. 31.3). For many chronic illnesses, symptom breakthrough can occur if the blood concentration falls below the minimum effective concentration, e.g. in asthma or depressive illness. This minimum level can also be critical for control of pain; consequently drugs such as opioid analgesics are often given as extended-release preparations.

Maintaining drug levels overnight. It is often not acceptable that patients be required to take medications during the night, with consequent loss of sleep. Overnight management of pain in terminally ill patients can be very important to maintain sleep.

Chronotherapy. Timing the drug release to coincide with when it is required is known as *chronotherapy.* For example, a modified-release dosage form may be tailored to enable drug release to occur in the morning around the time of wakening, when symptoms of, for example, arthritis, asthma or allergies are often at their worst. A clinical study has shown that patients with arthritis had a better reduction in morning joint stiffness when they received modified-release prednisolone rather than a conventional dosage form.

Reducing side effects. Immediate-release formulations can often have a high maximum concentration in the blood (C_{max}). If C_{max} is above the maximum safe concentration of the drug, adverse events may be more likely. Using modified-release formulations to reduce C_{max} can reduce the incidence and severity of the side effects of some drugs. Additionally, some drugs, such as potassium chloride, can be irritating to the gastrointestinal tract if delivered in an immediate-release bolus. A slow, sustained release is required to minimize the build-up of irritant concentrations.

Improving patient adherence. A significant driver to developing a modified-release dosage form comes from trying to achieve once-daily dosing. Once-daily dosing is considered to be more convenient for patients and reduces the risk of missed doses throughout the day.

Treatment of local areas in the gastrointestinal tract. Some conditions, such as inflammatory bowel disease, require topical treatment (e.g. with steroids) at the inflamed intestinal surface. Site-specific drug targeting (e.g. to the colon) can deliver the drug directly to its site of action.

What modified-release drug delivery means for health care professionals and the pharmaceutical industry

Provides physician, pharmacist and patient choice. Health care professionals will be primarily concerned with the therapeutic advantages outlined so far, but increasingly there is concern for personalized medicines and health services. A choice of immediate-release dosage forms and modified-release dosage forms can allow health care professionals to tailor treatment to their patients' needs.

Product life extension. Improving on current marketed formulations by employing modified-release technologies can sometimes enable pharmaceutical companies to extend a product's patent life.

Higher development costs. For pharmaceutical companies the development costs for a modified-release formulation are much higher than those for a conventional immediate-release dosage form.

Cost savings for health care providers. Cost savings may be achieved from better disease management.

Sites of action for modified-release dosage forms and biopharmaceutical considerations

The gastrointestinal tract

Biopharmaceutical factors (i.e. the effect of the gastrointestinal tract physiology and environment on drugs and dosages forms) are considered in more detail in Chapter 19. Here some of the key biological factors that influence the in vivo behaviour of modified-release dosage forms are summarized and discussed. To understand these, the factors limiting drug bioavailability should be noted. The overall process of drug release and absorption will only be as fast as the slowest of many processes. The most common possible rate-limiting steps following oral administration of a solid dosage form are (1) drug release from the dosage form, (2) dissolution of the drug and (3) absorption of drug molecules.

pH

The stomach generally has a low pH and is therefore acidic. Gastro-resistant coated dosage forms are designed to be acid resistant. Some patients can have a higher stomach pH because of age, disease or ethnic origin which can affect dosage form disintegration and dissolution. This can result in premature drug release and/or dose dumping (dose dumping is the release of all of the drug in one bolus).

Gastrointestinal pH generally increases in the small intestine, due to bicarbonate secretion. This is often used as a trigger for small intestinal drug delivery via gastro-resistant coating. The pH gradually increases to a maximum of approximately 7 at the ileocaecal junction. In the colon the pH drops slightly because of the production of short-chain fatty acids by bacteria there, but gradually rises again distally. In some people the pH does not get as high as 7 (and this may change from day to day). Therefore if a polymer is used which dissolves at pH 7 (see later), then there is a good chance that the dosage form using this polymer will not dissolve, leaving a tablet intact and the patient without the dose. This has been observed in the clinic with some patients with ulcerative colitis.

Transit time

The time that a dosage form spends in the stomach, small intestine and colon can be critical for some modified-release systems. In the fasted state, the stomach will empty a nondisintegrating (i.e. nonimmediate release) dosage form within 1–2 hours (via a clearing motility mechanism known as the migrating myoelectric complex). Ingestion of food delays this mechanism, and modified-release dosage forms can sometime be trapped in the stomach as long as food is present.

The small intestine is the site of absorption for most drugs, and although the transit time of a dosage form through this region is normally around 3–4 hours, it can actually be highly variable (from 0.5 h to 9 h has been recorded). A modified-release dosage form which releases the drug very slowly needs to take into account that it may only be at its site of absorption for a few hours.

The colon has a very variable transit time (1 h to 72 h). Often modified-release dosage forms reach the colon (as they may not have disintegrated in the stomach or small intestine). How effective they will be at this point depends on whether or not the drug is absorbed in the colon.

The clinical implications of this are seen in a study in which an OROS (osmotic extended-release system) tablet was administered (see later for more details on this type of device). In one instance, it travelled slowly through the intestine and the patient received a suitable dose (i.e. blood levels were adequate and maintained). In another instance, it travelled through the intestine in less than 10 hours, and very little drug was available to be absorbed by the patient, leaving the patient with subtherapeutic blood drug levels (Fig. 31.4).

Fluid

Fluid levels can be highly variable in the stomach, small intestine and colon. In the stomach there may be approximately 100 mL of total fluid. In

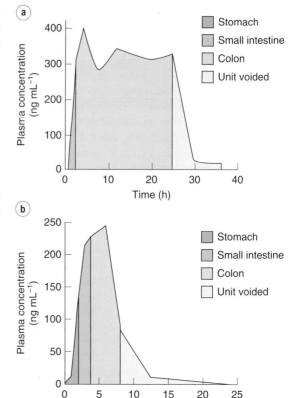

Fig. 31.4 • Plasma concentration–time profiles for oxprenolol delivered from an OROS device in an individual with a long **(a)** and a short **(b)** colon transit time. Adapted from Washington et al., 2001, with permission.

the small intestine there is approximately 50 mL to 100 mL of *free* fluid (i.e. that not bound up with digested material, and thus free to dissolve drugs or dosage forms). The colonic contents can be very viscous, with only approximately 10 mL of free fluid actually available. All modified-release dosage forms require the presence of fluid in order for drug release to occur. Less free liquid is available as the modified-release dosage form travels down the gut.

Fluid composition (beyond pH) is also important. The presence of ions, fats, enzymes and salts can all affect the mechanisms of drug release from modified-release dosage forms. For example, fats may slow down release from swelling matrix systems, meaning that the required blood levels may not be achieved as quickly in their presence. Sugars can sometimes disrupt controlled-release gels.

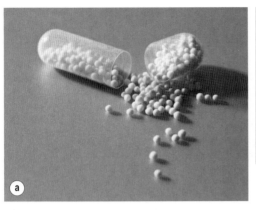
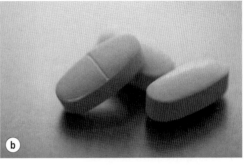

Fig. 31.5 • The use of multiple-unit pellets in a capsule **(a)** or a single-unit tablet **(b)** for modified-release drug delivery.

Designing a modified-release formulation: factors to consider

There are several decisions that need to be taken when designing a modified-release formulation. Assuming it has been established that a drug is a suitable candidate for modified-release drug delivery, the points discussed in the following sections should be considered.

Single-unit dosage form or multiple-unit dosage form

A modified-release formulation can be designed as a single entity (usually a tablet) (Fig. 31.5b). Single-unit tablets are sometimes known as *monolithic* dosage forms. A single-unit dosage form is advantageous from a manufacturing standpoint, as it can often be manufactured using conventional techniques, such as compaction and film coating. There may be some biopharmaceutical disadvantages to tablet formulations however. For example, as they do not disintegrate in the stomach, the dosage form could become trapped in the stomach for a long time (with food). For drugs targeted to the small or large intestine, this could prevent them reaching their site of action. Multiple-unit systems (e.g. pellets or granules filled into a hard capsule shell; Fig. 31.5a) may have more reproducible gastric emptying and have a reduced risk of dose dumping. However, these can be more difficult to manufacture (requiring extrusion–spheronization or drug loading onto seed cores) and to scale up.

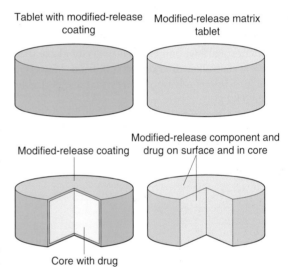

Fig. 31.6 • Coated and matrix tablets for modified release.

Matrix formulation or coated formulation

The release of an active pharmaceutical ingredient can be modified by two main methods (Fig. 31.6). Firstly, the release-modifying ingredients can be incorporated throughout the matrix of the dosage form, wherein the whole dosage form encompasses the modified-release element. The second option is the application of a modified-release coating to a dosage form, wherein the drug is usually contained in the core and is released through, or via the dissolution of, the modified-release coat. There are slight deviations from these two techniques however, as will be seen in later sections (e.g. with osmotic systems).

Type of release rate

Two basic mechanisms can control the rate and extent of drug release. These are (1) dissolution of the active drug component and (2) diffusion of dissolved species. Four processes operate in a modified-release dosage form to facilitate this:

1. Hydration of the device (either swelling or dissolution of some component of the modified-release dosage form).
2. Diffusion of water into the device.
3. Dissolution of the drug.
4. Diffusion of the dissolved drug out of the device. However, drug that is in contact with the surface of the dosage form does not need to diffuse and is often quickly dissolved in a 'burst release'.

Given the multistep process of drug release from modified-release dosage forms, and the complex gastrointestinal environment, it is understandable that precisely controlling drug release is difficult. However, there are various release patterns that are desirable (Table 31.1).

There are various strategies which have been adopted in an attempt to control and manipulate drug release patterns. These are summarized in Table 31.2 and are discussed in more detail in the following sections.

Extended release

Before an extended-release dosage form is developed, the suitability of the drug in question should be considered. The solubility of a drug in aqueous media, and its ability to permeate the intestine, are key considerations when one is assessing whether a drug may be suitable for modified release. There are three potential rate-limiting steps in the bioavailability of a drug from a dosage form:

1. release from the dosage form;
2. dissolution of the drug; and
3. absorption through the gastrointestinal mucosa.

Drugs are categorized according to steps 2 and 3. The Biopharmaceutics Classification System of drugs (see Chapter 21 for details) classifies drugs into four categories:

- type I: high solubility, high permeability;
- type II: low solubility, high permeability;
- type III: high solubility, low permeability; and
- type IV: low solubility, low permeability.

High-solubility and high-permeability drugs (class I) are most suitable for extended-release delivery (ideally by passive diffusion). These properties mean that drug release from dosage forms can be the rate-limiting step in the process, and this can then be tailored by the dosage form design. For drugs with low solubility (< 1 mg/mL), the low rate of dissolution can already give some inherent sustained-release behaviour of the pure drug molecule, and dissolution of drug particles in the gut can be the rate-limiting step. After drug release and dissolution have occurred, absorption must occur. Drugs with low permeability ($< 0.5 \times 10^{-6}$ mm s^{-1} through CaCo-2 tissue culture; see Chapter 21) are unlikely to be suitable for extended-release preparations. This is because they are already rate limited in their absorption. Class IV drugs have low solubility and low permeability, and these are the most challenging to formulate as modified-release products.

Other considerations as to the suitability of a drug for extended release include how quickly a drug is eliminated once it is in the bloodstream. The most suitable drugs may have relatively short half-lives ($t_{1/2}$ = 4 h to 6 h). Drugs with long half-lives may achieve pseudo-sustained-release blood levels despite being formulated as immediate-release forms, whereas for drugs with shorter half-lives, very high doses may be needed to maintain blood levels.

Dose is another factor to consider. To limit the size of the dosage form, the potency of the drug in the modified-release form can be critical. Up to 1000 mg potency tablets are available in extended-release formulations, but this is only achieved by using very large tablets, which may not always be acceptable for some patient populations (especially paediatric or geriatric patients; see Chapter 45).

Hydrophilic matrix systems

Hydrophilic matrix systems can also be referred to as swellable soluble matrices. They are used for extended (sustained) release. The drug is mixed with a water-swellable, hydrophilic polymer (usually along with some other excipient materials) and compressed into a tablet. The polymer is usually in the form of a powder or granule, and tablets will be manufactured by direct compression or roller compaction (dry granulation processes). The resulting tablet has drug material interspersed between polymer particles. On exposure to fluid, the polymer material in the tablet starts to swell, producing a gel matrix. The gel can then allow drug release by dissolution of the gel and

Table 31.1 Release patterns for modified release

Release patterns for modified release include:

(a) constant release rates (Fig. 31.7a)   (c) delayed release (Fig. 31.7c) and
(b) declining drug release profile (Fig. 31.7b)   (d) bimodal release (Fig. 31.7d).

Drug release profiles show how the drug is released in a simple system, e.g. into dissolution media, and the figures (left graphs) show a cumulative release over time (ideally 100% of drug should be released) and are influenced only by drug release from the dosage form. Drug in blood profiles (right graphs) are influenced by drug release, but also by absorption, distribution, metabolism and excretion and so drug levels in the blood rise and fall according to all these parameters combined. Thus drugs with the same release profile may have different blood drug profiles. An example blood drug profile for each is shown.

(a) Constant release

Drug release profile   **Drug in blood profile**

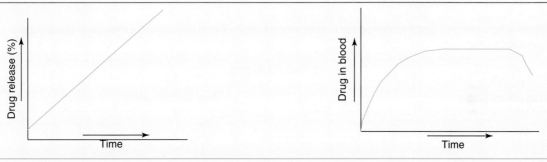

To maintain constant drug blood concentrations a constant release rate is preferred. These follow zero-order kinetics. In the human body, these drug levels take time to build up in the blood to a stable level.

(b) Declining release

Drug release profile   **Drug in blood profile**

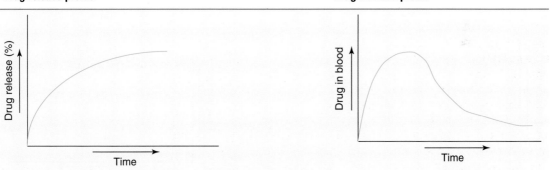

Drug release from these types of systems is often a function of the square root of time or follows first-order kinetics. They do not maintain a constant blood drug concentration but can provide a sustained release.

Continued

Table 31.1 Release patterns for modified release—cont'd

(c) Delayed release

Drug release profile   **Drug in blood profile**

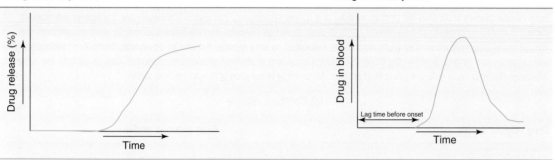

This could be considered a type of bimodal release in which zero or negligible drug is released until a desired time or site in the gastrointestinal tract.

(d) Bimodal release

Drug release profile   **Drug in blood profile**

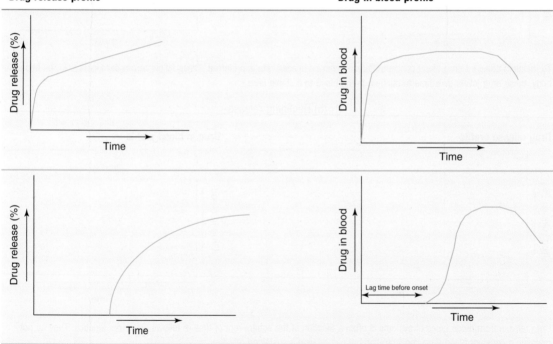

Extended release dosage forms often aim to achieve an initial primer dose of drug to achieve prompt therapeutic response. This primer dose could be an immediate-release layer or coating. This can then be followed by a slow release of the remaining drug (the maintenance dose) which should sustain the blood levels in the therapeutic range. First-order release kinetics can be used to achieve the primer dose in a rapid fashion. Dose maintenance will follow zero-order kinetics.
Another example of bimodal release is delayed release followed by extended release.

Table 31.2 The different types of modified-release dosage form used commercially and being investigated for oral drug delivery

Type of dosage form	Extended release					Delayed release	
	Hydrophilic matrix	Insoluble polymer matrix	Membrane-controlled extended release	Osmotic pump system	Gastroretentive system	pH-controlled delayed release	Bacterially triggered delayed release
Single or multiple units?	Monolithic tablet	Monolithic tablet	Monolithic coated tablet/coated pellet	Single unit	Monolithic tablet/coated pellet	Monolithic coated tablet or coated pellet	Monolithic coated tablet or coated pellet
Type of drug release	Zero order, first order, bimodal	First order	First order	Zero order, first order	First order	Delayed, then first order	Delayed, then first order
Key features	Slow/sustained release of drug is achieved by diffusion through a swollen polymer gel	Slow/sustained release of drug is achieved by diffusion through a nondissolving sponge-like polymer scaffold	Slow/sustained release of drug is achieved by diffusion through a polymer coat (modified by film thickness and/or pore formers)	Water diffusion through a semipermeable coat increases osmotic pressure in the device, forcing drug out through a hole	Various: sticking to stomach wall (mucoadhesion), avoiding gastric emptying by large size or floating on stomach contents	Coating dissolves on exposure to small intestinal or colonic environment by virtue of sensitivity to pH	Coating digested on exposure to colonic environment by virtue of sensitivity to digestion by colonic bacteria
Key ingredients	Swelling polymers (e.g. hydroxypropyl cellulose, polyethylene oxide)	Insoluble polymers (e.g. ethylcellulose)	Water-insoluble polymers (e.g. ethylcellulose, acrylic copolymers), pore formers (e.g. polyethylene glycol)	Osmotically active filler (e.g. lactose–fructose), semipermeable membrane (e.g. cellulose acetate)	Mucoadhesive polymers (e.g. chitosan), swelling polymers, gas-generating bicarbonates)	pH-responsive polymers (acrylic copolymers, phthalate polymers)	Polysaccharides which are digested only by colonic bacteria (e.g. some starches, pectin)
Eroding?	Yes	No	No	No	Yes, but slowly	Yes	Yes
Pharmaceutical technology	Tableting	Tableting	Tableting/pelletization and coating	Tableting, coating and laser drilling	Tableting/pelletization	Tableting/pelletization and coating	Tableting/pelletization and coating
Status	Commercial products	Commercial products	Commercial products	Commercial products	Some commercial products but mainly experimental/clinical trial stages	Commercial products	Experimental/clinical trials
Use	Drugs requiring extended-release action to achieve once-daily dosing, reduced toxicity, etc.				Drugs which have poor colonic absorption, local delivery to the stomach	Acid-sensitive drugs, stomach irritants, colonic delivery, small intestinal delivery	Colonic delivery

the drug trapped within it or erosion of the gel and release and dissolution of drug particles trapped within it.

The rate at which water can diffuse through the tablet – and later through the hydrated gel – affects the drug release rate. The rate of hydration is affected by the structure of the gel. Hydrophilic gels can be regarded as a network of interlinked/interspersed polymer stands. In the interstitial spaces between the strands is a continuous phase through which water and drug may diffuse. The interstices connect together to form a tortuous pathway through the gel. The tortuosity of this pathway is therefore critical for drug release. This can be affected by using polymers of different molecular weights or by using cross-linked gels, and so the release rate can be modified by these factors. Increasing the polymer concentration can also reduce the number of 'pathways', and slows down drug release.

Polymers, such as hydroxypropyl methylcellulose or polyethylene oxide (which are commonly used for modified-release matrix systems), do not actually form true gels and are better described as forming very viscous solutions. Their structure is more dynamic than that of true gels (e.g. cross-linked alginic acid) as the chains can move relative to one another, so the interstitial continuum is not fixed. The mechanism

of drug release is depicted in Fig. 31.7. Diffusion-based release mechanisms usually follow zero-order or first-order kinetics (assuming sink conditions in the gastrointestinal tract and sufficient fluid), but additional erosion of the matrix due to gastrointestinal motility and hydrodynamics can complicate the true in vivo release rate. Often polymer type and concentration are used to control drug release, which can be tailored (faster and slower) as required (Fig. 31.8).

Hydrophilic matrix systems would generally be selected where a sustained drug release is required.

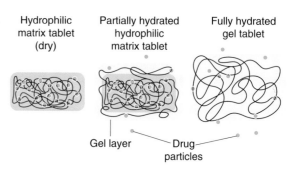

Hydrophilic matrix tablet (dry)   Partially hydrated hydrophilic matrix tablet   Fully hydrated gel tablet

Gel layer   Drug particles

Fig. 31.7 • Process of drug release from a hydrophilic matrix. Water has to penetrate the dry matrix tablet. As the tablet becomes hydrated, drug can diffuse out.

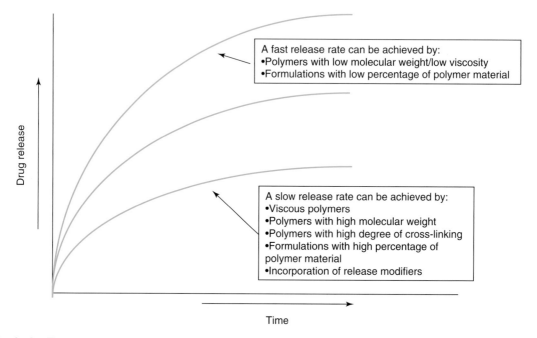

A fast release rate can be achieved by:
•Polymers with low molecular weight/low viscosity
•Formulations with low percentage of polymer material

A slow release rate can be achieved by:
•Viscous polymers
•Polymers with high molecular weight
•Polymers with high degree of cross-linking
•Formulations with high percentage of polymer material
•Incorporation of release modifiers

Drug release

Time

Fig. 31.8 • Theoretical release profiles for hydrophilic matrix tablets for extended release (fast, medium and slow profiles).

They have the advantage of using standard safe excipients, use standard technologies, are well established and can attain high drug loads. They do have the risk of 'food effects', whereby different blood profiles are attained in the fed and fasted states. This often results from the challenge of the gastrointestinal environment, which is variable with respect to fluid, food and transit. These can be challenging factors for a hydrophilic matrix tablet.

Insoluble polymer matrix

These are far less commonly used than their water-soluble/water-swellable counterparts. They consist of an inert matrix system in which the drug is embedded in an inert polymer. Their structure has been likened to that of a sponge. If drug molecules were interspersed throughout a sponge and water were applied, drug could leach out via the water-filled channels (Fig. 31.9). In contrast to hydrophilic matrices, these systems stay intact throughout the gastrointestinal tract.

The rate of drug release from insoluble polymer matrices is controlled by the pore size and number of pores, and the tortuosity of the matrix. Pore-forming agents can be added to increase tortuosity and facilitate drug release. The release mechanism will also depend greatly on how the drug is dispersed within the system (dissolved, molecularly dissolved, or dispersed). The drug release does not follow zero-order kinetics; drug release decreases with time owing to the increasing distance drug molecules have to travel to reach the surface of the device.

Like their hydrophilic counterparts, insoluble matrices are a relatively simple concept which uses standard tableting technology. However, they can also suffer from some food effects, in particular related to rapid transit through the small intestine, or entrapment in the stomach in the fed state.

Membrane-controlled systems

Membrane-controlled delivery systems differ from the matrix formulations in that the rate-controlling part of the system is a membrane through which the drug must diffuse, rather than diffusing through the whole matrix. Generally, drug is concentrated in the core, and must traverse a polymeric membrane or film, which slows down the release rate. Important criteria for such a dosage form are that the drug should not diffuse in the solid state. On exposure to an aqueous environment, water should be able to diffuse into the system and form a continuous phase through which drug diffusion and release can occur (Fig. 31.10). Drug release through a membrane is controlled by the thickness and the porosity of the membrane, as well as the solubility of the drug in the gastrointestinal fluids.

The biopharmaceutical considerations of transit and fluid are much the same as for monolithic matrix tablets. However, membrane-controlled drug delivery systems may be more likely to be in the form of pellets than monolithic systems. Pellets and tablets have different biopharmaceutical considerations. For example, tablets are more likely to become trapped in the stomach if administered with food (especially with a high-calorie meal). Pellets can get trapped too, but there is an increased chance of fortuitous emptying through the pyloric sphincter. Pellets will tend to distribute themselves through the small intestine. They also have less risk of dose dumping; if a tablet coating fails, then the whole dose can be dumped; with a pellet formulation, the disruption

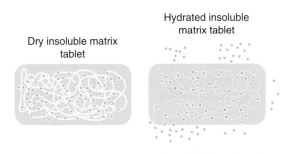

Fig. 31.9 • A dry insoluble matrix tablet has channels *(white)* interspersed within the polymer. These channels hydrate and the drug can diffuse out.

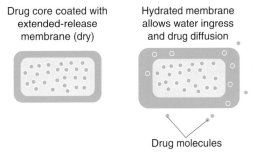

Drug molecules

Fig. 31.10 • Drug release mechanism for a dosage form coated with a modified-release membrane.

of one pellet coating may release only a small fraction of the total drug dose.

Osmotic systems

Osmotic pump systems are another form of membrane-controlled release drug delivery system but work in a different way to that described previously. A drug is included in a tablet core which is water soluble, and which will dissolve (or suspend) the drug in the presence of water. The tablet core is coated with a semipermeable membrane which will allow water to pass into the core. As the core components dissolve, a hydrostatic pressure builds up and forces (pumps) drug solution (or suspension) through a hole drilled in the coating (Fig. 31.11). The rate at which water is able to pass through the membrane and how quickly the drug solution (or suspension) can pass out of the hole govern the rate of drug release. The orifice needs to be small enough to prevent diffusion but large enough to minimize hydrostatic pressure (600 µm to 1 mm diameter is normal). The orifice can be made by laser drilling, indentations in the tablet (not fully covered by coating) or the use of leachable substances (pore formers).

The rate at which the drug solution/suspension is forced out can be modified by changes in the viscosity of the solution formed inside the system. The essential difference between an osmotic pump system and a 'classic' membrane-controlled system is that for the osmotic pump, only one diffusion process is required (in this case 'water in').

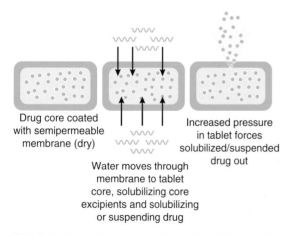

Drug core coated with semipermeable membrane (dry)

Water moves through membrane to tablet core, solubilizing core excipients and solubilizing or suspending drug

Increased pressure in tablet forces solubilized/suspended drug out

Fig. 31.11 • Release mechanisms for an osmotic pump delivery system.

Osmotic pump systems require exposure to sufficient fluid in order to build up an internal osmotic pressure. This will depend on fluid levels in the gut. Like any other nondisintegrating dosage form, they are reliant on being at the site of drug absorption for sufficient time to release their drug load. For example, if the osmotic system was designed to have drug release over 12 hours, it needs to be in the stomach and intestine for this amount of time, otherwise drug release will be incomplete.

Gastroretention

Gastroretention is the mechanism by which a dosage form is retained in the stomach, generally for the purposes of improving drug delivery. It has been proposed as a mechanism by which drug absorption in the upper gastrointestinal tract can be maximized. Gastroretentive approaches to drug delivery aim to overcome the physiological mechanisms in the stomach which would normally enable gastric emptying, so that a modified-release dosage form is retained for longer in the stomach. Drugs which may benefit from gastroretention include those for local action in the stomach (e.g. to treat *Helicobacter pylori* infection), drugs which have a narrow absorption window in the small intestine and drugs which are degraded in the colon.

Several approaches have been investigated, but none deliver true gastroretention. The approaches which have been used to try to achieve gastroretention are very varied and are summarized in Table 31.3. Success with gastroretention has been limited, mainly due to the challenge presented by the stomach and gastric emptying, which is incredibly difficult to overcome by formulation methods alone.

Delayed release

Gastro-resistant coatings

The concept here is similar to that of membrane-controlled extended release, except that the membrane is designed to disintegrate or dissolve at a predetermined point. The most common trigger for delayed-release coatings is pH. Gastro-resistant coatings are polymer coatings which are insoluble at low pH but are soluble at higher pH (e.g. somewhere between pH 5 and pH 7 depending on the polymer). The drug release rate is controlled by its exposure to the correct pH (Fig. 31.12). Generally, this will require sufficient time to allow full coat dissolution.

Table 31.3 Overview of some of the popular research areas for achieving gastroretention (including some formulation and biopharmaceutical considerations)

Approach to achieve gastroretention	Concept	Formulation considerations	Biopharmaceutical comments
Mucoadhesion Tablet sticks to stomach wall Stomach contents	Mucoadhesive polymers could theoretically cause a dosage form to adhere to the stomach mucosa to retain it in the stomach	Chitosan, Carbopol and polycarbophil are mucoadhesive polymers which have been investigated (with limited success)	Although animal studies suggest this to be a sound concept, it has not been realized in humans, probably because of the fast mucus turnover and high motility of the stomach
Floating Tablet floats on stomach contents Pylorus	Dosage form should float on the stomach contents, thus avoiding gastric emptying	Gas-generating agents, such as bicarbonate, or lipids can be used	Requires food to be present in the stomach. Has not shown clinical success for drug delivery but agents such as Gaviscon® which form a raft on stomach contents have been used for treatment of heartburn and indigestion
Size-increasing systems Tablet expands, making it difficult to pass through pylorus. 	A dosage form that swells and increases in size as soon as it reaches the stomach to avoid being able to pass through the pyloric sphincter	Swellable polymers such as hydroxypropyl methylcellulose, polyethylene oxide and xanthan gum have been investigated	Some marketed products use this approach but need to be given in the fed state and gastric emptying is delayed primarily by the effect of food on the stomach. The resting size of the pylorus (open) is approximately 10 mm to 11 mm but it can stretch further than this

This approach is most commonly used for releasing drug in the small intestine. A similar concept can be used for the colon. The highest pH in the gastrointestinal tract is generally at the ileocaecal junction, just before the colon. Here the pH can be around 7. Using polymers which dissolve at pH 7 should theoretically dissolve a dosage form here and release drug as the device moves into the colon. This approach has been used to deliver anti-inflammatory medications, including budesonide, beclometasone and mesalazine to treat ulcerative colitis in the large intestine.

Gastro-resistant coating of formulations has two functions: (1) to protect the stomach from the drug and (2) to protect acid-sensitive drugs from the stomach environment. They can be used to eliminate

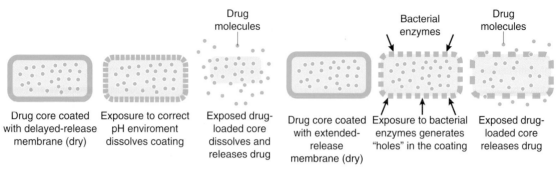

Fig. 31.12 • Drug release mechanism for a dosage form with a gastro-resistant coating.

Fig. 31.13 • Release mechanisms for bacterially triggered colonic targeting.

drug release in the stomach in order to target the small intestine or colon. Although the concept of gastro-resistant coating has been used for many years, and there are many products on the market, there are some shortcomings based on the fact that gastrointestinal pH is not always predictable and reproducible in vivo. For instance, in patients with a higher than normal stomach pH (achlorhydria), there is a risk of premature drug release.

Colonic drug delivery

Colonic drug delivery can be achieved by the utilization of pH-responsive polymers (e.g. Eudragit S, which dissolves at around pH 7) to target the colon. Targeting the colon is difficult as a tablet or pellet may be in the region of highest pH (at the ileocaecal junction) for only a short time, and the target pH (often pH 7) may not be reached. This can lead to dosage form failure (i.e. it does not disintegrate and is passed intact in the stools, consequently not releasing the drug).

An alternative approach is the use of the gut bacteria as a trigger for drug release. A coating is prepared from a material which is insoluble in the gastrointestinal fluids (e.g. ethylcellulose), but it will also contain a component that can be digested only by colonic bacteria (not by pancreatic enzymes). An example of a material that can be used is the polysaccharide known as 'resistant starch'. This type of starch can only be broken down by bacterial enzymes in the colon. When the dosage form reaches the colon, the starch component of the coat is digested and dissolves, leaving pores through which drug can be released (Fig. 31.13).

Bacterially triggered systems tend to be more reproducible in terms of consistent drug release than pH-responsive systems. However, there may be some

patient populations in which gastrointestinal microorganism (microbiota) levels are affected by disease, and the effect on such modified-release drug delivery systems is not fully known. Being a relatively recent development, this technology has also not advanced as far clinically as pH-responsive colonic drug delivery, and is still in the experimental and clinical testing stages. Other new systems have also been proposed which combine Eudragit S as the polymer and resistant starch to give a dual-release mechanism (i.e. release is triggered by both the pH change and the bacteria). This is said to ensure rapid and consistent drug release.

3D printing

Three-dimensional (3D) printing, or additive manufacturing, is a new technique that creates solid objects layer-by-layer using computer-aided design. 3D printing is now used as a production tool or for rapid prototyping in many diverse fields, including the aerospace industry, architecture, nanosystems, fashion and biomedical research. In the pharmaceutical field, this represents a shift in medicine design and manufacture away from the established industrial production of tablets/capsules of limited dose range towards in situ fabrication of unit dosage forms with doses and drug combinations tailored to the patient. In 2015, the first 3D printed formulation (Spritam®), based on powder bed liquid 3D printing technology (ZipDose®), was approved by the US Food and Drug Administration (FDA). Spritam® (levetiracetam) is a fast-dissolving tablet formulation indicated for the treatment of epileptic seizures. 3D printing, whilst a new technology, has been used to fabricate complex tablet geometries, not otherwise possible using conventional technology, and to create modified-release formulations with extended-release characteristics (Goyanes et al., 2015a) and delayed-release characteristics (Goyanes et al., 2015b).

Conclusions

Modified-release drug delivery can be broken down into two main categories: delayed release and extended release. Within these, there are different strategies and formulation techniques which can be employed to meet the desired treatment criteria. Furthermore, the release mechanisms can be combined to give bimodal release (e.g. delayed and sustained release). Choosing which approach is most suitable will depend on the drug molecule, the type of release that is required and the condition the drug is treating. There is no 'one size fits all' solution for tailoring drug release, and significant resources have to be employed to develop these formulations successfully. Continued research into this area and understanding of the biopharmaceutical implications are necessary to develop quality products to improve patient treatment.

Please check your eBook at **https://studentconsult. inkling.com/** for self-assessment questions. See inside cover for registration details.

References

Goyanes, A., Wang, J., Buanz, A., et al., 2015a. 3D printing of medicines: engineering novel oral devices with unique design and drug release characteristics. Mol. Pharm. 12, 4077–4084.

Goyanes, A., Chang, H., Sedough, D., et al., 2015b. Fabrication of controlled-release budesonide tablets via desktop (FDM) 3D printing. Int. J. Pharm. 496, 414–420.

Washington, N., Washington, C., Wilson, C.G., 2001. Drug delivery to the large intestine and rectum. In: Physiological Pharmaceutics: Barriers to Drug Absorption, second ed. CRC Press, Boca Raton.

Bibliography

Davis, S.S., 2005. Formulation strategies for absorption windows. Drug Discov. Today 10, 249–257.

Varum, F.J.O., Merchant, H.A., Basit, A.W., 2010. Modified-release formulations in motion: the relationship between gastrointestinal transit and drug absorption. Int. J. Pharm. 395, 26–36.

Varum, F.J., Hatton, G.B., Basit, A.W., 2013. Food, physiology and drug delivery. Int. J. Pharm. 457, 446–460.

Coating of tablets and multiparticulates

Stuart C. Porter

CHAPTER CONTENTS

KEY POINTS

- Coating, especially film coating, of pharmaceutical tablets and multiparticulates is commonplace.
- Coatings are applied for many reasons, e.g. improving product appearance, making swallowing easier and modifying drug release.
- Pan-coating techniques are usually used for coating tablets, while fluid-bed processes are often preferred for coating multiparticulates.
- Sugar coating is a multistep, time-consuming process, while film coating is generally a faster, single-step process.
- As film coating has become the dominant process used in the global pharmaceutical industry today, the once common use of organic solvents (with their many associated hazards) has been replaced with the preferred use of aqueous coating formulations.
- All coating processes can be considered stressful (in the mechanical sense), thus placing stringent demands on the robustness of

the core (the tablets or multiparticulates being coated) to help minimize defects.

Introduction

Coatings may be applied to a wide range of oral solid dosage forms, including tablets, capsules, multiparticulates and drug crystals. While tablets represent the class of dosage form that is most commonly coated, coated multiparticulates are also popular.

Definition of coating

Coating is a process by which an essentially dry, outer layer of coating material is applied to the surface of a dosage form in order to confer specific benefits that broadly range from facilitating product identification to modifying drug release from the dosage form.

Reasons for coating

The reasons for coating pharmaceutical oral solid dosage forms are quite varied. The more common reasons include (no order of importance implied):

1. Providing a means of protecting the drug substance (active pharmaceutical ingredient) from the environment, particularly light and moisture, and thus potentially improving product stability.
2. Masking the taste of drug substances that may be bitter or otherwise unpleasant.
3. Improving the ease of swallowing large dosage forms, especially tablets. Tablets that are coated are considered by patients to be somewhat easier to swallow than uncoated tablets.
4. Masking any batch differences in the appearance of raw materials and hence allaying patient concern over products that would otherwise appear different each time a prescription is dispensed or product purchased (in the case of over-the-counter products).
5. Providing a means of improving product appearance and aiding in brand identification.
6. Facilitating the rapid identification of a product by the manufacturer, the dispensing pharmacist and the patient. In this case the coatings would almost certainly be coloured. It is important here to emphasize that efficient labelling and the associated procedures are the only sure way

of identifying a product. However, product colour is a useful secondary check.

7. Enabling the coated product (especially tablets) to be more easily handled on high-speed automatic filling and packaging equipment. In this respect the coating often improves product flow, increases the mechanical strength of the product and reduces the risk of cross-contamination by minimizing 'dusting' problems.
8. Imparting modified-release characteristics that allow the drug to be delivered in a more effective manner.

Types of coating processes

Three main types of process are used in the pharmaceutical industry today:

- film coating;
- sugar coating; and
- compression coating.

Film coating is the most popular technique, and virtually all new coated products introduced to the market are film coated. Film coating involves the deposition, usually by the spraying of a liquid coating system, of a thin film of a polymer-based formulation onto the surface of a tablet, capsule or multiparticulate core.

Sugar coating is a more traditional process closely resembling that used for coating confectionery products. It has been used in the pharmaceutical industry since the late 19th century. It involves the successive application of sucrose-based coating formulations, usually to tablet cores, in suitable coating equipment. The water evaporates from the syrup, leaving a thick sugar layer around each tablet. Sugar coats are often shiny and highly coloured.

Compression coating, although traditionally a less popular process, has gained increased interest in recent years as a means of creating specialized modified-release products. It involves the compaction of granular material around a preformed tablet core using specially designed tableting equipment. Compression coating is essentially a dry process.

Each of these processes will now be considered in turn and an overview of relevant coating processes and materials will be given.

Table 32.1 Major differences between sugar coating and film coating

Features	Sugar coating	Film coating
Tablets		
Appearance	Rounded with high degree of polish	Retains contour of original core Usually not as shiny as sugar coat types
Weight increase due to coating materials	30% to 50%	2% to 3%
Logo or 'break lines'	Not possible	Possible
Other solid dosage forms	Coating possible but little industrial importance	Coating of multiparticulates very important in modified-release forms
Process		
Stages	Multistage process	Usually single stage
Typical batch coating time	8 h, but easily longer	1.5 h to 2 h
Functional coatings	Not usually possible apart from gastro-resistant (enteric) coating	Easily adaptable for controlled release

Film coating

Film coating is the more contemporary and thus commonly used process for coating oral solid dosage forms. As described already, it involves the application of a thin film to the surface of a tablet, capsule or multiparticulate core. Currently all newly launched coated products are film coated rather than sugar coated, often for many of the reasons given in Table 32.1.

Types of film coatings

Film coatings may be classified in a number of ways but it is common practice to do so in terms of the intended effect of the applied coating on drug release characteristics. Hence film coatings may be designated as either:

- *Immediate-release film coatings*, also known as 'nonfunctional' coatings. This is something of a misnomer as this terminology refers to the fact that the coating has no measurable effect on biopharmaceutical properties; however, all coatings, as explained earlier, have many other properties and functions.
- *Modified-release film coatings*, also known as 'functional' coatings. These may be further categorized as either delayed-release (e.g. gastro-resistant) or extended-release coatings. Note that the newer term 'gastro-resistant'

coating is replacing the older term 'enteric' coating in pharmacopoeias.

Immediate-release coatings are usually readily soluble in water, while gastro-resistant coatings are only soluble in water at pH values in excess of 5–6 and are intended to either protect the drug while the dosage form is in the stomach (in the case of acid-labile drugs) or prevent release of the drug in the stomach (in the case of drugs that are gastric irritants). More recently, gastro-resistant coatings have been employed as an integral part of colonic drug delivery systems (Alvarez-Fuentes et al., 2004). For the most part, extended-release coatings are insoluble in water. They are designed to ensure that the drug is released in a consistent manner over a relatively long period of time (typically 6 h to 12 h) and thus reduce the number of doses that a patient needs to take in each 24-hour period. Additionally, extended-release film coatings are used to modify drug release in such a way that desired therapeutic benefits can more easily be achieved and thus drug efficacy can be improved.

Description of the film-coating process

Film coating involves the application of liquid, polymer-based formulations to the surface of the tablets (for the sake of brevity, the term 'tablet' will be used here to represent any form of dosage unit that is to be coated). It is possible to use conventional panning equipment but more usually specialized equipment is employed to take advantage of the fast coating times and high degree of automation possible.

The coating liquid (solution or suspension) contains a polymer in a suitable liquid medium, together with other ingredients such as pigments and plasticizers. This solution is sprayed onto a rotating, or fluidized, mass of tablets. The drying conditions employed in the process result in the removal of the solvent, leaving a thin deposit of coating material around each tablet core.

Process equipment

The vast majority of film-coated tablets are produced by a process which involves the atomization (spraying) of the coating solution or suspension onto the surface of tablets.

Modern pan-coating equipment is of the side-vented type (as shown in Fig. 32.1) and some typical examples include:

- Accela-Cota – Thomas Engineering (USA);
- Premier – Bosch-Manesty (UK);
- Hi-Coater – Freund-Vector (Japan and USA);
- Driacoater – Driam Metallprodukt (Germany);
- HTF/150 – GS (Italy);
- IDA – Dumoulin (France);
- BCF – Bohle (Germany); and
- FastCoat – O'Hara (Canada).

Manufacturers of units that operate on a fluidized-bed principle include:

- GEA (Aeromatic-Fielder) (Switzerland, USA and UK)
- Glatt (Switzerland, Germany and USA)
- Vector-Freund (Japan and USA)
- Innojet (Germany).

Depending on the particular film-coating application involved, fluidized-bed equipment may be further divided into one of the three operating principles shown in Fig. 32.2.

The coating formulation is invariably added as a solution or suspension via a spray gun. The design and operation of film-coating spray guns are similar in both perforated-pan and fluidized-bed coaters, although differences in the performance of spray guns provided by different vendors, especially in perforated-pan processes, have been noted (Macleod & Fell,

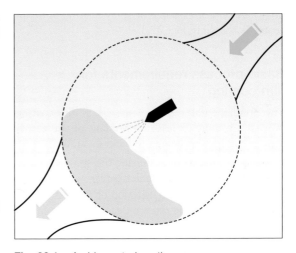

Fig. 32.1 • A side-vented coating pan.

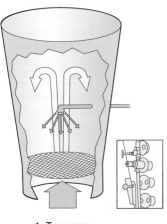

1. Top spray

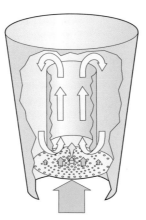

2. Bottom spray

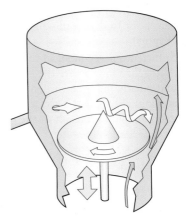

3. Tangential

Fig. 32.2 • Fluidized-bed coating equipment.

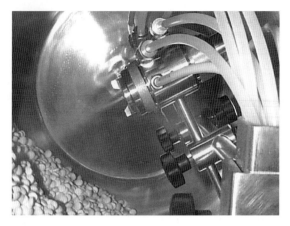

Fig. 32.3 • Example of spray coating in a pan coater.

2002). A typical example of spray coating in a pan coater is shown in Fig. 32.3.

Basic process requirements for film coating

The fundamental requirements of a film-coating process are more or less independent of the actual type of equipment being used and include:

- Adequate means of atomizing the spray liquid for application to the tablet cores.
- Adequate mixing and agitation of the tablet bed. Spray coating relies on each core passing through the area of spraying (commonly called the spray zone) an equal number of times throughout the process. This is distinct from sugar coating, where each application of syrup is spread from tablet to tablet, as a result of tablet contact during tumbling in the coating pan, prior to drying (discussed later in this chapter).
- Sufficient energy input in the form of heated drying air to evaporate the solvent. This is particularly important when aqueous-based coatings are applied because they require more energy input as a result of the higher latent heat of vaporization of water.
- Good exhaust facilities to remove dust- and solvent-laden air.

Film-coating formulations

Currently, the majority of film-coating processes involve the application of a coating liquid where a

significant proportion of the main component (the solvent/vehicle) is removed by means of a drying process that is concurrent with the application of that coating liquid. Film-coating formulations typically comprise:

- polymer;
- plasticizer;
- colourants; and
- solvent/vehicle.

There are certain types of coating process that differ from this common approach. For example, some processes involve the application of hot-melt coatings that congeal on cooling (Jozwiakowski et al., 1990), while others take advantage of recent developments in powder application technologies (Porter, 1999).

It should be mentioned that all ingredients used in film-coating formulations must comply with the current relevant regulatory and pharmacopoeial requirements in the intended marketing area.

Film-coating polymers

The ideal characteristics of a film-coating polymer are discussed in the following sections. These properties differ widely between the various polymers that might be considered for film-coating formulations.

Solubility

Polymer solubility is important for two reasons:

- It determines the behaviour of the coated product in the gastrointestinal tract (i.e. the rate at which the drug will be released, and whether there will be any delay in the onset of drug release).
- It determines the solubility of the coating in a chosen solvent system (a factor that can have great influence on the functional properties of the final coating).

Film coatings that are used on immediate-release products should utilize polymers that have good solubility in aqueous fluids to facilitate the rapid dissolution of the active ingredient from the finished dosage form following ingestion. Such coatings are usually applied as solutions in an appropriate solvent system (with a strong preference being shown for water). However, film coatings used to modify the rate or onset of drug release from the dosage form tend to have limited or no solubility in aqueous media; such coatings are usually applied either as polymer solutions in organic solvents or as aqueous polymer dispersions (discussed later in this chapter).

Viscosity

Viscosity is very much a limiting factor with regard to the ease with which a film coating can be applied. High viscosity (typically that exceeding approximately 500 mPa s) complicates transfer of the coating liquid from the storage vessel to the spray guns, and subsequent atomization of that coating liquid into fine droplets. Ideally, therefore, polymers applied as solutions in a selected solvent should exhibit relatively low viscosities (ideally less than 300 mPa s) at the preferred concentration. This will help to facilitate easy, trouble-free spray application of the coating solution, especially in production-scale film-coating equipment.

Permeability

Appropriate permeability (to which the chosen polymer makes a significant contribution) is a key attribute when considering the various functional properties that film coatings are expected to possess. For example, coating permeability is of significant importance when the film coating is intended to:

- mask the unpleasant taste of the active ingredient in the dosage form;
- improve stability of the dosage form by limiting exposure to atmospheric vapours and gases, particularly water vapour and oxygen; and
- modify the rate at which the active ingredient will be released from the dosage form.

Mechanical properties

In order to perform effectively for the purpose intended, a film coating must exist as a discrete, continuous coating around the surface of the product to be coated, and must be free from defects typically caused by the stresses to which the coating is likely to be exposed during the coating process, during packaging and during the subsequent distribution of the final product.

Consequently, film-coating polymers should possess suitable characteristics with respect to:

- *film strength*, which greatly affects the ability of the coating to resist the mechanical stresses to which it will be exposed during the coating process and during subsequent handling of the coated product;
- *film flexibility*, which imparts benefits similar to those of film strength and minimizes film cracking during handling or subsequent storage; and
- *film adhesion*, which is necessary to ensure that the coating remains adherent to the surface of the dosage form right up to the point of being taken by the patient.

The generation and minimization of film-coating defects are discussed more fully later in this chapter.

Types of film-coating polymers: immediate-release coatings

Cellulose derivatives

Most cellulosic polymers used in film-coating formulations are substituted ethers of cellulose.

Hydroxypropyl methylcellulose is the most widely used of the cellulosic polymers. Its molecular structure is shown in Fig. 32.4. It is readily soluble in aqueous media and forms films that have suitable mechanical properties and coatings that are relatively easy to apply. Coatings that utilize this polymer may be clear or coloured with permitted pigments. The polymer

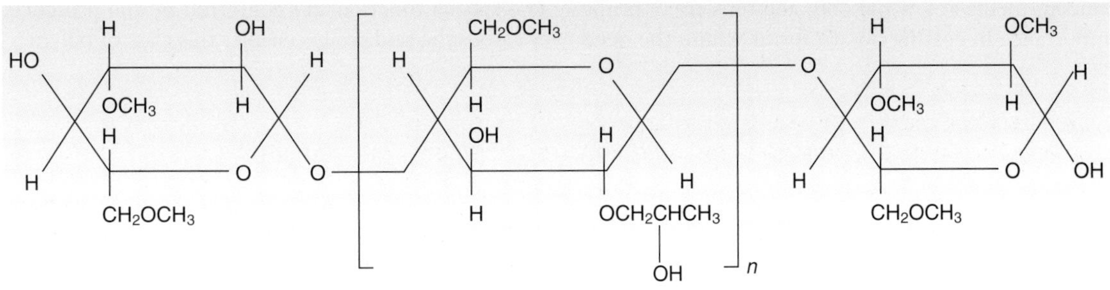

Fig. 32.4 • Hydroxypropyl methylcellulose.

is the subject of monographs in the major international pharmacopoeias.

Other cellulosic derivatives used in film coatings which have properties similar to those of hydroxypropyl methylcellulose include *methylcellulose* and *hydroxypropyl cellulose*.

Vinyl derivatives

The most commonly used vinyl polymer in pharmaceutical applications is *polyvinylpyrrolidone*. Unfortunately, this polymer has limited use in film-coating formulations because of its inherent tackiness. A copolymer of vinylpyrrolidone and vinyl acetate, *copovidone*, is considered a better film former than polyvinylpyrrolidone. Another useful vinyl polymer is poly(vinyl alcohol) (PVA), a partial hydrolysate of poly(vinyl acetate), which can be used to produce film coatings that have suitable mechanical properties and are highly adherent to pharmaceutical tablets. In addition, PVA exhibits good barrier properties with regard to environmental gases (Okhamafe & York, 1983) and water vapour (Jordan et al., 1995).

Film coatings that use PVA as the primary polymer have mainly been exploited as special barrier coatings, helping to improve the stability of drug substances that are either sensitive to moisture (especially in countries that have humid climates) or readily oxidized when exposed to atmospheric oxygen.

Recently, film coatings based on a copolymer of vinyl alcohol and ethylene glycol (Ziegler & Koller, 2003) have become available. These coatings are less tacky than traditional PVA coatings and have the additional benefit of being extremely flexible, thus improving film robustness and allowing greater expansion capabilities should the tablet cores expand slightly during the coating process.

Aminoalkyl methacrylate copolymers

These acrylic copolymers are readily soluble in aqueous media at low pH only, and thus are of prime importance in coating dosage forms where the need

to achieve effective taste masking is a critical attribute (Dittgen et al., 1997). These polymers are typically applied as solutions in organic solvents, although special forms may also be used to prepare aqueous polymer dispersions. An example of the molecular structure of this type of acrylic polymer is shown in Fig. 32.5.

Types of film-coating polymers: modified-release coatings

Cellulose derivatives

As is the case with cellulosic polymers used in immediate-release applications, cellulosic polymers used for modified-release purposes are typically substituted ethers of cellulose. However, the level of substitution in this case is usually much higher, thus rendering the polymer insoluble in water. A typical example of such a cellulosic polymer is *ethylcellulose* (EC), which is preferred for many extended-release applications (Porter, 1989). Historically, ethylcellulose has been applied as solutions in organic solvents, although aqueous polymer dispersions are commercially available.

Other cellulose derivatives used for modified-release applications include cellulose esters such as *cellulose acetate* (CA).

Methylmethacrylate copolymers

Acrylic ester polymers are typically insoluble in water but can be prepared with varying degrees of permeability to render them suitable for a variety of extended-release applications (Dittgen et al., 1997). Originally intended for use as solutions in organic solvents, these polymers are commonly used today as aqueous polymer dispersions.

Methacrylic acid copolymers

The special functionality conferred by the presence of carboxylic acid groups enables this class of polymer

$$[-CH_2-C(R_1)(R_2)-CH_2-C(R_1)(R_3)-CH_2-C(R_1)(R_4)-CH_2-C(R_1)(R_4)-]_n$$

Where $R_1 = CH_3$ $R_2 = COOC_4H_9$ $R_3 = COOCH_3$
$R_4 = COOCH_2-CH_2-N(C_2H_2)_2$

Fig. 32.5 • Aminoalkyl methacrylate copolymer.

$$[—CH_2—C(CH_3)(COOH)—CH_2—C(CH_3)(COOH_3)—]_n$$

Fig. 32.6 • Methacrylic acid copolymer.

to function as gastro-resistant coatings (Dittgen et al., 1997). This is because the polymer is insoluble in water at the low pH that typifies conditions in the stomach but gradually becomes soluble as the pH rises towards neutrality, a condition that is more typical of the upper part of the small intestine. Currently, methacrylic acid copolymers are commonly used as aqueous polymer dispersions. An example of the molecular structure of this type of acrylic polymer is shown in Fig. 32.6.

Phthalate esters

In terms of functionality, phthalate ester polymers exhibit properties similar to those of methacrylic acid copolymers (Chang, 1990), in that they are most suited to delayed-release applications. Chemically, they are formed by the substitution of phthalic acid (or similar) groups into polymers that have been commonly used in other film-coating applications. Thus some common examples of phthalate ester polymers are *hydroxypropyl methylcellulose phthalate* (HPMCP), *cellulose acetate phthalate* (CAP), and *poly(vinyl acetate phthalate (PVAP)*. Phthalate ester polymers may be applied as solutions in organic solvents or as aqueous polymer dispersions.

Plasticizers

Plasticizers are generally added to film-coating formulations to modify the physical properties of the polymer. This is necessary because most acceptable film-coating polymers can be brittle and inflexible. It is generally accepted that the mechanism by which plasticizers exert their effect is for plasticizer molecules to interpose themselves between the polymer molecules, thus increasing free volume and facilitating increased polymer chain motion within the structure of the coating. The positive benefits of this interaction include:

- increased film flexibility; and
- reduced residual stresses within the coating as it shrinks around the core during drying.

Some examples of commonly used plasticizers are:

- polyols, such as polyethylene glycols and propylene glycol;

- organic esters, such as diethyl phthalate and triethyl citrate; and
- oils/glycerides, such as fractionated coconut oil.

For a given application, it is generally desirable to use plasticizers that are soluble in the solvent system being used.

Colourants

Pharmaceutically acceptable colourants are available in both water-soluble form (known as *dyes*) and water-insoluble form (known as *pigments*). The insoluble form is preferred in film-coating formulations, because pigments tend to be more chemically stable towards light, provide better opacity and covering power, and provide a means of optimizing the permeability properties of the applied film coating. In addition, water-insoluble pigments will not suffer from the disadvantageous phenomenon of mottling (caused by solute migration, as discussed in Chapter 29) that can be observed with water-soluble dyes.

Some examples of colourants are:

- iron oxide pigments;
- titanium dioxide; and
- aluminium lakes (a pigment formed by bonding of water-soluble colourants to approved substrata, such as fine alumina hydrate particles).

Whilst the selection of a colourant is typically based on the need to achieve a certain visual effect and, to a lesser extent, the potential influence on film mechanical properties, an underlying selection criterion is that of regulatory acceptance. Whereas there are many colourants that can be used, few have the full global regulatory acceptance required to facilitate the worldwide use of the same coating formulation.

Solvents

Initially, film-coating processes were very much dependent on the use of organic solvents (such as *methanol–dichloromethane* combinations or *acetone*) in order to achieve the rapid drying characteristics demanded by the process. Unfortunately, organic solvents possess many disadvantages (Hogan, 1982) that are related to the following factors:

1. *Environmental issues*. The venting of untreated organic solvent vapour into the atmosphere is ecologically unacceptable, and efficient solvent vapour removal from gaseous effluent of coating processes is expensive.

2. *Safety issues.* Organic solvents may be flammable (and thus explosive hazards) or expose plant operators to toxic hazards.

3. *Financial issues.* Potentially unacceptable cost factors associated with the use of organic solvents are related to the need to build explosion-proof processing areas and provide suitable storage areas for hazardous materials. In addition, the relative expense of organic solvents as a raw material has to be considered.

4. *Solvent residue issues.* For a given process, the amount of organic solvent retained in the film coat must be investigated, especially since there is increasing regulatory pressure to quantify and limit the residue levels.

Such disadvantages have provided the momentum for the current utilization of aqueous coating formulations as the preferred option. However, as a result of improved efficiency and decreased costs associated with solvent recovery, there has been an upsurge in interest in solvent coating but almost exclusively in modified-release coating applications.

Aqueous polymer dispersions

Essentially, all polymers used in modified-release film-coating applications are, in order to achieve their intended functionality, generally insoluble in water. Hence they have been applied as solutions in organic solvents. The growing demand for aqueous formulations in modern film-coating processes thus initially caused a dilemma for pharmaceutical formulators, a dilemma that has ultimately been resolved by creating aqueous polymer dispersions of many of these polymers. The term 'aqueous polymer dispersion' is broadly used to describe polymer systems that are supplied as lattices, as well as those that have been formed into aqueous suspensions, and their use has been comprehensively reviewed in Felton & McGinity (2008).

Ideal characteristics of film-coated products

A film-coated product *and* its associated manufacturing process should be designed and controlled to ensure that the following characteristics are evident:

- even coverage and colour of the coating across the surface of each dosage unit within a batch, and from batch to batch;
- absence of defects that detract from the finished product appearance, or which affect dosage form functionality and stability; and
- compliance with finished product specifications and any relevant compendial requirements.

When designing film-coating formulations, formulators often find it useful to use specialized assessment techniques that allow the properties of the individual ingredients being considered (including their potential beneficial interactions), of the coating formulations, and of the final coated product to be evaluated. A review of many of these useful assessment techniques has been provided by Porter & Felton (2010).

Film-coating defects

Film coating is not a perfect process. Defects and imperfections in the coat can occur if the formulation of the coat and the core, or the coating process, is not adequately designed and controlled. The defects that are commonly attributed to film coating are usually:

- visual defects (usually seen with film-coated tablets); and
- defects that affect functional properties (such as those influencing drug release, and thus these are usually associated with modified-release products).

By far the most common defects are those in the former category, and these have been described in detail by Rowe (1992), with suggestions for their resolution. Visual defects can be categorized as those relating to:

- *Processing issues.* These are typically associated with an imbalance between the rate of delivery of the coating liquid and the rate of evaporation during the drying process. This imbalance results in either overwetting (where tablets or multiparticulates might become stuck together) or overdrying, when surface erosion of the tablets, as well as chipping of the tablet edges, may result.
- *Formulation issues.* These are usually associated with some deficiency in the core (tablet or multiparticulate) or the coating. Core formulation issues often result in mechanical defects, such that the core is not able to

withstand the attritional effects of the coating process, leading to tablet breakage and erosion. Coating formulation issues often result in a film of inadequate mechanical strength, leading to film cracking and chipping, or inadequate film adhesion, resulting in film peeling and logo bridging.

Sugar coating

Sugar coating has long been the traditional method for coating pharmaceutical products (usually tablets). It involves the successive application of sucrose-based coating formulations to tablet cores in suitable coating equipment. Conventional panning equipment with manual application of syrup has been extensively used, although more specialized equipment and automated methods are now making an impact on the process. A comparison between sugar coating and film coating is given in Table 32.1 and illustrated in Fig. 32.7.

Types of sugar coatings

Sugar coatings are composed of ingredients that are readily soluble, or disintegrate rapidly, in water. Although it is technically feasible to apply sugar coatings to a wide range of pharmaceutical core materials, it is almost exclusively reserved for coating tablets. In general, sugar-coated tablets are intended to exhibit immediate-release attributes. However, one of the stages of the sugar-coating process, the sealing step (discussed later), involves the deposition of a polymer-based coating on the surface of the uncoated tablets. At this stage, it is possible to use some of the speciality polymers (described earlier in the section entitled 'Film coating') that are either partially or completely insoluble in water, thus enabling the sugar-coated product to exhibit delayed (gastro-resistant)-release or extended-release characteristics.

Ideal characteristics of sugar-coated tablets

Sugar-coated tablets should possess a smooth, rounded contour, with even colour coverage and a glossy finish. Those tablets that have been imprinted should exhibit high print quality (clear distinct print with no

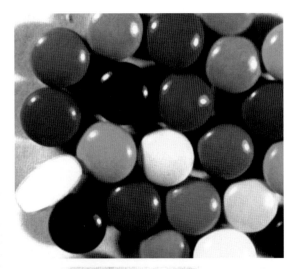
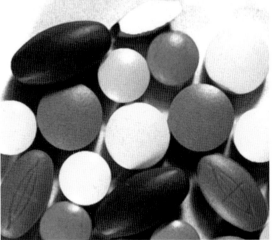

Fig. 32.7 • Sugar-coated tablets *(top)* and film-coated tablets *(bottom)*.

smudging or missing print). As is the case with film-coated tablets, sugar-coated tablets must be compliant with finished product specifications and any relevant compendial requirements.

Process equipment

Typically, tablets are sugar coated by a panning technique, using a traditional rotating sugar-coating pan with a supply of drying air (preferably capable of being thermostatically controlled), and an extraction system to remove dust- and moisture-laden air (illustrated in Fig. 32.8).

Traditional sugar-coating processes involve manual application techniques, whereby the coating liquid

589

At each stage of the coating process, multiple applications of the specified coating formulation are made by a sequential approach that involves:

* applying a predetermined amount of coating liquid;
* allowing the coating liquid to be distributed throughout the tablet mass as the tablets tumble in the rotating pan;
* drying by directing air of the desired temperature onto the surface of the rolling mass of tablets; and
* repeating each of these steps the required number of times.

Each of these substeps of a typical sugar-coating process is now discussed in turn.

Sealing

Sugar coatings are aqueous formulations that are, quite literally, poured directly onto the tumbling tablets. Hence water has an opportunity to penetrate directly into the tablet cores, potentially affecting product stability and possibly causing premature tablet disintegration. To prevent these problems, the cores are usually sealed initially with a water-proofing or sealing coat. Traditionally, alcoholic solutions of *shellac* were used for this purpose although the use of synthetic polymers, such as *cellulose acetate phthalate* or *poly(vinyl acetate phthalate)*, is now favoured. Unless a modified-release feature needs to be introduced, the amount of sealing coat applied has to be carefully calculated so that there is no negative influence on drug release characteristics for what should otherwise be an immediate-release product.

Subcoating

Sugar coatings are usually applied in quite substantial quantities to the tablet core (typically increasing the weight by as much as 50% to 100%) in order to round off the tablet edges. Much of this material build-up occurs during the subcoating stage and is achieved by adding bulking agents such as *calcium carbonate* to the sucrose solutions. In addition, antiadherents such as *talc* may be used to prevent tablets sticking together, and polysaccharide gums, such as *gum acacia*, may also be added as a binder in order to reduce brittleness.

Smoothing

The subcoating stage is notorious for producing a surface finish that is somewhat rough. To facilitate

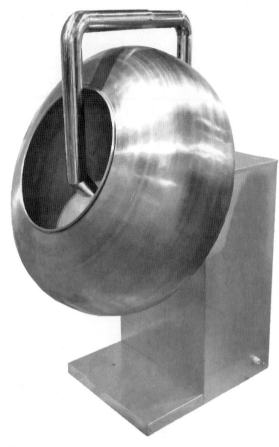

Fig. 32.8 • Traditional sugar-coating pan.

is ladled directly onto the surface of the cascading bed of tablets. In efforts to improve control and to speed up the sugar-coating process, many of the process equipment improvements discussed in the section entitled 'Film coating' are used. Automated dosing techniques and control procedures can also now be used to great effect.

Description of the sugar-coating process

Sugar coating is a multistage process and can be divided into the following steps:

1. sealing of the tablet cores;
2. subcoating;
3. smoothing;
4. colouring;
5. polishing; and
6. printing.

the application of the colouring layer (which requires a smooth surface), subcoated tablets are usually smoothed out by applying a sucrose coating that is often coloured with titanium dioxide to achieve the desired level of whiteness.

Colouring

Nearly all sugar-coated tablets are coloured because visual elegance is usually considered to be of great importance with this type of coated dosage form. Colour coatings usually consist of sucrose syrups containing the requisite colouring materials. As with film-coating colours, sugar-coating colourants may be subdivided into either water-soluble dyes or water-insoluble pigments. Traditionally, water-soluble dyes have been used, but in order to speed up the coating process and minimize colour migration problems, dyes have gradually been replaced with pigments. The actual colourants used must comply with regulations promulgated by the national legislation of the country where the products are to be marketed.

Polishing

Once the colour coating layers have been applied and dried, the tablet surface tends to be smooth but somewhat dull in appearance. To achieve the glossy finish that typifies sugar-coated products, a final stage involving the application of waxes is employed. Suitable waxes include *beeswax, carnauba wax* or *candelilla wax* applied as finely ground powders or as suspensions/solutions in an appropriate organic solvent.

Printing

It is common practice to identify all oral solid dosage forms with a manufacturer's logo, product name, dosage strength or other appropriate code. For sugar-coated products, such identification can be achieved only by means of a printing process, which is typically an offset gravure process using special edible inks. However, alternative printing processes, such as ink-jet and pad-printing processes, have also gained acceptance.

Sugar-coating defects

Sugar coating is technically and practically a difficult process that requires a great deal of skill and experience. Defects in the coating can occur without adequate process control. Although they may well have drug release or stability implications, defects associated with sugar-coated tablets are likely to be visual in nature. Common sugar-coat defects include:

- tablets that are rough in appearance (in which case the surface may also exhibit a marbled appearance as surface pits can become filled with wax during the polishing stage);
- tablets that are smooth but dull in appearance;
- tablets that have pieces of debris (usually from broken tablets from the same batch) stuck to the surface;
- tablets exhibiting poor colour uniformity; and
- tablets that split on storage as a result of inadequate drying (causing the tablets to swell).

Compression coating

Compression coating differs radically from film coating and sugar coating. The process involves the compaction of granular material around preformed tablet cores (Fig. 32.9) using specially designed tableting equipment. Compression coating is essentially a dry process (although the coating formulation may have been produced by a wet-granulation process).

Description of the compression-coating process

Compression coating is based on a modification of the traditional tableting process. Tablet cores are first prepared and then mechanically transferred, on the same machine, to another, slightly larger die that has been partially filled with the coating powder. The tablet core is positioned centrally into this partially filled die, more coating powder is added on top of the core and the whole composite mass undergoes a second compaction event. A detailed description

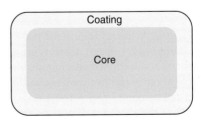

Fig. 32.9 • Representation of a compression-coated tablet.

of the compression-coating process has been given by Gunsel & Dusel (1990).

Traditionally, compression coating has been used to separate incompatible materials (one contained in the tablet core and the second contained in the coating). With the traditional compression-coating process, there is still an interface layer (between the two layers) that may potentially compromise product stability. Thus it is also possible to apply two coating layers where the first coating layer is an inert, placebo formulation that effectively separates the core and the final coating layer, each of which contains a drug substance that is incompatible with the other.

Compression coating is a mechanically complex process that requires careful formulation and processing of the coating layer. Large or irregularly shaped granules will cause the core to tilt in the second die used for compression of the coating, increasing the likelihood of compressing an uneven or incomplete coating, with the core occasionally being visible at the tablet surface.

Types of compression coatings

Compression coatings are generally made from powdered ingredients that either dissolve or readily disintegrate in aqueous media, and thus have commonly been used for immediate-release tablet products. There has been increased use of compression coatings for the purpose of creating modified-release products (Chopra, 2003; Waterman & Fergione, 2003).

Coating of tablets

Overview of coating of tablets

Tablets are by far the most common type of oral solid dosage form that is coated. They may be coated with both immediate-release and modified-release coatings. Of the techniques available for applying coatings to tablets, the following are the most likely to be used:

- *Sugar coating*. Whereas traditional pan-coating methods are often utilized, there is growing preference for automated techniques involving the application of thinner coatings so that batches can be completed within one work day (rather than the more traditional 3–5 days).
- *Film coating*. Typically, pan-coating processes are preferred, although limited interest in using

fluidized-bed processes for small tablets is also evident.

- *Compression coating*. This is more often used today for novel drug delivery applications, especially when partial coatings (e.g. those applied only to the upper and lower faces of the tablets) are required.

Standards for coated tablets

In general, pharmacopoeias have similar requirements for coated and uncoated tablets, the differences being that:

- Film-coated tablets must comply with the uniformity of mass test unless otherwise justified and authorized.
- Film-coated tablets must comply with the disintegration test for uncoated tablets except that the apparatus is operated for 30 minutes. The requirement for coated tablets other than those that are film coated is modified to include a 60-minute operating time. Furthermore, the test may be repeated using 0.1 N HCl in the event that any tablets fail to disintegrate in the presence of water.

Coating of multiparticulates

Coated multiparticulates, often referred to as 'pellets' or 'beads', commonly form the basis for a wide range of modified-release dosage forms (as described by Tang et al., 2005 and in Chapter 31). This dosage form is typically used for extended-release products, but interest has grown in its use for delayed-release (gastro-resistant) applications as well. Coated multiparticulates possess many benefits compared with conventional nondisintegrating tablets (coated or otherwise) for a broad range of modified-release applications. These benefits are discussed more fully in Chapters 22 and 31 but are summarized here:

1. *Capitalizing on small size (typically 0.5 mm to 2.0 mm)*. Gastrointestinal tract transit times can be somewhat erratic for nondisintegrating tablets (especially as a result of food effects); particles smaller than approximately 2.0 mm can pass through the constricted pyloric sphincter even during the gastric phase of the digestion process and distribute themselves more readily throughout the distal part of the gastrointestinal tract.

2. *Minimizing irritant effects.* Whole, nondisintegrating tablets can potentially lodge in restrictions within the gastrointestinal tract, causing the release of drug to be localized and therefore cause mucosal damage should the drug possess irritant properties. This potentially harmful effect can be minimized with multiparticulates because their small size reduces the likelihood of such entrapment, and the drug concentration is spread out over a larger number of discrete particles.

3. *Reducing the consequences of imperfect coatings.* Film coatings, deposited using a spray technique, can potentially possess imperfections (such as pores) that could compromise the performance of modified-release dosage forms. Traditional coated tablets can be problematic in this regard, as the whole dose could potentially be released quite rapidly if such imperfections (in the coating) exist. With multiparticulates, such a risk is greatly reduced because an imperfect coating on one or two pellets (out of 50–200 that constitute a single dosage unit) is likely to have little effect in terms of lack of benefit, or even harm, to the patient.

4. *Reducing the impact of poor coating uniformity.* Film-coating processes are incapable of ensuring that every entity (tablet, pellet, etc.) within a batch of product will receive exactly the same amount of coating. With a tablet, the complete dose of drug is contained in that dosage unit, so any tablet-to-tablet variation in the amount of coating applied can result in variable drug release from dosage unit to dosage unit. The types of process used for coating multiparticulates are renowned for achieving better uniformity of distribution of the coating material. A further advantage relates to the possible problem of 'dose dumping' resulting from a defect in a film coat. With multiparticulates, because the total dosage unit is made up of a large number of discretely coated particles, a defect in one pellet will 'dump' only a small fraction, say 1/200, of the total unit dosage. This is likely to have no pharmacological consequences. In contrast, a defect in a coated monolithic tablet could release 24 hours' worth of drug into a patient in just a few minutes.

Most commonly, two-piece, hard gelatin capsules are filled with coated multiparticulates to form the final dosage unit, although coated multiparticulates may also be compacted (as long as appropriate formulation and processing strategies are used to avoid rupturing of the coating) into tablets.

Types of multiparticulates

A number of different types of multiparticulates are illustrated in Fig. 32.10. They are commonly film coated in order to create modified-release products.

Drug crystals. Drug crystals, as long as they are of the appropriate size and shape (elongated or acicular crystals should be avoided), can be directly coated with a modified-release film coating.

Irregular granules. Granulates, such as those regularly used to prepare tablets, can be film coated, but variation in particle size distribution (from batch to batch), as well as the angular nature of such particles, can make it difficult to achieve a uniform coating thickness around each particle.

Spheronized granules. Spheroidal particles simplify the coating process. The production of the spheroidal cores is detailed in Chapter 28.

Drug-loaded nonpareils. Another process for producing spheroidal particles involves the application of the drug to the surface of placebo pellets, often called *nonpareils.* These are preformed spherical particles approximately 1 mm in diameter consisting primarily of sucrose and starch, although some such particles may also be prepared using microcrystalline cellulose. Application of the drug uses either:

- a powder-dosing technique involving alternate dosing of powder (containing the drug substance) and binder liquid onto the surface of the nonpareils until the required dose of drug has been achieved; or
- spray application of the drug, either suspended or dissolved in a suitable solvent (usually water) containing also a polymer binder (such as hydroxypropyl methylcellulose or polyvinylpyrrolidone), onto the surface of the nonpareils.

Mini tablets. Many of the other types of multiparticulates described so far suffer from two potential drawbacks, namely:

- variation in particle size distribution; and
- variation in particle shape and surface roughness.

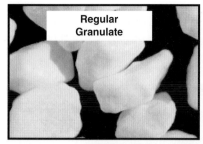
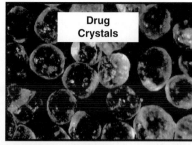
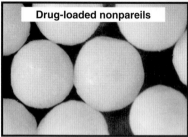
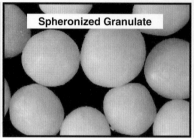
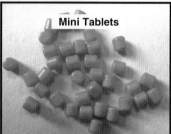

Fig. 32.10 • Examples of film-coated multiparticulates.

Such variability can result in variable coating thickness and thus product performance. This problem can be overcome by using mini compressed tablets (typically in the size range from 1 mm to 2 mm) produced using a modification of traditional tableting processes.

Mechanisms of drug release from multiparticulates

There are many factors that influence drug release from coated multiparticulates, some of which are related to the formulations used and others to the various manufacturing processes employed. Irrespective of the actual number of factors involved, it is generally accepted that the mechanisms of drug release (Ozturk et al., 1990; Zhang et al., 1991) can generally be ascribed to specific conditions.

Diffusion

Diffusion is primarily a process whereby a drug will partition into the film coat membrane and permeate it. The rate at which the drug is released by this mechanism is primarily influenced by the drug concentration gradient across the membrane, the thickness of the membrane, the solubility of the drug in the membrane and the permeability coefficient governing passage of the drug through the membrane.

Osmosis

Once water has passed through the film coating, dissolution of soluble components (excipients and drug) within the core can allow an osmotic pressure to be generated inside the coated particle that will influence the rate at which the drug will be pushed out through pores or a preformed aperture in the membrane.

Dialysis

Dialytic effects describe conditions where water-filled channels are formed in a microporous membrane (often created by the imperfections common to many applied film coatings) through which drug in solution can pass. The key factors influencing drug release by this mechanism include the length and tortuosity of these channels, as well as the solubility of the drug in water.

Erosion

Some coatings are designed to erode gradually with time, thereby releasing the drug contained within the pellet in a controlled manner. Examples of these types of coating are usually those that consist of natural materials such as shellac (the solubility of which in water increases with increasing pH) or waxes and fats that become soft enough to facilitate erosion as the coated multiparticulates are subjected to intense agitation as they pass through the gastrointestinal tract.

Processes for coating multiparticulates

Traditionally, multiparticulates were coated using pan-coating processes, often employing techniques very similar to those used in sugar coating. As coating processes evolved, spray application techniques became more prevalent, and today fluidized-bed processes are preferred because of their ability to:

- enable discrete coatings to be applied to small particles while minimizing the risk of agglomeration; and
- ensure that coatings are uniformly deposited on the surface of each multiparticulate in the batch.

All the polymeric film-coating procedures described so far in this chapter can be used for the coating of multiparticulates. The fluidized bed is used in preference to the perforated pan. Another coating technique that is finding favour for the coating of modified-release pellets is hot-melt coating.

Hot-melt coating

Hot-melt coatings are usually applied to multiparticulates in order to mask taste and modify drug release. They consist of waxy materials (such as beeswax, synthetic spermaceti and other synthetic monoglycerides/diglycerides) that have melting points in the range from 55 °C to 65 °C and exhibit melt viscosities that are typically less than 100 mPa s (to allow the formation of smooth coatings on the surfaces of particles). Hot-melt coatings are preferably applied to multiparticulates by fluidized-bed coating processes, as described by Kennedy & Niebergall (1996).

Please check your eBook at **https://studentconsult. inkling.com/** for self-assessment questions. See inside cover for registration details.

References

Alvarez-Fuentes, J., Fernandez-Arevalo, M., Gonzalez-Rodriguez, M.L., et al., 2004. Development of enteric-coated timed-release matrix tablets for colon targeting. J. Drug Target. 12, 607–612.

Chang, R.-K., 1990. A comparison of rheological and enteric properties among organic solutions, ammonium salt aqueous solutions, and latex systems of some enteric polymers. Pharm. Technol. 14, 62–70.

Chopra, S.K., 2003. Procise: drug delivery systems based on geometric configuration. In: Rathbone, M.J., Hadgraft, J.Roberts, M.S. (Eds.), Modified-Release Drug Delivery Technology, vol. 184. Drugs and the Pharmaceutical Sciences. Marcel Dekker, New York.

Dittgen, M., Durrani, M., Lehmann, K., 1997. Acrylic polymers: a review of pharmaceutical applications. S.T.P. Pharma Sci. 7, 403–437.

Felton, L.A., McGinity, J.W. (Eds.), 2008. Aqueous Polymeric Coatings for Pharmaceutical Dosage Forms, third ed. Informa, New York.

Gunsel, W.C., Dusel, R.G., 1990. Compression-coated and layer tablets. In: Lieberman, H.A., Lachman, L.Schwartz, J.B. (Eds.), Pharmaceutical Dosage Forms: Tablets, vol. 1, second ed. Marcel Dekker, New York.

Hogan, J.E., 1982. Aqueous versus organic solvent film coating. Int. J. Pharm. Technol. Prod. Manufact. 3, 17–20.

Jordan, M.P., Easterbrook, M.G., Hogan, J.E., 1995. Investigations into the moisture barrier properties of polyvinyl alcohol (PVA) tablet film coatings. Proceedings of 1st World Meeting, APGI.APV, Budapest, 9–11 May.

Jozwiakowski, M.J., Jones, D.M., Franz, R.M., 1990. Characterization of a holt-melt fluid bed coating process for fine granules. Pharm. Res. 7, 1119–1126.

Kennedy, J.P., Niebergall, P.J., 1996. Development and optimization of a solid dispersion hot-melt fluid bed coating method. Pharm. Dev. Technol. 1 (1), 51–62.

Macleod, G.S., Fell, J.T., 2002. Comparison of atomization conditions between different spray guns used in pharmaceutical film coating. Pharm. Technol. Eur. 1, 247–284.

Okhamafe, A.O., York, P., 1983. Analysis of the permeation and mechanical properties of some aqueous-based film coating systems. J. Pharm. Pharmacol. 35, 409–415.

Ozturk, A.G., Ozturk, S.S., Palsson, B.O., et al., 1990. Mechanism of release from pellets coated with an ethylcellulose-based film. J. Control. Release 14, 203–213.

Porter, S.C., 1989. Controlled-release film coatings based on ethylcellulose. Drug Dev. Ind. Pharm. 15, 1495–1521.

Porter, S.C., 1999. A review of trends in film-coating technology. Am. Pharm. Rev. 2 (1), 32.

Porter, S.C., Felton, L.A., 2010. Techniques to assess film coatings and evaluate film-coated products. Drug Dev. Ind. Pharm. 36, 128–142.

Rowe, R.C., 1992. Defects in film-coated tablets: aetiology and solutions. In: Ganderton, D., Jones, T.M. (Eds.), Advances in Pharmaceutical Sciences. Academic Press, London.

Tang, E.S.K., Chan, L.W., Heng, P.W.S., 2005. Coating of multiparticulates for sustained release. Am. J. Drug. Deliv. 3, 17–28.

Waterman, K.C., Fergione, M.B., 2003. Press-coating of immediate-release powders onto coated

controlled-release tablets with adhesives. J. Control. Release 89, 387–395.

Zhang, G., Schwartz, J.B., Schnaare, R.L., 1991. Bead coating. I. Change in release kinetics (and mechanism) due to coating levels. Pharm. Res. 8, 331–335.

Ziegler, R., Koller, J., 2003. Protection of light-sensitive active ingredients by instant-release coatings based on Kollicoat IR. Poster presented *at AAPS Annual Meeting and Exposition*, Salt Lake City, 26–30 October.

Bibliography

Aliseda, A., Berchielli, A., Doshi, P., et al., 2010. Spray atomization modelling for tablet film coating processes. In: am Ende, D.J. (Ed.), Chemical Engineering in the Pharmaceutical Industry: R&D to Manufacture. John Wiley & Sons (in conjunction with AIChE), Hoboken.

Cole, G.C., Hogan, J.E., Aulton, M.E., 1995. Pharmaceutical Coating Technology. Taylor & Francis, London.

Jones, D., 2009. Development, optimization and scale-up of process parameters: Wurster coating. In: Qui, Y., Chen, Y.Zhang, G.G.Z. (Eds.), Developing Solid Oral Dosage Forms: Pharmaceutical Theory and Practice. Academic Press, Burlington.

Porter, S.C., Sackett, G., Liu, L., 2009. Development, optimization and scale-up of process parameters: Pan coating. In: Qui, Y., Chen, Y.Zhang,

G.G.Z. (Eds.), Developing Solid Oral Dosage Forms: Pharmaceutical Theory and Practice. Academic Press, Burlington.

Rowe, R.C., Sheskey, P.J., Cook, W.G., et al., 2016. Handbook of Pharmaceutical Excipients, eighth ed. Pharmaceutical Press, London.

33

Hard capsules

Brian E. Jones

KEY POINTS

- Hard capsules are a popular solid oral dosage form consisting of two pieces, a cap and body.
- Good patient adherence is achieved through the use of colour for identification, an easy to swallow shape and a shell that masks the taste of the contents.
- Manufacture involves dipping metal mould pins into solution of polymers: films form on the mould surfaces, are dried, cut to length and two parts assembled.
- Traditionally hard capsules are made from gelatin and now also from hypromellose (hydroxypropyl methylcellulose).
- They can be filled with formulations having a wide range of properties, from dry solids to nonaqueous liquids.
- Powder mixtures are the principal formulation type; involving a simple two-step manufacturing process, mix and fill.
- All filling machines, manual and automatic, use volumetric devices to measure the correct fill weight.
- Dosing of the powder is either 'dependent', using the capsule body to measure the powder, or 'independent', with the powder measured using a dosing mechanism, most frequently forming a soft plug of powder.
- The powder formulation objective is to produce stable mixtures of active ingredients plus excipients with good flow and packing properties.
- Standard capsules release contents in the stomach. Release lower in the gastrointestinal tract is achieved by modifying the fill formulation or by coating of the capsule.

Introduction

The word 'capsule' is derived from the Latin *capsula*, meaning a small box. In current English usage it is applied to many different objects, ranging from flowers to spacecraft. In pharmacy, the word is used to describe an edible package made from gelatin or other suitable material which is filled with drug(s) to produce a unit dosage, mainly for oral use. There are two types of capsule, 'hard' and 'soft'; better adjectives would be 'two-piece' in place of 'hard' and 'one-piece' in place of 'soft'. The hard capsule consists of two pieces in the form of cylinders closed at one end; the shorter piece, called the 'cap', fits over the open end of the longer piece, called the 'body'. Soft capsules are discussed in Chapter 34.

Raw materials

Similar raw materials have been used in the manufacture of both types of capsule. Traditionally both contain gelatin, water, colourants and optional materials, such as process aids and preservatives; in addition, soft capsules contain various plasticizers, such as glycerine and sorbitol. The major pharmacopoeias (European, Japanese and US) permit the use of gelatin or other suitable material. Since the late 1990s, hard capsules have also been manufactured from hypromellose (hydroxypropyl methylcellulose) in order to produce a shell with low moisture content.

Gelatin and hypromellose

Gelatin is still the major component used for capsules, but many new products, particularly those used in dry powder inhalers, are made from hypromellose. All polymer systems need to have the same basic properties for the manufacture of capsules:

1. They are nontoxic (gelatin is widely used in foodstuffs, and hypromellose is used in tablets for film coating) and are acceptable for use worldwide.
2. They are readily soluble in biological fluids at body temperature.
3. They are good film-forming materials, producing strong flexible films. The wall thickness of a hard gelatin capsule is approximately 100 μm.
4. Solutions of high concentration (e.g. 40% w/v) are mobile at 50 °C. Other biological polymers, such as agar, are not mobile.
5. A solution in water undergoes a reversible change from a sol to a gel at temperatures only a few degrees above ambient temperature. This is in contrast to other films formed on dosage forms, where either volatile solvents or large quantities of heat are required to cause this

change of state (e.g. tablet film coating). These types of film are formed by spraying and have a structure that could be described as formed of overlapping plates, whereas the shell of capsules is homogeneous in structure, which gives them their strength.

Gelatin is a substance of natural origin that does not occur as such in nature. It is prepared by the hydrolysis of collagen, which is the main protein constituent of connective tissues (Jones, 2004). Animal skins and bones are the raw materials used for its manufacture. There are two main types of gelatin: type A, which is produced by acid hydrolysis, and type B, which is produced by basic hydrolysis. The acid process takes approximately 7–10 days and is used mainly for porcine skins, because they require less pretreatment than bones. The basic process takes about 10 times as long and is used mainly for bovine bones. The bones must first be decalcified by washing in acid to give a soft sponge-like material, called ossein, and calcium phosphates are produced as a by-product. The ossein is then soaked in lime pits for several weeks.

After hydrolysis, the gelatin is extracted from the treated material using hot water. The first extracts contain the gelatin with the best physical properties, and as the temperature is raised, the quality falls. The resulting weak solution of gelatin is concentrated in a series of evaporators and then chilled to form a gel. This gel is extruded to form strands, which are then dried in a fluidized-bed system. The dried material is graded and then blended to meet the various specifications required.

The properties of gelatin that are most important for capsule manufacturers are the Bloom strength and viscosity. The Bloom strength is a measure of gel rigidity. It is determined by preparing a standard gel (6.66% w/v) and maturing it at 10 °C. It is defined as the load in grams required to push a standard plunger 4 mm into the gel. The gelatin used in hard capsule manufacture is of a higher Bloom strength (200 g to 250 g) than that used for soft capsules (150 g) because a more rigid film is required for the manufacturing process.

Many materials used in the manufacture of pharmaceuticals are manufactured from raw materials of bovine origin (e.g. stearates and gelatin). The outbreak of bovine spongiform encephalopathy (BSE), which started in the UK, has led to strict rules being introduced by the EU to minimize the risks posed by animal transmissible spongiform encephalopathy

(TSE) agents. The *European Pharmacopoeia* has a general chapter on minimizing the risk of transmitting TSE agents via medicinal products and guidance on products at risk. Manufacturers of relevant materials have to submit data to the European Directorate for the Quality of Medicines & HealthCare, which will review the data and issue a certificate of suitability for the product. This must then be submitted to the national regulatory authorities for medicinal products that contain these materials. The Scientific Steering Committee of the EU has collected data from many countries and has assigned to each a geographical BSE risk (GBR). There are four categories, ranging from GBR I, which is for a country in which BSE has never been detected and has in place a surveillance programme (e.g. New Zealand), to GBR IV, which is for a country in which the disease is prevalent (e.g. as was the case in the UK). Currently, gelatin for use in pharmaceuticals in the EU is sourced from bovine bones obtained from GBR I countries.

Hypromellose is manufactured from cotton linters or wood by treatment with sodium hydroxide solutions and further chemicals to produce methyl hydroxypropyl ethers. These are treated with hydrochloric acid to produce different viscosity grades (Rogers, 2012).

Colourants

The colourants that can be used are of two types: water-soluble dyes or insoluble pigments. To make a range of colours, dyes and pigments are mixed together as solutions or suspensions. The dyes used are mostly synthetic in origin and can be subdivided into the azo dyes (those that have an –N=N– linkage) and the non-azo dyes, which come from a variety of chemical classes. Most dyes used currently are non-azo dyes, and the three most widely used are erythrosine (E127), indigo carmine (E132) and quinoline yellow (E104). Two types of pigment are used: black, red and yellow iron oxides (E172) and titanium dioxide (E171), which is white and is used to make the capsule opaque. The colourants that can be used to colour medicines are governed by legislation, which varies from country to country despite the fact that it is based on toxicological testing (Jones, 1993). In the last 20 years there has been a move away from soluble dyes to pigments, particularly the iron oxides, because they are not absorbed on ingestion.

Process aids

The *United States Pharmacopeia–National Formulary* describes the use of gelatin containing not more than 0.15% w/w sodium lauryl sulfate for use in hard gelatin capsule manufacture. This functions as a wetting agent, to ensure that the lubricated metal moulds are uniformly covered when dipped into the gelatin solution.

Preservatives were formerly added to hard capsules as an in-process aid in order to prevent microbiological contamination during manufacture. Manufacturers operating their plants to good manufacturing practice (GMP) guidelines no longer use them. In the finished capsules, the moisture levels, 13% to 16% w/v, are such that the water activity will not support bacterial growth because the moisture is too strongly bound to the gelatin molecule. Hypromellose, because of its raw materials and processing, has low microbial levels, and capsules manufactured using it have a lower moisture specification than gelatin.

Manufacture

The process in use today is the same as that described in the original patent of 1846. Metal moulds at room temperature are dipped into a hot gelatin solution, which gels to form a film. This is dried, cut to length and removed from the moulds, and the two parts are joined together. The difference today is that the operation is now fully automated, and is performed as a continuous process on large machines housed in air-conditioned buildings. There are a limited number of specialist companies that manufacture empty capsule shells for supply to the pharmaceutical and health food industries, which fill them with their own products.

The first step in the process is the preparation of the raw materials. A concentrated solution of gelatin, 35% to 40%, is prepared using demineralized hot water, 60 °C to 70 °C, in jacketed pressure vessels. This is stirred until the gelatin has dissolved, and then a vacuum is applied to remove any entrapped air bubbles. Aliquots of this solution are dispensed into suitable containers, and the required amounts of dye solutions and pigment suspensions are added. The viscosity is measured and adjusted to a target value by the addition of hot water. This latter parameter is used to control the thickness of capsule shells during production: the higher the viscosity, the thicker the shell wall produced. The prepared mixes are then transferred to a heated holding hopper on the manufacturing machine. Hypromellose solutions can be converted into a gelling system by the addition of a gelling agent, such as carrageenan, and a co-gelling agent, such as potassium chloride, and used to manufacture capsules on standard unmodified machines using the same conditions as for gelatin. Hypromellose capsules can also be made by the hot mould dip process, which relies on the property that the viscosity of solutions increases with temperature. In this case, hot mould pins (~70 °C) are dipped into hypromellose solutions at 22 °C; these solutions do not have gelling agents added.

The manufacturing machines are approximately 10 m long, 2 m wide and 3 m high. They consist of two parts, which are mirror images of each other: on one half the capsule cap is made and on the other the capsule body is made. The machines are also divided into two levels, an upper and a lower level. The moulds, commonly referred to as 'pins', are made of stainless steel and are mounted in sets on metal strips, called 'bars'. There are approximately 50 000 mould pins per machine. The machines are housed in large rooms, where the humidity and temperature are closely controlled.

The sequence of events in the manufacturing process is shown in Fig. 33.1. At the front end of the machine is a hopper, called a 'dip pan' or 'pot'.

This holds a fixed quantity of gelatin at a constant temperature, between 45 °C and 55 °C. The level of solution is maintained automatically by a feed from the holding hopper. Capsules are formed by the dipping of sets of moulds, which are at room temperature, 22 °C, into this solution. A film is formed by gelling on the surface of each mould. The moulds are slowly withdrawn from the solution and then rotated during their transfer to the upper level of the machine, in order to form a film of uniform thickness. Groups of 'pin bars' are then passed through a series of drying kilns, in which large volumes of controlled-humidity air are blown over them. When they reach the rear of the machine, the bars are transferred back to the lower level and pass through further drying kilns until they reach the front of the machine. Here, the dried films are removed from the moulds and cut to the correct length, the two parts are joined together and the complete capsule is delivered from the machine. The mould pins are then cleaned and lubricated for the start of the next cycle. The lubricant used is a release aid to enable the dried capsules to be removed from the mould pins without damage. It is an essential part of the process, and capsules cannot be made without it. Hypromellose solutions behave in a similar way to gelatin, except that the speed of gelling is slower and thus the machine output is reduced.

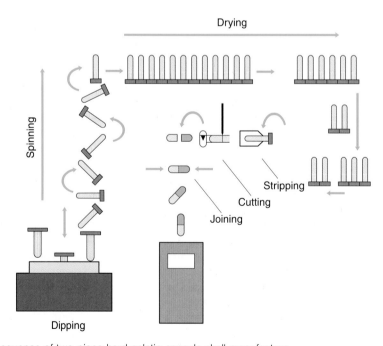

Fig. 33.1 • The sequence of two-piece hard gelatin capsule shell manufacture.

The machines are normally operated on a 24-hour basis, 7 days per week, stopping only for maintenance. The output per machine is more than 1 million capsules per day, depending on the size: the smaller the capsule, the higher the output.

The assembled capsules are not fully closed at this stage and are in a 'prelocked' position, held together by indentations on the inside of the cap walls, which prevents them falling apart before they reach the filling machine. The capsules now pass through a series of sorting and checking processes, which can be either mechanical or electronic, to remove as many defective ones as possible. The quality levels are checked throughout the process using standard statistical sampling plans based on military inspection standards. If required, capsules can be printed at this stage. This is done by an offset gravure roll printing process using edible inks based on shellac. The information printed is typically the product name or strength, a company name or logo, or an identification code. The capsules are finally packed for shipment in moisture-proof liners, preferably heat-sealed aluminium foil bags, in cardboard cartons. In these containers they can be stored for long periods without deterioration in quality, provided they are not subjected to localized heating or sudden temperature changes that will affect their moisture content and dimensions.

Empty capsule properties

Empty gelatin capsules contain a significant amount of water that acts as a plasticizer for the film and is essential for their function. During industrial filling and packaging operations, they are subjected to mechanical handling, and because the gelatin walls can flex, these forces can be absorbed without any adverse effect. The standard moisture content specification for hard gelatin capsules is between 13% and 16% w/w. This value can vary depending on the conditions to which the capsules are exposed: at low humidities they will lose moisture and become brittle, and at high humidities they will gain moisture and soften. The moisture content can be maintained within the correct specification by storing them in sealed containers at an even temperature. The standard moisture content for hypromellose capsules is 3% to 6%, and when they lose moisture, they do not become brittle.

Gelatin capsules are readily soluble in water at 37 °C. Their rate of dissolution decreases when the temperature falls below this. Below approximately 26 °C they are insoluble and simply absorb water, swell and distort. This is an important factor to take into account during disintegration and dissolution testing. Because of this, most pharmacopoeias have set a limit of (37 ± 2) °C for the media in which these tests are performed. Capsules made from hypromellose have a different solubility profile, being soluble at temperatures as low as 10 °C (Chiwele et al., 2000).

Capsule filling

Capsule sizes

Hard capsules are made in a range of sizes; the standard industrial ones in use today for human medicines range in size from 0 to 4 (Table 33.1). To estimate the fill weight for a powder, the simplest way is to multiply the body volume by its tapped bulk density. The fill weight for liquids is calculated by multiplying the specific gravity of the liquid by the capsule body volume multiplied by 0.9. This is to prevent overfilling and spillage of liquid during machine movement.

To accommodate special requirements, some intermediate sizes are produced, termed 'elongated sizes', that typically have an extra 10% fill volume compared with the standard sizes; for example, for 500 mg doses of antibiotics, elongated size 0 capsules are commonly used. The shape of the capsule has remained virtually unchanged since its invention more than 160 years ago, except for the development of the self-locking capsule during the 1960s, when automatic filling and packaging machines were introduced. Filled capsules were subjected to vibration during this process, causing some to come apart and spill their contents. To overcome this, modern capsule shells have a series of indentations on the inside of the cap and on the external surface of the body, which, when the capsule is closed after filling, form

Table 33.1 Capsule size and body volumes

Capsule size	Body volume (mL)
0	0.69
1	0.50
2	0.37
3	0.28
4	0.20

an interference fit sufficiently strong to hold them together during mechanical handling. The manufacturer of the empty shells can be identified from the indentations, which are specific to each one.

Capsule shell filling

Hard capsules can be filled with a large variety of materials of different physicochemical properties. The limitations in the types of material that can be used to fill hard capsules are shown in Table 33.2. Gelatin and hypromellose are relatively inert materials. The substances to be avoided are those which are known to react with gelatin, e.g. formaldehyde, which causes a cross-linking reaction that makes the capsule insoluble, or those that interfere with the integrity of the shells, e.g. substances containing free water, which can be absorbed by the gelatin or hypromellose, causing them to soften and distort. There is also a limitation on the size of capsule that can be easily swallowed, and thus large doses of low-density formulations cannot be used.

The materials that have been used to fill hard capsules are given in Table 33.3. The reason why such a range of materials can be handled is the nature of the capsule-filling process. Empty hard capsules are supplied in bulk containers. First, it is necessary for the filling machine to orient them so that they are all pointing in the same direction, i.e. body first. To do this, they are loaded into a hopper and from there fall randomly through tubes to a rectification section. Here the capsules are held in tight-fitting slots. Metal fingers strike them in the middle, and because the bodies have the smaller diameter, they rotate away from the direction of impact. Next the capsules are sucked into pairs of bushings that trap the caps in the upper pair, because of their greater diameter, thus separating them from the bodies. The bodies are then passed under the dosing mechanism and filled with material. Thus if a substance can be measured and dosed, capsules can be filled with it. The caps are then repositioned over the bodies and metal fingers push the bodies up into them to rejoin the two parts to the correct length so that the locking features of the capsule are engaged.

Capsule-filling machines

The same set of basic operations is performed whether capsules are being filled on the bench for extemporaneous dispensing or on high-speed automatic machines for industrial products. The major difference between the many methods available is the way in which the dose of material is measured into the capsule body.

Filling of capsules with powder formulations

Bench-scale filling

There is a requirement for filling small quantities of capsules, from 50 to 10 000, in hospital pharmacies or in industry for special prescriptions or trials. There are several simple pieces of equipment available, e.g. the Feton filling machine, which consists of sets of plastic plates with predrilled holes to take either 30 or 100 capsules of a specific size. Empty capsules are fed into the holes, either manually or with a simple loading device. The bodies are locked in their plate by means of a screw, and the caps in their plate are removed. The bodies are released and drop below their plate surface. Powder is placed onto this surface and is spread with a spatula so that it fills the bodies. The uniformity of fill weight is very dependent on good flow properties of the powder. The cap plate is then repositioned over the body plate, and the capsules are rejoined using manual pressure. Stainless steel versions of these devices are now available (e.g.

Table 33.2 Limitations in properties of materials for filling of capsules

Must not react with gelatin or alternative shell component

Must not contain a high level of 'free' moisture

The volume of the unit dose must not exceed the sizes of capsule available

---

Table 33.3 Types of material for filling of hard gelatin capsules

Dry solids
  Powders
  Pellets
  Granules
  Tablets
Semisolids
  Thermosoftening mixtures
  Thixotropic mixtures
  Pastes
Liquids
  Nonaqueous liquids

Profill, Torpac, USA) that can be cleaned and auto-claved to comply with GMP requirements.

Industrial-scale filling

The machines for the industrial-scale filling of hard capsules come in great variety of shapes and sizes, ranging from semiautomatic to fully automatic and ranging in output from 3000 to 150 000 per hour. Automatic machines can be either continuous in motion, like a rotary tablet press, or intermittent in motion, where the machine stops to perform a func-tion and then indexes round to the next position to repeat the operation on a further set of capsules.

The dosing systems can be divided into two groups:

- *Dependent* – dosing systems that use the capsule body directly to measure the powder. Uniformity of fill weight can only be achieved if the capsule is completely filled.
- *Independent* – dosing systems whereby the powder is measured independently of the body in a special measuring device. Weight uniformity is not dependent on filling the body completely. With this system capsules can be part filled.

Dependent dosing systems

The auger. Empty capsules are fed into a pair of ring holders (Fig. 33.2), the caps being retained in one half and the bodies being retained in the other half. The body holder is placed on a variable-speed revolving turntable; the powder hopper is pulled over the top of this plate, which revolves underneath it. In the hopper, a revolving auger forces powder down into the capsule bodies. The weight of powder with

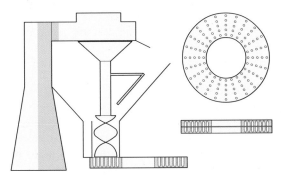

Fig. 33.2 • An auger filling machine using the ring system, Model no. 8. Modified from Jones, 2007, with permission.

which the body is filled is dependent mainly on the time the body is underneath the hopper during the revolution of the plate holder.

These machines are semiautomatic, requiring an operator to transfer the capsule holders from one position to the next. They were first developed for large-scale use during the first half of the 20th century and are still widely used in many countries. The contact parts of these machines were originally made from cast iron but are now made from stainless steel to comply with GMP requirements. Their output varies between 15 000 and 25 000 per hour, which is dependent on the skill of the operator, and they are widely used by the herbal and nutraceutical industries.

Independent dosing systems

Most industrial machines in Europe and the USA are fully automatic and use dosing mechanisms that form a 'plug' of powder. This is a soft compact formed at low compression forces, between 10 N and 100 N, which are significantly less than those used in tableting (10 kN to 100 kN). The reason the plug is soft is because it is not the final dosage form, unlike the tablet, as the material will be contained inside a capsule shell and can be handled without problems. There are two types of plug-forming machine: the 'dosator' system and the 'dosing disc and tamping finger' system.

Dosator. This consists of a dosing tube inside which there is a movable spring-loaded piston, thus forming a variable-volume chamber in the bottom of the tube (Fig. 33.3). This is lowered open end first into a bed of powder, which enters the tube to fill the chamber and forms a plug. This can be further consolidated by applying a compression force with the piston. The assembly is then raised from the powder bed and positioned over the capsule body. The piston is lowered, ejecting the powder plug into the capsule body. The weight of powder added can be adjusted by altering the position of the piston inside the tube, i.e. increasing or decreasing the volume, and by changing the depth of the powder bed.

This system is the most widely used and is the one most described in the literature. Some examples of machines that use this system are:

- *Intermittent motion machines* – Zanasi (IMA Pharma), Pedini, Macophar, Bonapace, ACG-PAM. Their outputs range from 3000 to 60 000 per hour.

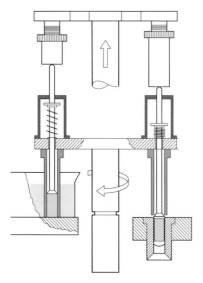

Fig. 33.3 • A dosing tube or dosator-type machine (Zanasi RM63). From Jones, 2007, with permission.

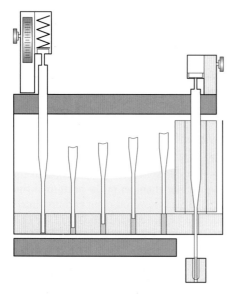

Fig. 33.4 • A dosing disc and tamping finger machine (Höfliger & Karg). From Jones 2007, with permission.

- *Continuous motion machines* – MG2, Imatic (IMA Pharma), ACG. Their outputs range from 30 000 to 150 000 per hour.

Dosing disc and tamping finger. The dosing disc forms the bottom of a revolving powder hopper (Fig. 33.4). This disc has several sets of accurately drilled holes in which powder plugs are formed by several sets of tamping fingers – stainless steel rods that are

lowered into them through the bed of powder. At each position the fingers compress the material in the holes, building up a plug before they index on to the next position. As the disc rotates, material flows into the holes. At the last position, fingers push the plugs through the disc into capsule bodies. The powder fill weight can be varied by the amount of insertion of the fingers into the disc, by the thickness of the dosing disc being changed, and by adjusting the amount of powder in the hopper.

The machines that use this system are all intermittent in motion. Some examples are manufactured by Robert Bosch, Harro Höfliger, ACG-PAM machinery and Qualicaps.

Instrumented capsule-filling machines and simulators

Unlike tablet machines, few workers have instrumented capsule-filling machines. This is for a variety of reasons. Capsules are used only in the pharmaceutical and health food industries, as opposed to tablets, which are widely used by many other industries and therefore there is more incentive to do fundamental research. The tablet press is simple to quantify: there are two punches and a die that holds a specific volume of material. On a capsule-filling machine there are a variety of moving parts involved in dosing, which occurs in an unconfined bed of powder. The forces involved are small. As a result of this, comparatively few articles have been published on the topic. Dosator machines have been studied the most. Strain gauges have been fixed to the piston and have enabled the compression forces (10 N to 250 N) and ejection forces (1 N to 20 N) in lubricated products to be measured. Distance transducers have been used to measure the relative movements of the piston and the dosator. Simulators have also been built to overcome the problem of the machine parts moving, but to date these have had limited application (Armstrong, 2004).

Filling of capsules with pellets

Preparations formulated to give modified-release patterns are often produced as granules or coated pellets. They are filled on an industrial scale by machines adapted from powder use. All have a dosing system based on a chamber with a volume that can easily be changed. Pellets are not compressed in the process and may have to be held inside the measuring devices by mechanical means (e.g. by applying suction to the dosing tube). In calculating the weight of particles that can be filled into a capsule, it is necessary to make an allowance for their size. Unlike powders, which have a much smaller size, they cannot fill as much of the available space within the capsule because of packing restrictions. The degree of this effect will be greater the smaller the capsule size and the larger the particle diameter.

Filling of capsules with tablets

Tablets are placed in hoppers and allowed to fall down tubes, at the bottom of which is a gate device that will allow a set number of tablets to pass. These fall by gravity into the capsule bodies as they pass underneath the hopper. Most machines have a mechanical probe that is inserted into the capsule to check that the correct number of tablets have been transferred. Tablets for capsule filling are normally film coated to prevent dust generation, and are sized so that they can fall freely into the capsule body but without turning on their sides. A recent innovation is the filling of capsules with coated mini tablets, which have a significantly smaller surface area than the equivalent quantity of pellets, thus reducing the amount of coating required and improving its uniformity.

Filling of capsules with semisolids and liquids

Liquids can easily be dosed into capsules by volumetric pumps (Rowley, 2004). The problem after filling is to stop leakage from the closed capsule. This can be done in one of two ways, either by formulation or by sealing of the capsule. Semisolid mixtures are formulations that are solid at ambient temperatures and can be liquefied for filling by either heating (thermosoftening mixtures) or stirring (thixotropic mixtures). After filling, they cool and solidify or revert to their resting state in the capsule to form a solid plug. Capsules are filled with both types of formulations as liquids with use of volumetric pumps. These formulations are similar to those that are used to fill soft gelatin capsules but differ in one important respect: they can have melting points higher than 35 °C, which is the maximum for soft capsules because this is the temperature used by the sealing rollers during their manufacture. Nonaqueous liquids, which

are mobile at ambient temperatures, require the capsules to be sealed after they have been filled. The industrially accepted method for making tamper-evident capsules (USA) is to seal the cap and body together by applying a gelatin solution around the centre of the capsule after it has been filled. When this has been dried, it forms a hermetic seal that prevents liquid leakage, contains odours inside the shell and significantly reduces oxygen permeation into the contents, protecting them from oxidation. An example is the Qualicaps Hicapseal machine, with output ranging from 40 000 to 100 000 per hour. Liquid-filled capsules can also be sealed by a liquid fusion method, which injects an ethanolic solution into the gap between the cap and body, which is then heated to fuse the walls together. An example is the CFS 1200 capsule filling and sealing machine.

Formulation

All formulations which are used to fill capsules have to meet the same basic requirements:

1. They must be capable of being filled uniformly to give a stable product.
2. They must release their active contents in a form that is available for absorption by the patient.
3. They must comply with the requirements of the pharmacopoeial and regulatory authorities, e.g. dissolution tests.

To formulate a formulation rationally, it is necessary to take into account the mechanics of the filling machines and how each type of product is handled.

Powder formulation

Most products that are used to fill capsules are formulated as powders. These are typically mixtures of the active pharmaceutical ingredient together with a combination of different types of excipients (Jones, 1995; Table 33.4). The ones selected depend on several factors:

- the properties of the active drug: its dose, solubility, particle size and shape;
- the filling machine to be used; and
- the size of capsule to be used.

The latter factor defines the free space inside the capsule that is available to the formulator (Jones, 1998). The active compounds that can be most easily

Table 33.4 Types of excipient used in powder-filled capsules

Diluents, which give plug-forming properties
Lubricants, which reduce powder-to-metal adhesion
Glidants, which improve powder flow
Wetting agents, which improve water penetration
Disintegrants, which produce disruption of the powder mass
Stabilizers, which improve product stability

formulated are low-dose potent ones, which in the final formulation occupy only a small percentage of the total volume (< 20%) and so the properties of the mixture will be governed by the excipients chosen. Those compounds with a high unit dose (e.g. 500 mg of an antibiotic) leave little free space within the capsule, and the excipients chosen must exert their effect at low concentrations (< 5%), and the properties of the mixture will be governed by those of the active ingredient.

Formulation for filling properties

There are three main factors in powder formulation:

- good flow (using a free-flowing diluent and glidant);
- no adhesion (using a lubricant); and
- cohesion (plug-forming diluent).

The factor that contributes most to the uniform filling of capsules is good powder flow, because all machines operate by measuring volumes of powders, and thus the formulator's objective is to make powders behave like liquids. The powder bed, from which the dose is measured, needs to be homogeneous and packed reproducibly in order to achieve uniform fill weights. Packing is assisted by mechanical devices or suction pads on the filling machines. Low-dose active ingredients can be made to flow well by mixing them with free-flowing diluents (e.g. lactose). The diluent is also chosen for its plug-forming properties: the diluents most frequently used are lactose, starch 1500 and microcrystalline cellulose. When space is limited, then either glidants, which are materials that reduce interparticulate friction, such as colloidal silicon dioxide, or lubricants, which are materials that reduce powder-to-metal adhesion (e.g. magnesium stearate), are added, enabling the dosing devices to function efficiently. Glidants exert their effect by coating the surfaces of the other ingredients, and thus the mixing

of them into the bulk powder has a significant effect on their functioning.

Formulation for release of active ingredients

The first stage in release from capsules is disintegration of the capsule shell. When gelatin capsules are placed in a suitable liquid at body temperature, 37 °C, they start to dissolve and within 1 minute the shell will split, usually at the ends. With a properly formulated product, the contents will start to empty out before all the gelatin has dissolved. The official tests for disintegration and dissolution were originally designed for tablets. Capsules have very different physical properties, and after the contents have emptied, the gelatin pieces remaining will adhere strongly to metal surfaces and may confuse the end point of the test. Hypromellose capsules take a longer time to the first split, but after this tend to disperse faster than gelatin capsules (Missaghi & Fasshi, 2006).

The literature shows that the rate-controlling step in capsule disintegration and product release is the formulation of the contents, which ideally should be hydrophilic and dispersible (Jones, 1987). The factors that can be modified to make the active ingredients readily available depend on their properties and those of any excipients being used. The active ingredients have a fixed set of physicochemical properties, which, except for the particle size, are out of the control of the formulator.

It has been shown that the particle size influences the rate of absorption for several compounds formulated into capsules. For sulfisoxazole (Fig. 33.5), three different particle sizes were filled into capsules and administered to dogs; the smallest particles gave the highest peak blood level. This can be explained simply by the fact that the dissolution rate is directly proportional to the surface area of the particles: the smaller the particle, the greater the relative surface area. However, this is not a panacea for formulation problems because small particles tend to aggregate and the effect is lost. It has been shown that the important factor with particle size is the 'effective surface area', which is the area of the active ingredient available to the dissolution fluid. This is related to the packing of particles and is a measure of how well the fluid can penetrate into the mass.

Diluents are the excipients that are usually present in the greatest concentration in a formulation. They were classically defined as inert materials added to

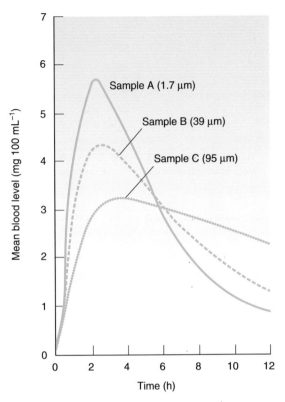

Fig. 33.5 • Effect of particle size on bioavailability of sulfisoxazole. Modified from Fincher et al., 1965.

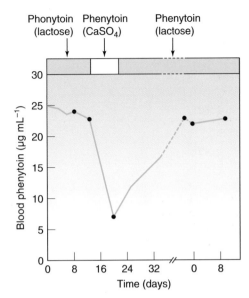

Fig. 33.6 • Effect of diluent on bioavailability of phenytoin. Modified from Tyrer et al., 1970.

a mixture to increase its bulk to a more manageable quantity. Although they are relatively inert chemically, they do play a role in release. The case that first demonstrated this occurred in Australia in the late 1960s. A capsule was reformulated that contained phenytoin (diphenylhydantoin), which is used for the treatment of epilepsy and is taken long term. The diluent used was changed from calcium sulfate to lactose. In the months following this change, there was an upsurge in reports of side effects similar to overdosing of product. It was demonstrated that the change had had a significant effect on the bioavailability of the active ingredient (Fig. 33.6). The change to lactose gave much higher blood levels of the drug, which was probably due to it being readily soluble whereas calcium sulfate is not.

Since this occurrence, the phenomenon has been shown to occur with other drugs. The diluent used should be chosen in relation to the solubility of the active ingredient. If a soluble diluent such as lactose is added to a poorly or insoluble compound, it will make the powder mass more hydrophilic, enabling it to break up more readily on capsule shell

disintegration. The converse is also true: drugs that are readily soluble are best mixed with insoluble diluents such as starch or microcrystalline cellulose, because they help the powder mass to break up without interfering with their solubility in the medium.

Some excipients, such as lubricants and glidants, are added to formulations to improve their filling properties and these can sometimes have an effect on release. The important thing to avoid in formulations is materials that tend to make the mass more hydrophobic. The most commonly used lubricant for both encapsulation and tableting is magnesium stearate. Simmons et al. (1972) studied the dissolution rate of chlordiazepoxide capsule formulations with three levels of magnesium stearate: 0%, 1% and 5% (Fig. 33.7). They found that the dissolution rate was greatly reduced at the highest level of magnesium stearate, which they explained was due to the poor wetting of the powder mass. However, hydrophobic additives are not always deleterious because they reduce the cohesiveness of the powder mass. This was first demonstrated by Nakagawa et al. (1980), who were studying the dissolution of different particle sizes of rifampicin with and without magnesium stearate (Fig. 33.8). They found that for the larger particles (180 μm to 355 μm), the addition of magnesium stearate reduced the rate, whilst for the smaller particles (< 75 μm), it increased the rate.

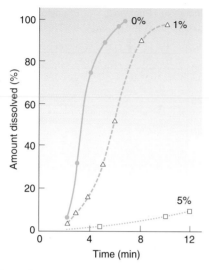

Fig. 33.7 • Effect of lubricant concentration (magnesium stearate) on release of chlordiazepoxide. Modified from Simmons et al., 1972.

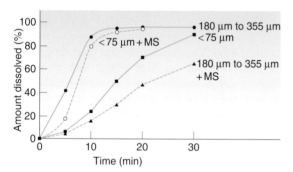

Fig. 33.8 • Effect of lubricant (magnesium stearate, MS) particle size on in vitro release of rifampicin. Modified from Nakagawa et al., 1980.

This is because magnesium stearate reduces the cohesiveness of the small particles so that they spread more rapidly through the dissolution medium than the unlubricated material. Augsburger (1988) studied the system comprising hydrochlorothiazide, micro-crystalline cellulose and various levels of magnesium stearate (Fig. 33.9). Capsules were filled on an instrumented machine using the same compression force and it was found that as the concentration of magnesium stearate increased, the dissolution rate increased to a maximum value at approximately 1% w/v, after which it fell. This was correlated to the hardness of the powder plug, which followed a similar pattern, becoming softer, i.e. easier to break apart, as the concentration of the lubricant increased. Above 1%, the plug becomes too hydrophobic for the increase in 'softness' to compensate for this.

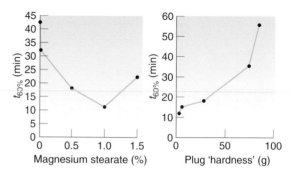

Fig. 33.9 • Effect of lubricant (magnesium stearate) and plug 'hardness' on in vitro release of hydrochlorothiazide. Modified from Mehta & Augsburger, 1981.

The increase in the use of dissolution testing for control purposes has led to products being formulated to improve dissolution properties. This has been achieved in two ways: by the addition of either surfactants or disintegrants. The addition of a wetting agent, sodium lauryl sulfate, has been studied by several workers. For poorly soluble drugs, the use of a soluble diluent together with 1% sodium lauryl sulfate gave the best results. Disintegrants were formerly never added to capsule formulations because starch, which was the most widely used tableting disintegrant, does not function well in this context. This is because the powder plug is much more porous than a tablet and the starch swells insufficiently to disrupt it. More recently, 'superdisintegrants' have been introduced that either swell manyfold on absorbing water (e.g. sodium starch glycolate) or act as wicks, attracting water into the plug (e.g. croscarmellose and crospovidone). These actions are sufficient to help break up the capsule plug. The choice of disintegrant is dependent on the solubility of the drug and the diluent, which governs whether either swelling or wicking is the main disruptive force required (Mehta & Augsburger, 1981).

Formulation optimization

The formulator has to produce a product that complies with the three formulation goals. Sometimes these are contradictory: for example, extra hydrophobic lubricant is required for filling machine performance, which could interfere with release. Therefore in the development stage, the formulation needs to be optimized so that it can meet the product specification. This can be done by using various statistical tools based on analysis of variance experiments that can identify the contribution of each excipient and process operation to the product performance (e.g. uniformity of fill weight and content, dissolution rate, disintegration, yield).

Computer-based expert systems which are based on neural networks coupled to a knowledge base can be used to aid the formulator (Lai et al., 1996). The systems are set up with use of rules that have been established through experience and research. They enable formulators to enter into the system the characteristics of the active ingredient and the type of product they would like to produce. The system then produces suggested formulations to try. This can significantly reduce the development time for a new product.

To summarize, the main factors in powder formulation release are:

- active ingredient, optimum particle size;
- hydrophilic mass, relating solubility of drug to excipients;
- dissolution aids, wetting agent, superdisintegrant; and
- optimum formulation for filling and release.

Formulation for position of release

Many products are formulated to release their contents in the stomach. However, this may not always be the best place for the absorption of the active ingredient, and capsule formulation can be readily manipulated so that the contents are released at various positions along the gastrointestinal tract (Jones. 1991).

A common problem with oral dosage forms is making them easy to swallow. Some people have great difficulty swallowing because the process is not a reflex and is controlled by the central nervous system. The capsule is a good shape for swallowing because the tongue will automatically align it with its long axis pointing towards the throat. Many tablets are now made in this shape – sometimes called a 'caplet' – in order to facilitate swallowing. Patients who have difficulty swallowing should be instructed to do so either standing or sitting, so as to make full use of gravity, and to drink water to lubricate the throat. They should drink a little water and hold it in the mouth. The capsule should be placed in the mouth and the head should be tilted forward. The capsule will now float on the water towards the back of the mouth, and when the head is lifted, the bolus of water and the capsule will go straight down the throat to the stomach.

In the stomach, drug release can be modified in a number of ways. It has been suggested that for some compounds the best way to improve their absorption is for the dosage form to be retained in the stomach so that it will dissolve slowly, releasing a continuous flow of solution into the intestines. 'Floating capsules' have been made which contain various hydrophilic polymers, such as hypromellose, that swell on contact with water and form a mass that can float on the gastric liquids. Some compounds are destroyed at acid pH values, and a gastro-resistant (enteric) product can be made by either coating the filled capsule with an enteric film in a similar manner to that for a tablet or, more usually, by formulating the contents as pellets and coating them with an enteric polymer before filling the capsule with them.

Much has been written in the literature about the advantages or disadvantages of making prolonged-release dosage forms as monolithic or as multiparticulate systems (see Chapter 31). The current consensus is that multiparticulates are better because they will be released in a stream from the stomach when the capsule shell disintegrates and will not be retained for variable periods, as would occur for a monolithic product. They improve safety by avoiding the risk of the dose being dumped at one point, which could cause problems of local gastric irritation.

Some compounds are absorbed only at specific locations along the intestines. If this window of absorption is known, then a formulation can be made to release its contents in that region. There is currently an interest in targeting compounds to the distal parts of the intestines. This has been achieved in two ways. Products can be formulated to give a prolonged release and filled into a capsule that is enteric coated, e.g. Colpermin (McNeil Products) an enteric-coated capsule filled with a prolonged-release formulation of peppermint oil. The capsule disintegrates in the duodenum and the contents slowly release the peppermint oil, which acts as a smooth muscle relaxant as it passes through the remainder of the tract. Products have also been prepared that have been coated with polymers that are soluble only at higher pH values, 6–7. This pH is not reached until further along the small intestine, and so the contents are delivered to the more distal parts. Currently, many new therapeutic entities are proteins or polypeptides, and to make an effective oral dosage form, it is necessary to deliver them to the colon, thereby avoiding the proteolytic enzymes in the stomach and small intestine. The release mechanisms for these capsules are based on specific colonic conditions, e.g. coatings that are disrupted by colon-specific enzymes or by pressure (Nagata & Jones, 2001).

Not all capsules are administered by the oral route. Capsules have been used successfully for many years for products for inhalation. The active ingredient, which is micronized, is filled into the capsule either 'as is' or dispersed on a carrier particle. The weight of the active ingredient with which the capsule is filled is much lower than for other types of product, typically less than 25 mg. Capsule are filled with these formulations on automatic machines that have microdosing devices, and the product is administered by use of a special dry powder inhaler delivery device.

A capsule is placed in the device and the powder is released by the capsule wall being punctured by sharp pins or cut by blades. Hypromellose capsules are the choice for this application because they puncture well and do not become brittle if they are stored incorrectly by patients (Torrisi et al., 2013). These devices are breath actuated. When the patient breathes in, the powder empties from the inhaler and the turbulent airflow dislodges the carrier particles (if present) and the drug powder is inhaled into the lungs (discussed further in Chapter 37).

Please check your eBook at **https://studentconsult. inkling.com/** for self-assessment questions. See inside cover for registration details.

References

Armstrong, N.A., 2004. Instrumented capsule-filling machines and simulators. In: Podczeck, F., Jones, B.E. (Eds.), Pharmaceutical Capsules. Pharmaceutical Press, London.

Augsburger, L.L., 1988. Instrumented capsule filling machines: methodology and application to product development. S.T.P. Pharma Sci. 4, 116–122.

Chiwele, I., Jones, B.E., Podczeck, F., 2000. The shell dissolution of various empty hard capsules. Chem. Pharm. Bull. 48, 951–956.

Fincher, J.H., Adams, H.M., Beal, H.M., 1965. Effect of particle size on gastrointestinal absorption of sulfisoxazole in dogs. J. Pharm. Sci. 54, 704–708.

Jones, B.E., 1987. Factors affecting drug release from powder formulations in hard gelatin capsules. S.T.P. Pharma Sci. 3, 777–783.

Jones, B.E., 1991. The two-piece gelatin capsule and the gastrointestinal tract. S.T.P. Pharma Sci. 2, 128–134.

Jones, B.E., 1993. Colours for pharmaceutical products. Pharm. Tech. Int. 5 (4), 14–20.

Jones, B.E., 1995. Two piece capsules: excipients for powder products.

European practice. Pharm. Tech. Eur. 7 (10), 25–34.

Jones, B.E., 1998. New thoughts on capsule filling. S.T.P. Pharma Sci. 8 (5), 277–283.

Jones, B.E., 2007. Hard capsules. In: Swarbrick, J., Boylan, J.C. (Eds.), Encyclopedia of Pharmaceutical Technology, vol. 1, 3rd ed. Marcel Dekker, New York.

Jones, R.T., 2004. Gelatin: manufacture and physico-chemical properties. In: Podczeck, F., Jones, B.E. (Eds.), Pharmaceutical Capsules. Pharmaceutical Press, London.

Lai, S., Podczeck, F., Newton, J.M., et al., 1996. An expert system to aid the development of capsule formulations. Pharm. Tech. Eur. 8 (9), 60–68.

Mehta, A.M., Augsburger, L.L., 1981. A preliminary study of the effect of slug hardness of drug dissolution from hard gelatin capsules filled on an automatic capsule-filling machine. Int. J. Pharm. 7, 327–334.

Missaghi, S., Fasshi, R., 2006. Evaluation and comparison of physicomechanical characteristics of gelatin and hypromellose capsules. Drug Dev. Ind. Pharm. 32, 829–838.

Nagata, S., Jones, B.E., 2001. Hard two-piece capsules and the control of drug delivery. Eur. Pharm. Rev. 5 (2), 41–46.

Nakagawa, H., Mohri, K., Nakashima, K., et al., 1980. Effects of particle size of rifampicin and addition of magnesium stearate on release of rifampicin from hard gelatin capsules. Yakugaku Zasshi 100, 1111–1117.

Rogers, T.L., 2012. Hypromellose. In: Rowe, C.R., Shesky, P.J., Cook, W.G., et al. (Eds.), Handbook of Pharmaceutical Excipients. Pharmaceutical Press, London.

Rowley, G., 2004. Filling of liquids and semi-solids into hard two-piece capsules. In: Podczeck, F., Jones, B.E. (Eds.), Pharmaceutical Capsules. Pharmaceutical Press, London.

Simmons, D.L., Frechette, M., Ranz, R.J., et al., 1972. A rotating compartmentalized disk for dissolution rate determinations. Can. J. Pharm. Sci. 7, 62–65.

Torrisi, B.M., Birchall, J.C., Jones, B.E., et al., 2013. The development of a sensitive methodology to characterise hard shell capsule puncture by dry powder inhaler pins. Int. J. Pharm. 466, 545–552.

Tyrer, J.M., Eadie, M.J., Sutherland, J.M., et al., 1970. Outbreak of anticonvulsant intoxication in an Australian city. Br. Med. J. 4, 271–273.

Bibliography

Armstrong, N.A., James, K.C., 1996. Pharmaceutical Experimental Design and Interpretation. Taylor and Francis, London.

Jones, B.E., 2004. The history of the medicinal capsule. In: Podczeck, F., Jones, B.E. (Eds.), Pharmaceutical Capsules. Pharmaceutical Press, London.

Newton, J.M., 2004. Drug release from capsules. In: Podczeck, F., Jones, B.E. (Eds.), Pharmaceutical Capsules. Pharmaceutical Press, London.

Ogura, T., Matsuura, S., 1998. HPMC capsules: an alternative to gelatin. Pharm. Tech. Eur. 10 (11), 32–42.

Podczeck, F., 2004. Dry filling of hard capsules. In: Podczeck, F., Jones, B.E. (Eds.), Pharmaceutical Capsules. Pharmaceutical Press, London.

34

Soft capsules

Keith G. Hutchison   Josephine Ferdinando

KEY POINTS

- Soft gelatin capsules (softgels) comprise a liquid or semisolid preparation inside a capsule that is formed in a single-step encapsulation process.
- They can be used as a formulation approach with the potential to:
  - increase the rate of drug absorption, increase the extent of bioavailability and reduce variability in drug plasma levels;
  - improve patient adherence and consumer preference;
  - improve manufacturing safety for potent and cytotoxic drugs; and
  - improve manufacturability of low melting point and low-dose drugs.
- Careful consideration should be given to any migration of the drug or other formulation components when one is formulating a softgel so as to achieve satisfactory product stability and shelf life.
- There are a number of fill formulation approaches which can be used, including suspensions and solutions, using hydrophilic or lipophilic excipients or a mixture of these, to produce emulsions or self-emulsifying microemulsions or nanoemulsions.

Introduction

When pharmaceutical formulation scientists are designing a solid oral dosage form for drug compounds, they have a number of choices which can be influenced by consumer preference/adherence, economics and technical feasibility. In recent years, new drug molecules tend to be less soluble in aqueous systems, and if they are intended for oral administration, this can present a considerable formulation challenge for delivering the drug to achieve the desired rate and extent of absorption. One approach is to make a liquid formulation containing the drug either in solution or suspended in a matrix that is more readily dissolved on contact with gastrointestinal media. In order to convert a liquid formula into a solid dosage form, it may be encapsulated into soft gelatin capsules, also known as softgels.

This chapter explains:

- why softgels are selected for formulation development;
- how they are formulated; and
- how they are manufactured and tested.

Description of the soft gelatin capsule dosage form (softgels)

Softgels consist of a liquid or a semisolid matrix inside a one-piece outer gelatin shell (Fig. 34.1). Ingredients that are solid at room temperature can also be encapsulated into softgels providing they are at least semisolid below approximately 40 °C. The drug compound itself may be either in solution or in suspension in the capsule-fill matrix. The characteristics of the fill matrix may be hydrophilic (e.g.

polyethylene glycols), lipophilic (e.g. triglyceride vegetable oils), or a combination of hydrophilic and lipophilic ingredients (see also Fig. 34.1).

Significant advances have been made in recent years regarding the formulation of softgel fill matrices (Gullapalli, 2010). These include self-emulsifying microemulsions and nanoemulsions encapsulated as preconcentrates in softgels. The term 'preconcentrate' means that the softgel fill matrix which is a combination of lipophilic and hydrophilic liquids as well as surfactant components disperses after oral administration to form an emulsion, with a droplet size in either the micrometre or the nanometre size range.

The softgel capsule shell consists of gelatin, water and a plasticizer. The shell may be transparent or opaque and can be coloured and flavoured if desired. Preservatives are not normally required owing to the low water activity in the finished product. The softgel can be coated with enteric-resistant or delayed-release coating materials. Although virtually any shape of softgel can be made, oval or oblong shapes are usually selected for oral administration.

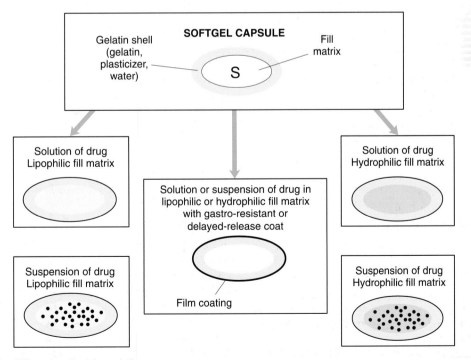

Fig. 34.1 • Different softgel formulations.

Softgels can be formulated and manufactured to produce a number of different drug delivery systems:

- *Orally administered softgels* containing solutions or suspensions that release their contents in the stomach in an easy-to-swallow, convenient unit dose form (Fig. 34.2).
- *Chewable softgels*, where a highly flavoured shell is chewed to release the drug liquid fill matrix. The drug(s) may be present in both the shell and the fill matrix.
- *Suckable softgels*, which consist of a gelatin shell containing the flavoured medicament to be sucked and a liquid matrix or just air inside the capsule.
- *Twist-off softgels*, which are designed with a tag to be twisted or snipped off, thereby allowing access to the fill material. This type of softgel can be used for unit dosing of topical medication, inhalations or oral dosing of a paediatric product (Fig. 34.3).
- *Meltable softgels* designed for use as pessaries or suppositories.

Rationale for the selection of softgels as a dosage form

Some of the reasons why softgels may be selected as the preferred formulation approach are summarized in Table 34.1, and a more detailed description follows. Whilst softgels can solve various technical formulation challenges not possible with tablets, consideration should be given to the fact that they can be more costly than tablet formulations and require specialized manufacturing equipment.

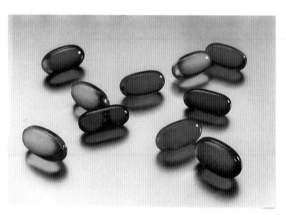

Fig. 34.2 • Swallowable softgel capsules.

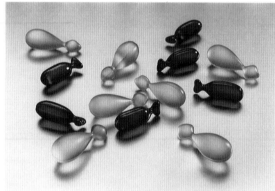

Fig. 34.3 • Twist-off softgel capsules.

Table 34.1 Key features and advantages of the softgel dosage form

Features	Advantages
Improved drug absorption	Increased rate and extent of absorption and/or reduced variability, mainly for poorly water-soluble drugs
Patient adherence and consumer preference	Easy to swallow. Absence of poor taste or other sensory problems. Convenient administration of a liquid-drug dosage form
Safety – potent and cytotoxic drugs	Avoids dust-handling problems during dosage form manufacture; better operator safety and environmental controls
Oils and low melting point drugs	Overcomes problems with manufacture as compressed tablet or hard capsules
Dose uniformity for low-dose drugs	Liquid flow during dosage form manufacture is more precise than powder flow. Drug solutions provide better homogeneity than powder or granule mixtures
Product stability	Drugs are protected against oxidative degradation by lipid vehicles and softgel capsule shells

Improved drug absorption characteristics

Increased rate of absorption

Major advances have been made in the area of developing softgel formulations to address drug absorption issues (Ferdinando, 2000; Perlman et al., 2008; Aboul-Einien, 2009). For poorly water-soluble drugs, ideally the dosage form would present the drug to the gastrointestinal tract in solution form, from which the drug can be rapidly absorbed. This can be achieved using a drug-solution matrix in a softgel formulation, and such formulations can provide faster absorption than from other solid oral dosage forms, such as compressed tablets (Lissy et al., 2010). This is probably because absorption of a poorly soluble drug from a tablet formulation requires time for disintegration of the tablet into granules, then drug dissolution into gastrointestinal fluid. With the solution–softgel approach, the shell ruptures within minutes to release the drug solution, which can be in a hydrophilic or highly dispersing vehicle that aids the rate of drug absorption. This may be beneficial for (1) therapeutic reasons, such as the treatment of migraine or acute pain, or (2) where there is a limited absorptive region or 'absorption window' high in the gastrointestinal tract. Fig. 34.4 shows the faster absorption that can be achieved using a solution–softgel formulation of ibuprofen compared with a tablet (Saano et al., 1991).

Increased bioavailability

As well as increasing the rate of absorption, softgels may increase the extent of absorption (Aboul-Einien, 2009). This can be particularly effective for drugs with poor aqueous solubility and a relatively high molecular weight. An example of such a product is the protease inhibitor saquinavir, which was formulated as a solution–softgel product (Perry & Noble, 1988). The solution–softgel formulation provided approximately three times greater bioavailability than a saquinavir nonliquid hard capsule formulation as measured by the area under the plasma concentration–time curve.

In some cases, a drug may be solubilized in vehicles that are capable of spontaneously dispersing into an emulsion on contact with gastrointestinal fluid. This is known as a *self-emulsifying drug delivery system (SEDDS)* (Gao et al., 2006). Drug may be dissolved in an oil/surfactant vehicle that produces a microemulsion or a nanoemulsion on contact with gastrointestinal fluids. A nanoemulsion of progesterone has been developed whereby the vehicle consists of oils and surfactants in appropriate proportions. On contact with aqueous fluids, it produces an emulsion with an average droplet size less than 100 nm. The solubility of the drug is maintained as long as possible, delivering solubilized drug directly to the enterocyte membrane. This can increase bioavailability compared with formulations in which the drug is dosed in the solid state. Fig. 34.5 shows the plasma concentration–time profile for progesterone absorbed from a softgel nanoemulsion formulation (Ferdinando, 2000).

Softgel formulations may contain excipients, for example one or more surfactants that can aid stability, aid wettability or even enhance the permeability of the drug (Aungst, 2000).

Decreased plasma variability

High variability in drug plasma levels is a common characteristic of drugs with limited bioavailability. By dosing a drug optimally in solution, one can significantly reduce the plasma level variability of the drug, particularly if absorption is limited by drug solubility. Self-emulsifying drug delivery systems have been shown to reduce variability of exposure to the lipophilic drug torcetrapib compared with a formulation in oil (Perlman et al., 2008). The cyclic polypeptide drug ciclosporin (Sandimmune Neoral®) benefits from such an approach by use of a microemulsion preconcentrate in a softgel (Drewe et al., 1992; Meinzer, 1993).

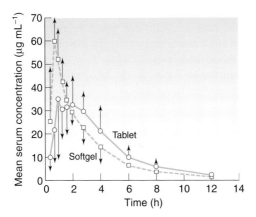

Fig. 34.4 • Pharmacokinetic evaluation of softgels and tablets containing 400 mg ibuprofen (in 12 volunteers). From Saano et al., 1991.

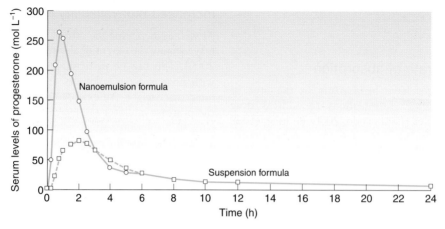

Fig. 34.5 • Pharmacokinetic evaluation of progesterone comparing a softgel nanoemulsion formulation of progesterone with a softgel containing a suspension of the drug in an oil following single dose administration in 12 healthy human volunteers. From Ferdinando, 2000.

Patient adherence and consumer preference

A number of self-medicating consumer preference studies have been conducted to gauge the user's perception of softgels relative to hard capsules and tablets. The results of the studies showed that consumers expressed their preference for softgels in terms of (1) ease of swallowing, (2) absence of taste and (3) convenience of use (Jones & Francis, 2000).

This expressed appeal of the softgel dosage form may have a positive impact on patient adherence. Patient adherence may be further enhanced if the softgel formulation enables dosing of smaller or fewer dosage units, as a result of increased bioavailability.

Safety for potent and cytotoxic drugs

The mixing, granulation and compression/filling processes used in preparing tablets and hard capsules can generate a significant quantity of airborne powders. This can be a cause of concern for the manufacture of highly potent or cytotoxic compounds because of safety considerations for the operator and environment.

If a solution or suspension of the drug is prepared where the active component is essentially protected from the environment by the liquid, these safety concerns can be reduced.

Oils and low melting point drugs

When the drug substance is an oily liquid, has a melting point lower than approximately 75 °C or is difficult to compress, liquid filling of softgels (with or without other diluents) can provide a successful approach to presenting it in a solid oral dosage form.

Dose uniformity of low-dose drugs

Presentation of low-dose drugs in a solution form can overcome the challenges of achieving dosage unit homogeneity compared with other solid oral dosage forms. Where the dose is in the order of micrograms, it can be difficult to mix with other powders sufficiently well to ensure an even distribution in the bulk materials prior to compression of tablets or filling of hard capsules. This can result in assay variation due to content inhomogeneity. By dissolving the drug in a liquid and encapsulating it in a softgel, such inhomogeneity concerns can be avoided.

Product stability

If a drug is subject to oxidative or hydrolytic degradation, the preparation of a liquid-filled softgel may prove beneficial. The liquid is prepared and encapsulated in a protective nitrogen atmosphere and the subsequent dried shell has very low oxygen permeability. By formulating in a lipophilic vehicle and packaging in well-designed blister packs using materials of low moisture transmission, the drug can be protected from moisture. As for all dosage forms, thorough stability evaluation is required, including excipient compatibility studies, to check against negative drug stability effects, caused, for example, by component migration between the fill formulation and the capsule shell, exposure to moisture during manufacture or interaction between the drug and the fill excipients. This may result in the requirement of refrigerated storage (Klein et al., 2007).

Manufacture of softgels

Softgels were used in the 19th century as a means of administering bitter-tasting or liquid medicines. These were manufactured individually by preparing a small sack of gelatin and allowing it to set. Each sack, or gelatin shell, was then filled with the medication and heat sealed. This method of manufacture was improved using a process that involved the sealing of two sheets of gelatin film between a pair of matching flat brass dies. Each die contained pockets into which the gelatin sheet was pressed and which were filled with the medication. The pressure between

the two plates enabled individual capsules to be cut out from the die mould, and these capsules were subsequently dried.

However, it was not until the invention of the rotary die encapsulation machine by Robert Pauli Scherer in 1933 that liquid-fill capsules could be manufactured on a production scale. The rotary die process involves continuous formation of a heat seal between two ribbons of gelatin simultaneous with dosing of the fill liquid into each capsule. Although the speed and efficiency of the manufacturing process have improved greatly in recent years, the basic manufacturing principle remains essentially unchanged. The overall layout of a soft gelatin encapsulation machine is shown in Fig. 34.6.

Before the encapsulation process occurs, two subprocesses are often performed simultaneously, yielding the two components of a softgel. These are (1) the gel mass which will provide the softgel shell and (2) the fill matrix for the softgel contents.

The gel mass is prepared by dissolving the gelatin in water at approximately 80°C under a vacuum, followed by the addition of the plasticizer (e.g. glycerol). Once the gelatin has fully dissolved, other

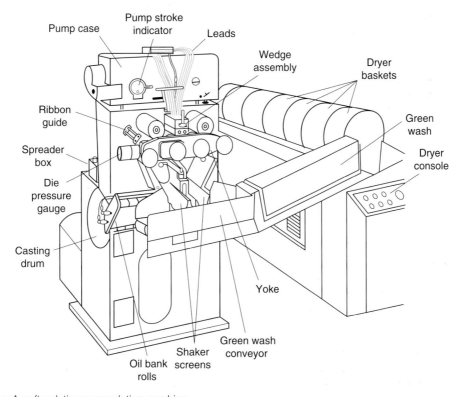

Fig. 34.6 • A soft gelatin encapsulation machine.

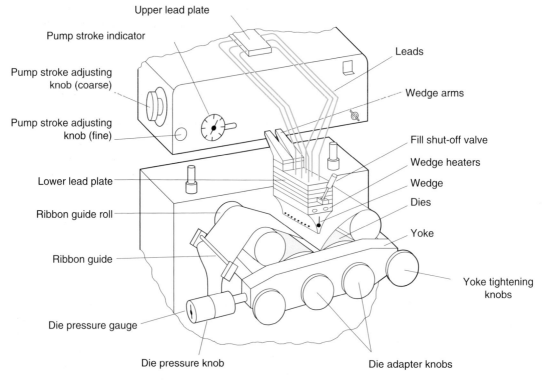

Upper lead plate

Pump stroke indicator

Pump stroke adjusting
knob (coarse)

Pump stroke adjusting
knob (fine)

Lower lead plate

Ribbon guide roll

Ribbon guide

Die pressure gauge

Die pressure knob

Leads

Wedge arms

Fill shut-off valve

Wedge heaters

Wedge

Dies

Yoke

Yoke tightening
knobs

Die adapter knobs

Fig. 34.7 • Detail of a soft gelatin encapsulation machine.

components such as colours, an opacifier and flavours may be added. The hot gel mass is then supplied to the encapsulation machine through heated transfer pipes by a casting method that forms two separate gelatin ribbons, each with a width of typically 150 mm. During the casting process, the gelatin passes through the sol–gel transition and the thickness of each gel ribbon is controlled to ±0.1 mm in the range from 0.5 mm to 1.5 mm. The thickness of the gel ribbons is checked regularly during the manufacturing process.

The two gel ribbons are then carried through rollers (at which a small quantity of vegetable oil lubricant is applied) and onwards to the rotary die encapsulation tooling (Fig. 34.7). Each gel ribbon provides one half of the softgel. It is possible to make bicoloured softgels using gel ribbons of two different colours.

The liquid fill matrix containing the active drug substance is manufactured separately from the preparation of the molten gel. Manufacture of the active fill matrix involves dispersing or dissolving the drug substance in the nonaqueous liquid vehicle using conventional mixer-homogenizers.

A number of different parameters are controlled during preparation of the active fill matrix, depending on the properties of the drug substance. For example,

oxygen-sensitive drugs are protected by mixing under a vacuum and/or inert gas; in some cases, an antioxidant component may be added to the formulation. Additionally, if the drug substance is present as a suspension in the liquid fill matrix, then it is important to ensure that the particle size of the drug does not exceed approximately 200 µm. By doing this, it is possible to ensure that drug particles do not become entrapped within the capsule seal, potentially leading to loss of integrity of the softgel.

In the rotary die encapsulation process, the gel ribbon and the unit dose of liquid fill matrix are combined to form the softgel. The process involves careful control of three parameters:

- *Temperature*. This controls the heat available for capsule seal formation.
- *Timing*. The timing of the dosing of unit quantities of liquid fill matrix into the softgel during its formation is critical.
- *Pressure*. The pressure exerted between the two rotary dies controls the softgel shape and the final cut-out from the gel ribbon.

Fig. 34.8 shows a simplified diagram representing the mechanism of softgel formation using

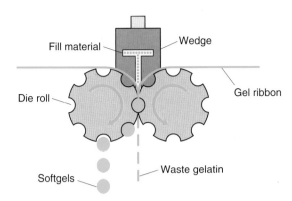

Fig. 34.8 • Softgel formation mechanism.

contrarotating dies and the wedge-shaped fill matrix injection system.

Accurately metered volumes of the liquid fill matrix are injected from the wedge device into the space between the gelatin ribbons as they pass between the die rolls. The wedge-shaped injection system is itself heated to approximately 40 °C. The injection of liquid between the gel ribbons forces the gel to expand into the pockets of the dies, which govern the size and shape of the softgels. The ribbon continues to flow past the heated wedge injection system and is then pressed between the die rolls. Here, the two softgel capsule halves are sealed together by the application of heat and pressure. The softgel capsules are cut automatically from the gel ribbon by raised rims around each die on the rollers.

After manufacture, the capsules are passed through a tumble dryer and then, to complete the drying process, they are spread onto trays and stacked in a tunnel dryer that supplies air at approximately 20% relative humidity. The tunnel drying process may take 2–3 days or possibly as long as 2 weeks, depending on the specific softgel shell formulation. Finally, the softgels are inspected and packed into bulk containers in order to prevent further drying, and for storage.

Formulation of softgels

Gelatin shell formulation

Typical softgel shells are made up of gelatin, a plasticizer and materials that impart the desired appearance (colourants and/or opacifiers) and sometimes flavours. The following sections describe each

of these materials, their functions, their types and the amounts most frequently used in manufacturing softgel shells.

Gelatin

A large number of different gelatin shell formulations are available depending on the nature of the liquid fill matrix. Most commonly, the gelatin is alkali-processed (or base-processed) (type B) gelatin and it normally constitutes 40% of the wet molten gel mass. Type A, acid-processed gelatin can also be used.

Plasticizers

Plasticizers are used to make the softgel shell elastic and pliable. They usually account for 20% to 30% of the wet gel formulation. The most common plasticizer used in softgels is glycerol, although sorbitol and propylene glycol are also frequently used, often in combination with glycerol. The amount and the choice of the plasticizer contribute to the hardness of the final product and may even affect the final product's dissolution or disintegration characteristics, as well as its physical and chemical stability. Plasticizers are selected on the basis of their compatibility with the fill formulation, their ease of processing and the desired properties of the final softgels, including hardness, appearance, handling characteristics and physical stability.

One of the most important aspects of softgel formulation is to ensure that there is minimum interaction or migration between the liquid fill matrix and the softgel shell. The choice of plasticizer type and concentration is important in ensuring optimum compatibility of the shell with the liquid fill matrix.

Water

Water usually accounts for 30% to 40% of the wet gel formulation, and its presence is important to ensure proper processing during gel preparation and softgel encapsulation. Following encapsulation, excess water is removed from the softgels through controlled drying. In dry softgels, the equilibrium water content is typically in the range of 5% to 8% w/w, which represents the proportion of water that is bound to the gelatin in the softgel shell. This level of water is important for good physical stability of softgels because in harsh storage conditions softgels will become either too soft and fuse together or too hard and brittle.

Colourants/opacifiers

Colourants (soluble dyes or insoluble pigments or lakes) and opacifiers are typically used at low concentrations in the wet gel formulation. Colourants can be either synthetic or natural and are used to impart the desired shell colour for product identification. An opacifier, usually titanium dioxide, may be added to produce an opaque shell when the fill formulation is a suspension or to prevent photodegradation of light-sensitive fill ingredients. Titanium dioxide can either be used alone to produce a white opaque shell or in combination with pigments to produce a coloured opaque shell.

Properties of soft gelatin shells

Oxygen permeability

The gelatin shell of a soft gelatin capsule provides a good barrier against the diffusion of oxygen into the contents of the product. The quantity of oxygen (q) that passes through the gelatin is governed by the permeability coefficient (P), the area (A), the thickness (h) of the shell, the pressure difference ($p_1 - p_2$) and the time of diffusion (t) by the following equation:

$$q = \frac{PAt(p_1 - p_2)}{h}$$

(34.1)

The permeability coefficient (P) is related to the diffusion coefficient (D) and the solubility coefficient (S) by the equation $P = DS$. This relationship, described by Henry's law, assumes no interaction between the gas and the polymeric film, but P is clearly affected by the formulation of the gelatin shell, as shown in Fig. 34.9.

Fig. 34.9 shows the relationship between the oxygen permeability coefficient and the glycerol concentration in the gelatin shell of softgels at room temperature and relative humidity from 31% to 80%. The oxygen permeability decreases with the relative humidity and the glycerol content in the gelatin shell formulation (Hom et al., 1975). For maximum protection against the ingress of oxygen, the gelatin shell should be dry and formulated to contain approximately 30% to 40% glycerol.

Residual water content

Softgels contain little residual water, and compounds which are susceptible to hydrolysis may be protected

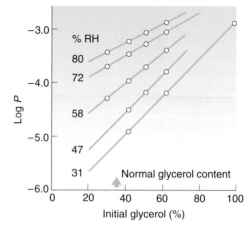

Fig. 34.9 • Relationship between oxygen permeability coefficient and the glycerol concentration in the shell of softgels at room temperature and a range of relative humidities. *RH*, relative humidity. From Hom et al., 1975.

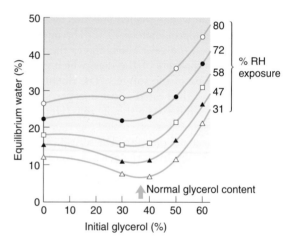

Fig. 34.10 • Relationship between equilibrium water content and the concentration of glycerol in the shell of soft gelatin capsules at room temperature and a range of relative humidities. *RH*, relative humidity. From Hom et al., 1975.

if they are dissolved or dispersed in an oily liquid fill material and encapsulated as a soft gelatin capsule. Fig. 34.10 shows the relationship between the equilibrium water content and the concentration of glycerol in the gelatin shell of a softgel, stored at room temperature and environmental relative humidities of between 31% and 80%. The data show that minimum water content is found at glycerol levels in the shell of between 30% and 40%. Such a formulation dried at 31% relative humidity has a water content in the shell of approximately 7% (Hom et al., 1975), and a water content in the fill in equilibrium with the atmosphere. The residual water content of most pharmaceutical compounds stored at 20% relative humidity (the drying condition for softgels) is low and the water levels in the fills of softgels therefore are very low.

Formulation of softgel fill materials

In terms of formulation requirements, the softgel should be considered as a biphasic dosage form: a solid-phase capsule shell and a liquid-phase capsule fill matrix. Although it is possible to incorporate a drug in the shell of a softgel, the overwhelming majority of products have the active ingredient(s) within the fill matrix. The liquid-phase fill matrix is selected from components with a wide range of different physicochemical properties. The choice of components is made according to one or more of a number of criteria, including the following:

- capacity to dissolve the drug (if a solution fill is required);
- rate of dispersion in the gastrointestinal tract after the softgel shell ruptures and releases the fill matrix;
- capacity to retain the drug in solution in the gastrointestinal fluid;
- compatibility with the softgel shell; and
- ability to optimize the rate, extent and consistency of drug absorption.

Types of softgel fill matrices

Lipophilic liquids/oils

Triglyceride oils, such as soya bean oil, are commonly used in softgels. When used alone, however, their capacity to dissolve drugs is limited. Nevertheless, active ingredients such as hydroxycholecalciferol and other vitamin D analogues and steroids such as oestradiol can be formulated into simple oily solutions for encapsulation in softgels. The drug may also be suspended in oils with appropriate excipients to ensure homogeneity during the manufacturing process.

Hydrophilic liquids

Polar liquids with a sufficiently high molecular weight are commonly used in softgel formulation either to dissolve or to suspend the drug. Polyethylene glycol (PEG) is the most frequently used, for example PEG 400, which has an average molecular mass of

approximately 400 Da. Smaller hydrophilic molecules, such as ethanol or indeed water, can be incorporated in the softgel fill matrix in low levels, typically below 10% by weight. If included at higher levels, they may cause physical instability as they can migrate into the shell. Additional excipients may be included with hydrophilic liquids to increase the drug solubility in the matrix, such as polyvinylpyrrolidone, (PVP) or using a counterion approach as developed for the enhanced solubility system for drugs such as ibuprofen (Seager, 1993).

Self-emulsifying drug delivery systems (SEDDS)

A combination of a pharmaceutical oil and a surfactant such as polyoxyethylene sorbitan monooleate can provide a formulation which emulsifies and disperses rapidly in the gastrointestinal fluid. The resulting droplets enable rapid transfer of the drug to the mucosa and subsequent drug absorption. If the droplets formed on contact with aqueous media are in the micrometre size range, then the emulsion formed is known as a microemulsion; if they are in the nanometre range, then it is known as a nanoemulsion.

In order to produce a microemulsion or a nanoemulsion in the gastrointestinal tract, a 'preconcentrate' is formulated in the softgel fill matrix. The preconcentrate fill matrix contains a lipid component and one or more surfactants, which spontaneously form a microemulsion or a nanoemulsion on dilution in an aqueous environment such as gastrointestinal fluid (Fig. 34.11).

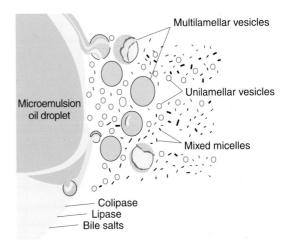

Fig. 34.11 • Proposed nanoemulsion/microemulsion dissolution mechanism.

Microemulsion and nanoemulsion systems have the advantage of a high capacity to solubilize drug compounds, and can retain the drug in solution even after dilution in gastrointestinal fluids. In addition, the microemulsion droplets have a high surface area, and are essentially surfactant micelles swollen with solubilized oil and drug. This high surface area facilitates the rapid diffusion of the drug from the dispersed oil phase into the aqueous intestinal fluids, until an equilibrium distribution is established. Thereafter, as the drug is removed from the intestinal fluids through absorption, it is quickly replenished by the flow of fresh material from the microemulsion droplets. Improved pharmacokinetic characteristics may be achieved with this formulation approach.

Lipolysis systems

In addition to promoting the solubility of drug compounds, lipid formulations can also facilitate dissolution by taking advantage of the natural process of lipolysis. Lipid components of a softgel fill matrix, which comprise triglycerides or a partial glyceride (monoglyceride/diglyceride), are often subject to intestinal fat digestion or lipolysis. Lipolysis is the action of the enzyme pancreatic lipase on triglycerides and partial glycerides to form 2-monoglycerides and fatty acids. These 2-monoglycerides and fatty acids, known as lipolytic products, then interact with bile salts to form small droplets or vesicles. These vesicles are broken down into smaller and smaller vesicles, ultimately resulting in the formation of mixed micelles that are approximately 3 nm to 10 nm in size.

If a drug substance possesses higher solubility in lipolytic products than in triglyceride oils, then it is advantageous for lipolysis to occur in the intestinal lumen. In this way the process of lipolysis promotes the formation of an excellent dissolution medium for the drug, namely lipolytic products. On the other hand, the absorption of a drug compound may be adversely affected by the presence of bile salts, and in such a case it may be advantageous for lipolysis to be reduced or blocked completely. It has been found that certain hydrophilic and lipophilic surfactants have the ability to block or promote lipolysis (MacGregor et al., 1997). These hydrophilic and lipophilic surfactants are often used in softgel fill matrix formulations.

Measurement of the rate and extent of lipolysis for a softgel fill matrix formulation can be achieved by an in vitro pH stat measurement technique. In this, lipolysis is quantified by the amount of free fatty acids liberated by enzymatic digestion of the lipids in the softgel fill matrix. The quantity of a 1.0 M sodium hydroxide titrant is directly proportional to the extent of lipolysis.

The mixed intestinal micelles produced as a result of this lipolysis process are of physiological importance because these structures can transport high concentrations of hydrophobic molecules across the aqueous boundary layer which separates the absorptive membrane from the intestinal lumen. Thus lipolytic products (i.e. fatty acids and monoglycerides) and hydrophobic drug, if present, reside in the hydrophobic core regions of mixed intestinal micelles. In contrast, the surface of the micelles remains hydrophilic, and this facilitates rapid micellar diffusion across the aqueous boundary layer to the intestinal membrane. In the microclimate adjacent to the intestinal membrane, the pH is lower than in the intestinal lumen. This promotes demicellization, leading to the formation of a supersaturated solution of lipolytic products (and hydrophobic drug, if present) close to the enterocyte surface. These materials are then readily absorbed across the cell membrane by passive diffusion.

Mixed intestinal micelles comprising bile salts and lipolytic products can enhance the bioavailability of hydrophobic drugs whose absorption is normally dissolution-rate limited. This is because mixed intestinal micelles can be very potent solubilizing agents for a wide range of hydrophobic drugs, much more so than simple bile salt micelles formed in the absence of lipolytic products. For example, under simulated physiological conditions, the aqueous solubility of cinnarizine in simple bile salt micelles is 4 μg mL^{-1}, compared with 0.5 μg mL^{-1} in aqueous buffer. However, in the presence of mixed micelles, the solubility of cinnarizine is further enhanced to approximately 44 μg mL^{-1} (Embleton et al., 1995).

Taking cinnarizine as an example, it would be advantageous to formulate a softgel fill matrix that allows lipolysis to occur in the intestinal lumen because of the high drug solubility in lipolytic products. If the inhibition of lipolysis by a hydrophobic surfactant were allowed to occur, then it is highly likely that cinnarizine absorption would be impaired because of the reduced flow of drug into mixed micelles. However, if certain lipophilic surfactants with a hydrophile–lipophile balance (HLB) less than 10 are added to the formulation, then the inhibitory effects of hydrophilic surfactants on lipolysis can be reduced or eliminated.

Two formulations containing cinnarizine, a hydrophobic drug whose absorption is normally

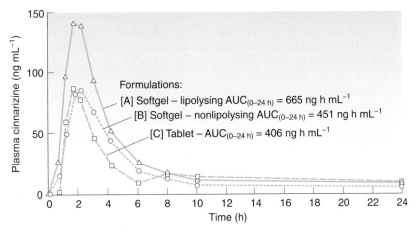

Fig. 34.12 • Plasma concentration versus time curves for three formulations of cinnarizine in the dog ($n = 6$). AUC, area under the plasma concentration versus time curve. From Embleton et al., 1995.

dissolution-rate limited, have been compared (Fig. 34.12; Embleton et al., 1995). Formulation A was prepared as a lipolysing formulation and formulation B was prepared as a nonlipolysing formulation, as demonstrated by the in vitro model. Formulation A was composed of a digestible triglyceride oil, a hydrophilic surfactant and a lipophilic surfactant, which was chosen on the basis of its ability to overcome the inhibitory effects of the hydrophilic surfactant on the in vitro triglyceride lipolysis. In vitro, this formulation exhibited 79% lipolysis after 60 minutes compared with the digestible oil alone. In contrast, formulation B contained a lipophilic surfactant that did not overcome the inhibitory effects of the hydrophilic surfactant on the lipolysis of the triglyceride oil and was shown to exhibit 3% lipolysis. It was proposed that the oil in formulation A, which forms a fine oil-in-water emulsion on aqueous dilution, is rapidly digested, forming mixed intestinal micelles with endogenous bile. These micelles transport the drug to the intestinal membrane, where the pH of the microclimate promotes micellar breakdown, facilitating enterocyte transport to the systemic circulation. In contrast, on dilution with aqueous fluids, formulation B forms a translucent microemulsion (as indicated by a blue tinge resulting from the Tyndall effect). As a result of this formulation failing to undergo lipolysis and thereby remaining unaffected by enzymic activity, the drug is maintained within the oil phase, inhibiting the production of mixed intestinal micelles, hence restricting absorption of the drug.

The significance of the lipolysis process in enhancing the bioavailability of hydrophobic drugs was investigated further in an in vivo study. This study compared the bioavailability of cinnarizine (30 mg) orally administered as a lipolysing formulation (formulation A) or a nonlipolysing formulation (formulation B) to six beagle dogs with a commercially available tablet (formulation C). The area under the plasma concentration–time curve (0 h to 24 h) for formulation A compared with the tablet preparation was significantly increased by 64% and for formulation A compared with formulation B was increased by 48%. C_{max} of formulation A was approximately 75% higher than that of both formulation B and formulation C (Fig. 34.12).

The results of this study have given valuable insight into the effect of the microemulsion formulation on absorption of a hydrophobic drug in the gastrointestinal tract, and information as to how the lipolysis process may influence bioavailability (Lacy et al., 2000). More recently, several studies have been performed to improve the understanding of drug disposition from lipid-based formulation systems (Porter et al., 2008). A lipid formulation classification system has been devised to organize drug–lipid compositions according to the type of excipients used (Pouton, 2006):

type I: oils (triglycerides or mixed monoglycerides and diglycerides);

type II: water-insoluble surfactants with HLB < 12;

type III: water-soluble surfactants with HLB > 12; and

type IV: hydrophilic cosolvents such as polyethylene glycol.

The tendency for drugs to precipitate from lipid formulas in gastrointestinal fluid can be mitigated by the presence of polymeric precipitation inhibitors such as cellulosic excipients (Warren et al., 2010).

Product quality considerations

Ingredient specifications

All the ingredients of a softgel dosage form are controlled and tested to ensure compliance with pharmacopoeial specifications. Additional specification tests may be added for certain excipients to ensure manufacture of a high-quality softgel product. For example, it is important to limit certain trace impurities such as aldehydes and peroxides that may be present in polyethylene glycol. The presence of high levels of these impurities gives rise to cross-linking of the gelatin polymer, leading to nonsolubilization through further polymerization. On prolonged storage, this can lead to slow dissolution of the capsule shell and subsequent retarded drug release.

Gelatin also requires careful control of quality to ensure a manufacturable and stable product. The quality of gelatin is controlled by parameters such as the viscosity of a hot solution and the Bloom strength of the gel. The Bloom strength is a measure of gel rigidity (see also Chapter 33).

In-process testing

During the encapsulation process, tests for the following parameters are performed:

- the gel ribbon thickness;
- softgel seal thickness at the time of encapsulation;
- fill matrix weight and capsule shell weight; and
- softgel shell moisture level and softgel hardness at the end of the drying stage.

Appropriate control levels for these parameters are established during process development for each softgel product, and are applied in routine production-scale manufacture.

Finished product testing

Finished softgels are subjected to a number of tests in accordance with compendial requirements for unit dose capsule products. These normally include capsule appearance, active ingredient assay and related substances assay, as well as fill weight, content uniformity, microbiological testing and dissolution testing. Development of a dissolution test using traditional media can be a challenge for certain softgel formulations, including those with oily fills or those which rely on physiological conditions to release the drug. Some have argued that disintegration testing may be more suitable for certain softgels (Han & Gallery, 2006), whilst others use surfactant-based or enzyme-based media to achieve full dissolution in vitro.

Please check your eBook at **https://studentconsult. inkling.com/** for self-assessment questions. See inside cover for registration details.

References

Aboul-Einien, M.H., 2009. Formulation and evaluation of felodipine in softgels with a solubilized core. Asian J. Pharm. Sci. 4, 144–160.

Aungst, B.J., 2000. Mini review: intestinal permeation enhancers. J. Pharm. Sci. 89, 429–442.

Drewe, J., Meier, R., Vonderscherer, J., et al., 1992. Enhancement of the oral absorption of cyclosporin in man. Br. J. Clin. Pharmacol. 34, 60–64.

Embleton, J., Hutchison, K.G., Lacy, J., 1995. The effect of in-vivo lipolysis in improving the bioavailability of

orally administered cinnarizine in self-emulsifying oily vehicles. *American Association of Pharmaceutical Sciences Conference*, Miami Beach.

Ferdinando, J.C., 2000. Formulation solutions – softgels. Pharm. Manuf. and Pack. Sourcer Spring Issue, 69–73.

Gao, P., Charton, M., Morozowich, W., 2006. Speeding development of poorly soluble/poorly permeable drugs by SEDDS/S-SEDDS formulations and prodrugs (part II). Amer. Pharm. Rev. 9, 16–23.

Gullapalli, R.P., 2010. Review: Soft gelatin capsules (softgels). J. Pharm. Sci. 99, 4107–4148.

Han, J.-H., Gallery, J., 2006. A risk based approach to in vitro performance testing: a case study on the use of dissolution vs. disintegration for liquid filled soft gelatine capsules. Amer. Pharm. Rev. 9, 152–157.

Hom, F.S., Veresh, S.A., Ebert, W.R., 1975. Soft gelatin capsules II: oxygen permeability study of capsule shells. J. Pharm. Sci. 64, 851–857.

Jones, W.J., Francis, J.J., 2000. Softgels: consumer perceptions and market impact relative to other oral dosage forms. Adv. Ther. 17 (5), 213–221.

Klein, C.E., Chiu, Y.-L., Awani, W., et al., 2007. The tablet formulation of lopinavir/ritonavir provides similar bioavailability to the soft-gelatin capsule formulation with less pharmacokinetic variability and diminished food effect. J. Acquir. Immune Defic. Syndr. 44, 401–410.

Lacy, J.E., Embleton, J.K., Perry, E.A., 2000. Delivery systems for hydrophobic drugs. US Patent 6,096,338.

Lissy, M., Scallion, R., Stiff, D.D., et al., 2010. Pharmacokinetic comparison of an oral diclofenac potassium liquid-filled soft gelatin capsule with a diclofenac potassium tablet. Expert Opin. Pharmacother. 11, 701–708.

MacGregor, K.J., Embleton, J.K., Lacy, J.E., 1997. Influence of lipolysis on drug absorption from the gastrointestinal tract. Adv. Drug Deliv. Rev. 25, 33–46.

Meinzer, A., 1993. Sandimmun® Neoral® soft gelatin capsules. International Industrial Pharmaceutical Research Conference, Wisconsin.

Perlman, M.E., Murdande, S.B., Gumkowski, M.J., et al., 2008. Development of a self-emulsifying formulation that reduces the food effect for torcetrapib. Int. J. Pharm. 351, 15–22.

Perry, C.M., Noble, S., 1988. Saquinavir softgel capsule formulation. Drugs 55, 461–486.

Porter, C.J., Pouton, C.W., Cuine, J.F., et al., 2008. Enhancing intestinal drug solubilization using lipid-based delivery systems. Adv. Drug Deliv. Rev. 60, 673–691.

Pouton, C.W., 2006. Formulation of poorly water-soluble drugs for oral administration: physicochemical and physiological issues and the lipid formulation classification system. Eur. J. Pharm. Sci. 29, 278–287.

Saano, V., Paronen, P., Peura, P., 1991. Relative pharmacokinetics of three oral 400 mg ibuprofen dosage forms in healthy volunteers. Int. J. Clin. Pharmacol. 29, 381–385.

Seager, H., 1993. Soft gelatin capsule technology – a route to improved drug delivery. Pharm. Manuf. Rev. 5, 9–10.

Warren, D.B., Benameur, H., Porter, C.J., et al., 2010. Using polymeric precipitation inhibitors to improve the absorption of poorly water soluble drugs: a mechanistic basis for utility. J. Drug Target. 18, 704–731.

35

Dissolution testing of solid dosage forms

Ana Cristina Freire   Abdul W. Basit

CHAPTER CONTENTS

KEY POINTS

- Dissolution is often the rate-limiting step in the absorption of drugs with limited water solubility.
- Drug dissolution can be correlated to oral bioavailability, whilst disintegration is generally a poor indicator of the drug's oral bioavailability.
- Dissolution test conditions are selected on the basis of the characteristics of the drug, the type of drug product and the objective of the test.
- Dissolution testing is a key quality control test.
- Dissolution tests can be conducted in simple buffer solutions or in more biorelevant dissolution media.
- Dissolution tests are normally performed under sink conditions.
- There are four types of compendial dissolution apparatus: the basket apparatus, the paddle apparatus, the reciprocating cylinder and the flow-through cell.
- Noncompendial dissolution apparatus usually better simulate the physiology of the gastrointestinal tract.

The relevance of drug dissolution and dissolution testing

The biological events that occur in the body following the administration of a drug are varied and complex. Before being absorbed into the bloodstream, an orally administered drug is exposed to the dynamic conditions of the gastrointestinal lumen, and much of what happens there will have a bearing on its therapeutic activity.

A drug can permeate the intestinal mucosa only in its dissolved state. If the solubility of the drug in the gastrointestinal aqueous fluids is limited, dissolution will be the rate-limiting step in absorption, and will dictate the rate and extent to which the drug becomes available in the bloodstream. Because of the link between oral bioavailability and dissolution, most oral drug products such as suspensions, granules, pellets, tablets and capsules are currently required to be tested for their dissolution characteristics. Disintegration measurements are also routinely performed on immediate-release products, although, for the most part, the results from such tests correlate poorly with bioavailability.

The concept of dissolution from a physical chemistry standpoint is well established; research into the mechanisms of dissolution of solids in liquids started more than a century ago with the pioneering work of Noyes and Whitney (discussed fully in Chapter 2). However, it took several decades before the link between dissolution and oral bioavailability in the context of a pharmaceutical product was fully appreciated. This is considered to have occurred in 1951, when Edwards studied the dissolution of aspirin tablets in different media. His conclusions from that study were that "the dissolution of an aspirin tablet in the stomach and intestine is the rate process controlling the absorption of aspirin into the bloodstream".

The clinical relevance of the observations of Edwards was realized only in the mid-1960s, when several reports linking dissolution data with clinical efficacy, inferior efficacy and even toxicity of some commercial oral solid drug products were made available. For example, clinical inadequacies with formulations of the oral antidiabetic and poorly water-soluble drug tolbutamide were documented. Ineffective tablets were shown to disintegrate and dissolve at a slower rate than those which were clinically effective (Fig. 35.1).

Reports of toxicity with a formulation of phenytoin available in Australia and New Zealand followed in 1968. The substitution of the more hydrophilic excipient lactose for calcium sulfate in an immediate-release hard gelatin capsule enhanced the dissolution rate and bioavailability of phenytoin, leading to numerous cases of anticonvulsant intoxication. This is further discussed in Chapter 33 (see Fig. 33.6 and the associated text).

However, undoubtedly the reference case for the impact of drug dissolution on oral bioavailability was that of digoxin tablets. In the early 1970s, several marketed formulations of digoxin were shown to yield up to sevenfold differences in blood levels of the drug. In the search for an explanation, digoxin tablet formulations were studied for their dissolution properties, exposing huge differences in this parameter. Interestingly, a good correlation was noted between the dissolution rate and digoxin blood levels. In other words, absorption of digoxin was higher for those formulations which dissolved more quickly (Fig. 35.2). In contrast, the disintegration time of the different tablets was very similar and bore no relation to digoxin blood levels, raising questions as to the value of the disintegration test in detecting differences in the oral bioavailability of solid drug products.

In light of these cases, it became clear that the formulation and manufacturing process was linked to the therapeutic efficacy of the drug. Dissolution, and not disintegration, became an accepted indicator of oral bioavailability of solid drug products. This prompted the US Food and Drug Administration(FDA) to make the use of dissolution testing official in 1970, and to introduce dissolution requirements in the pharmacopoeial monographs of tablets and capsules. By 1995, four different dissolution apparatus had been included in the *United States Pharmacopeia* (USP).

General requirements for in vitro dissolution testing

Today, in vitro dissolution studies are performed for several reasons:

- most often to ensure that preparations comply with product specifications;
- to evaluate the potential effect of formulation and process variables on the bioavailability of a drug during product development; and
- to provide an indication of the performance of the preparation in vivo.

Changes to the release profile and/or dissolution rate of the drug can be brought about by the characteristics of the dosage form and by its method of manufacture. However, dissolution becomes more complicated if

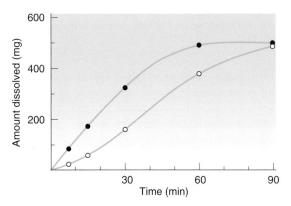

Fig. 35.1 Dissolution of tolbutamide from clinically effective tablets *(closed circles)* and clinically ineffective tablets *(open circles)* as a function of time. From Levy, 1964.

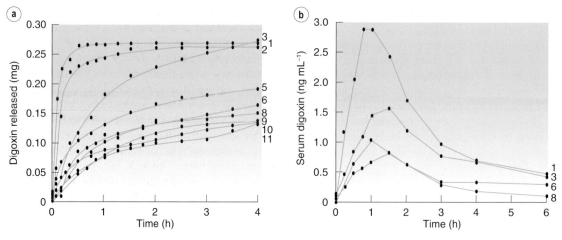

Fig. 35.2 Dissolution rates of different brands of digoxin tablets available on the UK market at the time of the study **(a)** and corresponding blood (serum) levels of digoxin **(b)**. Formulation 1 ('new Lanoxin') and formulation 8 ('old Lanoxin') are from the same brand, prepared by different manufacturing methods. Adapted from Fraser et al., 1973.

the physiological properties of the gastrointestinal tract are taken into consideration (see Chapter 19). These must be reflected in any efficient in vitro test.

pH of the gastrointestinal luminal fluids

As it travels through the gastrointestinal tract, a drug is exposed to conditions of increasing pH. Such pH conditions play an important role in the solubility of ionizable drugs, with pK_a values within the pH physiological range (1–7.5), and may affect their bioavailability (discussed fully in Chapter 20). This must be simulated, particularly in predictive dissolution testing (see later).

Composition of the gastrointestinal luminal fluids

Whilst pH may be sufficiently simulated with buffered solutions, the composition of the gastrointestinal tract fluids is not. Gastrointestinal luminal fluids are enriched with amphiphilic bile components, such as bile salts and lecithin. These substances enhance the dissolution rate of drugs either via an increase in wettability or, at higher concentrations, through the formation of micelles. Although fasted-state fluids already have wetting and solubilizing effects, these are further increased after a meal, owing to increased secretion of bile and the presence of degradation products of lipids contained in the meal (i.e. fatty acids and monoglycerides). For this reason, the dissolution of poorly soluble drugs is generally higher

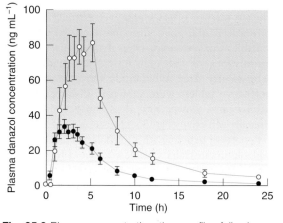

Fig. 35.3 Plasma concentration–time profiles following administration of 100 mg danazol in a hard gelatin capsule in the fed state *(open circles)* and the fasted state *(closed circles)* in humans. Adapted from Charman et al., 1993.

in fed conditions than in fasted conditions. This is well exemplified by the lipophilic drug danazol; as seen in Fig. 35.3, the bioavailability of this compound is considerably higher in the fed state.

Two main uses of in vitro dissolution testing are now discussed further. These are:

- to assess the quality of solid drug products (i.e. using in vitro dissolution testing as a quality control tool); and
- as a prognostic tool for the performance of solid drug products in the gastrointestinal tract (known as predictive dissolution).

As a quality control tool

Before a drug product is released onto the market (and routinely once it has been marketed), it must be subjected to rigorous control to ensure that the quality and performance (with regard to both safety and efficacy) of the final product are acceptable. Currently, almost all solid oral drug products require in vitro dissolution testing as part of their quality control (QC) assessment. This involves analysing the drug-release profile of different batches of the same drug product with a view to either confirming manufacturing and product consistency or to verify the stability of the product during its shelf life.

Predictive dissolution testing

Dissolution data can also be used as a prognostic tool to predict the behaviour and performance of oral solid drug products in the gastrointestinal tract. The aim is to correlate as closely as possible measured in vitro parameters with oral bioavailability. This type of dissolution testing is known as *predictive dissolution testing*. Unlike QC dissolution testing, it may require dissolution test methods which reflect more closely the physiological make-up of the gastrointestinal tract. Such test conditions are not easy to devise, but if they are devised appropriately, they will enable the development of in vitro/in vivo predictions.

These predictions can be simple qualitative or semiquantitative relationships (in vitro–in vivo relationships) or quantitative correlations established using mathematical models (in vitro–in vivo correlations, IVIVCs). In its simplest definition, an IVIVC is a correlation (preferably linear) between an in vitro feature of the drug product (in the present context, its dissolution characteristics) and a biological parameter (e.g. the uptake of the drug in vivo and subsequent drug blood levels). The establishment of such a correlation during predictive dissolution testing is one of the most important aspects of a dissolution test for a preparation undergoing formulation development.

Predictive dissolution data have two main applications. Firstly, they can guide the early development of a new drug product by selecting formulations that yield the desired in vivo dissolution characteristics. Secondly, they serve as a surrogate for clinical studies. In order to introduce new generic drug products onto the market, companies are required to demonstrate that the generic product yields rates and extents of drug absorption statistically similar to those of the innovator (or branded) drug product – in other words, that the two products are bioequivalent.

Bioequivalence has traditionally been demonstrated in appropriately designed clinical studies, which are both time-consuming and expensive. However, following the introduction of the Biopharmaceutics Classification System in 1995 (see Chapter 21), it became apparent that the dissolution data of some drug products can be correlated to oral bioavailability. Since 2000, bioequivalence between immediate-release products of highly water-soluble and easily absorbed drugs can be established on the basis of dissolution data, provided that the excipients present in the formulation do not affect the absorption of the drug.

Dissolution testing

The aim of any dissolution test is to measure the rate at which the drug substance is released from the dosage form and dissolves in a particular dissolution medium. It is necessary for such tests to be performed under well-defined conditions to allow comparison of observed data. Various guidelines and protocols are available. However, in many instances it is left to the scientists to decide the best conditions. Choosing these conditions is never an easy task. Protocols tend to vary greatly amongst drug products, and often the same product is tested under different conditions, depending on whether the test is conducted for QC purposes or to predict the performance of the drug product in the gastrointestinal tract. Key variables to consider when designing dissolution tests are described in the following paragraphs.

Type of dissolution apparatus used. Although many types of dissolution apparatus are available, the most commonly used are compendial dissolution apparatus. These are standardized and robust dissolution testers described by pharmacopoeias.

Volume and composition of the dissolution medium. The selection of the medium and its volume is guided by the aim of the dissolution test, the solubility of the drug and the type of apparatus used. All tests are conducted at 37 °C to mimic body temperature.

Hydrodynamics. This refers to the mechanical agitation provided by the dissolution apparatus which will aid in the dissolution of the drug. The various dissolution apparatus offer different hydrodynamics, and these may be varied to allow the best results to be obtained.

Number of units to be tested. Dissolution tests designed to assess the quality of a batch of tablets are normally repeated for at least six units per batch or formulation, depending on test variability.

The design of suitable dissolution tests; quality control versus predictive dissolution testing

QC dissolution methods are often easier to design; these make use of established compendial equipment, and the composition and volume of the dissolution medium is generally chosen according to the solubility of the drug. Devising a predictive dissolution test is more challenging as biorelevant conditions need to be sought to mimic the physiological parameters which affect the dissolution of the drug in the gastrointestinal tract. The major considerations in designing both types of dissolution test methods are described in the following sections.

Dissolution testing for quality control

QC methods are described in the monograph of the product in the various pharmacopoeias. As a general rule, these methods are of simple execution, reliable, reproducible, yet sufficiently discriminatory to be able to detect small product deviations. From a QC point of view, an overdiscriminatory method is sometimes preferred so as to detect any product changes before the performance in the gastrointestinal tract is affected. The other prime concern of a QC test is to use conditions under which at least 80% of the drug can be dissolved.

Compendial dissolution apparatus

Four dissolution apparatus are currently described in the US and European pharmacopoeias for the testing of oral solid drug products. These are the basket apparatus (Fig. 35.4), the paddle apparatus (Fig. 35.5), the reciprocating cylinder (Fig. 35.6) and the flow-through cell (Fig. 35.7). The selection of a dissolution apparatus depends mainly on the solubility of the drug and the type of dosage form. The first-choice equipment for QC dissolution testing is the basket apparatus and the paddle apparatus because their simple design makes them ideal for routine use. However, because of the limited volume of the

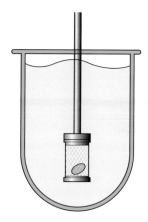

Fig. 35.4 Basket apparatus (*United States Pharmacopeia* Apparatus 1).

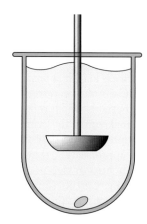

Fig. 35.5 Paddle apparatus (*United States Pharmacopeia* Apparatus 2).

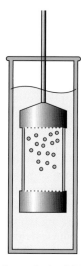

Fig. 35.6 Reciprocating cylinder (*United States Pharmacopeia* Apparatus 3).

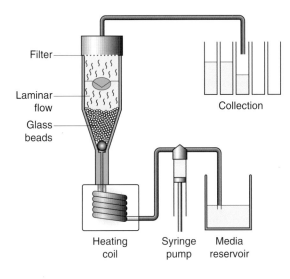

Fig. 35.7 Flow-through cell (*United States Pharmacopeia* Apparatus 4).

medium and operational difficulties in changing the medium, these apparatus are often more suited to immediate-release products than to modified-release products, and in particular immediate-release formulations of soluble drugs.

The reciprocating cylinder and flow-through cell systems are particularly useful for the testing of modified-release dosage forms and poorly soluble drugs respectively. A brief description of each apparatus is given in the following sections. Advantages and disadvantages of their use are summarized in Table 35.1.

Many pharmacopoeias worldwide define detailed specifications for standard dissolution apparatus and methods. As a result of harmonization of these standards, most pharmacopoeial specifications are extremely similar. For brevity, this chapter will refer to the USP specifications. All major pharmacopoeias are very similar, but even if the detail differs, the

Table 35.1 Advantages and disadvantages of compendial dissolution apparatus

Apparatus	Advantages	Disadvantages
Basket (USP Apparatus 1)	Suited for QC dissolution testing Broad experience Easy to operate Standardized Robust	Fixed (limited) volume of medium makes it unsuitable for testing of poorly soluble drugs Formulation may clog the basket mesh Small disintegrated particles may fall out
Paddle (USP Apparatus 2)	First-choice apparatus for QC dissolution testing Broad experience Easy to operate Standardized Robust	Fixed (limited) volume of medium makes it unsuitable for testing of poorly soluble drugs Floating dosage forms (e.g. capsules) require sinkers Positioning of the dosage form in the vessel is important
Reciprocating cylinder (USP Apparatus 3)	Change of media fully automated Ease of sampling Suitable for QC testing of modified-release products Small volumes of media suitable for predictive dissolution Hydrodynamics more similar to those in the gastrointestinal tract	Not suitable for dosage forms that disintegrate into small particles The use of surfactants is discouraged as they can cause foaming Small volumes of media unsuitable for QC dissolution testing of poorly soluble drugs Evaporation of media in tests of long duration
Flow-through cell (USP Apparatus 4)	Unlimited fluid supply makes it ideal for testing poorly soluble drugs Gentle hydrodynamic conditions and possibility of varying hydrodynamics during the test Allows rapid change of media Continuous sampling	Limited experience Complex design makes it inappropriate for QC dissolution testing Results very dependent on the type of pump used

QC, Quality control; *USP*, United States Pharmacopeia.

principle of operation and interpretation of the results is the same.

Basket apparatus (USP Apparatus 1)

The basket apparatus was the first official dissolution tester to be described in the USP, in 1970, and remains one of the most commonly used methods for testing the dissolution of capsules and tablets.

In this apparatus the dosage form is placed inside a rotating basket made of a stainless steel wire mesh and immersed in dissolution medium, which has been prewarmed, at 37 °C. An outline of the apparatus is shown in Fig. 35.4, with a more detailed diagram shown in Fig. 30.20. During the test the basket rotates at a constant speed, typically set between 50 and 100 rpm. The dissolution medium is contained in a glass cylindrical vessel with a spherical bottom and with a nominal capacity of no less than 1 L. The dissolution medium volume used with this method is normally 0.9 L, although lower (0.5 L) and higher (4 L) volumes may also be used. The composition and/or pH of the medium may be changed by manual replacement of the medium or by adding media of different composition. At predetermined times, samples of the dissolution medium are removed and analysed for drug content.

Paddle apparatus (USP Apparatus 2)

Following its introduction in the USP in 1978, the paddle apparatus became the most widely used dissolution tester. It uses the same dissolution vessels as the basket apparatus but here the dosage form is positioned at the centre bottom of the vessel. An outline of the apparatus is shown in Fig. 35.5, with a more detailed diagram shown in Fig. 30.21. Agitation is provided by a metallic paddle which rotates at speeds between 50 and 150 rpm (most often 50–75 rpm). To prevent dosage forms from floating (this normally occurs with capsules), the use of sinkers is recommended. Sinkers are a wire helix made of nonreactive material wherein the dosage form is placed. Changes of the dissolution medium during the test are done manually, as described for the basket apparatus.

Reciprocating cylinder (USP Apparatus 3)

In 1991, driven by the need to provide a controlled and automated pH and volume change of the dissolution medium during the test, the USP introduced the reciprocating cylinder apparatus. Current designs of this equipment allow up to six automated medium changes per test, as well as changes to the agitation speed. This feature makes it particularly suited to estimate the drug release profile in different parts of the gastrointestinal tract as needed in the case of modified-release formulations, such as extended-release or gastro-resistant coated products. It also represents a step closer to biorelevant conditions and to developing IVIVCs.

The apparatus (Fig. 35.6) comprises two cylinders: an inner cylinder containing the dosage form and an outer cylinder vessel, which holds approximately 200 mL to 300 mL of dissolution medium. During the test the inner cylinder is dipped vertically into the dissolution medium several times, creating convective forces for dissolution. It is generally considered that five dips per minute is equivalent to 50 rpm in the paddle apparatus. The inner cylinder is fitted with a mesh screen at the bottom and top which allows the medium to circulate freely inside it, yet prevents losses of finely disintegrated material.

Flow-through cell (USP Apparatus 4)

The flow-through cell was adopted by the USP in 1995, primarily for the testing of modified-release products. In this apparatus the dosage form is positioned in a small-volume cell, on a glass bead bed or on a clip holder. The sample under test is subjected to a continuous flow of media in an upward direction. The medium is pumped from a reservoir at a flow rate which may range from 5 mL min^{-1} to 20 mL min^{-1}. The pulsating movement of the pump creates gentler hydrodynamics compared with other compendial apparatus (arguably more similar to the movement that would be experienced by a dosage form in the gut). The dissolution medium can be changed during the test by exchanging the media reservoirs.

This apparatus (Fig. 35.7) can be configured to use a fixed volume (closed system) or unlimited volumes of the dissolution medium (open system). In the latter set-up, fresh dissolution medium is delivered continuously by the pump and collected for analysis after it has passed though the sample cell; this system is particularly suitable for testing the dissolution of poorly soluble drugs.

Volume and composition of the dissolution medium

The choice of the volume and composition of the dissolution medium is very much dependent on the solubility of the drug. As previously mentioned, a QC dissolution method must allow for at least 80% of the drug to dissolve during the duration of the test. To achieve this, QC methods are normally operated under 'sink conditions'. A dissolution test is said to be performed under sink conditions if the concentration of the drug in the bulk of the dissolution medium does not exceed 10% of the solubility of the drug. Under sink conditions the concentration gradient between the diffusion layer surrounding the solid drug particles and the dissolution medium is assumed to be constant (see Chapter 2). Sink conditions may represent an important deviation from what happens in the gastrointestinal tract, where such conditions are not always present and dissolution of poorly soluble drugs is often incomplete.

Sink conditions are easy to achieve with highly water-soluble drugs but pose a considerable problem for those drugs which have limited aqueous solubility. The basket and paddle apparatus are normally operated with a volume of 0.9 L, and although this may be increased to 4 L, it may still not permit sink conditions to be reached for some drugs. Increasing the volume beyond 4 L is possible only with the flow-through cell system. However, this apparatus is unsuitable for routine use; therefore, choosing a medium in which the drug is soluble is of paramount importance. Other considerations in choosing a QC dissolution medium are:

- it must not affect the stability of the drug;
- simple composition is required to permit automation of the method;
- it must be easy to be prepare;
- it must be inexpensive; and
- it should preferably be nonorganic.

Not surprisingly, very few media meet such requirements to be regarded as suitable for QC dissolution testing. Although pure water would appear to be an obvious choice, its use is discouraged because of the inability of this medium to withstand pH changes. The most commonly used dissolution media are either dilute acid solutions or aqueous buffers of a higher pH. Weakly basic drugs, by virtue of their higher solubility under acid conditions, are most often tested in diluted acid solutions (e.g. 0.1 M hydrochloric acid or simulated gastric fluids). These are also the media of choice for immediate-release dosage forms of highly soluble drugs. Phosphate buffer solutions (which can be manipulated to have a pH between 5.0 and 8.0) are suited for the testing of weakly acidic drugs. If the solubility of the drug in these media is low, surfactants can be added to the media to enhance drug solubility and meet sink conditions.

Dissolution limits

Performing the dissolution test is only one part of QC testing. The data obtained must be checked against set dissolution limits to ensure that the drug product meets the required specifications. Dissolution limits for immediate-release and gastro-resistant coated products are defined in the pharmacopoeias, with slight variations between the various pharmacopoeias.

For immediate-release products, a single-point specification is used to ensure prompt dissolution; normally no less than 75% of the drug must be dissolved within 45 minutes.

Dissolution limits for gastro-resistant products are based on a two-point specification to ensure limited drug dissolution in the acidic conditions of the stomach and fast dissolution in the conditions of the small intestine. The specifications are typically no more than 10% of the drug dissolved in 0.1 M hydrochloric acid within 2 hours (the typical maximum residence time of nondisintegrating tablets in the fasted stomach), followed by no less than 75% dissolution within 45 minutes in phosphate buffer (pH 6.8).

As for extended-release products, the specifications may be set by the product's manufacturer. A minimum of two specification points are normally required; the earlier specification point provides assurance against premature drug dissolution, while the second should ensure complete drug dissolution.

Predictive dissolution testing

Predictive dissolution tests are designed to give a close account of the product's performance in the gastrointestinal tract (rather than a simple yes/no result as in the case of QC dissolution tests). The best way to achieve this is by using dissolution conditions which mirror, as closely as possible, the physiology of the gastrointestinal tract. However, recreating such conditions is a great challenge. This is because the gastrointestinal tract is a very complex and dynamic environment; its physiology changes every day and throughout our lives, is affected by a number of diseases and by the food we consume, and above all, it is still poorly understood.

Dissolution data indicative of performance in the gastrointestinal tract can be obtained by adding surfactants to the dissolution medium to better simulate the solubility of the drug in the gastrointestinal luminal fluids. Although this is a very common strategy, it must be tested carefully, as many artificial surfactants, when used in high concentrations, may solubilize the drug too well and overestimate the solubility of the drug in the gastrointestinal luminal fluids. For extended-release drug products and whenever the solubility of the drug is pH dependent, use of different buffered solutions with various pH values so as to simulate transit through different segments of the gastrointestinal tract may be useful. These changing pH conditions are easy to recreate with USP Apparatus 3 and USP Apparatus 4 but not with USP Apparatus 1 and USP Apparatus 2. When these simple test methods fail, more advanced ones are required. Next we discuss the biorelevant media and noncompendial dissolution apparatus that are being used increasingly to develop predictive dissolution tests.

Biorelevant dissolution media

The composition of the gastrointestinal tract luminal fluids could not be any more different from that of the simple buffered aqueous solutions that are used for the QC dissolution testing of drugs. Ingested food and endogenous fluids are mixed together in the lumen of the gastrointestinal tract, yielding a compositionally complex medium, the pH, composition and volume thereof are constantly changing in response to external and internal stimuli. Understandably its complexity and dynamic nature cannot be completely simulated; rather only a few parameters which are more likely to affect the solubility of drugs are often incorporated into the design of a biorelevant dissolution medium.

Milk and nutritional liquid products

Dissolution testing may be performed in media simulating the contents of a meal with a view to predicting food effects. For example, full-fat milk (with 3.5% fat) and Ensure® Plus have been successfully used to simulate the initial stages of the fed stomach. Both media contain protein, fat and carbohydrates in ratios which are comparable to those found in the typical Western diet. Fat and proteins aid the dissolution of poorly soluble drugs, whereas the higher pH of these media favours the dissolution of weak acidic drugs. Apart from the effect on solubility, milk may also delay the disintegration of slow-disintegrating tablets.

Simulated gastric and intestinal fluids

Simulated gastric or intestinal fluids are aqueous-based solutions containing one or more biological components which are known to influence the dissolution of drugs in vivo.

Media containing enzymes (pepsin or pancreatin) and artificial surfactants, in concentrations greater than those found in the gastrointestinal tract, were amongst the first to be developed to simulate the fasted gastric and small intestinal fluids. These media were soon found to overestimate the solubility of many drugs in the gastrointestinal fluids.

In a later development, fasted-state gastric and intestinal simulated media containing physiological concentrations of natural bile salts (sodium taurocholate) and lecithin were introduced. The fed-state versions of these media are more complex; they contain milk or lipolysis products to simulate adequately the influence of meal digestion on the solubility of drugs. The full compositions of these media are given in Tables 35.2 and 35.3.

Bicarbonate buffers

Bicarbonate is the main buffer species in the luminal fluids of the small intestine. However, thus far its use in dissolution media has been very limited. Dissolution media are typically composed of phosphate ions, whose presence in the gastrointestinal luminal fluids is insignificant. A change from phosphate-based to bicarbonate-based buffers should therefore better resemble the ionic composition and buffer capacity of the fasted jejunal and ileal fluids. The few dissolution studies that have used bicarbonate buffers found these to be superior to phosphate buffers in predicting the dissolution behaviour of gastro-resistant polymers and the solubility of ionizable drugs in the gastrointestinal tract (Liu et al., 2011).

Unlike the fasted-state and fed-state simulated fluids, these buffers are easy to prepare and their composition is very simple. However, because of the difficulty in stabilizing the pH, bicarbonate buffers must be continuously purged with carbon dioxide, making the experimental set-up more difficult. Nevertheless, in recent years computer-controlled dynamic dissolution systems based on bicarbonate buffers have been developed, showing good IVIVCs

Table 35.2 Composition of fasted-state and fed-state state simulated gastric fluids

FaSSGF		FeSSGF	
Sodium taurocholate (mmol L^{-1})	0.08	Sodium chloride (mmol L^{-1})	237.02
Lecithin (mmol L^{-1})	0.02	Acetic acid (mmol L^{-1})	17.12
Pepsin (mg mL^{-1})	0.1	Sodium acetate (mmol L^{-1})	29.75
Sodium chloride (mmol L^{-1})	34.2	Milk and buffer	1:1
		Hydrochloric acid/sodium hydroxide	qs to pH 5
pH	1.6	pH	5.0
Osmolality (mOsm kg^{-1})	120.7 ± 2.5	Osmolality (mOsm kg^{-1})	400
Buffer capacity (mmol L^{-1} ΔpH^{-1})	–	Buffer capacity (mmol L^{-1} ΔpH^{-1})	25

FaSSGF, Fasted-state simulated gastric fluid; *FeSSGF*, fed-state simulated gastric fluid.
Data from Jantratid et al. (2008).

Table 35.3 Composition of fasted-state and fed-state simulated intestinal fluids

FaSSIF		FeSSIF	
Sodium taurocholate (mmol L^{-1})	3	Sodium taurocholate (mmol L^{-1})	10
Lecithin (mmol L^{-1})	0.2	Lecithin (mmol L^{-1})	2
Maleic acid (mmol L^{-1})	19.12	Glyceryl monooleate (mmol L^{-1})	5
Sodium hydroxide (mmol L^{-1})	34.8	Sodium oleate (mmol L^{-1})	0.8
Sodium chloride (mmol L^{-1})	68.62	Maleic acid (mmol L^{-1})	55.02
		Sodium hydroxide (mmol L^{-1})	81.65
		Sodium chloride (mmol L^{-1})	125.5
pH	6.5	pH	5.8
Osmolality (mOsm kg^{-1})	180±10	Osmolality (mOsm kg^{-1})	390 ± 10
Buffer capacity (mmol L^{-1} ΔpH^{-1})	10	Buffer capacity (mmol L^{-1} ΔpH^{-1})	25

FaSSIF, Fasted-state simulated intestinal fluid; *FeSSIF*, fed-state simulated intestinal fluid.
Data from Jantratid et al. (2008).

for modified-release products (Merchant et al., 2014; Goyanes et al., 2015).

Noncompendial apparatus

The various compendial dissolution apparatus bear little resemblance to the gastrointestinal tract physiology, and recreating such complexity in vitro may be too great a task. The gastrointestinal tract simply does not 'paddle' in the same way or at the same speed as the compendial dissolution apparatus. Attempts to render flow rates more biorelevant led to the development of USP Apparatus 4. However, its unidirectional flow pattern does not account for retropulsion, and the flow patterns used may still be too strong compared with those in the gastrointestinal tract. Apart from poor hydrodynamics, the closed and static environment of compendial dissolution apparatus does not account for drug transport across the intestinal mucosa. Combining drug dissolution with absorption may improve the predictive power of dissolution testing. Some examples of noncompendial apparatus, which are increasingly being used to establish IVIVCs, are described in the following sections.

Stress test apparatus

This novel apparatus simulates the irregular motility patterns of the gastrointestinal tract and the physical stress experienced by the dosage form during gastric emptying and transit through the gut. Its design allows the dosage form to be either submerged in liquid or exposed to air in an attempt to recreate the discontinuous distribution of fluid in the intestines.

This apparatus has been shown to successfully reproduce the dissolution profile of an extended-release formulation of diclofenac in the gastrointestinal tract, which was not possible with USP Apparatus 2 (Garbacz et al., 2008).

Dynamic Gastric Model

The Dynamic Gastric Model (DGM) is a computer-controlled simulator of the digestion patterns of the stomach. It consists of three mains parts: the main body (or fundus), the valve assembly and the distal region of the stomach or antrum. The simulator models the mechanical and enzymatic events occurring in these regions and which lead to the digestion of meals. Heterogeneous gastric mixing in the main body of the stomach is provided by gentle contractions. Gastric secretions (acid and enzymes) are delivered via a dispenser, from the sides of the simulator to recreate the secretion of these compounds by the gastrointestinal mucosa. The rate at which secretions are released into the main body is controlled by the volume and pH of the contents in a manner similar to that in the gastrointestinal tract (Vardakou et al., 2011).

The contents are moved from the main body into the antrum and vice versa through the valve assembly. The forces which coexist in the antrum are considerably stronger than those in the main body; these represent the physiological grinding forces responsible for the breakdown of food particles. Once ready, the processed bolus is ejected through a valve and collected for further analysis.

As stand-alone equipment, the DGM is unlikely to give a useful estimate of the performance of dosage forms in the gastrointestinal tract. However, if it is combined with an equally biorelevant simulator of the small intestine, the DGM may provide good correlations to oral bioavailability.

Simulator of the gastrointestinal tract (TIM-1)

The dynamic system known as TIM-1 is the most complete simulator of the gastrointestinal tract. TIM-1 models the upper gastrointestinal tract and is composed of interconnected segments representing the stomach, duodenum, jejunum and ileum. Most physiological parameters such as body temperature, pH, peristaltic mixing, gastrointestinal tract transit and main secretions (saliva, lipase, pepsin, HCl, pancreatic juice, bile and sodium bicarbonate) are simulated with this system. Transit is regulated by peristaltic valves which exist at the end of each segment, and mixing is generated by consecutive cycles of compression and relaxation (Blanquet et al., 2004).

Its unique feature is the ability to simulate passive absorption of water and small molecules, such as dissolved drug, via dialysis membranes. Although this represents a vast improvement compared with most simulators which do not account for absorption, it is still far from the conditions present in the gastrointestinal tract, where active transport, efflux and intestinal wall metabolism are also present.

TIM-1 can be used to predict the performance of dosage forms in the gastrointestinal tract, yet this is not without some technical problems. For instance, each experiment takes considerably longer than a standard dissolution test, and the conditions in which the test is conducted are often drug specific and formulation specific. Problems aside, this simulator has successfully established IVIVCs where compendial dissolution apparatus have failed.

Conclusions

Testing of the dissolution properties of oral solid drug products has been practised in the pharmaceutical industry for many decades, yet the role of such tests is still very much evolving. What was once a simple test to differentiate a 'good' batch of a drug product from a 'bad' one is now developing into a key tool for predicting bioavailability. In early-stage research and development, dissolution data aid in the selection of candidate formulations for further development, a role of increasing relevance because of the growing number of poorly water-soluble investigational drugs. From a regulatory point of view, dissolution testing may be used to establish equivalence between drug products, obviating the need for expensive and lengthy clinical studies.

Given the many uses and benefits of dissolution testing in various stages of the drug product's lifecycle, it is not surprising that considerable efforts have been made into developing appropriate dissolution methods. As there is no absolute method for dissolution testing, pharmaceutical scientists are constantly being challenged to design new methods based on the goal of the test (i.e. QC, establishing IVIVC or demonstrating bioequivalence) and on the characteristics of the drug product. The key challenge remains that of designing predictive dissolution tests because of the difficulties in simulating the interactions between the drug and the complex environment of the gastrointestinal tract. However, as understanding of these interactions improves, so does the predictive power of dissolution tests. The recent development of biorelevant dissolution media and the design of sophisticated simulators of the gastrointestinal tract are key examples of this.

Please check your eBook at **https://studentconsult.inkling.com/** for self-assessment questions. See inside cover for registration details.

References

Blanquet, S., Zeijdner, E., Beyssac, E., et al., 2004. A dynamic artificial gastrointestinal system for studying the behavior of orally administered drug dosage forms under various physiological conditions. Pharm. Res. 21, 585–591.

Charman, W.N., Rogge, M.C., Boddy, A.H., et al., 1993. Effect of food and a monoglyceride emulsion formulation on danazol bioavailability. J. Clin. Pharmacol. 33, 381–386.

Fraser, E.J., Leach, R.H., Poston, J.W., et al., 1973. Dissolution and bioavailability of digoxin tablets. J. Pharm. Pharmacol. 25, 968–973.

Garbacz, G., Wedemeyer, R.-S., Nagel, S., et al., 2008. Irregular absorption profiles observed from diclofenac extended release tablets can be predicted using a dissolution test apparatus that mimics in vivo physical stresses. Eur. J. Pharm. Biopharm. 70, 421–428.

Goyanes, A., Hatton, G.B., Merchant, H.A., et al., 2015. Gastrointestinal release behaviour of modified-release drug products: dynamic dissolution testing of mesalazine formulations. Int. J. Pharm. 484, 103–108.

Jantratid, E., Janssen, N., Reppas, C., et al., 2008. Dissolution media simulating conditions in the proximal human gastrointestinal tract: an update. Pharm. Res. 25, 1663–1676.

Levy, G., 1964. Effect of dosage form properties on therapeutic efficacy of tolbutamide tablets. Can. Med. Assoc. J. 90, 978–979.

Liu, F., Merchant, H.A., Kulkarni, R.P., et al., 2011. Evolution of a physiological pH 6.8 bicarbonate buffer system: application to the dissolution testing of enteric coated products. Eur. J. Pharm. Biopharm. 78, 151–157.

Merchant, H.A., Goyanes, A., Parashar, N., et al., 2014. Predicting the gastrointestinal behaviour of modified-release products: utility of a novel dynamic dissolution test apparatus involving the use of bicarbonate buffers. Int. J. Pharm. 475, 585–591.

Vardakou, M., Mercuri, A., Naylor, T.A., et al., 2011. Predicting the human in vivo performance of different oral capsule shell types using a novel in vitro dynamic gastric model. Int. J. Pharm. 419, 192–199.

Bibliography

Dokoumetzidis, A., Macheras, P., 2006. A century of dissolution research: From Noyes and Whitney to the Biopharmaceutics Classification System. Int. J. Pharm. 321, 1–11.

Freire, A.C., Basit, A.W., Choudhary, R., et al., 2011. Does sex matter? The influence of gender on gastrointestinal physiology and drug delivery. Int. J. Pharm. 415, 15–28.

Limberg, J., Potthast, H., 2013. Regulatory status on the role of in vitro dissolution testing in quality control and biopharmaceutics in Europe. Biopharm. Drug Dispos. 34, 247–253.

McAllister, M., 2010. Dynamic dissolution: a step closer to predictive dissolution testing? Mol. Pharm. 7, 1374–1387.

Mudie, D.M., Amidon, G.L., Amidon, G.E., 2010. Physiological parameters for oral delivery and in vitro testing. Mol. Pharm. 7, 1388–1405.

Varum, F.J., Hatton, G.B., Basit, A.W., 2013. Food, physiology and drug delivery. Int. J. Pharm. 457, 446–460.

36

Parenteral drug delivery

Robert Lowe

CHAPTER CONTENTS

KEY POINTS

- Parenteral preparations are administered to a patient by injection.
- The medicine may be injected into the vascular system, into muscle or soft tissue to provide a systemic action, or into an anatomical space (such as a joint), or into a particular organ to provide a local action.
- Medicines are administered by injection because the drug substance may not be absorbed orally, because a rapid effect may be required in an emergency, because a prolonged and controlled effect may be required or because the oral route of administration is not available (e.g. the patient is unconscious).
- There are both general pharmacopoeial standards and category-specific pharmacopoeial standards (injections, infusions, etc.) with which parenteral products must comply.
- All parenteral products must be sterile.
- The formulation of a parenteral preparation can affect how rapidly or slowly the drug is absorbed from the site of injection.
- Excipients may be added to parenteral preparations to adjust the pH and tonicity of the preparation to mimic human plasma values. Excipients can be added to increase the stability or solubility of the drug.
- Parenteral preparations intended for multiple use must contain an antimicrobial preservative.
- Containers for parenteral preparations should be made, where possible, from transparent, inert materials such as glass or plastic. They must be airtight to maintain the sterility of the preparation before use.

Introduction

In medicine and pharmacy, *enteral administration* is the term used to describe drug administration via the gastrointestinal tract. Most medicines are administered orally via this route in the form of tablets, capsules or liquids. The enteral route also encompasses rectal administration using dosage forms such as suppositories, enemas or rectal ointments. In contrast to this, the term *parenteral administration* literally means any method of drug administration which does not use the gastrointestinal tract, such as by inhalation or application to the skin. In practice, however, parenteral administration is commonly taken to mean drug administration by injection, and this is how the term is interpreted in this chapter.

In this chapter we will explore why the parenteral route of administration may be chosen by the clinician or the manufacturer of a medicine. The routes available for parenteral administration and the tissues, organs and anatomical spaces that can be accessed by injection are outlined. The various forms, or types, of parenteral product commonly manufactured are described and the pharmacopoeial standards for injectable products are discussed. The ingredients of formulated injectable products with regard to vehicles or solvents, excipients and preservatives are described along with physiological considerations, such as the pH and tonicity of the product before administration. Finally, the containers, closures and primary packaging commonly used for parenteral products are described.

Reasons for choosing parenteral administration

The vast majority of patients would prefer to receive their medication as an oral tablet or liquid to swallow, or as a cream, ointment or transdermal patch to apply to the skin rather than receive treatment via injection, which can be painful or stressful (indeed some patients have needle phobia). From a manufacturer's point of view, it is often simpler and much cheaper to prepare medicines such as tablets or liquids, particularly given the less stringent requirements for manufacturing premises for these nonsterile products, compared with the costs associated with manufacturing sterile medicines, such as injections, in highly specialized, controlled, clean environments. There are, however, several clinical advantages associated with parenteral administration.

Many medicines are administered parenterally simply because the drug molecule itself would be rapidly broken down in the gastrointestinal tract and would thus become inactivated before it could be absorbed into the circulatory system. Good examples of this are aminoglycoside antibiotics, such as gentamicin. The injectable route may be chosen to provide a highly localized effect. This is particularly true when the injection route accesses a particular anatomical area or organ system. Examples of this include the injection of drugs, such as steroids, into joint spaces (intra-articular injection), intraocular injections to treat eye diseases or intrathecal injections where medicines are administered into the spinal column to deliver drugs into the cerebrospinal fluid that otherwise might not accumulate sufficiently in the brain to achieve the desired effect.

Intravenous injection delivers the drug directly into the circulatory system, where it is then rapidly distributed around the body. This is important clinically as the drug will rapidly produce an effect, whereas peak blood levels may not be achieved for 1–2 hours after a drug is administered orally. This rapid onset of action for an intravenously administered drug may be critical in emergency situations. Conversely, if a drug is administered by intramuscular injection, the release of the medicine from the injection site into the circulation can be delayed and prolonged. Indeed, as will be seen later, by manipulation of the formulation of intramuscular injections it is possible to provide prolonged drug release allowing doses to be required at once-monthly intervals. Finally, the intravenous route of injection is routinely used to administer medication to the unconscious patient who is unable to swallow. This route is also used in conscious or unconscious patients if the gastrointestinal tract is not working. In this scenario, not only medicines but also fluids for hydration and electrolyte replacement, plus all the nutrients, vitamins and trace elements normally obtained from a healthy diet supplied by parenteral nutrition are provided intravenously.

Routes of parenteral administration

As noted already, medicines are injected by many different routes, and the choice of route is governed by the purpose of the treatment and the volume of medicine to be administered.

Intravenous injections and infusions

Intravenous injections and infusions are administered into an easily accessible prominent vein near the surface of the skin, typically on the back of the hand or in the internal flexure of the elbow. The volumes administered can range from 1 mL for an intravenous injection up to several litres for an intravenous infusion. Medicines administered by intravenous injection (or intravenous bolus dose) will rapidly increase the concentration of the drug in the plasma and produce a rapid effect. If the medicine is first added to a large volume of fluid (500 mL to 1 L infusion bag) and then administered by intravenous infusion at a slow and controlled rate, often with use of a pump, the drug will enter the circulation at a much slower and controlled rate. By altering the infusion rate, the clinician can titrate the dose against the effect required, e.g. controlling blood pressure, by manipulating the infusion rate of, for example, an inotropic drug such as dobutamine.

Drug solutions at high or low pH or highly concentrated hypertonic solutions (see later) will damage the cells lining the vein and cause localized pain and inflammation (thrombophlebitis). To avoid this problem a *central line* may be inserted. This is a long, indwelling catheter inserted into a vein in the neck or forearm with the end of the catheter sited in the superior vena cava close to the right atrium of the heart (Fig. 36.1). Medicines administered intravenously, via a central line, become rapidly diluted in a large volume of blood and do not cause local irritation to the blood vessel. Injections which are formulated either as water-in-oil emulsions or suspensions must not be administered by the intravenous route. This is because the suspended drug particles can physically block blood capillaries and the oil phase

of a water-in-oil injection could cause a fat embolism, again blocking blood vessels.

Intra-arterial and intracardiac injections

The large majority of drugs that are administered parenterally are given intravenously. As noted already, this delivers the drug directly into the bloodstream to provide a rapid and predictable clinical effect. However, it is not the only way that medicines can be administered into the vascular system.

Intra-arterial administration is essentially the same as intravenous administration except that the drug is administered into an artery rather than a vein. Arteries are not as readily accessible as veins, and this technique is much more invasive, and carries a greater risk than simple intravenous administration. For this reason, it is seldom used. Intra-arterial administration is sometimes used when intravenous access cannot easily be established, such as in very premature infants, because of the very small size of their veins in relation to the catheter tubes used to maintain vascular access. Intra-arterial administration has also been used in the treatment of some cancers (such as liver cancer) where the anticancer medicines are injected into an artery upstream of the tumour site to ensure the maximum amount of drug reaches the tumour before distribution elsewhere around the body. Distribution of the drug to the tumour site can be improved by the anticancer drug being absorbed into biodegradable polymer beads which lodge in the vascular system of the tumour and release the drug as the beads break down. However, the benefits of this method of intra-arterial administration do not currently appear to outweigh the risks to any significant degree, so therefore this method of administration is not commonplace.

Intracardiac injections are used to administer a drug (a common example being an aqueous solution of adrenaline) directly into either cardiac muscle or a ventricle of the heart. This is undertaken only in life-threatening emergencies to produce a rapid, local effect in the heart during a myocardial infarction or in circulatory collapse.

Intradermal injections

Intradermal injections are given into the skin between the epidermal and dermal layers (Fig. 36.2). Volumes

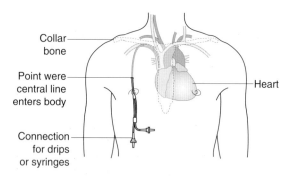

Collar bone

Point were central line enters body

Connection for drips or syringes

Heart

Fig. 36.1 • Central-line placement.

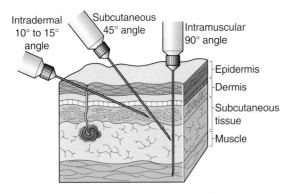

Fig. 36.2 • Intradermal, subcutaneous and intramuscular injection routes.

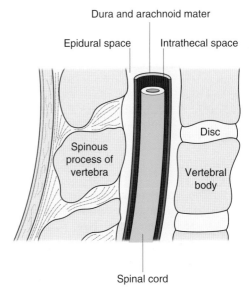

Fig. 36.3 • Spinal anatomy.

of up to 0.2 mL can be given by this route, and absorption from the intradermal injection site is slow. This route is used for immunological diagnostic tests, such as allergy tests, or the injection of tuberculin protein to determine immunity against tuberculosis. Some vaccines such as BCG (tuberculosis) are administered by intradermal injection.

Subcutaneous injections

Subcutaneous (also called hypodermic) injections are administered into the loose connective and adipose tissues immediately beneath the dermal skin layer (see Fig. 36.2). Typical injection sites are the abdomen, upper arms and upper legs. Volumes of up to 1 mL can be administered comfortably, and aqueous solutions or suspensions of drugs are administered by this route. As this tissue is highly vascular, drugs administered by the subcutaneous route are fairly rapidly and predictably absorbed from this site. A common example of a drug administered by subcutaneous injection is insulin.

Intramuscular injections

Intramuscular injections are preferably administered into the tissue of a relaxed muscle (see Fig. 36.2). The muscle sites commonly used for intramuscular injection are the buttock, thigh or shoulder muscles. Aqueous or oily solutions or suspensions can be administered in volumes of up to 4 mL. In adults the gluteal, or buttock, muscle will be used for larger-volume injections, whereas in children the thigh muscle is usually larger and thus preferred. Drugs administered by the intramuscular route are more

slowly absorbed from the injection site into the systemic circulation compared with those administered by the subcutaneous route.

Intraspinal injections

Intraspinal injections are given between the vertebrae of the spine into the area of the spinal column (Fig. 36.3). Only drugs in aqueous solution are administered by this route. Intrathecal injections are administered into the cerebrospinal fluid (CSF) in the subarachnoid space between the arachnoid mater and the pia mater, the two innermost protective membranes surrounding the spinal cord. This route can be used for spinal anaesthesia, and in this case the specific gravity of the injection can be manipulated to localize the site of action and thus the area of the body anaesthetized. Intrathecal injections are also given to introduce drug substances into the CSF that would otherwise not diffuse across the blood–brain barrier. Typically, these could be antibiotics to treat meningitis, or anticancer agents such as methotrexate or cytarabine. Volumes up to 10 mL can be administered by intrathecal injection.

Epidural injections or infusions are given into the epidural space between the dura mater (the outermost protective membrane covering the spinal cord) and the vertebrae. This route is commonly used for spinal anaesthesia, for example during childbirth.

Intra-articular injections

Intra-articular injections are given into the synovial fluid of joint cavities such as the knee. Aqueous solutions or suspensions can be administered by this route. This route of injection produces a local effect, and typically anti-inflammatory drugs are administered to treat arthritic conditions or sports injuries.

Ophthalmic injections

Ophthalmic injections are administered either around or into the eye; in the latter case these are referred to as intraocular injections (see Chapter 39). Subconjunctival injections usually of 1 mL or less are administered under the conjunctiva or into the skin surrounding the eye (e.g. inside the eyelid). Intraocular injections can be further classified as intracameral injections into the anterior chamber of the eye (in front of the lens) or intravitreal injections into the vitreous chamber (into the main body of the eye behind the lens). The volume of intracameral injections can be from 0.1 mL to 1 mL, depending on whether the drug is left in the eye or administered during surgery on the open eye. This route has been used to administer antibiotics or local anaesthetics during eye surgery (e.g. cataract surgery). Intravitreal injections are used to administer several different drugs used to treat various ocular diseases. Because of the danger caused by rising intraocular pressure which can damage the retina, a maximum volume of only 0.1 mL can be administered by the intravitreal route. Ophthalmic drug delivery by injection is discussed further in Chapter 39.

Pharmacopoeial requirements

General requirements

Almost all pharmacopoeias lay down the requirements for parenteral products in a series of general monographs, with which all parenterally administered medicines are expected to comply. Most pharmacopoeias are very similar in their requirements, although details do differ and these need to be checked closely. Several different categories of parenteral preparation are described and further requirements specific to a given medicinal form are specified. This is discussed in the following sections.

Sterility

All parenteral preparations are sterile preparations intended for injection, infusion or implantation into the body. The requirement for sterility is vital as the method of administration of these products bypasses the body's natural defence systems and barriers (such as the skin or gastrointestinal system), and introduces the medicine directly into the bloodstream or other body tissues. The methods for sterilization of parenteral medications are discussed in Chapters 16 and 17.

Excipients

Excipients may be added to parenteral preparations to serve a number of purposes. They can be added to make the preparation isotonic in relation to human blood, to adjust the pH, to increase the solubility of the drug substance, to increase the stability of the drug substance and increase the shelf life of the product or to act as a preservative. The use of such excipients will be discussed more fully later. However, it is worth noting here that the use of excipients should not adversely affect the action of the drug substance, or cause any side effects or toxicity at the concentrations used in a given formulation.

Containers

Containers for parenteral preparations should be made, wherever possible, from materials that are sufficiently transparent to allow the contents to be visually inspected for particles, before use. Containers can be made from glass or plastic. Whatever the type of container, it should be effectively sealed to prevent the enclosed medicine becoming contaminated with microorganisms or other contaminants during storage before use. Containers should therefore be airtight and also preferably tamper evident. The types of containers and closures will be discussed further later.

Endotoxins and pyrogens

As well as being sterile, parenteral preparations must be practically free from endotoxins and pyrogens. These substances are bacterial products that may be released from certain types of bacteria when they are alive, or after they die. They may therefore be present in sterile products as a by-product of the sterilization process which kills the bacteria during manufacture. When they are injected into a patient, they can cause fever, and even shock if present in sufficient quantities. Therefore parenteral products must comply with the test for bacterial endotoxins or the test for pyrogens. For further information on endotoxins and pyrogens, and on depyrogenation of containers, equipment and raw materials, see Chapters 16 and 17.

Particulates

The final general test with which certain parenteral products much comply is for particulate contamination. They must be free of visible particles and contain only very low numbers of subvisible particles. This is of particular importance for medicines administered intravenously. Particles inadvertently injected with a medicine will travel through the venous system to the heart and from there to the lungs. In the lungs, the vascular system narrows to a network of capillaries around each alveolus, and any suspended particles may become entrapped at this point, preventing blood from flowing, resulting in a pulmonary embolism.

Pharmacopoeias have standards for particulate matter in injections for intravenous use; for example the *European Pharmacopoeia* has limits on the number of 10 μm and 25 μm particles per container of injectable product. The *European Pharmacopoeia* notes that these levels would not be appropriate for suspensions for injection. Suspensions for injection are meant to be administered by the intramuscular, intra-articular or subcutaneous routes.

Obviously, suspensions are not (supposed to be) injected intravenously for the reasons noted earlier, but when injected intramuscularly or subcutaneously or into a joint space, the suspended particles will dissolve slowly and provide a prolonged effect. This may be many hours in the case of subcutaneous insulin suspension, or perhaps many weeks for a steroid suspension injected into a joint. The required dissolution characteristics will, to a great extent, determine the size and nature of the solid drug particles (e.g. amorphous or crystalline).

Emulsions can be injected intravenously, but here the maximum droplet size will be linked to capillary diameter. The droplet size must be controlled and is usually less than 3 μm in diameter to prevent oil embolisms forming in the bloodstream. However, there is evidence that certain oil droplets may deform to some extent, to pass through a capillary without occluding it, such that oil droplets slightly larger than the diameter of a capillary can be administered.

Category-specific requirements

Pharmacopoeias usually recognize several distinct categories of parenteral product. These are injections, infusions, concentrates for injection or infusion, powders for injection or infusion and gels for injection.

Injections

Injections can be sterile solutions, emulsions or suspensions. One prepares these by dissolving, emulsifying or suspending the drug substance (or substances), together with any required excipients, in water or nonaqueous liquid or a mixture of aqueous and nonaqueous vehicles. Solutions for injection are clear and free from visible particles. Emulsions for injection must not show any evidence of phase separation (creaming or cracking; see Chapter 27). Suspensions for injection may undergo sedimentation, but if so the particles must be readily resuspended on shaking to give a suspension that is sufficiently stable to allow a uniform dose to be withdrawn from the container.

With regard to the resuspension of sedimented injections in practice, it is not usual for particle size to be tested in a quantitative manner on a routine basis before use. Indeed, resuspended injections can be administered in patients' homes or at GP clinics where particle size determination apparatus is not available. Thus it is the responsibility of the original formulator/manufacturer of the suspension to provide the necessary data to convince the regulatory authorities that resuspension can be readily achieved by a patient, medical practitioner or nurse by simple shaking before administration.

Aqueous injections that are designed for multiple dosing must contain an antimicrobial preservative, unless it can be shown that the preparation itself has sufficient antimicrobial properties to be self-preserving. Preservatives must not be used when the volume to be routinely administered in a single dose exceeds 15 mL. Preservatives must not be used if the product is intended to be injected epidurally or intrathecally (or by any other route giving access to the CSF), or if it is to be injected into the eye. Unpreserved injections should preferably be presented in single-dose containers (ampoules or prefilled syringes) rather than vials. This is because vials allow more than one dose to be withdrawn and therefore may become contaminated with microorganisms if used for multiple doses.

Infusions

Infusions are sterile aqueous solutions or emulsions with water as the continuous phase. They are usually made isotonic with respect to blood. They are large-volume parenteral products, typically ranging in volume from 100 mL to 1000 mL, but they may be larger. Infusions do not contain antimicrobial preservatives. Solutions for infusion are clear and free from visible particles. Emulsions do not show any sign of phase separation.

Concentrates for injection or infusions

Concentrates for injection or infusion are sterile solutions intended for injection or infusion only after dilution. They are diluted to a prescribed volume usually with an aqueous liquid such as saline (0.9% w/v sodium chloride) or water before administration. After dilution, they comply with the requirements for injections or infusions given earlier.

Powders for injection or infusion

Powders for injection or infusion are dry solid, sterile substances sealed in their final container. When they are dispensed, a volume of the prescribed sterile diluent (usually an aqueous liquid) is added and shaken with the powder. This mixture should rapidly form either a clear, particle-free solution or a uniform suspension. After dissolution or suspension, they comply with the requirements for injections or infusions.

Freeze-dried (lyophilized) products for parenteral use are considered to be powders for injection or infusion. Freeze-drying is often used for drug substances that are not stable in solution (e.g. they degrade by hydrolysis). In this process, a solution of the drug is prepared and then sterilized by filtration and the final container (usually a vial) is filled with it. The solution is then freeze-dried by reduction of the temperature and application of a vacuum, so that the water in the drug solution is removed by sublimation, leaving a sterile plug of the drug substance in the vial, which is then closed and sealed. For further details of this process, see Chapters 17 and 29.

Absorption from injection sites

Factors affecting absorption from the injection site

For a drug to exert its pharmacological effect (i.e. provide a clinical action) it must be able to reach its appropriate site of action. The movement of a drug from the site of administration (injection site) into the bloodstream is the process of drug absorption. From this it can be seen that there is no absorption process if the drug is injected intravenously into the bloodstream or into a similar fluid of distribution such as the cerebrospinal fluid or ocular fluid (intrathecal and intraocular injections), or directly into the site of action (e.g. intra-articular or intraocular injections). In contrast, drugs that are injected intradermally, subcutaneously or intramuscularly must undergo absorption to reach the systemic circulation. This occurs by diffusion of the drug through the tissues surrounding the injection site followed by penetration through the walls of blood capillaries or the lymphatic system. Both the subcutaneous area and muscle tissue are richly supplied with blood capillaries. Lymph vessels are found extensively in subcutaneous tissue and in connective tissue sheaths around muscles but are found only in small numbers within muscle tissue itself.

Subcutaneous and intramuscular injections may be either solutions or suspensions. Intradermal injections are usually solutions, but generally are only used for diagnostic purposes (e.g. allergy testing) and act locally at the site of administration. When aqueous solutions of drugs are administered by subcutaneous or intramuscular injection, drug absorption is usually comparable to that seen with oral administration, and absorption is usually complete within 30 minutes, although the lipid solubility of the drug can play a role and delay the absorption of a drug injected into subcutaneous fatty tissue. The fairly rapid absorption of aqueous injections from subcutaneous or intramuscular injection sites depends on an unimpaired blood flow surrounding the injection site. Vasoconstrictors such as adrenaline may be incorporated into the formulation of other drugs to prolong their retention at the injection site. This is commonly used to prolong the action of local anaesthetic drugs at and around the injection site (e.g. during dental surgery). Large molecules such as proteins and peptides (e.g. insulin) and colloidal particles (e.g. injectable iron complexes) with molecular masses greater than 20 000 Da are absorbed by lymph vessels rather than the capillary network at subcutaneous or intramuscular injection sites. The speed of lymphatic flow and thus systemic uptake can be increased by exercise of the injected muscle or massage of the injection site for subcutaneous injections.

Formulation factors

If a drug is formulated as a suspension, the suspended drug must first dissolve from its solid state before it can be absorbed from the injection site. This means that drug absorption from an injected suspension is much slower than from a solution injected into the same site. This slow and prolonged release from the site of action can be used to reduce the frequency of dosing that might otherwise be required if a drug were administered intravenously or orally. Drugs salts with low aqueous solubility may be specifically chosen for intramuscular injection to provide a prolonged effect. Benzathine penicillin injected intramuscularly as a suspension forms a depot from which the active penicillin is slowly released. Such a product is used in the treatment of early syphilis. Procaine penicillin is another depot-forming salt of penicillin.

Several corticosteroids, such as hydrocortisone acetate, prednisolone acetate and triamcinolone acetonide, are formulated as suspensions for intramuscular injection. When given by this route, they release the drug into the systemic circulation over a period of 2 days to 1 week depending on the dose given. Corticosteroid aqueous suspensions can also be given by intra-articular injection into joint spaces to produce a prolonged anti-inflammatory action over many weeks, usually to treat arthritic conditions. However, as the suspended drug substance can irritate the joint cartilage, a joint should be treated in this manner no more than three times a year.

The rate of release of a drug from a suspension is governed by the solubility of the drug in the tissue fluids and the surface area of the suspended drug particles. Differences in particle size and crystal structure have been used to alter the rate of absorption of drugs from subcutaneous injection sites. Most notably this has been used with insulin to give a range of insulin injections with different times for the onset and different durations of action. Subcutaneous injection of insulin causes few problems, but lipodystrophy may occur if injections are given repeatedly into the same area. Aside from causing subcutaneous indentations, there is a reduction of vascularity in the affected area and therefore slower absorption of the insulin from the injection site. This can be avoided if the site of subsequent injections is moved around the body.

Soluble insulin is the short-acting form of the drug, and is usually injected 15–30 minutes before eating. When injected subcutaneously, it has an onset of action of 30–60 minutes, a maximal effect between 2 and 4 hours after injection, and a duration of action of up to 8 hours. Soluble insulin can also be injected intravenously in response to diabetic emergencies, such as diabetic ketoacidosis. When injected intravenously, soluble insulin is rapidly eliminated and its effect disappears within 30 minutes. In the treatment of the unconscious diabetic patient, a slow intravenous infusion of soluble insulin may be more appropriate.

Intermediate-acting and long-acting insulins have an onset of action approximately 1–2 hours after subcutaneous injection, a maximal effect 4–12 hours after injection and duration of 16–35 hours. They are administered once or twice daily in conjunction with short-acting insulin. Isophane insulin is an intermediate-acting insulin in the form of a suspension of soluble insulin complexed with protamine sulfate. The insulin protamine complex forms rod-shaped crystals longer than 1 μm but rarely exceeding 60 μm. Insulin Zinc Suspension (Mixed) is a long-acting insulin and is a mixture of amorphous and regular crystals. The amorphous crystals dissolve more rapidly than the regular crystals. The ratio of the amorphous and crystalline insulin must be controlled. The *British Pharmacopoeia* and the *European Pharmacopoeia*, for example, direct that Insulin Zinc Suspension consists of 30% amorphous crystals of no uniform shape but not exceeding 2 μm in size, and 70% crystalline insulin consisting of rhombohedral crystals between 10 μm and 40 μm in size. Insulin Zinc Suspension is obtained by addition of a suitable zinc salt such as zinc chloride to soluble insulin.

Oily intramuscular injections are solutions or suspensions of drug substances, often steroids, hormones or fat-soluble vitamins in a suitable metabolizable oil, such as arachis oil or sesame oil, as the vehicle. This approach can be used to administer drugs that are insoluble in water, or water-soluble drug substances can be chemically modified to produce an oil-soluble compound specifically for administration in an oily injection. The use of undecanoate, enanthate or propionate esters to obtain the oil-soluble form of a drug is commonplace. As oily injections are much more viscous than aqueous injections, the injected solution does not spread along the muscle fascias when injected intramuscularly. This means a depot is formed in the muscle tissue. The drug must undergo partition from the oil into the aqueous tissue fluid before it can be absorbed; therefore release from oily intramuscular injections is very slow. Many antipsychotic medicines are given as oily intramuscular injections as they require dosing only every 2–4 weeks rather than daily oral dosing; thus adherence to treatment can be better managed.

Excipients

It is very unusual for an injectable medicine to be composed entirely of the drug substance and no other ingredient. The drug, unless presented as a dried powder for reconstitution before use, will be dissolved or suspended in a vehicle such as water or a saline solution (0.9% sodium chloride) or a nonaqueous liquid. Other ingredients (excipients) may be present in the formulation to aid the dissolution or suspension of the drug in the vehicle. Other excipients may be incorporated to comply with pharmacopoeial requirements such as the incorporation of a preservative if the preparation is for multiple use rather than a single dose product. Excipients are often included in parenteral products to prevent, reduce or delay the degradation of the drug product over time and thus increase the product's shelf life. Finally, excipients are frequently added to adjust the pH and tonicity of the product to make them comparable to the physiological pH and tonicity of the tissue into which it is being injected (usually comparable to human plasma values). This is done to reduce pain and irritation that may otherwise be caused to blood vessels or tissues by the administration process.

Vehicles for injections

Water for Injections is the most common vehicle used for parenteral products. Water for Injections is a highly purified grade of water which is subject to pharmacopoeial standards with respect to production methods and purity. Water is, of course, well tolerated by the body and it is a solvent for a wide range of drug substances. For those drugs which are poorly soluble in water, water-miscible nonaqueous solvents such as ethanol, glycerol or propylene glycol may be added as cosolvents to improve the solubility of a drug substance.

Solubilizing agents may be added to an injection formulation to aid the dissolution of drugs with poor aqueous solubility. Polyoxyethylene castor oil derivatives will solubilize hydrophobic drugs into aqueous solutions for injections and are used, for instance, for formulations of paclitaxel, diazepam and cisplatin. Cyclodextrins are cyclic oligosaccharide molecules (see Fig. 24.1) with a bucket-like structure containing a hydrophobic central cavity, whilst the outer surface is hydrophilic. Cyclodextrins can form inclusion complexes with a variety of poorly water-soluble drug molecules. The 'hydrophobic' drugs are held within the cyclodextrin 'bucket', with the outer surface of the complex remaining hydrophilic. Both α-cyclodextrin and γ-cyclodextrin can be used in parenteral products, but β-cyclodextrin should not be used as it causes severe kidney damage.

Water-insoluble drugs may be administered parenterally by dissolution of the drug in a suitable oil and formation of an oil-in-water emulsion with use of a suitable emulsifying agent to stabilize the emulsion (see Chapter 27 for further details on emulsions). Droplet size must be controlled and is usually less than 3 μm in diameter to prevent oil embolisms forming in the bloodstream. Lecithin and various sorbitan fatty acid esters have been used as emulsifying agents in parenteral products. Finally, oils such as arachis oil or sesame oil may be chosen as a vehicle for intramuscular injections, for drug release over a prolonged period (depot injections).

Preservatives

Antimicrobial preservatives are added to injections which are designed for multiple use. Such products are usually packaged in glass vials or cartridges with a synthetic rubber septum that can be punctured on several occasions to withdraw a dose of the drug for administration (see the section entitled 'Containers'). A preservative is included to inhibit the growth of any microorganisms that may be inadvertently introduced into the product during repeated use by the patient or health care professional.

Excipients such as ethanol, glycerol and propylene glycol which may be added to a formulation as cosolvents to aid drug dissolution will also provide an antimicrobial effect. Ethanol is effective at concentrations above 10% v/v, glycerol at 10% to 20% v/v and propylene glycol at 15% to 30% v/v. Some of the commonly used antimicrobial preservatives suitable for parenteral administration are given in Table 36.1. Fatal toxic reactions in low-birth-weight newborn babies have been linked to injections preserved with benzyl alcohol. Thus parenteral products preserved with benzyl alcohol should not be administered to newborn babies. In addition, as noted earlier, preservatives should not be added to large-volume parenteral products (infusions), or products intended for intraspinal or intraocular injection. Preservation of pharmaceutical products, including injections, is discussed in detail in Chapter 48.

Table 36.1 Preservatives used in parenteral products

Preservative	Typical concentration (% w/v)
Benzalkonium chloride	0.01
Benzoic acid	0.17
Benzyl alcohol	1–2
Chlorobutanol	0.1–0.5
Chlorocresol	0.1
Cresol	0.15–0.3

Antioxidants

If the drug substance to be injected is prone to degradation by oxidation, a number of formulation processes and excipients can be used to reduce the rate of drug degradation in the product and thus increase the shelf life or extend the expiry date.

It is common practice to use pharmaceutical-grade compressed nitrogen gas (filtered through a 0.2 μm pore size filter) during the manufacturing process. Nitrogen is bubbled through the solution containing the drug before the final packaging is filled. The nitrogen gas displaces any dissolved oxygen from the drug solution. This process is known as 'sparging'. A nitrogen overlay may also be applied during the filling operation before the final containers of the drug product are sealed. This will displace air from the headspace between the surface of the product and the top of the container (e.g. in a vial or ampoule), thereby removing oxygen.

An antioxidant may also be included in the formulation. Antioxidants are chemicals that have a lower oxidation potential than the drug substance and thus will react with any oxygen present in the product in preference to the drug. Vitamin C (ascorbic acid) and vitamin E (α-tocopherol) can be used for this purpose, both in pharmaceutical products and in food. α-Tocopherol is highly lipophilic and can be used in oil-based parenteral products usually in the range from 0.001% to 0.05% v/v. Ascorbic acid is used in aqueous parenteral products at a concentration of 0.01% to 0.1% w/v. Ascorbic acid can also be used to adjust the pH of the formulation (see later). Butylated hydroxyanisole (BHA) and butylated hydroxytoluene (BHT) are structurally similar antioxidants used in parenteral preparations either separately or in combination. For intramuscular injections, they are usually used at a concentration

of 0.03% w/v and for intravenous injections, 0.0002% to 0.002% w/v is used. The most commonly used antioxidants are the sulfite salts. Sodium metabisulfite is used at concentrations between 0.01% and 0.1% w/v, and also has some preservative properties. It is used as an antioxidant for acidic parenteral products. If the product is of neutral pH, sodium bisulfite is used, whereas sodium sulfite is used as an antioxidant in alkali parenteral products.

The activity of an antioxidant can be enhanced by the inclusion of an antioxidant synergist, also referred to as a chelating or sequestering agent. Antioxidant synergists reduce oxidation by removing trace levels of metal ions from the product by forming chelates with them. Metal ions, particularly copper, iron and manganese ions, are believed to catalyse oxidation reactions between oxygen and drug substances. Examples of chelating agents used in parenteral products include citric acid at concentrations between 0.3% and 2.0% w/v and derivatives of edetic acid (ethylenediaminetetraacetic acid [EDTA]) at concentrations of 0.0005% to 0.01% w/v. Citric acid can also be used to adjust the pH of formulations, and edetate compounds possess preservative properties.

If the primary mechanism of drug degradation in the product over time is hydrolysis rather than oxidation, then the shelf life of the product will be increased by removal of all water from the product. Injectable products which are presented as freeze-dried powders (see Chapter 29 for the freeze-drying process and Chapter 17 for the sterilization of these powders) are usually formulated in this manner to improve the stability of a readily hydrolysed drug substance.

pH adjustment and buffers

The physiological pH of plasma and extracellular fluid is 7.4; therefore, ideally all injectable products should be formulated to this pH. However, there is likely to be an optimum pH at which the drug substance is most stable. The solubility of the drug in the vehicle may also be dependent on pH. Therefore the pH chosen for a parenteral product is likely to be a compromise between the requirements for stability, solubility and physiological compatibility. Injectable products should have a pH between 3.0 and 9.0 before administration; pH values above or below this range are too corrosive and will cause tissue damage at the site of injection. The pH of a parenteral formulation can be adjusted with acidifying or alkalizing agents. Acidifying agents include hydrochloric, citric and sulfuric acids. Alkalizing agents include sodium bicarbonate, sodium citrate and sodium hydroxide.

Buffers are included in parenteral products to maintain the pH of the product at the desired optimum value. Changes in pH may arise because of interactions between an ingredient in the formulation and the container, or from changes in storage temperature. The buffer ingredients commonly used in parenteral products include combinations of citric acid, sodium citrate, sodium acetate, sodium lactate and monobasic and dibasic sodium phosphate.

Tonicity-adjusting agents

An aqueous solution of sodium chloride at a concentration of 0.9% w/v or 9 g L^{-1} has a measured osmolarity of 286 mmol L^{-1} and is isotonic (meaning it has the same osmotic pressure; see Chapter 3) with human plasma, which has an osmolality of between 280 mmol kg^{-1} and 295 mmol kg^{-1}.

Hypotonic solutions have a lower osmotic pressure than plasma. If mixed with blood, they would cause the blood cells to swell and burst as water would be driven into the cells by osmosis. Hypertonic solutions have a higher osmotic pressure than plasma. If mixed with blood, they would cause the blood cells to lose water by osmosis and shrink.

Hypotonic injection solutions are made isotonic by the addition of sodium chloride, dextrose or mannitol. Hypertonic injection solutions must be made isotonic by dilution before administration. Pharmacopoeias direct that intravenous infusions should be made isotonic with human plasma. Whilst not a pharmacopoeial requirement, it is considered desirable for subcutaneous, intradermal and intramuscular injections also to be isotonic. Intrathecal and intraocular injections should also be isotonic to avoid serious changes in osmotic pressure in the CSF and the eye.

There are a number of methods available for calculating the amount of additional substance to be added to a hypotonic drug solution to render it isotonic, including freezing point depression, the use of sodium chloride equivalents, molar concentrations and calculations based on serum osmolarity. One method is demonstrated in the next section:

Isotonicity calculation based on freezing point depression

The presence of solutes in water will increase osmolarity and depress the freezing point of water. These

effects (colligative properties; see Chapter 3) are dependent on the concentration of solute particles. Consequently, the freezing point of a solution can be used as a measure of its osmolarity. The freezing point of blood serum/plasma and tears is −0.52°C. Therefore an aqueous solution that freezes at −0.52°C is isotonic. For high concentrations of electrolytes there may be a slight deviation in the direct relationship between concentration and freezing point depression, but in most cases the relationship holds true. Reference sources, such as the *Pharmaceutical Codex*, give the freezing point depressions produced by a wide range of soluble materials.

The required amount of adjusting substance required to make a hypotonic solution isotonic is given by the equation

$$w = \frac{0.52 - a}{b}$$

(36.1)

where W is the weight/volume percentage of adjusting substance in the final solution, a is the freezing point depression of unadjusted solution (i.e. freezing point depression of 1% solution × strength in weight/volume percentage) and b is the freezing point depression of water due to 1% w/v of adjusting substance, usually sodium chloride or glucose. A worked example is presented in Box 36.1.

Suspending agents

Drugs presented as suspensions for injection may require a suspending agent to ensure that the drug can be readily and uniformly resuspended before use. A water-soluble cellulose derivative such as methylcellulose can be used in intramuscular and intra-articular injectable suspensions. Povidone was used in the past for this purpose, but safety concerns about this compound when injected intramuscularly have led to it falling out of favour. A suitable nonionic injectable surfactant such as a polysorbate may also be included in a suspension formulation to aid the uniform dispersion of the suspended drug substance.

Containers

As noted already (see the section entitled 'Pharmacopoeial requirements') the container or primary packaging of a parenteral product should ideally be transparent to allow the product to be examined

Box 36.1

Use of freezing point depression to adjust solutions to isotonicity

You are requested to make a solution containing 0.28% w/v potassium chloride isotonic by the addition of anhydrous glucose. From the literature, the freezing point depression of a 1% solution of potassium chloride is 0.439 °C and for anhydrous glucose it is 0.101 °C.

Use Eq. 36.1:

- A 1% solution of potassium chloride depresses the freezing point of water by 0.439 °C. Therefore the freezing point depression of unadjusted solution = 0.28 × 0.439 = 0.123 °C.
- A 1% solution of anhydrous glucose depresses the freezing point of water by 0.101 °C.

$$w = \frac{0.52 - 0.123}{0.101} = \frac{0.397}{0.101} = 3.93$$

Thus you require the addition of 3.93% w/v anhydrous glucose (i.e. 3.93 g anhydrous glucose per 100 mL) to make the potassium chloride solution isotonic with plasma.

---

before use. This is particularly important for injections supplied as powders for reconstitution, as the health care practitioner needs to be able to see that the drug substance has completely dissolved in the diluent before withdrawal of the dose. Large-volume infusion fluids often have other drugs added to them, so again the clarity of the container is important to allow the proper mixing of the product to be assessed and to check that large particles (e.g. from the rubber closure) have not been inadvertently introduced.

Whatever type of container is used, it must be tightly sealed to maintain the sterility of the injection before use and to prevent other contaminants (e.g. oxygen) entering the product which may lead to degradation of the drug substance. The container should not interact with the drug product or other excipients it contains. It should also be robust enough to withstand the sterilization process chosen. In preference, parenteral products are manufactured and added to the primary container, which is then sealed and the product is then terminally sterilized inside the container, for example by use of moist heat in an autoclave (see Chapters 16 and 17). If the drug substance cannot withstand this process, then the containers will be sterilized first, the drug product will be sterilized by filtration, and then the

containers will be filled under conditions of strict asepsis and sealed. This latter method of aseptic production obviously carries the risk of microbial contamination of the product during the filling and sealing process, hence the preference for sterilization of the drug product inside the sealed container after filling (terminal sterilization).

Ampoules

Small-volume parenteral products are often packaged in glass or plastic ampoules. The use of glass and plastics as packaging materials for pharmaceutical products is discussed in Chapter 46. Ampoules are used for single-use, unpreserved products. Glass ampoules range in size typically from 1 mL to 10 mL in volume, although larger sizes are available. The glass chosen is referred to as type I or borosilicate glass, which is less alkaline than the glass usually used for beverages and other purposes. Ampoules are supplied as open-necked containers that are sealed by fusion of the narrow glass neck after filling (Fig. 36.4). Usually the neck of the ampoule has a painted ceramic ring on it. Because of the baking process required to fuse the ceramic to the glass, this acts as a weak point at which the ampoule can be easily snapped open by hand. The main disadvantages of glass ampoules are the fragility of the container, the potential for deposition of glass particles into the drug product on opening and the potential for injury to the fingers of the person opening the ampoule. The problem of fragility is overcome by use of robust

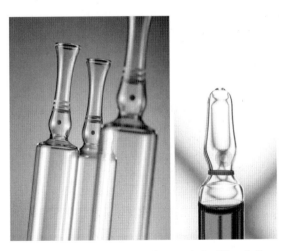

Fig. 36.4 • Open glass ampoules ready for filling *(left)* and a filled sealed glass ampoule *(right)*.

secondary packaging. Glass particles can be removed from the product by the contents of the ampoule being drawn through a filter straw or quill into a syringe. The advantages of glass ampoules are low cost and (if type I glass is used) very little interaction between the container and the product.

Plastic ampoules are prepared by a highly automated blow–fill–seal product process. The filling machine is loaded with the drug solution and with plastic granules (polyethylene and/or polypropylene), which are then melted. The molten plastic is blown into the ampoule-shaped mould of the machine to form the body of the ampoule, the body of the ampoule is filled with product and then the lid of the ampoule is moulded onto the top of the ampoule to form a seal. All of this happens as a single process which can take less than 1 second to complete (Fig. 36.5). The sealed ampoule is opened by the lid being twisted off, and very few particles are generated to contaminate the product. Plastic ampoules are much more robust than glass ampoules. The disadvantages are that this is a more costly process, and is suitable only for drug products formulated as simple solutions (e.g. freeze-drying processes cannot be undertaken with plastic ampoules). A full comparison of glass and plastics as materials for pharmaceutical packaging is provided in Chapter 46.

Vials

Vials are containers usually made of type I glass with a reusable synthetic rubber closure. Vials have advantages as containers as they permit multiple withdrawals and are made in sizes usually ranging from 5 mL to 100 mL. Vials are sealed with a bromobutyl or chlorobutyl synthetic rubber (elastomer) closure held in place by an aluminium seal crimped around the neck of the glass vial. The rubber closure

(or septum) is usually protected by a plastic flip-off cap (Fig. 36.6). This acts purely as a dust cap and does not provide a covering that maintains the sterility of the septum before use.

To withdraw a dose from a vial, the cap is removed and the septum disinfected with a sterile alcohol wipe. A syringe and needle is used to puncture the rubber closure and remove the required amount of product. The rubber septum is self-sealing to a high degree, and so more than one withdrawal can be made from a vial. However, only a limited number of punctures can be made through the rubber closure before it will lose its integrity as a seal. Products packaged in vials for multiple use will therefore incorporate a preservative to prevent any

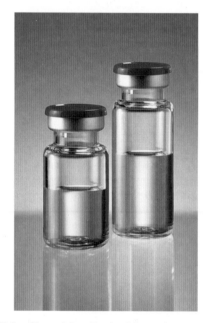

Fig. 36.6 • Glass vials with aluminium crimp seal and cap in place.

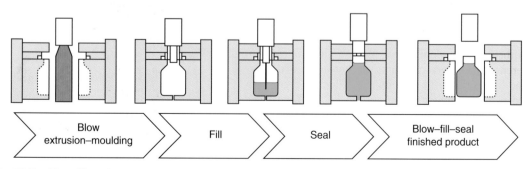

Fig. 36.5 • Blow–fill–seal process.

Blow extrusion–moulding

Fill

Seal

Blow–fill–seal finished product

microorganisms accidentally introduced into the product during use from proliferating.

The glass is inert and does not interact with the drug, and the use of synthetic rubber closures reduces the likelihood of the drug or other excipients reacting with, or being sorbed by, the rubber on storage. Synthetic rubber is also latex-free, which is important as sensitization to latex is an increasing problem for health care workers. The main disadvantage is that puncturing the rubber closure can cause large rubber particles to be introduced into the drug product.

Infusion bags and bottles

Large-volume parenteral products are packaged in glass bottles, collapsible plastic bags and semirigid plastic bottles, although the use of glass bottles for large-volume parenteral products is becoming much less commonplace. These products range in size from 100 mL to 1000 mL, although larger sizes (e.g. 3000 mL) can be used, particularly for parenteral nutrition products.

Collapsible bag presentations are the most common form of container (Fig. 36.7). They are manufactured from PVC or more increasingly polyolefin plastic. Collapsible bags usually have an additive port to allow other injectable drugs to be added to the infusion fluid. The main advantage of collapsible bags is that they collapse under atmospheric pressure as the contents are removed from them; therefore they do not require an air inlet system to equilibrate air pressure between the outside and the inside of the container, as do rigid glass bottles. The main disadvantage of PVC bags is that drugs may become adsorbed onto the plastic (e.g. insulin) or react with the plastic (e.g. etoposide). Additionally, components can leach out of the plastic, such as monomers and phthalate plasticizers, which may be toxic on long-term exposure. Polyolefin is much less reactive and is now replacing PVC for this reason in infusion bags.

Semirigid plastic containers are often made of polyethylene (Fig. 36.8). These containers may have an additive port to allow other drugs to be added to them. As they do not fully collapse during use, air equilibration may be required. Large-volume glass bottles are essentially the same as glass vials but on a larger scale. All large-volume parenteral products are meant for single use only.

Nowadays, parenteral products may be packaged in syringes, and may thus be presented to the health care professional or patient in a ready-to-use format. This requires aseptic filling with specialist equipment. Various types of infusion device are also available, although it is more common for these to be purchased empty and filled within the hospital pharmacy or health care setting before use on an individual patient basis. Such infusion devices are used to administer drugs intravenously over a prolonged period (e.g. from 1 day to 1 week). They are used for the administration of analgesia postoperatively (which the patient may control on demand) or as part of palliative care. Other applications for portable infusion devices include the

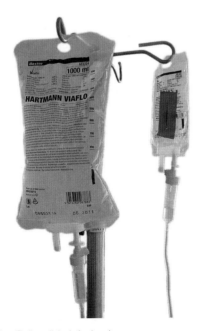

Fig. 36.7 • Collapsible infusion bag.

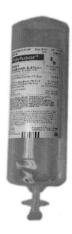

Fig. 36.8 • Semirigid infusion container.

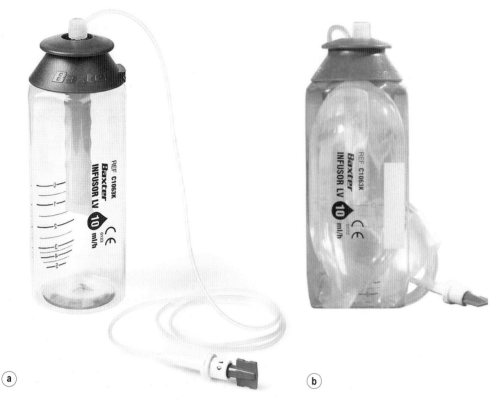

Fig. 36.9 • An elastomeric infusion device **(a)** empty and **(b)** filled. (Courtesy of Baxter Healthcare.)

delivery of anticancer chemotherapy or antibiotics over a period of several days. Infusion devices can be battery-powered pumps which infuse medication from an attached plastic reservoir. However, it is now much more common to use elastomeric infusion devices (Fig. 36.9). These elastomeric devices contain a balloon which acts as the drug reservoir. When filled, the balloon is greatly expanded and the drug solution inside is under pressure. The rate of administration is controlled by a simple restriction valve set in place in the device's outlet tubing, which allows a very small flow of drug solution from the reservoir (e.g. 1 mL h^{-1}, 2 mL h^{-1} or 5 mL h^{-1} depending on the device chosen). The advantage of elastomeric devices is that the mechanical pressure from the inflated reservoir powers the device and no batteries are required. The disadvantage is that the flow rate through the restriction valve is temperature sensitive, so can be altered dependent on how the device is worn by the patient. If the restriction valve is placed next to the skin of the patient, a higher than expected flow rate is seen.

Please check your eBook at **https://studentconsult. inkling.com/** for self-assessment questions. See inside cover for registration details.

Bibliography

Ansel, H.C., Allen, L.V. Jr., Popovich, N.G., 1999. Pharmaceutical Dosage Forms and Drug Delivery Systems, 7th ed. Lippincott Williams & Wilkins, Baltimore.

British Pharmacopoeia Commission, 2017. British Pharmacopoeia. Stationery Office, London.

Lund, W. (Ed.), 1994. Pharmaceutical Codex, 12th ed. Pharmaceutical Press, London.

Rees, J.A., Smith, I., Watson, J. (Eds.), 2014. Pharmaceutical Practice, 5th ed. Churchill Livingstone, Edinburgh.

Rowe, R.C., Sheskey, P.J., Cook, W.G., et al. (Eds.), 2016. Handbook of Pharmaceutical Excipients, 8th ed. Pharmaceutical Press, London.

Wade, A., 1980. Pharmaceutical Handbook, 19th ed. Pharmaceutical Press, London.

Pulmonary drug delivery

Kevin M. G. Taylor

CHAPTER CONTENTS

KEY POINTS

- Pulmonary delivery may be used for drugs having local or systemic activity.
- Effective drug delivery to the lungs is dependent on the formulation, the delivery device and the patient.
- The structure of the airways is effective in preventing entry of materials, including therapeutic aerosols.
- There are three principal mechanisms of particle deposition in the airways: inertial impaction, gravitational sedimentation and Brownian diffusion.
- The aerodynamic particle size of an inhaled particle or droplet, which depends primarily on physical size and density, is the critical parameter in determining its fate within the lung.

- There are three main categories of devices available for pulmonary drug delivery: pressurized metered-dose inhalers, dry powder inhalers and nebulizers.
- Pressurized metered-dose inhaler formulations may be solutions or suspensions and include a liquefied gas (a hydrofluoroalkane) as a propellant, and may also include surfactants and cosolvents.
- Dry powder inhalers deliver the drug as a fine powder. Formulations often include carrier particles, usually lactose, to aid dispersion of the drug powder, so that is becomes available for inhalation by patients.
- Nebulizers deliver relatively large doses of drugs as aerosols, generated from aqueous solutions or suspensions.
- In vitro measurement of the aerosol properties of inhalation products is usually carried out using cascade impactors, which fractionate aerosols according to their aerodynamic size distribution.

Inhaled drug delivery

Therapeutic agents for the treatment or prophylaxis of diseases of the airways, such as asthma, chronic obstructive pulmonary disease (COPD) and cystic fibrosis, are usually delivered directly to the respiratory tract. The administration of a drug at its site of action can result in a rapid onset of activity, which may be highly desirable, for instance when bronchodilating drugs for the treatment of asthma are being delivered. Additionally, smaller doses can be administered locally compared with delivery by the oral or parenteral routes, thereby reducing the potential incidence of adverse systemic effects and reducing drug costs. The pulmonary route is also useful where a drug is poorly absorbed orally (e.g. sodium cromoglicate) or where it is rapidly metabolized orally (e.g. isoprenaline). The avoidance of first-pass (presystemic) metabolism in the liver may also be advantageous, although the lung itself has some metabolic capability.

The lung may also be used as a route for delivering drugs having systemic activity, because of its large surface area, the abundance of capillaries and the thinness of the air–blood barrier. This has been exploited in the treatment of migraine with ergotamine and diabetes with insulin, and the potential for delivering biopharmaceuticals, such as insulin, vaccines and growth hormone, via the airways is now well established.

Lung anatomy

The lung is the organ of external respiration, in which oxygen and carbon dioxide are exchanged between blood and inhaled air. The structure of the airways also efficiently prevents the entry and promotes the removal of airborne foreign particles, including microorganisms.

The respiratory tract can be considered as comprising conducting (central) regions (trachea, bronchi, bronchioles, terminal and respiratory bronchioles) and respiratory (peripheral) regions (respiratory bronchioles and alveolar regions), although there is no clear demarcation between them (Fig. 37.1). The upper respiratory tract includes the nose, throat, pharynx and larynx; the lower respiratory tract comprises the trachea, bronchi, bronchioles and the alveolar regions. Simplistically, the airways can be described by a symmetrical model in which each airway divides into two equivalent branches or generations. In fact, the trachea (generation 0) branches into two main bronchi (generation 1), of which the right bronchus is wider and leaves the trachea at a smaller angle than the left bronchus, and hence is more likely to receive inhaled material. Further branching of the airways ultimately results in terminal bronchioles. These divide to produce respiratory bronchioles, which connect with alveolar ducts leading to the alveolar sacs (generation 23). These contain approximately 2×10^8–6×10^8 alveoli, producing a surface area of 100 m^2 to 140 m^2 in an adult male.

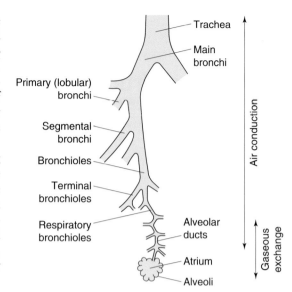

Fig. 37.1 • The human airways.

The conducting airways are lined with ciliated epithelial cells. Insoluble particles deposited on the walls of the airways in this region are trapped by the mucus, swept upwards from the lungs by the beating cilia to the throat, and swallowed.

Inhalation aerosols and the importance of particle size distribution

To deliver a drug into the airways, it must be presented as an aerosol (with the exception of medical gases and vapours). In pharmacy, an aerosol is defined as a two-phase system of solid particles or liquid droplets dispersed in air or another gas, having sufficiently small size to display considerable stability as a suspension.

The deposition of a drug/aerosol in the airways is dependent on four factors: the physicochemical properties of the drug, the formulation, the delivery/liberating device and the patient (breathing patterns and clinical status).

The most fundamentally important physical property of an aerosol for inhalation is its size. The particle size of an aerosol is usually standardized by calculation of its aerodynamic diameter, d_a, which is the physical diameter of a unit density sphere which settles through air with a velocity equal to that of the particle in question. Therapeutic aerosols are heterodisperse (polydisperse) and the distribution of sizes is generally represented by the geometric standard deviation (σ_g), when the size is log-normally distributed.

For approximately spherical particles

$$d_a = d_p(\rho/\rho_0)^{1/2}$$

(37.1)

where d_p is the physical diameter, ρ is the particle density and ρ_0 is unit density (i.e. 1 g cm^{-3}).

When d_p is the mass median diameter, d_a is termed the mass median aerodynamic diameter.

Porous particles, with large physical diameters of the order of 20 μm, are efficiently delivered to, and deposited in, the lungs. Their low density, due to the porous or hollow nature of their structure, means such particles have a small aerodynamic diameter and are thus carried in the inspired air, deep into the lungs. Additionally, large particles are less prone to aggregation than smaller ones (see later), offering formulation advantages, and the particles are too large to be cleared from the airways by alveolar macrophages.

Influence of environmental humidity on particle size

As a particle enters the respiratory tract, the change from ambient to high relative humidity (~99%) results in condensation of water onto the particle surface, which continues until the vapour pressure of the water equals that of the surrounding atmosphere. For water-insoluble materials, this results in a negligibly thin film of water; however, with water-soluble materials a solution is formed on the particle surface. As the vapour pressure of the solution is lower than that of pure solvent at the same temperature, water will continue to condense until equilibrium between the vapour pressures is reached (i.e. the particle will increase in size). The final equilibrium diameter is constrained by the Kelvin effect, i.e. the vapour pressure of a droplet solution is higher than that for a planar surface, and is a function of the particle's original diameter. Hygroscopic growth will affect the deposition of particles, resulting in deposition higher in the respiratory tract than would have been predicted from measurements of their initial size.

Particle deposition in the airways

The efficacy of a therapeutic aerosol is dependent on its ability to penetrate the respiratory tract and

be deposited. To penetrate to the peripheral (respiratory) regions, aerosols require a size smaller than approximately 5 μm or 6 μm, with less than 2 μm being preferable for alveolar deposition. Literature values for 'respirable' size vary and must be considered alongside the environmental changes in size described earlier and the heterodisperse nature of inhalation aerosol size distributions. Larger particles or droplets are deposited in the upper respiratory tract and are rapidly removed from the lung by the mucociliary clearance process. As a consequence, the drug becomes available for systemic absorption and may potentially cause adverse effects. Corticosteroid aerosols of sufficiently large size may deposit in the mouth and throat, with the potential to cause adverse effects, including oral candidiasis. The size of aerosolized drug may be especially important in the treatment of certain conditions where penetration to the peripheral airways is particularly desirable; for instance, the treatment and prophylaxis of the alveolar infection *Pneumocystis carinii* pneumonia.

Three mechanisms are mainly responsible for particulate deposition in the lung: gravitational sedimentation, impaction and diffusion.

Inertial impaction

The airstream changes direction in the throat, or where a bifurcation occurs in the respiratory tract. Particles within the airstream, having sufficiently high momentum, will impact on the airways' walls rather than following the changing airstream. This deposition mechanism is particularly important for large particles having a diameter greater than 5 μm, and particularly greater than 10 μm, and is common in the upper airways, being the principal mechanism for deposition in the nose, mouth, pharynx, larynx and the large conducting airways. With the continuous branching of the conducting airways, the velocity of the airstream decreases and impaction becomes a less important mechanism for deposition.

The probability of impaction is proportional to

$$\frac{V_t V \sin\theta}{gr}$$

(37.2)

where θ is the change in direction of the airways, r is the airway's radius, V is the airstream velocity and V_t is the terminal settling velocity (see Eqn 37.3).

Gravitational sedimentation

From Stokes's law, a particle settling under gravity will attain a constant terminal settling velocity, V_t:

$$V_t = \frac{\rho g d^2}{18\eta}$$

(37.3)

where ρ is the particle density, g is the gravitational constant, d is the particle diameter and η is the air viscosity.

Thus gravitational sedimentation of an inhaled particle is dependent on its size and density, in addition to its residence time in the airways. Sedimentation is an important deposition mechanism for particles in the size range from 0.5 μm to 3 μm, in the small airways and alveoli, for particles that have escaped deposition by impaction.

Brownian diffusion

Collision and bombardment of small particles by molecules in the respiratory tract produce Brownian motion. The resultant movement of particles from high to low concentrations causes them to move from the aerosol cloud to the airways' walls. Diffusion is inversely proportional to particle size. It is the predominant mechanism for particles smaller than 0.5 μm, with the rate of diffusion given by the Stokes–Einstein equation:

$$D = \frac{k_B T}{3\pi\eta d}$$

(37.4)

where D is the diffusion coefficient, k_B is Boltzmann's constant, T is the absolute temperature, η is the viscosity and d is the particle diameter.

Other mechanisms of deposition

Although impaction, sedimentation and diffusion are the most important mechanisms for drug deposition in the respiratory tract, other mechanisms may occur. These include interception, whereby particles having extreme shapes, such as fibres, physically catch on to the airways' walls as they pass through the respiratory tract, and electrostatic attraction, whereby an electrostatic charge on a particle induces an opposing charge on the walls of the respiratory tract, resulting in attraction between the particle and the walls.

Effect of particle size on deposition mechanism

Different deposition mechanisms are important for different-sized particles. Those larger than 5 μm will deposit predominantly by inertial impaction in the upper airways. Particles of size between 1 μm and 5 μm deposit primarily by gravitational sedimentation in the lower airways, especially during slow, deep breathing, and particles smaller than 1 μm deposit by Brownian diffusion in the stagnant air of the lower airways. Particles of approximately 0.5 μm are inefficiently deposited, being too large for effective deposition by Brownian diffusion and too small for effective impaction or sedimentation, and they are often quickly exhaled. This size of minimum deposition should thus be considered during formulation, although for the reasons of environmental humidity discussed previously, the equilibrium diameter in the airways may be significantly larger than the original particle size in the formulation.

Breathing patterns

Patient-dependent factors, such as breathing patterns, lung physiology and the presence of pulmonary disease, also affect particle deposition. For instance, the larger the inhaled volume, the greater the peripheral distribution of particles in the lung, whilst increasing the inhalation flow rate enhances deposition in the larger airways by inertial impaction. Breath-holding after inhalation increases the deposition of particles by sedimentation and diffusion. Optimal aerosol deposition occurs with slow, deep inhalations to total lung capacity, followed by breath-holding prior to exhalation. It should be noted that changes in the airways resulting from disease states (e.g. obstruction of the airways) may affect the deposition profile of an inhaled aerosol.

Clearance of inhaled particles and drug absorption

Particles deposited in the ciliated conducting airways are cleared by mucociliary clearance within 24 hours and are ultimately swallowed. The composition of mucus and the process of mucociliary clearance are discussed in Chapter 38. Insoluble particles penetrating to the alveolar regions and which are not solubilized in situ are removed more slowly. Alveolar macrophages engulf such particles and may then migrate to the bottom of the mucociliary escalator, or may be removed via the lymphatics. The clearance of particle-loaded macrophages occurs over a period of days or weeks.

Hydrophobic compounds are usually absorbed at a rate dependent on their oil–water partition coefficients, whereas hydrophilic materials are poorly absorbed through membrane pores at rates inversely proportional to molecular size. Thus the airways' membrane, like the gastrointestinal tract, is preferably permeable to the un-ionized form of a drug. Some drugs, such as sodium cromoglicate, are partly absorbed by a saturable active transport mechanism, whilst large macromolecules may be absorbed by transcytosis. The rate of drug absorption, and consequently drug action, can be influenced by the formulation. Rapid drug action can generally be achieved using solutions or powders of aqueous soluble salts, whereas slower or prolonged absorption may be achieved with suspension formulations, powders of less soluble salts or novel drug delivery systems such as liposomes, microspheres and nanocarriers.

Formulating and delivering therapeutic inhalation aerosols

There are currently three main types of aerosol-generating device for use in inhaled drug therapy: pressurized metered-dose inhalers (pMDIs), dry powder inhalers (DPIs) and nebulizers.

Pressurized metered-dose inhalers

Pressurized metered-dose inhalers (pMDIs), sometimes referred to as metered-dose inhalers, were introduced in the mid-1950s and are the most commonly used inhalation drug delivery devices. In pMDIs, the drug is either dissolved or suspended in liquid propellant(s) together with other excipients, including surfactants, and is presented in a pressurized canister fitted with a metering valve (Fig. 37.2). A predetermined dose is released as a spray on actuation of the metering valve. When released from the canister, the formulation undergoes volume expansion in the passage within the valve and forms a mixture of gas and liquid before discharge from the orifice. The high-speed gas flow helps to break up the liquid into a fine spray of droplets.

Containers

Pharmaceutical aerosols may be packaged in tin-plated steel, plastic-coated glass or aluminium containers.

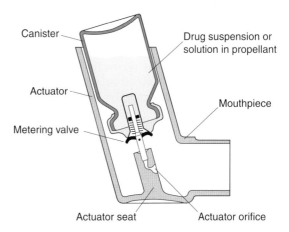

Fig. 37.2 • The pressurized metered-dose inhaler.

In practice, pMDIs are generally presented in aluminium canisters, produced by extrusion to give seamless containers with a capacity of 10 mL to 30 mL. Aluminium is relatively inert and may be used uncoated where there is no chemical instability between the container and the contents. Alternatively, aluminium containers with an internal coating of a chemically resistant organic material, such as an epoxy resin or polytetrafluoroethylene (PTFE), can be used.

Propellants

The propellants used in pMDI formulations are liquefied gases, traditionally chlorofluorocarbons (CFCs), although in recent years these have been replaced by hydrofluoroalkanes (HFAs). At room temperature and pressure, these are gases but they are readily liquefied by decreasing temperature or increasing pressure. The head space of the aerosol canister is filled with propellant vapour, producing the saturation vapour pressure of the propellant at that temperature. On spraying, medicament and propellant are expelled, and the head volume increases. To reestablish the equilibrium, more propellant evaporates, and so a constant-pressure system with consistent spray characteristics is produced.

The reaction of CFCs with the ozone in Earth's stratosphere, which absorbs UV radiation at 300 nm, was a major environmental concern towards the end of the 20th century. CFCs pass to the stratosphere, where in the presence of UV radiation they liberate chlorine, which reacts with ozone. The depletion of stratospheric ozone results in increased exposure to the UV-B part of the UV spectrum, resulting in several adverse effects, in particular an increased incidence of skin cancer. The Montreal Protocol of 1987 was a global ban on the production of the five worst ozone-depleting CFCs by the year 2000. This was amended in 1992 so that production of CFCs in developed countries was phased out by January 1996. In the European Union and the USA, all ozone-depleting CFCs were banned by the end of 1995, except for an 'essential use exemption' whilst manufacturers developed medically acceptable non-ozone-depleting alternatives to the remaining CFC-based pMDIs. This exemption remained in place for several years, but now CFC-based inhalers are no longer produced for use in Europe and the USA. In household and cosmetic aerosols, CFCs have been replaced by hydrocarbons, such as propane and butane. Alternatively, nontoxic compressed gases such as nitrogen dioxide, nitrogen and carbon dioxide may be used (e.g. in food products). However, compressed gases do not maintain a constant pressure within the canister throughout its use, as the internal pressure is inversely proportional to the head volume, and so product performance changes with use. For reasons of toxicity and inflammability, hydrocarbons were not considered appropriate alternatives to CFCs for inhalation products, and so non-ozone-depleting alternatives to CFCs have been developed.

The propellants HFA-134a (trifluoromonofluoroethane) and HFA-227 (heptafluoropropane) are non-ozone-depleting, nonflammable HFAs, also called hydrofluorocarbons (HFCs), which are now used as inhaler propellants (see Table 37.1).

The introduction of HFA-134a and HFA-227 as replacement, non-ozone-depleting propellants in the past 2 decades presented major formulation challenges to the pharmaceutical industry; in particular, they are poor solvents for the surfactants which had received regulatory approval for use in CFC-based pMDI formulations, as suspending agents and to lubricate the valve. Ethanol is approved for use in formulations containing HFAs to allow dissolution of surfactants, and is included in some marketed HFA-based pMDI products. However, ethanol has low volatility, and its inclusion may, depending on its concentration, increase the droplet size of the emitted aerosols.

The Kigali agreement of 2016 amended the 1987 Montreal Protocol with the objective of the gradual complete phase out of HFC usage to begin 2019. This will impact on pMDI formulation and production in the future.

Metering valve

The metering valve of a pMDI permits the reproducible delivery of small volumes (25 μL to 100 μL) of product. Compared with the nonmetering continuous-spray valve of conventional pressurized aerosols, the metering valve in pMDIs is used in the inverted position (Fig. 37.3). Depression of the valve stem allows the contents of the metering chamber to be discharged through the orifice in the valve stem and made available to the patient. After actuation, the metering chamber refills with liquid from the bulk and is ready to dispense the next dose. A corollary of this is that the pMDI needs to be primed, i.e. the metering chamber must be filled, prior to the first use by a patient (and subsequently if the device is

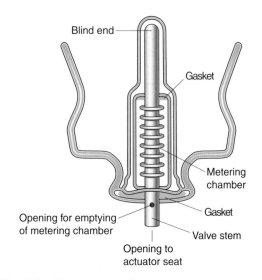

Fig. 37.3 • The metering valve.

Table 37.1 Formulae and physicochemical properties of hydrofluoroalkanes used as propellants in pressurized metered-dose inhaler formulations

Number	Formula	Boiling point (°C)	Vapour pressure (kPa) at 20 °C	Density (g mL⁻¹) at 20 °C
134a	$C_2F_4H_2$	−26.5	660 (6.6 bar)	1.23
227	C_3F_7H	−17.3	398 (3.98 bar)	1.41

stored for a length of time). The valves of pMDIs are complex in design and must protect the product from the environment, whilst also protecting against product loss during repeated use. The introduction of HFA propellants with different solvent properties necessitated the development of new valve elastomers. The valve stem fits into the actuator, which is made of polyethylene or polypropylene. The dimensions of the orifice in the actuator play a crucial role, along with the propellant vapour pressure, in determining the shape and speed of the emitted aerosol plume.

Formulating pMDIs

Pressurized aerosols may be formulated as either solutions or suspensions of drug in the liquefied propellant. Solution preparations are two-phase systems. However, the propellants are poor solvents for most drugs. A cosolvent such as ethanol or 2-propanol may be used, although their low volatility retards propellant evaporation. In practice, the large majority of pressurized inhaler formulations have been suspensions. These three-phase systems are harder to formulate, and all the problems of conventional suspension formulation, such as caking, agglomeration and particle growth, need to be considered. Careful consideration must also be given to the particle size of the solid (usually micronized to between 2 μm and 5 μm), valve clogging, moisture content, the solubility of the drug substance in the propellant (a salt may be desirable), the relative densities of the propellant and the drug, and the use of surfactants as suspending agents, e.g. lecithin, oleic acid and sorbitan trioleate (usually included at concentrations between 0.1% and 2.0% w/w). These surfactants are very poorly soluble (< 0.02% w/w) in HFAs, and so ethanol is usually used as a cosolvent, although alternative surfactants are being developed. Solution formulations of some drugs, such as beclometasone dipropionate, are now available. Evaporation of HFA propellant following actuation of these formulations results in smaller particle sizes than with conventional suspension formulations of the same drug, with consequent changes in its pulmonary distribution and bioavailability. The dose may be adjusted accordingly or the volatility of the product may be modified by the addition of a less volatile component, such as glycerol. The difference in performance of beclomethasone dipropionate pMDIs from different manufacturers, resulting from differences in their formulation, means that they are not considered interchangeable and they should consequently be prescribed by brand name.

Filling pMDI canisters

Canisters are filled either by liquefying the propellant by reducing its temperature (cold filling) or by filling the vapour at elevated pressure (pressure filling).

In cold filling, drug substance, excipients and propellant are chilled, and the canister is filled with them at approximately −60°C. Additional propellant is then added at the same temperature, and the canister is sealed with the valve. In pressure filling, most frequently employed for inhalation aerosols, a concentrated solution or suspension of drug in propellant, under pressure, is filled into canisters through the valve, followed by addition of further propellant.

Once filled, the canisters are leak tested, often by placing them in a water bath at elevated temperature, usually 50°C to 60°C. Following storage to allow equilibration of the formulation and valve components, the containers are weighed to check them for further leakage, prior to insertion into actuators and spray testing.

Advantages and disadvantages of pMDIs

The major advantages of pMDIs are their portability, low cost and disposability. Many doses (up to 200) are stored in the small canister, which may also have a dose counter, and dose delivery is reproducible. The inert conditions created by the propellant vapour, together with the hermetically sealed container, protect drugs from oxidative degradation and microbiological contamination. However, pMDIs have disadvantages. They are inefficient at drug delivery. On actuation, the first propellant droplets exit at a high velocity, which may exceed 30 m s^{-1}. Consequently, much of the drug is lost through impaction of these droplets in the oropharyngeal areas. The mean emitted droplet size typically exceeds 40 μm, and propellants may not evaporate sufficiently rapidly for their size to decrease to that suitable for deep lung deposition. Evaporation, such that the aerodynamic diameter of the particles is close to that of the original micronized drug, may not occur until 5 seconds after actuation.

An additional problem with pMDIs, which is beyond the control of the formulator and manufacturer, is their incorrect use by patients. Reported problems include:

- failure to remove the protective cap covering the mouthpiece;
- the inhaler being used in an inverted position;

- failure to shake the canister;
- failure to inhale slowly and deeply;
- inadequate breath-holding following inhalation; and
- poor inhalation–actuation synchronization.

Correct use by patients is vital for effective drug deposition and therapeutic action. Ideally, the pMDI should be actuated during the course of a slow, deep inhalation, followed by a period of breath-holding. Many patients find this difficult, especially children and the elderly. The misuse of pMDIs through poor inhalation–actuation coordination can be significantly reduced with appropriate instruction and counselling. However, it should be noted that even using the correct inhalation technique, only 10% to 20% of the stated emitted dose may be delivered to the site of action.

Spacers, valved-holding chambers and breath-actuated metered-dose inhalers

Some of the disadvantages of pMDIs, namely inhalation–actuation coordination and the premature deposition of high velocity, large droplets high in the airways, can be overcome by using extension devices, referred to as 'spacers' or valved holding chambers, positioned between the pMDI and the patient (Fig. 37.4). These are frequently employed with a pMDI, for administering aerosol medications to young children (see also Chapter 45) and for those with poor inhalation technique. The dose from a pMDI is discharged directly into the reservoir prior to inhalation, from which the patient inhales via a one-way valve. This reduces the initial droplet velocity, large droplets may be removed by impaction, efficient propellant evaporation occurs and the need for actuation–inhalation coordination is removed. The disadvantage of traditional spacers, though highly effective, is that they may be cumbersome because

of their large volume (e.g. Volumatic®, GlaxoSmith-Kline), although smaller, medium-volume spacers are now available (e.g. AeroChamber Plus®, GlaxoSmith-Kline). Alternatively, extension tubes may be built into the design of the pMDI itself as an extended mouthpiece (e.g. Syncroner®, Sanofi-Aventis). Breath-actuated pMDIs do not release the drug until inspiration occurs. In the Autohaler® (3M), an inspiratory demand valve triggers a spring mechanism to release the drug, whilst in the Easi-Breathe® (Teva), a vacuum in the device is released on inspiration to trigger the actuation. Breath-actuated devices overcome the actuation–inhalation coordination problems associated with conventional pMDIs and are easy to use without adding bulk to the device.

Dry powder inhalers

In dry powder inhaler (DPI) systems, the drug is inhaled as a cloud of fine particles. The drug is either preloaded in an inhalation device or filled into hard gelatin or hypromellose capsules which are loaded into a device prior to use.

DPIs have several advantages over pMDIs. DPI formulations are propellant-free and usually do not contain any excipient, other than a carrier (see later), which is usually lactose. They are breath-actuated, avoiding the problems of inhalation–actuation coordination encountered with pMDIs. DPIs can also deliver larger drug doses than pMDIs, which are limited by the volume of the metering valve and the maximum suspension concentration that can be employed without causing valve clogging. However, DPIs have several disadvantages. Liberation of powders from the device and the deaggregation of particles are limited by the patient's ability to inhale, which in the case of respiratory disease may be impaired. An increase in turbulent airflow created by an increase in inhaled air velocity increases the deaggregation of the emerging particles but also increases the potential for inertial impaction in the upper airways and throat, and so a compromise has to be found. Furthermore, DPIs are exposed to ambient atmospheric conditions, which may reduce formulation stability. For instance, elevated humidity may cause powders to aggregate.

Formulating DPIs

To produce particles of a suitable size (preferably less than 5 μm), drug powders for use in inhalation systems are usually micronized. Alternatives are

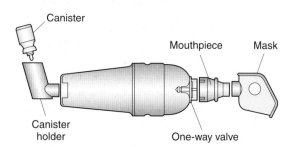

Fig. 37.4 • Spacer device, fitted with a facemask for use by a child.

Labels in figure: Canister, Mouthpiece, Mask, Canister holder, One-way valve spray-drying, spray–freeze-drying and supercritical fluid technology. The high-energy powders produced by micronization have poor flow properties because of their static, cohesive and adhesive nature. The flowability of a powder is affected by its physical properties, including particle size and shape, density, surface roughness, hardness, moisture content and bulk density.

To improve their flow properties, poorly flowing drug particles are generally mixed with larger 'carrier' particles (median size usually 30 μm to 150 μm) of an inert excipient, usually lactose (α-lactose monohydrate). The drug and carrier particles are mixed to produce an ordered mix in which the small drug particles attach to the surface of the larger carrier particles. This not only increases liberation of the drug from the inhalation device by improving powder flow but also increases the uniformity of capsule or device filling. Once liberated from the device, the turbulent airflow generated within the inhalation device should be sufficient for the deaggregation of the drug–carrier aggregates. The larger carrier particles impact in the throat, whereas smaller drug particles are carried in the inhaled air deeper into the respiratory tract.

The success of DPI formulations depends on the adhesion of the drug and carrier during mixing and filling of devices or hard capsules, followed by the ability of the drug to detach from the carrier during inhalation, such that free drug is available to penetrate to the peripheral airways. Adhesion and detachment will depend on the morphology of the particle surfaces and surface energies, which may be influenced by the chemical nature of the materials involved and the nature of powder processing. Assessment of the balance between adhesive and cohesive forces between particles, using techniques such as atomic force microscopy, has been employed to characterize powder blends used in DPI formulation. Additionally, a ternary mix may be employed. Thus fine particle size lactose can be added to larger, conventional carrier lactose to occupy the high-energy sites on the larger carrier particles. Only low-energy sites remain for drug–carrier interaction, enhancing the detachment of drug particles during inhalation of the formulation. Likewise, materials such as leucine and magnesium stearate may be included in formulations to modify the adhesion properties of the drug and carrier particles. The interactions between micronized drugs, fine carrier particles and large carrier particles in DPI formulations are discussed in Chapter 8.

The performance of DPI systems is thus strongly dependent on formulation factors. Other factors affecting aerosol delivery and deposition include the design of the delivery device and the patient's inhalation technique.

Unit-dose devices with drug in hard gelatin capsules

The first DPI device developed was the Spinhaler® for the delivery of sodium cromoglicate. Each dose, contained in a hard gelatin capsule, was placed individually into the device, in a loose-fitting rotor. The capsule was pierced by two metal needles on either side of the capsule, and inhaled airflow though the device caused a turbovibratory air pattern as the rotor rotated rapidly, resulting in the powder being dispersed to the capsule walls and out through the perforations into the inspired air. Although the tendency nowadays is to develop multiple-dosing devices, other hard-capsule-based devices, working on similar principles are still available, e.g. the HandiHaler® (Boehringer Ingelheim/Pfizer) and the Aerolizer®/Cyclohaler® (Novartis/Teva; Fig. 37.5).

Multidose devices with drug preloaded in the inhaler

The evolution of an earlier device, the Diskhaler® in which a drug/lactose mix was filled into aluminium foil blister disks for loading into the device, led to the Accuhaler®, also called Diskus® inhaler (GlaxoSmithKline). Here the drug–carrier mix is premetered, i.e. it is preloaded into the device in foil-covered blister pockets containing 60 doses (Fig. 37.6). The foil lid is peeled off the drug-containing pockets as each dose is advanced, with the blisters and lids being wound up separately within the device, which is discarded at the end of use. As each dose is packaged separately and only momentarily exposed to ambient conditions prior to inhalation, the Accuhaler is relatively insensitive to humidity compared with hard-capsule-based systems. The Ellipta® inhaler (Glaxo SmithKline) is a similar blister-based device.

An alternative approach is a reservoir-based device, in which a dose is accurately measured and delivered from a drug reservoir. In the Clickhaler® DPI (Innovata Biomed), a drug–lactose blend is stored in a reservoir. Metering cups are filled by gravity from this reservoir and delivered to an inhalation passage, from which the dose is inhaled. The device is shaken

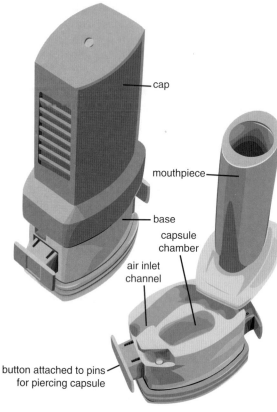

Fig. 37.5 • The Aerolizer®/Cyclohaler® dry powder inhaler.

before use. The device is capable of holding up to 200 doses and incorporates a dose counter which indicates the number of metered doses and informs patients when the device, which is discarded after use, is nearly empty. After the final dose has been dispensed, the push button locks to prevent further use.

The Turbohaler® (AstraZeneca) has overcome the need for both a carrier (in some formulations) and the loading of individual doses (Fig. 37.7). The device contains a large number of doses (up to 200) of loosely aggregated micronized drug, which is stored in a reservoir, from which it flows on to a rotating disc in the dosing unit. The fine holes in the disc are filled, and excess drug is removed by scrapers. As the disc is rotated, by moving a turning grip back and forth, one metered dose is presented to the inhalation channel, and this is inhaled by the patient, with the turbulent airflow created within the device breaking up any drug aggregates. A dose indicator is incorporated.

Breath-assisted devices

Several devices have been developed which reduce or eliminate the reliance on the patient's inspiratory effort to disperse the drug. This is advantageous as inspiratory effort may be affected by the patient's age and/or clinical condition. For instance, Nektar Therapeutics produced a device for the delivery of insulin as a very fine powder in which compressed air was used to disperse drug from a unit-dose package into a large holding chamber, from which it was inhaled by the patient. The device was marketed briefly by Pfizer for the delivery of insulin by inhalation, but was withdrawn for many reasons, including cost, the cumbersome design of the delivery device and the need for injections of insulin to supplement inhaled drug.

Nebulizers

Nebulizers are devices which convert liquids into aerosols; they deliver relatively large volumes of drug solutions and suspensions over an extended period, and are frequently used for drugs that cannot be conveniently formulated into pMDIs or DPIs, or where the therapeutic dose is too large for delivery with these alternative systems. Nebulizers also have the advantage over pMDI and DPI systems in that the drug may be inhaled during normal tidal breathing through a mouthpiece or facemask, and thus they are useful for patients such as young children, the elderly and patients with arthritis, who experience difficulties with pMDIs.

There are three categories of commercially available nebulizer: jet, ultrasonic and mesh.

Jet nebulizers

Jet nebulizers (also called air-jet or air-blast nebulizers) use compressed air from a compressed gas cylinder, hospital air line or electrical compressor to convert a liquid (usually an aqueous solution) into a spray. The jet of high-velocity gas is passed either tangentially or coaxially through a narrow Venturi nozzle, typically 0.3 mm to 0.7 mm in diameter. An area of negative pressure, where the air jet emerges, causes liquid to be drawn up a feed tube from a fluid reservoir by the Bernoulli effect (Fig. 37.8). Liquid emerges as fine filaments, which collapse into droplets as a result of surface tension. A proportion of the resultant (primary) aerosol leaves the nebulizer directly; the remaining large, nonrespirable droplets impact on

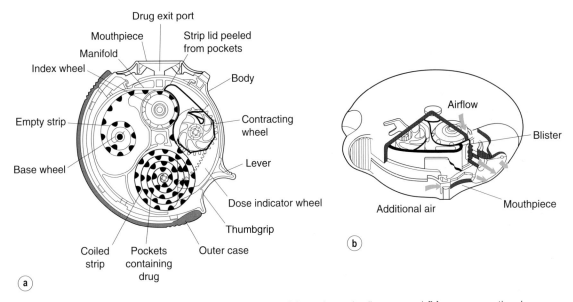

Fig. 37.6 • The Accuhaler®/Diskus® dry powder inhaler: **(a)** a schematic diagram and **(b)** a cross-sectional representation of the device. From Prime et al., 1996, with permission.

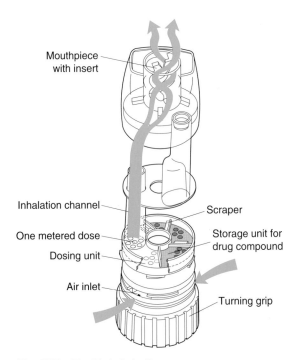

Fig. 37.7 • The Turbohaler®. Courtesy of AstraZeneca.

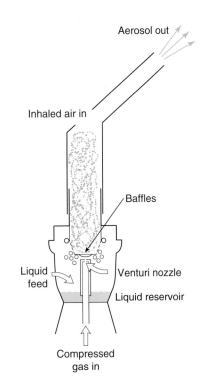

Fig. 37.8 • A jet nebulizer. Compressed gas passes through a Venturi nozzle, where an area of negative pressure is created. Liquid is drawn up a feed tube and is fragmented into droplets. Large droplets impact on baffles, and small droplets are carried away in the inhaled airstream.

baffles or the walls of the nebulizer chamber and are recycled into the reservoir fluid.

Nebulizers are operated continuously, and because the inspiratory phase of breathing constitutes approximately one-third of the breathing cycle, a large proportion of the emitted aerosol is not inhaled but is released into the environment. Open-vent nebulizers, incorporating inhalation and exhalation valves (e.g. the Pari LC® nebulizer), have been developed in which the patient's own breath boosts nebulizer performance, with aerosol production matching the patient's tidal volume and greatly enhancing drug delivery. On exhalation, the aerosol being produced is generated only from the compressor gas source, thereby minimizing drug wastage.

The rate of gas flow driving atomization is the major determinant of the aerosol droplet size and rate of drug delivery for jet nebulizers; for instance, there may be up to a 50% reduction in the mass median aerodynamic diameter when the flow rate is increased from 4 L min^{-1} to 8 L min^{-1}, with a linear increase in the proportion of droplets smaller than 5 μm.

Ultrasonic nebulizers

In ultrasonic nebulizers, the energy necessary to atomize liquids comes from a piezoelectric crystal vibrating at high frequency. At sufficiently high ultrasonic intensities, a fountain of liquid is formed in the nebulizer chamber. Large droplets are emitted from the apex, and a 'fog' of small droplets is emitted from the lower part (Fig. 37.9). Some models have a fan to blow the inhalable droplets out of the device, whereas in others the aerosol becomes available to the patient only during inhalation.

Mesh nebulizers

More recently, mesh nebulizers have become commercially available, in which aerosols are generated by passing liquids through a vibrating mesh or plate with multiple apertures. The energy of vibration comes from a vibrating piezoelectric crystal attached to a horn transducer which transmits vibrations to a perforated plate with up to 6000 tapered holes (Fig. 37.10) or from an aerosol generator comprising a domed aperture plate, with up to 10 000 tapered holes and a vibrational element which contracts and expands to generate the aerosol. These devices generate aerosols with a high fine particle fraction, deliver fluids very rapidly and have very small residual

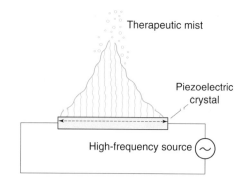

Fig. 37.9 • An ultrasonic nebulizer.

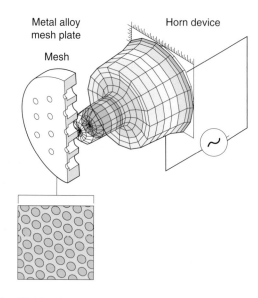

Fig. 37.10 • Aerosol production in a vibrating-mesh nebulizer. Courtesy of Omron Healthcare.

volumes (see later) compared with jet and ultrasonic nebulizers. A recent development is the 'adaptive aerosol delivery' (AAD) system employed in the I-neb® AAD® mesh nebulizer (Philips Respironics), which analyses the patient's breathing pattern and emits aerosol only during inhalation, thus eliminating wastage during exhalation.

Formulating nebulizer fluids

Nebulizer fluids are formulated in water, occasionally with the addition of a cosolvent such as ethanol, and with the addition of surfactants for suspension formulations. Because hypoosmotic and hyperosmotic solutions may cause bronchoconstriction, as may high hydrogen ion concentrations, isoosmotic solutions of pH not lower than 3 and not higher than 10 are usually employed. Stabilizers such as antioxidants and preservatives may also be included, although these may also cause bronchospasm, and for this reason sulfites, in particular, are generally avoided as antioxidants in such formulations. Although chemically preserved multidose preparations are commercially available, nebulizer formulations are generally presented as sterile, isotonic unit doses (usually 1 mL to 2.5 mL) without a preservative.

Whilst most nebulizer formulations are solutions, suspensions of micronized drug are also available for delivery from nebulizers. In general, suspensions are poorly delivered from ultrasonic nebulizers, whilst mesh nebulizers are considered suitable for delivering suspensions. With jet nebulizers, the efficiency of drug delivery increases as the size of the suspended drug is decreased, with little or no delivery of particles when they exceed the droplet size of the nebulized aerosol.

As the formulation of fluids for delivery by nebulizers is relatively simple, these devices are frequently the first to be employed when investigating the pulmonary delivery of new drug entities in clinical trials. Recently, they have been used for the delivery of biopharmaceuticals and drug delivery systems, such as liposomes. In general, ultrasonic nebulizers have not been successful for delivering either biopharmaceuticals or liposomes, because of denaturation resulting from the elevated temperatures produced. Consequently, ultrasonic nebulizers are expressly excluded for the delivery of recombinant human deoxyribonuclease in the management of cystic fibrosis. Mesh and jet nebulizers have been successfully used to deliver some peptides, nucleic acids and liposome formulations, although the shearing forces that occur in jet nebulizers may produce time-dependent damage to some materials.

Physicochemical properties of nebulizer fluids

The viscosity and surface tension of a liquid being nebulized may affect the output of nebulizers, as energy is required to overcome viscous forces and to create a new surface. However, the size selectivity of the nebulizer design and dimensions, with large primary aerosol droplets being recycled into the reservoir liquid, means that changes in the size distribution of the primary aerosol, resulting from changes in the properties of the solution being atomized, may not be reflected in the size distribution of the emitted aerosol. In general, the size of aerosol droplets is inversely proportional to viscosity for jet and mesh nebulizers and directly proportional to viscosity for ultrasonic nebulizers, with more viscous solutions requiring longer to be nebulized to dryness and leaving larger residual volumes in the nebulizer following atomization. Surface tension effects are more complex, but usually a decrease in surface tension is associated with a reduction in mean aerosol size.

Temperature effects during nebulization

The aerosol output from a jet nebulizer comprises drug solution and solvent vapour, which saturates the outgoing air. This causes the solute concentration to increase with time and results in a rapid decrease in the temperature of the liquid being nebulized by approximately 10 °C to 15 °C. This temperature decrease may be important clinically, as some asthma sufferers experience bronchoconstriction on inhalation of cold solutions. Furthermore, the cooling effect within the reservoir fluid will reduce drug solubility and result in increased liquid surface tension and viscosity. Precipitation is uncommon with bronchodilators, which have high aqueous solubility, but problems may arise with less soluble drugs. In such instances the use of an ultrasonic nebulizer may be appropriate, as the operation of such devices may increase the solution temperature by up to 15 °C depending on the device design. As indicated already, this temperature increase may have detrimental effects on heat-sensitive materials intended for nebulization. Mesh nebulizers have a negligible effect on fluid temperature.

Duration of nebulization and residual volume

Clinically, liquids may be nebulized for a specified period or, more commonly, they may be nebulized to 'dryness', which may be interpreted as the *sputtering time*, which is the time when air is drawn up the feed tube and nebulization becomes erratic, although agitation/tapping of the nebulizer permits treatment to be continued; the *clinical time*, which is the time at which therapy is ceased following sputtering; or the *total time*, which is the time at which the production of aerosol ceases.

Regardless of the duration of nebulization, not all the fluid in the nebulizer can be atomized. Some liquid, usually approximately 1 mL for jet and ultrasonic nebulizers, remains as the 'dead' or 'residual' volume, associated with the baffles, internal structures and walls of the nebulizer. The proportion of drug retained as residual volume is more marked for smaller fill volumes; hence for a 2-mL fill volume, approximately 50% of fluid will remain associated with the nebulizer and be unavailable for delivery to the patient. This reduces to approximately 25% with a 4-mL fill volume, although there is a commensurate increase in the time necessary to nebulize the liquid to dryness. For this reason small-volume nebulizer fluids may be diluted to a larger volume by addition of a suitable diluent, usually sterile 0.9% sodium chloride solution. Vibrating-mesh nebulizers have a much smaller residual volume than jet or ultrasonic devices, which may mean that the nominal dose or dose volume used with a mesh nebulizer should be reduced compared with that employed with a conventional nebulizer.

Variability between nebulizers

Many different models of nebulizer and compressor are commercially available, and the size of the aerosols produced and the dose delivered can vary considerably. Variability may not only exist between different nebulizers but also between individual nebulizers of the same type, and repeated use of a single nebulizer may cause variability due to baffle wear and nonuniformity of assembly. Nebulizers, unlike the DPI and pMDI devices, are not manufactured by the producers of nebulizer solutions and suspensions. The choice of nebulizer employed for their delivery is thus usually beyond the influence of the pharmaceutical manufacturer.

Novel delivery devices

A number of new inhalation devices have been developed which do not fit neatly into the traditional categories of pMDIs, DPIs and nebulizers, because they operate on alternative principles. Two metered-dose liquid inhalers are The Respimat® (Boehringer Ingelheim; Fig. 37.11) and the AERx® pulmonary delivery system (Aradigm; Fig. 37.12). The Respimat Soft Mist™ inhaler, which is described as a nonpressurized metered-dose system, is a handheld device with a multidose reservoir releasing a cloud of 1.5 seconds' duration. This is much slower than for conventional pMDIs, allowing more time for coordination between actuation and inhalation. The device is

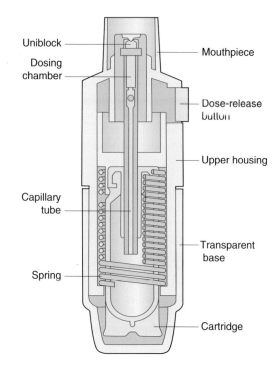

Fig. 37.11 • The Respimat® Soft Mist™ inhaler. Courtesy of Boehringer Ingelheim International.

mechanically actuated without use of a propellant. The aerosol generated by the device has lower velocity and smaller particle size than that generated with a conventional pMDI, resulting in superior peripheral lung deposition. The AERx® pulmonary delivery system has drug contained in unit-dose blister packs. Drug delivery is electronically controlled and involves extrusion of liquid through a single-use nozzle containing numerous spherical holes, with exits approximately 1 μm in diameter. This produces very fine aerosols, suitable for delivery of biopharmaceuticals, such as insulin, to the peripheral airways. The device electronically monitors the patient's inspiratory flow rate, and releases drug at the inspiratory flow rate determined to be optimal for drug delivery.

Methods of aerosol size analysis

The regional distribution of aerosols in the airways can be measured directly by γ-scintigraphy, by the radiolabelling of droplets or particles, usually with the short half-life γ-emitter technetium-99m. However, more commonly, in vitro measurements

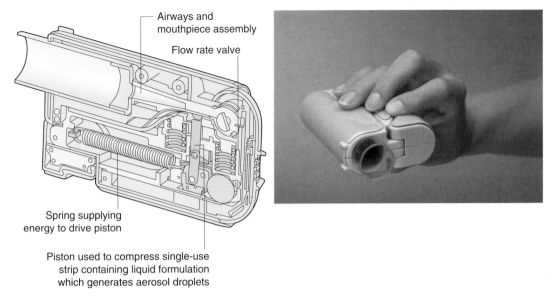

Fig. 37.12 • The AERx® pulmonary delivery system. Courtesy of Aradigm.

of aerosol size are used to "predict" clinical performance. They also have widespread use in research and development and in routine quality control of inhalation products. The principal methods that have been employed for size characterization of aerosols are microscopy, laser diffraction and cascade impaction.

Optical methods for measuring the physical size of deposited aerosols using microscopy are laborious and do not give an indication of their likely deposition within the humid airways while being carried in an airstream. With methods of analysis based on laser diffraction, aerosolized droplets or particles are sized as they traverse a laser beam to give a volume median diameter. This method has been used routinely to characterize aerosols generated by nebulizers. However, again, the aerodynamic properties of an aerosol are not being measured. In addition, the spraying of droplets into a beam exposes them to ambient conditions of temperature and humidity, which may result in solvent evaporation and consequently size reduction.

Cascade impactors and impingers

Cascade impactors comprise a series of progressively finer jets and collection plates, allowing fractionation of aerosols according to their aerodynamic size distribution as the aerosol is drawn through the device at a known flow rate. Large, denser particles will deposit higher in the impactor, whereas smaller, less

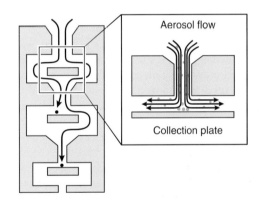

Fig. 37.13 • Principle of operation of a cascade impactor. Courtesy of Copley Instruments.

dense particles will follow the airflow and deposit only when they have been given sufficient momentum as they are accelerated through the finer jets lower in the impactor (Fig. 37.13). The first stage of the impactor is usually preceded by a 90° bend, usually metal to mimic the human throat. These 'throats', or induction ports, are described in pharmacopoeias, whilst research is ongoing to develop designs which more closely mimic the human anatomy. Traditional cascade impactors are constructed from metal. The two most commonly used are (1) the Andersen Cascade Impactor (ACI), which comprises eight impaction stages, with metal collection plates followed by a terminal filter, and (2) the Next Generation

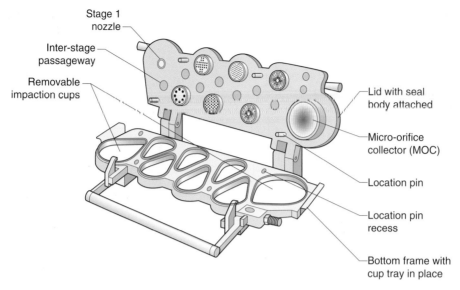

Stage 1 nozzle

Inter-stage passageway

Removable impaction cups

Lid with seal body attached

Micro-orifice collector (MOC)

Location pin

Location pin recess

Bottom frame with cup tray in place

Fig. 37.14 • The Next Generation Impactor. Courtesy of Copley Instruments.

Impactor (NGI), which consists of seven impaction stages followed by a micro-orifice collector, which can be used in place of a terminal filter in most cases. The NGI uses collection cups rather than plates and can be used with flow rates from 15 L min^{-1} to 100 L min^{-1} (Fig. 37.14). The cut-off diameters for each stage at a particular airflow rate can be determined using monodisperse aerosols or calculated using calibration curves. When determining the size of an aerosol, cumulative percentage undersize of deposited aerosol on each stage is plotted against the cut-off diameter for that stage to allow calculation of the mass median aerodynamic diameter. The ACI and NGI are used for aerodynamic assessment of pMDIs and DPIs (*United States Pharmacopeia* and *European Pharmacopoeia*) and the NGI is used for aerodynamic assessment of nebulizers (*United States Pharmacopeia* and *European Pharmacopoeia*).

Multistage liquid impingers work on the same principle of cascade impaction. They are constructed from glass or glass and metal and have three, four or five stages, with wet sintered glass collection plates followed by a terminal filter. The five-stage liquid impinger (Fig. 37.15), with an appropriate induction port and mouthpiece adapter, is used to determine the aerodynamic size of DPIs (*United States Pharmacopeia* and *European Pharmacopoeia*) and pMDIs (*European Pharmacopoeia*). The multistage liquid impinger may be operated at a flow rate between 30 L min^{-1} and 100 L min^{-1}. At 60 L min^{-1} (i.e.

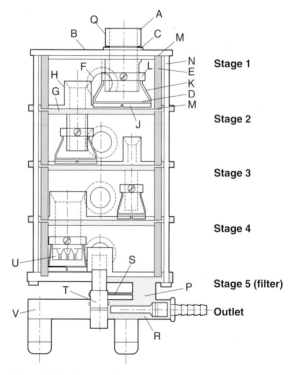

Stage 1

Stage 2

Stage 3

Stage 4

Stage 5 (filter)

Outlet

Fig. 37.15 • The multistage liquid impinger. Courtesy of AstraZeneca.

1 L s⁻¹), the effective cut-off diameters of stages 1, 2, 3 and 4 are 13.0 μm, 6.8 μm, 3.1 μm and 1.7 μm respectively. The fifth stage comprises an integral filter which captures particles smaller than 1.7 μm.

When testing DPIs to pharmacopoeial requirements, an airflow rate (Q) calculated to produce a pressure drop of 4.0 kPa over the inhaler is employed. If this exceeds 100 L min⁻¹, then 100 L min⁻¹ is used. The cut-off diameters of each stage at a given flow rate (Q) can be calculated from

$$D_{50'Q} = D_{50'Q_n}(Q_n/Q)^{1/2}$$

(37.5)

where $D_{50'Q}$ is the cut-off diameter at flow rate Q and $D_{50'Q_n}$ refers to the nominal cut-off values determined when Q_n is 60 L min⁻¹ (values given earlier).

The use of cascade impaction methods to determine the aerodynamic size of aerosols has a number of disadvantages. The high flow rates employed (typically 28.3 L min⁻¹ to 100 L min⁻¹) result in rapid solvent evaporation from droplets, whilst particles may 'bounce off' metal collection plates and pass to lower stages, although this latter effect may be reduced by coating the collection surface, for instance, a silicone fluid or glycerol. These effects can result in a significant decrease in the measured aerosol size. In addition, these measuring devices are operated at a constant airflow rate. However, the dispersion of dry powder formulations and the deposition profile of inhaled aerosols will vary considerably with the flow rate. To overcome the limitations of measurement at a single flow rate, a 'breath simulator' can be used, whereby a computer-controlled piston draws air through the inhaler and into an impaction sizer, following a predetermined inhalation profile.

Cascade impactor methods are invasive, laborious and time-consuming but necessary to derive information about median aerodynamic size and the polydispersity of the aerosol. To ensure that inhalation products are likely to be clinically effective, in addition to size properties, the emitted dose is calculated together with the 'fine particle fraction' (that fraction of the emitted dose smaller than a stated size, usually 5 μm), which are combined to give a 'therapeutically useful' or 'respirable' dose or mass (fine particle dose/fine particle mass).

For routine analysis, a simplified glass two-stage (twin) glass impinger may be employed (Fig. 37.16). Aerosol collected in the throat and the upper stage (stage 1) is considered 'nonrespirable', whereas that

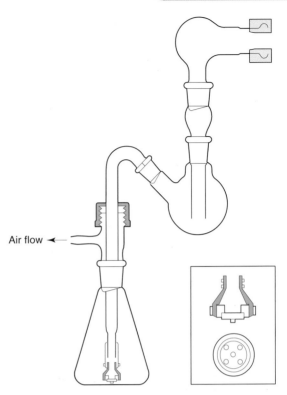

Fig. 37.16 • The two-stage (twin) impinger. Courtesy of Copley Instruments.

collected in the lower stage (stage 2) is considered 'respirable'. For this glass device, the cut-off diameter for stage 2 is 6.4 μm, i.e. aerosols collected in this stage have an aerodynamic diameter less than 6.4 μm and for this measurement technique constitute the fine particle fraction. This two-stage impinger may be used for fine particle assessment of aerosols generated from pMDIs, DPIs and nebulizers (*European Pharmacopoeia*) but gives much less information about aerosol particle size distribution than a full multistage impactor or impinger.

Work is under way to establish the use of 'abbreviated impactor measurement', whereby only two or three stages of the ACI or NGI are used for routine research and development or quality control functions, by fractionating the collected aerosol into the coarse particle mass (usually larger than 5 μm) and fine particle mass (smaller than 5 μm), and where a third stage is used, an extrafine particle mass (smaller than 1 μm).

Please check your eBook at **https://studentconsult. inkling.com/** for self-assessment questions. See inside cover for registration details.

Reference

Prime, D., Slater, A.L., Haywood, P.A., et al., 1996. Assessing dose delivery from the Flixotide Diskus Inhaler – a multidose powder inhaler. Pharm. Technol. Eur. 8 (3), 23–34.

Bibliography

Begat, P., Morton, D.A., Staniforth, J.N., et al., 2004. The cohesive-adhesive balances in dry powder inhaler formulations I: direct quantification by atomic force microscopy. Pharm. Res. 21, 1591–1597.

Campen, L.V., Venthoye, G., 2006. Inhalation: dry powder. In: Swarbrick, J. (Ed.), Encyclopedia of Pharmaceutical Technology, third ed. Informa Healthcare, New York.

Carvalho, T.C., Peters, J.I., Williams, R.O. III, 2011. Influence of particle size on regional lung deposition – what evidence is there? Int. J. Pharm. 406, 1–10.

Colombo, P., Traini, D., Buttini, F. (Eds.), 2013. Inhalation Drug Delivery: Techniques and Products. Wiley-Blackwell, Chichester.

Hickey, A.S.J. (Ed.), 2003. Pharmaceutical Inhalation Aerosol Technology, second ed. Marcel Dekker, New York.

Munro, S.J.M., Cripps, A.L., 2006. Metered dose inhalers. In: Swarbrick, J. (Ed.), Encyclopedia of Pharmaceutical Technology, third ed. Informa Healthcare, New York.

Nichols, S.C., Mitchell, J.P., Sandell, D., et al., 2016. A multi-laboratory in vitro study to compare data from abbreviated and pharmacopoeial impactor measurements for orally inhaled products: a report of the European Aerosol Group. AAPS PharmSciTech. doi:10.1208/s12249-015-0476-9.

Placke, M.E., Ding, J., Zimlich, W.C., 2006. Inhalation, liquids. In: Swarbrick, J. (Ed.), Encyclopedia of Pharmaceutical Technology, third ed. Informa Healthcare, New York.

Taylor, G., Kellaway, I., 2001. Pulmonary drug delivery. In: Hillery, A.M., Lloyd, A.W., Swarbrick, J. (Eds.), Drug Delivery and Targeting for Pharmaceutical Scientists. Taylor and Francis, London.

Taylor, K.M.G., McCallion, O.N.M., 2006. Ultrasonic nebulizers. In: Swarbrick, J. (Ed.), Encyclopedia of Pharmaceutical Technology, third ed. Informa Healthcare, New York.

Nasal drug delivery

38

Gary P. Martin   Alison B. Lansley

KEY POINTS

- Drugs are administered to the nasal cavity for (1) localized effect, (2) systemic action, (3) vaccine delivery and (4) possible direct nose–brain delivery.
- Some exemplar drugs administered via the nose are (1) corticosteroids, antihistamines and antibacterials (localized delivery), (2) polypeptide hormones, 5-HT$_1$ agonists and alkaloids (systemic delivery) and (3) influenza vaccine.
- The nasal cavity (volume 15 mL, surface area 160 cm^2, pH 5.5–6.5) contains mucus which is propelled by cilia towards the nasopharynx. This mechanism, termed mucociliary clearance, removes drugs from the nasal cavity.
- The nasal cavity contains a broad range of enzymes, which can provide a metabolic barrier to the absorption of both low molecular weight drugs and peptides, and inactivate locally acting drugs.
- The formulation strategies to improve absorption into the systemic circulation include (1) increase

of aqueous solubility (e.g. cosolvents and cyclodextrins), (2) reduction of enzymatic degradation (e.g. encapsulation, use of prodrugs and inclusion of enzyme inhibitors), (3) increase of mucosal contact time (e.g. incorporation of mucoadhesives) and (4) promotion of permeability through membranes (e.g. by increasing solubility, or by using permeation enhancers).
- The efficiency of direct nose–brain transport is generally low (usually less than 1% of the administered dose).
- Nasal drops and sprays are traditional delivery forms but currently devices are being developed that use (1) breath actuation, (2) electronic atomization and (3) pressurized metered dosing.
- The dosage forms comprise solutions, suspensions, semisolids and powders.

Introduction

The most common reason for introducing a drug into the nasal cavity is to provide a convenient and accessible route for rapidly and efficiently managing the localized symptoms associated with allergic rhinitis, nasal congestion and nasal infection. The drugs applied topically for such purposes include antihistamines, corticosteroids, sodium cromoglicate, sympathomimetics and antiseptics/antibiotics (Table 38.1). These drugs are administered either in liquid form (from a spray or as drops) or as creams/ointments.

The intranasal route has also been exploited for the delivery of drugs to the systemic circulation (Table 38.1). There are several possible reasons for pharmaceutical companies to consider using this route

Table 38.1 Examples of medicines administered into the nasal cavity

Drug	Drug class	Use	Delivery system
Locally acting preparations			
Azelastine hydrochloride	Antihistamine	Allergic rhinitis	Metered spray
Fluticasone propionate/furoate, beclometasone dipropionate, betamethasone sodium phosphate, budesonide, ciclesonide, flunisolide, mometasone furoate and triamcinolone acetonide	Corticosteroid	Allergic/perennial rhinitis	Nasal drops/metered spray
Ephedrine hydrochloride and xylometazoline hydrochloride	Sympathomimetic	Nasal congestion	Nasal drops
Sodium cromoglicate	Cromoglicate	Allergic rhinitis	Metered spray
Ipratropium bromide	Antimuscarinic	Rhinorrhea	Metered spray
Chlorhexidine and neomycin	Antibacterial	Elimination of *Staphylococci*	Cream
Mupirocin	Antibacterial	MRSA[b] elimination	Ointment
Preparations administered for systemic effects			
Desmopressin acetate	Pituitary hormone	Diabetes insipidus/mild haemophilia	Metered spray
Fentanyl citrate	Opioid analgesic	Moderate/severe pain	Metered spray
Nafarelin acetate	A gonadotropin-releasing hormone agonist	Management of endometriosis	Metered spray
Naloxone hydrochloride	Competitive opioid antagonist	Emergency treatment of opioid overdose	Unit-dose spray
Nicotine	Alkaloid	Smoking cessation	Metered spray
Salmon calcitonin[a]	Polypeptide hormone (calcium regulator)	Postmenopausal osteoporosis	Metered spray
Buserelin	Gonadorelin analogue	Prostate cancer/endometriosis	Metered spray
Sumatriptan	5-HT$_1$ agonist	Migraine	Unit-dose spray
Nasal vaccines			
Influenza	Live attenuated virus	Vaccination	Prefilled unit-dose syringe

[a]No longer available in some markets (including Europe and Canada) because of a reported increased risk of associated cancer.
[b]*MRSA*, meticillin-resistant *Staphylococcus aureus*.

for marketed medicines rather than the much more popular oral route. These include:

- the potential to elicit a rapid onset of action (e.g. in the treatment of breakthrough pain, opioid overdose, migraine and erectile dysfunction);
- the avoidance of gastrointestinal and hepatic presystemic metabolism (e.g. for susceptible peptides, such as desmopressin and other drugs such as hyoscine and morphine), despite the

nasal cavity containing inherent enzymatic activity;

- the willingness of patients to use this route for systemic therapies rather than some of the other alternatives to the oral route (such as parenteral and rectal) because of its ease of access (discovered from a young age!) and the noninvasiveness and consequent lack of pain associated with the application of the medicine;

- the lower costs incurred by the pharmaceutical industry (in comparison with those for parenteral products) as there is no requirement for sterilization of the final product; and

- the management of chronic disorders; providing the medicine does not induce irritation, it can be used for prolonged periods (perhaps with alternate use of the nostrils).

The nasal cavity has also been used, or proposed, as a portal for the delivery of vaccines, particularly for vaccines against infections associated with the respiratory tract such as influenza and possibly, eventually, tuberculosis. The presentation of an antigen, in combination with an acceptable adjuvant to the nasal-associated lymphoid tissue (NALT) can promote both cellular and humoral responses. However, human vaccinations need not be restricted to airway infections, and systemic immune responses are demonstrable after introduction of appropriate antigens via this route. Intranasal vaccination has been studied with a view to combating noroviruses, measles virus, herpes viruses, and the microorganisms that cause diphtheria and tetanus. An intranasal vaccine containing live attenuated influenza virus has been marketed (Table 38.1).

Currently, there is much research aimed at establishing whether the olfactory region, positioned in the upper reaches of the nasal cavity (Fig. 38.1), offers a potential means, in humans, of circumventing the obstacles imposed by the blood–brain barrier (BBB) to the access of many drugs from the

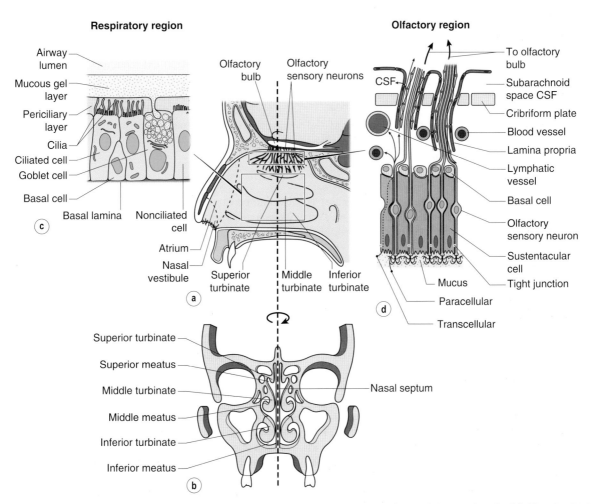

Fig. 38.1 • Lateral wall of the nasal cavity (a) and cross-section through the middle of the nasal cavity (b). The respiratory epithelium (c) and the olfactory epithelium (d). CSF, Cerebrospinal fluid.

bloodstream to the brain. This region contains a direct physiological link between the environment and the central nervous system (CNS). Clearly, if such a route could be established conclusively as being viable for the delivery of therapeutic quantities of drugs in humans, then this would have great potential in treating conditions such as Alzheimer's disease, brain tumours, epilepsy, pain and sleep disorders. However, although there are several studies that suggest that drugs may be absorbed from the olfactory region, the true significance of many findings is confounded by the use of animal models, with the data often being extrapolated uncritically to humans.

To appreciate fully the potential of the nasal cavity for drug delivery, it is pertinent to review the relevant anatomy and physiology, consider in more detail the applications of using the route, review the physicochemical properties of administered drugs and factors that might affect the choice of formulation and discuss the devices that can be used to deliver nasal medicines.

Anatomy and physiology

The nasal cavity is 120 mm to 140 mm from the nostrils to the nasopharynx (Fig. 38.1) and is divided in two by the nasal septum. The total surface area of both cavities is approximately 160 cm^2, and the total volume is approximately 15 mL. The first part of the nasal cavity (termed the nasal vestibule) is the narrowest part, with a cross-sectional area of 30 mm^2 on each side. The lining of the vestibule changes from skin at the entrance to a stratified squamous epithelium which extends over the anterior third of the entire nasal cavity. The nasal vestibule contains vibrissae (hairs) which filter out inhaled particles with an aerodynamic particle size greater than approximately 10 μm. Progression through the nasal cavity leads to the turbinate region. The turbinates are convoluted projections from the nasal septum which are lined with a pseudostratified columnar epithelium (80% to 90% of the total surface area of the nasal epithelium in humans) composed of mucus-secreting goblet cells, ciliated and nonciliated cells and basal cells (Fig. 38.1). The apical surfaces of the ciliated and nonciliated cells are covered with nonmotile microvilli, which serve to increase the surface area of the epithelial cells. There are also approximately 100 motile cilia on each ciliated cell which are responsible for mucus transport. Serous and seromucous glands also contribute to nasal secretions. As air moves through the turbinate region via the meatuses (Fig. 38.1), the low rate of airflow in combination with the turbulence created by the shape of the turbinates encourages the air to make contact with the highly vascularized walls, enabling it to be warmed and humidified. Particulates (5 μm to 10 μm) within the airstream, such as dust, pollen, microorganisms and pollutants, have the potential to deposit on the viscoelastic mucous gel lining the turbinate walls. The cilia, beating within the periciliary fluid, engage with the underside of the mucus and propel the gel and the deposited particles to the nasopharynx, where they are either swallowed or expectorated. This process is termed mucociliary clearance and is able to clear mucus at a rate of approximately 7 mm min^{-1}. Approximately 20% of the inspired air is directed to the top of the turbinates, where the olfactory region is located (Fig. 38.1). This is an area of approximately 12.5 cm^2 (~8% of the total surface area of the nasal epithelium in humans) of nonciliated pseudostratified columnar epithelium traversed by 6 million to 10 million olfactory sensory neurons which pass from the nasal cavity, between the epithelial (sustentacular) cells and through the cribriform plate to the olfactory bulb of the brain.

Drug delivery

Certain constraints are imposed on the formulation of preparations for the nasal route, and two case studies, one a locally acting drug (budesonide) and a second systemically acting peptide drug (desmopressin), are given in Table 38.2.

As with the formulation of any medicine, the information obtained from preformulation studies (see Chapter 23) is an essential prerequisite in the design of an intranasally delivered medicine. The solubility (see Chapter 2) of the drug to be administered is a key determinant in the final formulation. The restricted volume that can be applied to the nasal cavity also impacts on the nature of the resultant formulation. Generally, the premise of presenting the drug in the simplest formulation, containing the fewest excipients possible to ensure a stable medicine with an adequate shelf life, is the course that should be followed in the development process. Currently, delivery devices are usually metered-dose manual pump sprays, because these are cheap, robust and reliable, but more sophisticated systems are now under development, as discussed later.

Table 38.2 Considerations in formulating nasal preparations

Considerations	General comments	Budesonide aqueous nasal spray	Desmopressin acetate nasal solution
Drug		Budesonide	Desmopressin acetate
Molar mass (g/mol)		430.5	1183.3
Dose of drug required		64 μg per spray (256 μg daily)	10 μg to 40 μg daily (i.e. 40 IU to 160 IU)
Vehicle		Purified water	Purified water
Volume of delivered dose	25 μL to 200 μL per nostril	50 μL (two actuations per nostril once a day or one actuation per nostril twice a day)	100 μL to 400 μL (one actuation contains 10 μg and the total dose should be divided evenly between the nostrils)
Aqueous solubility of drug	Dictates whether suspension or solution is formulated	Practically insoluble in water (20 μg mL^{-1}), formulated as a micronized suspension	Completely soluble at the required dose
Wetting agent	If suspension	Polysorbate 80	None
Solubilizer	If solution is required		Not required
Chelating agent	To optimize stability	Disodium edetate	None
Antioxidant	To optimize stability	Ascorbic acid	None
pH	pH should favour optimal drug stability, other considerations include maximizing amount of drug in un-ionized form and avoidance of irritation of nasal mucosa	4.5 adjusted with concentrated hydrochloric acid	3.5–6.0 adjusted with either hydrochloric acid or with citric acid/disodium phosphate buffer
Viscosity	Increasing viscosity increases residence time in the nasal cavity and reduces postnasal drip	Dispersible cellulose (microcrystalline cellulose and sodium carboxymethylcellulose, 89:11, w/w)	None
Tonicity	Should be adjusted to approximately the same osmotic pressure as that of the body fluids	Anhydrous glucose	Sodium chloride
Preservative	Should be nonirritant	Potassium sorbate	One of: benzalkonium chloride, chlorobutanol or potassium sorbate
Humectant	To minimize irritation, e.g. glycerol		
Flavouring/taste-masking agent	To improve taste as formulation is cleared to throat		
Delivery device	Drops or spray (squeeze bottle or metered dose)	Metered-dose, manual pump spray	Metered spray pump and/or calibrated rhinal tube (see Table 38.8)

Local delivery

For conditions affecting the nose, it is logical to deliver the drug directly to its site of action. This permits the rapid relief of symptoms with a much lower dose of drug than would be necessary if it were delivered by the oral route, and reduces the chance of systemic side effects. For example, this is particularly pertinent in the delivery of corticosteroids to reduce local inflammation of the nasal mucosa and sinuses, without causing pituitary–adrenal suppression, or when using localized antihistamine therapy without inducing drowsiness.

Systemic delivery

The rationale for the use of the nasal cavity for systemic delivery includes its accessibility, avoidance of presystemic metabolism and potential to provide a rapid onset of action for drugs with the appropriate physicochemical properties. Its use for peptides (Tables 38.1 and 38.2) has been successful as, although only a very low percentage of administered drug is absorbed (i.e. low bioavailability), the plasma levels attained are sufficient for therapeutic efficacy. Many of the marketed nasally administered peptides have wide therapeutic windows. Therefore, providing the minimum therapeutic level of drug is exceeded in the bloodstream, a large variability in the final plasma level attained can be tolerated, without the occurrence of systemic toxicity. Any potential localized toxicity can be minimized in long-term administration by alternating nostrils with daily dosing (Table 38.2). Intranasal delivery can also be useful in emergency situations, such as in the treatment of opioid overdose (with use of naloxone) or in the treatment of intractable childhood seizures (with use of benzodiazepines). Drug delivery via this route is also well suited to drugs that, when administered orally, cause emesis (e.g. galantamine used to treat dementia).

Anatomical and physiological factors affecting intranasal systemic delivery

For a drug molecule to enter the systemic circulation it must first be absorbed across the nasal epithelium.

This may occur via the mechanism of passive diffusion via the transcellular route or the paracellular route (see Chapter 19). The transcellular pathway is the principal route of absorption for lipophilic molecules, whilst small, hydrophilic molecules diffuse *between* the epithelial cells (paracellularly) via the tight junctions, which are dynamic structures responsible for the integrity of the nasal epithelium. This latter pathway avoids the need for the drug molecules to pass into and out of the lipophilic membrane of the epithelial cells, but imposes a size restriction of between 0.39 nm and 0.84 nm. Transcellular absorption can also occur via endocytosis, the route believed to be exploited by some large hydrophilic molecules (> 1 kDa), and via active transport mechanisms where drug molecules with a structure similar to that of a natural substrate can interact with a carrier protein to cross the epithelial cells.

Because most drug absorption occurs by passive diffusion, the relatively large surface area of the nasal cavity and its rich blood supply (which helps to maintain the concentration gradient across the epithelium) aid this process. Working against these positive attributes of the nasal cavity are the barriers presented by mucus and the epithelium itself and the nasal clearance mechanisms, including mucociliary clearance and metabolism. The advantages and disadvantages of the nasal cavity for systemic drug delivery are summarized in Table 38.3.

Mucociliary clearance

The main drug absorption site is the respiratory epithelium of the nasal turbinates, which is where mucociliary clearance dominates. Drug deposited anterior to this region will remain in the nasal cavity for longer than drug deposited in the turbinates, but absorption from this site is less. Once drug particles (if formulated as a suspension) or molecules (if in solution) find their way on to the mucociliary 'conveyor belt', they will be cleared from the nasal cavity and therefore have a limited contact time with the absorption site. For drugs which are in solution and rapidly absorbed (lipophilic, low molecular weight), the limited contact time is likely to be well in excess of that required for complete absorption. However, for drug particles needing time to dissolve before absorption, and for polar drug molecules with a low rate of absorption once in solution, mucociliary clearance is likely to play a significant role in limiting the extent of absorption.

Barrier provided by mucus

The nasal mucosa is protected from the external environment by a layer of mucus. In the nasal cavity

Table 38.3 Advantages and disadvantages of intranasal drug delivery for systemic activity

Advantages	Disadvantages
Large surface area for absorption (~ 160 cm^2)	Limited to small delivery volumes (25 μL to 200 μL), therefore potent drugs are required
Good blood supply and lymphatic system	Mucociliary clearance and/or barrier provided by mucus decrease absorption of some drugs
Avoids hepatic first-pass metabolism of oral route	Enzymatic activity (pseudo first-pass effect)
Epithelium is permeable to small, lipophilic drug molecules; rapid absorption and onset of action	Low epithelial permeability for hydrophilic drugs; absorption enhancers and/or large doses are required
Noninvasive, so minimal infection risk during application and low risk of disease transmission (unlike parenteral route)	
Easy to self-administer and adjust dose	

this exists as a gel phase which is approximately 1 μm to 10 μm thick and found above a watery, sol phase surrounding the cilia (periciliary layer) which is approximately 7 μm deep (Fig. 38.1). Mucus is secreted continuously by the goblet cells and submucosal glands. Normal mucus is 97% water and 3% solids, with the latter comprising (1) mucins (approximately 30% of the solid content), (2) non-mucin proteins (e.g. albumin, immunoglobulins, lysozyme and lactoferrin), (2) inorganic salts and (4) lipids. Mucins are extremely large glycoproteins (up to 3×10^6 Da per monomer) with protein regions rich in serine and threonine which are linked, by their hydroxyl side groups, to sugar chains (O-glycosylation). They are anionic (negatively charged) because most of their terminal sugars contain carboxyl or sulfate groups. These glycosylated (sugar-rich) regions are separated by regions of nonglycosylated, 'naked' protein, rich in cysteine residues, which are believed to form globular domains stabilized by disulfide bonds. These 'naked' domains are the most hydrophobic regions of mucins and probably adsorb significant amounts of lipids. They are also the most antigenic sites on mucins. Entanglement of mucin polymers leads to the formation of a mucous gel and the generation of a mesh which is stabilized by noncovalent calcium-dependent cross-linking of adjacent polymers. The sugar side chains bind large amounts of water, allowing the mucus to act as a lubricant and a reservoir for the periciliary fluid within which the cilia beat. Mucus is a viscoelastic gel with the properties of both a deformable solid (elasticity) and a viscous fluid (see Chapter 6). Cilia can transport mucus only of the appropriate viscoelasticity, and this is controlled by the level of mucus hydration.

The presence of mucus at the epithelial surface of the nasal cavity provides an additional potential diffusion barrier to drug delivery. The ability of a molecule to diffuse through the gel is a function of the size of the drug molecule, the effective mesh size of the mucous gel formed by the mucin molecules and any interactions between the drug and the components of the mucous gel. The diffusion of small, uncharged molecules appears to be less affected by a mucous barrier than the diffusion of larger, cationic molecules. However, several high molecular weight, globular proteins (e.g. bovine serum albumin) and even 500 nm polyethylene glycol (PEG) nanoparticles have been observed to readily diffuse through mucus (cervical) at a rate comparable to their rate of diffusion through water. Mucus seems to present a barrier to the permeation of small, relatively hydrophobic molecules such as testosterone and this is believed to result from their interaction with the lipid component of the mucous gel or the hydrophobic (nonglycosylated) region of the mucin molecules. It is thought that such small molecules are only able to form low-affinity, monovalent bonds with the mucins which persist for just a short time. A number of studies indicate that positively charged (cationic), low molecular weight drugs, such as amikacin, gentamicin, tobramycin and some β-lactam antibiotics, bind electrostatically to negatively charged components in mucus. It is believed that such molecules bind tightly and polyvalently to the negatively charged sugar residues of the mucins. Large positively charged nanoparticles, such as those coated with chitosan, bind especially tightly to mucous gels by a similar mechanism.

Enzymatic activity

A broad range of enzymes are present in the nasal cavity, including those involved with phase 1 metabolism (e.g. monooxygenase, carboxyl esterases, epoxide hydrolases and cytochrome P450 isoenzymes) and also conjugative phase II metabolism (e.g. UDP-glucuronyltransferase and glutathione S-transferase). In addition, proteolytic enzymes (proteases and aminopeptidases) provide a potential barrier to the absorption of certain peptides. Drugs may be metabolized in the lumen of the nasal cavity or as they pass across the nasal epithelium. However, the metabolic activity of the nasal cavity is less than that of the gastrointestinal tract (on a nanomole per milligram of protein basis) and, in addition, there are a number of factors that will affect the relevance of metabolism to drug absorption. These include the amount of drug applied to the nasal surface area, the chemical nature of the drug, the rate of removal of the drug from the cavity and its rate of absorption across the mucosa.

Epithelial barrier – efflux transporters

The absorption of certain drugs across the nasal epithelium can be limited by the presence of efflux transporters. One such transporter, belonging to the superfamily of adenosine triphosphate (ATP)-binding cassette (ABC) transporters, has been found in the nasal respiratory mucosa and is termed P-glycoprotein 1 (P-gp), multidrug resistance protein 1 (MDR1), or ABC subfamily B member 1 (ABCB1). This transporter is also expressed by cells within the intestine and poses a similar barrier to drugs that are orally administered (see Chapter 19). P-gp is a 170 kDa glycosylated transmembrane protein found in the apical membranes of the cells. It is able to bind a wide variety of hydrophobic and amphiphilic substrates, including certain peptides, to its binding site, which is located cytoplasmically at the inner leaflet of the apical cell membrane, and actively pump them from the cell, back into the nasal cavity. Hence drugs that are substrates for P-gp will be less well absorbed across the nasal epithelium than their physicochemical properties (molecular size, lipophilicity, degree of ionization) might predict. Active transport/efflux operates against a concentration gradient, is saturable and can be competitively inhibited by other substrates for the binding site. Thus coadministration of an inhibitor of P-gp, such as rifampicin or verapamil, can enhance drug absorption. P-gp is also found in the olfactory epithelium, at a higher concentration than is found in the respiratory epithelium, where it reduces drug absorption into the brain.

Physicochemical properties of drugs affecting intranasal systemic delivery

In general, for a drug to be absorbed it must be in solution (molecularly dispersed). Because the volume of liquid that can be administered intranasally is relatively low (25 μL to 200 μL), drugs with low aqueous solubility and/or those for which a high dose is required can be problematic. Such issues can be overcome by formulation of the drug as a suspension or powder (generally with particles in the micrometre size range), in which case the drug will be required to dissolve in the fluid of the nasal cavity before absorption. There is some evidence that nanoparticles (which are an order of magnitude smaller) can be transported from the nasal cavity into the systemic circulation without dissolving, and it is possible that uptake may involve the NALT.

Solubility

The strategies to increase the solubility of a drug can involve (1) selection of a different salt form, (2) modification of its molecular form (including the use of a prodrug) and (3) the use of appropriate excipients, such as cosolvents, when the drug is formulated (considered later).

Prodrugs are often developed to increase the lipophilicity of a drug molecule and hence its absorption across a biological membrane. However, in the case of nasal delivery, the principle has been explored to increase the aqueous solubility of the parent drug to enable a clinically relevant dose of the drug to be dissolved in less than 150 μL of solution, and has been successful for several drugs. For instance, the solubility of L-dopa (aqueous solubility 1.65 mg mL^{-1}) is increased 400-fold if it is produced as a butyl ester prodrug, enabling an effective dose of 10 mg to be delivered in 125 μL. The prodrug is rapidly converted to the active parent drug once it enters the bloodstream.

The appropriate choice of the salt form of an ionizable drug can be used to increase its aqueous solubility. This is an empirical process because it is hard to predict reliably the effect of a particular counterion on the solubility of the resulting salt. Nevertheless, examples exist where this approach has been successful. For instance, the solubilities of galantamine hydrobromide and morphine sulfate have been increased sufficiently by exchange of the bromide or sulfate ions for gluconate to make nasal delivery feasible for these compounds. However, a change in salt form can result in irritancy to the nasal mucosa and this has to be considered when an appropriate counterion is being chosen.

Lipophilicity/hydrophilicity and molecular size

Once in solution, lipophilic drugs such as propranolol, progesterone and fentanyl are rapidly absorbed from the nasal cavity by the transcellular route and have a nasal bioavailability similar to that obtained after intravenous administration (almost 100%). The absorption of hydrophilic (polar) drugs occurs via the paracellular route (between the epithelial cells via the tight junctions), and the rate and extent of absorption is inversely proportional to the molecular weight of the drug. The paracellular route provides a much smaller area for absorption than the transcellular route. In the gastrointestinal tract, the area for the paracellular route is about 0.01% of that for the transcellular route. Thus the absorption of hydrophilic compounds is much slower than that of lipophilic drugs.

For both lipophilic and hydrophilic molecules, absorption is relatively efficient for drugs with a molecular mass below 1 kDa but then declines as molecular mass increases. Nevertheless, calcitonin (salmon) has been successfully used to reduce the risk of vertebral fractures in postmenopausal osteoporosis despite being a hydrophilic peptide with a molecular mass of 3432 Da and having a nasal bioavailability that is just 3% of its bioavailability when it is delivered intramuscularly. With regard to dose reproducibility from the nasal cavity, dosing is relatively consistent for low molecular weight drugs when compared with the oral or parenteral routes, whereas for compounds with a high molecular weight, such as peptides and proteins, relatively high variability is exhibited compared with injections.

Degree of ionization

For drugs that are weak acids or bases, the pH of the nasal cavity will affect the degree of ionization of the drug. The pH at the surface of the nasal mucosa has been reported to be 7.4, whilst the pH of the mucus is in the range 5.5–6.5. In addition, the pH of the formulation itself can alter the local pH, particularly if buffered vehicles are used. Studies have indicated that the un-ionized form of a drug, which has a higher oil–water partition coefficient than its ionized counterpart, is better absorbed than the ionized form (pH-partition hypothesis) (see Chapter 20). The ionized form of the drug also shows some permeation ability, the degree of which may be dependent on the nature of the counterion.

Formulation factors affecting intranasal systemic delivery

The same general formulation considerations apply to drugs formulated for systemic action as for local action, as indicated by the examples shown in Table 38.2. However, additional strategies can be used to increase absorption across the nasal epithelium. In essence, the bioavailability of nasally administered drugs can be limited by:

- low aqueous solubility;
- rapid and extensive enzymatic degradation of the drug in the nasal cavity;
- short contact time between the drug and the absorptive epithelium of the turbinates because of mucociliary clearance; and
- poor permeation of the drug across the respiratory epithelium.

The approaches that have been used to overcome these limitations are summarized in Table 38.4 and include the use of prodrugs (see earlier), enzyme inhibitors, mucoadhesive formulations and permeation enhancers which affect the epithelial barrier.

Increasing aqueous solubility

As discussed already, for a drug to be absorbed, it should normally be in solution. Drug solubility can be increased by use of a mixed solvent system or a cosolvent in the formulation. The solvents used with water for nasal delivery include glycerol, ethanol, propylene glycol and PEG. It is important that any cosolvents do not irritate the nasal mucosa, and it is likely that ethanol, used at high concentrations, would not be well tolerated. However, PEG 300 has been used successfully to increase the solubility of buprenorphine hydrochloride and melatonin, and has enabled clinically relevant doses to be administered, with low nasal irritation being observed in humans.

Cyclodextrins (see Chapter 24) are cyclic compounds composed of α-D-glucopyranose units. They tend to be water soluble because of their hydrophilic/polar outer surface, but have a hydrophobic/less polar

Table 38.4 Common problems associated with poor nasal bioavailability and possible solutions

Problem	Challenge	Possible solutions
Low aqueous solubility of drug	Increase aqueous solubility of drug	Prodrugs Cosolvents Cyclodextrins Novel drug delivery systems
Enzymatic degradation of drug	Reduce affinity of drug for nasal enzymes Inhibit nasal enzymes Limit access of nasal enzymes to drug	Prodrugs Enzyme inhibitors Encapsulation, e.g. liposomes, microspheres, nanoparticles
Short contact time	Increase residence time of drug in turbinates	Increase viscosity of formulation Use mucoadhesive formulations
Low permeation across the nasal epithelium	Increase permeability Increase solubility	Prodrugs (with increased lipophilicity) Prodrugs (with increased hydrophilicity) Cosolvents Cyclodextrins Novel drug delivery systems
	Modify nasal epithelium	Permeation enhancers

centre. They are able to increase the aqueous solubility of lipophilic compounds by forming dynamic inclusion complexes where the lipophilic part of the drug molecule is incorporated into the lipophilic central cavity of the cyclodextrin ring. An intranasal formulation containing 17β-estradiol solubilized in dimethyl-β-cyclodextrin (seven glucopyranose units) was available for the treatment of menopausal symptoms, until it was withdrawn in 2006. The formulation was well-tolerated and as effective as transdermal and oral formulations of estradiol. The dimethyl-β-cyclodextrin was reported to increase absorption of the drug by both enhancing its solubility and increasing the permeability of the nasal epithelium.

pH of the formulation

Many drugs are weak acids or bases, and their degree of absorption will depend on their pK_a and the pH of the absorption site. The pH of a formulation is generally dictated by the stability of the drug but, within these constraints, a pH favouring more un-ionized molecules would be expected to enhance absorption. It is important to recognize that the formulation should be nonirritant to the nasal mucosa, and formulation at a pH close to that of the nasal cavity (5.0–6.5) may also be desirable, although, unexpectedly, it has been shown that pH values ranging from 3 to 10 can be tolerated by the nasal mucosa (Table 38.2).

Use of enzyme inhibitors

Should peptides be administered via the nasal cavity, they are potentially prone to degradation by the enzymes of the nasal mucus and epithelium. Proteolytic enzyme inhibitors could prevent the hydrolysis of peptide and protein drugs in the nasal cavity, improving their stability at the absorption site. As examples, the aminopeptidase and trypsin inhibitor camostat mesilate increased the nasal absorption of the peptide vasopressin and its analogue desmopressin, and the absorption of calcitonin can also be enhanced by the use of trypsin inhibitors. However, proteolytic enzyme inhibitors do not improve the ability of peptide and protein drugs to cross the epithelium of the nasal cavity and therefore do not dramatically increase nasal bioavailability, as clearance mechanisms continue to operate to remove the drug from the absorption site.

Increasing nasal residence time

Unless a drug molecule possesses the ideal characteristics for rapid absorption, the percentage of the administered dose entering the systemic circulation is likely to be affected by the residence time of the nasal formulation in the turbinates. One way of increasing the time that the formulation is in contact with the absorptive mucosa is by the use of mucoadhesive polymers, such as cellulose derivatives, polyacrylates, starch and chitosan. Most of these polymers are 'generally recognized as safe' (i.e. given GRAS status as categorized by the US Food and Drug Administration) and if included as pharmaceutical excipients within the vehicle have been shown to increase the absorption of hydrophilic macromolecules. The polymers themselves are not absorbed and therefore would not be expected to cause any systemic toxicity.

Polymeric material can adhere to both the nasal epithelial surface (bioadhesion) and nasal mucus (mucoadhesion). Mucoadhesive formulations can be administered to the nasal cavity in the form of solid powders or particulates, gels or liquids. For good mucoadhesion, the formulation should spread well on the nasal mucosa (solid formulations should flow well and be readily wettable), after which the hydration of the polymer and the intimate contact it has with the nasal mucosa is very important. Mucoadhesives can increase absorption by three mechanisms:

- Optimum hydration will promote the extension of polymer chains which will interact with the nasal tissue and resist the removal of the

formulation by mucociliary clearance, thus increasing its retention time in the nasal cavity.
- By acting as carriers, they can reduce the contact between the drug and the enzymes of the nasal mucosa and protect the drug from any potential degradation.
- Some polymers can affect the tight junctions between the epithelial cells. As the polymer becomes hydrated, it causes dehydration of the epithelial cells, which can temporarily open the tight junctions, so increasing permeability of the epithelium with regard to drugs using the paracellular route.

With time, the continuous production of mucus will cause further hydration of the polymer (beyond the optimum required for mucoadhesion), the strength of mucoadhesion will diminish and normal mucociliary clearance will resume, so clearing the polymer from the nasal cavity.

Examples of polymers and drugs that have been used in studies of nasal mucoadhesion are given in Table 38.5. When the polymers are formulated in solution, the viscosity of the preparation will be greater than that of a simple solution. Whilst an

Table 38.5 Mucoadhesive polymers proposed/used for nasal delivery

Polymer type	Examples of mucoadhesive polymers studied	Dosage forms	Examples of drugs studied
Cellulose derivatives (soluble)	Hydroxypropyl methylcellulose, hydroxypropyl cellulose, methylcellulose, carboxymethylcellulose	Gel Powder Liquid	Apomorphine Insulin Ciprofloxacin
Cellulose derivatives (insoluble)	Ethyl cellulose, microcrystalline cellulose	Powder Spray	Leuprolide Calcitonin
Polyacrylates	Carbopol 971P, Carbopol 934P, Carbopol 981P	Powder Liquid Gel	Apomorphine Metoclopramide
Starch	Drum-dried waxy maize starch Degradable starch microspheres Starch nanoparticles Starch microspheres	Liquid Powder	Apomorphine Desmopressin Gentamicin Human growth hormone Insulin Metoclopramide
Chitosan	Chitosan Chitosan microspheres Chitosan glutamate	Liquid Powder	Insulin Human growth hormone Morphine hydrochloride Gentamicin Metoclopramide
Pectin	Low-methoxyl (LM) pectin (PecSys™)	Liquid turning to gel in situ	Fentanyl (PecFent™)

increased formulation viscosity leads to a prolonged residence time, it does not always result in increased absorption. This might be due to the decreased rate of diffusion of the drug molecules through a solution of higher viscosity. However, the viscosity of a solution for nasal delivery has to be limited to approximately 500 mPa s because, although more viscous solutions show better mucoadhesion, they are too viscous to be instilled easily and accurately into the nasal cavity. To overcome this problem a type of gel has been developed (in situ gel) that is liquid before administration (allowing convenient and accurate dosing) but forms a gel once in contact with the nasal mucosa (in situ). The temperature or pH of the mucus promotes the transition from liquid to gel. In studies, this approach has been used successfully to increase the nasal absorption of metoclopramide, sumatripan and insulin. A marketed product (PecFent™) containing the analgesic fentanyl and low-methoxyl (LM) pectins is administered to the nasal cavity as a solution, but then the pectins interact with calcium ions in nasal secretions to form a mucoadhesive/bioadhesive gel. Fentanyl is a low molecular weight, lipophilic molecule that readily crosses the nasal epithelium and is useful for the treatment of breakthrough pain, with a more rapid onset of action and better bioavailability from the nasal cavity than from the oral transmucosal route (buccal or sublingual). Nevertheless, it has a relatively short duration of action. The LM pectin in the formulation causes a slight delay in the onset of action compared with a nasal formulation without LM pectin (greater t_{max} and lower C_{max}) (see Chapter 21) but prolongs the residence time of the fentanyl in the nasal cavity, extending its duration of action until the product is cleared.

Polymers can also be formulated as dry powders; these are not mucoadhesive when dry, which allows them to be easily administered by metered-dose insufflations, but they become mucoadhesive once in contact with the nasal mucosa by absorbing water from the nasal mucus. Powders have certain advantages over liquid formulations, and these include:

- A larger amount of drug can be delivered.
- There is no need for preservatives as they do not support microbial growth.
- There is no requirement for storage at reduced temperatures because of better stability.

These advantages make the study of dry powder formulations for the administration of small hydrophobic drugs, peptides and vaccines popular. The disadvantages of powder administration include the possible irritation of the nasal mucosa and a possible gritty texture. The aerodynamic size of the particles (see Chapter 37) will affect the deposition site in the nasal cavity, and manufacturing particles of the correct aerodynamic particle size to deposit in the respiratory region of the nasal cavity, where maximum absorption occurs, can be expensive.

Polymers can also be formulated as microparticles/microspheres and nanoparticles (see Chapter 44). These systems can protect the drug from enzymatic degradation, increase contact with the absorptive epithelium and enhance uptake. Nanoparticulate systems are taken up by the NALT, suggesting potential application for the delivery of vaccines.

Enhancing the permeability of the nasal epithelium

It is possible to increase the absorption of both small and large hydrophilic drug molecules by administering them with permeation enhancers which modify the structure of the nasal epithelium. However, it is important that any alteration to the barrier function of the epithelium is short term and reversible, because the epithelium constitutes one of the body's primary defence mechanisms against insult from the external environment. A range of nasal products is on the market, none of which contain a permeation enhancer. This is either because the drug molecules are both small and lipophilic, and have adequate absorption without the need for a permeation enhancer, e.g. sumatriptan, fentanyl and nicotine, or because the nasal bioavailability, although low, is still sufficient for the drug to exert a therapeutic effect, as is the case for the peptides calcitonin, desmopressin, buserelin and nafarelin (when bioavailability is often below 5%). For this latter group, it is also likely that the permeation enhancers available at the time of marketing were too toxic for use. Thus there is a need for safe and efficient permeation enhancers to enable less potent biological drugs to be delivered intranasally and to increase the bioavailability of those currently on the market.

The requirements of an ideal permeation enhancer include the following:

- rapidly acting with a transient and reversible effect on the nasal epithelium;
- not absorbed systemically;
- nontoxic, nonirritant and nonallergenic;
- does not permit entry of dangerous environmental material;

Table 38.6 Examples of permeation enhancers

Type of permeation enhancer	Examples	Proposed mechanism(s) of action	Toxicity
Cationic polymers	Chitosan Poly(L-arginine) Cationized gelatin	Ionic interaction with negatively charged nasal epithelium and nasal mucus Transiently open tight junctions Bioadhesion	Well tolerated Negligible mucosal damage
Cell-penetrating peptides (also called protein transduction domains)	Penetratin Octa-arginine	Various hypotheses which are largely unsupported	Variable
Cyclodextrins	Modified derivatives	Protection of drug from enzymatic degradation either directly or by shielding susceptible portions of molecules in hydrophobic cavity Removal of lipids from cell membranes leading to increase in membrane permeability Change distribution of tight junctions causing increased paracellular permeability Interaction of cyclodextrins with hydrophobic portions of large molecules, e.g. peptides and proteins, can increase their permeability	Considered safe
Tight junction modulating lipids	Glycosylated sphingosines Alkylglucosides Oxidized lipids Ether lipids	Interaction with lipid raft associated with tight junctions to modulate their properties	Alkylglucosides are cytotoxic
Tight junction modulating peptides	PN159 (a peptide sequence) AT1002 (a hexamer peptide)	Various	Low toxicity
Nitric oxide donors	S-Nitroso-N-acetyl-DL-penicillamine Sodium nitroprusside	Unknown	Negligible cytotoxicity
N-acetylcysteine		Reduction of mucus viscosity	Used clinically, shows low toxicity and no local irritation

- compatible with drugs and other excipients in the formulation; and
- safe for long-term use (depending on the condition to be treated).

Examples of permeation enhancers that have been studied to increase the absorption from the nasal cavity include surfactants (such as bile salts and their derivatives) and certain phospholipids. These have proved effective in promoting absorption by a variety of different mechanisms, including solubilization of the drug, inhibition of enzymatic activity, extraction of lipid or protein from the cell membrane, alteration of the mucus layer and alteration of tight junctions. However, many of these enhancers severely irritate and damage the nasal mucosa at the concentrations required to promote nasal absorption. Some of the materials able to enhance permeability whilst possessing a better toxicity profile are detailed in Table 38.6.

A number of permeation enhancers are currently being developed commercially for clinical use (Table 38.7). These have achieved a better balance between efficacy and safety/toxicity and have been assessed in humans in clinical trials. The permeation enhancers are generally being developed for use with peptide and protein drugs, but none of these products have yet reached the market. The most developed product is that containing the small hydrophilic molecule morphine in a formulation with chitosan (Rylomine™), which reached phase III trials in the United States.

Table 38.7 Some permeation enhancers currently in development

Permeation enhancer	Nasal product	Proposed mechanism of action	Toxicity
Cyclopentadecalactone (azone) (CPE-215®)	Desmopressin (SER120™)	No published information, but has surfactant properties which are likely to increase fluidity of cell membrane and increase transcellular permeability	Considered safe On US FDA's list of inactive ingredients approved for use in drug applications SER120 Is undergoing phase III trials in the US
Alkylsaccharides (Intravail™)	Sumatriptan Diazepam Insulin	Surfactant-like. Molecules have a polar sugar head group esterified with a nonpolar alkyl chain which can be of various lengths	Promising safety profile, in phase I trials of parathyroid hormone (1–34) but the formulation is no longer in development
Chitosan (ChiSys™)	Granisetron (ALM 101) Influenza A virus H5N1 (avian influenza) Anthrax vaccine	Transiently opens tight junctions Bioadhesion	Well tolerated in phase I, II and III clinical trials of morphine (US) is no longer in development
Macrogol 15 hydroxystearate/Solutol HS 15 (CriticalSorb™)	Human growth hormone (CP024) Parathyroid hormone (1–34) (CP046)	Increases permeability of paracellular and transcellular routes	Generally recognized as safe (GRAS status – US FDA) Well tolerated by the nasal mucosa in both short-term (14 day) and long-term (6 month) repeated-dose preclinical toxicity studies Well tolerated in phase I trials (UK)

FDA, Food and Drug Administration.

A high plasma bioavailability for nasal formulations intended to act locally is undesirable because of the potential to cause systemic side effects. For example, the bioavailability of budesonide from a nasal spray (Table 38.2) can be 23% to 37%.

Patient factors affecting intranasal systemic delivery

Patient adherence. If a patient does not use a medication appropriately, then it cannot be expected to be effective. Thus good patient adherence is paramount for successful treatment. For systemic treatment the nasal route is usually chosen when the oral route is not available. Thus use of the nasal route is generally compared with parenteral delivery, or with use of other transmucosal routes. The nasal route is accessible to the patient using simple dosage forms (sprays and drops) permitting self-medication over extended periods. Unlike parenteral delivery, it is noninvasive and therefore has a reduced risk of introducing infection on application and a low risk of disease transmission. In addition, provided that the formulation does not cause irritation, it should be comfortable to use. In studies comparing intranasal delivery with parenteral delivery, fewer patients preferred the parenteral route. When compared with another transmucosal route, e.g. rectal, intranasal administration of midazolam for the treatment of childhood seizures was found to be safe and effective, easier for care-givers and more dignified for the patient than rectal administration, which is commonly used to control breakthrough seizures in the home.

Disease. A number of nasal diseases might be expected to affect the absorption of drugs into the systemic circulation, either by altering nasal mucociliary clearance (e.g. the common cold) or by affecting the permeability of the nasal epithelium (e.g. allergic rhinitis). However, there is little information in the literature to substantiate this. This is possibly because for those drugs that are rapidly absorbed, the effect is negligible, and for those that are poorly absorbed, provided they have a sufficiently wide therapeutic window, the variability is acceptable. Clearly, for a poorly absorbed drug with a narrow therapeutic window, the potential unpredictability in absorption caused by such diseases would be undesirable.

Nasal vaccines

Mucosal tissues are attractive sites for vaccination because of their accessibility and immunological competence and because local immune responses can be elicited which can protect against infection at the point of virus entry. Intranasal vaccination targets the NALT, which is situated beneath the nasal epithelium and consists of groups of dendritic cells, T cells and B cells.

So far, the intranasal route has been successfully used (Table 38.1) for a commercial influenza (live-attenuated) vaccine (called Fluenz Tetra™ in the UK and Europe and Flumist Quadrivalent™ in the US). Conventional needle-based intramuscular vaccinations are able to induce the production of serum antibodies (IgG) which, by transudation to the lungs, protect the lower respiratory tract against influenza infection and the more severe complications of influenza. However, vaccines given intranasally can induce local IgA responses in the upper respiratory tract (as well as systemic IgG responses) which can neutralize the target virus immediately after it is inspired and protect against early disease symptoms. Secretory IgA is also more cross-reactive than IgG and can provide protection against different strains of the virus. Nevertheless, because the nasal mucosa is exposed to a multitude of antigens present in the environment, tolerance mechanisms limit the resultant immune reaction. Consequently, these mechanisms have to be overcome for successful vaccination and, unless the vaccine contains live attenuated viruses, it is essential to incorporate an effective mucosal adjuvant within the final formulation. The benefits of nasal vaccination when compared with needle-based delivery systems include a reduced risk of needle-stick injuries and risk of infection from the reuse of needles, increased patient adherence among patients with needle phobia, a decreased need for vaccines to be administered by trained health care professionals and possibly a decreased need for cold chain storage and distribution, if vaccines can be formulated as dry powders. In addition, use of the route provides a ready means of vaccinating large population groups. Vaccine formulation and delivery is described in greater detail in Chapter 43.

CNS delivery

The BBB restricts the entry of potentially harmful substances into the brain but also limits the access of potentially useful drugs. It exists at the level of the cerebral microvasculature. In contrast to the leaky barrier presented by the endothelial cells of the capillaries in the peripheral circulation, the endothelial cells in the brain exhibit low rates of pinocytosis and are joined by tight junctions which limit the paracellular diffusion of hydrophilic solutes from the blood into the brain. In addition, the BBB expresses a high number of efflux transporters, such as P-gp, which further reduce access to the brain for those molecules that might otherwise be predicted to be well absorbed based on their size and lipophilicity.

Drugs delivered intranasally that enter the systemic circulation would have to cross the BBB to enter the CNS. However, it has been proposed that there is a route from the olfactory region of the nasal cavity (Fig. 38.1) to the brain that avoids the BBB and which can be exploited to deliver drugs *directly* to the brain. This is currently an area of great research interest, and studies have shown that both low molecular weight drugs and high molecular weight peptides and proteins appear to be able to access the brain following intranasal delivery. It is possible that a drug will gain access to the brain following its absorption into the systemic circulation and not via a direct route, and it is important to eliminate or account for this possibility in the design of studies seeking to establish or quantify direct nose-to-brain transport. It should also be noted that many of the studies of direct nose-to-brain transport have been undertaken in rats, which differ in their nasal anatomy compared with humans; the nasal passages of the rat have a higher surface area to volume ratio than those of humans (51.5 and 6.4 respectively), mucociliary clearance in the rat is in the anterior direction whereas mucus is moved posteriorly in humans and a significantly higher percentage of the nasal epithelium is concerned with olfaction in the rat (50%) than in humans (8%). In addition, the experimental conditions used in some studies could not be considered applicable to humans; formulations containing penetration enhancers at concentrations damaging to the nasal mucosa have been used, and some formulations have been applied to the nasal cavity in a manner that would be inappropriate in humans (too large a volume or application at too high a pressure over an extended time which might be expected to damage the epithelium). Nevertheless, studies in rats are important and provide useful information on the pathways and mechanisms of drug absorption both into the systemic circulation and into the CNS.

The olfactory mucosa is composed of the olfactory epithelium and its underlying lamina propria. The routes by which the molecules cross the olfactory epithelium have yet to be fully elucidated, but a number of possible pathways have been suggested (Fig. 38.1). An intracellular, axonal pathway has been proposed where substances are taken into the olfactory sensory neurons (OSNs) via adsorptive, receptor-mediated or nonspecific fluid-phase endocytosis and transported within the cell along the axon to the olfactory bulb. Another pathway involves substances crossing the other cells of the olfactory epithelium (e.g. sustentacular (supporting) cells) via transcellular or paracellular passive diffusion to reach the lamina propria. Tight junctions exist between cells in the olfactory epithelium, but the regular turnover of cells in the epithelium may lead to loosening of the tight junctions, helping the paracellular transport of higher molecular weight substances.

Once molecules are at the lamina propria, entry into the CNS is believed to occur, via diffusion or convection, extracellularly along the perineural space (which is the space surrounding the olfactory nerve bundles), through the cribriform plate and into the CSF or olfactory bulb. However, some of the molecules are also likely to enter the blood vessels of the systemic circulation or lymphatic vessels and will therefore be prevented from entering the CNS by this direct route. Of the two routes into the CNS, it has been suggested that intracellular transport along the axon of the OSN would be too slow to account for the experimental results observed and that the other, extracellular, perineural pathway is the most likely.

Immunohistochemical studies have found the efflux transporter P-gp localized to the endothelial cells lining the olfactory bulb and the olfactory epithelium. P-gp is able to reduce entry into the CNS of those drugs which are substrates for the transporter. Because drugs need to be inside the epithelial cell to interact with the binding site of P-gp, this will mainly affect those drugs crossing the supporting cells of the olfactory epithelium via the transcellular route.

The trigeminal nerve, which innervates the respiratory epithelium of the nasal cavity, also feeds into various areas of the brain and could potentially be exploited for nose-to-brain drug delivery. However, so far, this route has not been implicated as providing a pathway for CNS drug delivery.

In the many studies of drug transport (low molecular weight drugs and peptides and proteins) from the nose to the brain, the amount of drug reaching the CNS is small compared with the amount administered to the nasal cavity, generally less than 1%. One major problem is the inaccessibility of the olfactory region of the nasal cavity coupled with the poor permeation ability of certain types of molecule (including peptides and proteins) across the olfactory epithelium. There is a need for a formulation containing an acceptable nasal permeation enhancer and a bioadhesive material which can be delivered from a nasal device that is able to target the formulation to the olfactory region.

Nasal delivery systems

Nasally administered medicines can be formulated as ointments or creams but most usually as a liquid (solution, gel or suspension) or as a powdered solid (Tables 38.1 and 38.2). The formulation issues with each of these dosage forms have been considered in Chapters 24, 26, 27 and 28. With multidose liquid dosage forms, the possibility of 'suck back' exists, which is when a portion of the administered dose is sucked back into the remaining liquid in the delivery device. As a consequence, multidose liquid dosage forms can require the inclusion of antimicrobial preservatives to prevent the growth of contaminating microorganisms. There is evidence that some of these preservatives can irritate the nasal mucosa and/or damage the cilia and therefore compromise mucociliary clearance, especially if used over a long period. The strategies to minimize or avoid such effects include the alternate use of the nostrils, if long-term daily dosage is required, and the use of pressurized containers or unit-dose delivery systems (Table 38.8), which do not require the inclusion of a preservative. There is a move towards delivery systems that deliver an accurate metered dose and away from dosage forms such as nasal drops, which require considerable skill, dexterity and even flexibility (in terms of mobility) to be applied uniformly across the mucosa. Smaller volumes (<100 μL) tend to persist longer than larger volumes, which may drip from the nostril after delivery.

Powdered solids tend to remain in the nasal cavity for longer than liquids, as a preliminary hydration step generally occurs before mucociliary clearance reaches maximal efficiency. This can prolong the time over which systemic drug absorption can occur or the duration of action of a locally acting drug. Creams and ointments can also be used to prolong retention in the nasal cavity. Moreover, the use of solids or

Table 38.8 Nasal dosage forms and some of the available delivery systems

Nasal dosage form	Dispensed form	Comments
Creams and ointments	Tube	For example, mupirocin, chlorhexidine hydrochloride/neomycin sulfate Applied with finger. Messy to apply Uncontrolled dose (only for drugs with large therapeutic window and high tolerability) For drugs with localized effects only
Liquids (solutions/ emulsions/ suspensions)	Dropper/ squeezed plastic bottle	Often used for nasal decongestants. Absence of valve system, so liquids introduced into the cavity can be 'sucked back' into the storage container as pressure is released, leading to contamination issues Application procedure for efficient coating of nasal mucosa is complex, involving the patient adopting a semi-recumbent or other unusual position Drops/liquid delivered too quickly causes formulation to enter throat, causing cough/gagging (or exit onto lip/mouth). Uncooperative patients can expel most of the dose by blowing through the nose Volume administered is subject to the technique of the user and this form is suitable only for drugs with a large therapeutic window
	Nasal spray	Spray nozzle (either metered-dose pump or syringe) produces fine droplets (usually 25 μm to 50 μm). Able to introduce single dose (25 μL to 200 μL) – spread across nasal mucosa. Available as unit dose or reservoir (multiple doses) (generally 3 mL to 50 mL) spray bottle. Unit dose used for paediatric patients, vaccination and short-term treatment (e.g. pain; opioids). Reservoir (bottle) used for longer-term treatment (e.g. inflammation; corticosteroids) Easier/faster (<60 s) to administer than drops but pump often requires priming (by actuation of a pump mechanism until a mist is produced)
	Breath-actuated delivery	For example: 1. Desmopressin Rhinal Tube. A calibrated tube for paediatric and adult use; involves one end of a tube containing the dose being placed in the nostril and the other in the mouth. The dose is delivered with 'a short sharp puff' 2. OptiNose™ liquid delivery. A tight-fitting nozzle is placed in one nostril and a metered dose (dispensed from a reservoir) is aerosolized by the patient blowing through a mouthpiece. The nasal cavity is sealed by this action, preventing drug loss to the mouth and throat, and droplets are carried beyond the nasal valve and spread throughout the cavity. Preservative-free formulations can be used. Clinical trials have been conducted for treatment of migraine, nasal polyps, sinusitis and autism
	Electronic atomization	For example, droplet size can be controlled (generally 8 μm to 30 μm) to maximize nasal deposition. Preservative-free formulations can be used (since there is no risk of container contamination). Deposition in paranasal sinuses is possible. Electronics can use 'lock out' to prevent drug abuse. Relatively expensive dosage form. Clinical trial for intranasal administration of insulin for treatment of Alzheimer's disease
Powders	Nasal pressurized metered-dose inhaler	Many were phased out and replaced by lower-cost aqueous formulations when chlorofluorocarbon propellants were replaced Hydrofluoroalkane propellants can be used. Preservative-free formulations can be used (e.g. glucocorticoids such as ciclesonide). Can generate a good dispersion throughout the nasal cavity
	Breath-actuated delivery	For example, OptiNose™ powder delivery. The OptiNose™ device is a multidose device which delivers metered doses using the principle by which air is blown from the mouth through one end of tube and exits the other end, which is placed in the nostril. Blowing activates the anatomical reflex that closes the air passage between the nasal and oral cavities, whilst the patient's input energy disperses the powder. Dry powder formulations generally tend to adhere better to the nasal mucosa, allowing a longer time for absorption. Sealing the cavity might enable smaller particles (5 μm) to be used to target olfactory mucosa whilst limiting pulmonary deposition

creams limits the rapid introduction of fluid to the throat and mouth, which can often initiate an unwelcome taste and possibly induce coughing and gagging. Control of particle size is important because particles smaller than 10 μm can move beyond the nasal turbinates towards the lung, whereas particles larger than 50 μm can be cleared more rapidly by mucociliary clearance and nose blowing.

An interesting advance in nasal delivery devices which shows useful potential in delivering nasal formulations involves breath-actuated bidirectional delivery (Table 38.8). The device is constructed such that the aerosolization of the powder is initiated by patients themselves exhaling through the mouth against a resistance. This action closes the soft palate and separates the nasal cavity from the oral cavity. A communication pathway remains between the two nostrils, located behind the nasal septum. The expired air (and aerosolized powder) blown into one nostril is turned through 180°, passes through the pathway and leaves via the second nostril, ensuring that powder deposits throughout the cavity.

Summary

The potential of delivering drugs and vaccines to the body via the nasal cavity is far from being fully realized. There are active programmes within a number of pharmaceutical and biotechnological companies seeking to use the route. The development of more nasal vaccines is almost certain. However, the use of the nose for systemic delivery is contemplated only if the oral route, for whatever reason, is not viable. It is limited in terms of the dose that can be delivered, either as a result of solubility of the drug (given the volume of liquid that can be delivered comfortably) or in terms of the quantity of powder or semisolid that can be tolerated per dose. Once drug is delivered, it must be absorbed rapidly otherwise the normal clearance mechanisms will remove it from the absorbing epithelium and result in reduced bioavailability. Strategies are therefore being used to either extend the absorption window (through the use of mucoadhesive excipients) or increase permeability (by a number of means, including the use of permeation enhancers). As with pulmonary delivery however, the primary packaging is an important component of the final medicine, as this also forms part of the delivery device. There is much scope to develop novel devices with improved dose dispensing and superior targeting (perhaps to the olfactory region) or more efficient coating of mucosa. Drug development programmes need to consider both the device and the formulation as a whole, taking into account the therapeutic purpose of the medicine. Finally, as with pulmonary dosage forms, patient counselling will be especially important in advising patients of their medicines to gain maximum effectiveness, because whatever formulation is marketed, it will not be as easy to administer as the swallowing of a solid dosage form.

Please check your eBook at **https://studentconsult. inkling.com/** for self-assessment questions. See inside cover for registration details.

Bibliography

Amorij, J.-P., Hinrichs, W.L.J., Frijlink, H.W., et al., 2010. Needle-free influenza vaccination. Lancet. Infect. Dis. 10, 699–711.

Cone, R.A., 2009. Barrier properties of mucus. Adv. Drug Deliv. Rev. 61, 75–85.

Costantino, H.R., Illum, L., Brandt, G., et al., 2007. Intranasal delivery: physicochemical and therapeutic aspects. Int. J. Pharm. 337, 1–24.

Djupesland, P.G., 2013. Nasal drug delivery devices: characteristics and performance in a clinical perspective—a review. Drug Deliv. Transl. Res. 3, 42–62.

Djupesland, P.G., Messina, J.C., Mahmoud, R.A., 2014. The nasal approach to delivering treatment for brain diseases: an anatomic, physiologic, and delivery technology overview. Ther. Deliv. 5, 709–733.

Duan, X., Mao, S., 2010. New strategies to improve the intranasal absorption of insulin. Drug Discov. Today 15, 416–427.

Fahy, J.V., Dickey, B.F., 2010. Airway mucus function and dysfunction. Medical progress. N. Engl. J. Med. 363, 2233–2247.

Fortuna, A., Alves, G., Serralheiro, A., et al., 2014. Intranasal delivery of systemic-acting drugs: small-molecules and biomacromolecules. Eur. J. Pharm. Biopharm. 88, 8–27.

Illum, L., 2012. Nasal drug delivery – recent developments and future prospects. J. Control. Release 161, 254–263.

Jiang, L., Gao, L., Wang, X., et al., 2010. The application of mucoadhesive polymers in nasal drug delivery. Drug Dev. Ind. Pharm. 36, 323–336.

Khanvilkar, K., Donovan, M.D., Flanagan, D.R., 2001. Drug transfer through mucus. Adv. Drug Deliv. Rev. 48, 173–193.

Lochhead, J.J., Thorne, R.G., 2012. Intranasal delivery of biologics to the central nervous system. Adv. Drug Deliv. Rev. 64, 614–628.

Malerba, F., Paoletti, F., Capsoni, S., et al., 2011. Intranasal delivery of therapeutic proteins for neurological diseases. Expert Opin. Drug Deliv. 8, 1277–1296.

Merkus, F.W.H.M., van den Berg, M.P., 2007. Can nasal drug delivery bypass the blood-brain barrier? Drugs R. D. 8, 133–144.

Pires, A., Fortuna, A., Alves, G., et al., 2009. Intranasal drug delivery: how, why and what for? J. Pharm. Pharm. Sci. 12, 288–311.

Zaman, M., Chandrudu, S., Toth, I., 2013. Strategies for intranasal delivery of vaccines. Drug Deliv. Transl. Res. 3, 100–109.

39

Ocular drug delivery

Hala Fadda   Ashkan Khalili   Peng Tee Khaw   Steve Brocchini

CHAPTER CONTENTS

KEY POINTS

- The drug delivery routes available for treating ocular conditions are the topical, systemic (oral or injection), intraocular and periocular (injection or implant) routes.
- Topical ophthalmic preparations can be classified into solutions, suspensions, ointments, gels and submicron emulsions.
- Designing ocular drug delivery formulations requires an understanding of what can be tolerated by the eye. Important considerations in the design of topical ophthalmic preparations include volume, osmolality, pH, surface tension and viscosity.
- The front of the eye can often be effectively treated with topical ophthalmic preparations. The main shortcoming of the topical route,

however, is its inefficiency whereby only 1% to 5% of the instilled dose reaches the aqueous humour.

- The highly efficient lacrimal drainage system, rapid absorption by conjunctiva blood vessels and corneal barrier to drug permeation are the mechanisms mainly responsible for low ocular drug bioavailability via the topical route.
- Ophthalmic drugs with modest lipophilicity and low molecular weight are absorbed more efficiently via the corneal route than are hydrophilic, ionized drugs.
- Phase I and phase II drug metabolism reactions occur in ocular tissue. These have been exploited in the design of prodrugs.
- Sustained-release intraocular implants are being developed to treat diseases affecting the back of the eye. Implants help achieve steady concentrations of the drug and avoid the need for very frequent repeated injections into the eye.
- Intraocular implants must be biocompatible and stable at the implant site. Intraocular implants can be bioerodible or nonbioerodible.
- It is a regulatory requirement that preparations intended for ophthalmic use, including those for cleansing the eyes, be sterile. Antimicrobial preservatives can irritate and damage tissue, and some formulations are provided preservative-free.

Introduction

Many eye diseases, if left untreated, can result in severe morbidity (blindness), having a significant impact on patient quality of life. Many leading causes of blindness worldwide, including glaucoma and age-related macular degeneration (AMD), are now better treated with topical drops or intraocular injection thanks to recent ocular drug delivery strategies which have evolved in the last 10 years. Drug delivery to the eye is one of the most important areas of modern ocular therapy and presents many opportunities and challenges. The current market for ophthalmic pharmaceuticals is worth many billions of dollars a year. The front of the eye is accessible, and conditions affecting it can be treated by simple topical eye drops. The back of the eye, however, is treated as an entirely separate ocular region, and more advanced delivery systems have been designed for its treatment, including intraocular injections and implants that can provide sustained drug release over 2 years. In addition to low molecular weight molecules such as steroids, antibiotics and antivirals, a range of new therapies have been and are being developed for treating ocular conditions including proteins, genes and cells.

This chapter will describe the anatomy and physiology of the eye as well as the most common conditions affecting the different ocular regions. The natural anatomical ocular barriers to drug bioavailability have a great impact on ocular pharmacokinetics. Understanding ocular physiology is essential for developing drug delivery systems that are effective, safe and acceptable to patients. The design of topical ophthalmic preparations ranging from solutions to ointments and in situ forming gels will be discussed. Although eye drops have been used since the time of Cleopatra and account for more than 90% of the ophthalmic preparations in the clinic, they have poor bioavailability and a short duration of action. The reason for these shortcomings and formulation efforts to overcome them will be described.

The remainder of the chapter will focus on intraocular systems, including injections and implants that deliver drugs directly to the back of the eye. This direct delivery approach increases drug bioavailability and is approved for the delivery of several drugs. The use of antibody-based drugs administered by intravitreal injection has revolutionized the treatment of AMD, which is the main cause of blindness in the elderly. Current treatment goals are to develop systems that provide therapeutic drug levels within the eye for prolonged periods and to minimize the invasiveness of drug delivery procedures. Intraocular implants, which have been developed through sophisticated pharmaceutical, material and biomedical engineering approaches, are helping to achieve these goals. There remains much unmet clinical need, and research in this area is flourishing.

Anatomy and physiology of the eye

The structure of the eye is shown in Fig. 39.1, which shows the layers and chambers of the eye and the routes of and barriers to ocular drug delivery. Each of these is discussed in the following sections.

Layers of the eye

The outer layer of the eye can be considered as segments of two spheres: sclera and cornea. The white opaque sclera constitutes the back five-sixths of the

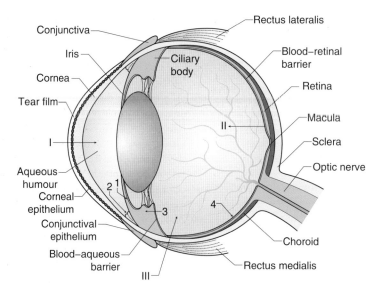

Fig. 39.1 • Structure of the eye . I–III routes of and barriers to ocular drug delivery, 1–4 ocular drug elimination pathways (see section 'Ocular drug delivery routes and elimination pathways' for details).

globe, and the transparent cornea provides the forward one-sixth of the globe. The sclera is a tough fibrous tissue that protects the eye from internal and external forces and maintains its shape. The front of the sclera is often referred to as the 'white' of the eye. The episclera is the outermost layer of the sclera and has a rich blood supply. The conjunctiva is a thin, transparent membrane (nonkeratinized, stratified columnar epithelium) that covers the visible part of the sclera and extends to the inside of the eyelids. The optic nerve emerges from the sclera in the posterior part of the eye.

The cornea is the most anterior part of the eye, in front of the iris and pupil. It is densely innervated by nerves, particularly sensory nerves. Whilst the central cornea is avascular, the region of the corneoscleral limbus is supplied by branches of the anterior ciliary arteries. The cornea refracts and transmits light to the lens and retina. It also protects the eye against infection and structural damage to the deeper parts. The cornea and sclera are connected at the limbus.

The surfaces of the cornea and conjunctiva are covered by a film of tears, produced mainly by the lacrimal gland. It lubricates the eye surface and protects it from chemicals, microbes and airborne solid particles. It comprises three layers: a mucous layer adhering to the epithelium (produced by goblet cells in the conjunctiva), an aqueous layer (produced by lacrimal glands) and a superficial lipid layer (produced by meibomian glands). The aqueous layer comprises electrolytes, proteins, glycoproteins, biopolymers,

glucose and urea, and has a thickness of 8 μm to 12 μm. The lipid layer is composed of sterol esters, wax esters and fatty acids. The mucous layer interacts with the epithelial cells of the cornea, and so each eyelid blink allows spread of the tear film over the eye surface. A dynamic equilibrium exists in the precorneal tear film as it goes through a continuous cycle of production, evaporation and drainage.

The middle layer of the eyeball consists of the iris, ciliary body and choroid. The ciliary body is a ring of tissue that extends from the base of the iris to the choroid. The ciliary muscle is its most prominent structure and is in a contracted state to allow the lens to become convex. The ciliary body is also the site of production of aqueous and vitreous humour. The turnover rate of aqueous humour production is approximately 2.2 μL min^{-1} to 3.1 μL min^{-1}. The iris is a fragile diaphragm with circular constrictor and radial dilator muscles positioned in front of the lens and ciliary body, which separates the anterior and posterior chambers. It controls the size of the pupil and thus the amount of light reaching the retina. The colour of the iris is determined by the amount of melanin expressed in it. The choroid is the vascular layer of the eye lying between the retina and sclera. It provides oxygen and nutrients to the outer layers of the retina and provides a dark chamber for a better quality image to be formed on the retina.

The inner layer of the eye is the retina, which is a complex network of neurons that process light. It consists of two layers: (1) the neural retina and (2) the retinal pigment epithelium (RPE). The layer of the retina surrounding the vitreous cavity is the neural retina, and the outer retinal wall surrounded by the choroid and sclera is the RPE. The neural cells of the retina are arranged in several parallel layers and the major classes present are photoreceptors (the rods and cones that are responsible for the conversion of light into an electrical signal through a complex mechanism), bipolar cells, horizontal cells, amacrine cells, ganglion cells (which transmit and process light signals) with their long axon bodies, which stretch all the way to the brain, and the Müller glia (which form the organizational backbone of the neural retina). The RPE comprises approximately 4.2 million to 6.1 million epithelial cells arranged in a hexagonal pattern. Their important functions include the maintenance of photoreceptor function, storage and metabolism of vitamin A, production of growth factors required by nearby tissue, and wound healing after injury or surgery. There are also two types of photoreceptors: cone and rod cells. Rods (115 million, mainly located in the peripheral retina) are the key cells for the detection of contrast, brightness and motion. The main functions of cones (6.5 million, mainly located in the central retina) are spatial resolution and colour vision. Both types of photoreceptors heavily rely on the support of RPE cells for their function and survival.

Chambers of the eye

The eye contains three main chambers: anterior chamber, posterior chamber and vitreous cavity. Aqueous humour fills the anterior and posterior chambers. It is a clear, colourless, watery fluid that comprises a vast array of electrolytes, organic solutes, growth factors and other proteins that nourish the nonvascularized tissue of the anterior chamber, particularly the trabecular meshwork, lens and corneal endothelium. It is produced by the ciliary body epithelium and flows into the anterior chamber. Aqueous humour leaves the anterior chamber through the trabecular meshwork into Schlemm's canal and episcleral veins (conventional pathway) or through the sclera and other downstream tissues (unconventional pathway). Aqueous outflow is the main source of mass transfer out of the eye. If the exit of aqueous humour from the eye is blocked, the amount of fluid within the eye increases, leading to an increase in intraocular pressure, which may lead to glaucoma and cause damage to the optic nerve. The trabecular

meshwork is made up of an extracellular matrix and specialized endothelial cells, forming a porous-like structure through which aqueous humour flows into Schlemm's canal. Schlemm's canal connects with the venous system through a network of 25 to 35 collector channels.

The vitreous cavity forms 80% of the volume of the eye. It weighs approximately 3.9 g and contains vitreous humour. This is a hydrogel containing approximately 98% water. The other 2% of vitreous components are predominantly collagen fibrils (collagen type II) and hyaluronic acid. Proteins, inorganic salts, glucose and ascorbic acid are also present. Vitreous humour has a pH of approximately 7.5 and a viscosity two to four times that of water. The presence of sodium hyaluronate is primarily responsible for the viscosity of the vitreous humour. Its viscous properties allow it to return to its normal shape when compressed. The vitreous body can be divided into cortical and central vitreous. The cortical vitreous humour is of higher density and has slower turnover, while the central vitreous humour is more liquid with higher turnover.

Ocular drug delivery routes and elimination pathways

The routes of and barriers to ocular drug delivery can be summarized with reference to Fig. 39.1 (see I, II and III):

I. The cornea is the main route through which ocular topically administered drugs reach the aqueous humour.

II. The blood–retinal barrier (RPE and retinal capillary endothelium) restricts entry of drugs from the systemic circulation into the posterior segment of the eye.

III. Intravitreal delivery route to directly reach the back of the eye.

Drug elimination occurs from the ocular surface via tear turnover, nasolacrimal drainage and absorption into conjunctiva blood vessels, leading to systemic clearance. Once the drug is in the aqueous or posterior segments (Fig. 39.1), drug elimination may occur:

1. from the aqueous humour into the systemic uveoscleral circulation;

2. from aqueous humour outflow through the trabecular meshwork and Schlemm's canal;

3. from the vitreous humour via diffusion into the anterior chamber; and

4. via the posterior route across the blood–retinal barrier.

Some common ocular conditions and pharmacological interventions

Ocular drug delivery is undertaken for treatment of local disease at different sites in the eye, and thus a brief introduction to common eye conditions is appropriate.

Dry eye syndrome. Dry eye is a common disease which occurs when either the tear volume is inadequate or of poor quality (poor functional tear). This often results in unstable tears and consequently ocular surface disease, which is a term now often used instead of dry eye to reflect the complex nature of a poor tear film and abnormal ocular surface. Dry eye and ocular surface disease is often difficult to control, depending on the underlying cause, and can become a chronic disease. The main management is to control the symptoms and protect the ocular surface from being damaged. The initial treatments include use of tear substitutes and mucolytic eye drops. In advanced cases, the use of anti-inflammatory eye drops, surgical intervention (e.g. to reduce lacrimal drainage by closure of the lacrimal punctum) and contact lenses have been shown to be beneficial. Management of associated eyelid disease with cleaning and unblocking of meibomian gland orifices, and systemic therapies to reduce inflammation may also be required.

Cataract. Cataract is the opacity of the lens, which often results from denaturation of the lens protein. Cataracts, which are usually age related, are the most common cause of treatable blindness worldwide. Surgery is the only proven treatment and is considered as the most successful surgery among all types of surgical interventions in humans. The procedure involves extraction of the clouded lens and implantation of a synthetically produced intraocular lens.

Glaucoma. Glaucoma is a group of diseases in which there is a specific type of damage to the optic nerve (optic disc cupping), resulting in a characteristic pattern of visual field loss: first peripheral and then central vision loss. Glaucoma, a lifelong condition, is the leading cause of irreversible blindness worldwide and is the second most common cause of blindness,

after cataract. The most important and only modifiable risk factor in this group of diseases is raised intraocular pressure. It has been shown that reduction of intraocular pressure, medically (eye drops), by laser or surgically, can decrease the progression of the visual field loss.

Age-related macular degeneration. AMD is a degenerative disorder that affects the macula, the most sensitive part of the retina, and consequently results in the loss of central vision. AMD is the leading cause of visual loss in industrialized countries and often occurs in the population older than 50 years. There are two forms of AMD: wet and dry. Wet AMD arises when abnormal new blood vessels grow underneath the macula and leak, thus causing scar tissue to develop in the macula, resulting in loss of central vision, often very quickly. With the more common dry AMD, RPE cells degenerate, causing the loss of photoreceptors (due to loss of support provided by the RPE). This causes atrophy and gradual blurring of central vision. Recent anti-vascular endothelial growth factor (anti-VEGF) treatments including pegaptanib (Macugen®, Pfizer), ranibizumab (Lucentis®, Genentech) and aflibercept (Eylea®, Regeneron Pharmaceuticals) have shown beneficial effects in the majority of patients with wet AMD. These treatments, however, require multiple intraocular injections, with up to 12 injections per year (this is discussed in detail later).

Endophthalmitis. Endophthalmitis is the inflammation of the internal layers of the eye. Infectious endophthalmitis most frequently occurs following ocular surgery and penetrating trauma, particularly with retained foreign body. Special care must be taken when injecting medicines into the back of the eye to ensure complete sterility is maintained. The most commonly cultured bacteria in postoperative endophthalmitis are Gram-positive bacteria (90%), including *Staphylococcus epidermidis*, *Staphylococcus aureus* and *Streptococcus* species. The most common bacteria found following trauma are staphylococcus and bacillus species. Noninfectious endophthalmitis may have many causes, including impurities or aggregation in intraocular injections (e.g. endotoxin, silicone oil precipitates). The main treatments are antibiotics and anti-inflammatory drugs administered via the periorbital, intraocular or parenteral routes, sometimes combined with removal of the infected vitreous humour (vitrectomy). The visual outcome is often very poor despite aggressive treatment.

Topical ophthalmic preparations

Topical ophthalmic preparations include solutions, suspensions, ointments/gels and the newer dispersion systems. These have traditionally been used for treating pathological diseases of the 'front of the eye'. Conditions affecting the anterior eye segment include infection (conjunctivitis), inflammation, allergy, dry eye, glaucoma and corneal ulceration.

Designing ocular drug delivery formulations requires an understanding of what can be tolerated by the eye. Physiological and biochemical mechanisms exist to protect the eye from harmful stimuli. Tears contain lysozymes and immunoglobulins, which impart an anti-infectious activity. While these mechanisms are protective, they do sometimes present a barrier to drug absorption. The lacrimal system of the eye is extremely dynamic. The tear volume in the normal eye is 5 µL to 9 µL. Basal tears are continuously secreted by the lacrimal glands at an average rate of 1.2 µL min^{-1}, thus giving a tear turnover rate of approximately 17% per minute. Reflex tears are triggered by irritants, and their secretion rate ranges from 3 µL min^{-1} to 400 µL min^{-1}, the intention being rapidly to eliminate the stimulus. Another protective mechanism is the eyelid movements associated with blinking. Blinking moves tear fluids and foreign matter to the nasal corner of the lid surface, where the liquid exits via the puncta and is then drained away by the nasolacrimal ducts into the inferior nasal passage – often called the lacrimal pump (Fig. 39.2). Some of the drug can end up rapidly entering the systemic circulation by absorption through the vascular nasal mucosa, being inhaled as an aerosol or through absorption from the gastrointestinal tract after being swallowed. The combined mechanisms of lacrimal drainage and blinking mean that administered eye drops are rapidly cleared, with residence times ranging from 4 to 23 minutes. Moreover, the rate of drainage from the eye has a positive, linear correlation with the instilled volume. It has been found that the conjunctival sacs are capable of accommodating only 20 µL to 30 µL of added fluid temporarily without spilling; however, the typical drop volume from eye drop bottles made by different manufacturers ranges from 34 µL to 63 µL. Not only is this variability large but it also exceeds the volume that can be accommodated by the eye if several drops are administered at once.

Ideally, administered eye drops should be spaced by at least 5 minutes to minimize washout. Punctal occlusion by the closing of the eye and gently pressing of the inside corner for at least 1 minute maximizes local absorption and minimizes systemic exposure by up to 70%. To reduce the elimination rate of administered eye drops, it is important that the topical preparations do not cause irritation. This can be achieved by designing their properties to be as close as possible to those of the lacrimal fluids covering the surface of the eye.

Formulating ophthalmic preparations

Osmolality

The concentration of salts in lacrimal fluids determines their osmolality. The predominant inorganic ions in tears are sodium, potassium, calcium, chloride and bicarbonate ions. These have an important function in controlling the osmotic pressure of the intercellular and extracellular fluids of the epithelial spaces of the cornea and conjunctiva. The osmolality in healthy, nondry eyes is on average 302 mmol kg^{-1} during daytime. Patients with dry eye syndrome have been found to present with tear film hyperosmolality, which contributes to the symptoms of the disease. When the eye is exposed to a hypotonic ophthalmic solution, the corneal epithelium becomes more permeable and water flows into the cornea, causing oedema. Hypertonic solutions have a dehydrating effect on the corneal epithelium. Hypotonic and hypertonic solutions are

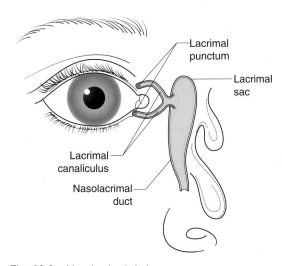

Fig. 39.2 • Nasolacrimal drainage.

irritating to the eye and therefore induce an increased production rate of tears. The rate of tear production increases to several hundred microlitres per minute through reflex tear secretion and reflex blinks. This increased tear turnover rate reduces the retention half-life of a solution that has been applied to the eye. Occasionally hypertonic eye drops (5% sodium chloride solution) are used for the treatment of eye conditions (e.g. corneal oedema due to a failing endothelial pump). The presence of hypertonic sodium chloride causes osmotic dehydration of the cornea, clearing some of the oedema and improving sight.

Normal tear osmotic pressure is equivalent to 0.9% to 1.0% sodium chloride solution. Solutions of osmotic pressure equivalent to 0.6% to 1.3% sodium chloride appear to be well tolerated by the eye. Ophthalmic solutions can be made isotonic by the use of tonicity agents such as sodium chloride, potassium chloride, buffering salts, dextrose, mannitol and glycerol, as long as they are compatible with the other ingredients in the formulation.

Hydrogen ion concentration (pH)

The pH of tears is close to neutral and is controlled by various substances dissolved in the aqueous layer of tears: carbon dioxide, bicarbonate, proteins, enzymes and fatty acids. The pH of tears is subject to diurnal variation and increases slowly from 6.9 to 7.5 during the waking hours of the day because of carbon dioxide evaporation. The buffer capacity of tear fluids is low but significant; it is predominantly controlled by the balance of bicarbonate and carbon dioxide, as well as proteins. Acidic or basic solutions instilled into the eye cannot be neutralized by the tears that are present, and therefore reflex tears are generated to dilute the administered drop and eliminate it. Strongly acidic or basic solutions should not be administered to the eye as they can damage the ocular tissue. The eye can generally tolerate topical ophthalmic preparations at a pH within the range of 3.5 to 9. However, it is preferable to formulate preparations as close to physiological tear pH as possible to reduce damage and discomfort and the associated increased lacrimation.

The pH is important in drug ionization and product shelf-life stability. Pilocarpine is a natural alkaloid used in the treatment of glaucoma. It undergoes pH-dependent hydrolytic degradation, and one of the ways to achieve stability of pilocarpine aqueous solution is to maintain the pH at 3.5–5.5 through the use of a weak acidic buffer (e.g. boric acid and sodium citrate). Because the pH deviates from the physiological pH of lacrimal fluids, the constituting buffer must be weak to reduce irritation and allow tear fluids to be restored to their normal pH within a short period without excessive lacrimation. Drug ionization is also important in determining drug solubility and permeation across the corneal epithelium. The extent of ionization can be manipulated through control of the pH of ophthalmic preparations.

Commonly used buffers in ophthalmic solutions include borate and phosphate buffers. To prepare solutions of lower pH, acetic acid/sodium acetate and citric acid/sodium citrate buffers are used. It is important that strong buffers are not used, and to use a low concentration of weak buffers.

Surface tension

The surface tension of tear fluid at physiological temperature in a healthy eye is 43.6 mN m^{-1} to 46.6 mN m^{-1}. Administration of solutions that have a surface tension much lower than that of the lacrimal fluid destabilizes the tear film and disperses the lipid layer into droplets that are solubilized by the drug or surfactants in the formulation. The oily film reduces the rate of evaporation of the underlying aqueous layer, and therefore once it is lost, dry spots are formed on the cornea which are painful and irritant. Surfactants are implicated in this disruption of the oily layer.

Surfactants are typically included in ophthalmic preparations to solubilize or disperse drugs. Nonionic surfactants are the least irritant and therefore the most commonly used; examples include polysorbate 20, polyoxyl 40 stearate and polyoxypropylene–polyoxyethylenediol. Despite being the least irritant, nonionic surfactants have been shown to remove the mucous layer and disrupt the tight junction complexes of the cornea, thereby increasing drug permeation. Surfactants may also interact with polymeric substances in the preparation and reduce the efficacy of preservatives. The concentration of surfactant is important not only in terms of drug solubility, safety and patient tolerance, but also because high concentrations can lead to foaming on product manufacture or shaking.

Viscosity

Viscosity-enhancing polymers are used in ophthalmic solutions to reduce the drainage rate, thus prolonging drug retention in the precorneal tear film and enhancing drug absorption. Water-soluble polymers that have been used to increase solution viscosity include poly(vinyl alcohol) (PVA), polyvinylpyrrolidone, and various cellulose derivatives, particularly methylcellulose, hydroxypropyl methylcellulose and carboxymethylcellulose (at concentrations of 0.2% to 2.5%) and polyethylene glycol (at concentrations of 0.2% to 1%). Tears are non-Newtonian fluids with shear-dependent viscosity. This is commonly seen with linear, multiple-charged polymers such as sodium hyaluronate and carbomers. Zero shear viscosity values of approximately 6.4 mPa s have been reported for normal tears. Acceptable viscosity of ophthalmic preparations is up to 15 mPa s; beyond that increased lacrimation and drainage occur to restore the tear film to its physiological viscosity. Furthermore, very viscous solutions can cause blurring of vision, potential blocking of the puncta and canaliculi, and pain on blinking.

Topical, liquid ophthalmic preparations

Solutions

Ophthalmic solutions are the most common topical ophthalmic preparation. They are typically the easiest to manufacture (have the lowest production cost) and are relatively easy for a patient or health care provider to administer. Ophthalmic solutions are also desirable where a rapid onset of action is required as they do not need to undergo dissolution. This would be the case for local anaesthetics (e.g. lignocaine, proxymetacaine hydrochloride), ocular diagnostics (fluorescein sodium) and ocular preoperative drugs. Moreover, solutions are homogeneous and therefore display a better dose uniformity. A limitation of solutions, however, is that they are rapidly drained out of the eye. Moreover, the rate of drainage is proportional to the size of the drop administered. The volume of eye drops administered from commercial eye dropper bottles has been reported to be in the range of 34 μL to 63 μL; this is dependent on the physical shape and orifice of the dropper opening, the physicochemical properties of the liquid and the manner in which the dropper is used.

Suspensions

Several ocular preparations are available as suspensions. This approach has been used to administer drugs which are sparingly soluble in water (e.g. steroids) or to prolong drug release. Particles tend to be retained in the conjunctival sac (pouch where the conjunctiva covering the inside of the lower eyelid and the sclera meet) and slowly go into solution, thus increasing the contact time. Particle size and shape need to be carefully selected as some particles can cause irritation of the sensory nerves in the epithelium. The *European Pharmacopoeia* and *United States Pharmacopeia* set limits for the maximum particle size permitted in ocular suspensions because large particles give rise to irritation and increased tearing. For a sample containing 10 μg of solid active substance, the *European Pharmacopoeia* states that 'not more than 20 particles should have a maximum dimension greater than 25 μm, and not more than two of these particles have a maximum dimension greater than 50 μm. None of the particles has a maximum dimension greater than 90 μm'.

The particles of a suspension need to be readily dispersible on shaking by the patient to ensure uniform dose administration. Homogeneity and dose uniformity need to be confirmed in multidose containers from first to last use. A problem that can arise with suspensions is conversion of the crystal structure of the drug (i.e. polymorphic changes during storage), which can lead to changes in drug solubility and dissolution behaviour. If the drug particle size is polydisperse, Ostwald ripening may occur on changes in storage temperature or prolonged storage. Cake formation can also be a problem, which may not be resolved by forming a flocculated suspension since large floccules can irritate the eye. Using a polymer solution as a viscosity-enhancing agent can prevent caking and allow particle resuspension by shaking. Betaxolol and brinzolamide are available as suspensions. The formulation of the former contains carbomer 934P and ion-exchange resins. Nepafenac is a nonsteroidal anti-inflammatory prodrug indicated for the treatment of pain and inflammation associated with cataract surgery. It is practically insoluble in water and is therefore formulated as suspension formulations: Nevanac® 0.1% dosed three times daily and Ilevro® 0.3% (Alcon Laboratories, USA) dosed once daily. The newer Ilevro formulation has a higher concentration of the active substance, 2.5-fold smaller drug particle size, and higher viscosity (through the use of carbomer–guar polymers) compared with the Nevanac formulation. These formulation changes have increased ocular bioavailability and allowed once daily administration, thus improving patient convenience/adherence.

Submicron emulsions

Ciclosporin is an immunomodulator with anti-inflammatory effects. It is available at a concentration of 0.05% as a submicron emulsion (Restasis®, Allergan) for topical application to the eye. Ciclosporin is hydrophobic (log P = 3.0) and has a very poor aqueous solubility of 6.6 µg mL^{-1} and cannot therefore be formulated in conventional aqueous ophthalmic vehicles. It has been successfully solubilized in an oil-in-water submicron emulsion formulated at a pH of 6.5–8.0. The oil phase in Restasis is castor oil and the emulsion is stabilized with the nonionic surfactant polysorbate 80 and glycerine, which behaves here as a cosurfactant. Ocular submicron emulsions with a droplet size of approximately 0.1 µm have also shown potential for prolonging drug release and achieving significantly higher drug concentrations in the cornea and aqueous humour compared with suspensions.

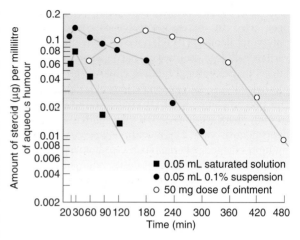

Fig. 39.3 • Comparison of aqueous humour levels of fluorometholone following administration of different dosage forms. From Sieg and Robinson, 1975.

Topical, semisolid ophthalmic preparations

Ointments

Ophthalmic ointments constitute approximately 10% of ophthalmic products and are usually used for the treatment of inflammation, infections and ocular surface disease. They offer the advantage of reducing drug drainage by tear flow, thereby increasing corneal residence time. Ointments can also be entrapped in the conjunctival sac, whereby they serve as a reservoir for the drug. Sustained drug release over 2–4 hours is usually observed. Ointments also have the advantage of allowing the incorporation of drugs with poor aqueous solubility. Hydrophobic ointments sometimes increase the stability of hydrolysable compounds, particularly peptides. Soft paraffin and liquid paraffin are commonly used as bases for ophthalmic ointments. Antibiotics, antifungals and steroids are the classes of drugs most available as ointments. Drug bioavailability usually peaks later with ointment vehicles than with solutions or suspensions. Total bioavailability in the aqueous humour can also be significantly greater than with solutions or suspensions (Fig. 39.3). Ointments are, however, more difficult to administer than solutions and may give rise to a more variable dose. In addition, blurring of vision arises, which tends to reduce patient adherence, making ointments more useful for night-time administration. Drug molecules may be entrapped within the ointment base because of favourable partitioning towards the base, therefore inhibiting drug release. The base is also sensitive to changes in temperature.

Gels

Gels, which are semisolid systems comprising water-soluble bases, are also available and are more favourable than ointments for water-soluble drugs. These utilize polymers such as PVA, poloxamer, hydroxypropyl methylcellulose, or carbomers dispersed in a liquid. Ganciclovir is an antiviral indicated for herpetic keratitis (eye ulcers caused by herpes virus which mainly affect the cornea). It is available as a gel (Zirgan, Bausch and Lomb) and utilizes carbomers. It is formulated at pH 7.4 which in addition to being well tolerated by the eye, allows polymer inter-chain repulsion and swelling to form a transparent gel.

Gels that are activated by ions, pH and temperature have also been developed. These undergo a phase transition from liquid to solid in the conjunctival sac to form a viscoelastic gel. These in situ forming gels have an advantage over the preformed gels in that the dose is more reproducible and administration is easier, thus improving patient adherence. Examples of polymers activated by temperature include poloxamers (e.g. poloxamer 407). Smart Hydrogel™ has been developed and is a graft copolymer of poly(acrylic acid) and a poloxamer which requires only 1% to 3% polymer concentration to undergo gelation at body temperature. Smart Hydrogel also has bioadhesive properties because of the presence of poly(acrylic acid).

Timolol is a nonselective beta-blocker licensed for treatment of glaucoma. Timolol maleate gel-forming solution (Timoptic-XE®, Merck) is clinically available and contains a purified anionic heteropolysaccharide derived from gellan gum. The gellan gum is in aqueous solution and forms a gel in the presence of cations which exist in the precorneal tear film. The cations neutralize the polymer, causing a reduction in its solubility. They also bridge the polymer chains, thus forming a structured polymer network. Timoptic-XE is administered once daily, compared with twice daily for the regular Timoptic® preparation to achieve a similar reduction in intraocular pressure. This gel is subsequently removed by the flow and drainage of tears. Alginates also undergo sol to gel phase transition when exposed to the ionic strength of ocular fluids. See Table 39.1 for examples of gel and gel-forming ophthalmic preparations. Carbomers have pK_a values of 4–5, and ophthalmic solutions of these polymers are prepared in this pH range. When these systems are exposed to the near-neutral pH of ocular fluids, the polymer solubility is reduced and the system undergoes gelation.

Mucoadhesive systems

Other ways to increase the contact time of topical ophthalmic solutions with the ocular surface have been through the use of mucoadhesive polymers. These polymers can associate with the mucin coat that covers the conjunctiva and cornea. Mucin has a protein or polypeptide core with carbohydrate chains branching off. The mucin coat serves to protect, hydrate and lubricate the surface of the eye. Mucoadhesive polymers are commonly macromolecular hydrocolloids with numerous hydrophilic functional groups possessing the correct charge density. They should also exhibit good wetting of the ocular surface to facilitate maximum interaction with the mucin coat. Electrostatic and hydrogen-bond interactions are the most common interactions between mucoadhesive polymers and mucin.

Mucoadhesive polymers can be natural, synthetic or semisynthetic. The synthetic polymers include poly(acrylic acid) and polycarbophil, as well as cellulose derivatives. The (semi)natural mucoadhesive polymers include chitosan and various gums, such as guar, xanthan, carrageenan, pectin and alginate. Chitosan is a cationic polymer which has shown promise for ophthalmic use. Besides being mucoadhesive, it has good wetting properties and is biodegradable, is biocompatible and has good ocular tolerance. It is positively charged at neutral pH and therefore electrostatic forces arise between it and the negatively charged sialic acid residues of the mucus glycoproteins, which contribute to its mechanism of mucoadhesion. Hyaluronic acid is another polymer which has also shown potential. It is a high molecular weight biological polymer consisting of linear polysaccharides and is present in the extracellular matrix, as well as being the main component of the vitreous humour. It has mucoadhesive and viscoelastic properties. as well as high water binding capacity. Hyaluronic acid is used in some ocular surgical procedures in the anterior chamber (e.g. cataract, glaucoma), subconjunctival space (e.g. glaucoma filtering surgery) or posterior chamber (retinal reattachment). Polycarbophil (poly(acrylic acid) cross-linked with divinyl glycol) has been used in a topical azithromycin formulation

Table 39.1 Examples of gel and gel-forming topical ophthalmic preparations

Active ingredient	Brand name and dosage form	Therapeutic class and indication	Release-controlling excipient
Timolol maleate	Timoptol-LA/Timoptic-XE (gel-forming solution)	Beta-blocker for treatment of glaucoma. To be applied once daily	Gellan gum
Betaxolol	Betoptic S (eye drops)	Beta-blocker for treatment of glaucoma. To be applied twice daily	Amberlite® IRP-69 (cation-exchange resin)
Loteprednol etabonate	Lotemax (gel)	Corticosteroids for treatment of post-operative pain and inflammation following ocular surgery. To be applied four times daily	Polycarbophil
Ganciclovir	Zirgan (gel)	Antiviral for eye ulcers. To be applied five times daily	Carbomer
Fusidic acid	Fucithalmic (eye drops)	Antibacterial. To be applied twice daily	Carbomer

which is available in the clinic under the name of AzaSite®/DuraDite® (Inspire Pharmaceuticals). It has been shown to have higher bioavailability than conventional aqueous eye drops. Therapeutic drug levels also persist for several days in the eyelids and conjunctiva following the administration of the last dose. Polycarbophil is insoluble in water, and its swelling is pH dependent. Swelling is greatest at pH 6–7, which is the pH range of lacrimal fluids. On exposure to tears, polycarbophil swells and entangles with mucin on the ocular surface. Hydrogen bonding also exists between the un-ionized carboxylic acid of polycarbophil and the mucin.

Ion-exchange resins

The concept of ion-exchange resins has existed for more than 50 years and they been used and marketed in various dosage forms to control drug delivery. The drug (acidic or basic) is ionically bound to an ion-exchange resin to form an insoluble complex. The drug can be released from the complex only through exchange of the bound drug ions with physiological ions in body fluids. The actual resin is an insoluble, ionic material composed of two parts, a structural portion comprising a polymer matrix, usually styrene cross-linked with divinylbenzene, and a functional portion, which is the ion-active group. The ion-active group can be either negatively or positively charged, thus functioning as either a cation exchanger or an anion exchanger. These drug–resin complexes are usually spherical and porous and usually hydrate on exposure to aqueous fluids. They are insoluble, nonabsorbable and considered safe for use in oral and ophthalmic preparations in humans. They have had several applications in pharmaceuticals, including taste masking, drug stabilization and sustained-release solid dosage forms as well as liquid suspensions.

Betaxolol hydrochloride (a cardioselective beta-blocker) is available as an ion-exchange resin suspension formulation (Betoptic S®, Alcon Laboratories, USA). The positively charged drug is bound to a cation-exchange resin (Amberlite® IRP69). The matrix of Amberlite IRP69 is styrene–divinylbenzene polymer and the functional portion is sodium polystyrene sulfonate. Sulfonic acid acts as a strong cation exchanger. The mobile, or exchangeable, cation is sodium; this can be exchanged for many cationic species (e.g. potassium or calcium present in lacrimal fluids). On ocular instillation of the suspension,

betaxolol is displaced from the resin by the sodium ions in the tear film. This exchange occurs over several minutes. The polar nature of betaxolol can cause ocular discomfort, and therefore formulating it as an ion-exchange resin reduces the rate of drug release and minimizes this discomfort.

Resin particle size is one of the factors that controls the rate of drug release. In Betoptic S, the resins have been finely milled to a diameter of 5 μm to achieve a fine suspension. A polymer, Carbomer 934P (a water-soluble acrylic polymer), is also included to increase the physical stability and ease of resuspension of the product, as well as to enhance the ocular residence time.

Barriers to topical ocular drug absorption

The topical route of drug delivery is the most common way of treating the anterior segment, and more than 90% of the ophthalmic medicines on the market are in the form of eye drops. The topical route provides selectivity with an enhanced therapeutic index, it also circumvents first-pass metabolism and drugs can be administered in a simple, noninvasive manner. Its main shortcoming, however, is its inefficiency, such that only 1% to 5% of the instilled dose reaches the aqueous humour. The highly efficient lacrimal drainage system taking drug away from the tear film to the nose, drug absorption by conjunctiva blood vessels into the systemic circulation, and the corneal barrier to drug permeation are the mechanisms mainly responsible for this low ocular drug bioavailability. Drug binding to proteins also reduces absorption, and protein levels of lacrimal fluids are higher in inflamed or infected eyes.

The corneal barrier

Drugs can permeate the cornea by passive diffusion, facilitated diffusion or active transport. Facilitated diffusion and active transport occur via transporter proteins expressed on the corneal epithelium. Passive diffusion does not require transporters; however, it is determined by the physicochemical properties of the drug. The cornea is divided into five layers: the epithelium, Bowman's membrane, the stroma, Descemet's membrane and the endothelium. The layers which form substantial barriers to drug permeation are the epithelium, stroma and endothelium

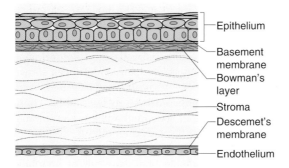

Fig. 39.4 • The human cornea in cross section.

Labels:
Epithelium
Basement membrane
Bowman's layer
Stroma
Descemet's membrane
Endothelium

(from the outer to the inner surface) (Fig. 39.4). The epithelium and endothelium are rich in lipids, while the stroma has high water content. The corneal epithelium is approximately 0.1 mm (six cells) thick and is considered to be the rate-limiting barrier to transcorneal drug permeation. It contributes approximately 90% of the barrier to hydrophilic drugs and approximately 10% of the barrier to lipophilic drugs. Drugs can penetrate this layer by passing through the cells (transcellular route) or between the cells (paracellular route). The epithelium, however, has tightly adherent cells with tight junctions and excludes macromolecules with a radius greater than 1 nm. Only small drugs with a molecular weight less than 350 and ions can permeate through the paracellular route. Most lipophilic compounds can pass through the corneal epithelium via the transcellular route. The cornea is considered a tight tissue, tighter than the intestine, lung and nasal mucosa, making drug absorption via the paracellular route more difficult than via these other organs. It is noteworthy, however, that in certain ocular circumstances affecting the epithelial cells of the cornea (e.g. contact-lens-related infectious keratitis and multiple applications of eye drops, e.g. local anaesthetics), drug permeation from ocular eye drops can be enhanced because of defects caused in the epithelial layer.

The stroma is a cellular, aqueous environment interdispersed with glycosaminoglycans and collagen fibrils (collagen types I and III) that are organized in parallel lamellae. It is open knit, allowing hydrophilic molecules to pass through relatively easily. However, it limits the penetration of highly lipophilic or high molecular weight compounds. The corneal endothelium is a single-cell layer with large intercellular junctions. It is in direct contact with the aqueous humour and partially resists the

permeation of lipophilic compounds, though not hydrophilic ones.

Ophthalmic drugs with modest lipophilicity and low molecular weight are absorbed more efficiently via the corneal route than are hydrophilic, ionized drugs. The optimal lipophilicity for the permeation of steroids and beta-blockers corresponds to log P of 2–3. Compounds with a higher lipophilicity (log $P > 3$) have been shown to have lower permeability as their permeation is rate limited by the slow transfer through the hydrophilic stroma. Drugs need to have an appropriate balance of lipid solubility and water solubility for good corneal permeation.

Good aqueous solubility is important as drugs must be in solution to permeate through the cornea, especially the stroma. It also creates a high drug concentration gradient between the tear film and corneal epithelium. Because the instilled drops are diluted by tear fluids and are in contact with the corneal epithelium for a very short time, making bioavailability low, high drug concentration is one important consideration, when possible, for ophthalmic solutions. For ionizable drugs, the pH of the formulation can be adjusted to obtain the optimum balance of solubility and transepithelial permeation. It is desirable for a drug to possess good aqueous solubility at the physiological pH of tears, without the loss of lipophilicity for corneal permeation.

Noncorneal routes of absorption

While the corneal route is the principal route of entry into the eye for topically administered drugs, studies have shown that absorption can also occur via the conjunctival-scleral layer, particularly for large hydrophilic molecules such as timolol maleate, and carbonic anhydrase inhibitors, as well as proteins and peptides which can be used as carriers. The conjunctiva has 5–15 layers of squamous epithelial cells with tight junctions at the apical end. It is more permeable or leaky than the cornea and allows drugs to permeate through both the paracellular route and the transcellular route. The conjunctiva is highly vascularized, so drug absorption often results in systemic distribution of the drug away from the eye. The cornea covers only approximately one-sixth of the surface area of the eye, so conjunctival absorption can readily occur. Efflux drug transporters on the epithelial cells have also been identified. The conjunctival stroma comprises blood vessels, nerves and lymphatics that attach to the sclera. Drug permeation through the sclera occurs through the aqueous intercellular space between the collagen fibres. Drug permeation through the sclera is not dependent on lipophilicity or size. Drugs with a molecular weight greater than 1000 are almost incapable of permeating through the cornea, whereas dextran (molecular weight 40 000) and albumin (molecular weight 69 000) have good ability to permeate through the sclera. Despite this, the conjunctival-scleral route is considered a nonproductive route because the blood vessels in the conjunctiva rapidly absorb the instilled drug, which dissipates into the systemic circulation rather than ending up in the aqueous humour. For this reason, significant drug interactions can occur between ocular and orally administered medicines, and some topical ocular preparations are contraindicated in patients with certain medical conditions (e.g. eye drops of beta-blockers in patients with either asthma or overt cardiac failure). Although topical ocular drug doses are far lower than oral doses, the direct access via the inhaled or nasal mucosal absorption route bypasses losses including intestinal absorption and liver first-pass effects.

Increasing drug solubility and absorption in topical ophthalmic preparations

Drug ionization, salts and esters

The pK_a of the drug (acid dissociation constant) and the pH determine its degree of ionization in solution. Whilst the pK_a can be altered only through structural changes in the molecule, the pH of the drug vehicle can be varied. Controlling the pH can increase drug solubility and thus increase the drug concentrations that can be accommodated in the product. A higher proportion of un-ionized species can increase transcorneal permeation. However, controlling drug ionization through the pH of the administered solution only has a short-lived effect as lacrimation restores the pH of the administered solution to the physiological pH of tear fluids, which ultimately determines the ionization pattern. Interestingly, however, carbonic anhydrase inhibitors display a greater pharmacological effect (reduction in intraocular pressure) in the ionized form than in the un-ionized form. This effect is observed not because of greater drug permeation but because of the ability of these inhibitors to be sequestered in the cornea and form a depot.

Chemical derivatization of the drug through formation of salts or hydrolysable esters affects drug solubility and lipophilicity and can therefore be an important determinant of ocular bioavailability. Prednisolone acetate formulated as a suspension has been shown to have higher corneal permeation and increased ocular bioavailability compared with its hydrophilic counterpart, prednisolone sodium phosphate. Dexamethasone acetate ester displays the optimum balance of solubility and corneal permeability compared with the very water-soluble phosphate salt or lipophilic free base.

Cyclodextrins

Cyclodextrins (CDs) have shown great potential in increasing the solubility of poorly water-soluble drugs (see Chapter 24). CDs are cyclical oligosaccharides with a lipophilic centre and a hydrophilic outer surface. They can complex lipophilic drugs in their interior, thus forming water-soluble complexes. This maintains the structure and lipophilicity and hence permeability of the compounds. The drug is noncovalently associated with CD by hydrogen bonding, hydrophobic interactions or van der Waals forces. The hydrophilic CD acts as a carrier, delivering water-insoluble molecules to the corneal membrane, where they can separate from the CD complex. A state of equilibrium exists between free and complexed drug which is dependent on the strength of the noncovalent interactions between the drug and CD. The relatively lipophilic membrane has low affinity for the large hydrophilic CD molecules, and the biological membrane is not disrupted as is observed with penetration enhancers. Moreover, this provides an opportunity for delivering irritant drugs as they are not freely available and are entrapped in the complex. Research with this formulation approach has shown it increases corneal penetration of dexamethasone, pilocarpine and carbonic anhydrase inhibitors.

Prodrugs

Increased corneal penetration can be gained through the use of prodrugs. A prodrug is a drug with added functionalities that converts to the active parent drug through enzymatic or chemical reactions. Approaches for enhancing corneal penetration through the use of prodrugs include optimization of lipophilicity, enhancement of aqueous solubility, increase of affinity for uptake transporters and evasion of efflux pumps.

Drugs with carboxylic acid groups, such as the prostaglandin analogues indicated for glaucoma, have low corneal permeation. This is due to the ionization of the carboxylic acid group at the near-neutral pH of tears, which reduces permeation through the lipophilic epithelium. One strategy to mitigate this has been esterification of the carboxylic acid group. Because the cornea has high esterase activity, these derivatives can easily revert to their parent form. However, one of the problems with ester prodrugs is their increased susceptibility to hydrolysis. Bulky isopropyl esters have been used to achieve stability in aqueous solutions. The prostaglandin analogues latanoprost and travoprost are isopropyl esters. These prodrugs have been shown to have increased corneal permeability and greater intraocular pressure lowering effects compared with their parent forms (i.e. free acids).

Dipivalyl adrenaline (dipivefrine) is also indicated for glaucoma and was the first marketed ophthalmic prodrug. It is metabolized to adrenaline, which was the drug originally used, though this was later found to give rise to severe side effects in patients. Adrenaline is a polar drug and was subject to rapid clearance from the ocular surface via nasal lacrimal drainage. Systemic absorption was therefore significant, giving rise to cardiac arrhythmias and blood pressure elevation. The prodrug, the dipivalyl ester of adrenaline, was designed to be more lipophilic than the parent drug for increased corneal permeation.

Other examples of prodrugs in the clinic include the beta-blocker levobunolol (log P = 2.4). Levobunolol is converted in the cornea to the active dihydrolevobunolol by metabolic reduction of its keto group. Dihydrolevobunolol is more lipophilic and has a longer half-life than its parent form. Active research is being pursued in designing prodrugs of the antivirals aciclovir and ganciclovir. Amino acid and peptide derivatives of these prodrugs target the amino acid and peptide transporters of the cornea.

Sterility of ophthalmic preparations

It is a regulatory requirement that preparations intended for ophthalmic use, including those for cleansing the eyes, be sterile. Ocular infections are extremely dangerous and can rapidly lead to the loss of vision. Eyebaths, droppers and all other dispensers should also be sterile and regulated if packaged with the drug product. For ophthalmic preparations, terminal sterilization of products in their final containers should be adopted wherever possible. If the product cannot withstand terminal sterilization, then filtration under aseptic conditions should be considered, usually performed using a filter pore size of 0.22 µm or less. Sterilization methods are discussed in greater detail in Chapters 16 and 17. The raw materials used for aseptic manufacture should be sterile, wherever possible, or should meet a low specified bioburden control limit. Ophthalmic preparations must furthermore be labelled with the duration of use once opened.

Preservatives are included in multidose containers to destroy and inhibit the growth of microorganisms that may have been accidentally introduced on opening of the container (see Chapter 48). They are not to be used in products for intraocular administration as they can lead to irritation. Ideally, a preservative should have a broad-spectrum antimicrobial activity, exhibit compatibility and stability with all the ingredients in the preparation and the container, and be innocuous to the ocular tissue. Benzalkonium chloride is the most commonly used preservative, at concentrations ranging from 0.004% to 0.02%. It is a quaternary ammonium surfactant and causes epithelial inflammation and cell damage on repeated administration. Poor tolerance to treatment has been associated with benzalkonium chloride, and chronic inflammation of the conjunctiva has been reported. Benzalkonium chloride is also found in other products, such as hand sanitizers and antiseptics such as Dettol. Newer alternatives have been developed, SofZia® and Purite®, for which tolerance is better. SofZia is found in travoprost ophthalmic solution (Travatan®, Alcon Laboratories, USA) and Purite is present in brimonidine tartrate (Alphagan® P, Allegan, USA). These newer preservatives work in a different way from benzalkonium chloride. SofZia is an ionic-buffered preservative comprising boric acid, propylene glycol, sorbitol and zinc chloride, while Purite is a stabilized oxychloro complex that breaks down into innocuous products on contact with air.

Single-dose units have been developed to circumvent the use of preservatives while maintaining stability. The manufacturing and packaging of these unit is, however, expensive and so they have not been embraced for all marketed ophthalmic solutions. Several multidose bottles have been developed that maintain sterility without the use of a preservative; one of these is the ABAK® patented filter system, which uses a 0.2 μm polyether sulphone membrane with both hydrophilic and hydrophobic properties to prevent bacteria from entering the bottle. The Airless Antibacterial Dispensing System (AADS™, Pfizer) works by preventing air, and therefore bacteria, from entering the container on dispensation. Furthermore, a silver coil is included in the bottle tip. Silver has antibacterial properties and therefore any bacteria contacting the tip do not contaminate the contents. This system guarantees 3 months of sterility.

Ocular drug pharmacokinetics

Drug half-life in the anterior chamber

Peak drug levels in the anterior chamber are reached 20–30 minutes after eye drop administration. These concentrations in the aqueous humour are typically, however, twofold less than the administered concentration. From the aqueous humour the drug can diffuse to the iris and ciliary body, where it may bind to melanin and form a reservoir allowing gradual drug release to the surrounding cells. The drug is eliminated from the aqueous humour by two main routes: aqueous turnover through the trabecular meshwork and Schlemm's canal (Fig. 39.1, route 2) and by the venous blood flow of the anterior uvea across the blood aqueous barrier (Fig. 39.1, route 2). Aqueous humour turnover is at a rate of 2.2 μL min^{-1} to 3.1 μL min^{-1}. For an individual with an average anterior chamber volume of 185 μL, the half-life of anterior chamber fluid is 43 minutes. Moreover, the directional flow of aqueous humour from the ciliary body towards the trabecular meshwork is often against the diffusion of the drug towards intraocular target tissues. The other mechanism of drug elimination by the uveal blood flow is dependent on the drug's ability to permeate the endothelial cells of the blood vessels and is therefore more favourable for lipophilic drugs. The clearance of lipophilic drugs can be in the range from 10 μL min^{-1} to 30 μL min^{-1}. Drug half-lives in the anterior chamber are typically short, approximately 1 hour. Drug distribution to the vitreous is extremely slow as the lens prohibits diffusion.

Active transporters of the cornea

Various uptake and efflux transporters have been shown to be present in the corneal epithelium. These transporters are also present in the epithelium of the intestine, blood–brain barrier and kidney tubuli. Efflux transporters protect cells from noxious stimuli and are also implicated in drug resistance. It is estimated that 25% of administered drugs are substrates for transporters. Because the cornea is in contact with the external environment, it is not surprising that it expresses efflux transporters as part of a protective mechanism.

Efflux transporters that have been identified on the corneal epithelium include P-glycoprotein (also known as multidrug resistance protein 1), breast cancer resistance protein (BCRP) and multidrug-resistance-associated protein (MRP) 5. P-glycoprotein was found to be implicated in the transport of ciclosporin (immunomodulator for treating dry eyes) in the cornea. The prostaglandin agonists used in the treatment of glaucoma (bimatoprost, latanoprost and travoprost) and their free acid forms are substrates of the MRP5 efflux pump on the cornea. Bimatoprost is also a substrate for P-glycoprotein. Coadministration of these prostaglandin agonists for the treatment of glaucoma has been proposed for overcoming efflux, as well as for achieving a synergistic pharmacological effect, since these molecules may act primarily at different receptors to reduce intraocular pressure.

One of the main groups of uptake transporters in the corneal epithelium is the amino acid transporters. The corneal epithelium is a highly regenerative tissue with continuous protein synthesis, thus placing a demand on amino acid transport. The aqueous humour is the main source of nutrient provision for the corneal epithelium. Oligopeptide transporters have also been identified and shown to be involved in the transport of valaciclovir (L-valyl ester of aciclovir) through the cornea. They are also being utilized in prodrug delivery. The organic anion transporting polypeptide (OATP) family has substrates of a mainly anionic, amphipathic nature. Their presence in the cornea may be implicated in the transport of thyroid hormone, which has a role in the development and transparency of the cornea. Its involvement in drug transport has not been determined.

The pharmacokinetic significance of the role of these ocular transporters still requires investigation. With respect to topical solutions, the contact time is short and most of the drug absorption occurs in 2–3 minutes after instillation. Hence these transporters may become saturated, and passive diffusion becomes the predominant mechanism.

Blood–retinal barrier

The blood–retinal barrier (Fig. 39.1, route II) restricts the entry of drugs from the systemic circulation into the posterior segment of the eye. It is composed of two parts: an outer part formed by the RPE and an inner part, comprising endothelial cells of the retinal vessels. These two parts are connected to each other by tight junctions which pose a barrier to the perfusion of hydrophilic drugs from the highly vascular choroid into the retina and vitreous humour, and vice versa. The blood–retinal barrier has some structural similarities to the blood–brain barrier.

Transporters that have been identified in the RPE include amino acid transporters, oligopeptide transporters, monocarboxylate transporters, folate transporters and vitamin C transporters, as well as glucose transporters, OATP, organic cation transporter (OCT) and organic anion transporter (OAT). The efflux transporters are P-glycoprotein, MRP1, MRP4, MRP5 and breast cancer resistance protein. Drugs that have been found to have interactions with transporters in the blood–retinal barrier are predominantly substrates of OAT, OCT or OATP. Substrates of OAT include various antibiotics (penicillin, erythromycin and tetracycline) and antivirals (aciclovir, zidovudine). The main substrates for OCT are the antiglaucoma drugs carbachol, dipivefrine, brimonidine and timolol. Penicillin, erythromycin, steroidal anti-inflammatory agents (dexamethasone, hydrocortisone, prednisolone) and ciclosporin are OATP substrates. Transporters seem to play an important role in drug delivery to the posterior segment of the eye. Moreover, drug concentrations are low at the blood–retinal barrier, which means that the transporters are unlikely to be saturated and therefore their role is unlikely to be significant.

Ocular metabolism

Another ocular defence mechanism which protects the eye from the outside environment is the metabolism of xenobiotics. A xenobiotic is a chemical compound foreign to a given biological system. For humans, xenobiotics include drugs, drug metabolites and environmental compounds such as pollutants that are not produced by the body. In the environment, xenobiotics include synthetic pesticides, herbicides and industrial pollutants that are not found in nature. Both phase I and phase II metabolism reactions occur in ocular tissue. Phase I is where a polar functional group is introduced into the molecule which makes it more susceptible to phase II conjugation reactions. In some cases, however, the products of phase I reactions are eliminated from the body without further changes. Studies show that the most active metabolic sites in the eye are the ciliary body and pigmented epithelium of the retina. This may be attributable to the high perfusion of these sites by the blood circulation and consequently exposure to the xenobiotics circulating in the blood. Moreover, the main function of the ciliary body is to produce aqueous humour through ultrafiltration of plasma. It should therefore have an increased capacity to handle the exogenous compounds to which it is exposed and convert them into harmless metabolites, which could otherwise have toxic effects on the lens and other internal organs of the eye. Alternatively, it is possible that these tissues may be more prone to long-term effects of xenobiotics (e.g. the products of cigarette smoke may have long-term effects on the RPE, which may become more susceptible to disease and may die more rapidly in people who smoke).

The enzymes involved in phase I reactions are the esterases, which have been identified in ocular tissue and include acetylcholinesterase, butyrylcholinesterase and carboxycholinesterases. This hydrolysis of compounds containing ester linkages has been exploited in prodrug design, including design of dipivalyl adrenaline and pilocarpine prodrugs. Various esterases have been identified in the cornea. Aldehyde and ketone reductases have also been reported in ocular tissue. Ketone reductase reduces levobunolol, a beta-blocker indicated for the treatment of glaucoma. Peptidase activity has also been determined. Cytochrome P450 (CYP) expression is considered marginal in the human cornea, iris–ciliary body and retina–choroid.

Several ocular drugs are substrates for CYPs and the expression levels of these enzymes in the liver have been implicated in the systemic response to these locally administered ophthalmic medicines. Timolol is a nonselective beta-blocker used as an antiglaucoma medication. Although it is topically administered into the eye, it is partially absorbed into the systemic circulation, where it is metabolized by the CYP2D6. Individuals who are poor metabolizers of timolol can be more prone to its adverse systemic effects, such as reductions in heart rate and blood pressure. Moreover, CYPs are inducible by several pharmacological agents, including phenobarbital, rifampicin and phenytoin. Such induction can increase drug metabolism. One of the phase II enzymes identified in the eye is glutathione *S*-transferase. This binds to lipophilic compounds, such as bilirubin and haematin, which is a critical step in the detoxification process. Glutathione *S*-transferase has been identified in the lens, and deficiency of it has been associated with cataract.

Targeting the posterior segment of the eye

Systemic drug delivery

Diseases affecting the posterior segment of the eye are currently the most important cause of irreversible vision impairment leading to blindness worldwide. These include AMD, diabetic retinopathy and optic nerve damage associated with glaucoma. The posterior segment can be reached by topical, systemic or direct drug delivery systems. The topical and systemic routes are, however, tortuous for the drug and several barriers need to be overcome. Topical administration presents a long diffusion pathway for the drug, and the administered dose may end up in the systemic circulation through the conjunctival and nasal blood vessels. A small amount of drug that might cross the conjunctiva, and then the sclera would also encounter washout by high choroid circulation (dynamic barrier). Adequate and reproducible concentrations are therefore not reached in the posterior segment.

Systemic delivery of a drug means it needs to be able to cross the blood–retinal barrier to reach the retina and vitreous humour. Moreover, only a small fraction of blood flow circulates through the posterior segment of the eye, and therefore high systemic doses need to be administered, which can lead to systemic side effects. Despite these absorption barriers, verteporfin (Visudyne®, Novartis) has been successfully developed and licensed for intravenous administration for the photodynamic treatment of wet AMD associated with predominantly classic subfoveal choroidal neovascularization. It is a liposomal drug delivery system available as a lyophilized cake which is reconstituted for intravenous injection. Liposomes are phospholipid vesicles with an aqueous core and phospholipid bilayers which allow the entrapment of hydrophilic and lipophilic drugs respectively. They are biocompatible and biodegradable and can vary in size from nanometres to tens of micrometres (see Chapter 44). Verteporfin is a water-insoluble drug

and is entrapped within lipid bilayers of liposomes. Following intravenous infusion, verteporfin is activated by local irradiation with a nonthermal red laser (low-energy laser) applied to the retina. Light is delivered to the retina as a single circular point, via a fibre optic. Cytotoxic derivatives are produced which cause local damage to the neovascular endothelium, thus occluding the targeted vessels. Treatment is administered to the patient every 3 months. This treatment has been largely superseded by intravitreal injections of anti-VEGF therapies.

Intraocular injections

Intravitreal injections provide the most efficient means of reproducible drug delivery to the back of the eye. The drug bypasses the blood–ocular barriers, thus achieving higher intraocular levels, which improve treatment efficacy. Systemic side effects are also minimized. Intravitreal injections have been shown to be effective in patients for a variety of low molecular weight drugs and monoclonal antibodies. The intravitreal route is approved for anti-VEGF agents indicated for the treatment of neovascular (or wet) AMD. Neovascular AMD can progress rapidly, leading to irreversible sight loss within days or weeks. VEGF induces angiogenesis and augments vascular permeation and inflammation, which are thought to contribute to the progression of the wet form of AMD. VEGF has also been implicated in blood–retinal barrier breakdown. The three approved treatments, pegaptanib sodium (Macugen®, Pfizer), ranibizumab (Lucentis®, Genentech) and aflibercept (Eylea®, Regeneron Genentech) are all large molecules that bind to and inhibit the activity of different isoforms of VEGF. Pegaptanib is a PEGylated modified oligonucleotide, ranibizumab is a fragment of a monoclonal antibody (Fab fragment of humanized immunoglobulin G1) and aflibercept is a recombinant fusion protein consisting of portions of VEGF receptors fused to the Fc portion of human immunoglobulin G1. They need to be injected into the vitreous humour approximately every 4–8 weeks. Drug retention in the vitreous space depends on the drug half-life, which in turn determines the frequency of administration. The half-lives of most drugs for the treatment of posterior segment disease range from a few hours to a few days, which have been estimated with different animal models. Dexamethasone phosphate has a vitreal half-life of 5.5 hours. The half-life of pegaptanib in the vitreous humour is 3–5 days, that of ranibizumab is 3–4 days and that of aflibercept is predicted to be 7 days because of its larger size. Triamcinolone acetonide is one of the few exceptions, with a long half-life of 18.6 days; the injections are therefore given only every 3–4 months. Triamcinolone acetonide is injected as a suspension, and its slow dissolution in the vitreous humour contributes to its long half-life.

Repeated intravitreal injections cause patient discomfort, and associated complications include retinal detachment, endophthalmitis, vitreous haemorrhage and infection. The lens can also be affected and cataracts may form. Elevation of intraocular pressure may also occur, especially with steroid injections. Small volumes of 0.05 mL to 0.10 mL are typically used for injection. Although these adverse events have a low incidence, they can be sight-threatening. Sustained-release implants are being developed to overcome these problems and to achieve steady concentrations of the drug while minimizing the peaks and troughs in drug levels. Table 39.2 summarizes the different approaches for targeting the posterior segment of the eye.

Intraocular implants

Implantable drug delivery systems can be classified into bioerodible and nonbioerodible systems. In both systems, drug-release kinetics are determined by the polymer system used, the drug physicochemical properties and diffusion of the drug through the polymer. Biocompatibility is an essential property for all systems; the components should not interact with the surrounding tissue and should not elicit foreign body reactions through inflammatory or immune responses. Moreover, implants must not be affected by the host and they need to be relatively stable at the implant site. The inside of the eye is a viable location for implantation as evidenced by the use of intraocular lenses which are implanted to replace the clouded-over natural lens during cataract surgery.

Nonbiodegradable intraocular implants

Nonbiodegradable systems are commonly 'reservoir' devices, whereby the drug core is coated by a semi-permeable polymer through which the drug can pass, or the polymer coating may have an opening of a fixed area through which the drug can diffuse out. The other type of nonbiodegradable system is the 'monolithic' type, which is a homogeneous mix of

drug and polymer. It is easier, however, to achieve zero-order kinetics from a reservoir system. Vitrasert® (ganciclovir 4.5 mg; Bausch and Lomb), the first implantable intravitreal device to be available in the clinic, was approved by the US Food and Drug Administration (FDA) in 1996. It is indicated for the local treatment of cytomegalovirus retinitis. Ganciclovir is embedded in a PVA and ethylene vinyl acetate polymer-based system. The drug is slowly released from this implant over 5–8 months. PVA is a hydrophilic polymer acting as the scaffold for the implant, as well as controlling the rate of drug diffusion. Ethylene vinyl acetate is hydrophobic polymer used to coat the implant to also control drug diffusion. Fluid is imbibed into the implant and dissolves the drug; a saturated solution is formed within the core and drug molecules diffuse out of the system under a concentration gradient. The advantages of this system are that as long as a saturated drug solution remains in the core, the release rate will be constant. Moreover, no initial burst release of drug is observed. Intraocular insertion of the implant requires surgery; a 4 mm to 5 mm sclerotomy at the pars plana is necessary for implantation. Further surgery is required to remove the implant depleted of drug. The risks associated with this invasive procedure include vitreous haemorrhage, cataract, retinal detachment and endophthalmitis.

Retisert® (fluocinolone acetonide 0.59 mg; Bausch and Lomb) was approved by the FDA in 2005 and is indicated for the treatment of chronic infectious uveitis affecting the posterior segment of the eye. The pure drug is compressed into a 1.5 mm tablet die and coated with a PVA membrane and silicone laminate which has a release orifice. The initial drug release rate is 0.6 µg per day, decreasing in the first month to a steady state of 0.3 µg to 0.4 µg per day in approximately 30 months. With this course of treatment, uveitis recurrence rates are reduced. However, studies have shown patients need cataract extraction and intraocular pressure lowering surgery.

Iluvien® (fluocinolone acetonide 0.19 mg; Alimera Sciences) was approved by the FDA in 2014 and is indicated for the treatment of diabetic macular oedema. It takes the shape of a 3.5 mm × 0.37 mm cylinder and the drug is in a PVA matrix which is encased in a polyimide tube (Fig. 39.5). One end of the tube is coated with silicon bioadhesive, and the other end is coated with PVA, which controls drug release. A human pharmacokinetic study (the FAMOUS study) was conducted over 36 months and measured drug concentrations in the aqueous

Table 39.2 Intravitreal drug delivery systems for treating the posterior segment of the eye

Drug	Brand name	Dose / frequency of administration	Pharmaceutical characteristics	Ocular indications
Injectable steroid suspensions				
Triamcinolone acetonide (80 mg mL^{-1})	Trivaris (Allergan)	Injection of 4 mg (50 μL of 80 mg mL^{-1} suspension) / approx. every 3–4 months	Sterile aqueous gel suspension in a vehicle containing 2.3% sodium hyaluronate, sodium chloride, sodium phosphate dibasic, sodium phosphate monobasic; pH adjusted to 7.0–7.4	Sympathetic ophthalmia Temporal arteritis Uveitis Ocular inflammatory conditions unresponsive to topical corticosteroids
Triamcinolone acetonide (40 mg mL^{-1})	Triesence (Alcon Laboratories)	Injection of 4 mg (100 μL of 40 mg mL^{-1} suspension) / approx. every 3–4 months	0.5% carboxymethylcellulose sodium, 0.015% polysorbate 80, sodium chloride (for isotonicity), potassium chloride, calcium chloride, magnesium chloride, sodium acetate, sodium citrate; pH of suspension adjusted to 6.0 to 7.5 with sodium hydroxide or hydrochloric acid	Sympathetic ophthalmia Temporal arteritis Uveitis Ocular inflammatory conditions unresponsive to topical corticosteroids
Injectable anti-VEGF solutions				
Ranibizumab (10 mg mL^{-1})	Lucentis (Genentech)	Injection of 0.5 mg (50 μL of 10 mg mL^{-1} solution) Injection of 0.3 mg (50 μL of 6 mg mL^{-1} solution) / approx. every 4 weeks	10 mM histidine hydrochloride, 10% α-trehalose dihydrate, polysorbate 20; pH adjusted to 5.5	Wet AMD Macular oedema following retinal vein occlusion Diabetic macular oedema Diabetic retinopathy in patients with diabetic macular oedema
Pegaptanib sodium (3.47 mg mL^{-1})	Macugen (Pfizer)	Injection of 0.31 mg (90 μL of 3.46 mg mL^{-1} solution) / approx. every 6 weeks	Sodium chloride, monobasic sodium phosphate, dibasic sodium phosphate, hydrochloric acid or sodium hydroxide for pH adjustment	Wet AMD
Aflibercept	Eylea (Regeneron Pharmaceuticals)	Injection of 2 mg (50 μL of 40 mg mL^{-1} solution) / approx. every 4–8 weeks	Sodium phosphate, sodium chloride, polysorbate 20, sucrose; pH adjusted to 6.2	Wet AMD Macular oedema following retinal vein occlusion Diabetic macular oedema Diabetic retinopathy in patients with Diabetic macular oedema
Sustained-release implants				
Ganciclovir 4.5 mg	Vitrasert (Bausch and Lomb)	5–8 months	Nonbiodegradable PVA–EVA polymer-based system	AIDS-related cytomegalovirus retinitis
Fluocinolone acetonide 0.59 mg	Retisert (Bausch and Lomb)	30 months	Nonbiodegradable implant with PVA membrane	Chronic infectious uveitis
Fluocinolone acetonide 0.19 mg	Iluvien (Alimera Sciences)	36 months	Nonbiodegradable implant of PVA matrix encased in a polyimide tube	Diabetic macular oedema
Dexamethasone 0.7 mg	Ozurdex (Allergan)	6 months	Biodegradable with PLGA copolymer	Macular oedema following retinal vein occlusion, diabetic macular oedema and uveitis

All intravitreal drug delivery systems are sterile and preservative-free. The suspensions and solutions contain sterile water for injections.
AMD, age-related macular degeneration; EVA, ethylene vinyl acetate; PLGA, poly(lactic-*co*-glycolic acid); PVA, poly(vinyl alcohol); VEGF, vascular endothelial growth factor.

humour of patients receiving treatment with the Iluvien implant. The highest concentrations were observed at week 1 after administration and then the concentrations gradually declined, remaining stable between 12 and 36 months (Fig. 39.6). The Iluvien implant can be inserted into the vitreous humour through a 25-gauge needle; this contrasts with the other implants on the market, which need to be surgically inserted.

Ongoing developments in this area include (1) a helical device, comprising a nonferrous metal scaffold coated with a polymer–drug matrix for the delivery of triamcinolone acetonide administered by transconjunctival injection for diabetic macular oedema and (2) an implant containing genetically modified cells which produce growth factors, including ciliary neurotrophic factor. The pore size of the implant allows the growth factors to diffuse outwards into the eye and nutritional molecules to enter, but prevents the entry of antibodies or inflammatory cells that would attack the foreign genetically modified cells.

Biodegradable intraocular implants

Biodegradable systems are composed of polymers that are metabolized by enzymatic or nonenzymatic (e.g. hydrolysis) reactions in vivo into more soluble forms that can be safely eliminated by the body. Their main advantage over nonbiodegradable systems is that they do not have to be removed from the body once the drug has been exhausted. Biodegradable polymers can be made into a variety of shapes and sizes, including pellets, sheets, discs and rods, through different processes. Hot melt extrusion has been used whereby the polymer and drug are subjected to elevated temperature and pressure, causing the polymer to undergo melting while being

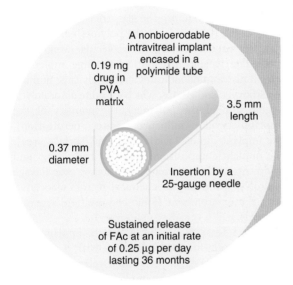

Fig. 39.5 • Nonbiodegradable intraocular implant: Iluvien® implant containing 0.19 mg fluocinolone acetonide (FAc). *PVA,* poly(vinyl alcohol). Courtesy of Alimera Sciences Ltd.

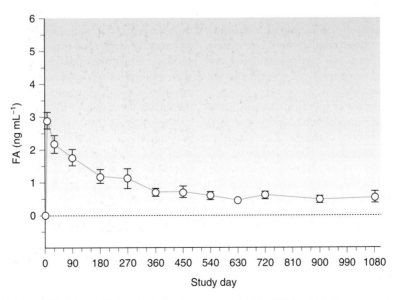

Fig. 39.6 • Nonbiodegradable intraocular implant: fluocinolone acetonide (FA) levels in human aqueous humour.

simultaneously propelled through a die to form uniform polymer strings or sheets. Solution casting has been used to produce polymer films. This involves the formation of a homogeneous solution or dispersion of the polymer and drug in a solvent which is spread onto a flat surface. The solvent is then allowed to evaporate and the dry film is peeled off.

Freeze-drying is another method employed, with the cake formed being subsequently shaped by heating and compression. Developing ocular biodegradable systems is, however, more complicated as a multitude of factors need to be taken into consideration, including device stability, as well as erosion of the polymer and surface area changes which will affect in vivo kinetics.

Ozurdex® (Allergan) is a dexamethasone (0.7 mg) bioerodible ocular implant with a 6-month duration of action. It is approved by the FDA for the treatment of macular oedema following retinal vein occlusion, diabetic macular oedema and uveitis. This implant is based on the copolymer poly(lactic-co-glycolic acid) (PLGA) which has been used for more than 30 years in biodegradable sutures for ophthalmic surgery. To prolong the duration of action of corticosteroids in the vitreous cavity, intravitreal injection of a suspension of triamcinolone acetonide (Kenalog®) has been used for many years off-label. Since the introduction of Ozurdex®, preservative-free triamcinolone acetonide intravitreal injections, Triesence® (Alcon Laboratories) and Trivaris® (Allergan), have been registered for use. One advantage of Ozurdex is that it displays a similar pharmacokinetic profile between vitrectomized and nonvitrectomized eyes, whereas suspensions of triamcinolone acetonide clear more quickly in vitrectomized eyes. Furthermore, the formulation of a corticosteroid in a PLGA matrix has the advantage that ocular pharmacokinetics can be better controlled compared with the dissolution of a free drug suspension.

PLGA is a copolymer of glycolic acid and lactic acid, which are also degradable and biocompatible. Hydrolysis of the ester bond of these PLGAs generates acid, which can catalyse the degradation of the polymer. This is known as autocatalysis. Generation of the acid during PLGA degradation can cause a local decrease in pH, which has been associated with localized inflammation. Complete polymer degradation results in conversion to the original monomers, lactic acid and/or glycolic acid, which are metabolized to carbon dioxide and water by the Krebs cycle. PLGA is a versatile copolymer; the lactide to glycolide ratio and the stereoisomeric composition (the amount of L-lactide vs the amount of DL-lactide) are the critical factors for PLGA degradation as they regulate polymer chain hydrophilicity and crystallinity. A 1:1 ratio of lactic acid to glycolic acid provides the fastest bio-degradation rate; an increase or decrease of the proportion of either monomer often prolongs the degradation time.

Several other factors can modulate the degradation behaviour of PLGA and other polyester polymer implants, including the morphology of the copolymer (extent of crystallinity), the glass transition temperature (which determines if the polymer exists in the glassy or rubbery state), the molecular weight and molecular weight distribution (a large molecular weight distribution indicates a relatively large number of carboxylic end groups, which expedite autocatalytic degradation of the polymer), the porosity of the implant (which influences water permeation), the implant dimensions (size, shape, surface area), the implant composition (acidic or basic drugs and excipients; basic compounds can catalyse ester linkage hydrolysis) and physicochemical factors associated with the environment (ionic composition, strength and pH).

Drug release from PLGA matrix implants can follow pseudo-first-order kinetics with a triphasic pattern. The first phase is burst release, whereby drug at the surface of the implant dissolves, creating a high rate of drug release in a short period. This burst release is likely to be exacerbated if the system has a large surface area (e.g. microparticles) and for systems with high drug loading and comprising hydrophilic drugs. The second phase is the diffusive phase involving drug dissolution and diffusion out of the matrix down a concentration gradient, which is governed by drug solubility in the surrounding fluid. As water penetrates into the core, the implant swells and random hydrolytic cleavage of the polymer chains can also occur. This creates pores, which increase the surface area available for drug diffusion. Eventually bulk erosion in the core of the matrix causes the polymer chains to lose their structural integrity and mass loss occurs. This third phase results in rapid release of the remaining drug load when hydrolysis of the polymers reaches a threshold. The implant shape changes and the implant finally fragments. This burst drug release is the main disadvantage of these PLGA biodegradable polymer implants over the nonbiodegradable ones. A recent study combined two PLGA polymers of different molecular weight and in different ratios to achieve a pseudo-first-order release with a minimum burst effect. The polymer with the higher molecular weight provides the scaffold

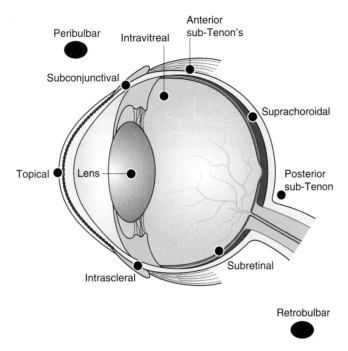

Fig. 39.7 • Different routes of ocular drug administration.

for the implant and the lower molecular weight polymer undergoes gradual hydrolysis and regulated drug dissolution and release.

In addition to PLGA, other aliphatic polyesters have also been investigated for their use in ocular implants. Poly(ε-caprolactone) is of particular interest as it has a slow rate of degradation and can therefore be used to achieve prolonged drug release for a year or more. It is a semicrystalline polymer with a melting point between 59 °C and 64 °C. It is currently used for sutures, artificial skin support and cellular regeneration. In a recent study, triamcinolone acetonide loaded poly(ε-caprolactone) implants were prepared by homogeneous mixing of the drug and polymer in solvent followed by solvent evaporation. The powder formed was then hot melt extruded into thin filaments using a syringe. The filaments formed were 150 μm in diameter and were cut into desired lengths of 2 mm. The rods were implanted into the subretinal space, and drug release was observed for at least 4 weeks. An initial phase of fast drug release followed by a pseudo-first-order release was observed.

Periocular drug delivery routes

The periocular routes have become increasingly popular for drug delivery to the posterior segment of the eye. The periocular route encompasses subconjunctival, sub-Tenon, peribulbar and retrobulbar routes of administration, which place the drug close to the sclera (Fig. 39.7). It is superior in safety compared with the systemic and intravitreal routes because of the lower systemic exposure and risks of injection respectively. With respect to efficacy, it lies at the middle to low end compared with the other (intravitreal, topical and systemic) delivery routes. It does achieve, however, better bioavailability in the outer and middle regions of the eye and is therefore currently the preferred route for treating diseases of the uveal tract, sclera and cornea. It is also well suited for the treatment of mild to moderate acute posterior segment disease and for preventative drug therapy. The dynamic physiological clearance mechanisms encountered by drugs administered by the periocular route compared with the intravitreal route are the subconjunctival–episcleral blood and lymph vessel flow and the choroidal vasculature.

The subconjunctival route bypasses the permeation barrier of the conjunctiva and cornea and can therefore achieve both anterior and posterior drug levels. It is a popular route for the administration of antibiotics (e.g. as prophylactic agents following cataract surgery). It is also used for the local delivery of cytotoxic injections of 5-fluorouracil and occasionally mitomycin C in conjunction with glaucoma filtration surgery. In glaucoma filtration surgery, a sclera flap is created, forming a new channel for outflow of aqueous humour to reduce the intraocular pressure. As is the case with all surgical procedures, a wound healing response occurs, resulting in the formation of scar tissue. Here, scar tissue forms in the subconjunctival space, which can gradually reduce and block the aqueous drainage, resulting in a rise in intraocular pressure. This makes it necessary in some cases to administer cytotoxic agents repeatedly following surgery for the prevention of scarring.

Sub-Tenon injection is between the sclera and Tenon's capsule. Tenon's capsule is a sheet of connective tissue between the eyeball (globe) and socket (orbit) which provides a smooth socket allowing free movement of the globe. This route allows prolonged contact of the drug with the sclera. The sclera has a relatively large surface area of 16.3 cm^2 and high permeation relative to the cornea. Molecules of size up to 70000 Da have been shown to readily permeate through it. The ability of a drug to permeate through the sclera is inversely proportional to the molecular size. Although no clear correlation exists between drug lipophilicity and the steady-state permeation coefficient for the sclera, drugs with higher lipophilicities exhibit stronger binding to the sclera and longer transport lag times. Injection via the sub-Tenon route is used to administer local anaesthetics, corticosteroids and anticancer agents.

Intravitreal pharmacokinetics

Drugs administered into the vitreous humour can be cleared by two routes: the anterior and posterior routes. The anterior route is where the drug diffuses into the anterior chamber and leaves with the aqueous humour, via the trabecular meshwork and Schlemm's canal. The posterior route is across the retinal surface. The physicochemical properties that influence drug clearance are the molecular weight, compound lipophilicity (measured by log P or log D) and dose number (dose/solubility at pH 7.4).

The logarithm of the molecular weight has been found to correlate positively with the vitreal half-life of molecules. This can be explained by the slow diffusion of high molecular weight compounds in the vitreous gel, as well as the observation that high molecular weight compounds are predominantly eliminated through the longer anterior pathway. Log D and log P correlate negatively with the vitreal half-life of the drug. Lipophilic compounds have a shorter half-life than hydrophilic ones. It has been proposed that hydrophilic molecules are predominantly eliminated by the anterior route. The posterior route is the main elimination pathway for lipophilic drugs and offers a large surface area and active transporter mechanisms, thus providing a faster route of elimination than the anterior route. Molecules that can permeate across the retina (e.g. steroids) will be cleared via both the retina and aqueous outflow on intravitreal injection. Soluble, low molecular weight drugs will have a vitreous half-life of several hours on intravitreal injection. In contrast, charged high molecular weight drugs such as the antibody-based therapeutic proteins display a longer vitreous half-life in the range of 3–7 days as they diffuse more slowly in the vitreous humour than do low molecular weight molecules. Moreover, therapeutic proteins cannot permeate the retina and are therefore eliminated by aqueous outflow only. Dose number also positively correlates with the vitreal half-life of molecules. If the dose administered exceeds the solubility of the molecule and is administered as a suspension, then the drug will need to undergo dissolution before it is absorbed and/or cleared, thus prolonging its half-life. This is the case for the administration of triamcinolone acetonide. Traditional in vitro models of ocular pharmacokinetics have been relatively simple, including simple test tube release. In vivo models can provide pharmacokinetic data, including in humans, for dosing with topical or systemic antibiotics before cataract surgery, when aqueous levels can be sampled. However, for therapeutic proteins and antibodies which require intravitreal injection, this cannot be done in humans, and in experimental models an antibody response to the human or humanized antibody makes longer-term pharmacokinetics impossible to determine. New in vitro models which mimic the human eye and produce a much more clinically relevant longer-term result are currently being developed (e.g. PK-Eye™).

Problems with traditional and new ocular drug delivery systems

Deposits of triamcinolone acetonide particles and crystals have been identified in the vitreous humour and retina of patients who have been treated with intravitreal triamcinolone acetonide injections. These deposits have been observed in patients months and even a couple of years after the last administration of a triamcinolone injection. It is speculated that these insoluble deposits arise from aggregation or clumping of drug particles. It could even be that a polymorphic conversion of the drug occurs in the ocular fluids, resulting in an extremely stable, and therefore insoluble, form of triamcinolone which persists in the posterior segment of the eye.

Countless numbers of intraocular implants have been shown to perform successfully in vitro during preclinical development; however, very few perform satisfactorily in vivo and make it to the clinic. One of the main reasons for this failure is nonbiocompatibility, which triggers the formation of a thick fibrotic capsule around implants, which is often referred to as a foreign body response. The fibrotic encapsulating tissue is an amalgamation of cells, fibrinogen, fibrin, collagen fibres and other proteins. It is predominantly an inflammatory response, orchestrated by interleukins and transforming growth factors synthesized by epithelial cells. This collagenous fibrotic tissue creates a diffusion barrier for drug molecules and retards biodegradation of the implant. Foreign body reactions are largely influenced by the surface properties of the implant, including contact angle, surface functional groups, water–polymer interactions, roughness, morphology, porosity and contact duration.

Repeated intravitreal injections are associated with an increased risk of scleral damage, toxic effects on the ocular tissue due to high peak drug concentrations, ocular infection, increase in intraocular pressure, incision-related subconjunctival and intravitreal haemorrhage and discomfort associated with foreign body sensation and pain in the patient.

A thorough characterization of the compatibility of excipients in the formulation with the active compound is absolutely necessary. Benzalkonium chloride is cationic and therefore is incompatible with anionic drugs. Its activity, and consequently preservative efficacy, is reduced in the presence of multivalent metal ions and anionic and nonionic surfactants. Despite these interactions of benzalkonium chloride with drugs and other excipients, it may still be necessary to use it in some cases. Examples of these include sodium cromoglicate and nedocromil sodium, which form insoluble emulsion complexes with benzalkonium chloride through ion pairing. These insoluble complexes are, however, removed by filtration during the manufacturing process.

Patient adherence and instillation of eye drops

The short half-life of drugs in the anterior chamber requires the frequent administration of eye drops. This presents problems with patient adherence to treatment regimens. Studies have shown that almost 50% of glaucoma patients were nonadherent with respect to their medication use for more than 75% of the time. Eye drops are challenging to administer and require coordination, manual dexterity and vision, necessitating clear instructions and patient counselling. Administration of eye drops requires relatively acceptable vision and the ability to open and squeeze the bottle. The self-application of drops is difficult for patients with limited vision. Elderly patients often suffer from joint disease such as arthritis and may also have poor coordination, which can result in the drop missing the eye or the tip of the bottle scratching the cornea. Most glaucoma patients are older individuals, and a study has shown that 17% of glaucoma sufferers rely on others to administer their eye drops. In addition, many patients have not had the necessary training for the appropriate method of drop administration, which often results in poor adherence. The easiest way to administer the drop efficiently is to pull the lower eyelid downwards and administer the drop into the lower ocular cul-de-sac. The patient can do this while looking in a mirror. Several devices are available for use in conjunction with different eye drop bottles to make this process easier. Dose timing and frequency have also been strongly associated with nonadherence to eye drop therapy. Patients with a three times daily regimen were more likely to experience missed doses and also had irregular timing of doses compared with patients with twice daily regimens. This illustrates the importance of designing ophthalmic preparations that provide a sustained drug release and which require less frequent dosing.

Please check your eBook at **https://studentconsult. inkling.com/** for self-assessment questions. See inside cover for registration details.

References

Daniels, J., Dart, J., Tuft, S., et al., 2001. Corneal stem cells in review. Wound Repair Regen. 9, 483–493.

Sieg, J.W., Robinson, J.R., 1975. Vehicle effects on ocular drug bioavailability.

I. Evaluation of fluoromethalone. J. Pharm. Sci. 64, 931–936.

Willoughby, C., Ponzin, D., Ferrari, S., et al., 2010. Anatomy and physiology of the human eye: effects

of mucopolysaccharidoses disease on structure and function – a review. Clin. Experiment. Ophthalmol. 38, 2–11.

Bibliography

Awwad, A., Lockwood, A., Brocchini, S., et al., 2015. The PK-Eye: a novel *in vitro* ocular flow model to optimise intraocular drug pharmacokinetics. J. Pharm. Sci. 104, 3330–3342.

Bravo-Osuna, I., Noiray, M., Briand, E., et al., 2012. Interfacial interactions between transmembrane ocular mucins and adhesive polymers and dendrimers analyzed by surface plasmon resonance. Pharm. Res. 29, 2329–2340.

Campochiaro, P.A., Nguyen, Q.D., Hafiz, G., et al., 2013. Aqueous levels of fluocinolone acetonide after administration of fluocinolone acetonide inserts or fluocinolone acetonide implants. Ophthalmology 120, 583–587.

Chang-Lin, J.-E., Burke, J.A., Peng, Q., et al., 2011. Pharmacokinetics of a sustained-release dexamethasone intravitreal implant in vitrectomized and nonvitrectomized eyes. Invest. Ophthalmol. Vis. Sci. 52, 4605–4609.

del Amo, E.M., Urtti, A., 2008. Current and future ophthalmic drug delivery systems: a shift to the posterior segment. Drug Discov. Today 13, 135–143.

Durairaj, C., Shah, J.C., Senapati, S., et al., 2009. Prediction of vitreal half-life based on drug

physicochemical properties: quantitative structure-pharmacokinetic relationships (QSPKR). Pharm. Res. 26, 1236–1260.

Durrani, A.M., Farr, S.J., Kellaway, I.W., 1995. Influence of molecular weight and formulation pH on the precorneal clearance rate of hyaluronic acid in the rabbit eye. Int. J. Pharm. 118, 243–250.

Edman, P., 1993. Biopharmaceutics of Ocular Drug Delivery. CRC Press, Boca Raton.

Furrer, P., Delie, F., Plazonnet, B., 2008. Ophthalmic drug delivery. In: Rathborne, M.J., Hadgraft, J., Roberts, M., et al. (Eds.), Modified-Release Drug Delivery Technology. Informa Healthcare, New York.

Gaudana, R., Jwala, J., Boddu, S.H., et al., 2009. Recent perspectives in ocular drug delivery. Pharm. Res. 26, 1197–1216.

German, E.J., Hurst, M.A., Wood, D., 1999. Reliability of drop size from multi-dose eye drop bottles: is it cause for concern? Eye (Lond.) 13, 93–100.

Ghate, D., Edelhauser, H., 2006. Ocular drug delivery. Expert Opin. Drug Deliv. 3, 275–287.

Guo, X., Chang, R.-K., Hussain, M.A., 2009. Ion-exchange resins as drug

delivery carriers. J. Pharm. Sci. 98, 3886–3902.

Lee, S., Hughes, P., Ross, A., et al., 2010. Biodegradable implants for sustained drug release in the eye. Pharm. Res. 27, 2043–2053.

Mannermaa, E., Vellonen, K.-S., Urtti, A., 2006. Drug transport in corneal epithelium and blood-retinal barrier: emerging role of transporters in ocular pharmacokinetics. Adv. Drug Deliv. Rev. 58, 1136–1163.

Reddy, I.K., 1995. Ocular Therapeutics and Drug Delivery. CRC Press, Boca Raton.

Robinson, J., Mlynek, G., 1995. Bioadhesive and phase-change polymers for ocular drug delivery. Adv. Drug Deliv. Rev. 16, 45–50.

Schindler, R.H., Chandler, D., Thresher, R., et al., 1982. The clearance of intravitreal triamcinolone acetonide. Am. J. Ophthalmol. 93, 415–417.

Shirasaki, Y., 2008. Molecular design for enhancement of ocular penetration. J. Pharm. Sci. 97, 2462–2496.

Weiner, A., 2008. Drug delivery systems in ophthalmic applications. In: Wax, M., Clark, A. Yorio, T. (Eds.), Ocular Therapeutics: Eye on New Discoveries. Academic Press, New York.

Topical and transdermal drug delivery

40

Adrian C. Williams

CHAPTER CONTENTS

KEY POINTS

- Human skin is a formidable barrier, but delivering drugs to and through the skin can be advantageous, for example by avoiding first-pass metabolism.
- Topical drug delivery treats a disorder at, or near, the site of application and aims to deliver the active pharmaceutical ingredient to the skin or underlying tissue.
- Transdermal drug delivery delivers the drug through the skin to the systemic circulation.
- Skin is a complex multilayered membrane but the outermost layer, the stratum corneum, provides the principal barrier to drug delivery.
- Drugs suitable for transdermal and topical drug delivery typically have a molecular weight of less than 500, $\log P_{water}^{octanol}$ between 1 and 4 and an effective daily dose of less than 10 mg.
- Drug transport through the skin is largely by passive diffusion and can be modelled by Fickian diffusion laws.
- Numerous formulation options are available for topical drug delivery, the most common of which are creams, gels, lotions, sprays and ointments.
- Patches, of varying complexities, are the most common transdermal drug delivery systems.
- Transdermal and topical drug delivery can be enhanced by some formulation strategies, such as using penetration enhancers or supersaturated systems.
- Because the nail is a hard keratinized structure, drug delivery through the nail is even more challenging than drug delivery through intact skin.

Introduction

Topical and transdermal formulations have a long history of use. More than 2000 years ago, Greek physicians used formulations containing salt, vinegar, honey and resins to treat skin lesions and ulcers. Chinese, Egyptian and Roman medical histories describe numerous remedies applied topically as pastes and poultices.

Topical and transdermal formulations are widely used for delivering drugs not only to the skin and underlying tissue but also through it for systemic action. Prescription Cost Analysis data show that in 2014 more than 40 million prescription items classified under "skin" (*British National Formulary*, BNF, Section 13) were dispensed by community pharmacy's in England, including 15.6 million emollient and barrier preparations (BNF Section 13.2) and 1.4 million preparations for eczema and psoriasis (BNF Section 13.5). In addition, many other products are dispensed for topical anaesthesia and antisepsis, for local and regional pain relief or for transdermal delivery, such as oestradiol patches. Additionally, 'over-the-counter' products are widely sought by patients, and range from emollients to nonsteroidal anti-inflammatory creams and gels, to treatments for warts, verrucae and fungal infections, such as tinea pedis (athlete's foot). Thus pharmacists often supply topical and transdermal formulations which contain a broad variety of active ingredients; indeed, it has been reported that up to 20% of all repeat prescriptions are for application to the skin. The efficacy of these products is critically dependent on biological factors, such as the integrity of the skin, on the physicochemical properties of the active ingredient and on the formulation designed to release and deliver the active ingredient into or across the skin.

Terminology

The literature occasionally contains different terminology relating to transdermal and topical drug delivery. For this chapter, it may be helpful to clarify some terms at this point.

Topical drug delivery. The application of a formulation to the skin to treat a local disorder, i.e. the active pharmaceutical ingredient acts within the skin or at the underlying tissue (e.g. a locally acting hydrocortisone cream).

Transdermal drug delivery. The application of a formulation to the skin to deliver a drug to the systemic circulation (e.g. fentanyl patches).

Locally acting. The active pharmaceutical ingredient acts directly on the skin.

Regionally acting. The active pharmaceutical ingredient acts in the area close to where the formulation is applied. This is often also described as locally

acting, but here the drug does not act directly on the skin (e.g. topically applied ibuprofen gels to treat musculoskeletal conditions).

Permeant. The chemical species that is moving into or through the tissue. This will be the active pharmaceutical ingredient, but may also be other ingredients within the formulation.

Permeation. Movement of the permeant through the membrane.

Penetration. Entry into the tissue. Penetration does not necessarily require the molecules to pass out of the tissue.

Diffusion. Movement of molecules through a domain, from high concentration to low concentration, by random molecular movement.

Diffusivity. This is a property of the permeant in the membrane and is a measure of how easily it will traverse through the tissue. It is expressed as area per unit time (usually cm^2/h or cm^2/s).

Diffusion coefficient (D). This is the diffusion coefficient of the permeant, and is sometimes a term used interchangeably with diffusivity. As with diffusivity, it is expressed as area per unit time (usually).

Permeability coefficient (k_p). Describes the speed of permeant transport, given as distance per unit time (usually centimetres per hour).

Partition coefficient (P). This is a measure of the distribution of molecules between two phases. For transdermal drug delivery studies, a partition coefficient (usually expressed as log_{10} value, hence 'log *P*') between octanol and water is often used as a guide to how well a molecule will distribute itself between water and stratum corneum lipids. In some texts, the symbol *K* is used for the partition coefficient; here, and to avoid confusion with the permeability coefficient (k_p), the symbol *P* (also widely used in the literature) has been employed.

Partitioning. The process of molecules distributing themselves between two domains. In transdermal drug delivery, partitioning is generally used to describe molecular redistribution from one domain to another, such as from an aqueous domain to a lipid domain.

Flux (J). The rate of a permeant crossing the skin (or entering the systemic circulation). It is given in units of mass/area/time (usually $\mu g/cm^2/h$).

Lag time (L). This is obtained from a permeation profile by extrapolating the steady-state flux line to the time axis. Some older texts used the symbol τ

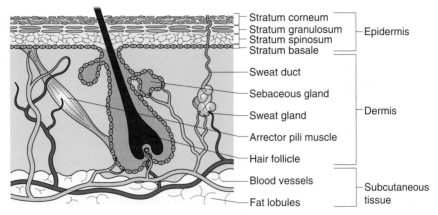

Fig. 40.1 • Cross-section through human skin showing the different skin layers and appendages.

whereas others used t_L for the lag time, but most modern texts use the letter L.

Vehicle. The base formulation in which the drug is applied to the skin.

Thermodynamic activity. Used here as a measure of the 'escaping tendency' of a molecule from its formulation. By definition, a thermodynamic activity of 1 equates to a saturated solution, or suspension, as the molecules in a saturated solution have the greatest 'escape tendency'.

Skin structure and function

Human skin is a highly complex multilayered organ designed to 'keep the outside out and the insides in'. It is the largest organ of the body, constituting approximately 10% of the body mass and covering an area of approximately 1.8 m² in a typical adult. As a self-repairing barrier, skin permits terrestrial life by preventing the ingress of microorganisms and chemicals, whilst regulating heat and water loss from the body. The body continually loses water, and transepidermal water loss is in the region of $1 \text{ mg cm}^{-2} \text{ h}^{-1}$, but its value varies with body site, external conditions (temperature, humidity) and skin integrity.

For drug delivery and therapy, the intact skin presents a formidable barrier and a difficult challenge to formulation scientists. The properties of the skin limit the range of active ingredients that can be delivered through the barrier to achieve therapeutic levels. However, skin can be relatively easily damaged through mechanical, chemical or microbiological assault and by radiation, such as sun damage. In these cases, drug delivery may be enhanced and could in fact lead to adverse reactions.

Structure of the skin

In terms of drug delivery, human skin can be considered as a series of layers which potentially provide a series of barriers to a molecule traversing the tissue (Fig. 40.1).

The subcutaneous layer

The inner subcutaneous fatty layer is typically several millimetres thick, except for some areas such as the eyelids, where it is mostly absent. This subcutaneous layer of adipose tissue provides mechanical protection against physical shock, insulates the body, provides a store of high-energy molecules and carries the principal blood vessels and nerves to the skin. The subcutaneous layer is seldom an important barrier to transdermal and topical drug delivery but may be a barrier to regionally targeted molecules such as ibuprofen for muscular pain relief.

The dermis

Overlying the fatty layer is the dermis, a layer typically 3 mm to 5 mm thick that is the major component of human skin. The dermis is composed of a network of mainly collagen and elastin in a mucopolysaccharide gel; essentially this combination provides an aqueous environment similar to a hydrogel. The dermis has several structures embedded within it, termed appendages, in particular nerve endings, pilosebaceous units (hair follicles and sebaceous glands) and eccrine and apocrine sweat glands (see later).

The dermis is metabolically active and requires extensive vasculature for this, as well as for regulation of body temperature, for wound repair, to deliver oxygen and nutrients to the tissue and to remove waste products. The blood supply reaches to approximately 0.2 mm below the skin surface, near the dermis–epidermis boundary, and so most molecules passing through the outer epidermal layer of the skin are rapidly diluted and are carried systemically by the blood. This rich blood flow keeps the dermal concentration of most transdermally delivered drugs low, which in turn provides a concentration gradient from the outside of the body into the skin; it is this concentration gradient (more accurately, it is the chemical potential gradient) that provides the driving force for drug delivery through the skin.

The epidermis

The epidermis overlies the dermis and is itself multiply layered and contains various cell types, including keratinocytes, melanocytes and Langerhans cells. Keratinocytes in the basal layer (stratum basale) undergo division and then differentiate as they migrate outwards, forming the stratum spinosum, then the stratum granulosum and finally the stratum corneum. Differentiation is complex and essentially changes the metabolically active basal cells that contain typical organelles, such as mitochondria and ribosomes, into stratum corneum that comprises anucleate flattened corneocytes packed into multiple lipid bilayers.

The stratum corneum

This outer skin layer is predominantly responsible for the barrier properties of human skin and limits drug delivery into and through the skin. The stratum corneum typically comprises only 10 to 15 cell layers and is approximately 10 μm thick when dry (although it can swell to several times this when wet). The stratum corneum is thinnest on the lips and eyelids and thickest on the load-bearing areas of the body, such as the soles of the feet and palms of the hands. The lipid bilayers in which the keratin-filled cells are embedded are uniquely different from other lipid bilayers in the body because they are comprised largely of ceramides, fatty acids, triglycerides and cholesterol/cholesterol sulphate, whilst phospholipids are largely absent. Longer-chain ceramides act as 'rivets' connecting bilayers together and corneodesmosomes interconnect corneocytes. The resulting structure can be likened to a brick wall (see Fig. 40.1) where the keratin-filled cells act as the bricks in a mortar of multiply bilayered lipids.

In normal skin it takes approximately 14 days for a daughter cell in the stratum basale to migrate and differentiate into a stratum corneum cell, and these cells are then retained in the stratum corneum for a further 2 weeks before they are shed.

The appendages

In terms of drug delivery the appendages can be viewed as shunt routes or 'shortcuts' through which molecules can pass across the stratum corneum barrier.

Specialized *apocrine glands* are found at specific body sites, such as the axillae and nipples, whereas *eccrine glands* are found over most of the body surface at a density of 100–200 glands per square centimetre. When stimulated by heat or emotional stress, eccrine glands secrete sweat, which is a dilute salt solution of around pH 5.

The largest appendages are the *hair follicles* and associated *sebaceous glands*, which secrete sebum, composed of fatty acids, waxes and triglycerides. These lubricate the skin surface and help to maintain the skin surface pH at around 5. Skin has variable numbers (and sizes) of follicles, with typically 50–100 hair follicles per cm^2 but the load-bearing areas of the soles and palms are largely devoid of these appendages.

Whilst these shunt routes offer a potential route through intact skin, the fractional area that they occupy is relatively small; for example, on the forearm, hair follicles occupy approximately 0.1% of the surface area, although on the forehead this may be as much as 13%. The ducts are seldom empty, being occupied by sweat or sebum flowing out of the body, which again inhibits drug delivery. However, formulators are able to target these structures, for example by delivering nanosized drug delivery systems, such as liposomes, to the follicles to treat acne.

The shunt routes are important for electrically enhanced transdermal drug delivery (iontophoresis) and also play a role in the early time course of passive drug delivery through the skin, where diffusion through the intact stratum corneum barrier has yet to reach the steady state.

Transport through the skin

From the previous discussion on the structure of skin, it is clear that delivery of drug molecules from a topically applied formulation into the systemic

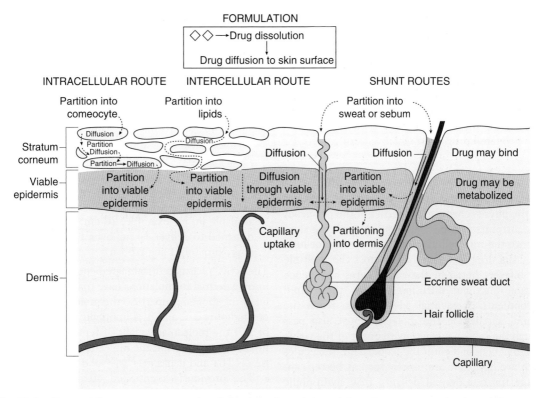

Fig. 40.2 • Some of the processes occurring during transdermal drug delivery from a suspension formulation.

circulation is complex, with numerous processes occurring and several routes of transport in operation, as illustrated in Fig. 40.2.

Initially, drug molecules must be presented to the skin surface. Consequently, if the formulation contains solid drug, then dissolution and diffusion through the formulation is the initial step in delivery. If the formulation contains dissolved drug, then as the molecules nearest to the skin surface enter the tissue, these must be replaced by other molecules diffusing within the formulation towards the skin surface. Once at the outer layer of the stratum corneum, the drug molecule has three potential routes to cross the skin. Firstly, it can pass via the shunt routes as described earlier. In this case molecules will partition into sweat or sebum before diffusing against the outflow from the glands.

More usually, the molecule encounters the intact stratum corneum 'brick wall', where transport can be via either an *intracellular* (also termed *transcellular*) route or an *intercellular* route.

For the intracellular route, the drug molecule initially partitions into a keratin-filled corneocyte, which is essentially an aqueous environment, then diffuses through the corneocyte before partitioning into the intercellular lipid domains. For transcellular transport to continue, the molecule must then diffuse through the lipoidal region before repeatedly partitioning into and diffusing through the aqueous keratin in corneocytes and then intercellular lipids.

In contrast, the intercellular route requires the molecule to partition into the lipid bilayers between the corneocytes, and then diffusion is via a tortuous route within the continuous lipid domain, i.e. following the mortar in the 'brick wall'.

Having travelled through the stratum corneum, molecules diffuse through the lower epidermal layers before being cleared by the capillaries at the epidermal–dermal junction. During transport, there is potential for the permeant to bind to skin components such as keratin, in which case it may not reach the systemic circulation but could be sloughed off. In addition, skin is metabolically active and contains esterases, peptidases and hydrolases that can reduce the bioavailability of topically applied drugs such that, for example, only approximately 70% of topically applied glyceryl trinitrate (nitroglycerine) may be bioavailable.

It is important to recognize that, whilst three different routes exist for drugs to cross the skin (intercellular, transcellular and shunt routes), for any permeant *all* three routes operate but the proportion of molecules crossing by the different routes will differ depending on the physicochemical properties of the permeant

Permeant properties affecting permeation

Considering the processes described so far, it is evident that the physicochemical properties of the permeant will control its transport into and through the skin. For both the transcellular route and the intercellular route, the drug molecule has to cross the multiple lipid bilayers between the corneocytes and hence partition into and diffusion through these lipid environments is essential. However, to reach the systemic circulation the molecule must also pass through the more aqueous environment of the viable epidermal cells and enter the blood. Thus molecules which are lipophilic are usually seen as better candidates for transdermal delivery than hydrophilic compounds, but high lipophilicity is problematic for clearance.

The molecular weight of the permeant also impacts dramatically on its transport through the skin. The skin is designed to act as a barrier to external chemicals and so prevents the entry of large molecules, such as larger peptides and proteins. Not only is molecular weight an important factor in diffusion, but molecular structure (in particular hydrogen-bonding potential) can control the extent of binding to skin constituents and hence affect bioavailability. Naturally, the drug must have some solubility in the formulation, and whilst transport through the stratum corneum is usually the rate-limiting step in transdermal delivery, low drug release from a formulation can occasionally limit drug transport. Finally, the effective dose of the drug must be relatively low to allow the application of appropriately sized patches/formulations.

These processes restrict the range of drugs that can be delivered transdermally to therapeutically useful levels, and some generic 'rules of thumb' can be used to predict whether transdermal delivery is viable for an active pharmaceutical ingredient. These include:

- Ideally the molecular weight of the drug should be less than 500, although effective delivery of larger molecules may be feasible if the therapeutic dose is very low.
- Ideally the log partition coefficient ($\log P^{\text{octanol}}_{\text{water}}$) should be in the range from 1 to 4, although more lipophilic molecules, such as fentanyl, may be effectively delivered.
- The drug should have an effective daily dose of approximately 10 mg. Typically, a 'very good' permeant will have a flux in the region of 1 mg cm^{-2} day^{-1}, and hence for a realistic patch size of 10 cm^2, a daily dose of approximately 10 mg can be delivered. Nicotine has near ideal properties for transdermal delivery and is available in, for example, 20 cm^2 patches designed to deliver 14 mg over 16 hours, i.e. approximately 1 mg cm^{-2} h^{-1}.

The active pharmaceutical ingredients currently used in transdermal formulations have many of the previously mentioned properties; the molecular weight of oestradiol is 272 and it is lipophilic, with $\log P^{\text{octanol}}_{\text{water}}$ of 2.7; the molecular weight of fentanyl is 336 and it has $\log P^{\text{octanol}}_{\text{water}}$ of 4.4; the molecular weight of nicotine is 162 and it has $\log P^{\text{octanol}}_{\text{water}}$ of 1.2.

The previously mentioned attributes relate to 'conventional' active pharmaceutical ingredients and reflect the properties of current commercially successful formulations. However, there is a growing body of evidence, supported by advances in assay sensitivity, to show that some larger biomacromolecules may passively penetrate into intact human skin. These include peptides and proteins, recombinant antigens, antisense oligonucleotides and aptamers. For these, whilst the rates of penetration into and permeation through skin may be extremely low, their high potencies may elicit pharmacological activity. Hence for both conventional and biological active ingredients, the effective dose must be considered, and whether this can be achieved by a highly potent but poorly permeating species.

Mathematics of skin permeation

With such a highly complex multilayered organ as skin, and numerous factors affecting transdermal drug delivery, it appears daunting to apply mathematical principles to describe this process. However, simple mathematical principles can be used to understand the basic principles of permeation through membranes, including skin, and these assist in designing dosage forms for transdermal and topical drug delivery.

Fick's laws of diffusion

For simple passive diffusion where molecules move by random motion from one region to another in the direction of decreasing concentration, transport can be described by Fick's first law of diffusion (see Chapter 2):

$$J = -D\delta C/\delta x$$

(40.1)

where J is the flux (the mass flow rate at which the material passes through unit area of the surface), C is the concentration of the diffusing substance, x is the space coordinate measured normal to the section and D is the diffusion coefficient of the permeant. The negative sign demonstrates that the flux of molecules is in the direction of decreasing concentration. When a topically applied drug enters the skin, it is usually assumed that the diffusion gradient is from the outer surface into the tissue, i.e. is unidirectional.

Fick's second law of diffusion gives

$$\delta C/\delta t = D\delta^2 C/\delta x^2$$

(40.2)

where t is time. Essentially, this equation shows that the rate of change of concentration with time at a point within a diffusional field is proportional to the rate of change in the concentration gradient at that point.

These laws assume that diffusion is through an isotropic material (i.e. one that has the same structural and diffusional properties in all directions); skin clearly is not isotropic, with multiple layers, different permeation routes, etc., and indeed it is remarkable that Fickian diffusion can be used to generate valuable approximations from transdermal drug delivery data.

Experimental estimation of skin penetration

Experimentally, it is usually difficult to study transdermal drug delivery in vivo, so most researchers use in vitro protocols to mimic as closely as possible the in vivo situation. Most commonly, a membrane (e.g. human epidermis) is used to separate two compartments in a diffusion cell. The drug in a vehicle (e.g. water, buffer or in a formulation) is then applied to the uppermost skin surface (stratum corneum). This is usually termed the 'donor' solution. The other compartment contains a 'receptor' (or receiver)

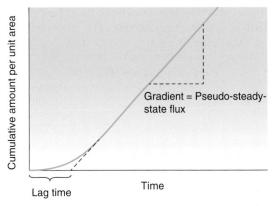

Fig. 40.3 • Typical permeation profile for an infinite-dose application to human skin, obtained from a plot of the cumulative amount per unit area of diffusant passing into the receptor compartment with time. Steady-state flux is seen when the gradient becomes linear. Extrapolation of this line to the time axis gives the lag time.

solution that is a good solvent for the drug but which will not affect the skin barrier. This receptor solution thus provides essentially sink conditions (near zero concentration) of the permeant and allows a concentration gradient to exist between the donor and the receptor phase, which in turn provides the driving force for diffusion across the membrane. If the cumulative mass of permeant that crosses the membrane is plotted as a function of time, then a typical permeation profile can be drawn, as illustrated in Fig. 40.3.

As can be seen, after sufficient time the plot approaches a straight line, and from the slope we can obtain the steady-state flux, dm/dt, and Eq. 40.2 can then be simplified to

$$dm/dt = DC_o/h$$

(40.3)

where dm/dt is the flux, usually termed J, which is the cumulative mass of permeant that passes per unit area of the membrane in time t, C_o is the concentration of the permeant in the first layer of the membrane (at the skin surface, in contact with the donor solution) and h is the membrane thickness.

It is difficult to measure C_o, the concentration of the permeant in the first layer of the skin, but the concentration of the drug in the vehicle (donor solution), termed C_v, which bathes the skin membrane is usually known or can be determined easily. Differences in drug concentration between the donor solution and the first skin layer arise because of partitioning of the molecule between the membrane and donor solution so

$$P = C_o/C_v \text{ and hence } C_o = PC_v$$

(40.4)

where P is the partition coefficient of the permeant between the membrane and the vehicle. Then, simply substituting Eq. 40.4 into Eq. 40.3 gives

$$dm/dt = \text{flux}(J) = DPC_v/h$$

(40.5)

Eq. 40.5 thus reiterates that the flux of a permeant through skin will be high for molecules with a high diffusion coefficient (e.g. generally having a relatively low molecular weight), will increase with increasing partitioning of the molecules between the donor solution and the membrane (e.g. for lipophilic molecules) and will increase with increasing effective concentration in the donor solution (which increases the chemical potential gradient), whereas the flux through thicker membranes is reduced.

Fig. 40.3 also shows that the lag time can be evaluated experimentally. The lag time (L) can be related to the diffusion coefficient by

$$L = h^2/6D$$

(40.6)

So if the thickness of the membrane (h) is known, then the diffusion coefficient can be calculated. This approach works well for relatively uniform and simple membranes such as polymers but, as seen earlier, skin is far from simple. The effective thickness of the skin membrane is very difficult to estimate; if molecules traverse it via the tortuous intercellular route, then a simple measure of membrane thickness does not reflect the diffusional pathway. Because of this difficulty, a composite parameter, the permeability coefficient k_p, is often used as

$$k_p = PD/h$$

(40.7)

Using Eq. 40.7, Eq. 40.5 can then be simplified to

$$J = k_p C_v$$

(40.8)

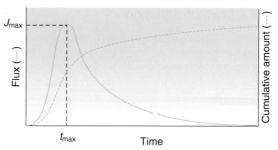

Fig. 40.4 • Typical permeation profile for a finite-dose application to human skin, showing increasing flux (amount transported per unit area with time) to a maximum value, beyond which it falls as the drug concentration in the donor solution declines, resulting in a drop in the concentration gradient across the membrane. The cumulative amount of drug passing the membrane thus reaches a plateau.

This considers transdermal delivery where the donor solution remains essentially at the same concentration during the time course of delivery, known as infinite-dose conditions, and sink conditions prevail in the receptor solution. When a finite dose is applied, such as the application of a small amount of gel or cream, then the amount of the drug in contact with the skin surface will diminish with time. In this case the permeation profile will typically resemble that in Fig. 40.4 where the flux initially increases to a maximum value (J_{max}), beyond which depletion of the drug in the donor solution means that the concentration difference across the membrane, which drives diffusion, starts to fall. Finite-dose profiles can be characterized by the time to maximum flux (t_{max}), by the maximum flux (J_{max}) and from the area under the curve.

Experimental methods for studying transdermal drug delivery

When designing and optimizing transdermal and topical formulations, most researchers begin with a review of:

- the physicochemical properties of the permeant (molecular weight, solubility, partition coefficient, pK_a, melting point, etc.);
- the desired dose;
- the skin site; and
- the skin condition (e.g. if a product is to be applied to broken skin or psoriatic plaques).

Various mathematical predictions have been constructed from databases of permeation experiments and relate potential flux to factors such as molecular weight, lipophilicity, aqueous solubility and hydrogen bond donor/acceptor groups. Such predictions can offer a useful guide to rule out molecules with unfavourable characteristics before time-consuming experimental studies are undertaken.

In vivo experiments

Clearly the gold standard evaluation of transdermal and topical delivery is to apply the formulation to patients and to assess drug levels at the target site. In practice this is difficult to achieve, except in cases where a local biological response can be recorded, for instance blanching of the skin in response to vasoconstriction, such as with corticosteroids. For systemically acting drugs as well as the majority of locally acting agents, formulation design and development uses in vitro tests.

Whilst most studies use in vitro techniques, some in vivo methods are available. One option is to determine plasma levels following transdermal delivery, allowing typical pharmacokinetic parameters such as C_{max} and the area under the curve to be determined, as for other routes of administration. However, for initial formulation development studies, such an approach is time-consuming and expensive and may not secure regulatory approval.

Microdialysis has been used where a semipermeable tube is inserted either underneath the skin or to a defined depth within the skin. The formulation is then applied to the skin surface and drug molecules permeating through the tissue are collected in the perfusate, which is continually pumped through the probe. This technique requires specialized training for probe insertion and can present analytical challenges but offers significant advantages in assaying the permeant that has travelled through the skin barrier (i.e. it can be very valuable for assessing metabolites).

An alternative in vivo approach is to measure the loss of material from the skin surface. Whilst it is relatively easy to assay the amount of drug remaining in a formulation, typically only a small fraction of the applied dose partitions into the skin, and this approach does not define the fraction of absorbed dose that is bioavailable (i.e. unbound and active at the target sites). As an extension to this approach, tape stripping of the skin in vivo is a useful technique

particularly for locally acting drugs. Essentially, a drug is applied to a defined skin area, left for a period and then that remaining at the surface is recovered. The stratum corneum is then sequentially removed using adhesive tape and the drug content in each strip is determined to build a drug profile through the tissue. As each strip can remove variable amounts of the skin, drug levels can be normalized to protein content in each strip, reflecting the amount of stratum corneum removed. More invasive is the removal of skin biopsy samples, but the depth of the biopsy can be varied such that a punch biopsy can provide data for drug levels within the stratum corneum, viable epidermis, dermis and fatty layer, whilst a simple suction blister can be used to remove only the stratum corneum and viable epidermis.

Finally, noninvasive analysis of drug content in different skin strata can be determined for locally acting drugs that elicit a pharmacological or physiological response. Typical responses may be an increase in sweat secretion, vasoconstriction, vasodilation, changes to pain thresholds or changes in blood flow that can be monitored by laser Doppler velocimetry.

In vitro diffusion cells

In principle, in vitro diffusion experiments are relatively simple, employing a two-chamber diffusion cell (examples of which are shown in Fig. 40.5) with the chambers separated by a membrane. Formulations can be applied in the donor compartment and samples can then be taken from the receptor compartment at intervals and the drug can be assayed before permeation profiles are constructed as in Figs 40.3 and 40.4.

In practice, each element of this experiment requires careful thought and consideration.

Selection of an appropriate membrane

Careful membrane selection is essential and needs to consider the purpose of the experiment. If, for example, the purpose is to compare release from a series of formulations or to assess stability on storage, then a simple artificial (e.g. polymeric) membrane may be appropriate. If the purpose is to assess the feasibility of delivering a drug through human skin, then which skin strata should be selected? Most commonly, epidermal membranes (from stratum corneum to the basal membrane) are chosen because the drug is cleared from the dermal–epidermal

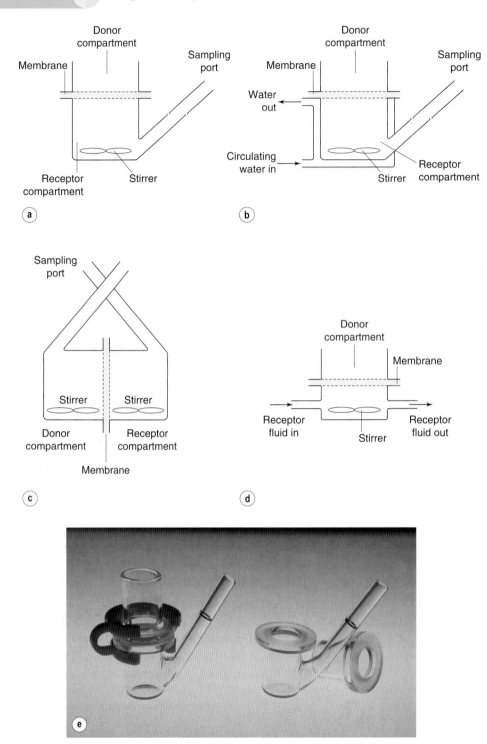

Fig. 40.5 • Examples of diffusion cells commonly used in transdermal and topical drug delivery studies.
(a) Franz-type cell. **(b)** Jacketed Franz-type cell. **(c)** Side-by-side cell. **(d)** Flow-through cell. **(e)** Photograph of assembled and disassembled Franz-type cell.

boundary in vivo. However, if metabolism is likely to be significant, then the conditions must maintain enzyme activity in the tissue. Many researchers use animal skin as a substitute for human tissue because of legal constraints in some countries or lack of availability of human samples. However, it is well established that drug diffusion through some animal skins differs significantly from that through human skin.

Receptor solution

Similar detailed consideration should be given to the choice of the receptor solution. This should be a good solvent for the permeant so that the drug does not violate sink conditions, usually taken to be less than 10% of the saturated concentration in the receptor phase at any time. The receptor fluid should not affect the integrity of the skin barrier, so the use of solvents such as ethanol at high concentrations should be avoided because they too could diffuse 'backwards' from the receptor solution into, for example, an aqueous solvent in the donor phase; not only could this damage the stratum corneum barrier but it could also alter the partitioning of the drug into the skin and/or affect drug release from the donor solution. A surfactant could be added but may also damage the integrity of the stratum corneum barrier. It is important to stir the receptor compartment to ensure there is appropriate mixing and to clear drug molecules from directly beneath the membrane.

Temperature

Diffusion is temperature dependent, so most researchers submerge their diffusion cells in a water bath or circulate water in a jacket around the cell. Typically, the aim is to maintain the skin surface temperature near 32 °C, and typically submerging the diffusion cells in a water bath at approximately 37 °C achieves this.

Other factors

Amongst other factors to consider is the amount of a formulation to apply to the membrane surface, selected to mimic in vivo use and so, for example, this may be either a finite dose for a locally acting cream or an infinite dose to mimic a 7-day patch application. The choice of vehicle from which a drug may be applied must also be considered; aqueous solutions are often used but buffering may be required

depending on ionization, or if solubility is low, then the solution may rapidly deplete as the drug crosses the membrane. As seen earlier, there is a lag time until pseudo-steady-state permeation is reached, so the experimental duration needs consideration. Steady-state flux is reached after approximately 2.7 times the lag time, so for a permeant with a long lag time (e.g. 10 h), the steady state is not reached until 27 hours, and then data need to be collected to evaluate the flux. Maintaining skin integrity for extended periods is thus necessary and may require the use of an antimicrobial agent. An appropriately accurate and sensitive method needs to be established to determine the amount of permeant in the receptor solution at defined time points, and analytical interference by skin components that leach from the tissue during the experiment must be avoided. The number of replicate experiments must be considered. If an artificial and well-characterized membrane is used, then reproducibility should be high, but when a biological membrane is selected, then natural variability usually dictates that a minimum of six replicates are needed, and best practice is to use more than one skin donor. The use of tissue from more than one source reduces potential errors arising from a damaged piece of skin, but the integrity of the membrane before the start of the permeation study should be verified.

Transdermal and topical preparations

A remarkably broad range of formulation options are available for topical and transdermal preparations, ranging from simple solutions and lotions, through commonly used creams (aqueous or oily), ointments, gels and patches to the less common aerosols and foams. When one is selecting and designing formulations, account must be taken of the physicochemical properties of the drug, such as its solubility and pK_a, as described earlier. Equally, the formulation must be stable, the drug and excipients must be compatible and drug must be released from the dosage form following application. Importantly, the formulation should be cosmetically acceptable, with a good skin feel, texture and fragrance. Ultimately, the product will be applied to human skin in vivo and so the pathophysiology of the tissue must be understood; the application of an alcoholic gel formulation to broken skin is unlikely to enhance patient adherence. Taking these factors into account, topical and transdermal formulations aim to deliver the drug to therapeutically active levels at the target site (either local or systemic). It has been estimated that for topical products such as creams and gels, typically only between 1% and 3% of the applied dose is bioavailable, whereas bioavailability from patches is typically 30% to 70% for drugs such as buprenorphine and fentanyl.

Formulation principles

Based on the consideration of skin structure and the mathematical theory explained earlier, some general principles are useful to guide the selection of a dosage form and excipients.

Principle 1: select a suitable drug molecule. As described already, large hydrophilic molecules are relatively poor candidates for delivery across intact skin. Ideally a drug should be moderately lipophilic ($\log P_{\text{water}}^{\text{octanol}} = 1–4$), of relatively low molecular weight (< 500) and effective at low dosages (< 10 mg day^{-1}) in vivo for transdermal delivery.

Principle 2: release of the drug. The formulation should be designed to ensure appropriate release of the drug; this may be rapid release for a locally acting drug, or sustained and slow release for a 7-day patch. If the formulation contains a moderately lipophilic drug in a lipophilic oily base, the drug is less likely to partition out of the formulation and enter the lipophilic skin barrier than if it is applied from a more aqueous base. Essentially, the vehicle should allow some solubility of the drug but should not retain the drug by being a very good solvent (see *principle 3*).

Principle 3: use thermodynamics. The driving force for diffusion is the chemical potential gradient across the membrane; often the term 'concentration gradient' is used but 'chemical potential gradient' is more accurate for complex membranes such as skin. Eq. 40.5 describes how transdermal flux is dependent on drug concentration, but in thermodynamic terms it can be shown that

$$\mathrm{d}m/\mathrm{d}t = \text{flux} = J = aD/\gamma h$$

$$(40.9)$$

where a is the thermodynamic activity of the drug in the donor formulation and γ is the effective activity coefficient in the skin barrier. Thus to achieve the highest flux, the drug in the vehicle should be at its maximum thermodynamic activity. By definition, a pure solid is at maximum thermodynamic activity and is given a value of 1. Thus a saturated solution which is in equilibrium with excess solid is also at maximum thermodynamic activity, and so the greatest flux can be achieved by using the drug at its solubility limit in the formulation.

For formulation development, thermodynamic activity can be considered as the 'escape tendency' of the drug from its vehicle; if a drug is at saturation, there is a strong thermodynamic drive for it to leave the formulation, and hence it will enter the skin and permeate, whereas if it is present at a small fraction of its solubility limit, then the drive to escape is low. In practice, a saturated system tends to be relatively unstable, and so a formulation with the drug near saturation is a useful compromise.

This principle has important formulation and clinical implications. Firstly, for example, a finely divided suspension formulation with saturated drug will provide the maximum flux. If further drug is then added to the formulation, the concentration of the drug in the system increases, but the thermodynamic active or 'effective' concentration (i.e. that of dissolved drug molecules) remains the same and so the flux remains the same. Conversely, if a suspension is diluted but the drug remains saturated, then the flux remains the same until dilution reduces the amount of the drug to below its saturation point, and for a subsaturated solution formulation, dilution will reduce the flux. Secondly, Eq. 40.9 illustrates that different formulations of any particular drug at the same thermodynamic activity will give the same flux (as long as the excipients do not modify any properties of skin). Thus by appropriate formulation it is possible to reduce the drug loading in a topical product whilst maintaining the same thermodynamic activity and hence delivering the same amount of drug; Dioderm® contains 0.1% hydrocortisone but is clinically equivalent to 1% Hydrocortisone Cream BP as the drug is at the same thermodynamic activity in both formulations despite differences in concentration.

Principle 4: alcohol can help. Many effective topical and transdermal products contain low molecular weight alcohols or other volatile ingredients. Alcohols themselves can partition into skin and can provide a transient 'reservoir' into which the drug can then partition. In addition, they may improve the diffusion coefficient of the drug in the stratum corneum. Further, whilst alcohols are typically 'good' solvents for most drugs, they evaporate from the

Table 40.1 A general classification scheme for topical and transdermal vehicles

System	Single phase	Two phase	Multiphase
Liquid	Nonpolar solutions (oils), e.g. liquid paraffin Polar solutions (lotions), e.g. aqueous solutions or volatile solvents	Dilute emulsions (o/w or w/o), found in some lotions Suspensions, e.g. some paints, often aqueous. Can deposit powder on skin	Dilute multiple emulsions (o/w/o or w/o/w) Suspensions
Semisolid	Ointments with dissolved medicaments Gels with dissolved medicaments	Emulsions (o/w or w/o) with dispersed medicaments. Includes creams Thick suspensions, e.g. pastes	Multiple emulsions with dispersed medicaments, e.g. cream pastes
Solid	Powders	Some transdermal patches	Some complex transdermal patches

o/w, oil in water; *o/w/o*, oil in water in oil; *w/o*, water in oil; *w/o/w*, water in oil in water.

skin surface when rubbed on it in a finite-dose application. Taking ibuprofen hydroalcoholic gels as an example, the drug has a low aqueous solubility of less than 1 mg mL^{-1}, whereas it is readily soluble in ethanol and in a 20:80 w/w ethanol–water system its solubility is nearly 10 mg mL^{-1}. If a gel containing 5 mg/mL is rubbed into the skin, initially the drug is dissolved in the formulation, but as the ethanol evaporates the formulation becomes steadily more aqueous until only water remains. At this point the ibuprofen is in excess of its solubility limit, so has maximum thermodynamic activity, resulting in increased delivery into the tissue (as described in *principle 3*).

Principle 5: occlusion increases delivery of most drugs. Occlusion (covering the skin with an impermeable barrier) hydrates the skin by blocking transepidermal water loss to the external environment. The water content of the stratum corneum can rise to up to 400% of the tissue's dry weight, and this increased hydration increases transdermal and topical delivery of most drugs. Some preparations require occlusion to deliver the required dose to therapeutic levels, such as EMLA cream (which contains lidocaine and prilocaine), which should be applied as a thick layer under an occlusive dressing. Alternatively, occlusion can be inadvertent, such as when applying hydrocortisone ointments or creams to treat nappy rash when tightly fitting waterproof pants can occlude the area.

Formulation options

Considering the broad range of topical and transdermal formulations, ranging from simple solutions to complex multiple emulsions, these systems can be classified in numerous ways. Most commonly, formulations are described in terms of their physical properties but, as seen earlier, these can be complex and changing, for example where a simple gel can lose solvent by evaporation to deposit a solid film on the skin surface. However, the scheme in Table 40.1 may be helpful when one is considering formulation options.

Generally, semisolid formulations are selected for increased residence on the skin, transdermal patches are selected for extended drug delivery through the skin and liquid formulations are selected for a rapid short-term input of permeant into the skin. In both the clinical domain and the cosmetic domain, skin type can affect the choice of formulation base, in that generally:

- For normal to oily skin types, gels are often preferred.
- For normal to dry skin types, lotions are often preferred.
- For dry skin, creams are often preferred.

In addition to skin type, the skin site to be treated can affect the selection of the vehicle, thus:

- For hairy areas, lotions, gels or sprays are usually preferable.
- For intertriginous areas (sites where skin may touch or rub such as the axilla of the arm), creams or lotions are usually preferred.

However, it is mainly clinical rationale as to which formulation type is selected for topical therapy. Dependent on the lesion type:

- For a wet, vesicular or weeping lesion, a 'wet' (usually aqueous-based) formulation is generally preferred, such as a cream, lotion or gel.

- For a dry, thickened scaly lesion, a 'dry' (usually fatty) formulation is preferred, such as an ointment or paste.

A simplified decision tree to illustrate how the clinical condition can influence the choice of formulation options and formulation design is given in Fig. 40.6.

Beyond the broad nature of the vehicle, specific formulation components may be required, dependent on the physicochemical properties of the drug (e.g. the drug pK_a and the need for a buffer, the stability of the drug and the need for an antioxidant), clinical considerations (e.g. intact or broken skin, duration of use) and to improve patient adherence. Commonly used components in topical and transdermal formulations include solvents, solubilizing agents, oils, thickening agents and pH modifiers, examples of which are given in Table 40.2. It should be borne in mind that the active pharmaceutical ingredient itself may have properties that can affect the formulation (e.g. chlorhexidine is surface active and forms micelles).

Common formulation types

Whilst Table 40.1 provides a broad classification scheme of topical and transdermal formulations, the most common systems are described in further detail in the following sections.

Liquid formulations

Liquid formulations for external application may be simple single-phase solutions using (1) an aqueous base, (2) a solvent, (3) a miscible cosolvent system (e.g. ethanol and water) or (4) an oil. Examples of single-phase solutions include soaks and paints, such as chlorhexidine solutions for skin disinfection, or lotions of malathion used to treat head lice. Liquid preparations generally have a short residence time on the skin, usually resulting in low drug delivery into the tissue and so tend to be used to treat surface conditions (e.g. disinfection). More viscous preparations can be generated to increase the residence time, for example by addition of glycerol, propylene glycol or polyethylene glycol, as employed in anti-infective ear drops. When simple solutions are applied to the skin, the solvent evaporates and can cool and soothe the skin, an effect that is more pronounced from alcoholic vehicles. The evaporation of a solvent can increase the thermodynamic activity of the drug in the evaporating vehicle, which can influence delivery as described in *principle 4*.

Low-viscosity 'thin' oil-in-water (o/w) or water-in-oil (w/o) emulsions and suspensions are two-phase liquid systems, whereas more complex o/w/o or w/o/w 'thin' emulsions are multiphase liquids. The distinction between a 'thin' emulsion that is a liquid formulation and a semisolid cream system is rather arbitrary, but emulsions are most widely used in creams as described later.

As with single-phase solutions, solvent can evaporate from an aqueous or solvent-based suspension when applied to intact skin, so providing a cooling sensation, although clearly alcoholic-based formulations should not be applied to broken skin. As the solvent evaporates, drug delivery can be enhanced because of increased thermodynamic activity of the permeant in the vehicle (as described earlier). Suspensions such as calamine lotion deposit drug powder on the skin, which increases the residence time of the active ingredient on the skin surface. If a suspension is used to deliver drug into the skin, then clearly any deposited solid on the skin surface must undergo dissolution to liberate molecules before their penetration into and permeation through the skin.

Table 40.2 Examples of some typical components found in topical and transdermal formulations

Component	Examples
Solvent	Water, propylene glycol, ethanol, isopropyl alcohol
Solubilizing agent	Surfactants: anionic (e.g. sodium lauryl sulfate); cationic (e.g. cetrimide); nonionic (e.g. nonoxynol series); zwitterionic (e.g. dodecyl betaine)
Oils	Mineral oil, liquid or soft paraffins, silicone oils
Thickening agents	Gums, celluloses (e.g. hydroxypropyl methylcellulose), carbomers, polyvinylpyrrolidone
Preservatives	Antioxidants (e.g. ascorbic acid, butylated hydroxyanisole); antimicrobial agents (e.g. parabens); chelating agents (e.g. ethylenediaminetetraacetic acid)
pH modifiers	Monoethanolamine, lactic acid

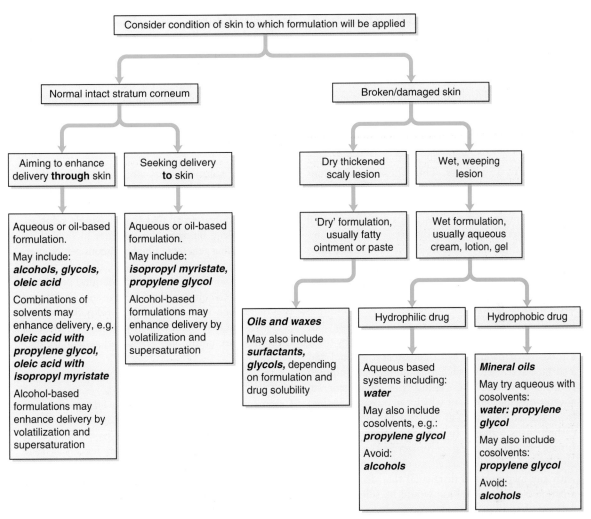

Fig. 40.6 • Simplified decision tree to assist selection of topical and transdermal formulations considering the state of the skin barrier.

Semisolid formulations

The vast majority of topically applied formulations are semisolids which offer a longer residence time on the skin than liquid formulations. There are numerous options available to the formulator, and semisolids are generally well accepted by patients. Single-phase semisolid systems include ointments and gels in which the active ingredient is dissolved, whereas ointments or gels containing drug powder (usually microcrystalline) are two-phase semisolids.

Ointments

Ointments are fatty preparations that are usually occlusive and are generally used on dry lesions.

Unmedicated ointments are used as emollients to soothe, smooth and hydrate dry skin conditions.

Commonly, ointments are produced from soft, hard and liquid paraffins (or similar excipients) to generate a hydrocarbon base. The bases are highly occlusive and so prevent transepidermal water loss; this, in turn, causes the skin to hydrate and hence their usefulness in dry skin disorders. Hydration of the stratum corneum also tends to increase transdermal drug flux and so, coupled with the long residence time of these formulations on the skin, can provide prolonged drug delivery. However, thick greasy ointments can be difficult to spread, particularly on damaged or broken skin, where they are commonly applied, and patients often find these formulations are messy to use.

Absorption bases

Absorption bases contain an emulsifying agent that allows the formulation to soak up water or aqueous secretions while remaining semisolid. Generally, they tend to contain a hydrocarbon, such as a paraffin, together with a miscible substance that is polar, such as sorbitan monooleate. This combined system can absorb up to 15% water. Thus these formulations provide some occlusion of the skin, hydrate the stratum corneum and can be left in contact with the tissue for prolonged periods. Because of potential allergic reactions and sensitization, wool fats and lanolin, traditionally used in absorption bases, have largely been replaced with purified lanolin or other excipients.

Emulsifying bases

Emulsifying bases are similar to absorption bases but can form an oil-in-water system, for example by using a mixture of paraffins with cetostearyl alcohol and a surface-active agent such as sodium lauryl sulphate (SLS) or cetrimide. These emulsifying agents generate a water-miscible ointment which can be easily washed from the skin surface, in contrast to greasy hydrocarbon bases. Anionic (e.g. SLS), cationic (e.g. cetrimide) or nonionic (e.g. cetomacrogol) emulsifying ointments can be formulated, to ensure compatibility with any incorporated drug such that, for example, a cationic or nonionic base would be selected for a cationic drug.

Water-soluble bases

Water-soluble bases are usually prepared from a mixture of water-soluble polyethylene glycols of varying molecular weights that can be blended to generate bases which soften or melt when applied to the skin surface. Water-soluble bases mix easily with skin secretions, spread well on the skin surface and can be readily washed off. However, they lose their semisolid consistency if approximately 10% water is taken into the ointment and they may be incompatible with several classes of compounds, including phenols and penicillin.

Gels

Gels are typically formed from a liquid phase that has been thickened with other components and may contain dissolved (single-phase) or dispersed (two-phase) drug in a semisolid system. The liquid in the gel essentially forms a continuous phase, with the thickening agent enhancing viscosity by providing the porous scaffold of the gel. As with solutions or suspensions, the liquid phase may be aqueous, alcoholic, miscible blends or a nonpolar solvent, and as described earlier, the solvent may evaporate, cooling the skin and increasing drug flux by enhancing the thermodynamic activity of the drug in the evaporating vehicle.

As gelled solutions, the continuous phase allows unhindered diffusion of dissolved molecules throughout the polymer scaffold and hence drug release should be equivalent to that from a simple solution, unless the drug binds to the polymer in the gel, or polymer loading generates a highly viscous gel. Numerous thickening agents are available, the selection of which is influenced by the physicochemical properties of the drug and compatibility with the solvent. Natural polymers such as carrageenans or refined/synthetic polymers such as hydroxypropyl methylcellulose or carbomers are commonly employed gelling agents.

Creams

Creams are the most common semisolid topical dosage form and are typically two-phase emulsions, either water-in-oil or oil-in-water (see Chapter 27). Oily creams (w/o semisolid emulsions) are less greasy than ointments, are easier to apply and can usually be simply washed off the skin surface, and hence are well accepted by patients. However, whilst water-in-oil creams can deposit a protective oily layer on the surface, they tend to be less occlusive than an ointment and so may not be as beneficial in dry skin conditions. Oil-in-water creams (also called 'washable' or 'vanishing' creams) with a continuous aqueous phase are often rubbed into skin and again can provide a cooling sensation. The processes occurring during delivery from a cream are complex and difficult to define; the cream changes as it is applied, rubbed in, the continuous phase evaporates (or if oily may penetrate the skin) and the emulsion breaks down. In addition, the active ingredient may be loaded in one phase but will partition between the continuous and dispersed phases or may become incorporated into micelles as the formulation collapses. Furthermore, creams usually include an antimicrobial preservative, which may have surface activity (as indeed may the medicament), a buffer, an antioxidant and fragrance materials. Considering this complexity, formulation for optimal release and delivery tends to be on an individual drug basis, taking the principles described earlier in this chapter into account.

Multiphase semisolid formulations

Multiphase semisolid formulations tend to use emulsions or multiple emulsions (oil-in-water-in-oil or water-in-oil-in-water emulsions) with the drug dispersed in a paste. Pastes (either two-phase or multiphase) are stiff preparations containing up to 50% solids, commonly in a fatty base. These preparations are useful for treatment of localized skin sites, as with Lassar's paste (zinc and salicylic acid) or dithranol paste. Pastes also lay down a thick impermeable film that can be cut and used in sub-blocks. Pastes tend to be less greasy than ointments as the powder may absorb some of the more mobile hydrocarbons from the fatty base.

Solid formulations

Powders. Powders are seldom applied directly to the skin for drug delivery because drug dissolution is necessary before permeation; without the use of a solvent, skin exudates are generally unable to dissolve the applied powder

Topical sprays. Topical sprays are available to deposit powders on the skin surface but generally incorporate a volatile solvent that dissolves some drug before evaporation (with consequent elevated thermodynamic activity).

Dusting powders. Dusting powders are used to reduce friction between skin surfaces, and antiseptic dusting powders are available, but do not aim to deliver drug into the skin.

Patches. These are solid dosage forms that range in complexity from simple two-phase systems to multiphase systems. Most simply, *in situ film-forming systems* are available that allow a patient to deposit a thin film on a diseased site for local therapy; these formulations contain polymers such as polyvinylpyrrolidone, poly(vinyl alcohol) or silicones in either an aqueous or a more volatile solvent system that can be applied by spraying onto the affected area. As the solvent evaporates, the film forms. It can be unmedicated for use as a wound dressing, or may contain an antimicrobial agent to prevent infection. In addition, for example, antifungal agents such as terbinafine can be incorporated to treat athlete's foot, with the spray offering simple dosing between toes.

In situ films remain at the affected site for extended periods and then can be designed to be easily washed off or to resist water. However, as described earlier, the drug must be in solution for absorption, and hence some residual solvent or nonvolatile solvent (such as an oil) may be incorporated into the formulation.

Prefabricated transdermal patches are an alternative delivery device. These merit more detailed consideration.

Transdermal delivery patches

Prefabricated transdermal patches are designed to deliver a constant and controlled dosage over extended periods for systemic therapy. They offer advantages over conventional oral dosage forms in that:

- Drug administration through the skin avoids the pH variations seen with gastrointestinal transit.
- The drug reaches the systemic circulation whilst avoiding first-pass hepatic metabolism (though the skin has some metabolic activity).
- Patches can be removed easily and quickly in cases where adverse drug reactions occur.
- Patient adherence is high.

However, because of the barrier properties of the skin, relatively few drug molecules have the appropriate physicochemical and therapeutic properties for sustained transdermal delivery.

Scopolamine patches for motion sickness were first approved by the United States Food and Drug Administration in 1979. Since then, buprenorphine, clonidine, oestradiol (alone or in combination with norethindrone, norelgestromin or levonorgestrel), fentanyl, lidocaine, nicotine, nitroglycerine, oxybutynin and testosterone patches have been commercialized. More recently, a methylphenidate transdermal patch has been developed to treat attention deficit–hyperactivity disorder, the monoamine oxidase inhibitor selegiline has been developed in patch form for management of Parkinson's disease and major depression, a rivastigmine patch is available for patients with Alzheimer's disease a rotigotine patch is commercialized for restless leg syndrome in Parkinson's disease and a granisetron patch is manufactured to treat nausea and vomiting following chemotherapy. It is notable that recent patches have aimed to meet a clinical need, for example to assist with adherence amongst patients with Alzheimer's disease rather than simply selecting a candidate drug based on its physiochemical properties.

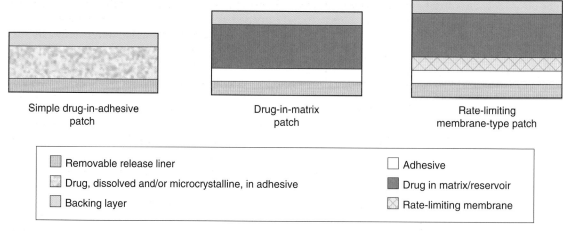

Simple drug-in-adhesive
patch

Drug-in-matrix
patch

Rate-limiting
membrane-type patch

Removable release liner

Drug, dissolved and/or microcrystalline, in adhesive

Backing layer

Adhesive

Drug in matrix/reservoir

Rate-limiting membrane

Fig. 40.7 • Common patch designs.

Designs of transdermal patches

Numerous patch designs exist; some are illustrated in Fig. 40.7. The simplest systems contain the drug in an adhesive, with more complexity introduced in matrix-type patches and reservoir systems.

Drug-in-adhesive patches are the simplest and most common patch design and are widely used to deliver nicotine, oestradiol and nitroglycerine. These patches are formed by dissolving or dispersing drug within an adhesive, which is then coated onto a backing layer before a release liner is applied. Drug-in-adhesive patches tend to be thinner and more flexible than other systems, and so may aid patient comfort and hence adherence. As with all patches, different daily dosages can easily be delivered by increasing the surface area of the patch; a 20 cm^2 patch will deliver double the daily dose of an equivalent 10 cm^2 patch. Drug-in-adhesive patches can be formulated to deliver their drug for up to 1 day (e.g. nicotine) to up to 7 days (e.g. granisetron, oestradiol and buprenorphine). Patches are typically intended to deliver the drug at a constant rate for the duration of use – i.e. zero order. In practice, for a patch where the drug is dissolved in an adhesive, the concentration of the drug in the patch drops as molecules leave and enter the skin. The reduction in the concentration gradient from the patch to the skin thus slows delivery, although initially to only a marginal extent. To mitigate against this, the adhesive layer can be made thicker and hence contains a greater drug loading so release of a given amount of drug is less marked, or additives can be added to the adhesive to increase drug solubility, in addition to excipients that may aid delivery or enhance drug stability.

Drug can be included in a separate matrix which can be formulated to increase the drug content in the system or to control drug release. The drug-containing matrix or reservoir is often a polymeric mixture, e.g. polyvinylpyrrolidone and poly(vinyl acetate), potentially with the addition of a plasticizer such as glycerol; hydrogels may also be used as the matrix. Clearly drug released from the matrix will partition into and diffuse through the underlying adhesive layer.

More complex rate-limiting membrane systems typically contain the drug in a reservoir but with release controlled through a semipermeable membrane. The reservoir may be liquid or more usually a gel, and can be designed to contain high drug loadings. More complex patch configurations based on the previously mentioned systems are feasible (e.g. multilayered drug-in-adhesive systems with a rate-limiting membrane separating two adhesive layers of different drug loadings).

For all the configurations mentioned, patches have a removable release liner, an adhesive and a backing layer, whilst the more complex patches may also have a matrix and/or a rate-controlling membrane.

Removable release liner. A release liner temporarily covers the adhesive and is the layer that is removed to allow the patch to be applied to the skin. Liners are often made from polymers such as poly(ethylene–vinyl acetate), or aluminium foil, dependent on the nature of the adhesive that it covers. The liner must easily peel away from the adhesive but must be bonded firmly enough to prevent accidental removal. Liners are usually occlusive to prevent the loss of volatile patch components, such as ethanol, before use.

Adhesive. The adhesive is a crucial component of all transdermal delivery patches, and pressure-sensitive adhesives, such as acrylates, polyisobutylene or poly-siloxane adhesives, are usually used. Clearly the adhesive must:

- stick to the skin for the patch's lifetime;
- be nonirritating and nonallergenic as it may be in place for up to 7 days;
- be compatible with the drug and other excipients; and
- allow the patch to be removed painlessly without leaving adhesive residue on the skin surface.

During formulation development, considerable effort is spent testing patch wear but the presence of a drug (or other excipients) in the adhesive can affect its properties; hence data from placebo tack, wearability and irritation studies may not truly reflect in vivo use of a medicated system.

Backing layer. Numerous materials can be used for patch backing layers, depending on the patch design, size and length of intended use. For relatively short-use small patches, an occlusive backing layer may be selected, and this will hydrate the underlying skin, which can increase delivery. Example materials include polyethylene or polyester films. For larger patches for longer-term use, backing layers that permit some vapour transmission are typically preferred, such as poly(vinyl chloride) films. In addition, the backing layer should allow multidirectional stretch and be pliable to allow the patch to move as the skin moves.

Matrix/reservoir. A drug matrix or reservoir is usually prepared by dissolving the drug and polymers in a common solvent before adding in other excipients such as plasticizers. The viscosity of the matrix can be modified by the amounts of polymers incorporated, or by cross-linking polymers in the matrix, and can consequently be used to control diffusion of the active ingredient through the matrix to the adhesive and then on to the skin surface. Reservoirs may use a viscous liquid, such as a silicone or a cosolvent system, occasionally with ethanol, into which the drug is dissolved and dispersed. In these cases, drug diffusion within the reservoir towards the skin surface is unhindered.

Rate-limiting membrane. Transdermal patches were originally designed so that the patch itself controlled the rate of delivery of the active ingredient to the skin surface, and so the patch would control drug flux. In practice, it is usually the stratum corneum barrier that limits the rate of drug input into the skin and hence provides the rate-limiting barrier.

However, semipermeable membranes are used to separate reservoirs from the underlying adhesive and can also be found separating multiple drug-in-adhesive layers. Various polymers can be used for such membranes, including poly(ethylene-vinyl acetate), with or without plasticizers. As with other patch components, the rate-limiting membrane must be compatible with the drug, nontoxic, stable and pliable.

Whilst this discussion has focused on transdermal delivery, patches are also used for local effects within the skin. Patches or plasters containing local anaesthetics such as lidocaine can be used before venipuncture or superficial dermatological procedures. An interesting development is a combination patch containing lidocaine and tetracaine and which includes a heating component; once the patch is removed from the pouch and is exposed to oxygen in the air, the patch begins to heat such that when it is applied to skin it may warm the tissue by approximately 5 °C. This warming enhances the delivery of the local anaesthetic. Additionally, transdermal drug delivery is not exclusively from patches; cutaneous solutions of oestradiol or testosterone delivered by metered or pump sprays for systemic action are commercially available.

Other formulations

Beyond the dosage forms described in Table 40.1, less common formulations are available for topical and transdermal drug delivery. These include those discussed in the following paragraphs.

Liposomes. These are spherical, bilayered structures, typically between 100 nm and 200 nm in diameter, that can be produced from phospholipids, and which are able to encapsulate a range of different drugs either in their aqueous core or within the lipid bilayer. The properties of the liposome are determined by their size, the number of bilayers and the component lipids; often materials such as dipalmitoyl phosphatidylcholine are used but cholesterol can be added to produce rigid vesicles, whereas addition of ethanol or surfactants can produce flexible liposomes.

Whilst liposomal formulations have been developed for parenteral administration of anticancer and antifungal agents, they are not widely used for topical and transdermal drug delivery, and are predominantly found in cosmetics and long-acting sunscreen formulations. The liposomes promote delivery of the active sunscreen into the stratum corneum and reduce wash off, as seen with surface-deposited agents. Liposomes as drug delivery vehicles are discussed further in Chapter 44.

Foams. Foams have been used to deliver various drugs to and through the skin (e.g. ibuprofen and betamethasone). Foams allow relatively easy dosing to the target site and, as dynamic systems where solvent evaporates and foams collapse on the skin surface, delivery can be enhanced beyond that seen for simple creams.

Solids or particulates. Solids can be used to target drug delivery to the hair follicles, as can liposomal products. The pore diameter of the follicle ranges from approximately 70 µm on the forehead to approximately 170 µm on the calf. Hair shaft diameters range from approximately 15 µm on the forehead to approximately 42 µm on the calf; these are usually filled with sebum. The volume of the follicular reservoir on the forehead has been estimated to be 0.19 mm³, into which microparticulates can be deposited to provide prolonged activity of materials such as benzoyl peroxide (which is highly insoluble), to manage acne vulgaris.

Enhancement of transdermal and topical drug delivery

The range of drugs that can be delivered transdermally to therapeutic levels is restricted because of the effective barrier provided by skin, in particular the stratum corneum, as discussed earlier. The factors influencing the magnitude of the permeant flux are summarized in Eq. 40.10, which is a reformulation of Eq. 40.5:

$$flux = \frac{\substack{\text{diffusion coefficient} \times \text{partition coefficient} \\ \times \text{concentration in the donor solution}}}{\text{membrane thickness}}$$

$$(40.10)$$

Consequently, various approaches have been used to modify the above parameters by manipulating the barrier properties of the skin (increasing diffusivity), the nature of the permeant or barrier (to increase partitioning) or to increase the concentration (or, more accurately, the thermodynamic activity) of the drug in its formulation. Manipulating skin thickness is difficult, although the application site can be selected as one where the stratum corneum is relatively thin, such as the scrotum, which is used to deliver testosterone. Additionally, external forces can be used effectively to circumvent the stratum corneum barrier.

Formulation manipulation

For a given drug in a defined formulation, maximum flux is achieved when the active ingredient is present at saturation (i.e. when C_o, in, for example, Eqn 40.3, is at its maximum). However, it is feasible to generate supersaturated systems where the drug is present in excess of its solubility limit. This occurs when, for example, a hydroalcoholic gel containing a poorly water-soluble compound is applied to the skin. As the alcohol (good solvent) evaporates, the drug can exceed its solubility limit in the remaining aqueous phase and so becomes supersaturated. Supersaturated states are inherently unstable, and the excess drug will tend to crystallize rapidly. However, if the formulation is viscous or antinucleating polymers are included, then drug crystallization can be inhibited for some time, in which case the drug remains in a supersaturated state and provides a greater flux than can be obtained from a saturated solution. In practice, many topically applied formulations are dynamic (gels, foams, creams, etc.), and patches can contain volatile ingredients that may either evaporate or partition into skin, resulting in transient supersaturated states.

Supersaturation can also be achieved from cosolvents as shown in Fig. 40.8; if solvent A is a 'poor' solvent for the permeant and solvent B is miscible with solvent A but is a 'good' solvent, then the solubility of the drug in mixtures of solvents A and B would follow the solid curve. If a solution of drug in solvent B is then diluted with the poor solvent A, the solubility of the drug follows the dotted line and generates supersaturated systems. With time, the drug will crystallize from this supersaturated state to equilibrate with the saturation curve, but crystallization can be

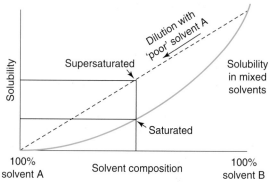

Fig. 40.8 • A method to generate supersaturated systems from mixed solvents.

inhibited by addition of some polymers, and this provides a transient increase in drug solubility beyond saturation, hence increasing drug flux.

Other formulation strategies can provide optimal transdermal delivery using the principles described earlier. For example, formulations should ensure optimal drug release and encourage partitioning of the drug into the stratum corneum by using a vehicle in which the drug is only moderately soluble. The active drug should have appropriate physicochemical properties, perhaps achieved by using a prodrug containing a lipophilic moiety which will enhance partitioning of the drug into the lipophilic stratum corneum; ester-linked fatty acids can serve this purpose, with the link then cleaved by esterases within the skin, liberating the active ingredient. Control of the pH in the formulation of ionizable drugs is important because ions permeate less well than neutral compounds, or ionic charges can be neutralized by employing ion pairs.

Skin modification

Numerous chemicals, collectively termed *penetration enhancers*, interact with stratum corneum components to increase transdermal drug delivery. These enhancers can act by disrupting the highly organized lipid bilayer packing, through interacting with intercellular proteins, by increasing partitioning of the drug into the membrane or by a combination of these mechanisms. Ideally, penetration enhancers will be pharmacologically inert, will modify the skin barrier in a reversible manner and will be nontoxic, nonirritating, compatible with drugs and excipients and acceptable to patients (good skin 'feel', odourless, colourless, etc.).

The safest and most widely used penetration enhancer is water, and the transdermal flux of most drugs is greater through hydrated skin than through dry tissue. Thus occlusion is an effective means of increasing the flux of most drugs. Ethanol and other low molecular weight alcohols that are often incorporated into topically applied formulations can also act as penetration enhancers (in addition to their other functions such as solvents). Ethanol can disrupt the intercellular lipid packing and so increase diffusivity through the stratum corneum but additionally can diffuse into the membrane and act as a solvent within the stratum corneum, into which drug can more easily undergo partition.

Small aprotic solvents, such as dimethyl sulfoxide, can interact with lipid bilayer head groups in the stratum corneum to disrupt their close packing and facilitate drug diffusion, whereas fatty acids (e.g. oleic acid) insert themselves along the stratum corneum lipid chains to disrupt packing. Bespoke penetration enhancers, such as Azone (1-dodecylazacyclopetan-2-one), have been designed to possess a bulky polar head group and a lipid chain. The molecule can insert itself within the lipid lamellae to disrupt the endogenous stratum corneum lipid bilayers at the head and chain regions. Other commonly used excipients with enhancer activities include terpenes (fragrance agent) and surfactants. Potential mechanisms by which penetration enhancers can disrupt the lipid bilayers of the stratum corneum are illustrated in Fig. 40.9.

External forces

Researchers have developed more active methods for increasing transdermal drug delivery, of which one approach is *iontophoresis*. An electrical potential gradient across the skin can be generated with relatively low current densities with an anode (positive electrode) and cathode (negative electrode) placed on the skin surface. A charged drug is placed under the electrode of the same polarity (e.g. anion placed under the cathode) such that when the current flows the anion is repelled by the cathode. As it attempts to migrate towards the anode, it enters the skin. In addition, as applied or endogenous ions migrate from one electrode to another (such as Na^+ migrating towards the cathode), water and neutral molecules can be transported along with the ions into the skin.

Devices designed to deliver liquids or particles into the skin using *needleless injectors* have also been developed. Using compressed gasses to propel particles or liquid at very high speed, the technology seeks to avoid needle phobia and deliver large molecules (e.g. vaccines) up to therapeutic levels in defined skin strata. As the particles are relatively small, when fired into the skin, they do not trigger the pain receptors, although the propellant gas may cause some sensation. Numerous factors can influence the efficiency of delivery from needleless injectors, ranging from the density of the particles to the thickness of the stratum corneum and the need to hold the device vertical to the skin surface to ensure that the particles penetrate the skin to the correct depth.

Alternatively, the stratum corneum barrier can be removed or reduced to enhance transdermal delivery. Thus *dermabrasion* or *laser ablation* has been used to facilitate transdermal drug delivery.

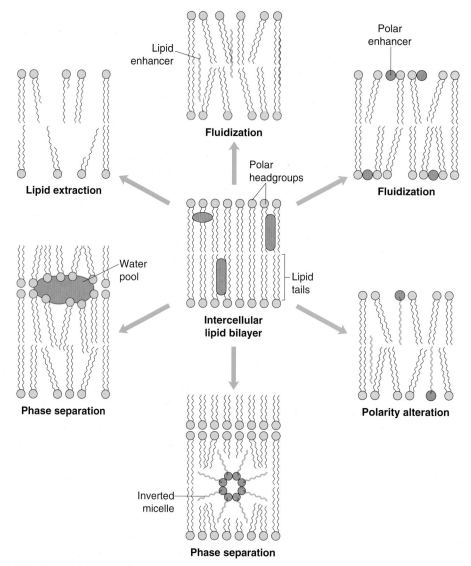

Fig. 40.9 • Potential mechanisms of action for penetration enhancers acting on the intercellular lipids of the stratum corneum.

Microneedles offer significant potential benefits for delivering both small and large molecules into and through the skin. These devices can be manufactured from a range of substances (stainless steel, silicon, plastic, dissolvable sugars and polymers), can be hollow or solid and can range in length from tens to hundreds of micrometres. Hundreds of microneedles can be produced in an array that is less than 1 cm² in area. The intact microneedles will puncture the stratum corneum before application of a dosage form, or the drug formulation can be delivered through hollow needles. Alternatively, the active drug can be administered within a dissolving microneedle array.

As microneedles are small and can be designed to puncture only the depth of the stratum corneum, pain receptors deeper in the skin are not stimulated, so delivery is painless. This technology is currently attracting considerable interest, particularly for delivery of vaccines, and it also offers potential for the sampling of body fluids, or disease biomarkers, for diagnosis or monitoring purposes.

Nail delivery

Despite significant anatomical differences, many of the principles described in this chapter apply to formulation design for drug delivery through nails (often termed *transungual delivery*). Human finger-nails consist of three main structures: the outermost nail plate, the underlying nail bed and the nail matrix (Fig. 40.10).

The *nail matrix*, sometimes called the nail root, contains onychocytes, a specialized version of the keratinocytes found in the stratum corneum. Much of the matrix is hidden, but the lunula, ('the moon') is the white crescent-shaped part of the matrix most clearly visible on the thumbs.

The *nail bed* is an extension of the matrix and contains blood vessels and nerves.

Overlying the nail bed is the protective *nail plate*, a translucent keratinized layer that appears pink because of the blood vessels in the nail bed. The nail plate comprises approximately 80–90 layers of keratinized cells and is 0.25 mm to 0.6 mm thick on the fingers, whereas toenails are up to 1.3 mm thick. Nail plate growth is variable, but is typically approximately 1 mm per month for toenails, whereas fingernails grow at approximately 3 mm per month. The nail plate has three distinct layers, an outer dorsal layer that is dense and hard, an intermediate layer that is fibrous with fibres aligned perpendicular to the direction of growth and a thin ventral layer that connects to the nail bed. The nail plate contains between 0.1% and 1% lipids, less than that found in the skin stratum corneum, and so is a more hydrophilic barrier than skin.

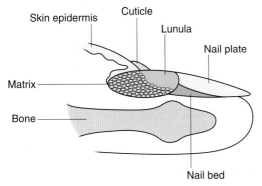

Fig. 40.10 • Simplified diagram of a cross-section through a human nail.

Diseases of the nail plate, bed and matrix are often unsightly and cause patient distress. Onycho-mycosis is a common fungal infection of the nail bed or plate and affects up to 5% of the population and can cause discolouration, thickening or crumbling of the nail plate. Nail psoriasis occurs in most patients with skin psoriasis and can cause pitting of the nail, discolouration and roughening or crumbling of the nail plate.

These and other nail disorders are difficult to treat, because the nail plate provides a formidable barrier to drug delivery, and so enhancement strategies have been sought. One approach is to simply abrade the nail, thinning it by filing or laser ablation or etching with acid, or creating pores with use of needles or microneedles. Alternatively, penetration enhancers can be included in formulations.

As with the stratum corneum, formulations can use a vehicle which encourages drug partitioning into the nail plate, with ethanol and other solvents also commonly used to increase delivery from supersaturated states and by interacting with the nail. Other chemical enhancers seek to disrupt the keratin fibres that are the main constituent of nail plates. As the nail plate has relatively low lipid levels, enhancers that work in skin by disrupting the lipid bilayers are ineffective in the nail. Thus kera-tolytic agents such as urea, oxidizing agents such as hydrogen peroxide and reducing agents such as thio-glycolic acid which disrupt disulfide bonds in keratins have been used to increase drug diffusivity through nail plates.

Antifungal agents such as terbinafine or itraconazole are commonly used orally to treat serious onycho-mycosis of the nail but can result in adverse reactions because orally delivered drugs must enter the systemic circulation before diffusing out to the infected area. Local delivery is thus clinically attractive but is limited by the nail plate barrier. Antifungal formulations of amorolfine, salicylic acid (which is keratolytic) and tioconazole for application to the nail are available as lacquers, paints and solutions. The excipients in the formulations include boric and tannic acids to etch the nail surface and alcoholic vehicles to enhance flux, and, notably, the patient information usually includes the instruction to file the nail before applica-tion. At present, topical formulations to manage nail psoriasis are not widely available.

Please check your eBook at **https://studentconsult. inkling.com/** for self-assessment questions. See inside cover for registration details.

Bibliography

Benson, H.A.E., Watkinson, A.C. (Eds.), 2012. Topical and Transdermal Drug Delivery: Principles and Practice. John Wiley & Sons, Hoboken.

Donnelly, R.F., Singh, T.R.R. (Eds.), 2015. Novel Delivery Systems for Transdermal and Intradermal Drug Delivery. John Wiley & Sons, Hoboken.

Dragicevic, N., Maibach, H.I. (Eds.), 2015. Percutaneous Penetration Enhancers: Chemical Methods in Penetration Enhancement. Springer-Verlag, Berlin.

Ita, K., 2015. Transdermal delivery of drugs with microneedles - potential and challenges. Pharmaceutics 7, 90–105.

Pastore, M.N., Kalia, Y.N., Horstmann, M., et al., 2015. Transdermal patches: history, development and pharmacology. Br. J. Pharmacol. 172, 2179–2209.

Patzelt, A., Lademann, J., 2013. Drug delivery to hair follicles. Expert Opinion in Drug Delivery 10, 787–797.

Shrama, A.M., Uetrecht, J., 2014. Bioactivation of drugs in the skin: relationship to cutaneous adverse drug reactions. Drug Metab. Rev. 46, 1–18.

Touitou, E., Barry, B.W. (Eds.), 2007. Enhancement in Drug Delivery. Taylor and Francis, London.

Williams, A.C., 2003. Transdermal and Topical Drug Delivery. Pharmaceutical Press, London.

Rectal and vaginal drug delivery

41

Kalliopi Dodou

CHAPTER CONTENTS

KEY POINTS

- The rectal and vaginal routes can be used for local as well as systemic drug delivery.
- These routes are transmucosal routes of drug delivery and thus offer the advantage of bypassing first-pass (presystemic) metabolism.
- The anogenital nature of the rectum and vagina can affect patient compliance especially for chronic ailments because of privacy and cultural aspects.
- Rectal dosage forms are used for local effect such as for the treatment of constipation and haemorrhoids.
- The rectal route can be ideal for systemic drug delivery for certain diseases and patient groups, such as unconscious, preoperative and postoperative patients, and paediatric and geriatric groups.
- Drug absorbed by the inferior and middle rectal veins bypasses the liver and enters the systemic circulation directly.
- The vaginal route is mainly used for contraception, labour induction, treatment of vaginal infections and management of local menopausal symptoms; however, this route can be exploited for diverse therapeutic applications, including vaccine delivery, chemotherapy and prophylaxis against sexually transmitted diseases.

Introduction

Rectal and vaginal dosage forms are useful when localized treatment of either the rectum or the vagina is required. For systemic drug delivery the oral route is most commonly used. Alternatives such as parenteral, transdermal and transmucosal (buccal, nasal, pulmonary, ocular, rectal and vaginal) routes are gaining popularity because they can bypass first-pass (presystemic) metabolism, avoid gastrointestinal side effects and often result in improved patient compliance.

The reasons for choosing the rectal route for systemic drug administration include the following:

- The patient is unable to swallow. This is the case with unconscious patients because of total anaesthesia, preoperatively and postoperatively, patients with gastrointestinal tract problems, such as nausea and vomiting, very young or very old patients, and patients with certain central nervous system (CNS) disorders, such as epilepsy.
- The drug under consideration is not well suited for oral administration; for example, drugs causing gastrointestinal side effects, unpalatable drugs and those which are susceptible to extensive first-pass metabolism and enzymatic degradation in the gastrointestinal tract.

Systemic drug delivery via the vaginal route is relatively unexploited because of its sex-specific nature. However, vaginal dosage forms have great potential in prophylaxis against sexually transmitted diseases (STDs) and in vaccine delivery and chemotherapy (e.g. for cervical neoplasias).

Common limitations and challenges for both the rectal route and the vaginal route include the following:

- Dosage form retention can be problematic because of peristalsis of the rectal wall and because of vaginal fluid clearance. This limitation can be overcome by the formulation of mucoadhesive dosage forms which can attach to the rectal and vaginal mucosal membranes.
- Patient compliance. The anogenital location, sexual and defecation associations, and potential for mucosal irritation render the rectal and vaginal routes less popular among patients who require medication for systemic minor ailments and chronic systemic drug delivery.

Consequently, the rectum and vagina are relatively uncommon routes of drug administration, and this is reflected in the market size of rectal and vaginal formulations being less than 1% of the total pharmaceutical market.

Rectal drug delivery

Anatomy and physiology of the rectum

The rectum is the caudal part of the gastrointestinal tract forming the final 15 to 20 cm of the large intestine. It can be subdivided into the ampulla and the anal canal, the former being approximately 80% of the organ. Rectal dosage forms are inserted into the body through the anus, which is a circular muscle at the end of the anal canal separating the rectum from the outside environment. The rectal wall surface is relatively flat, without villi and with only three major folds, called rectal valves. The rectal wall is composed of epithelium, which is one cell-layer thick and contains cylindrical cells and goblet cells that secrete mucus (rectal fluids).

Part of the rectal wall and the rectum's arterial supply and venous drainage are shown in Fig. 41.1. Arterial blood supply to the rectum is mainly via the superior rectal artery, assisted by the middle and inferior rectal arteries and the median sacral artery. Knowledge of the venous drainage from the rectum is important for the understanding of drug absorption. As can be seen from Fig. 41.1, there are three separate veins. The lower (or inferior) and middle rectal haemorrhoidal veins drain into the inferior vena cava, and hence this blood goes directly to the heart and into the systemic circulation. In contrast, the upper (or superior) rectal haemorrhoidal vein drains into the portal vein, and hence this blood passes through the liver before reaching the heart. Therefore drug absorbed by the middle and lower part of the rectum will enter the systemic circulation directly and avoid first-pass metabolism in the liver. The temperature within the rectum is approximately 37°C and the total volume of rectal fluids (rectal mucus) is estimated at approximately 3 mL, spread over a total surface area of approximately 300 cm^2. The pH of the rectal fluids is approximately 7.2–7.5 (i.e. close to neutral) in adults and alkaline (7.2–12.1) in most children. Rectal fluids have little buffering capacity; therefore, the drug can change the pH of the fluids. Under normal circumstances the rectum is empty. When faecal matter arrives from the colon, it provokes

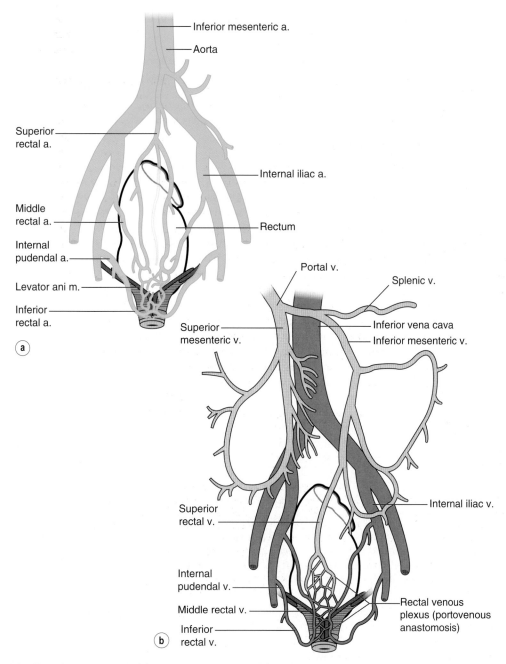

Fig. 41.1 • Rectal arterial supply **(a)** and venous drainage **(b)** of the human rectum. *a.*, artery; *m.*, muscle; *v.*, vein. From http://accessmedicine.mhmedical.com/data/books/mort/mort_c012f005.gif.

a defecation reflex, i.e. waves of contractions run over the wall of the colon in a caudal direction. This faecal matter is either expelled or transported back into the colon, depending on voluntary control of the anal sphincter. Insertion of the dosage form into the rectum can also stimulate peristalsis of the rectal wall and thus lead to dosage form expulsion.

Absorption of drugs from the rectum

Insertion of the dosage form into the rectum results in a chain of events leading to the absorption of the drug by passive diffusion. Dissolved drug molecules in the dosage form will diffuse out towards the rectal membrane. Suspended drugs will first need to leave the vehicle (if it is water immiscible) under the influence of either gravity or motility movements and then begin to dissolve in the rectal fluid. Dissolved drug molecules will diffuse through the rectal mucus and then into and through the epithelium of the rectal wall membrane. The process of absorption is by passive diffusion, as it is throughout the whole of the gastrointestinal tract for almost all drugs. Active transport processes, as found in the upper regions of the gastrointestinal tract, have not been shown to be present in the rectal area.

The rate and extent of drug absorption in the rectum is lower than for the oral route, mainly due to the smaller surface area for absorption compared with that of the small intestine. However, the rectum's rich blood supply enables uptake of drug molecules into the systemic circulation.

The bioavailability of drugs following rectal administration can be unpredictable as it depends on the positioning of the dosage form in the rectal cavity and on interpatient variations in rectal content. By keeping the dosage form in the lower part of the rectum, drug absorption is via the middle or inferior rectal veins, avoiding first-pass metabolism, and thus leading to increased drug bioavailability compared with the oral route. The bioavailability of drugs absorbed from the upper part of the rectum may be low because the drugs will potentially be metabolized by the liver during its 'first pass' and only a proportion of the drug molecules will enter the general circulation intact.

Box 41.1 provides a summary of the physiological factors that are important in rectal absorption. As indicated already, the quantity of rectal fluid available for drug dissolution is very small (~3 mL), spread

Box 41.1

Physiological factors affecting absorption from the rectum

Volume of rectal fluid
Composition, viscosity and thickness of rectal mucus lining
Contents in the rectum
Motility of the rectal wall

---

in a layer approximately 100 μm thick over the organ. Thus the dissolution of poorly water-soluble drugs is often the rate-limiting step in the absorption process.

Only under nonphysiological circumstances is this volume enlarged, e.g. by osmotic attraction by water-soluble vehicles or during diarrhoea. The properties of the rectal fluid, such as composition, viscosity and surface tension, are essentially unknown and have to be estimated from data available for other parts of the gastrointestinal tract.

The rectal wall exerts pressure on a dosage form present in the lumen, because of the motility of the rectal muscles. This pressure from the rectal wall stimulates spreading of the dosage form and thus promotes absorption.

In contrast with the upper part of the gastrointestinal tract, no esterase or peptidase activity is present in the rectum, resulting in a much greater stability of peptide-like drugs (thus allowing attempts at their delivery by this route). Administration of these compounds via the rectal route has been satisfactory when absorption enhancers such as polyoxyethylene lauryl alcohol ether are included in the formulation. One major drawback of absorption enhancers is the irritation they can cause to the rectal mucosa in the long term.

Rectal dosage forms

The advantages and limitations of rectal drug administration are outlined in Box 41.2. As explained already, the rectal route can be used for either local or systemic effect.

Local action

Rectal dosage forms for local effect are intended for the management of pain, itching and excoriation

Box 41.2

Advantages and limitations of rectal administration

Advantages

1. Safe route of drug administration allowing removal of the dosage form and discontinuation of drug delivery.
2. Suitable for drugs liable to degrade in the gastrointestinal tract or with high hepatic first-pass elimination.
3. Immediate-release and modified-release formulations can be administered.
4. Suitable route of drug delivery for elderly and terminally ill patients.
5. Suitable route of drug delivery for paediatric and neonatal patients who are unwilling or unable to swallow oral dosage forms.
6. Useful for preoperative and postoperative or unconscious patients and those who are nauseous or vomiting.

Limitations

1. Patient acceptability and adherence is poor, especially for long-term therapy.
2. Incorrect positioning of the dosage form can increase first-pass metabolism.
3. Dosage form retention can be problematic.
4. Dosage form expulsion is possible because of the motility of the rectal wall.

---

associated with haemorrhoids (painful, swollen veins in the lower part of the rectum and anus), anal fissures, colitis and proctitis (inflammation of the anus and rectum). Locally active drugs include astringents, antiseptics, local anaesthetics, vasoconstrictors, anti-inflammatory compounds and soothing and protective agents. Rectal stimulant laxatives are used for the local treatment of constipation or as colonic cleansers to empty the rectum of its contents before surgery. Topical antifungal preparations are applied in the anal area for the treatment of perianal thrush.

Systemic action

All drugs which are orally administered can be given by this route. Antiasthmatic, anti-inflammatory and analgesic drugs are widely administered by the rectal route. Rectal preparations may also be used for *diagnostic* purposes.

Several categories of rectal preparations for drug delivery are available: suppositories, rectal capsules,

rectal tablets, rectal solutions (including enemas), suspensions and emulsions, powders and tablets for rectal solutions and suspensions, semisolids (ointments and creams), rectal foams and rectal tampons. Of these, suppositories are the most commonly used. For the treatment of *local* conditions, such as haemorrhoids, fatty ointments are used widely. For the *systemic* administration of drugs, suppositories, tablets, capsules and microenemas are employed.

Rectal preparations may contain a number of excipients, such as viscosity enhancers, buffers, solubilizing agents, antimicrobial agents and antioxidants. Addition of absorption enhancers, such as surfactants, can be used to promote bioavailability. As in all drug delivery, the safety of excipients should be evaluated carefully. Local irritation with rectal formulations is frequently reported.

Suppositories

Suppositories are single-dose preparations with a shape, volume and consistency appropriate for rectal administration. Rectal suppositories are formulated in different sizes (usually 1 g to 4 g). They contain one or more active substances dispersed or dissolved in a suitable base that may be soluble or dispersible in water or may melt at body temperature. Excipients such as diluents, adsorbents, surface-active agents, lubricants, antimicrobial preservatives and colouring agents may be added if necessary. Their drug content varies widely from less than 0.1% up to almost 40%.

Vehicle (suppository base)

An ideal suppository vehicle or base should melt, dissolve or disperse at body temperature. It should be nonirritating, chemically and physically stable during storage and after preparation into a suppository, and pharmacologically inert. It should be compatible with a range of drugs and allow optimal drug release. It should also be convenient to handle during manufacturing and storage. Leakage following administration is likely to be less problematic if the viscosity of the vehicle after melting or dispersion is high.

There are two main classes of vehicles in use: glyceride-type lipophilic (fatty) bases and water-soluble bases. As a rule, hydrophilic drugs tend to be formulated in fatty bases and lipophilic drugs tend to be formulated in water-soluble bases so that they retain a high thermodynamic activity and thus high drug release from the dosage form.

Oleaginous (fatty) base

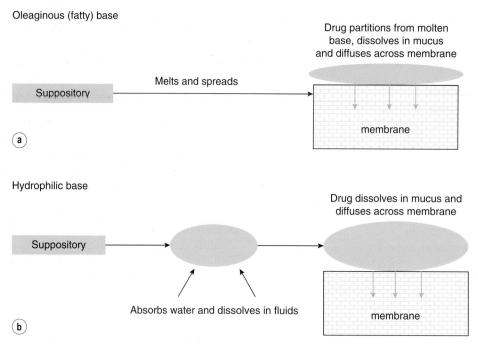

Fig. 41.2 • Process of drug release from a suppository in which the drug is in suspension. **(a)** Oleaginous (fatty) base. **(b)** Hydrophilic base.

Fatty vehicles

After insertion in the rectum, a fatty suppository vehicle will melt and spread along the rectal membrane (Fig. 41.2). The *melting point* of the base should therefore be slightly lower than body temperature, bearing in mind that the body temperature might be as low as 36°C at night. The fatty vehicle should have a sufficiently narrow melting temperature range so that it solidifies promptly after preparation, thus preventing agglomeration or sedimentation of suspended drug particles, especially of particles with high density.

The cooling rate of the molten vehicle should be slow to allow homogeneous solidification. A rapid cooling rate may result in fissures in the suppository, which is a quality defect. The melting temperature range should also be sufficiently wide to permit easy preparation, which may take a considerable length of time on an industrial scale. During solidification, a suppository should exhibit sufficient volume contraction to permit removal from the mould or plastic former.

The *viscosity* of the molten base plays an important role from both a technological/manufacturing viewpoint and a biopharmaceutical one:

• During manufacture, the viscosity of the molten base will affect flow into the moulds and also the sedimentation rate of suspended drug particles. A highly viscous molten base will flow with difficulty into the moulds but will also hinder particle sedimentation in the case of suspension suppositories.

• During and after melting in the rectal cavity, the suppository mass will spread over the rectal membrane. The rate of spreading is determined partly by the viscosity of the suppository at body temperature. The rate of transportation of suspended drug particles from within the base to the interface with the rectal fluid for them to be released and absorbed will also be affected by the viscosity of the molten base. The diffusion coefficient of dissolved drug particles in the molten base and hence the drug release rate will be affected by the viscosity of the molten base.

The fatty vehicles in use nowadays are almost exclusively semisynthetic or fully synthetic. Theobroma oil (also known as cocoa butter) – once a very commonly used base – is no longer used because of its many disadvantages, such as its polymorphic behaviour, insufficient contraction during cooling, low softening point, chemical instability, poor water-absorptive power and high cost.

Several substitutes have been developed, and are becoming increasingly popular because they have few or none of the problems mentioned previously. Commercial examples include Cotmar®, Dehydag®, Fattibase®, Suppocire® and Witepsol®. These are mixtures of natural or synthetic vegetable oils, consisting of mixed triglycerides of C_{12}–C_{18} saturated fatty acids, waxes and fatty alcohols. By using a combination of components, they can be designed to have a range of melting temperatures, e.g. different grades of Witepsol have melting points ranging from 29°C to 44°C.

The 'hydroxyl number' of these bases is a parameter that refers directly to the amount of monoglycerides and diglycerides present in the fatty base. A high number means that the base is less hydrophobic and has the ability to absorb water. This could also lead to the formation of a w/o emulsion in the rectum, which could slow down the drug release rate. Moisture absorption during storage can cause physicochemical instability because of an increased rate of decomposition of drugs that are easily hydrolysed. On the other hand, a high hydroxyl number may indicate high capacity for hydrogen bonding between the drug and the suppository base, which can enhance drug stability by preventing drug crystallization in the vehicle. An advantage of a high hydroxyl number is the wider melting and solidifying ranges, which permit easier manufacture.

Water-soluble vehicles

After insertion in the rectum, a water-soluble suppository vehicle will dissolve in the available volume of rectal fluid (Fig. 41.2). Hydrophilic water-soluble (or miscible) vehicles include the classic glycerinated gelatin (glycerol–gelatin) and polyethylene glycol (PEG; macrogol) bases. Glycerol–gelatin bases are mostly used for laxative purposes and in vaginal dosage forms (see later).

Because the volume of rectal fluid is small, complete dissolution of the water-soluble vehicle may be difficult. Additional water may be attracted from the rectal mucosa because of the osmotic effect of the dissolving vehicle. Depletion of rectal fluid will result in drying and irritation of the rectal membrane, which is an unpleasant sensation for the patient. Incorporation of water in the formulation, as in the case of glycerinated gelatin bases, will enable complete dissolution of the base in the rectal cavity and will also prevent irritation of the rectal membrane.

Glycerinated gelatin is a mixture of glycerol, gelatin and water. The mixture forms a translucent, gelatinous mixture which is dispersible in the rectum. The ratio of glycerol, gelatin and water can affect the dispersion time and thus the rate of drug release. A higher proportion of gelatin in the mixture makes it more rigid and longer acting. An example composition of the base is 20 g gelatin, 70 g glycerol and 10 g purified water.

Because of the water content of the formulation, preservatives such as methyl and/or propyl parabens are usually added to prevent bacterial growth. Formulations made with gelatin and glycerol tend to be hygroscopic and require well-closed containers for packaging.

PEGs are versatile polymers with regard to their properties and applications. They consist of mixtures of PEGs of different molecular weight. Their melting point depends on their molecular weight; low molecular weight PEGs (PEG 300 and PEG 600) are liquid at room temperature, those with a molecular weight of approximately 1000 are semisolid and those with a molecular weight above 3000 are waxy solids with melting points above 50°C. PEGs with different molecular weights can be combined to produce a range of melting points and the desired properties, as shown in Table 41.1.

Considering that the melting point of solid PEG vehicles is well above body temperature, they need to mix with the rectal fluid and dissolve. PEGs of all molecular weights are miscible with water and rectal fluids, thereby releasing drug by dispersion; the available volume of rectal fluid is too small for true dissolution. Because of their high melting points compared with those of fatty suppository vehicles, PEG-based formulations are especially suited for use in tropical climates.

However, the following disadvantages have to be considered. PEG-based formulations are hygroscopic and therefore attract water after administration,

Table 41.1 Compositions of polyethylene glycol bases with different physical characteristics

	Base A	Base B
PEG 1000	95%	75%
PEG 4000	5%	25%
Properties	Low melting temperature, immediate drug release	Higher melting temperature, sustained drug release

PEG, polyethylene glycol.

resulting in an uncomfortable sensation for the patient. Incorporation of at least 20% water in the base and moistening before insertion can help to reduce this problem. A considerable number of incompatibilities with various drugs, such as ibuprofen, indometacin and aspirin, have been reported on storage. PEGs are efficient cosolvents for drugs; because of their solubilizing effect, drugs may tend to remain in the base, and drug release may be slow.

PEG bases can develop peroxides when exposed to light and high temperatures; therefore, airtight packaging is recommended, and the formulation should be monitored for peroxides during stability studies when ascertaining shelf-life.

Formulation considerations for suppositories

Properties of the suppository base

A summary of the suppository base properties which should be considered at the preformulation stage is given in Box 41.3.

For fatty bases, the melting temperature and rheological properties of the molten base should be recorded at the preformulation stage, bearing in mind that drugs miscible with the base will suppress its melting point and therefore lower its viscosity. If the viscosity at 37 °C is low, hardening agents can be added to the formulation, such as beeswax and cetyl esters wax. Suppositories for adults are usually 2 mL in volume and those for children are usually 1 mL. It has been suggested that a larger volume may provoke a reaction of the rectal wall, thus helping to spread the molten base over a larger area. For example, an increase in volume of paracetamol suppositories results in faster and more complete absorption of the drug.

For water-soluble suppository bases, water solubility should be established and also the extent of dissolution in the volume of rectal fluid.

Drug properties

Box 41.4 lists the factors relating to the drug substance that should be considered at the preformulation stage.

Drug solubility in rectal fluid. The drug solubility in the rectal fluid determines the maximum attainable concentration and thus the driving force for absorption. The small volume of rectal fluid will prevent the dissolution of highly lipophilic compounds. For example, tamoxifen, which is a Biopharmaceutics Classification System class II drug (low aqueous solubility and high permeability; see Chapter 21), shows a marked decrease of its oral availability to 10% after rectal dosing, because of incomplete dissolution in the rectum. This example illustrates that switching from oral to rectal dosing should be done with caution. Wetting agents or surfactants can be added to the formulation to increase the solubility of lipophilic drugs in the rectal fluid.

Drug permeation ability in the rectal membrane. The drug should have some lipid solubility so that it can diffuse through the rectal membrane. Because of the limited rectal surface area for absorption, the rectum is thought to be unsuitable for the delivery of very hydrophilic compounds, as they will not diffuse across the lipophilic rectal membrane at therapeutically effective concentrations. For the delivery of Biopharmaceutics Classification System class III drugs (high solubility/low permeability), absorption (permeation) enhancers can be added to the formulation.

Drug solubility in the vehicle. The drug solubility in the vehicle determines the type of product, i.e.

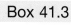

Box 41.3

Formulation parameters of suppository bases

Melting point
Rheological properties of molten or softened base
Aqueous solubility and extent of dissolution of
    water-soluble bases

Box 41.4

Drug-substance-related factors

Solubility in rectal fluids
Solubility in vehicle
Permeation ability in rectal membrane
Particle size
Displacement value
pK_a

solution or suspension suppository. When a drug has a high vehicle–water partition coefficient, it is likely to be in solution to an appreciable extent in the suppository. This generally means that the tendency to leave the dosage form will be low and thus the release rate into the rectal fluid will be slow. This is obviously unfavourable for rapid absorption.

The optimal balance between solubility in the vehicle and release from the vehicle is usually found using the rules listed in Table 41.2. Fatty bases are chosen for hydrophilic compounds and water-soluble bases are chosen for lipophilic compounds. These rules assume that the release from the dosage form is considered to be the rate-limiting step, and thus the tendency of the drug to remain in the base should be lowered as much as possible (rules 1 and 2). When the drug solubility is low in both fat and water, no definite rule can be given. It may be that the dissolution rate of the drug will become the controlling step, and thus it seems advisable to use micronized drug particles.

Drug particle size. The particle size of the drug is an important parameter for suspension suppositories. To prevent undue sedimentation during or after preparation, the drug should be incorporated in the base as fine (median size 125 μm to 180 μm) or very fine (median size ≤125 μm) powder.

Also, as dissolution rate is inversely proportional to particle size, drugs with low water solubility should be dispersed as small, preferably micronized, particles. A size range of 50 μm to 100 μm has been found ideal; the lower limit of 50 μm enables increased transport through the molten vehicle (Fig. 41.2), and the upper limit of 100 μm is a precaution against undue sedimentation during preparation.

Particle size should be considered alongside the density of the particle. The spreading suppository mass should take with it the suspended particles, so as to maximize the surface area for absorption. For dense particles, this can be problematic. It has been shown that particle density should range between 1.2 g cm^{-3} and 1.4 g cm^{-3} to allow particle flow in the molten base, even for particle sizes as large as 150 μm.

From a manufacturing perspective, small particles are more challenging to handle because of increased interparticulate van der Waals forces and thus increased tendency to agglomerate to a cohesive mass during powder flow. An additional complicating factor is the amount of drug present in a suppository. If the number of particles increases, the rate of agglomerate formation will increase. Another consequence of the presence of suspended particles is the increased viscosity of the molten base.

From the patient's perspective, the smaller the particles, the lower the probability of mechanical irritation of the rectal membrane (especially if the particle size is less than 50 μm).

Displacement value. A drug property which should be considered during the formulation of suspension suppositories, where the drug is dispersed in the molten base, is the displacement value. The displacement value is the mass of drug that displaces 1 g of base, and it allows calculation of the required amount of base in the suppository formulation. An example calculation is shown in Box 41.5.

Additives

Viscosity-increasing (hardening) agents. These excipients are required in the following cases:

- when the drug suppresses the melting point of the base and thus reduces its viscosity at 37 °C; and
- to increase the viscosity of the molten or dispersed suppository base without affecting its melting temperature.

Box 41.5

Worked example of displacement value

Prepare eight suppositories (1g each), each containing 200 mg bismuth subgallate:

For eight suppositories, 0.2 g × 8 = 1.6 g drug.

The displacement value for bismuth subgallate is 3.0 g.

Three grams of drug displaces 1 g base; therefore 1.6 g drug displaces (1.6/3) 0.53 g base.

The amount of base required for eight medicated suppositories is 8 g – 0.53 g = 7.47 g.

Table 41.2 Drug solubility and suppository formulation

Solubility in		Choice of base
Fat	Water	
Low	High	Fatty base (rule 1)
High	Low	Aqueous base (rule 2)
Low	Low	Indeterminate

Beeswax, colloidal silicon dioxide (Aerosil®) aluminium monostearate, hydroxypropyl methylcellulose and polyvinylpyrrolidone are examples of viscosity-increasing additives. These will create a gel-like system of high viscosity and confer on the formulation modified drug-release properties. In theory, the higher viscosity of the formulation will decrease the drug's diffusion coefficient and release from the vehicle; however, the in vivo drug release behaviour will also be determined by rectal motility, which tends to promote drug release.

Deagglomerators. Deagglomerators are excipients added in the formulation of suspension suppositories to prevent agglomeration of the drug particles, which in turn would render drug release erratic. Lecithin, for example, decreases the attraction between the drug particles and improves the flow properties of the dispersion. Surfactants may also act as deagglomerators, by preventing the formation of a cake in the melting suppository.

Drug solubility enhancers. Such excipients can be added to increase the aqueous solubility of lipophilic drugs in the rectal fluids, thereby enabling complete drug dissolution. Buffering agents alter the pH of the rectal fluid to enable drug ionization, thus increasing the aqueous solubility, of weakly acidic or basic compounds. Nonionic surfactants, such as poloxamers, can be used as wetting agents. However, the presence of surfactants in amounts higher than the critical micelle concentration can retard the release of some drugs from suppositories.

Surfactants may also act as spreading enhancers by enabling disintegration of the suppository vehicle with the occurrence of rectal motility. In the case of fatty bases, surfactants may create water-in-oil emulsions on mixing of the suppository with the rectal fluid; this should be strongly discouraged because transfer of drug molecules present in a dissolved state in the inner (globules) aqueous phase will be very slow and thus drug absorption will be very much retarded.

Absorption (permeation) enhancers. Fatty acids, surfactants, bile salts, nitric oxide donors, phenothiazines and salicylates are all classes of permeation enhancers which can enhance the rectal absorption of drugs. They have varying mechanisms of action. For example, salicylates and phenothiazines are calmodulin antagonists and disrupt rectal wall integrity by opening calcium tight junctions, thus increasing wall permeability. Nitric oxide donors increase blood flow to the rectal membrane, causing dilation of the tight junctions. Fatty acids intercalate within the lipid and protein fraction of the rectal membrane, creating pores.

Antimicrobial preservatives. Preservatives are required in water-soluble suppository base formulations to prevent microbial growth.

Other rectal preparations

Rectal capsules and tablets

Rectal capsules are solid, single-dose preparations generally similar in shape and appearance to soft capsules (see Chapter 34). They are filled with a solution or suspension of the drug in vegetable oil or liquid paraffin. There is limited experience with this dosage form, but it seems there are no striking differences in the bioavailability of drugs from rectal capsules and fatty suppositories.

Tablets are not common rectal dosage forms because they cannot disintegrate rapidly in the small volume of rectal fluid. Rectal tablets releasing carbon dioxide after insertion can be used, stimulating defecation.

Rectal enemas

Enemas are liquid preparations intended for rectal use and may be formulated as solutions, emulsions, foams and suspensions. The advantage of this delivery system is that no melting and dissolution is necessary before drug release can begin. Solutions, emulsions and suspensions are packaged into single-dose containers (plastic rectal tubes or bottles, depending on their volume) and are administered/emptied into the rectal cavity by compression via a nozzle/applicator. Administration cannot be performed easily by patients themselves, and sometimes delivery of the total content of the plastic container can be problematic. Rectal foams are packaged into pressurized metered-dose containers, which deliver the dose on actuation, and are thus easier to administer.

These liquid formulations are used for systemic effect (e.g. diazepam rectal tubes are used for the management of epileptic convulsions), for local effect to evacuate, cleanse or treat the lower parts of the gastrointestinal tract (e.g. mesalazine foam or enema) and for diagnostic purposes (e.g. barium enema).

For local treatment of the rectum, such as in the treatment of rectocolitis, enemas of relatively large volume (~100 mL) are used to enable the drug to reach the upper part of the rectum and the sigmoid colon. Even larger volumes are used for colon cleansing or colonic irrigation. Solutions or dispersions of the drug in a small volume (~3 mL) of liquid are called microenemas.

The formulation of enemas/microenemas comprises either an oily vehicle (e.g. arachis oil enema) or one or more active substances dissolved or dispersed in water, glycerol, macrogols (PEGs) or other suitable solvent. Rectal solutions, emulsions and suspensions may contain viscosity modifiers, buffers to adjust or stabilize the pH, and cosolvents to increase the solubility of the active substance(s) or to chemically stabilize the drug in the preparation. These excipients should not adversely affect the intended clinical effect or cause undue local irritation.

Powders and tablets for rectal solutions and suspensions

The powders and tablets intended for the preparation of rectal solutions or suspensions are single-dose solid preparations that are dissolved or dispersed in water or other suitable solvents at the time of administration. They may contain excipients to facilitate dissolution or dispersion, or to prevent aggregation of the particles. Such powders are often produced by freeze-drying (lyophilization). Freeze-dried powders have a large surface area and dissolve rapidly.

Semisolid rectal preparations

Semisolid rectal preparations are ointments, creams or gels. They are often supplied as single-dose preparations with a suitable applicator. They are intended for the symptomatic relief of haemorrhoids and anal fissures, e.g. heparinoid in lauromacrogol (Anacal®) rectal ointment.

Rectal tampons

Rectal tampons are solid, single-dose preparations intended to be inserted into the lower part of the rectum for a limited time and then removed. An example is Peristeen® anal plug, which is inserted in the rectum for up to 12 hours for the management of faecal incontinence.

Recent advances in rectal dosage forms

Research and development on rectal dosage forms focuses on two areas:

- the enhancement of patient adherence by enabling easier insertion of the dosage form into the rectum; and

- the design of mucoadhesive formulations that can allow retention and better positioning of the dosage form in the rectal cavity, together with prolonged-drug release.

In situ *thermoreversible mucoadhesive rectal gels* (also called thermoreversible 'liquid suppositories') are liquid formulations during storage at room temperature that form a gel at 37°C when inserted in the rectum. Once in the gel state, such formulations adhere to the rectal mucosa, preventing dosage form leakage, which is a common disadvantage with enemas. Lipophilic active ingredients require the incorporation of a solubility enhancer in the formulation, which will enable complete drug dissolution in the rectal fluid. For example, flurbiprofen liquid suppositories consisting of a poloxamer (thermoreversible polymer), sodium alginate (mucoadhesive polymer) and hydroxypropyl-β-cyclodextrin (solubility enhancer) have shown bioavailability comparable to that of a commercial intravenous flurbiprofen formulation (Kim et al., 2009). Thermosensitive, bioadhesive micellar rectal gels loaded with the chemotherapeutic agent docetaxel (Seo et al., 2013) showed a significant antitumour effect, sustained plasma levels and reduced toxicity profile compared with the oral formulation.

Vaginal drug delivery

Anatomy and physiology of the vagina

The human vagina is a fibromuscular tube structure that connects the uterus to the external environment. It is approximately 100 mm long and its anatomic location is between the rectum and the bladder. The vaginal wall is coated with mucus (cervicovaginal fluid), which provides lubrication and protection against infections. Clearance of vaginal fluid can affect dosage form retention in the vaginal cavity. The volume of the vaginal fluid is estimated to be approximately 0.75 mL at any time, with an overall average daily production of 6 mL.

The composition and volume of vaginal fluids varies significantly with age, stage of the menstrual cycle, pregnancy, sexual activity and infections. In healthy adult women, vaginal fluid is slightly acidic (with a pH range between 4 and 5) because of the presence of microflora, consisting primarily of lactobacillus bacteria, which convert glycogen from epithelial cells into lactic acid. The acidic pH provides natural protection from infections, including those which are sexually transmitted. During pregnancy, the pH is even lower, between 3.8 and 4.4. The pH tends to rise during local infections and in postmenopausal women, because of changes in the vaginal ecology and cellular glycogen levels. Human semen, which is highly buffered and slightly alkaline in pH, causes a transient increase in pH, which is necessary for sperm survival and to achieve fertilization.

Blood supply to the vagina is via the uterine and vaginal arteries. Blood drainage is via the vaginal venus plexus, a network of small veins, which drains to the iliac vein (inferior vena cava), which can easily transport drugs to the systemic circulation, avoiding first-pass metabolism by the liver. Veins at the upper region of the vagina are closely located to the arteries of the uterus, allowing vein-to-artery drug diffusion. This direct transport mechanism between the vagina and the uterus is called the "first uterine pass effect" and can be useful for drug delivery to the uterus after vaginal administration.

Absorption of drugs from the vagina

Drug absorption from the vagina is via passive diffusion. The vaginal wall is very well suited for the systemic absorption of drugs because of its vast network of blood vessels. A number of physiological factors such as volume, viscosity and pH of vaginal fluid can influence drug absorption. Drug-related factors that influence absorption include drug solubility in vaginal fluid, ionization behaviour at vaginal pH, characteristics of release from the formulation and molecular weight, as this will affect the diffusion coefficient via the vaginal membrane.

The advantages and limitations of drug delivery by vaginal administration are shown in Box 41.6.

Vaginal dosage forms

Vaginal dosage forms are used for both local and systemic effects, although applications for local effects are far more common.

Local action. Vaginal dosage forms are intended for a range of local effects:

- Treatment of certain bacterial infections such as bacterial vaginosis (clindamycin, metronidazole, dequalinium chloride), fungal infections such as candida infection (clotrimazole, miconazole,

---

Box 41.6

Advantages and limitations of vaginal administration

Advantages

1. Can be used for local and systemic delivery of drugs. Relatively large surface area and good drug absorption makes it useful for the systemic absorption of a range of drugs, including proteins and peptides.
2. Avoids hepatic first-pass metabolism.
3. The vaginal route has the potential for preferential delivery to the uterus, known as the 'first uterine pass effect'. The phenomenon is useful for uterine targeting of drugs such as progesterone and danazol.
4. Suitable for vaccine administration as it provokes an immune response.
5. Suitable for microbicide delivery.
6. Self-administration and removal of dosage forms is relatively easy.

Limitations

1. The vaginal route is sex specific.
2. Menstrual cycle and hormonal variations affect the rate and extent of absorption of drugs intended for systemic administration.
3. Drug release and availability of locally acting drugs can be influenced by interpatient variations in the volume of cervicovaginal fluids.
4. Dosage form retention can be problematic.
5. User preferences for vaginal drug delivery differ depending on cultural norms, partners, socioeconomic conditions and geographical locations.
6. Damage to the vaginal epithelium by the formulation can lead to infections.

---

econazole, fenticonazole) and viral infections such as infections with herpes simplex virus and human papillomavirus (e.g. aciclovir). Treatment of vaginal infections can be achieved with a much lower dose applied vaginally compared with oral administration.

- Local delivery of hormones for labour induction.
- Contraception via the delivery of spermicides such as nonoxynol 9.
- Local delivery of microbicides (compounds which can prevent transmission of sexually transmitted infections, including HIV).
- To adjust vaginal pH for the prevention and treatment of nonbacterial vaginosis.

Systemic action. The vagina is an underutilized route for systemic drug delivery. Some drugs can have a higher bioavailability via the intravaginal route than via the oral route, because of avoidance of first-pass metabolism. For example, oestrogens, progesterone and prostaglandin analogues are poorly absorbed after oral administration and also undergo extensive first-pass metabolism. As such, commercial vaginal formulations deliver progesterone as part of the assisted reproductive technology treatment program for infertile women, and oestradiol for the development of uterine lining to combat vaginal atrophy in postmenopausal women (hormone replacement therapy). Current research and development focuses on the vaginal delivery of vaccines, chemotherapeutic agents and microbicides.

Formulation design for vaginal dosage forms is similar in many respects to that for rectal preparations. A range of vaginal dosage forms are currently available and used in practice. These include vaginal pessaries (suppositories, tablets and capsules), liquids (vaginal solutions, emulsions and suspensions), semisolids (creams and gels), vaginal films, vaginal rings, tablets for vaginal solutions and suspensions, gaseous preparations (sprays and foams) and medicated vaginal tampons. An ideal vaginal dosage form should be easy to insert, be odourless, not cause irritation, burning or itching of the vaginal membrane and not leak after administration.

Pessaries

Vaginal pessaries are solid or semisolid, oval-shaped, single-dose preparations for vaginal insertion, and encompass formulations such as suppositories, tablets and capsules. Pessaries are supplied with an auxiliary device/applicator which enables insertion of the dosage form in the vagina.

Vaginal suppositories. Vaginal suppositories are similar formulations to rectal suppositories. They weigh approximately 1 g and contain one or more active substances dissolved or dispersed in a suitable base that may be soluble or dispersible in water, or may be fatty and melt at body temperature. Multiphase suppositories containing mucoadhesive polymers mixed in the base are also common. For example, Gyno-Pevaryl Once (econazole nitrate) pessaries contain Witepsol and Wecobee fatty bases mixed with Polygel, which retains the molten base attached to the vaginal wall.

The formulation considerations and drug release mechanisms from vaginal suppositories are similar to those for rectal suppositories (see earlier). Drug solubility in the suppository base is established at the preformulation stage, and the particle size of the active ingredient and excipients, if suspended in the vehicle, should be controlled to avoid any irritation of the vaginal membrane.

Vaginal tablets. Vaginal tablets are coated or uncoated solid, single-dose preparations, similar to oral tablets with respect to their formulation and manufacture. Tablet formulations offer the advantages of ease of storage, ease of use, low cost and well-controlled large-scale manufacturing. These are especially suitable for drugs susceptible to degradation in the presence of moisture. In tropical countries, vaginal tablets are the most commonly used vaginal dosage form.

Dissolution of the formulation in the small volume of vaginal fluid is one of the limiting factors for drug release from vaginal tablets. For this reason, vaginal tablets should be inserted as high as possible into the vagina. Excipients such as bicarbonate, together with an organic acid for carbon dioxide release, can be added to increase tablet disintegration, if necessary.

A good filler in the formulation and manufacture of vaginal tablets is lactose, because it is a natural substrate for the vaginal microflora that converts lactose into lactic acid, retaining the vaginal pH within its normal range. For example, Canesten® (clotrimazole) pessaries contain lactose monohydrate and lactic acid.

Other excipients used in vaginal tablet formulations include lubricants, glidants, binders and polymers for modified drug release, as for oral tablets (see Chapter 30). The inclusion of mucoadhesive polymers such as Carbopol® and xanthan gum in the formulation is desirable to minimize leakage and increase retention of the dispersed or dissolved tablet.

Vaginal capsules. Vaginal capsules are similar to rectal capsules, containing the drug as a solution or suspension in vegetable oil or liquid paraffin within a soft capsule shell. For example, Canesten® Soft Gel Pessary (vaginal capsule) consists of a mixture of liquid paraffin, white soft paraffin and medium-chain triglycerides as the oily vehicle in a soft gelatin capsule.

Semisolid vaginal preparations

Semisolid vaginal preparations are usually creams or gels. As with rectal semisolid preparations, they are supplied in multidose, collapsible tubes with a suitable applicator, or in prefilled single-dose applicators. They are intended for local or systemic drug delivery, prevention of bacterial vaginosis by restoring the pH balance (lactic acid gel) and also for personal care of the vaginal region. For example, Canesintima® Intimate Moisturiser is an aqueous gel enriched with *Camellia japonica* and hyaluronic acid for vaginal moisturization and lubrication intended for menopausal and postmenopausal women.

Semisolid formulations, because of their water content, are less likely to cause irritation of the vaginal wall than pessaries. However, they require the inclusion of an antimicrobial preservative in the formulation and are not suitable for drugs susceptible to hydrolysis. Mucoadhesive polymers, such as Carbopol, are often included in the formulation to enable dosage form retention in the vaginal wall and prolonged drug release.

Recent advances include:

- Thermoreversible mucoadhesive gels to allow easy insertion of the dosage form.
- Intravaginal vaccination. Clinical trials have demonstrated a greater immune response from a vaginal gel than for an orally administered cholera vaccine (Wassen et al., 1996).

Rheological properties of the semisolid, spreading behaviour, volume, pH, osmolarity, ease of insertion and retention and patient acceptability are all parameters that need to be considered for these preparations.

Vaginal films

Vaginal films are small, thin polymeric layers, designed to dissolve in the vaginal fluids and release the drug. They are single-dose preparations and can be easily inserted into the vaginal cavity without the need for an applicator. Because of their ease of administration, vaginal films tend to demonstrate higher patient acceptability than pessaries, semisolid vaginal formulations and vaginal rings.

In terms of composition, the films contain polymers which can confer mucoadhesive and modified-release properties on the formulation. When in contact with the vaginal fluids, they rapidly dissolve and turn to a mucoadhesive viscous solution that attaches to the vaginal wall. Vaginal Contraceptive Film® (VCF®), containing nonoxynol 9 (spermicide) as an active

ingredient in a water-soluble polymeric film, is an example of a marketed product.

Current research and development on vaginal films focuses on:

- Reformulation of antifungal drugs.
- Microbiocide delivery. Vaginal films containing antiretroviral-loaded nanoparticles have shown promising results in the prevention of HIV transmission.

Vaginal rings

Vaginal rings, also called intravaginal rings, are ring-shaped with a diameter of approximately 40 mm; they are flexible and often colourless dosage forms made from elastomeric polymers. They contain a drug reservoir within the polymer network and allow controlled drug release over a prolonged period. Vaginal rings can be inserted in the vagina with the aid of an applicator and should be removed at the end of the drug administration period if they are made from nonbiodegradable polymers such as silicone. The first vaginal rings were developed in the 1970s as contraceptive devices (NuvaRing®) and for the treatment of atrophic vaginitis (Estring®) as part of hormone replacement therapy. NuvaRing® is a poly(ethylene–vinyl acetate) (PEVA) ring that releases oestrogen and progestin for 3 weeks. Estring® is a silicone ring that releases oestradiol hemihydrate for 90 days.

Current research on vaginal rings aims to replace silicone and PEVA with biodegradable polymers, which will not require removal of the ring from the vagina, thus improving patient adherence, and which are also environmentally friendly. However, biodegradable polymers tend to have limited flexibility and cannot form robust rings.

In recent years, vaginal rings have attracted a lot of attention as promising microbicide delivery systems. A silicone vaginal ring designed to provide sustained dapivirine release over 28 days (Nel et al., 2016) was evaluated in phase III clinical trials against placebo amongst African women and was found to be effective in preventing HIV infection. More advanced formulations include multisegment vaginal rings (with hydrophilic and lipophilic polymer segments) which incorporate a combination of drugs with different physicochemical properties; this can be a combination of two antiretroviral active ingredients or a combination of an antiretroviral with a contraceptive (so-called dual-protection rings).

Vaginal solutions, emulsions, foams and suspensions

These are liquid preparations intended for personal care and cosmetic purposes (e.g. irrigation and cleansing of the vaginal cavity) and for local drug delivery. They are supplied in single-dose containers designed to deliver the preparation to the vagina, or are accompanied by a suitable applicator.

Excipients may be added to adjust the viscosity of the preparation and to adjust the pH so as to increase the solubility of the active substance(s). The excipients should not adversely affect the therapeutic activity of the active substance nor cause local irritation. Vaginal emulsions may show evidence of phase separation but are readily redispersed on shaking. Vaginal suspensions may show particle sedimentation during storage that is readily redispersed on shaking before administration.

Tablets for vaginal solutions and suspensions

The tablets intended for the preparation of vaginal solutions and suspensions are single-dose preparations that are dissolved or dispersed in water at the time of administration. They may contain excipients to facilitate dissolution or dispersion, or to prevent caking.

Medicated vaginal tampons

Medicated vaginal tampons are solid, single-dose polymeric preparations intended to be inserted in the vagina for a limited time and then removed. The drug is present in a matrix made from a suitable polymer such as silicone, cellulose or gelatin.

Manufacture of rectal and vaginal dosage forms

Rectal and vaginal suppositories

Suppositories are manufactured by hand on a small scale, in batches of 6–50, and on a (semi) automatic scale in batches of up to 20 000 per hour. There are two methods for manufacturing suppositories: *moulding* and *compression*.

Moulding

Moulding requires melting of the suppository base in a heat tank and comprises the following steps:

1. Lubrication of the mould. This is required only for water-soluble suppository bases. Fatty bases are inherently lubricating in nature.
2. Calibration of the mould.
3. Melting of the base in a temperature-controlled heat tank (200 L to 500 L capacity) and addition of drugs and excipients. The container has stirring and mixing devices to ensure a uniformly mixed mass during and after the addition of drug and excipients. If the active ingredient remains in suspension, the viscosity of the molten base and the drug particle size should be optimized during preformulation to ensure a homogeneous particle distribution during cooling.
4. Filling of moulds with medicated molten mass. Most equipment for manufacturing suppositories is now designed to use preformed moulded packaging. Here, the plastic pack acts as both the mould and the primary packaging. The molten mass from step 3 is poured into a continuously moving strip of moulds with high precision to achieve mass uniformity.
5. Cooling of filled moulds. The filled moulds are passed through a cooling tunnel to allow solidification of the molten mass. The cooling temperature and time are monitored.
6. The filled moulds are sealed, checked and labelled. The strips are then cut to the required pack size.
7. The cut strips are placed into cardboard secondary packs and are sometimes supplied with an applicator.

Compression

Compression is appropriate for heat-sensitive drugs or/and excipients which would degrade at the high temperatures used in the moulding method. The compression method involves the following steps:

1. Suppository base and drug(s) are mixed and heated simultaneously to produce a soft paste. High-shear mixers are required to ensure homogeneous mixing of the viscous paste.
2. The paste is forced through a cylinder to fill the preformed packaging.

The level of automation and scale of manufacturing differ significantly in machines from different manufacturers. Suppositories are packed individually in plastic (PVC) or aluminium foil strip packs. Packaging material which is impermeable to moisture and oxygen is chosen for drugs that are prone to hydrolysis.

Vaginal films

Vaginal films can be manufactured via either *solvent casting* or *hot-melt extrusion*.

Solvent casting

Solvent casting involves the following steps:

1. The active ingredient is either dissolved or dispersed in a solution of a water-soluble polymer (e.g. polyethylene oxide, polyvinylpyrrolidone, hydroxypropyl methylcellulose) in an appropriate solvent. A plasticizer (such as PEG, propylene glycol, or glycerol) can be added to the viscous solution, as it enhances the mechanical strength and flexibility of the film.
2. The liquid mixture is cast and then dried. The thickness of the cast film and the drying conditions (time and temperature) must be monitored.
3. The dried film is cut to strips of the required size; these are then packaged individually in blister packs or sachets. When organic solvents are used in the process, solvent residues in the dried films must be measured and controlled to ensure they are within safe limits.

Hot-melt extrusion

Hot-melt extrusion involves the following steps:

1. Drug and excipients are heated together and mixed within the extruder until molten.
2. The molten mass (extrudate) is forced into thin films of required thickness, via a flat extrusion die.
3. The films are cooled, cut to the required surface area and packaged individually.

The hot-melt extrusion method is not suitable for heat-sensitive drugs.

The parameters that should be optimized during the pharmaceutical development of films include dissolution and release behaviour in small volumes of fluids, mechanical strength, thickness, content uniformity, texture, and process parameters such as the drying time.

Vaginal rings

Vaginal rings containing silicone or thermoplastic (PEVA) polymers are manufactured via hot-melt extrusion of the drug–polymer mixture, followed by injection moulding into ring-holds to form the ring-shaped dosage form. Multisegment rings require extra manufacturing steps, where the moulded medicated polymer segments are glued together to form the final ring structure.

Rectal and vaginal tablets

Compaction of rectal and vaginal tablets, for direct application to the membrane or for reconstitution to solutions and suspensions before administration, is similar to the manufacture of oral tablets using punch and die tableting machines to produce tablets of the appropriate dimensions (see Chapter 30).

Other rectal and vaginal dosage forms

The industrial manufacture of many other types of rectal and vaginal dosage forms (solutions, emulsions, suspensions, creams, gels, etc.) differs little or not at all from that described in Chapters 24, 26, 27 and 40 of this book.

Quality control of rectal and vaginal dosage forms

Rectal and vaginal formulations are evaluated by in vitro and in vivo tests for quality, safety and effectiveness. Quality control tests form part of the product release and expiry (shelf-life) specifications of the dosage form. A list of properties that should be controlled is given in Box 41.7. These properties include appearance (shape, colour and surface properties) and odour (by organoleptic evaluation), release characteristics, melting and solubility, stability, pH, viscosity, spreading, mucoadhesion and mechanical

Box 41.7

Quality control tests for rectal and vaginal dosage forms

Appearance
Content of active ingredient
Weight
Disintegration
Melting (dissolution) behaviour
Mechanical strength
Antimicrobial preservation
Drug release
Safety – mucosal irritation

strength. Some of the tests are pharmacopoeial requirements for the finished product, whereas other tests are performed during the development phase and as in-process quality control testing. Formulations are also required to comply with the requirements of the pharmacopoeial monographs for the particular dosage form. For example, medicated vaginal tampons must comply with the requirements of the specific monograph on medicated tampons.

A number of tests for rectal and vaginal dosage forms are included in pharmacopoeias. For instance, the British and European pharmacopoeias include tests for:

- uniformity of dosage units;
- uniformity of content;
- uniformity of mass;
- disintegration;
- softening time of lipophilic suppositories;
- mechanical strength;
- dissolution; and
- antimicrobial preservative efficacy.

Assessment of drug release from suppositories

In vitro testing considerations

The parameters that should be considered and optimized for in vitro testing of drug release from suppositories are the temperature of the release medium, the type of release medium, the design of the apparatus and the use of an appropriate membrane.

The temperature of the release medium is usually set at 37 °C to mimic body temperature. Because body temperature may be as low as 36 °C at night and considering the drug release rate is temperature dependent, release data measured at 37 °C may be overestimates. Special attention should therefore be given to the testing temperature employed. In the apparatus shown in Fig. 41.3, the temperature at the surface of the release medium inside the tube, where molten suppository is gathered, may be a few degrees lower than the bulk temperature. Choosing the correct dimensions and closing the tube at the upper side would eliminate this problem.

Another important test parameter is the type of release medium. The composition and structure of rectal and vaginal fluids have to be considered to design physiologically appropriate simulation fluids.

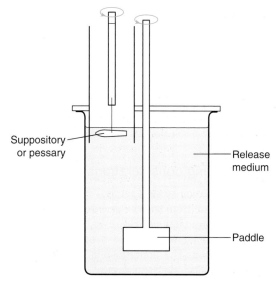

Fig. 41.3 • Dissolution tube apparatus for suppositories using the paddle method.

As the rate-limiting step in drug bioavailability is dissolution or/and drug diffusion in the viscous rectal and vaginal mucus, mucins are often included in the release medium. Buffer salts are also added to adjust the pH. The volume of the release medium in in vitro testing is usually relatively large (~900 mL) compared with the volumes of rectal and vaginal fluid.

The design of the dissolution apparatus is another important aspect considering that the contact area in the rectum or vagina over which spreading occurs cannot be easily standardized. Drug release from water-soluble and fatty suppositories can be assessed with the paddle, basket and flow-through cell apparatus designs (see Chapter 35). In the paddle apparatus shown in Fig. 41.3 the contact area is relatively small (~10 cm^2) compared with the total surface area of the rectum or vagina. Such apparatus is therefore intended to be used only for comparative studies and determination of batch-to-batch uniformity and not for in vivo simulation. No method is available which closely mimics the in vivo situation.

Synthetic membranes, which envelop the suppository in a smaller volume of release medium, are often used with the apparatus for assessing drug release from rectal and vaginal suppositories. Their use should, however, be discouraged as drug release measured in the outer compartment is not equal to the actual release occurring in the inner compartment, and the membrane itself may form a barrier to diffusing drug molecules, resulting in underestimation of drug release.

In the case of testing of drug release from rectal formulations, interest has been directed towards ways of incorporating a pressure feature, in consideration of the fact that rectal motility has an effect on dosage form spreading and drug partitioning from the formulation and thus may influence drug bioavailability.

In vivo testing considerations

In vitro dissolution studies act as a surrogate for in vivo drug release from and the performance of rectal and vaginal formulations. However, correlation of the data obtained with in vivo behaviour has not been established. The limitations in establishing in vivo behaviour include the biological complexities of the rectal and vaginal routes, interpatient variability and the lack of appropriate animal models. A number of different systems have been explored by scientists, but there is a lack of universally accepted or compendial models. For example, ex vivo studies using Franz diffusion cells to determine drug permeation via an animal rectal or vaginal membrane are commonly used. Tests for assessing systemic distribution, dosage form spreading and retention (mucoadhesion) are also performed in animal models, such as rabbits, monkeys and sheep. Whenever possible, data should

be obtained from clinical trials using human volunteers because no animal model is sufficiently reliable.

For a more detailed discussion of the general aspects of bioavailability testing, and in vitro–in vivo correlations, see Chapter 21.

Tests for vaginal irritation

Vaginal irritation from pharmaceutical, cosmetic and personal care products must be avoided as it can lead to easier acquisition of microbial infections, including sexually transmitted diseases. An in vivo safety test for vaginal irritation is usually performed in whole-animal test systems using rabbits, monkeys or pigs as a screening test in developing a new drug, excipient or formulation.

The current need to replace animal testing, because of animal welfare concerns and poor correlation between animal and human responses to the formulation, has led to the development of a set of in vitro vaginal irritation tests. These in vitro tests can be cell cultures (e.g. normal human ectocervical cells), reconstructed vaginal epithelium or tissue explants; the assessment of irritation is based on inflammation biomarkers such as cytokine release.

Please check your eBook at **https://studentconsult.inkling.com/** for self-assessment questions. See inside cover for registration details.

References

Kim, J.-K., Kim, M.-S., Park, J.-S., et al., 2009. Thermo-reversible flurbiprofen liquid suppository with HP-β-CD as a solubility enhancer: improvement of rectal bioavailability. J. Inclusion Phenom. Macrocyclic Chem. 64, 265–272.

Nel, A., Kapiga, S., Bekker, L.-G., et al., 2016. Safety and efficacy of dapivirine vaginal ring for HIV-1 prevention in African women. Conference on retroviruses and opportunistic infections 2016, 22–25 February 2016, Boston.

Seo, Y.G., Kim, D.-W., Yeo, W.H., et al., 2013. Docetaxel-loaded thermosensitive and bioadhesive nanomicelles as a rectal drug delivery system for enhanced chemotherapeutic effect. Pharm. Res. 30, 1860–1870.

Wassen, L., Schon, K., Holmgren, J., et al., 1996. Local intravaginal vaccination of the female genital tract. Scand. J. Immunol. 44, 408–414.

Bibliography

Acartürk, F., 2009. Mucoadhesive vaginal drug delivery systems. Recent Pat. Drug Deliv. Formul. 3, 193–205.

Bharate, S.S., Bharate, S.B., Bajaj, A.N., 2010. Interactions and incompatibilities of pharmaceutical excipients with active pharmaceutical ingredients: a comprehensive review. Journal of Excipients and Food Chemicals 1, 3–26.

Cicinelli, E., de Ziegler, D., Morgese, S., et al., 2004. "First uterine pass effect" is observed when estradiol is placed in the upper but not lower third of the vagina. Fertil. Steril. 81, 1414–1416.

Costin, G.-E., Raabe, H.A., Priston, R., et al., 2011. Vaginal irritation models: the current status of available alternative and in vitro tests. Altern. Lab. Anim. 39, 317–337.

Dodou, K., 2012. Exploring the unconventional routes — rectal and vaginal dosage formulations. The

Pharmaceutical Journal 289, 238–239.

Gupta, J., Tao, J.Q., Garg, S., et al., 2011. Design and development of an *in vitro* assay for evaluation of solid vaginal dosage forms. Pharmacology & Pharmacy 2, 289–298.

Jannin, V., Lemagnen, G., Gueroult, P., et al., 2014. Rectal route in the 21st century to treat children. Adv. Drug Deliv. Rev. 73, 34–49.

Kumar, V., Kalonia, D.S., 2006. Removal of peroxides in polyethylene glycols by vacuum drying: Implications in the stability of biotech and pharmaceutical formulations. AAPS Pharm. Sci. Tech. 7, E47–E53.

Malcolm, R.K., Fetherston, S.M., McCoy, C.F., et al., 2012. Vaginal rings for delivery of HIV microbicides. Int. J. Womens Health 4, 595–605.

Marques, M.R.C., Loebenberg, R., Almukainzi, M., 2011. Simulated biological fluids with possible application in dissolution testing. Dissolut. Technol. 18, 15–28.

Rowe, R.C., Sheskey, P.J., Cook, W.G., et al. (Eds.), 2016. Handbook of Pharmaceutical Excipients, eighth ed. Pharmaceutical Press, London.

Sharma, S., Kulkarni, J., Pawar, A.P., 2006. Permeation enhancers in the transmucosal delivery of macromolecules. Pharmazie 61, 495–504.

Touitou, E., Barry, B.W., 2011. Enhancement in drug delivery. CRC Press, Boca Raton.

Tukker, J.J., Blankenstein, M.A., Nortier, J.W.R., 1986. Comparison of bioavailability of tamoxifen after oral and rectal administration. J. Pharm. Pharmacol. 38, 888–892.

42

The formulation and manufacture of plant medicines

G. Brian Lockwood

CHAPTER CONTENTS

KEY POINTS

- Plant constituents are components in a number of modern conventional and complementary health care products.
- Quality control of crude plant drugs is more complex than for single chemical entities.
- The production methods used for plant-derived medicines are necessarily more involved than those used for single chemical entities.
- Because of the complex nature of plant-derived materials as drugs, they present a wide range of formulation problems.

- A wide range of formulations of plant medicines are increasingly available.
- There are a number of pharmaceutical issues related to plant medicines, including variability, quality, bioequivalence and adverse effects.

Introduction

Drugs obtained directly from plant sources are notably alkaloids, glycosides and phenolic compounds. Plant material is also a favoured source of volatile (essential) oils. They are used in a number of different dosage forms: conventional plant-derived pharmaceuticals, over-the-counter preparations for minor ailments, herbal remedies, homoeopathic mother tinctures and medicines, volatile (essential) oils used medicinally and in aromatherapy, nutraceuticals (single and complex entities), antioxidants plus a vast array of traditional usage forms worldwide.

Up until 2009 the *European Pharmacopoeia* contained over 166 monographs for herbal drugs and 77 for herbal preparations. Further monographs are continually being added (Vlietinck et al., 2009).

The number of legally authorized traditional herbal medicines available on the UK market has steadily increased over the last 10 years. During this period more than 100 licence applications have been submitted, and these include both single-component products and some products containing up to 20 different components. Authorizations for both single-herbal and multiherbal homoeopathic medicinal products were usually in single figures per year during the same period.

Plant-based products in medicinal use

A wide range of plant derivatives are used for the manufacture of medicinal products. These include fresh and dried plant material, acellular products, a wide range of types of extracts, including standardized extracts, and pure and in vitro biotechnology derived individual compounds. Examples of conventional single-component pharmaceuticals derived from plants are listed in Table 42.1.

The problems involved with the use of collected wild plant material include dramatic variability in quality as a result of the genetic variability of the wild stock, poor knowledge of the life cycles of plants and the effects of differing habitats on the levels of active constituents. Uncontrolled collection from the wild has led to devastation of certain supplies.

To control the influences of agroecological factors on the levels of active constituents in the plant, cultivation is used for production of the best quality raw materials. Medicinal plants should ideally be grown from homogeneous, genetically selected strains chosen for high yield of the relevant constituent(s) or other useful traits such as insect/fungal resistance.

Transport delays between collection and processing are a particular problem with the use of fresh plant material, and further compromise quality, leading to the possibility of degradation of the active constituent(s) as a result of microbial infestation, oxidation, reduction, hydrolysis and numerous other reactions. In spite of these disadvantages, herbalists are still convinced of the benefits of plant-based products.

Quality control of crude plant drugs

Quality control techniques are described in a range of monographs in national and international pharmacopoeias, as well as in herbal and homoeopathic pharmacopoeias. Quality control procedures should be applied to the herbal starting materials, their extracts and the finished products. Quality control techniques used for plants and their extracts are outlined in Table 42.2. Modern chromatographic techniques are also used for separation and quantification of specific individual constituents. This chapter will not detail the specific analytical techniques described, and the reader is referred to other texts for this information.

Plant preparations are often considered to be active because of their *combination* of constituents, and these often complex mixtures can be identified by a semiquantitative proof of content, such as a chromatographic fingerprint in combination with an appropriate assay of major constituents (Vlietinck et al., 2009). Combination of data from three types of chromatography is able to provide much qualitative and quantitative information.

Thin-layer chromatography is a semiquantitative technique using specified standards. By determination of R_f (retardation factor) values, this technique allows comparison between extracts of different origins and composition and known standards. This will give evidence for the presence of the components of the standards, plus indicative quantitative data as to their levels in the materials being tested.

To obtain true quantitative data, either high-performance liquid chromatography or gas chromatography should be used. These techniques are predominantly used for assays of either polar or

Table 42.1 Single chemical entities available after extraction from plant sources

Chemical entity	Current prescription medicine application	Plant source
Atropine	Antispasmodic, ophthalmic	*Atropa belladonna*
Codeine, morphine	Analgesic	*Papaver somniferum*
Colchicine	Gout treatment	*Colchicum autumnale*
Digoxin	Cardiac glycoside	*Digitalis lanata*
Ephedrine	Bronchospasm, nasal congestion treatment	*Ephedra* spp.
Galanthamine	Alleviation of Alzheimer's disease	*Narcissus* spp.
Pilocarpine	Treatment of xerostomia, myotic	*Pilocarpus jaborandi*
Quinine	Antimalarial	*Cinchona succiruba*
Sennosides	Laxative	*Cassia senna*
Vinblastine, vincristine	Anticancer agents	*Catharanthus roseus*

Table 42.2 Classic techniques for quality control

Standard	Technique	Purpose
Sampling	Selecting representative samples for analysis. Pharmacopoeias may suggest the number of samples from large consignments	To ensure all analytical data obtained truly represent the characteristics of the batch
Preliminary investigation	Organoleptic testing; observation of colour, odour, taste	Observation for evidence of poor quality or adulteration, to ensure high quality of final product
Foreign matter	Observation for excreta, mould, etc.	To ensure high quality of final product
Moisture content	Loss on drying at 100 °C to 105 °C, Dean–Stark measurement, GC, Karl Fischer method, IR, UV and NMR spectroscopy	Inhibit or minimize enzymic or microbial degradation
Extractive values	Water-soluble extractive, ethanol (45% to 90%) extractives, range of nonpolar solvent extractives	To determine whether low levels of compounds of specific polarity are present or even absent
Ash values	Incineration at 450 °C for total ash	Indication of level of inorganic matter or silica
Insoluble ash values	Water- and acid-insoluble ash contents	Indication of level of contamination with earth or silica
Crude fibre	Defatting followed by boiling	Confirmation of normal level or detection of excess material (e.g. stalk)
Macroscopical analysis	Comparison with botanical description	Initial identity of material
Microscopical analysis	Description of cells, inclusions and structures	Identification of material
Tannin content, bitterness value, swelling index	Quantitative measurements	Used for specific plants, containing tannins, bitter substances or those used for swelling ability (e.g. laxatives)
Microbiological contamination	Limits for levels of specific organisms	Check for levels of organisms greater than 10^3–10^4 per gram

From Evans (2009), with permission.
GC, gas chromatography; *IR*, infrared; *NMR*, nuclear magnetic resonance; *UV*, ultraviolet.

volatile constituents respectively. Gas chromatography is increasingly widely available coupled with mass spectrometry. This combination of gas chromatography and mass spectrometry allows identification and quantification of a wide range of components without the need for standards.

In addition to these chromatographic techniques, a number of spectroscopic techniques are widely used, such as visible, infrared and ultraviolet spectroscopy for determination of semiquantitative levels of constituents. In addition to these latter techniques, assays for specific constituents have been devised that use nuclear magnetic resonance spectroscopy, immunoassay, radioimmunoassay, enzyme-linked immunosorbent assay and fluorescence analysis. Near-infrared spectroscopy has recently been used for routine analysis of dry plant material and formulated products (both liquid and solid) and has the added advantage that it is noninvasive and can therefore be used for quality control in production and in packaging lines.

Herbal remedies often contain numerous herbal extracts, in many examples more than 10. This creates analytical difficulties, and this challenge, associated with the increasing use of all herbal remedies, particularly traditional and complementary medicines, has inspired analysts to produce more inclusive techniques, such as chemical pattern recognition and spectral correlation (Liang et al., 2004). DNA fingerprinting has recently been used to establish the identity of highly expensive raw materials, particularly those prone to substitution.

Production methods used to obtain plant-derived active constituents

The wide variety of medicinal plants, types of plant parts and various textures of material makes it impossible to standardize mechanical procedures, from harvesting through to drying, size reduction, or even essential oil extraction. The fibrous texture of in vivo or field-grown plant material and also unorganized crude drugs often requires severe mechanical disruption before extraction. Table 42.3 outlines the basic processes involved in production of plant extracts. These are applied to both conventional plant-based pharmaceuticals and complementary herbal medicines.

Harvesting

The first stage, harvesting, is strictly an agricultural and not a pharmaceutical process but it can have a great influence on the quality of the final product. Each procedure requires specialized equipment, often modified versions of commercial agricultural machinery.

Further mechanical processing techniques are often required, which may include cleaning or washing. Procedures are needed to eliminate unwanted foreign matter, such as other plant material, minerals, any other organisms and agrochemical residues. In some instances, manual techniques are still superior to mechanization.

Drying

Drying is usually an essential process, as medicinal plant material contains water. This water must be removed to maintain the quality of the raw plant material. Often this degradation is simply monitored by macroscopic investigation of colour, form and absence of microbiological and fungal growth. The moisture content of the raw material is affected by the prevailing humidity; hence there is a greater risk of degradation in crops grown in tropical climates that are subject to higher humidity and high temperature.

Drying is necessary in almost all cases to protect the active constituent content. The three main techniques used for drying of plant material are:

- *Natural drying.* Direct sunlight, which may have adverse effects.
- *Hot air drying.* The operational temperature depends on the nature of the active constituents and may range from 40 °C for essential oils to 100 °C for glycoside-containing material. Equipment similar to that used in pharmaceutical operations is used (see Chapter 29).
- *Microwave drying.* This is often used in combination with hot air drying. It may cause browning of the material, but it is useful in reduction of microbial contamination (Oztekin & Martinov, 2007).

Size reduction

The main aim of size reduction of the dried material is to create particles of similar size, which permits

Table 42.3 The major stages in the conversion of plant material into a concentrated extract

Production process	Purpose	Constraints
Harvesting	Stop metabolism at optimum time	Weather
Drying	Inactivate enzymes, inhibit microbial infestation	Plant part and temperature determine speed. Essential in tropical conditions
Size reduction (comminution)	Increase surface area for effective solvent extraction	Solvent flow impeded if particles are too small, possible release of excessive mucilage, which hinders later filtration
Extraction of active constituents	Production of most active base for formulation	Financial constraints to complete (100%) extraction
Extract concentration	Minimize volume/weight of extract, for ease of transport, storage, and ease of distribution in the final formulation	As above, but extra investment

uniform and maximum extraction of the required plant material. The rate of extraction is dependent on the rate of diffusion of solvent into the plant material and of solutes from the material into the surrounding solvent. Hence reasonably fine powders, with diameters approaching 0.5 mm, are preferred.

Care must be taken during size reduction of fresh (undried) material as in some cases it can lead to degradation of constituents via a number of chemical reactions and also endogenous enzymatic action. Low temperature can be used to reduce these possibilities, and deep-freezing may be required during storage of fresh materials before comminution (Bombardelli, 1991).

Size reduction can be performed with a variety of crushers and mills, usually fitted to a magnetic separator to collect extraneous metal particles. Dust collection devices are imperative for this process. Typical types of size reduction apparatus (see Chapter 10) used for plant material include:

- cutting and shredding mills for leaves and herbs;
- hammer and pin mills for herbs with high fat content;
- shredding and hammer mills for roots and barks; and
- further specialized mills for difficult samples.

Size reduction of plant material is a very inefficient operation, with only approximately 1% of the energy input directly responsible for the size reduction (Chaudhri, 1996).

Extraction of active constituents

Types of extracts

The next step in the process is to remove the active constituents from the dried and powdered plant. This is achieved mainly by the process of *extraction*. In its most common form, extraction consists of soaking the powdered material in a liquid (usually aqueous or ethanolic) solvent. The solvent diffuses into the powdered material and dissolves the ingredients, which then diffuse out into the liquid. Decreasing the particle size of the plant matrix, within limits, will therefore decrease the extraction time.

The major types of liquid product obtained by this process and then used in the manufacture of medicines include (Bonati, 1980; Vlietinck et al., 2009):

- decoctions and infusions;
- liquid extracts and tinctures;

- soft and dry extracts;
- purified (refined), standardized and quantified extracts; and
- single chemical entities.

Each of these products has particular advantages and disadvantages.

Liquid extracts are preferred over decoctions (plant boiled with water) and infusions (plant stood in hot or cold water) because of the higher concentration of active constituents in the extract. Liquid extracts are produced by extraction of 1 part of plant material with 1–2 parts of solvent, whilst tinctures require 1 part of plant material with 5–10 parts of solvent. These liquid extracts can be incorporated directly into semisolid formulations such as ointments or into liquid formulations such as drops or solutions (Vlietinck et al., 2009).

The choice of extract type depends on the intended application: dry extracts (liquid extracts that have subsequently been dried) are suitable for tablet/capsule formulations, whilst solvent extracts are more widely used in liquid formulations.

Purified (refined) and standardized extracts are intermediate between crude extracts and single chemical entities and as such have widespread application. They avoid the need to separate complex mixtures, but provide knowledge of the levels of constituents.

It is important to appreciate that with many plant materials a single chemical entity usually has the greatest activity, although synergistic interactions may increase the activity of complex mixtures.

All types of extracts need to be made with knowledge of the polarity of the targeted constituents, which may impact on the cost of the most appropriate solvent for the process, waste solvent disposal, extract stability, etc. The composition of most end materials is highly dependent on the procedures used for extraction, and often the most valuable constituents are produced by the most sophisticated processes.

Extraction procedures

Table 42.4 lists the types of extraction procedures that are widely used.

Removal of acellular products. This technique is really a collection method specific to a few plant products, but is also classed by some as a method of 'extraction'. As shown in Table 42.4, it is used only for a few specific examples of materials obtained by simple traditional techniques. Although crude in

Table 42.4 Extraction procedures

Technique	Advantage	Disadvantage	Description
Removal of acellular products (unorganized drugs)	Simple	High risk of microbial and extraneous contamination	Traditional plant products, e.g. opium (incision), certain essential oils such as citrus (applying pressure)
Distillation	Suitable for volatile oils		Water or steam diffusion at 100 °C causing volatilization and condensation
Maceration	Simple	Time-consuming, incomplete extraction	Prolonged infusion
Percolation	More concentrated extract	Time-consuming, expensive	Maceration followed by flow of fresh solvent
Countercurrent extraction	Can be used on large scale. Wide array of extractives possible	Often complex operating procedures need to be devised. Costly to run	Separation by bidirectional flow of two immiscible solvents
Supercritical fluid extraction	Main solvent is CO_2, no toxic residue	Costly industrial plant	Supercritical CO_2 plus cosolvent/modifier is forced through plant matrix

design, the products are the commercially available material, and often need highly specialized treatment before their incorporation into formulated products.

Distillation. If the active constituent is a volatile oil, it is most often removed by the process of distillation. Whist this 'extracts' the active constituents, it is not, in a chemical engineering sense (as described earlier), a true extraction process. Three different types of distillation processes are used for the removal of volatile oils from plant material:

Water distillation. The raw material and water are heated to boiling and oil is collected. This technique is slow, produces poor-quality oil and is labour-intensive.

Water and steam distillation. This involves direct contact between steam and raw material. Plant material is held above, not in, the water present for steam generation.

Steam distillation. This involves direct contact between the steam and raw material. Here the steam is generated externally as opposed to in the still. It is rapid and the rate of distillation is controlled.

Maceration. Maceration involves the steeping of raw material in a solvent, which is later strained out. It is widely used for the preparation of tinctures, but is very inefficient for the collection of solutes.

Percolation. Percolation involves the subjection of raw material to continuous flow of fresh solvent. This produces stronger extracts but at increased solvent cost. Repeated percolation with use of a number of extractors with solution percolates (solvent already containing extracted components) partially decreases the problem.

Countercurrent extraction. Countercurrent extraction is effected by continuous distribution of solutes from raw material between moving tubes of immiscible upper and lower phases (basically a series of interconnected separating funnels). This gives increased extraction yields, but the equipment is expensive and lengthy extraction times are needed for the best results.

Newer extraction techniques. A number of alternative techniques can be used in laboratory conditions. These include:

- supercritical fluid extraction;
- subcritical water extraction, which can be used from 100 °C to 374 °C under pressure;
- sonication-assisted extraction;
- microwave-assisted extraction, which is used for fast, selective heating of raw material in solvent, and removes the need for prior drying of material; and
- Phytol/Florasol extraction using hydrofluoroalkane 134a performed at −26 °C, which is useful for thermolabile materials (Oztekin & Martinov, 2007).

The supercritical fluid extraction technique involves elevating the temperature and pressure of the solvent above its critical point. It is now widely used in industrial-scale procedures. Supercritical CO_2 is a good solvent for nonpolar compounds but not for most plant compounds with biological activity (notably alkaloids, glycosides and phenolics), which are polar. For these, a cosolvent or modifier must be added to the CO_2. Industrial processes have been reported for naringin, colchicine and oleoresins (Wang & Weller, 2006).

Choice of extraction technique

Usually the method of choice is determined by the size of the batch of plant material to be extracted. Solvent extraction may include risks of toxicity when particular solvents are used.

The solubility of plant entities determines the choice of the best medium, but this is usually fixed by formulation constraints, resulting in either partial or complete lack of solubility. This problem is confounded by extracts containing ranges of chemicals of differing solubilities (Bonati, 1980). Alternative solvents may result in lower solute recoveries; therefore, cosolvents may be added to polar solvents to increase recovery.

Concentration, purification and drying of extracts

Concentration of extracts

Liquid extracts typically contain 2% to 5% of the plant constituents, and further concentration by evaporation is required. The Roberts concentrator was once commonly used but it is slow and inefficient. It is being replaced by either the descending film concentrator or the plate concentrator, both of which are fast acting and thus reduce the risk of degradation. If water is the solvent, no solvent recovery is required, although some degree of clean-up may be necessary before disposal. With other solvents, evaporated solvent must be collected by condensation under cooled conditions and the collection vessel must be enclosed to avoid evaporative losses.

Purification of extracts

Following concentration of the original extracts, further purification is often required. A number of procedures are available to remove extraneous plant material or undesirable material formed during extraction. These include decantation, pressure filtration, vacuum filtration, centrifugation and drying.

Many extracts are sticky because they are hygroscopic, and this causes processing problems. A number of crude plant drugs may need to undergo preliminary treatment such as defatting to avoid high fat levels in the extract, or enzyme inactivation to avoid degradation of active constituents (Bonati, 1991).

Drying of extracts

After purification, extracts may be dried, and several types of equipment are available to do this. The range of dryer types available is outlined in Table 42.5 (see Chapter 29 for further details).

Dry extracts have a superior stability profile over time and are likely to have lower levels of microbiological contamination. In addition to this, gamma irradiation can easily be used, if necessary, to eradicate any remaining microbiological contamination.

Table 42.5 Equipment for drying extracts

Type	Comments
Heated tray dryers	Deterioration due to long time in contact with heat, possible risk of oxidation of active constituents, labour-intensive
Cabinet vacuum dryers	Oven temperatures 60 °C to 80 °C, heterogeneous drying, possible risk of oxidation of active constituents, labour-intensive tray layout, uncertain end point
Drum/belt dryers	Evaporation provided by hot air stream, uncertain end point, possible risk of oxidation of active constituents, large-scale possibilities, requires regranulation stage
Atomizers/spray dryers	Lower temperatures used, less time in contact with heat, cheaper than freeze-drying, product in powder form, widely used
Freeze dryers	Low temperature, expensive to buy and operate, high-quality product in layer form, requiring regranulation

Formulation and manufacture of plant-based medicines

Active-constituent considerations

Purity of active constituent(s)

Production and formulation of plant-based medicines involves technology and stability problems far greater than those for single, natural isolated chemicals or synthetic compounds. One major cause of the problem is inclusion of compounds which are either pharmacologically inactive or are active but possess additive, synergistic or even opposite or dissimilar activities. Ideally, these constituents should have been removed during primary production, but this is often unrealistic because of constraints of cost, lack of knowledge of their identities, and technical inability to remove them. Formulation with plant extracts requires complete knowledge of the composition of the extract so that the formulator can choose the most suitable excipients and formulation. Ideally, only one plant extract should be included in any formulation but there are many examples where there are more than one. This may cause formulation problems due to interaction of components of one extract with the components of the other extract(s), causing instability.

The problems associated with converting fresh or dried plant material into medicinal products are highlighted in the third column of Table 42.3. This lists the constraints to producing the best quality products. In addition to these general problems, there are additional problems relating to specific plants and their constituents.

Standardized extracts are essential to get as many of the constituents actually present in the extract (and hence) into the formulation as possible. A number of these constituents are exceedingly unstable (e.g. valepotriates from valerian) when in acidic or basic medium in combination with water. Turbidity of reconstituted solutions is a widespread problem, sometimes dealt with by incorporation of polyvinylpyr-rolidone. Emulsions of particular extracts containing saponins (widespread in plant extracts) are often found to exhibit phase separation (Crippa, 1980)

Drying plant material inactivates endogenous enzymes, but extracts which contain glycosides are then subject to degradation when formulated into aqueous media, as the enzymes are reactivated.

The greatest risk to the quality of constituents is heating during manufacture, but the quality of water is also important. The pH has a major effect on the stability of a number of types or formulations and their active constituents. Both acidic and basic conditions have been shown to have detrimental effects.

As a direct result of these problems, there is a growing trend for manufacturers to substitute single chemical entities derived from the plant extracts, often commercially available, so as to eliminate or at least reduce the possibility of degradation. One example of this is the use of purified sennoside B in place of total sennoside extracts, as is the case in Senokot® preparations.

Variability of crude drug material

Supply of raw material is a major problem, owing to wide-scale variations in composition. Published surveys show that there can be a distinct difference in constituent levels even between batches from the same supplier.

Adulteration (deliberate or accidental substitution of inferior material) has long been a problem with herbal remedies. Traditional quality control procedures have been adopted to detect this situation, with a number of parameters specifically designed to identify the problem of adulteration with inferior material.

With the increased use of herbal remedies, the causes may be more sophisticated; for example attempts to improve the characteristics of the extracts with material not detected by standard assays. Bilberry extracts have been found adulterated with the food dye amaranth added specifically to make their colour appear more intense.

Finished-product considerations

A wide range of typical formulations are widely used for plant extracts, which include most of the types used for conventional pharmaceuticals. Most conventional dosage forms can be produced from plant liquid or dried extracts by conventional techniques.

As with conventional pharmaceuticals, solid dosage forms are the preferred type of formulation, whilst liquids such as syrups are losing favour because of lack of patient acceptability and poor stability during storage. Controlled-release solid dosage forms of plant-based material can also be manufactured.

Preparation of solid dosage forms

Approximately 75% of European herbal medicines are constituted from dry extracts. These dry extracts are invariably hygroscopic. A high-porosity excipient, such as microcrystalline cellulose, is usually added to the formulation, together with a cellulose derivative binder. As is the case with conventional tablets (see Chapter 30), these extra excipients are responsible for improved physical characteristics of the tablets, notably hardness, friability and disintegration, when used in the correct proportions for a particular plant extract (Crippa, 1978).

Freeze-dried extracts have been shown to have far greater solubility than powdered plant material, with a direct effect on bioavailability.

Pharmaceutical parameters, such as flowability and hygroscopicity, can differ widely depending on the source of the raw plant material. Likewise, compactability differs considerably, and all these factors may affect tablet/capsule weights and the levels of active constituents (Jin et al., 2008).

Preparation of liquid dosage forms

Nearly all types of extracts can be used in formulating liquid dosage forms. If dry extracts are used, the material must be redissolved, which may result in precipitation of components or at least the presence of turbidity. To avoid these issues, it is advisable to redissolve the material at precisely the same concentration in the solvent as that which was used to prepare the extract. On some occasions the downstream processing of the initial extract may modify the composition of the extract so that dissolution does not occur, in which case cosolvents or surfactants may need to be added. The solubility and stability of some extracts can be increased by pH manipulation, particularly when reduction favours salt formation for the active constituent, such as in the case of an alkaloid. The stability of these dosage forms is adversely affected by fermentation, which is prone to occur in extracts containing nutritive plant constituents, but this can be reduced by regulation of the alcohol content or by use of traditional preservatives, such as p-hydroxybenzoic acid esters (Bonati, 1991).

Two claimed advantages of plant-based liquid formulations is that they have improved bioavailability, and that unique formulations can be produced for individual patients (Bone, 2003).

Newer delivery systems

Methods used to manufacture liposomes, nanoparticles, phytosomes, emulsions and microspheres from numerous plant extracts are regularly reported in the scientific literature. Liposomes have been produced for markedly different products, including paclitaxel, curcumin, garlic and quercetin.

Herbal medicines are now being formulated and administered via the most up-to-date delivery technologies available. Transferosomes and ethosomes are being used for a range of topical applications. A range of herbal entities have also been formulated into microspheres, as small as 6 μm, which can be ingested or injected and targeted to specific organs of the body (Saraf, 2010).

Numerous applications of novel formulations on the laboratory scale have been published (Saraf, 2010) but there is little evidence of uptake at the commercial manufacturing level from published data.

Excipients

Preservatives. The p-hydroxybenzoic acid esters, such as the methyl and propyl esters (parabens), are widely used. However, in a number of formulations such as herbal cosmetics and external medicaments, bronopol is also widely used. The possibility of manufacturing 'organic products' without addition of preservatives has been commercially exploited in a number of herbal products. This strategy normally results in products having a reduced shelf life.

Antioxidants. The use of antioxidants to limit oxidation in pharmaceuticals and foods is widespread; ascorbate is widely used for this purpose.

Colouring materials. As concerns about the dangers of artificial colours continue worldwide, plant-derived colours are increasingly being used because their use obviates the use of synthetic dyes. An example is turmeric from the roots of *Curcuma longa*, which contains curcuminoids that have a yellow or orange colour. β-Carotene is another example, and is orange-yellow. Commercial β-carotene is derived from algae or is synthesized and is oil soluble, but it can also be made into a water-dispersible emulsion. These natural yellow to orange colours are an alternative to synthetic yellow dyes. Other plant-based colours include anthocyanins and tomato extract, which can produce a range of red colours in place of synthetic red dyes.

The possible use of plant extracts for colouring formulations has been extensively researched for a number of years, but the major problem is that they usually tend to be unstable in varying pH conditions, and are particularly prone to degradation.

Flavours. Plant extracts are often bitter or astringent, and such characteristics are often masked with sweeteners or flavours. Flavours are invariably included in liquid oral formulations to mask these bitter or unpleasant tastes, to improve patient adherence. Apart from volatile oils, which are selectively used for flavouring formulations designed for different patient groups, a wide range of soft fruit flavours, such as banana and strawberry, either natural or synthetic, are also used for flavouring.

Biotechnological production of plant products

A number of major prescription medicines are produced by in vitro techniques. Currently, digoxin, paclitaxel and vincristine, amongst a small number of medicines, are derived from plant cell culture techniques, and commercially manufactured and extracted in a complete 'in-house' procedure. These procedures are excessively expensive, and consequently only products with the highest value can be commercially exploited by plant cell culture.

Because of commercial sensitivity, biotechnology procedures are not published in detail; however, they are similar to those used for whole plant material, without the need for drying and size reduction, but involve simply leaching out the active constituents followed by purification and later formulation as for single chemical entities.

Quality of finished products

Quality of formulated herbal products

Unlike prescription products, there are few agreed standards for formulated herbal remedies. A survey of a large number of herbal products from a range of manufacturers found incorrect/inadequate labelling and products with wide ranging content claims, wide ranging recommended daily dosage, a range of different plant parts used and from a number of claimed sources of botanical origins. Wide ranging values for active constituent content have been reported for parthenolide in feverfew and for the active constituent(s) in, for example, ginseng, gingko, echinacea and St John's wort (Ruparel and Lockwood, 2011). This demonstrates the possible risk to patients and the urgent need for standards (Heptinstall et al., 1992).

Shelf life of formulated products

Labelling of products with the shelf life or expiry date is presently not mandatory for all formulated plant products. Scientific knowledge of degradation and acceptable shelf life is obviously necessary for these complex products. Improved packaging designs are now being used to limit degradation, but control of storage conditions from the warehouse to the point of sale is of major importance. There are a number of difficulties in conducting shelf-life determinations with complex products, and often simplistic parameters are used, such as the colour and consistency of the formulation, in addition to chemical evaluation. Further, detailed real-time and accelerated testing may be performed at specific temperature and humidities, as for conventional pharmaceuticals. These techniques are particularly useful to speed up data collection and for determining suitable formulations (Houghton and Mukherjee, 2009).

Bioequivalence of different formulations

The issue of bioequivalence of different formulations of conventional pharmaceuticals is well researched. However, such information is less detailed when comparing different formulations of plant medicines. Data from a limited number of single-component herbal medicines, showing variable plasma concentrations for each, are available. However, major complications occur when a herbal medicine's activity is derived from a range of components. In this instance, plasma concentrations are often insufficient to determine the levels of activity, and therefore assays for effects on biomarkers are required to show comparative activities of different formulations. Further problems are clearly evident when the active constituents of a plant-based product are unknown, which is often the case (Loew and Kaszkin, 2002).

Adverse effects and drug interactions

The public are slowly appreciating the fact that complementary medicines are not necessarily safe plant products simply because they are 'natural'. An increasing number of potential and actual adverse effects have been reported.

Synergy. Synergy is enhancement of the activity of one constituent by more than simple addition of the two individual activities. The chance of synergy occurring is increasingly likely with these complex products. The degree of synergy will depend on the concentrations of the entities involved; therefore product variability has increased consequences.

Drug interactions. Drug interactions with herbal medicines are poorly researched; however, there is always the possibility that one medicine will react with the active constituents of another, especially when they have marked pharmacological activity. The plants most likely to be involved are those which are metabolized by the cytochrome P450 enzyme system. Echinacea, garlic, cloves, evening primrose oil and soy constituents are examples of the major herbs responsible for these interactions. St John's wort is responsible for the largest amount of data on interactions, and it has proven hepatic enzyme-inducing properties (Williamson et al., 2009).

Summary

This chapter has discussed the use of plant products, featuring conventional and complementary medicines, herbal, homoeopathic and aromatherapy products, and their levels of use and the numerous forms of plants in use.

Production methods used for plant-derived conventional pharmaceuticals and complementary medicines were outlined. Formulation techniques and problems specific to plant products have been discussed.

Please check your eBook at **https://studentconsult. inkling.com/** for self-assessment questions. See inside cover for registration details.

References

Bombardelli, E., 1991. Technologies for the processing of medicinal plants. In: Wijesekera, R.O.B. (Ed.), The Medicinal Plant Industry. CRC Press, Boca Raton.

Bonati, A., 1980. Medicinal plants and industry. J. Ethnopharmacol. 2, 167–171.

Bonati, A., 1991. Formulation of plant extracts into dosage forms. In: Wijesekera, R.O.B. (Ed.), The Medicinal Plant Industry. CRC Press, Boca Raton.

Bone, K., 2003. A Clinical Guide to Blending Liquid Herbs: Herbal Formulations for the Individual Patient. Churchill Livingstone, Edinburgh.

Chaudhri, R.D. (Ed.), 1996. Herbal Drugs Industry. Eastern Publishers, New Delhi.

Crippa, F., 1978. Problems of pharmaceutical techniques with plant extracts. Fitoterapia 49, 257–263.

Crippa, F., 1980. Problems involved in pharmaceutical and cosmetic formulations containing extracts. Fitoterapia 51, 59–66.

Evans, W.C., 2009. Trease and Evans' Pharmacognosy, sixteenth ed. Saunders, Edinburgh.

Heptinstall, S., Awang, D.V.C., Dawson, B.A., et al., 1992. Parthenolide content and bioactivity of feverfew (Tanacetum parthenium (L.) Schultz-Bip.). Estimation of commercial and authenticated feverfew products. J. Pharm. Pharmacol. 44, 391–395.

Houghton, P., Mukherjee, P.K., 2009. Evaluation of Herbal Medicines. Pharmaceutical Press, London.

Jin, P., Madieh, S., Augsburger, L., 2008. Selected physical and chemical properties of Feverfew (Tanacetum parthenium) extracts important for formulated product quality and performance. AAPS PharmSciTech 9, 22–30.

Liang, Y.-Z., Xie, P., Chan, K., 2004. Quality control of herbal medicines. J. Chromatogr. B 812, 53–70.

Loew, D., Kaszkin, M., 2002. Approaching the problem of bioequivalence of herbal medicinal products. Phytother. Res. 16, 705–711.

Oztekin, S., Martinov, M., 2007. Medicinal and Aromatic Crops: Harvesting, Drying and Processing. Haworth Food and Agricultural Products Press, Binghampton.

Ruparel, P., Lockwood, B., 2011. The quality of commercially available herbal products. Nat. Prod. Commun. 6, 1–12.

Saraf, A.S., 2010. Applications of novel drug delivery system for herbal formulations. Fitoterapia 81, 680–689.

Vlietinck, A., Pieters, L., Apers, S., 2009. Legal requirements for the quality of herbal substances and herbal preparations for the manufacturing of herbal medicinal products in the European Union. Planta Med. 75, 683–688.

Wang, L., Weller, C.L., 2006. Recent advances in extraction of nutraceuticals from plants. Trends Food Sci. Technol. 17, 300–312.

Williamson, E.M., Driver, S., Baxter, K., 2009. Stockley's Herbal Medicines Interactions. Pharmaceutical Press, London.

Bibliography

Lockwood, G.B., 2009. Complementary and alternative medicine. In: Rees, J., Smith, I., Wingfield, A.J. (eds.), Pharmaceutical Practice, fourth ed. Churchill Livingstone, Edinburgh.

Delivery of biopharmaceuticals

43

Ijeoma F. Uchegbu   Andreas G. Schätzlein

CHAPTER CONTENTS

KEY POINTS

- Biopharmaceuticals are medicines which contain active agents of biological origin, and the following substances fall into this class: enzymes, monoclonal antibodies, cytokines, haematopoietic blood factors, peptides, genes, small interfering RNA, oligonucleotides, vaccines and carbohydrates.
- Biopharmaceuticals are usually commercially produced in mammalian cell bioreactors, purified by centrifugation and/or filtration and characterized by various spectroscopic, chromatographic and calorimetric techniques
- Biopharmaceuticals have specific formulation and delivery issues: (1) they are easily degraded/ inactivated on storage and (2) they are easily cleared in vivo and thus have difficulty reaching their therapeutic target.
- The delivery strategies for this class of medicines involve the use of polyethylene glycol conjugates to prolong the activity of proteins, polymer matrices to sustain the activity of peptides, vaccine delivery systems and vaccine adjuvants to enhance the prophylactic immune response and viral vectors to deliver gene therapies.

Introduction

Biopharmaceuticals, also known as biologicals or biologics, are medicines in which the active ingredient is derived from a biological (usually nonplant) source (Table 43.1). Vaccines are also considered here, even though they are constituted from whole attenuated/ inactivated organisms, as well as antigen subunits. The biopharmaceutical class of drugs includes proteins and peptides, nucleic acid drugs and carbohydrates (e.g. heparin), all chemical components that exist in nature (Fig. 43.1). There are a few carbohydrate drugs derived from biological sources, with heparin being the most well known, and whilst carbohydrate therapeutics are now being studied more intensely, they will not be treated in detail here because of the paucity of commercial products and information available. Other biopharmaceuticals include cell types such as transplanted stem cells and engineered tissues. Tissues and transplanted cells are beyond the

Table 43.1 Biopharmaceuticals

Biopharmaceutical class	Example
Peptides	Oxytocin
Proteins	
Enzymes	Pancreatic lipase
Monoclonal antibodies	Bevacizumab
Cytokines	Interferon beta-1b
Hormones	Human growth hormone
Haematopoietic growth factors	Epoetin
Vaccines	Diphtheria–pertussis–tetanus vaccine
Nucleic acid drugs	
Genes	Gendicine
Oligonucleotides	Vitravene
Small interfering RNA	No marketed products
Cell-based therapies	Platelets Cytomegalovirus-specific T cells
Carbohydrates	Low molecular weight heparin

scope of this chapter, and the interested reader is recommended to consult the scientific literature for information on tissue engineering and the associated drug delivery issues.

Since the 1990s there has been huge growth in the area of biopharmaceuticals, and this growth is predicted to continue, largely fuelled by the difficulty in identifying small-molecule candidates for the diseases that still have less than optimal treatment regimens or no treatments at all. The biopharmaceuticals market is dominated by three classes of drugs: protein and peptide hormones (e.g. insulin), monoclonal antibodies (e.g. trastuzumab) and vaccines (e.g. the influenza and the diphtheria–pertussis–tetanus vaccines). Other biopharmaceuticals include haematopoietic factors such as erythropoietin (epoetin), cytokines (e.g. the interferons) and enzymes such as the pancreatic enzyme pancrealipase. Gene therapeutics currently constitute only a tiny fraction of the market, in essence limited to three approved products: Gendicine®, marketed in China; Glybera®, approved in Europe; and Oncorine®, approved in Russia. RNA gene silencing agents, commonly known as small interfering RNAs (siRNAs), whilst an area

of active scientific endeavour, are yet to make their market debut.

One aspect that unites these drug molecules is that by and large they are still administered by a syringe and needle, despite the extensive efforts that have been made to deliver these compounds by nonparenteral means. Biopharmaceuticals are largely high molecular mass molecules (>5000 Da), with the exception of the short peptides, and they suffer from instability problems, either on storage or after being administered. These properties make the administration of these compounds by nonparenteral means problematic at best, and usually impossible.

This chapter will serve as an introduction to the delivery issues associated with key members of this class of drugs as well as providing an introduction to the established and emerging delivery solutions.

Protein and peptide drugs

Introduction

Proteins are composed of individual amino acids linked by amide bonds. The 20 essential amino acids (Fig. 43.1) are the constituent parts of proteins. Amino acids are chiral compounds and amino acids of biological origin are L-amino acids. Peptides differ from proteins mainly in the number of amino acids contained within each molecule. The amino acid residue distinction between peptides and proteins is not exact however; for example, *peptides* are defined as having fewer than 50 amino acids, whilst *proteins* usually contain hundreds of amino acids and have a tertiary (folded) structure. However, insulin, with 51 amino acids, is defined as a peptide.

Endogenous proteins are synthesized in the cell in an amino acid sequence that is defined by a specific nucleotide base pair sequence. Following the synthesis of the protein, there is posttranslational modification, including glycosylation and protein folding, to give the functional three-dimensional structure. Endogenous bioactive peptides are also synthesized within the cell and are normally the result of cleavage of larger proteins to give the peptide active. There are a number of therapeutic classes of proteins on the market (Table 43.1). The peptide therapeutic classes mostly comprise peptide hormones such as insulin and calcitonin as well as endogenous peptide analogues such as goserelin.

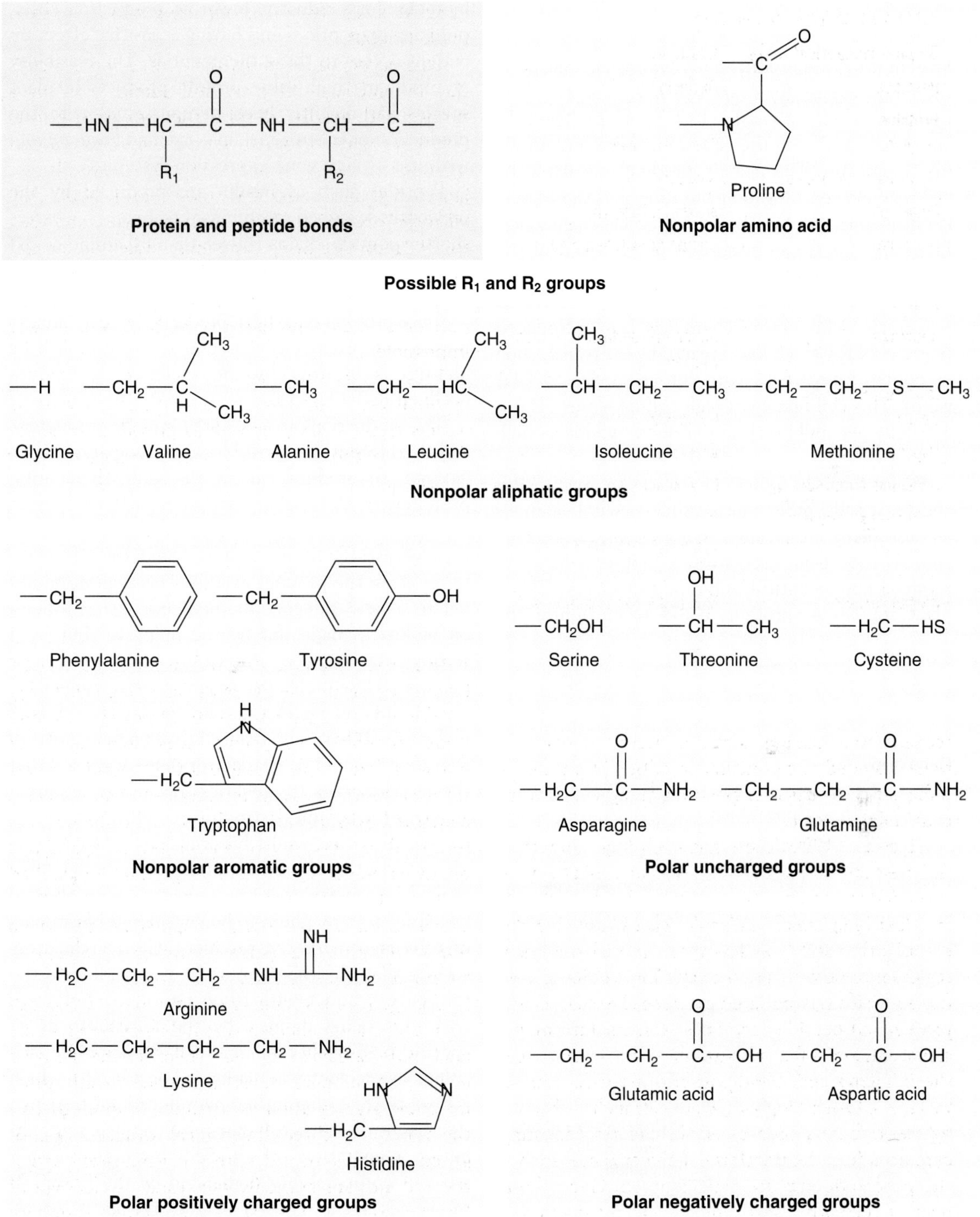

Fig. 43.1 • Amide bonds and amino acids found in proteins and peptides. The molecular structure at the *top left* is the base protein and peptide structure. The other groups shown are possible R_1 and R_2 groups that may be attached to the base structure.

Production

Protein drugs are produced in mammalian cells (e.g. the Chinese hamster ovary cell line), bacteria (e.g. *Escherichia coli*) or yeast cells (Fig. 43.2). The cells are transfected with the gene of interest and grown in a bioreactor. The protein product is isolated by cell lysis and centrifugation/filtration, and the protein itself is purified by chromatographic techniques. Protein yields are an important determinant of the efficiency of the process, and in Chinese hamster ovary cells are approximately 5 g L^{-1}. In an attempt to increase yields, new cell lines have been introduced (e.g. the PER.C6 cell line, created by the transfection of human retinal cells with the adenovirus 5 E1A gene). This cell line gives high cell densities (160 × 10^6 cells per millilitre) and antibody yields as high as 25 g L^{-1}.

Whilst the usual sources of proteins are mammalian and yeast cells, other sources such as whole animals are also being investigated. For example, transgenic animals have been used by GT Biotherapeutics to produce human antithrombin in goat's milk. Cheap plant sources of proteins could revolutionize the

biotechnology industry, lowering production costs, reducing drug prices and having a positive effect on patient access to these therapeutics. The feasibility of producing high-value protein products in plant species has recently been demonstrated with the production of trastuzumab in *Nicotiana benthamiana* with use of viral gene expression systems.

Peptides such as insulin are produced by the previously described recombinant techniques, whereas shorter peptide chains (fewer than 50 amino acids) are synthesized by relatively expensive and laborious solid-phase synthetic techniques.

Once proteins have been produced by recombinant means, the product is characterized to establish its identity and purity by the analytical techniques outlined in Table 43.2.

The production processes are normally proprietary, and therefore it is impossible, once the patents have expired, to produce exactly the same therapeutic protein with identical glycosylation patterns without access to the original bioreactor procedures. It is thus very difficult for a subsequent manufacturer to replicate the product exactly. This realization has led to a new category of medicine – the 'follow-on biologic', made not by the innovator but by a separate manufacturer, after patent expiry, in a similar manner to low molecular weight generic medicines. Such follow-on products are known as biosimilars or biobetters. It was soon realized that a new regulatory framework would be needed for these drugs and that the existing rules for generics specifically requiring an identical chemical structure could not apply. It was decided that whilst biosimilars would never be identical to the reference (innovator) product, they must be *comparable* with respect to a number of key indicators for them to be considered biosimilars of reference marketed products. Hence regulators specify that biosimilars must be comparable to the reference product with respect to clinical efficacy, with this being defined by the measurement of specific high-quality biomarkers. For example, for granulocyte colony stimulating factor (GCSF), which is used to treat chemotherapy-induced neutropenia, a measure of absolute neutrophil count is required before registration of a GCSF biosimilar. Other areas of comparability demanded by the European Medicines Agency (EMA) include preclinical toxicology, pharmacokinetics after a single dose and safety as demonstrated in a clinical trial. As a change in glycosylation pattern could impact on the immune response to the biosimilar, there is also a requirement

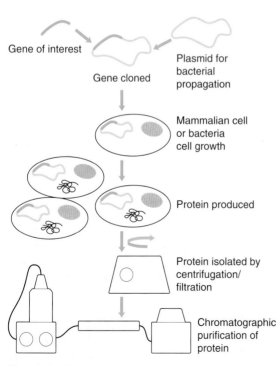

Fig. 43.2 • The production of biopharmaceuticals.

Table 43.2 Protein characterization techniques

Analytical technique	Physical/chemical basis of the technique	Protein characterization
Sodium dodecyl sulfate–polyacrylamide gel electrophoresis (SDS-PAGE) analysis – a qualitative evaluation of molecular weight against molecular weight markers	Separates proteins according to their electrophoretic mobility and molecular weight	Provides a qualitative evaluation of protein molecular weight and detects proteolysis and dimerization impurities
Isoelectric focusing	Separates proteins according to their charge, as a function of pH	Characterizes the homogeneity of the protein product
Capillary zone electrophoresis	Separates proteins according to hydrodynamic radius, friction and charge	Characterization of glycosylation patterns
Size-exclusion chromatography plus light scattering	Separates proteins according to hydrodynamic radius and measures molecular weight	Determines protein molecular weight
High-performance liquid chromatography	Separates molecules according to polarity and quantifies protein levels	Demonstrates protein purity and used to analyse impurity levels
Spectroscopic methods: nuclear magnetic resonance spectroscopy; ultraviolet absorption spectroscopy; circular dichroism infrared spectroscopy	Record electronic and molecular transitions in response to electromagnetic energy	Primary structure from nuclear magnetic resonance spectroscopy Reference material characteristics (e.g. from the infrared fingerprint region) Secondary structure from circular dichroism and infrared spectroscopy
Liquid chromatography–mass spectrometry	Separation according to hydrophobic–hydrophilic balance and the detection of mass fragments	Peptide mapping
Differential scanning calorimetry	Measures the enthalpy change of protein thermal transitions (e.g. protein folding)	Data on protein stability
Epitope mapping	Identifies antibody binding sites on a protein – these may be linear peptide epitopes or conformational epitopes arising from protein folding Requires synthesis of the epitope followed by binding studies	Measures efficacy and immunogenicity

for immunogenicity testing for all biosimilars and the obligation for the manufacturer to instigate a pharmacovigilance programme after marketing. These stringent requirements are borne out of the recently witnessed immunogenic reaction to epoetin alfa, in which epoetin alfa caused pure red cell aplasia when human serum albumin in the original formulation was removed and replaced with polysorbate 80 and glycine as stabilizers.

Several biosimilars have been introduced in India and Europe; the biosimilars currently available in Europe are listed in Table 43.3. In Europe, biosimilars are currently not interchangeable with the reference product, a fact that limits their market penetration.

Delivery issues

The delivery issues surrounding protein and peptide drugs are divided into two main categories: (1) maintenance of stability on storage and (2) the optimization of in vivo efficacy. Storage stability issues may be classified according to the chemical and physical origins of protein instability. Of the chemical origins of protein instability, deamination (Fig. 43.3) is arguably the most intensely studied and occurs with the most frequency. Deamination is the result of base-catalysed hydrolysis of asparagine (usually) and glutamine side chain amides to give aspartic acid and glutamic acid respectively. The reaction

Table 43.3 Biosimilars available in Europe

Therapeutic	Biosimilar	Biosimilar manufacturer	Reference product	Reference product manufacturer
Human growth hormone	Omnitrope Valropin	Sandoz Biopartners	Genotropin	Pfizer
Epoetin	Abseamed Retacrit Binocrit Epoetin alfa Hexal Silapo	Medice Arzneimittel Pütter Hospira Sandoz Hexal Biotech STADA Arzneimittel	Eprex	Janssen-Cilag
Granulocyte colony stimulating factor	Filagrastim Hexal Biogarastim Nevestim Zarzio Ratiograstim and filagrastim Tevagrastim	Hexal Biotech CT Arzneimittel Hospira Sandoz Ratiopharm Teva Pharma	Neupogen	Amgen

Adapted from Dranitsaris et al. (2011).

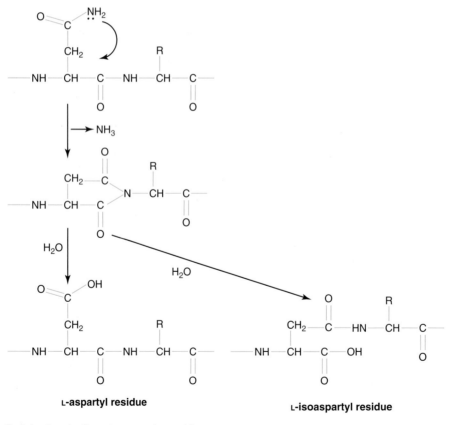

Fig. 43.3 • Protein deamination at asparagine residues.

mechanism, which proceeds via the five-membered cyclic ring, is the more prevalent mechanism, and the loss of ammonia on cyclization effectively makes the process irreversible. On deamination of asparagine, both aspartic acid and L-isoaspartic acid are formed.

Peptide bond hydrolysis is also a source of instability, and this occurs at aspartic acid and tryptophan sites and the hinge region of antibodies. Racemization of amino acids to convert them from the L-form to the nonnatural D-form also occurs at aspartic acid residues. Additionally, base-catalysed nucleophilic-attack-mediated amine-terminal cyclization to give diketopiperazine groups, occasionally with the loss of the first two amino acids, or an amine-terminal attack on the side chain of glutamic acid groups to produce a cyclic pyroglutamic acid residue are both promoted at basic pH. Oxidation of proteins by reactive oxygen species occurs at histidine, methionine, cysteine, tyrosine and tryptophan residues, and disulfide bond formation between cysteine residues is also a source of protein chemical instability. Base-catalysed protein degradation may be controlled by storage at acid pH (pH 3–6).

Care must be taken when one is selecting excipients for protein formulations as glycation of proteins may occur if proteins are placed in contact with reducing sugars, the net result being the reaction of a side chain lysine with the reducing sugar to form a Schiff's base – the Maillard reaction. Hence protein stabilization with sugars should not be attempted using reducing sugars.

Proteins are also susceptible to physical instabilities. From a physical instability perspective, proteins are prone to denature (alter their native secondary or tertiary structure) on exposure to heat, extremes of pH or organic solvents. One of the most important challenges associated with protein formulation is to prevent protein aggregation in solution. Protein aggregation to form non-native aggregates, whilst not completely understood, is known to be mediated by either hydrophobic attraction between the less polar parts of the protein molecule or covalent bonding between two protein molecules. Partial unfolding to reveal hydrophobic faces has been implicated in protein aggregation, and hence methods which stabilize the protein in its native state prevent protein aggregation. The administration of non-native aggregates is undesirable, as protein aggregates are known, specifically, to provoke an unwanted immune response, as well as to compromise the efficacy of the drug.

When one is optimizing the in vivo efficacy of proteins, the source of poor in vivo efficacy must first be thoroughly understood. One major source of

poor efficacy is the actual protein/peptide chemical structure. Protein and peptide drugs are composed of hydrolysable bonds (Fig. 43.1) and are generally large molecules (molecular masses greater than 1000 Da). Proteins have molecular masses of tens of thousands of daltons, and peptides usually have molecular masses of 1000 Da to 5000 Da. These molecules are highly water soluble, and the combination of a high molecular weight, high propensity for degradation and hydrophilic character means that these molecules have difficulty traversing biological, lipid-rich membranes (Fig. 43.4), such as those found in the gastrointestinal tract and brain capillary endothelial cells. There are certain delivery routes that are precluded because proteins are easily hydrolysed, and the oral delivery of proteins is not currently a possibility.

Whilst there has been a huge effort aimed at making peptides orally active, there are only two oral peptide drugs on the market, and both are cyclic peptides: ciclosporin and desmopressin, with desmopressin having unnatural amino acids. Cyclisation, unnatural amino acids and/or deamination undoubtedly makes these peptides less susceptible to gut aminopeptidases and carboxypeptidases.

Delivery of proteins to the brain by intravenous administration is not currently a clinical reality. Other delivery routes that have been attempted include the nasal route, which is useful experimentally for delivering peptides to the brain and has been used commercially for the systemic (not specifically brain-targeted) delivery of calcitonin, a 32-amino acid peptide used to treat osteoporosis. However, the dose volumes via this route are limited to approximately 150 µL, and a dose of approximately 25 mg is the upper limit (see Chapter 38). Despite these limitations, the exploitation of the nose-to-brain route of

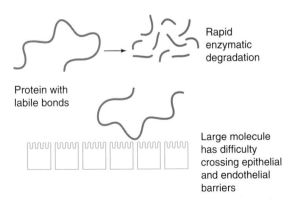

Rapid enzymatic degradation

Protein with labile bonds

Large molecule has difficulty crossing epithelial and endothelial barriers

Fig. 43.4 • The poor transport of proteins and peptides across biological membranes.

Table 43.4 Intravenous plasma half-lives of some therapeutic proteins

Protein	Plasma half-life following intravenous administration (h)
Arginine deaminase	2.8
Granulocyte colony stimulating factor	1.8
Human growth hormone	0.34
Interferon alfa-2a	0.7
Interferon beta-1a	0.98
Interferon beta-1b	1.1
Interleukin-6	0.05
Tumour necrosis factor alpha	0.07

Adapted from Veronese (2009).

administration cannot be ruled out, because there is a real therapeutic unmet need to deliver biopharmaceuticals to the brain.

Even when injected parenterally (e.g. intravenously) therapeutic proteins are cleared rapidly from the blood (Table 43.4), and this rapid clearance adversely affects the therapeutic outcomes. A further delivery challenge for therapeutic proteins in particular is their immunogenicity, whereby proteins generate neutralizing antibodies, which make subsequent doses of the drug ineffective.

Delivery systems

Protein stabilization

The formulation of proteins and peptides involves prevention of chemical degradation and enhancement of in vivo activity. To prevent chemical degradation a low pH is preferred (pH 3–6) as this limits the reactivity of nucleophiles. Nucleophilic attack leads to deamination or amine-terminal cyclization. Furthermore, drying, especially freeze-drying, may be used to stabilize proteins against a variety of degradative influences (e.g. hydrolytic peptide bond cleavage and protein unfolding), although on freeze-drying, cryoprotectants such as trehalose and sucrose must be added to the protein formulation to replace the hydrogen bonding of the protein that is lost on removal of water. To prevent oxidative damage, limiting access to oxygen is an obvious step, and this is achieved by reduction of the head space

in the final vial. Additionally, metal chelating agents (e.g. ethylenediaminetetraacetic acid) may be added to prevent metal-catalysed oxidation. Various sugars (e.g. trehalose and sucrose) have proven effective in preventing protein denaturation (protein unfolding). Protein aggregation may also be prevented by the inclusion of various sugars, glycerol, arginine and urea, and although the mechanism of action of these stabilizers is not entirely clear, they appear to prevent the interprotein interaction of protein hydrophobic faces. Such hydrophobic faces may be exposed on protein unfolding, and there is evidence that polyols such as glycerol preferentially bind to the exposed hydrophobic faces, preventing interprotein binding.

Protein delivery

Protein therapeutics are formulated with a number of excipients. As an illustrative example, the antiangiogenic monoclonal antibody bevacizumab is formulated with trehalose (a cryoprotectant and preventer of aggregation), phosphate buffer (for pH maintenance) and polysorbate 20 (for stabilization against interaction with surfaces, unfolding and aggregation).

Protein therapeutics are administered parenterally, usually intravenously, although sometimes subcutaneously or intramuscularly. Other nonparenteral routes, such as the nasal route and the pulmonary route, have also been attempted. There have been reports of the experimental administration of human growth hormone via the nasal route and interferon alfa via the pulmonary route; proteins are not administered via the oral route. Following intravenous administration, pharmaceutical proteins are generally rapidly cleared from the blood with short plasma half-lives (Table 43.4).

One method of prolonging the circulation time of proteins is by the use of polyethylene glycol (PEG) conjugation. Conjugation of PEG to the protein therapeutic typically reduces the activity of the protein but markedly extends the biological half-life of the protein and in essence extends its duration of action, leading to longer dosing intervals. For example, the activity of pegylated human growth hormone is reduced by 75% when compared with that of the native hormone but its intravenous half-life is increased 30-fold from 20 minutes to 10 hours. It is widely accepted that PEG acts by increasing the protein's molecular volume above the glomerular filtration threshold of approximately 122 nm^3 or 40 kDa, increasing the molecular volume substantially. For example, the conjugation of haemoglobin to two chains of intermediate molecular mass PEG (10 kDa) or two chains of higher molecular mass PEG (20 kDa) results in a molecular volume of 712 nm^3 or 1436 nm^3 respectively. PEG conjugation also reduces the immunogenicity of therapeutic proteins such as interferon beta-1b and recombinant human erythropoietin (epoetin) and masks sensitive degradation sites, preventing premature degradation. Several PEG conjugates are available commercially, including PEG-asparaginase, PegIntron® (interferon alfa-2b) and Pegasys® (interferon alfa-2a).

Whilst intravenous delivery of proteins is the norm, to increase patient adherence a subcutaneous formulation of trastuzumab has been developed in which the monoclonal antibody was formulated with recombinant human hyaluronidase to enable the subcutaneous administration of a comparatively large volume (5 mL).

Antibody–drug conjugates

Antibodies covalently bound to highly potent therapeutic active ingredients are a new class of therapeutic: the antibody–drug conjugate. Kadcyla® is an example of such an antibody–drug conjugate, and is formed by the covalent linkage of trastuzumab, a monoclonal antibody targeting human epidermal receptor 2 (HER2) on tumour cells, with emtansine. This new therapeutic enables the targeting of emtansine to tumours that are positive for HER2.

Peptide delivery

Peptides, containing 2–50 amino acid residues, are largely administered parenterally, although there are a few products on the market in which peptides are administered via the nasal route (e.g. calcitonin nasal spray – 32 amino acids), and an inhalation product, Afrezza®, has been approved for the pulmonary administration of insulin.

For the past 3 decades there has been a huge focus on alternative forms of insulin delivery because of the increasing prevalence of type II diabetes and the desirability of noninvasive means of administering insulin. It is estimated that there are 366 million people with diabetes worldwide, and all insulin-dependent diabetes patients administer their insulin, or their insulin is administered, via parenteral routes. There have been hundreds of studies examining the feasibility of delivering insulin via the oral route, but there are no commercially available insulin oral dosage forms. Insulin is administered subcutaneously in fast-acting

and long-acting forms. Insulin is composed of A and B chains. Rapidly acting insulin (Novolog®) contains a mutation in the B28 proline, which is replaced with an aspartic acid residue; this prevents insulin from forming hexamers because of charge repulsion, allowing the monomers to be rapidly absorbed. Long-acting insulin (e.g. Levemir®) is prepared by a decrease of the solubility of insulin such that insulin forms a depot. With Levemir, this is achieved by the conjugation of a C_{14} fatty acid chain to the B29 amino acid residue and the omission of threonine; the net result is that the molecules associate with albumin and have prolonged activity. An alternative method of reducing insulin's solubility involves the substitution of amino acids, such that insulin achieves its isoelectric point at neutral pH and forms an insoluble depot when injected subcutaneously, e.g. insulin glargine (Lantus®), where the A21 glycine is substituted for asparagine and a further two arginines are added to the carboxy terminal of the B chain.

An inhalable form of insulin has now been approved, marketed as Afrezza®. In this formulation, insulin is stabilized on porous inhalable 2 μm to 3 μm fumaryl diketopiperazine crystals, with insulin adsorbed on the surface (Technosphere® technology). The insulin particles have a high surface area, are deposited in the deep lung and dissolve in the lung, allowing insulin to diffuse across the alveolar epithelium. The formulation has a time to maximum plasma concentration (t_{max}) of 15 minutes, and therapeutic levels are maintained for 3 hours; hence the formulation is suitable for controlling postprandial glucose levels and is superior, in this regard, to subcutaneous insulin, which has t_{max} of 2 hours.

Long-acting peptides are required in certain disease states, such as for the treatment of prostate cancer via chemical castration. In this therapeutic regimen, a luteinizing hormone releasing hormone agonist, goserelin, needs to be administered for several weeks to achieve its therapeutic effect. Initial doses of goserelin lead to an increase in plasma testosterone levels. These elevated testosterone levels ultimately create a negative feedback loop within 14–21 days and eventually diminished levels of testosterone are achieved, a process termed chemical castration. The mechanism of action of goserelin is best suited to a long-acting formulation. Goserelin is hence formulated within poly(DL-lactide-co-glycolide) microspheres (see Chapter 44) as a 1-month or 3-month depot, known commercially as Zoladex®. The 1-month formulation contains 3.6 mg goserelin in a poly(DL-lactide-co-glycolide) matrix consisting of 50% lactide and 50%

glycolide, whilst the 3-month depot contains 10.8 mg goserelin in a poly(DL-lactide-*co*-glycolide) matrix consisting of 95% lactide and 5% glycolide. The higher level of the less soluble lactide in the 3-month depot formulation ensures that matrix erosion/degradation and drug release occur at a slower rate.

Vaccines

Introduction

Vaccines are administered prophylactically to patients to protect against infectious diseases. Mass immunization programmes at the start of the 20th century coupled with access to clean water and the invention of antibiotics have had the most profound effect on human health ever witnessed. UK death rates from infectious diseases fell from a high of 300 deaths per 100 000 population in 1917 to a low of 4 deaths per 100 000 population in 2010. Smallpox has been eradicated by vaccination, and the disease burden for

a number of infectious diseases has been significantly reduced in the United States (US). For example, the number of US cases of diphtheria, pertussis, tetanus, measles, rubella and mumps were all reduced in the 21st century from their peak levels in the 20th century by 99.95%, 98.2%, 98.34%, 99.99%, 99.97% and 99.86% respectively. Additionally, polio is all but eradicated in the Western Hemisphere. Vaccination is thus undeniably a success story.

Vaccines consist of antigens, which activate the immune system, produce antibodies against the antigen and induce immunological memory, enabling the immune system to recognize and destroy specific pathogens if it is exposed to the pathogenic molecules a second time (Fig. 43.5). There are three types of vaccines: live organisms, which have been attenuated to ensure that they do not cause disease; inactivated vaccines (inactivated by heat or chemical means); and subunit vaccines.

Prophylaxis against disease stems from innate and adaptive immune responses. The innate immune response is rapid and nonspecific, and is a response

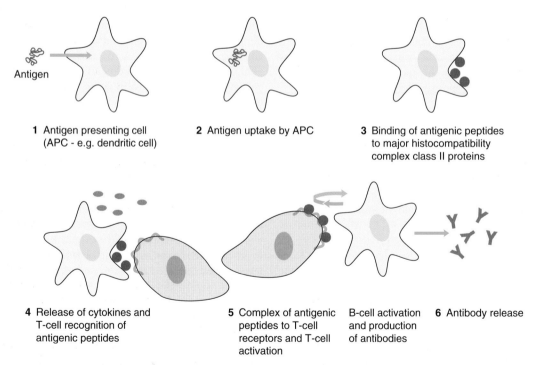

1 Antigen presenting cell (APC - e.g. dendritic cell)

2 Antigen uptake by APC

3 Binding of antigenic peptides to major histocompatibility complex class II proteins

4 Release of cytokines and T-cell recognition of antigenic peptides

5 Complex of antigenic peptides to T-cell receptors and T-cell activation

B-cell activation and production of antibodies

6 Antibody release

Fig. 43.5 • Vaccines generate an immune response by being taken up by antigen-presenting cells (APCs) such as dendritic cells, the activation and expansion of T cells by the antigenic peptide–major histocompatibility complex class II interactions and the expansion and antibody production by B cells. There is also stimulation of the innate immune response by the vaccine, which results in the release of cytokines; this cytokines release is required for the activation of T cells.

to pathogen-associated molecular patterns (PAMPs) on a vaccine or pathogen via pattern recognition receptors (PRRs) on antigen-presenting cells (APCs). The most studied PRRs are the Toll-like receptors. The innate immune response involves an activation of the immune system, the removal of foreign cells and proteins and an activation of the adaptive immune response. This early immune response provides a rapid and generic defence against threats and is vital for the initiation of the adaptive and longer-lasting immune response, which leads to immunological memory and to the antigen-specific removal of the pathogen. On application, vaccines are taken up by APCs, the most abundant of which are the dendritic cells. The antigenic peptides are then presented on the major histocompatibility complex class II proteins of the APCs and there is recognition of this complex by the T cells bearing T-cell receptors, which bind the complex. The result is T-cell activation and expansion. The release of costimulatory molecules and cytokines as part of the innate immune response also contributes to the activation of T cells. T-cell activation is followed by B-cell activation and expansion and the release of antibodies specific for the antigen. The mechanism by which vaccines stimulate an immune response has largely informed the development of vaccine delivery systems.

Production

Bacterial vaccines are grown in bioreactors, whilst viral vaccines are produced in fertilized chicken eggs, although there has recently been a move towards the manufacture of viral vaccines in mammalian cell lines such as the Madin–Darby canine kidney (MDCK) cell line. When viral vaccines are grown in MDCK cells, there is initially cell multiplication, followed by viral infection. The virus is taken up by the cell and the viral genomic material enters the nucleus, where multiple copies of the virus are produced; the virus then infects other cells, and when viral titres are sufficient, the viruses are harvested. Once the viral or bacterial vaccine has been harvested, it is inactivated by chemical methods or heat, before formulation. Alternatively, vaccine recombinant subunits are grown in host mammalian cells, by insertion of the gene for the antigen into bacterial, yeast or mammalian cells and the growing of multiple copies of the antigen. Subunit vaccines, e.g. the hepatitis B vaccine or the human papillomavirus vaccine (which consists of the viral capsid devoid of genetic material), are usually composed of the viral antigenic coat proteins. The antigen is isolated from the cells by ultracentrifugation and chromatographic means.

Delivery issues

The foremost delivery challenge surrounding vaccines is the maintenance of the cold chain (from manufacture to administration) to prevent antigen degradation and ensure potency. It is also desirable to prevent unwanted bacterial growth and to ensure a sufficiently high and prolonged immune response, as this will reduce the number of vaccination events. With subunit vaccines, it is necessary to present the antigenic proteins in particulate form to enable efficient uptake by APCs.

Delivery systems

Most multiple-use vaccines contain a preservative such as the mercury compound thiomersal. Vaccines may also contain antibiotics to prevent unwanted bacterial contamination and stabilizers such as 2-phenoxy esters. Furthermore, as stated already, all vaccines must be stored in a continuous cold chain to maintain antigen potency. This is a requirement, and this need for refrigeration contributes significantly to the costs of vaccine distribution and prevents low-resource communities from accessing vaccines. To circumvent the considerable expense associated with the maintenance of a cold chain, researchers have prepared vaccine–sugar glasses in which a vaccine is mixed with trehalose and sucrose and dried on a membrane to be hydrated when required.

To produce vaccines with a prolonged and enhanced immune response, huge efforts have been put into designing vaccine formulations. Vaccine formulation excipients may work in one or both of two ways: as delivery systems which present the antigen to APCs, and as adjuvants or immunopotentiators which stimulate innate immunity and ensure T-cell activation. Particulate vaccine delivery systems such as emulsions, liposomes and virosomes enable the subunit vaccines to be presented in a particle as it would be if it were still part of an infectious organism, allowing the antigen to then be taken up by APCs. Immunopotentiators include the imidazoquinolones, which have been shown to enhance the immune response in preclinical studies, and the potassium aluminium salts (e.g. $KAl(SO_4)_2 \cdot 12H_2O$, commonly known as alum), which are adjuvants which stimulate dendritic cells to release cytokines. Alum is licensed for human use as an adjuvant, as are the microemulsions MS59 and AS03, which both contain squalene as the oil and have been used in influenza and avian influenza vaccines respectively. Both these microemulsions potentiate the immune response.

There are various innovative approaches to vaccine delivery, one of which is the dry vaccine formulation mentioned earlier. A second innovation is intradermal vaccination using microneedles; this offers the two advantages of painless delivery and the ability to vaccinate large populations rapidly. Microneedles, which are 500 μm to 750 μm long, deliver their cargo into the epidermis or just below it and do not penetrate to the nerve endings, making the injection painless. The pores formed on insertion of the microneedles into the epidermis rapidly and painlessly reseal on withdrawal of the microneedles. Microneedles may be fabricated from solid, hollow or dissolvable materials; dissolvable microneedles have been fabricated from maltose and amylopectin. These devices, if adopted, could greatly change the way in which populations are vaccinated as they may be used for mass vaccination in the event of a pandemic, with patients vaccinating themselves in their own homes, having received the vaccines by post.

Nucleic acid drugs

Introduction

Nucleic acid based drugs fall into three classes: antisense oligonucleotides, siRNAs and genes. DNA is the constituent material of genes and RNA is the constituent material of messenger and transfer RNA. These nucleic acids consist of double-stranded chains of nucleotides (Fig. 43.6). Genes are an information repository for the cell and organism, containing genetic information which is established at conception. Genes are usually faithfully copied during the billions of cell division events that occur throughout a lifetime. However, a number of diseases may be traced to the mutation of various genes and thus have a genetic basis. Mutations may be present at conception or may occur later, e.g. as a result of environmental pollutants, such as those contained in tobacco smoke, or following excessive exposure to the sun's ultraviolet radiation. Genes give rise to the cell's proteins via transcription (messenger RNA synthesis) and translation – protein synthesis

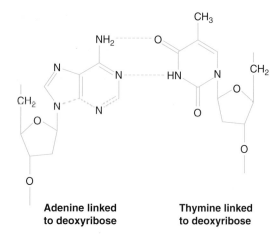

Adenine linked to deoxyribose   **Thymine linked to deoxyribose**

Fig. 43.6 • DNA is composed of four bases (adenine, thymine, guanine and cytosine) all arranged as base pairs, with adenine linked by hydrogen bonds to thymine (indicated by the *dotted lines*) and guanine (not shown) linked by hydrogen bonds to cytosine (not shown). The bases are, in turn, linked via a phosphodiester bond, e.g. linking the 3′ hydroxy group of deoxyribose to the 5′ hydroxy group of the adjacent deoxyribose molecule.

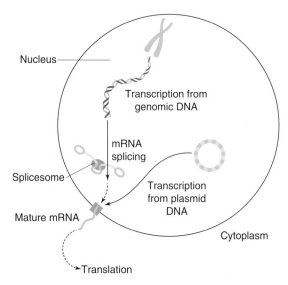

Fig. 43.7 • Gene transcription and translation to produce a functional protein. *mRNA*, messenger RNA.

(Fig. 43.7); proteins are the functional components of the cell. Gene mutations will thus alter the resulting protein, and such alterations may lead to disease. Disease-linked gene mutations, as in cystic fibrosis, result in a nonfunctioning protein – the nonfunctioning cystic fibrosis transmembrane regulator. The mutated cystic fibrosis transmembrane regulator gives rise to poor ion and fluid transport across membranes and specifically the poor-quality lung function observed in cystic fibrosis patients. Theoretically, gene therapy may be used to replace a mutated gene and thus achieve a functioning protein. However, gene replacement therapy is not straightforward as delivery vectors are required to achieve the gene therapy goal. Proof of this therapeutic concept has been demonstrated in humans via the licensed gene medicine Gendicine®. Gendicine contains wild-type p53 to replace mutated p53 in cancer cells and is delivered in an adenoviral vector.

Oligouncleotides, e.g. fomivirsen (Vitravene®), are single-stranded chains of nucleotides which inhibit translation, and in the case of fomivirsen, inhibit translation of viral messenger RNA, thus providing a treatment for cytomegalovirus ocular infections. Small interfering RNA (siRNA) sequences inhibit translation by combining with the RNA-induced silencing complex (RISC) to selectively and specifically cause the hydrolytic degradation of messenger RNA. The RISC precursor complex (~250 kDa) is transformed in the presence of adenosine triphosphate into the active 100 kDa complex that cleaves the substrate messenger RNA in regions homologous to the siRNA template. Small interfering RNA (siRNA) therapies are still largely experimental, and there are no siRNA therapeutics on the market at present.

Production

For genes to be used as therapeutics there is an absolute requirement for a delivery system. The three approved gene therapeutics (Gendicine®, Glybera® and Oncorine®) are delivered by viral vectors. Gendicine, which is delivered in an adenovirus vector, is produced as a viral particle. The Gendicine adenovirus consists of an E1 gene deleted adenoviral vector, with E1 gene deletion necessary to prevent replication. The adenovirus is produced in SBN-Cells, which supply the E1 proteins, necessary for replication. As there are some limitations associated with viral vectors for gene therapy, notable amongst these being their limited use as systemic therapeutics, a number of studies have looked at the development of synthetic vectors. If synthetic (chemical compound) vectors are used for gene therapy, the gene product is delivered as a bacterial plasmid. Plasmids containing the gene of interest are grown in *Escherichia coli* cell lines and purified by cell lysis, filtration, chromatographic separation and centrifugation.

Small interfering RNA (siRNA) and oligonucleotides are synthesized chemically, with many companies offering custom synthesis for particular siRNA or oligonucleotide sequences.

Delivery issues

The main delivery issues surrounding nucleic acid drugs are (1) poor plasma stability of DNA, siRNA and oligonucleotides and (2) the inability of a large polar (negatively charged at physiological pH) molecule such as DNA or even double-stranded siRNA to cross the lipid-rich plasma cell membrane. A further issue surrounding DNA delivery is that therapeutic DNA must gain entry to the cell nucleus to produce its therapeutic product, the functional protein. Entry to the nucleus is limited largely to cell division events. These delivery issues mean that gene and siRNA therapeutics have an absolute requirement for a delivery system.

Delivery systems

The delivery of genes in commercial gene therapies has so far been achieved with use of viruses, despite the fact that one-third of the more than 2000 gene therapy trials conducted to date used synthetic (nonviral) vectors or no vectors at all. Gendicine, the world's first gene therapeutic and currently only licensed for use in China, comprises the wild-type p53 gene within an E1 gene deleted adenovirus for the treatment of head and neck cancers. This replication-incompetent virus performs a mutation compensation function and is administered intratumorally. The need for intratumoral injections is a severe limitation of the therapy as it may not be easily used to treat metastatic cancers. Patients receive one injection per week for 4–8 weeks, and each injection consists of 10^{12} viral particles in 1 mL of water for injections containing glycerol (to maintain tonicity).

Normally p53 is upregulated in cancer cells and causes cell apoptosis, antiangiogensis, an activation of an antitumour immune response and a downregulation of the expression of the multidrug resistance genes. However, p53 is mutated in 50% to 70% of human tumours. On intratumoral administration of Gendicine, the adenovirus enters the cancer cell via the Coxsackie virus and adenovirus receptor and the cell then begins to overexpress wild-type p53, causing apoptosis. Gendicine is effective only when administered alongside radiotherapy.

Glybera is the first gene therapeutic to be approved in the European Union. The drug is indicated for the treatment of lipoprotein lipase deficiency, a rare disease in which patients present with hyperlipidemia and pancreatitis, the latter of which is fatal. The lipoprotein lipase gene is delivered by an adeno-associated virus vector. Administration of Glybera is problematic and requires intramuscular administration to 30–70 sites at any one time.

Viral delivery systems for gene therapy have had a turbulent history, with the high-profile death of an otherwise healthy patient in one adenovirus gene therapy trial, and patients developing leukaemia, stemming from insertional mutagenesis, in a trial involving ex vivo retroviral gene therapy for the treatment of severe combined immunodeficiency syndrome. As a result, a number of synthetic gene vectors have been explored, using poly(propylenimine) dendrimers, poly(ethylenimine) polymers, liposomes and naked DNA. Good preclinical efficacy (tumour regression) data have been obtained with the poly(propylenimine) dendrimer gene therapy system.

The delivery of siRNA has been accomplished clinically with a cyclodextrin-based nanoparticle carrier covered with PEG. Gene silencing of the M2 subunit of ribonuclease reductase was achieved in human melanoma tissue in this pivotal human study.

Summary

Biopharmaceuticals (peptides, proteins, vaccines and nucleic acid medicines) are varied in chemical structure but have in common the presence of labile covalent bonds that are prone to hydrolysis either on storage or following administration. A further factor confounding the long-term stability of these medicines is the functional tertiary structure of the protein class of molecules, a structure that is prone to unfolding at extremes of temperature or pH or in the presence of various chemical agents, such as metal ions. Stabilization of the functional protein entity on storage requires a fundamental understanding of the instability profile (e.g. the underlying mechanisms of protein unfolding and protein aggregations), and extreme care during production, processing and storage. A complete understanding of the mechanisms underpinning protein unfolding and aggregation is yet to be realized. This knowledge gap prevents formulators from adopting a rational set of steps towards protein formulation.

The most important factors to consider when one is formulating protein, peptide and gene biopharmaceuticals are the in vivo delivery challenges, i.e. the rapid clearance and degradation of the active agent in vivo and the active agent's difficulty in traversing cell membranes and cells. Solutions to these formulation/delivery difficulties include the attachment of PEG chains to proteins to reduce protein clearance and degradation, and the fabrication of poly(lactide-*co*-glycolide) matrices for the controlled and prolonged release of peptides. To enable genes to cross cell membranes and arrive at the cell nucleus, the commercial gene medicines are delivered by adenoviral and adeno-associated viral vectors.

From the foregoing it is clear that, if at all possible, the formulation of new biopharmaceuticals should be approached systematically by consideration of the nature of the source of the active agent's instability both on storage and on administration and a desire to match the drug to the disease, without introducing unwanted toxic effects.

Please check your eBook at **https://studentconsult. inkling.com/** for self-assessment questions. See inside cover for registration details.

References

Dranitsaris, G., Amir, E., Dorward, K., 2011. Biosimilars of biological drug therapies, regulatory, clinical and commercial considerations. Drugs 71, 1527–1536.

Veronese, F. (Ed.), 2009. PEGylated Protein Drugs: Basic Science and Clincial Applications. Birkhäuser, Berlin.

Bibliography

Dufes, C., Keith, W.N., Bilsland, A., et al., 2005. Synthetic anticancer gene medicine exploits intrinsic antitumor activity of cationic vector to cure established tumours. Cancer Res. 65, 8079–8084.

Falconer, R.J., Jackson-Matthews, D., Mahler, S.M., 2011. Analytical strategies for assessing the comparability of biosimilars. J. Chem. Technol. Biotechnol. 86, 915–922.

Hedge, N.R., Srivnas, V.K., Bayry, J., 2011. Recent advances in the administration of vaccines for infectious diseases: microneedles as painless delivery devices for mass vaccination. Drug Discov. Today 16, 1061–1067.

Hou, J.J.C., Codamo, J., Pilborough, W., et al., 2011. New frontiers in cell line development: challenges for biosimilars. J. Chem. Technol. Biotechnol. 86, 895–904.

Illum, L., 2012. Nasal drug delivery – recent developments and future prospects. J. Control. Release 161, 254–263.

Manning, M.C., Chou, D.K., Murphy, B.M., et al., 2010. Stability of pharmaceutical proteins. Pharm. Res. 27, 544–575.

Nelson, D.L., Cox, M.M., 2005. Lehninger Principles of Biochemistry, fourth ed. W.H. Freeman and Company, New York.

O'Hagen, D.T., Valiante, N.M., 2003. Recent advances in the discovery and delivery of vaccine adjuvants. Nat. Rev. Drug Discov. 2, 727–735.

Peng, Z., 2005. Current status of Gendicine in China – recombinant Ad-p53 agent for treatment of cancers. Hum. Gene Ther. 16, 1016–1027.

Shukla, D., Schneider, C.P., Trout, B.L., 2011. Molecular level insight into intra-solvent interaction effects on protein stability and aggregation. Adv. Drug Deliv. Rev. 63, 1074–1085.

Uchegbu, I.F., Schätzlein, A.G. (Eds.), 2006. Polymers in Drug Delivery. CRC Press, Boca Raton.

44

Pharmaceutical nanotechnology and nanomedicines

Yvonne Perrie

CHAPTER CONTENTS

KEY POINTS

- Pharmaceutical nanotechnology generally refers to pharmaceutical materials, structures and products of approximately 1 nm to 100 nm; however, an upper limit of 1000 nm is often considered.
- Systems that can be considered as nanomedicines include antibodies, polymer–drug conjugates, dendrimers, nanoparticles and liposomes.
- Because of the small size and high surface area to volume ratio of nanomedicines, formulation of drugs into nanomedicines can increase drug potency and efficacy by enhancing solubility and the dissolution rate, modifying drug distribution and improving drug targeting.
- To improve solubility and dissolution, drugs can be conjugated to water-soluble conjugates, formulated as nanosized drug particles, or incorporated into nanocarriers (e.g. dendrimers, micelles, liposomes or nanoparticles).
- Nanoparticles can enhance bioavailability by preventing renal clearance of drugs and protecting against clearance by the mononuclear phagocytic system.
- Nanoparticles can passively target tumour sites and the sites of inflammation through the 'enhanced permeability and retention effect', or these can be actively targeted through receptor–ligand interactions.

Introduction

In general terms, *pharmaceutical nanotechnology* is a term applied to the design, characterization and production of pharmaceutical materials, structures and products that have one or more dimensions between approximately 1 nm and 100 nm. However, this classification remains open to debate, and a degree of ambiguity remains over what is considered nanotechnology, particularly regarding the size range considered. An internationally accepted definition of nanotechnology is lacking, and frequently particles in larger size ranges are considered as nanotechnology; e.g. the US Food and Drug Administration (FDA) often considers 1000 nm as an appropriate upper limit regarding the screening of materials for consideration as nanotechnology. However, with the use of nanotechnology growing, both the European Medicines Agency and the FDA continue to refine their regulatory guidelines concerning nanotechnology in recognition of the key properties that nanomedicines can offer, i.e. their small size and high surface area to volume ratio. Yet it is generally agreed that use of size alone as the defining

factor for nanomedicines may be misleading. It is also useful to consider if a product exhibits different physical, chemical or biological properties that are attributed to its dimensions, even if these dimensions fall outside the nanoscale range. It is important to be aware that the functional effects of the product, such as bioavailability, toxicity and/or potency, may be influenced by the product's dimensions.

By application of this general definition, pharmaceutical nanotechnology can encompass many systems, from macromolecules, such as antibodies (e.g. Herceptin®) and polymer–protein conjugates (e.g. PegIntron®), to nanoscale particles (e.g. Emend®), through to colloidal and particulate constructs in the nanosize range, such as liposomal formulations (e.g. Ambisome®) and nanoparticle systems (e.g. Abraxane®). Examples of the range of such pharmaceutical nanotechnologies, sometimes referred to as nanomedicines, are shown in Fig. 44.1.

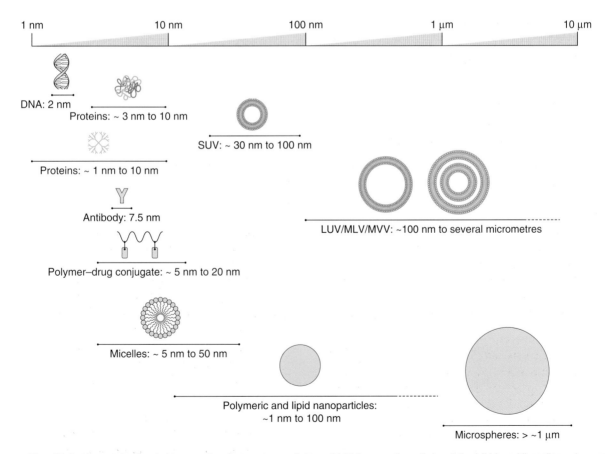

Fig. 44.1 • Approximate size range of various nanomedicines. *LUV*, large unilamellar vesicle; *MLV*, multilamellar vesicle; *MVV*, multivesicular vesicle; *SUV*, small unilamellar vesicle.

Applications of pharmaceutical nanotechnology

The application of nanotechnology encompasses the formulation and development of nanomedicines to increase drug potency and efficacy, and the use of nanomaterials in tissue engineering and implants to fabricate structures to support tissue regeneration within the body. Nanotechnology can also include the development of devices in the nanosize range such as implantable sensory systems (nanodiagnostics) for improved diagnostic measurements. This chapter will focus on the use of nanotechnology in drug formulation, which can offer particular advantages, including:

1. *enhanced solubility and dissolution*. Because of the high surface area to volume ratio offered by nanoparticles, the solubility and rate of dissolution of drugs can be increased.
2. *enhanced drug delivery*. The small particle size can prolong a drug's residence in the systemic circulation, it can modify drug distribution and it may permit drug targeting and transport across biological barriers.

There are already several products authorized for clinical use that can be classified as nanomedicines (Table 44.1). Some of these products have been approved for several years, having been originally approved for registration before the recognized classification of nanotechnology products. This includes some of the liposome-based products which have been licensed for clinical use since the mid-1990s. For example, the liposome formulation of doxorubicin (licensed in the US as Doxil® and marketed in Europe as Caelyx®) was the first liposomal product approved by the FDA. This product is a suspension of polyethylene glycol (PEG)-coated liposomes entrapping doxorubicin. Because of the ability of the liposome formulation to enhance targeting of doxorubicin to tumour sites, it was first developed for the treatment of AIDS-related Kaposi's sarcoma, and is now licensed for other antitumour indications, including metastatic breast cancer, advanced ovarian cancer and relapsed/refractory multiple myeloma. Table 44.1 shows that nanotechnology systems can offer a variety of attributes, and each of these types of system is discussed in further detail in this chapter.

Polymer–drug conjugates

To improve drug solubility and/or the delivery of drugs, drug molecules may be conjugated to polymers, producing *polymer–drug conjugates*. These polymer–drug

Table 44.1 Examples of licensed products that can be considered as nanomedicines

Product	Drug	Type of system	Attributes offered by the nanotechnology
Abraxane®	Paclitaxel	Nanoparticles	These albumin-bound nanoparticles increase the delivery of paclitaxel by overcoming the low solubility of paclitaxel and improving tumour cell drug delivery
Caelyx®/Doxil®	Doxorubicin	Liposomes	This formulation contains PEGylated liposomes, which can increase systemic circulation times and enhance delivery to tumour sites
Emend®	Aprepitant	Nanoparticles	These nanoparticles are prepared by a wet milling method and increase drug solubility and bioavailability
Mepact®	Mifamurtide	Liposomes	Entrapment of the drug within liposomes facilitates drug delivery and activation of macrophages
Myocet®	Doxorubicin	Liposomes	Incorporation of doxorubicin into liposomes increases tumour tissue distribution and reduces cardiac toxicity
Pegasys®	Peginterferon alfa-2a	Polymer–protein conjugate	PEGylation increases the stability of the protein
Rapamune®	Sirolimus	Nanoparticles	The formulation of a nanodispersion stabilized with poloxamer offers increased stability and bioavailability
Zevalin®	Ibritumomab tiuxetan	Antibody conjugate	Conjugation of a radioisotope to the antibody promotes targeting and destruction of B cells

conjugates are considered as new chemical entities in their own right and, as their overall size is generally smaller than 100 nm, these systems can be classified within the general area of nanotechnology. To build polymer–drug conjugates, many synthetic polymers can be produced that can offer appropriate quality and stability attributes, and they can be custom-made to have distinct characteristics, including specified molecular weight, size, charge, etc. As these polymers are synthetic, they are generally less immunogenic than naturally derived macromolecules. For the production of polymer–drug conjugates for parenteral administration, water-soluble polymers are used.

A polymer–drug conjugate can be described as being built of three basic components, as described in the following paragraphs.

A water-soluble polymer backbone. This can include synthetic polymers such as PEG, poly(ethyleneimine), polyvinylpyrrolidone, poly(vinyl alcohol), poly(glutamic acid) and hydroxypropyl methacrylate copolymers. Alternatively, natural polymers such as dextran, chitosans, hyaluronic acid and proteins can be used. Of the polymers, PEG is the most widely used; it is approved by the FDA for human use and offers properties including low immunogenicity, antigenicity and toxicity. PEG chains also offer high hydration and flexibility, which is useful in increasing solubility and improving drug delivery. Another important property of PEGs is their low polydispersity (in terms of molecular weight). The ease with which PEG can be modified and conjugated to drugs and proteins also offers an advantage. However, conjugation of PEG to proteins may in some instances reduce their biological activity, so the conjugation site of the PEG on the protein is an important consideration. Within clinically approved products, PEG molecular weights of 5000–40 000 are used.

A linker group. Whilst a drug can be directly covalently bonded to a polymer, it is more common to attach the drug via a *linker* or *spacer group*, to help avoid the therapeutic action of the drug being blocked by the polymer. The linker can also be designed to be cleaved under certain conditions, such as changes in pH, enzymatic degradation or hydrolysis. This property can be used to promote the triggered release of the drug from the polymer conjugate under suitable conditions, thereby enhancing drug targeting. Examples of linker groups that can be used include amine, carbamate and ester groups, with an amide linker being the most common option.

Drug. Commonly, drugs delivered by these conjugates are those used in anticancer chemotherapy, such as doxorubicin and paclitaxel. This is because polymer conjugates can improve delivery and reduce unwanted side effects for these drugs, which have narrow therapeutic windows. A second group of drugs that benefits from formulation as polymer conjugates is proteins, e.g. L-asparaginase or interferons. Generally, proteins have short half-lives and low stability after administration into the body. By conjugating proteins to polymers, one can increase their half-life by protecting the proteins from enzyme degradation and reducing clearance rates.

In addition to the three components of the system, targeting groups can be added to the polymer conjugate with the aim of enhancing specificity and cellular uptake. However, there are no licensed products currently on the market which adopt this active targeting method. Examples of polymer–drug conjugates on the market are given in Table 44.2. As can be seen, PEG is used in several of these formulations as the polymer backbone, and most of the systems are used to deliver protein therapeutics.

Rationale for polymer conjugation

As noted already, the conjugation of drugs to polymers can improve the therapeutic action of the drug by increasing solubility, protecting the drug from enzyme degradation, enhancing plasma circulation times and/ or enhancing drug targeting. This is achieved through various actions.

Increasing solubility

The conjugation of low-solubility drugs (e.g. paclitaxel, camptothecin or palatinate derivatives) to water-soluble polymers can enhance the solubility of the overall system; e.g., OPAXIO®, a polymer conjugate currently under development, comprising paclitaxel conjugated to poly(L-glutamic acid). The paclitaxel conjugate has enhanced solubility compared with paclitaxel, and therefore the conjugate can be administered without further solubilizing agents.

Enhancing bioavailability and plasma half-life

The increased hydrodynamic volume of the polymer–drug conjugate compared with the free drug can reduce rates of excretion via the kidneys. The renal clearance of compounds from the circulation is

Table 44.2 Examples of drug-polymer conjugates on the market

Name	Polymer–drug conjugate	Indication
Adagen®	PEG–adenosine deaminase	SCID syndrome
Cimzia®	PEG–anti TNF Fab' fragment	Crohn's disease and rheumatoid arthritis
Oncaspar®	PEG–asparaginase	Acute lymphoblastic leukaemia
PEGIntron®	Peginterferon alfa-2b	Hepatitis C
Pegasys®	Peginterferon alfa-2a	Hepatitis B and hepatitis C
Neulastra®	PEG–granulocyte colony stimulating factor	Prevention of neutropenia associated with cancer chemotherapy
Macugen®	PEG–anti-VEGF aptamer	Age-related macular degeneration
Somavert®	PEG–growth hormone receptor antagonist	Acromegaly
Zinostatin® Stimalamer®	Styrene–maleic anhydride copolymer–neocarzinostatin	Hepatocellular carcinoma

PEG, polyethylene glycol; *SCID*, severe combined immunodeficiency; *TNF*, tumour necrosis factor, *VEGF*, vascular endothelial growth factor.

dictated by their molecular weight, with clearance rates decreasing with increasing molecular weight up to a threshold of approximately 45 000. Above a molecular weight 45 000, renal excretion cannot occur, and larger polymers are more susceptible to clearance by the mononuclear phagocytic system (MPS). So, for example, the conjugation of molecules such as paclitaxel (molecular weight ~850), and proteins such as interferon (molecular weight ~20 000) to water-soluble polymers increases their overall molecular weight, enhancing drug circulation times and reducing kidney clearance rates.

Protecting against degradation after administration

The polymeric chains in the polymer–drug conjugate can also prevent the approach of antibodies and proteolytic enzymes to the drug. Water-soluble polymers become strongly hydrated, and these hydrated polymer strands can promote steric hindrance, and block enzymes and antibodies from reaching the drug. This protects the drug from degradation and enhances its plasma half-life and bioavailability. This is of particular advantage for protein-based therapeutic agents that are rapidly degraded by enzymes. However, it has been reported that antibodies against PEG can be generated in vivo, and these can remove and neutralize PEG conjugate products.

Reducing aggregation, immunogenicity and antigenicity

The hydrophilic coating offered by the polymers to the conjugate compound is the key to this property. The hydrated polymer chains can mask the hydrophobic regions in the protein, increase solubility and provide a steric shield that can help prevent protein–protein association, and reduce aggregation. For example, the native proteins in Neulasta® and PegIntron® have a high tendency to aggregate; however, PEG conjugation (referred to as *PEGylation or pegylation*) of these proteins can reduce aggregation and subsequently reduce associated immunogenic and antigenic problems. As already noted, the presence of the hydrated polymer in the conjugate can reduce antibody interactions, also reducing immunogenicity. PEGylation of proteins can also help stabilize proteins during lyophilization, so helping to produce products with acceptable storage conditions.

Promoting targeting to specific organs, tissue or cells

By conjugation of drugs or proteins to water-soluble polymers, not only can their half-lives be increased, but the specific accumulation of the drug or protein can also be promoted in certain tissues. This can be achieved through the use of targeting groups or the phenomenon known as the *enhanced permeability and retention (EPR) effect*. This EPR effect can be described as *passive targeting*, whereby the distribution of the conjugate is dictated by local physiological conditions at the target site. Normally after a drug enters the systemic circulation, the drug is required to cross the endothelial lining of the vasculature before it can reach the target site. In most parts of the body, the endothelial lining is continuous with the endothelial cells situated on a basal membrane, and tight junctions between adjacent cells. This makes transport across this barrier difficult. However, the structure of the blood capillary wall differs in different organs and tissues, with three general types of endothelial cells being recognized.

Continuous endothelial cells. Continuous endothelial cells are the most common. These cells have tight junctions and a continuous basement membrane. Continuous endothelial lining is found in areas such as capillaries in the brain, lung and muscles.

Fenestrated endothelial cells. This type of endothelial cells has gaps of between 20 nm and 80 nm between them, and this can allow the passage of small molecules out of the systemic circulation. Fenestrated endothelial linings are found in the capillaries in the kidneys and gastrointestinal tract.

Sinusoidal endothelial cells. Here there are gaps between the endothelial cells of up to 150 nm. The basement membrane is either discontinuous, as in the capillaries in the spleen, or absent altogether, as in the case of the capillaries in the liver.

Additionally, the integrity of the endothelial barrier can be disturbed by inflammatory processes or by tumour growth. This can result in defective hypervasculature, leading to endothelial fenestrations as large as 200 nm to 300 nm being present in the endothelial lining. In addition, because of rapid tumour growth, deficient lymphatic drainage is also an issue. This modified permeability of the endothelium at such sites allows nanomedicines, including polymer conjugates, to escape from the central circulation into the tumour site, where they are retained because of the poor tumour lymphatic drainage. This phenomenon is the EPR effect described earlier. Thus conjugation of a drug or protein to an appropriate soluble polymer will result in a construct with a large hydrodynamic volume which will have reduced kidney excretion and therefore an enhanced systemic circulation time. Because of the EPR effect the polymer conjugates can escape from the systemic circulation into tumour sites, where they will accumulate, enhancing drug action at the tumour site and reducing unwanted side effects elsewhere in the body.

The use of targeting groups to dictate the distribution of drugs and drug carriers can also be considered to promote targeting to a specific site. This is commonly referred to as *active targeting*. Here, the designer of the drug delivery system is relying on the interactions between a targeting group, which can be covalently attached to the polymer, and a corresponding receptor to facilitate the targeting of the system to a specific site. Examples of targeting groups include the use of antibodies because of their ability to specifically recognize and bind specific antigens (see later) and folate to target folate receptors, which are overexpressed in tumour cells. Similarly, lectins are overexpressed on the surface of many tumour cells and can be targeted via the use of glycoproteins.

Polymer–drug conjugates: case studies

OPAXIO® – a small-molecule conjugate. In this polymer–drug conjugate, paclitaxel is conjugated to poly(L-glutamic acid) (PGA) via an ester linker. Conjugating paclitaxel to the water-soluble PGA overcomes the poor aqueous solubility of paclitaxel, and the conjugate can be infused into the body without the addition of solvents. This conjugate has high drug content (~37% w/w) and is stable in the circulation, and whilst it remains bound to the polymer, paclitaxel is inactive. Because of its construct, the conjugate can passively target tumour sites via the EPR effect. The drug is then released intracellularly via degradation of PGA by lysosomal proteases, and the ester linker is degraded by esterases or acid hydrolysis. OPAXIO® is currently undergoing clinical trials as a potential treatment for non-small-cell lung cancer and ovarian cancer.

Oncaspar® – a protein conjugate. In this conjugate, L-asparaginase is bound to nonbiodegradable monomethoxylpolyethylene glycol (5000 g mol⁻¹) via an amide linker. This conjugate is used in the treatment of acute lymphoblastic leukaemia, and its mechanism of action is based on selective killing of leukaemic cells due to the depletion of plasma asparagine. Asparaginase is an enzyme which breaks downs the amino acid L-asparagine. This interferes with the growth of malignant cells, which, unlike most healthy cells, are unable to synthesize L-asparagine for their metabolism. PEGylation of the enzyme enhances the circulation time of the enzyme, allowing less frequent dosing. It can also be given to patients with a history of hypersensitivity to native L-asparaginase.

Antibodies and antibody-drug conjugates

Antibodies are large Y-shaped protein macromolecules produced by B cells. Antibodies can specifically bind

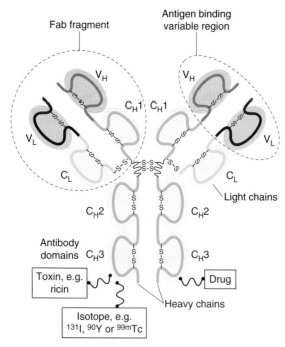

Fig. 44.2 • An IgG antibody that can be used as a drug, or as a carrier. Drugs, isotopes or toxins can be conjugated to the IgG molecules that can selectively target cells through their antigen binding region at the end of the Fab region.

to a range of pathogens, including bacteria and viruses, through their ability to specifically bind to antigens. There are several classes (or isotypes) of antibodies, with the five main types being IgG, IgA, IgM, IgE and IgD. Of these, IgG is the most abundant in the body. The basic structure of IgG comprises two identical heavy (50 kDa) polypeptide chains and two identical light (23 kDa) polypeptide chains. These chains are held together by disulfide bonds. The ability of antibodies to specifically target antigens is due to their amino acid sequence at the tips of the protein, which are the antigen binding sites (Fig. 44.2).

Antibody therapies

Given their ability to target a range of specific antigens and cell types, antibodies can be used for drug targeting, either as drugs in their own right or as targeting groups for drugs or delivery systems. To achieve this, IgG monoclonal antibodies have been developed. There are already several monoclonal antibodies

available as therapeutic agents (Table 44.3). As is the case with other nanotechnology systems, these therapies are generally focused on oncology. In the case of antibody therapies, the antibody is designed to actively target tumour cells. By the antibody binding to tumour cells, cell death can then occur via two types of mechanisms:

1. The antibody binds to the tumour cell and then acts as a marker for other components or cells of the immune system to destroy the tumour cell. For example, the binding of Trastuzumab acts as a marker to promote cells of the immune system to destroy the cancer cells.

2. The binding of the antibody can initiate signalling mechanisms in the target cell that block cell growth and/or lead to the target cell's self-destruction. For example, rituximab binds to the CD20 molecules on tumour cells and triggers cell apoptosis.

Alternatively, the antibody can bind to a protein and thereby block its ability to bind to a receptor, as in the case of adalimumab, which binds to tumour necrosis factor alpha (TNFα), thereby blocking its ability to bind to activate tumour necrosis factor receptors. In addition to whole antibodies, antibody fragments can be used. Fab fragments of monoclonal antibodies retain the targeting specificity of whole monoclonal antibodies, and may even offer stronger binding; however, the fragments can be produced more economically. Examples of antibody fragments licensed for use include ReoPro® and Lucentis® (see Table 44.3).

Antibody conjugates

Similar to polymer–drug conjugates, antibodies can also function as carriers for drugs and other agents, including radioisotopes and toxins. These antibody conjugates are sometimes referred to as immunoconjugates. By conjugation of a molecule to an appropriate monoclonal antibody, the molecules actively target the drug to the required site of action. Unfortunately, most antibody conjugates have a relatively low capacity for drugs; however, their high target specificity allows them to be used effectively in the clinical environment. Examples of antibody conjugates are given in Table 44.4. These either target radioisotopes, which can be used to promote cell death (e.g. Bexxar® and Zevalin®), or can be used for diagnostic imaging (e.g. ProstaScint®). Alternatively, the antibodies can

Table 44.3 Examples of clinically approved antibodies and antibody fragment therapies

Product name	Drug	Description	Indications
Avastin®	Bevacizumab	IgG targeted against VEGF-A. By binding to VEGF, it blocks angiogenesis (the growth of new blood vessels)	Metastatic colorectal cancer Advanced nonsquamous non-small-cell lung cancer Metastatic kidney cancer Glioblastoma
Herceptin®	Trastuzumab	IgG that binds to HER2 on the surface of cells. HER proteins regulate cell growth. In tumour cells, HER2 is overexpressed. By IgG binding to the cells, it blocks growth factor binding to receptors. This stops the cells from dividing. Binding of trastuzumab also acts as a marker to promote cells of the immune system to destroy the cancer cells	Breast cancer Metastatic cancer
Humira®	Adalimumab	IgG that binds to TNF-α, and prevents TNF-α from activating TNF receptors. This downregulates inflammatory reactions	Rheumatoid arthritis Crohn's disease Plaque psoriasis Psoriatic arthritis Ankylosing spondylitis Juvenile idiopathic arthritis
Lucentis®	Ranibizumab	A Fab antibody fragment derived from the antibody of bevacizumab. This offers stronger binding to VEGF-A than the parent antibody	Age-related macular degeneration
ReoPro®	Abciximab	This is a Fab fragment that binds to the IIb/IIIa receptor on the platelet, blocking interaction of fibrogen with the IIb/IIIa receptor, which blocks platelet aggregation	Prevention of cardiac ischaemic complications in patients undergoing percutaneous coronary intervention
Rituxan®	Rituximab	IgG directed against CD20 molecules. Binding of rituximab to the CD20 molecules on tumour cells triggers cell apoptosis	Non-Hodgkin's lymphoma Chronic lymphocytic leukaemia Rheumatoid arthritis Wegener's granulomatosis Microscopic polyangiitis
Synagis®	Palivizumab	IgG directed against an epitope of the A antigenic site of the F protein of respiratory syncytial virus	Prevention of serious lower respiratory tract diseases caused by respiratory syncytial virus in paediatric patients at high risk of respiratory syncytial virus infection

HER2, human epidermal growth factor receptor 2; *TNF*, tumour necrosis factor; *VEGF*, vascular endothelial growth factor.

be used to target toxins which can kill cells (e.g. Mylotarg®).

Dendrimers

Dendrimers are highly branched polymeric, star-shaped macromolecules which can be prepared in the nanosize range. Dendrimers are built by a controlled chemical synthesis, and they have three main elements (Fig. 44.3):

1. a central core;
2. the internal dendritic structure, which is composed of the branched polymeric structure built onto the central core; and
3. the exterior surface of the dendrimer.

By varying the construction of the dendrimer around the core unit, one can build dendrimers of different shapes and sizes, which can offer the ability to carry drugs within the construct, or one can conjugate drugs to the surface of the dendrimer. The surface

Table 44.4 Clinically approved antibody conjugate systems

Product name	Drug	Description	Indications
Bexxar®	Tositumomab	^{131}I conjugated to IgG targeted against CD20 protein on B cells. The binding of the antibodies and the radioisotopes work in combination to target and kill B cells	B-cell non-Hodgkin's lymphoma
Mylotarg®	Gemtuzumab ozogamicin	Ozogamicin conjugated to IgG which targets CD33. Ozogamicin is a cytotoxin. After binding to CD33, the conjugate enters the cells through the endocytic/lysosomal pathway. The antibody is then degraded and the cytotoxin is released into the cytosol, resulting in cell death	Acute myeloid leukaemia
ProstaScint®	Capromab pendetide	^{111}In–IgG antibody conjugate directed against the glycoprotein prostate-specific membrane antigen expressed by prostate epithelium	Imaging agent for metastatic prostate cancer
Zevalin®	Ibritumomab tiuxetan	^{90}Y–IgG conjugate directed against CD20 on B-cell lymphomas. The antibody binding to the CD20 protein and the targeted radioisotopes work in combination to target and kill B cells	B-cell non-Hodgkin's lymphoma

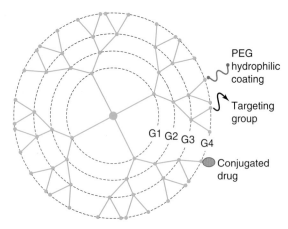

Fig. 44.3 • A dendrimer *(blue)* with four generations labelled G1 to G4 respectively. Drug molecules and targeting groups can be conjugated to the exterior of the dendrimer. Polyethylene glycol (PEG) can also be added to the exterior surface to provide a hydrophilic coating.

of the dendrimer can also be modified with targeting groups, or a hydrophilic coating to enhance solubility. Depending on their design, dendrimers can be built to be biodegradable or nonbiodegradable, similarly to the polymer–drug conjugates. These branched polymeric structures are synthesized by stepwise addition of layers of polymer branching, referred to as generations (termed G1, G2, etc.). In general, as the number of layers or generations increases, the structure of the dendrimer moves from the open structures of the low-generation dendrimer to an increasingly more globular and dense structure. In all cases, the resulting constructs are built to have a specific size, a high degree of molecular uniformity and a narrow molecular weight distribution. Whilst dendrimers can be considered as an evolution of branched polymers, they offer the advantage that they can be prepared with a very narrow size distribution. Furthermore, the large number of peripheral groups on the exterior surface of the dendrimer, which increase exponentially with each generation added, allows higher drug-loading capacities compared with the linear or branched polymers used in polymer–drug conjugates.

Applications of dendrimers

In general, the attributes offered by polymer conjugates discussed in previous sections apply to dendrimers; dendrimers can be designed to increase drug solubility and bioavailability, and can enhance drug delivery and targeting. The additional advantages of dendrimers over polymer conjugates include their near monodisperse size range and high drug-loading capacity. Dendrimers have been investigated for their potential to encapsulate drug molecules within the construct or by conjugation of the drug to the dendrimer. Encapsulation of the drug within the dendrimer can be exploited to protect labile drugs which are quickly degraded. Similarly, dendrimers can act as a solubilizing agent for low-solubility drugs (similar to micelles) by encapsulating the drug within the dendrimer construct, which offers a hydrophobic core and a hydrophilic exterior. The drug can be entrapped within the dendrimer either by simple physical entrapment or by nonbonding interactions, such as electrostatic interactions. When the drug is encapsulated within the dendrimer, controlled drug release can be achieved by design of the dendrimer to have triggered degradation. However, the ability to incorporate drugs within the system is heavily dictated by the architecture of the dendrimer.

Alternatively, drug molecules can also be loaded onto the surface of the dendrimers via electrostatic interactions or via conjugation of the drug to the surface groups on the dendrimer. Conjugation of the drug to the exterior of the dendrimer generally offers high drug loading because of the large number of peripheral end groups available on each dendrimer molecule. Drugs can be covalently attached through hydrolysable or biodegradable linkers, thereby offering greater control over drug release compared with electrostatic interactions. However, the addition of molecules to the surface of the dendrimer can also influence the dendrimer properties. For example, the addition of PEG to the surface of dendrimers allows their pharmacokinetic profile to be modified, with clearance via the liver being reduced and plasma circulation time increased. This can promote passive dendrimer–drug targeting via the EPR effect, similar to PEGylated protein constructs. Alternatively, active targeting can be considered by the conjugation of targeting groups to the surface of the dendrimer (Fig. 44.3).

Dendrimer systems: case studies

VivaGel® formulation, developed by Starpharma, is a microbicide gel which uses dendrimers. In this formulation, the dendrimer is the active ingredient in its own right rather than being used as a delivery system. The dendrimer has antiviral properties because of its ability to bind to viruses and thereby block their ability to infect cells. VivaGel® BV has EU market approval for the treatment and rapid relief of bacterial vaginosis.

Whilst not approved for clinical use, there are a range of commercially available dendrimers such as polyamidoamine (Starburst®) and poly(propylenimine) (Astramol®) dendrimers which have been widely studied for drug delivery.

Micelle systems

Micelles are widely used to formulate low-solubility drugs in colloidal solutions. Micelles form because of the ability of surfactant molecules to self-assemble into micelles in an aqueous environment. Whilst not a new type of formulation (see Chapter 5), their size (often <100 nm) means that micelles can be considered within the nanotechnology classification. As a consequence of the micellar structure, which offers a hydrophobic core and a hydrophilic surface, micelles are commonly used as solubilizing agents. For example, Fugizone® is a mixed micellar formulation which is used to solubilize amphotericin B, an antifungal agent used to treat invasive fungal infections, such as systemic candidiasis and histoplasmosis.

Polymeric micelles

Copolymers with surfactant characteristics can also be used to formulate micelles. Micelles formed from copolymers tend to have a relatively narrow size distribution compared with standard surfactant micelles. Generally, they also have a lower critical micelle concentration (CMC) and are more stable. Because of their low CMCs, polymeric micelles are relatively insensitive to dilution, thus preventing their rapid dissociation and enhancing their systemic circulation time compared with surfactant micelles. Polymeric micelles are built from copolymers with hydrophobic components comprising poly(propylene oxide), poly(D,L-lactic acid), poly(ε-caprolactone), poly(L-aspartate) and poloxamers. For the hydrophilic component, which forms the outer hydrophilic shell of the micelle, PEG is commonly used. The use of PEG as the hydrophilic component supports the formation of the micelles. The hydrated PEG surface created on the micelles enhances their plasma half-life by promoting steric hindrance and blocking enzymes and antibodies from reaching the drug, thereby offering protection to the drug, and blocking interactions with the MPS. As the micelles are sufficiently large (> 50 kDa) to avoid renal excretion yet small enough (< 200 nm) to avoid clearance by the liver and spleen, they are able to specifically accumulate at tumour sites and sites of inflammation because of passive targeting.

As for dendrimers, the outer surface of polymeric micelles can be further functionalized with targeting groups (such as folate, sugar residues or proteins) to promote their application in drug delivery and targeting. The attachment of monoclonal antibodies to reactive groups incorporated in the hydrophilic coating of polymeric micelles has also been investigated and shown to promote specific interaction of the micelles with antigens corresponding to the antibodies. These micelles are often referred to as *immunomicelles*.

Polymeric micelles: case studies

Estrasorb®. This is an oestradiol topical formulation designed to deliver oestradiol to the blood circulation following topical application. Oestradiol hemihydrate is encapsulated in a micellar nanoparticle drug delivery system (which comprises soybean oil, water, polysorbate 80 and ethanol). The formulation is used to treat menopausal symptoms, including hot flushes and night sweats.

Genexol®-PM. This is a polymeric micelle formulation of paclitaxel prepared with methoxypolyethylene glycol–poly(D,L-lactide) which is approved in South Korea for treatment of metastatic breast cancer. In vivo antitumour efficacy of the micellar formulation has been shown to be significantly higher than that of Taxol®.

Solid nanoparticles

Solid nanoparticles are solid constructs in the nanometre range, and can be prepared by a number of different manufacturing methods which generally involve either size reduction of particles (e.g. by milling) to within the nanoparticle range or molecular agglomeration (e.g. by precipitation methods) to form nanoparticles. The former is used to prepare drug particles in the nanosize range where there is no carrier material added, whilst the latter is more commonly used to prepare nanoparticle carriers in which drug is loaded.

Nanosized drug particles and drug nanocrystals

Reducing the size of drug particles to within the nanosize range substantially increases the total surface area of the system, hence increasing the solubility of the drug. This attribute can be exploited to increase the dissolution ability and bioavailability of drugs delivered by the oral route. The use of nanosized drug particles in oral drug delivery can also avoid variations in drug bioavailability caused by the fed/fasted state of a patient. However, nanosized drug particles, owing to their high surface area and subsequent high interfacial energy, tend to be unstable and prone to particle aggregation. To reduce this problem, surface-active agents can be used, as in the case of NanoCrystal technology, developed by Elan Corporation. NanoCrystals are prepared from 100% drug with no carrier, and stabilizers (nonionic and anionic surfactants) are added during the size-reduction process to increase stability. Within nanoparticle systems, the drug can be either crystalline or amorphous. The small particle size increases dissolution and saturation solubility. For oral delivery, nanocrystals are normally formulated into tablets or capsules. With these systems, a key consideration is drug loading, as a high nanocrystal loading in tablets could result in contact between nanocrystals, promoting potential fusion of the crystals during tablet compression. There are several drug nanoparticle products on the market which exploit this NanoCrystal technology (Table 44.5).

Solid polymeric nanoparticles

In addition to their production by size reduction of drug particles, solid nanoparticles can be formed from polymers with the drug incorporated within the polymer matrix or attached to the particle surface. As such, the delivery system can be loaded with a wide range of drugs (e.g. water-soluble and low-aqueous-solubility drugs, low and high molecular weight drugs, small molecules and proteins) and can offer protection to the drug. Incorporation of the drug into solid polymeric nanoparticles also allows modified drug biodistribution as the drug pharmacokinetic profile will be dictated by the properties of the nanoparticle attributes rather than those of the drug.

Polymeric nanoparticles are generally formulated from natural or synthetic polymers, with the most commonly studied polymers being those which are biodegradable, such as poly(lactide-*co*-glycolide) (PLGA), poly(lactic acid), poly(ε-caprolactone) and polysaccharides (particularly chitosan). The advantage of these polymers is that they are well characterized and used in a range of clinical products, particularly PLGA. In terms of drug delivery, the main areas in which polymeric nanoparticles are being considered

Table 44.5 Examples of products developed with drug nanoparticles

Product	Drug	Attributes
Emend®	Aprepitant	An oral capsule form of the poorly soluble drug aprepitant which is only absorbed in the upper gastrointestinal tract. Therefore the rapid dissolution offered by the nanocrystals supports fast absorption and increased bioavailability
Megace® ES	Megesterol acetate	The ES in the product name stands for enhanced stability. This product is a liquid dosage form, and the nanosized version of the drug allows the drug to be formulated in a smaller volume. The reduced dose volume, reduced dissolution times, and enhanced bioavailability are beneficial for drug compliance
Rapamume®	Sirolimus	This is an oral tablet of the poorly soluble drug, which is an immunosuppressant. The oral tablet offers higher bioavailability and can be more user-friendly than a liquid product
TriCor®	Fenofibrate	Generally, fenofibrate uptake is from the gut lumen region and therefore bioavailability is influenced by the patient's fed/nonfed state. By formulation of the drug as nanocrystals, the lipophilic drug has increased solubility and therefore uptake of the drug is not influenced by solubilization of the drug in food components

are related to their ability to promote passive targeting of drugs to tumour sites via the EPR effect. Similar to the other nanotechnology systems discussed, the surface coating of PEG on these nanoparticles produces so-called stealth nanoparticles, with the hydrated PEG surface coating prohibiting protein and antibody binding, thereby reducing recognition and clearance from the circulation. By increasing the plasma circulation time of the polymeric nanoparticles, this supports their accumulation at sites of leaky vasculature, including tumour sites. To formulate these 'stealth' systems, PEG–PLGA copolymers are often used. Alternatively, active targeting of these systems can be achieved by the attachment of targeting groups to the nanoparticles.

Solid-lipid nanoparticles

These are nanoparticles made from solid (high melting point) lipids dispersed in an aqueous phase. Examples of lipids used include solid triglycerides, saturated phospholipids and fatty acids, which are well tolerated by the body. Because of their composition, they are sometimes described as *solidified oil-in-water emulsions* in which the oil globule is replaced by solidified lipid. Much like the solid polymeric nanoparticles, solid-lipid nanoparticles can be used as drug delivery systems, with the drug being incorporated within the lipid matrix of the particle or by attachment of the drug to the lipid nanoparticle surface. Lipid particles are normally larger than 50 nm and can be prepared on a large scale by homogenization to disperse the lipid into an aqueous environment.

Solid-lipid nanoparticle dispersions have been developed for parenteral, oral, ocular, dermal and cosmetic applications. As with the polymeric nanoparticles, PEG coating of these systems has been shown to passively target tumour sites via the EPR effect. To actively target cancer cells, covalent coupling of targeting groups such as ferritin or galactose to the lipids used in the formulation has been investigated. Currently, there are a range of cosmetic products which use lipid nanoparticles loaded with cosmetic components such as ascorbyl palmitate, β-carotene and coenzyme Q_{10}. As these are all lipophilic, they are efficiently incorporated within lipid nanoparticles.

Protein nanoparticles

In addition to polymers and lipids, nanoparticles can also be prepared from proteins. The first commercial product based on protein nanotechnology was Abraxane® (nab-paclitaxel). Abraxane® is approved for the treatment of breast cancer in patients who do not respond to combination chemotherapy for metastatic disease or who relapse within 6 months of adjuvant chemotherapy. Abraxane® consists of 130 nm particles of albumin-bound paclitaxel. The drug, paclitaxel, has low water solubility and requires addition of solubility-enhancing agents to allow its clinical use. Before the development of Abraxane®, paclitaxel was only available as Taxol®. This is a liquid product with paclitaxel solubilized in polyethoxylated castor oil (Cremophor® EL) and ethanol. However, this formulation requires special infusion sets and prolonged infusion times and has toxicity issues associated with its use. By incorporation of paclitaxel into albumin nanoparticles, the albumin functions to coat the paclitaxel and provide colloidal stabilization to the drug. This circumvents both the low solubility and the Cremophor®-associated side effects.

Targeting mechanisms of Abraxane®

The albumin within the nanoparticle–albumin technology used in Abraxane® serves as more than a solubility-enhancing agent: albumin also promotes active targeting of the paclitaxel to tumour cells. As highlighted earlier, drug targeting of nanoparticles to tumours may be enhanced as a result of the EPR effect; the dense and highly permeable endothelial microvascular structure of tumours (which is a result of angiogenesis) allows large macromolecules and nanoparticles to leak into the underlying tumour tissue. The impaired lymphatic drainage at the tumour site slows drainage of these nanoparticles and macromolecules from the tumour site, resulting in the particles becoming trapped.

In the case of Abraxane®, a second mechanism has also been associated with the targeting and uptake of the albumin nanoparticles to tumour sites. This is the *albumin-activated glycoprotein 60 (gp60) pathway*. Within the body, albumin is able to transport hydrophobic molecules, such as vitamins, hormones and other plasma constituents, across the endothelial lining and out of the blood circulation. This is achieved by albumin binding to gp60 albumin receptors found on the surface of vasculature endothelial cells. These gp60 receptors are then responsible for the transport of albumin across blood vessel walls. The binding of albumin to the gp60 receptors activates the membrane protein caveolin 1. The activation of caveolin 1 subsequently results in the internalization of the cell membrane and the formation of transcytotic vesicles (known as caveolae). These caveolae then transport their contents across the endothelial cell cytoplasm, and release their contents into the cell's interstitium. In the case of tumours, this transport system is thought to be upregulated. Therefore, Abraxane® is able to exploit this albumin-activated gp60 transport mechanism to target the tumour site. After entering the systemic circulation, the albumin-bound paclitaxel can bind to the gp60 albumin receptors and be carried across the endothelial cells via transcytosis in the same way as albumin.

After crossing the endothelial lining, the drug must cross the tumour cell membrane and enter the tumour cells. Once the albumin-bound paclitaxel reaches the interstitium, the albumin may bind to an extracellular matrix glycoprotein known as SPARC (for 'secreted protein acid and rich in cysteine') which is also overexpressed in tumour cells. This can trigger the release of the paclitaxel from the albumin, allowing the free drug to diffuse to the nucleus of tumour cells, initiating cell death. Given that this mechanism of tumour targeting is an attribute of the albumin carrier system and not the drug, it is conceivable that it may be applied to the delivery of other low-solubility anticancer agents.

Inorganic nanoparticles

Nanoparticles can be fabricated from inorganic materials, including metal oxides, metal sulfides, carbon nanotubes, calcium phosphate and ceramics. These nanoparticles are generally not biodegradable and so have a more limited application. Abdoscan® is an example (albeit no longer available in Europe) of a metal oxide nanoparticle product. Abdoscan® can be used for magnetic resonance imaging (MRI) diagnostics of the bowel, as it is a superparamagnetic iron oxide nanoparticle formulation which is administered orally. The particles have a mean diameter no smaller than 300 nm. It is a negative contrast agent used for peroral bowel MRI diagnosis because of its high magnetic signal strength and decreased cytotoxicity. The particles are suspended in viscosity-increasing agents, such as starch, to prevent aggregation of the particles in vivo.

Liposomes and bilayer vesicles

Liposomes are closed spherical vesicles consisting of an aqueous core surrounded by one or more bilayer membranes (lamellae) alternating with aqueous compartments (Fig. 44.4). These bilayer membranes can be composed of natural or synthetic amphiphilic lipids, and commonly phospholipids are used for the formulation of liposomes; however, a range of amphiphilic lipids can be used. Liposomes form when the lipids (which are surface active with a hydrophilic head group and a hydrophobic chain(s) at opposing ends of the molecule) are exposed to an aqueous environment. At the appropriate lipid-to-water ratio and temperature, the lipids will arrange themselves into bilayer vesicles. Unlike micelle formation which

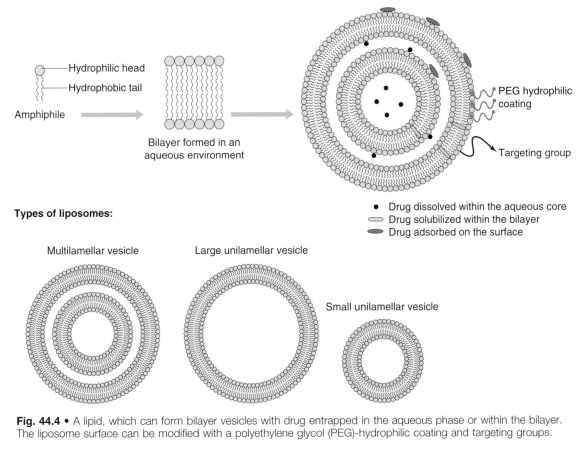

Fig. 44.4 • A lipid, which can form bilayer vesicles with drug entrapped in the aqueous phase or within the bilayer. The liposome surface can be modified with a polyethylene glycol (PEG)-hydrophilic coating and targeting groups.

occurs spontaneously, energy must be added to the system to drive the formation of liposomes.

Liposomes are able to carry both water-soluble and lipophilic moieties, with water-soluble drugs being incorporated within the aqueous compartments and lipid-soluble drugs being incorporated within the bilayer (similar to the solubilization of drugs within the core of micelles). In addition, some drugs and molecules can be adsorbed onto the surface of the liposomes through electrostatic interactions, e.g. nucleic acids and many proteins are anionic and can be electrostatically bound to the surface of cationic liposomes.

Liposomes can be formulated in a range of diameters from approximately 30 nm up to several micrometres, and therefore they can be considered as nanotechnology. Generally, liposomes are classified based on their size and number of lamellae (Fig. 44.4).

Small unilamellar vesicles. These are single-bilayer vesicles, approximately 30 nm to 100 nm in size.

They are generally easier to prepare in a homogeneous size range than other types of vesicles and are the most commonly used in clinically approved products. Because of their small size there is a low ratio of internal aqueous volume per mole of lipid.

Large unilamellar vesicles. These are large single-bilayer vesicles of 100 nm or greater. These vesicles offer a larger aqueous compartment than small unilamellar vesicles.

Multilamellar vesicles. These vesicles have multiple concentric bilayers and are 100 nm to several micrometres in size, depending on their composition and their method of preparation. Their low aqueous volume (due to the multiple bilayers) reduces their capacity for carrying water-soluble drugs.

Multivesicular vesicles. Multivesicular vesicles are of size similar to multilamellar vesicles; however, rather than having multiple concentric bilayers, they have vesicles within vesicles.

Clinical application of liposomes

Examples of liposome formulations on the market are given in Table 44.6. These include formulations which are prescribed for the treatment of certain cancers (e.g. Caelyx® and DaunoXome®), systemic fungal infections (e.g. AmBisome®), vaccines (e.g. Inflexal® V) and macular degeneration (e.g. Visudyne®); most of the products are designed for intravenous injection.

These formulations exploit the ability of liposomes to control the pharmacokinetic profile of their incorporated drug. Early in the development of liposomes as drug delivery vehicles it was established that intravenously injected liposomes interact with blood opsonins, which cause their removal from the blood circulation at rates that are dictated by vesicle size, lipid composition and surface charge. Because of this interaction with opsonins, liposomes end up (via opsonin recognition by appropriate cell receptors) in the tissues of the MPS,

Table 44.6 Examples of clinically approved liposome products

Product name	Drug	Formulation	Clinical indications
AmBisome®	Amphotericin B	SUV liposomes composed of hydrogenated soy phosphatidylcholine, cholesterol, distearoyl phosphatidylglycerol and α-tocopherol. The vesicles are smaller than 100 nm. Amphotericin B is intercalated within the liposome membrane	An antifungal agent given intravenously for the treatment of systemic fungal infections
Caelyx®/Doxil®	Doxorubicin	SUV liposomes 80 nm to 100 nm in size and composed of PEGylated distearoyl phosphatidylethanolamine, hydrogenated soy phosphatidylcholine and cholesterol. Doxorubicin is located within the aqueous core of the liposomes. It is present as a doxorubicin–sulfate complex, which is a gel-like precipitate within the vesicles helping to retain the drug within the liposomes with more than 90% loading efficiency	Advanced ovarian cancer, advanced breast cancer and AIDS-related Kaposi's sarcoma
DaunoXome®	Daunorubicin	SUV liposomes composed of distearoyl phosphatidylcholine and cholesterol and with a diameter of 45 nm. Daunorubicin is located in the aqueous core of the liposome in a manner similar to doxorubicin	Kaposi's sarcoma
Definity®	Octafluoropropane	This does not contain liposomes in the strictest sense of the term but contains lipid microspheres. They contain dipalmitoylphosphatidic acid, dipalmitoyl phosphatidylcholine and PEG 500 dipalmitoyl phosphatidylethanolamine. The mean diameter of these particles is 1.1 μm to 3.3 μm. Sparingly soluble octafluoropropane is incorporated within these constructs	This is used as a contrast agent for echocardiograms
DepoCyte®	Cytarabine	Multivesicular vesicles composed of dioleoyl phosphatidylcholine, cholesterol, dipalmitoyl phosphatidylglycerol and triolein. The vesicles are 3 μm to 30 μm in size. Cytarabine is entrapped in the aqueous compartments of the liposomes	Intrathecal treatment of lymphomatous meningitis
DepoDur®	Morphine sulfate	Multivesicular liposomes composed of dioleoyl phosphatidylcholine, dipalmitoyl phosphatidylglycerol, cholesterol and triolein. The morphine is incorporated within the aqueous regions of the vesicles; similar to DepoCyte®	Extended postoperative pain relief after major surgery. This is a single epidural injection

Continued

Table 44.6 Examples of clinically approved liposome products—cont'd

Product name	Drug	Formulation	Clinical indications
Epaxal®	Inactivated hepatitis A virus	The vesicles in this formulation are known as virosomes as the bilayer structures are built from phosphatidylcholine, cephalin and purified influenza virus surface antigens. The subunit antigens are incorporated within the bilayer lipid membrane and the vesicles are approximately 150 nm in size	Hepatitis A vaccine
Inflexal® V	Influenza haemagglutinin glycoprotein and neuraminidase	Similar to Epaxal®, the virosomes are prepared from phosphatidylcholine. The subunit antigens are incorporated within the bilayer lipid membrane	Influenza vaccine
Myocet®	Doxorubicin	Liposomes approximately 180 nm in size and composed of egg phosphatidylcholine and cholesterol. Doxorubicin is loaded into the aqueous core of the liposomes, where it forms a doxorubicin citrate complex	First-line treatment of metastatic breast cancer in women
Visudyne®	Vereporfin	Dimyristoyl phosphatidylcholine and egg phosphatidylglycerol. The sparingly soluble photosensitizer verteporfin is incorporated in the liposomes	Photodynamic therapy for macular degeneration

SUV, small unilamellar vesicle.

mostly fixed to macrophages in the liver and spleen. This property allows liposomes to be used for passive targeting of such sites. Alternatively, when administered via the intramuscular route or subcutaneous route, liposomes reach the lymphatic system, including the local lymph nodes. This provides the opportunity for liposomes to be used for the delivery of vaccines. However, to use liposomes for drug delivery to sites other than the MPS, the stability of liposomes in blood or interstitial fluids, vesicle clearance rates, and tissue distribution are key factors.

Formulation considerations that can improve this aspect include coating liposomes with hydrophilic polymers, such as polysialic acids and PEG; these polymers provide a hydrophilic surface which helps to repel opsonins and thus contribute to longer vesicle circulation times and, therefore, provide opportunities for the liposomes to interact with target cells other than those of the MPS. By avoiding MPS uptake, liposomes can accumulate in pathological sites with leaky vasculature, including tumour sites and sites of inflammation, through the EPR effect.

The application of liposomes in cancer chemotherapy

There are several liposome products designed for the delivery of cancer chemotherapy, and they can promote improved drug delivery via a range of different mechanisms. For example, Myocet® is a liposomal formulation of doxorubicin. The liposomes within Myocet® are approximately 180 nm in size and composed of egg phosphatidylcholine and cholesterol. Because of their larger size and lack of PEG coating, the liposomes in Myocet® are rapidly taken up by the MPS. This is thought to create an 'MPS depot', which results in slow release of the drug into the blood circulation, mimicking a slow transfusion.

Alternatively, liposomes can be formulated to exploit the EPR effect, thereby allowing them to target anticancer agents to tumour sites via passive targeting. To achieve this, the liposomes can be prepared with a PEGylated surface coating, as in Caelyx® (also marketed as Doxil®). Within this formulation the liposomes are smaller than 100 nm and incorporate PEG 2000–distearoyl phosphatidylethanolamine within their bilayer, which provides a hydrophilic PEG coating on the surface of the liposomes. This hydrophilic coating inhibits opsonization of the liposomes, avoids their clearance by the MPS, and therefore increases their circulation half-life. Subsequently, the liposomes are able to accumulate at tumour sites via the EPR effect. Targeting via the EPR effect is driven by the plasma concentration of liposomes. The liposomes retained in the tumour subsequently break down and release doxorubicin, which acts locally on cells.

DaunoXome®, a liposome formulation of daunorubicin, is also able to selectively deliver the entrapped drug to tumour sites. Unlike Caelyx®, in DaunoXome® the liposomes do not have a PEGylated hydrophilic coating. DaunoXome® liposomes are formulated from high transition temperature lipids and cholesterol, which makes the liposome bilayer resistant to opsonization. This, combined with their small size (45 nm), supports prolonged blood residence times and tumour targeting.

The established nature of liposomes in the field of anticancer agent drug delivery is demonstrated by the approval of a generic version of doxorubicin hydrochloride PEGylated liposomes. The generic is made by Sun Pharma Global FZE and was approved by the FDA in 2013 in response to a lack of availability of Doxil®.

The application of liposomes in the treatment of systemic fungal infections

AmBisome® is an antifungal preparation, administered by intravenous injection, consisting of amphotericin B incorporated in liposomes which are approximately 80 nm in diameter. Amphotericin B is generally the first-line drug used for the treatment of life-threatening systemic fungal and protozoal infections. However, its application is limited by its adverse side effects. There are three lipid-based formulations, with AmBisome® being the only liposome formulation, having an aqueous core within a bilayer system. Within AmBisome®, the liposomes are composed of hydrogenated soy phosphatidylcholine, cholesterol, distearoyl phosphatidylglycerol and α-tocopherol. In these liposomes, the amphotericin B is intercalated within the liposomal membrane because of its low solubility.

Abelcet® and Amphotec® are two alternative lipid-based formulations of amphotericin B. Abelcet® is formulated from dimyristoyl phosphatidylcholine and dimyristoyl phosphatidylglycerol, and the resultant constructs are ribbon-like complexes which are approximately 1.6 μm to 11 μm in diameter. Amphotec® consists of a complex of amphotericin B with cholesteryl sulfate which is disc-like in structure, with a diameter approximately 100 nm to 140 nm. Given the difference in their physical structures, these three formulations have different pharmacokinetic profiles, including differences in clearance rates and the volume of distribution, and therefore may not be considered directly interchangeable.

Liposomal delivery of vaccines

In addition to the ability of liposomes to passively target tumour sites, the natural tendency for liposomes to be taken up by phagocytic cells can be exploited to target cells of the immune system, such as dendritic cells, and thereby enhance the delivery of antigens. A range of bilayer vesicle systems have been shown to induce humoral and cellular immunity to a wide range of antigens. This is particularly useful for the delivery of soluble antigens which have a good safety profile but are weak at inducing immune responses. There are currently two liposome-type constructs, which are built from viral components and phospholipids, that are licensed as vaccine delivery systems (Table 44.6). These virosomes use viral components, such as influenza haemagglutinin, which enhances antigen delivery and targeting to the immune cells.

Sustained drug release from liposomes

Sustained drug release, multivesicle liposomes have been developed for clinical use. Both DepoCyte® and DepoDur® comprise large multivesicular vesicles which achieve sustained drug release through their slow clearance from the administration site and their slow breakdown. DepoDur® is administered as a single epidural injection and can give relief from postoperative pain for up to 48 hours.

Formulation design considerations for liposomes

When one is designing liposomes for drug delivery, in addition to consideration of the vesicle size and lamellarity, the lipid bilayer composition can play an important role in dictating the properties of the vesicles, and there are a wide range of options available for formulating liposomes.

Choice of lipid

Most clinically approved products use phosphatidylcholines (e.g. egg or soy phosphatidylcholine, dioleoyl phosphatidylcholine, dimyristoyl phosphatidylcholine) as the lipid within the formulation. It is used to give a structural framework in the liposome bilayers (Table 44.6). By varying the structure of the lipid fatty acid tails, one can manipulate the characteristics of the liposomes. By increasing the length of the carbon tails and the degree of saturation of the lipids, one can design the liposomes to have a more rigid and less permeable bilayer. This is useful for improving drug retention and avoiding opsonization. For example, DaunoXome® is formulated with distearoyl phosphatidylcholine, which has two fatty acid tails that are 18 carbons in length, and both are fully saturated. This allows strong hydrophobic interactions between the lipid tails and dense packing of them within the bilayer, which enhances the stability of the liposomes.

In addition to phospholipids, a range of other lipid/ amphiphilic molecules can be used to form liposomes. These include nonionic surfactants and amphiphilic synthetic block copolymers which form vesicles referred to as *niosomes* and *polymersomes* respectively. There are also *bilosomes* which are synthetic vesicles that include bile salts within the vesicle bilayer. Whilst each of these variations on liposomes may offer some differences in physicochemical characteristics, they all offer the bilayer structure which can incorporate drugs within the aqueous phase or within the bilayer depending on the drug attributes.

The key factor that dictates the aggregation of amphiphilic molecules into bilayer vesicles rather than, for example, micelles or liquid crystals is the molecular shape of the amphiphile as this will influence their geometrical packing within a given solution environment. The shape of an amphiphile may be expressed as its critical packing parameter (CPP), which is related to the ratio of the volume of the molecule (v) to the area of the head group (S_0) and the hydrophobic chain length (l_c), i.e.

$$CPP = v/S_0 l_c$$

$$(44.1)$$

Amphiphiles with a CPP of less than 1/3 (i.e. a cone shape) tend to form micelles, as in the case of, for example, sodium dodecyl sulfate (sodium lauryl sulfate). Amphiphiles with a CPP of between 0.5 and 1 (a truncated cone, e.g. phosphatidylcholine) will form vesicles. If the CPP of the molecule increases to more than 1 (e.g. dioleoyl phosphatidylethanolamine) inverted micelles tend to form. Whilst the use of CPP can provide a useful approach for predicting which structure amphiphiles may form, it is important to consider that changes in pH, temperature and lipid concentration can also have an influence. With lipid mixtures, the overall CPP of the system must be considered.

Cholesterol content

Cholesterol is also a common component of liposome formulations. Although cholesterol does not form bilayers on its own, it can be incorporated into liposome bilayers at concentrations up to 50% of total lipid. The presence of cholesterol in the bilayer can reduce the bilayer permeability of the liposomes and thus increase drug retention within liposomes. This has been attributed to the ability of cholesterol to reduce the mobility of the phospholipids and improve lipid packing within the bilayer.

Surface characteristics

A third consideration for liposomes is their surface properties. In addition to considering a PEGylated hydrophilic coating, one can also formulate liposomes to have an anionic or cationic surface charge. Cationic liposomes are currently being considered for the delivery of nucleic acid based therapies such as DNA and small interfering RNA, which are anionic and can electrostatically bind to cationic liposomes. Cationic liposomes are also being considered for the delivery of subunit vaccines, which are often anionic in nature. CAF01 is a cationic vesicle formulation, developed by Statens Serum Institut, Denmark. It is currently in clinical trials as a vaccine for the prevention of tuberculosis.

The conjugation of targeting groups to the surface of liposomes to promote their active targeting has also been investigated. Similar to the polymer-based systems, targeting groups such as folate or glycoproteins for targeting of tumour cells and the attachment of antibodies to liposomes have been investigated. Presently none of these are used clinically.

Drug characteristics

In addition to the design of the liposomal bilayer, the characteristics of the drug to be loaded into the vesicles require consideration. Drugs with high aqueous solubility (log $P < \sim1.7$) can be incorporated and retained within the aqueous compartments of the liposomes, whereas lipophilic drugs (log $P > 5$) are incorporated and retained within the liposome bilayers. Drugs with intermediate log P values are more difficult to incorporate within liposomes as they can partition between the aqueous phase and the bilayers, resulting in loss of the drug from the liposomes.

To address this issue and improve drug loading, remote drug loading has been developed. This is used in some marketed products, such as Caelyx® and DaunoXome®. In these formulations the liposomes are first prepared within an aqueous core containing ammonium sulfate. This results in an ammonium sulfate gradient across the liposome bilayer. When doxorubicin is added to the external aqueous phase, surrounding the liposomes during manufacture, doxorubicin diffuses across the liposomal membrane and enters the internal aqueous compartment of the liposomes. When inside the liposomes, because of the concentration of ammonium sulfate, the doxorubicin forms a drug–sulfate complex and becomes trapped within the vesicles. With use of this method, high drug loading efficiencies of more than 90% can be achieved.

Microcapsules and microspheres

Even though, as the name suggests, these particles are generally in the micrometre size range and therefore can fall outside the nanoparticle definition, these systems merit consideration here, given their clinical application in drug delivery. They are essentially spherical particles that can be manufactured to be solid or porous (often termed microparticles or microspheres) or they can be hollow (microcapsules). Their composition is basically the same as that of nanoparticles in that they can be formulated from polymers, lipids, proteins, etc. Polymers such as poly(lactic acid) and PLGA are commonly used. Drugs can be incorporated within the matrix systems, and therefore drug release is dictated by the degradation rate of the matrix. There are a number of polymeric microparticles approved for clinical use. Examples include the following:

- Lupron Depot® is a suspension of PLGA microspheres which are injected subcutaneously and act as a drug depot after administration, giving controlled release of leuprolide acetate for up to 6 months. This system is used for the palliative treatment of advanced prostate cancer, management of endometriosis, treatment of fibroids and the treatment of children with central precocious puberty. Other commercialized PLGA microsphere formulations containing leuprolide include Enantone® Depot, Enantone®-Gyn and Trenantone®.
- Decapeptyl® offers sustained release of triptorelin from microspheres prepared from PLGA. The active ingredient is triptorelin

acetate, a gonadorelin (luteinizing hormone releasing hormone) analogue, and it is prescribed for the treatment of advanced prostate cancer and endometriosis. The microsphere formulation is injected intramuscularly, and the bioavailability of triptorelin is reported as approximately 50%. Alternative microsphere formulations of triptorelin include Trelstar® Depot.

- Parlodel® LA is a PLGA microsphere formulation of bromocriptine mesilate which is a dopamine receptor agonist that reduces plasma levels of prolactin and is used in the treatment of Parkinson's disease.
- Sandostatin® LAR is administered by intramuscular injection and gives sustained release of octreotide, a synthetic form of the peptide hormone somatostatin. It is used in patients to help control symptoms of acromegaly and for the treatment of gastroenteropancreatic neuroendocrine tumours. It is formulated from PLGA microspheres of approximately 30 μm which offer steady-state drug release over 28 days.

Ongoing developments

Within the field of nanotechnology there are a large number of formulation options to enhance the delivery of a drug. There are several systems that are already licensed for clinical use, and many more are in various stages of clinical trials. Most of these systems are being considered for their application in oncology. However, nanotechnology is not limited to this area, and the application of these delivery systems is also being considered for peptide-based therapies and the delivery of DNA and small interfering RNA. Given the range of functional attributes of nanotechnology, it is likely that the application of this evolving technology will continue to expand, providing new and reformulated therapeutics which offer better clinical outcomes and improved patient-focused formulations.

Please check your eBook at **https://studentconsult. inkling.com/** for self-assessment questions. See inside cover for registration details.

Bibliography

Duncan, R., 2011. Polymer therapeutics as nanomedicines: new perspectives. Curr. Opin. Biotechnol. 22, 392–501.

Gregoriadis, G., Perrie, Y., 2010. Liposomes. In: Encyclopedia of Life Sciences (ELS). John Wiley & Sons, Chichester.

Lee, C.L., MacKay, J.A., Frechet, J.M.J., et al., 2005. Designing dendrimers for biological applications. Nat. Biotechnol. 23, 1517–1526.

Perrie, Y., Rades, T., 2012. FASTtrack Pharmaceutics – Drug Delivery and Targeting, second ed. Pharmaceutical Press, London.

Uchegbu, I.F. (Ed.), 2000. Synthetic Surfactant Vesicles, Niosomes and Other Non-Phospholipid Vesicular Systems. Harwood Academic Publishers, Amsterdam.

Veronese, F.M. (Ed.), 2009. PEGylated Protein Drugs: Basic Science and Clinical Applications. Birkhäuser, Berlin.

45

Design and administration of medicines for paediatric and geriatric patients

Catherine Tuleu   Mine Orlu   David Wright

CHAPTER CONTENTS

KEY POINTS

- In deciding on the appropriateness of a dosage form, one needs to assess the vulnerability and capability of the patient, young or old.
- The swallowing process is affected by a child's development and for adults by the ageing process. For some patients, administration of tablets/capsules may be problematic, if possible at all. This includes neonates and patients with conditions commonly associated with ageing, such as dementia, stroke, Parkinson's disease and cancer, which can cause difficulties when medicines are administered via the oral route.
- In children, manipulation of adult medicines and/ or addition of them to food is a common occurrence, even if this is not always appropriate practice.
- In certain cases, enteral feed tubes may be used to administer food, liquids and drugs to patients, but these can cause significant problems when oral formulations are administered.
- The permeability of the skin to drugs is affected by the development and ageing process.
- Inhalation devices provide clear examples of where the design of the administration device limits its suitability in relation to the patient's ability to use it correctly.
- The pharmacist is the only health care professional who has sufficient knowledge of the science of medicines formulation to provide informed advice regarding alternative options and the possible consequences of formulation manipulation with regard to a patient with swallowing problems.

Human development, ageing and drug administration

Whilst early development and ageing processes can affect the acceptability and appropriateness of different dosage forms for administration to either paediatric or geriatric populations, each patient should be considered on an individual basis. The fact that someone is young or old does not necessarily mean that that person will experience the problems commonly associated with his or her 'physical age'. It is, however, important for the designers of dosage forms to be aware of potential age-related problems and how these affect the suitability of different formulations depending on the 'behavioural age' or 'developmental age' of the patient. Furthermore, pharmacists and pharmaceutical scientists should be aware of the different options available to them, and be able to provide suitable products and advice on the most appropriate dosage form, formulation or method of administration.

Paediatric and geriatric populations

The *paediatric* population is generally classified into five age groups (International Conference on Harmonisation of Technical Requirements for Registration of Pharmaceuticals for Human Use, 1999):

- *preterm newborn infants* – those who are born before 38 weeks of pregnancy;
- *term newborn infants* – those who are less than 1 month old;
- *infants and toddlers* – those who are aged between 1 month and 2 years;
- *children* – those who are aged between 2 and 11 years; and
- *adolescents* – those who are aged 12 years to 16–18 years (dependent on regional definitions).

The *geriatric* population is arbitrarily defined as comprising patients aged 65 years or older (International Conference on Harmonisation of Technical Requirements for Registration of Pharmaceuticals for Human Use, 1995). The true representation of older people (e.g. age ranges, clinical condition) is important in the clinical drug product development. Thus in clinical testing programmes, data are recommended to be collected and presented for three individual age categories: 65–74 years, 75–84 years and 85 years or older (International Conference on Harmonisation of Technical Requirements for Registration of Pharmaceuticals for Human Use, 1995). Nevertheless, chronological age is not the only indicator to define older people. The geriatric population is a heterogeneous group mainly because of the presence of comorbidities as well as physical and cognitive decline which occurs with advanced age. Consequently, older patients with comorbidities, sensory deficits and frailty should be considered during both the design and the administration of medicines.

Swallowing oral dosage forms

Tablets and capsules are the most commonly prescribed solid dosage forms because they are relatively cheap to produce, are portable, can be coated to mask unpleasant taste or can be formulated to modify the drug release profile. Furthermore, their dry nature provides a stable environment for the drug, and hence allows the final product to have a relatively long shelf life. Whilst such medicines are popular with prescribers, they are not always the most suitable for patients with swallowing difficulties that can result from either a psychological aversion to swallowing tablets or a physical impairment to swallowing (*dysphagia*). Psychological aversion to swallowing tablets, which usually originates in childhood, is prevalent in all age groups, whereas dysphagia is much more common in older people.

The swallowing process

The swallowing process comprises three phases: the oral, pharyngeal and oesophageal phases (Fig. 45.1). Within the *oral phase* (Fig. 45.1b) the bolus is manipulated by the tongue in preparation for swallowing, usually breaking larger objects into smaller ones and mixing with saliva to make the bolus both soft and less adhesive. During the *pharyngeal phase* (Fig. 45.1c) muscle control is subconscious and the bolus is moved into the pharynx, where the passage to the lungs is automatically closed via movement of the epiglottis. Within the *oesophageal phase* (Fig. 45.1d) the bolus passes beyond the upper oesophageal sphincter and into the oesophagus. Although movement of the bolus is mainly due to gravity, it is partially controlled by peristaltic waves within the oesophagus which occur automatically in response to swallowing. Consequently, tablets and capsules are most easily swallowed by a person in an upright position (with the person sitting or standing up) and this advice is commonly given to patients for tablets or capsules which are known to cause oesophageal irritation (e.g. doxycycline).

Paediatric populations

Swallowing problems are common in young children. Before 4 or 5 months of age, infants possess an extrusion reflex which enables them to swallow only liquids. Moreover, a gag reflex of varying degrees can last up until approximately 7–9 months of age. Hence eating requires active effort, and the child must be

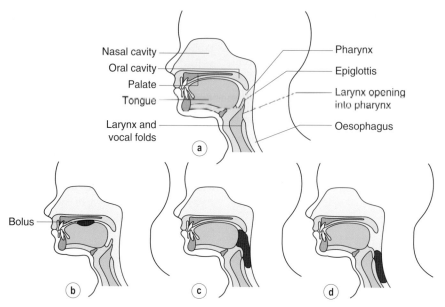

Fig. 45.1 • Anatomy of the mouth and phases of bolus swallowing. **(a)** Anatomy of the mouth. **(b)** Oral phase. **(c)** Pharyngeal phase. **(d)** Oesophageal phase.

able to coordinate sucking, swallowing and breathing. Infants are ready for spoon-feeding of semisolids by 4–6 months of age. Although they are not capable at that age of swallowing a monolithic dosage form (e.g. a tablet), multiparticulates (powders, granules, pellets, minitablets < 3 mm) might be given sprinkled onto a vehicle, e.g. soft food (if compatible). At ages greater than approximately 6 years, children are considered able to swallow conventional tablets or capsules. Generally, the smaller the solid dosage form, the easier it is for children to swallow, but interindividual differences in swallowing ability should be considered.

Geriatric populations

The loss of muscle control associated with the swallowing process is of concern for the administration of tablets and capsules to the elderly. As people get older, saliva production generally reduces, and this can make it more difficult to swallow tablets or capsules, which require some lubrication before swallowing. This can, however, be easily overcome if the tablets or capsules are taken with a glass of water; reduction in saliva production should not in itself be a reason for patients not to be prescribed such solid dosage forms. Furthermore, tablets or capsules administered without water can be held in the pharynx or oesophagus, and this can increase the

likelihood of local erosion or irritation, and therefore all patients, irrespective of age, should be told to take tablets and capsules with water.

Loss of muscle control during the oral phase of swallowing can make it difficult to create a manageable bolus for swallowing, may cause the 'loss' of small tablets within the oral cavity or can make it more difficult psychologically to overcome the gag reflex that is necessary to swallow tablets or capsules. Loss of muscle control during the pharyngeal phase, which is controlled subconsciously, can increase the likelihood of choking, or at least the anticipation of choking, if it is not possible to propel the bolus through this phase. During the pharyngeal phase the airway is temporarily closed to allow the safe passage of food or liquids into the stomach. If solid dosage forms lodge in this area, the epiglottis will not open and the patient will asphyxiate.

Loss of control of the epiglottis during the pharyngeal phase can result in it not closing as the bolus passes, and consequently the contents may inadvertently be aspirated into the lungs. The main defence mechanism within the lungs is the cough reflex, whereby contents are forcibly removed under pressure. A natural and background production of mucus which transports materials out of the lungs is another mechanism of removing foreign and waste products. However, this has limited capacity and is restricted to small particles. Consequently, unintended aspiration of nonsterile foods or medicines can increase the likelihood of pulmonary infections, which are more likely to be fatal in an older person.

In addition to the ageing process, conditions commonly associated with ageing such as dementia, stroke, gastro-oesophageal reflex disease (GORD), Parkinson's disease and cancer can all cause difficulties when tablets and capsules are administered orally. The loss of muscle control associated with the progression of Parkinson's disease and dementia results in dysphagia in most patients with these diagnoses. It is estimated that almost 70% of people who have a stroke will have some form of dysphagia immediately after the stroke. However, in most patients the normal swallow returns and less than 10% of people who experience a stroke are found to have permanent dysphagia. Dementia, stroke and Parkinson's disease have greatest impact on the oral and pharyngeal phases of swallowing, and therefore patients with these conditions become concerned about choking and aspiration. Head, neck and gastrointestinal tract cancers can all cause dysphagia by blocking access to the stomach, whilst radiotherapy and chemotherapy can affect the oral and gastrointestinal mucosa, thereby making swallowing more difficult. Persistent GORD can cause inflammation within the oesophagus, and this can result in patients describing foods and medicines as 'sticking in the back of their throats,' with a consequential struggle to swallow.

The nature of the dysphagia is therefore important when one is deciding on the best approach for the patient. For patients who are struggling to manipulate oral doses, increasing the bulk of a medicine or the addition of water to the swallow may make it easier for the patient, whereas those patients who have dysphagia due to a blockage may require physically very small doses or low-viscosity liquids. In those patients who are at risk of aspiration it may be inappropriate to administer tablets with water as the mixed consistencies may increase the likelihood of aspiration. Consequently, a single bolus of a thicker consistency may be more appropriate for such patients.

Assessment of swallowing ability

Speech and language therapists are usually the most appropriate professionals to assess the swallowing process. This may involve a brief bedside assessment via questioning and a test requiring the patient to drink a glass of water. More invasive procedures include use of a nasogastric camera (fibre-optic endoscopic examination) or an X-ray of the swallow of a radio-opaque liquid material (videofluoroscopy). The assessment should determine whether the oral route is appropriate and if so what the optimal texture of administered foods and medicines should be. This should provide some insight into the best pharmaceutical formulation for that patient.

If dysphagia is not identified in a patient and an inappropriate formulation is prescribed, then this may affect the patient's ability or willingness to self-administer the formulation perorally. Evidence suggests that older people frequently deny or ignore swallowing problems as this is indicative of ageing. An older person's ability to swallow oral medicines should, however, always be ascertained by the prescriber to ensure that he or she is given the most appropriate formulation.

Helping patients with swallowing difficulties

Where patients with dysphagia are still able to use the oral route, the prescriber or pharmacist has three main options available to him or her:

- determine whether the medicine is still required or whether its use can be safely discontinued;
- identify a suitable formulation which can be swallowed; and
- identify an alternative route of administration.

In reviewing the ongoing need for the medicine, the pharmacist, together with the prescriber, should determine if the medicine is effective and if so whether the benefits of the therapy outweigh any risks during administration. Additionally, if the dysphagia is likely to be acute, as may be seen immediately following a stroke, then use of medicines may be temporarily stopped until the swallow mechanism reappears.

Formulation design for paediatric and geriatric patients

Liquid peroral dosage forms

Formulating liquid, rather than solid medicines provides some particular problems for the pharmaceutical industry because of the need to keep the drug stable in the usually aqueous environment, to ensure that the final mixture is palatable and to ensure dosing consistency. Selection of a suitable liquid vehicle and manufacturing facilities requires significant investment, as does the selection of appropriate antimicrobials, stabilizers, suspending agents and flavourings (see Chapter 24). The combination of complex formulation science, relatively short shelf lives (compared with those of tablets and capsules) and the relatively small market size results in a lack of availability of licensed liquid medicines for many drugs. Moreover, liquid formulations often cost significantly more than their solid dosage form counterparts. Where licensed liquid medicines are available, the thickness may not always be appropriate, and therefore this also requires consideration.

Paediatric considerations

With children, liquids are actually easy to administer and offer flexible yet accurate dosing with an appropriate dosing device. The most suitable of these are oral syringes, graduated in millilitres, which can cater for the heterogeneous paediatric population and for a single child as it grows. However, the taste or smell of the drug can sometimes be difficult to mask in a liquid formulation, and this is a strong deterrent to patient adherence.

Selection of appropriate excipients

Formulation of liquids usually requires many excipients. These excipients can present a significant toxicological risk to a patient, depending on numerous factors, including the age of the child and the clinical condition, the route of administration, the exposure (dose and dosing frequency) and the safety profile of the excipient (allergies and sensitization, acute and cumulative toxicity), as illustrated in Table 45.1. The formulator of a liquid medicine needs to make rational choices regarding added excipients, deciding on their purpose, and if their use is inappropriate, an alternative must be sought. A striking example is the case of elixirs; these liquid formulations generally contain an appreciable percentage content of ethanol and have historically been used (and some still are) in neonates and infants. The inclusion of ethanol in paediatric medicines should be avoided, especially for babies and vulnerable patients, who are not able to metabolize it as efficiently as adults.

Sweeteners and flavouring agents. These are used to mask the taste of liquids and tablets, such as chewable and dispersible tablets. A sweet flavour

can be achieved by using sweeteners that may be categorized as follows:

1. Nutritive
   - sugars (e.g. sucrose, dextrose, fructose, lactose);
   - corn syrup;
   - high-fructose corn syrup; and
   - sugar alcohols (polyols, e.g. hydrogenated glucose syrup, maltitol, mannitol, sorbitol, and xylitol).
2. Nonnutritive
   - high-intensity 'artificial' sweeteners (e.g. acesulfame potassium, sucralose, aspartame, neotame, saccharin); and
   - natural intense sweeteners (e.g. glycyrrhizin, thaumatin, rebaudioside A).

Not all sweeteners have received regulatory authority approval in all countries, and this, alongside consideration of the safety profile, is an important factor when a formulator is selecting which of them to include in a formulation. By blending different sweeteners in combination with other ingredients, such as flavours and texture enhancers, the formulator can optimize the sensory characteristics of a drug product. For example, a sugar-free product can be prepared that is comparable in properties and taste with a sugar-containing version. However, this is not a simple task and requires very specific sensory expertise.

Sugar-free sweeteners. Because of the cariogenic (causing dental caries) nature of the sugars traditionally used as sweeteners, 'sugar-free' alternatives are now increasingly used in liquid medicines. Products that do not contain fructose, glucose or sucrose are considered to be 'sugar-free'. In addition, preparations containing hydrogenated glucose syrup (Lycasin), maltitol, sorbitol or xylitol may also be considered as 'sugar-free', as there is evidence that they do not cause dental caries (i.e. they are noncariogenic). However, preparations containing hydrogenated glucose syrup or maltitol, although they are noncariogenic, are not strictly 'sugar-free' as they are both metabolized to glucose.

Polyols can cause problems of digestive intolerance. These effects are dose dependent, and particular care must be taken when these are used in medicines for children with a low body weight.

If it is necessary to give a sugar-containing product to a child at bedtime, it is recommended to subsequently rinse the child's mouth.

Table 45.1 Excipients with elevated toxicological risk for the subpopulations of paediatric and geriatric patients

Excipient	Administration	Adverse reaction
Preterm and term neonates, infants ≤6 months		
Benzyl alcohol	Oral, parenteral	Neurotoxicity, metabolic acidosis
Ethanol	Oral, parenteral	Neurotoxicity
Polyethylene glycol	Parenteral	Metabolic acidosis
Polysorbate 20 and polysorbate 80	Parenteral	Liver and kidney failure
Propylene glycol	Oral, parenteral	Seizures, neurotoxicity, hyperosmolarity
Patients with reduced kidney function		
Aluminium salts	Oral, parenteral	Encephalopathy, microcytic anaemia, osteodystrophy
Polyethylene glycol	Parenteral	Metabolic acidosis
Propylene glycol	Oral, parenteral	Neurotoxicity, hyperosmolarity
Hypersensitive patients		
Azo dyes	Oral	Urticaria, bronchoconstriction, angioedema
Benzalkonium chloride	Oral, nasal, ocular	Bronchoconstriction
Chlorocresol	Parenteral	Anaphylactic reactions
Dextran	Parenteral	Anaphylactic reactions
Macrogolglycerol ricinoleate (Cremophor EL)	Parenteral	Anaphylactic reactions
Parabens	Oral, parenteral, ocular, topical	Allergies, contact dermatitis
Sorbic acid	Topical	Contact dermatitis (rarely)
Starches	Oral	Gluten-induced coeliac disease
Sulfites, bisulfites	Oral, parenteral	Asthma attacks, rashes, abdominal upset
Wool wax	Topical	Contact dermatitis, urticaria
Patients with metabolic disorders		
Aspartame	Oral	Phenylketonuria
Fructose	Oral, parenteral	Hereditary fructose intolerance
Lactose	Oral	Lactose intolerance, diarrhoea
Sorbitol	Oral	Hereditary fructose intolerance
Sucrose	Oral, parenteral	Hereditary fructose intolerance

Data from Breitkreutz & Tuleu, 2009.

Colouring agents. The use of colouring agents in medicines, particularly those intended for use by children, is widely debated. Colouring agents (colourants) are largely incorporated into pharmaceutical products to improve their appearance and/or sometimes to match the colour of a medicine with its taste, examples being the addition of a red colour with red-fruit flavours, yellow with lemon, purple with blackcurrant, etc. By default, paediatric medicines should normally not be coloured, except in some very specific and justifiable cases. Colouring agents permitted for use in foodstuffs are also allowed in medicines (providing they are approved by the relevant local regulatory bodies). However, azo dyes are not considered acceptable.

Geriatric considerations

Liquid medicines are the logical alternative to tablets and capsules for patients with swallowing difficulties and are recommended where a swallow mechanism via the oral route is still available, and when a suitable texture which minimizes the likelihood of aspiration can be obtained.

Clearly many of the formulation issues pertaining to liquid paediatric medicines, described already, equally apply to medicines for use by elderly patients. Particular attention should be paid to the suitability of any excipients used in liquid or dispersible medicines.

For instance, sorbitol is commonly used as a sweetener in liquid formulations, and a dosage exceeding 15 g per day in adults can result in bloating, flatulence and diarrhoea. This is the case for many polyols. In adults, their intake can lead to usually mild and temporary gastrointestinal symptoms. The cumulative amount administered should be checked when the patient is polymedicated. Medicines taken concomitantly, especially if they are liquids, should be checked for their polyol content. Gastrointestinal tract transit may be accelerated by these excipients, and there is the potential for drug absorption to be decreased.

When dispersible tablet formulations are used, the sodium content may be clinically important. For example, 4 g of paracetamol daily, administered as eight dispersible 500 mg tablets, provides up to 160 mmol of sodium.

Diabetes is common in the older population. Diabetes UK advises that when medicines are taken in small quantities, for limited periods, the sugar content is unlikely to cause problems for patients with diabetes. This is because the sugar content of medicines is low in relation to the total carbohydrate content of a normal diet. Sugar-free alternatives should be recommended if the medicine is for long-term use. Care should be taken with preparations containing hydrogenated glucose syrup or maltitol because, as mentioned already, they are both metabolized to glucose. Additionally, they offer no real advantage to patients with diabetes as they contain significant amounts of calories and carbohydrates. Therefore patients with diabetes should treat these products as if they contain sugar. Artificial sweeteners are virtually free of calories, and do not raise blood glucose levels.

Older patients often have multiple morbidities and are hence prescribed multiple drugs, which is described by the term 'polypharmacy'. It is important to provide the appropriate formulations and packaging to ensure patients with comorbidities are able to maintain self-administration of their medicines. The presentation of multiple drugs in a single entity, known as 'fixed-dose combinations', has potential in managing complex therapies and improving patient adherence.

Other oral dosage forms

Alternative presentations can be administered directly in, or to, the oral cavity. These include buccal tablets, (oro)dispersible, soluble or chewable tablets, sprinkle capsules or 'stickpacks'. However, because of the relatively small size of the market, the range of such options is still limited.

Nonperoral dosage forms

Parenteral routes

Parenteral routes of administration are discussed in Chapter 36. As the oral route is not usable in seriously ill patients, including neonates, intravenous administration via peripheral, umbilical or 'long' peripheral lines is frequently used. The addition of medications needs to be taken into account (i.e. their volume and ion contribution) in the context of the patient's complex fluid, electrolyte and nutrition management. Intramuscular administration is not recommended when muscle mass and perfusion is not optimal (e.g. in neonates) as this may lead to erratic bioavailability and importantly to pain during injection and risk of tissue damage. Moreover, children tend to be needle phobic. Most of the reconstitution of injectable drugs is done immediately before administration to the patient, and the risks and errors related to the preparation and administration of injectable drugs are numerous in paediatric settings. The formulation characteristics (pH, viscosity, osmolarity), the use of inappropriate concentrations requiring complex calculation and serial dilutions or measurement of small volumes, the site of injection and, if relevant, the needle thickness and needle length and the infusion rate all have to be scrutinized closely. The importance of being aware of the excipients to which the patient will be exposed cannot be overemphasized (Table 45.1).

Older people tend to have more fragile veins, largely due to muscle wasting and loss of supportive tissues. Consequently, siting and maintaining injection lines can be harder than in a younger person. Furthermore, the risk of vein rupture and extravasation is higher in the elderly. Similarly, subcutaneous injections are more difficult to administer to this patient group, because of loss of cutaneous tissue and collagen. The subcutaneous space is harder to find when the skin is pinched because of the overall skin structure lacking thickness and because of the fragility of the epidermis resulting from collagen loss.

Pulmonary route

There are many aerosol-generating medical devices. Apart from the formulation itself, the ability of the patient to use the device must be taken in account.

Inhalation (see Chapter 37) is the preferred route of administration in the treatment of asthma – the most common long-term medical condition, affecting almost 10% of children in the UK. It is important that the choice of the appropriate inhaler device and interface for patients is informed by the age of the patient, as presented in Table 45.2.

For children younger than 5 years, the preferred inhalation device would be a pressurized metered-dose inhaler (pMDI) with a mouthpiece and spacer (see later) or with a facemask for younger patients. The same applies for nebulizers, with modern designs tending to be smaller, more portable and more appealing to children than in the past. Dry powder inhalers are suitable only if sufficient inspiratory flow is achievable by patients, which are typically school-aged children. Spacers (valved-holding chambers) are large plastic containers, often in two halves that click together with a mouthpiece or facemask at one end and a hole for insertion of the mouthpiece of an inhalation device at the other end (Fig. 45. 2; see also Fig. 37.4). They are used without the need to coordinate breathing and actuation of a pMDI to ease administration, to decrease oropharyngeal

Table 45.2 Choosing an inhaler device and interface for patients of different ages

| | Age | | | |
	Birth to 4 years	4–5 years	6–12 years	≥13 years
Inhaler device	Nebulizer or pMDI with VHC and facemask	Nebulizer, pMDI with VHC, DPI or breath-actuated pMDI (at the age of 5 years)	Nebulizer, pMDI with VHC, DPI, breath-actuated pMDI or breath-actuated nebulizer	All devices
Interface	Mask, hood or high-flow nasal cannula	Facemask or mouthpiece	Mouthpiece or facemask	Mouthpiece or facemask

DPI, dry powder inhaler; pMDI, pressurized metered-dose inhaler; VHC, valved holding chamber.
Data from Ari & Fink, 2011.

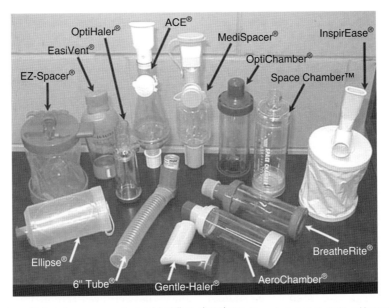

Fig. 45.2 • Examples of inhalation spacers/valved holding chambers. From Asmus et al., 2004, with permission.

impaction and increase deposition of the drug in the lungs (see also Chapter 37).

The ageing process can result in reduced visual acuity, reduced ability to manipulate small objects and cognitive impairment. All three can affect how a person uses any medicine and/or delivery device and should therefore always be considered when one is selecting the most appropriate formulation for an older person. Muscle wasting in the older person results in a lack of ability to use accessory muscles (intercostals) effectively when breath-actuated or nonpassive inhalation devices are used. Similarly, an older person with poor manual dexterity may have difficulties in coordinating inhalation technique because of visual/auditory/cognitive impairment. Finally, standard measures of lung function naturally decline over time (forced expiratory volume in the first second of expiration, forced vital capacity, etc.), suggesting loss of elastic recoil, loss of pulmonary volume and loss of muscular control, which would affect the ability to use an inhalation device or medication effectively. Devices exist (e.g. Haleraid®) which are placed over a conventional pMDI, to allow patients to actuate the device when strength in the hands is impaired (e.g. in arthritis).

Nasal route

Nasal administration (see Chapter 38) can also be difficult, but this needle-free approach may be used as an alternative to parenteral administration in acute situations before intravenous catheter insertion, or in situations where intravenous access is not likely to be required. Recent applications are for analgesic, anxiolytic and antiepileptic drugs. For example, diamorphine and fentanyl nasal formulations have been administered to treat acute pain in children as an alternative to parenteral administration. The taste of nasal formulations can be an issue as nasally administered preparations are partially swallowed. An appropriate device and formulation can increase nasal retention (see Chapter 38). The limited nasal capacity restricts the volumes that can be instilled, especially in children. Formulators need to ensure the tolerability and safety of any excipients, such as preservatives, used in these products.

Delivery to and through the skin

Delivery to and through the skin is discussed in Chapter 40. If babies are born at term, their stratum corneum is fully functional, but during the first years after birth the skin is more perfused and hydrated than in adults. Great care should be taken in preterm neonates, whose skin barrier is not efficient, and which could permit the absorption of undesirable materials. Another consideration is the reduced *body surface to body mass ratio* (cm^2/kg) and the smaller volume of distribution for very young children, which explains why absorption can be especially enhanced in neonates and infants, even more so if there is unintentional occlusion (e.g. by the use of nappies).

The transdermal route of administration is potentially useful, as it is passive. However, drugs suitable for delivery by this route need particular characteristics (see Chapter 40), and few products are currently available. Transdermal patches are easy to use, but adapting the dosage requirements for children over a range of body weights is a possible limitation of their use. The nature of patch design (see Chapter 40) means that patches intended for use in adults cannot simply be cut to modify the dose for administration to a child.

Self-administration of patches by older people can create problems because of difficulties in removing them from their packaging and removal of their backing strips, as well as difficulties in applying them to appropriate areas in rotation. Remembering to remove one patch before applying the next may be a problem in the cognitively impaired, and patients may have difficulties physically reaching patches which have been applied by a carer.

Rectal route

The acceptability of preparations such as suppositories to older people must be taken into account. Rectal administration (see Chapter 41) has many inherent limitations but can be an option for paediatric patients, especially to avoid the oral route or when this route is not usable because of, for example, vomiting or unconsciousness. The rectal route has been used for treatment of epilepsy, constipation, analgesia, inflammatory bowel disease, malaria, fever and nausea. In younger children, lack of self-control of retention of the dosage form can be a drawback.

Other routes of drug administration

The ocular (see Chapter 39) and otic/aural routes of administration are complicated by the difficulties associated with handling of administration devices, and often self-administration is not possible. Although usually not very well accepted, use of these routes is frequently unavoidable as products administered via these routes are for a local therapeutic effect. A balance between the manual dexterity of the person administering the dose and the cooperation of the patient needs to be struck and this is often problematic for the young and the old.

Alternative dosage forms and routes of administration which avoid the need to swallow are increasingly being made available.

Adaptation of existing dosage forms

If a specific paediatric or geriatric product is not available, then the manipulation of existing products, usually tablets or capsules, before administration has to be considered. The process of tablet crushing or capsule opening and mixing with food or water is a form of unlicensed manufacture (i.e. the procedure has not received approval by the appropriate regulatory authority) and therefore can be authorized only by a prescriber. Whilst in some situations it may be safe to undertake this practice, there are many tablet and capsule formulations where it would generally be considered unwise to tamper with the product before administration.

Firstly, it is unsafe to recommend that cytotoxic or hormonal products (e.g. finasteride, tamoxifen, methotrexate) are tampered with before administration. Hormonal and cytotoxic products can be aerosolized and inhaled, or absorbed through the skin, and therefore the administrator can be exposed to a dose of the drug, however small, which may be unsafe. Similarly, products which can cause contact skin sensitization, such as chlorpromazine, should not be crushed before administration. Consequently, when the prescriber is considering either recommending or authorizing the manipulation of an existing dosage form, the potential danger to the individual tampering with the product and the individual administering it should always be considered.

Such procedures should be considered as a last resort, and all reasonable steps should be taken to obtain an appropriate formulation, or change to an alternative medication that is available in an appropriate formulation.

Unlicensed products

Where suitable licensed alternative formulations are not available, it may be necessary to prepare, by extemporaneous compounding or by outsourcing ('specials'), unlicensed formulations to ensure that a patient obtains access to a prescribed drug. However, the quality of unlicensed products, patient acceptability, shelf life and cost can differ considerably. It is therefore necessary for pharmacists to have some understanding of the quality of the available products, as frequently there may be a choice available to them.

Pharmacy compounding includes the preparation, mixing, assembling, packaging or labelling of a drug in response to a prescription written by an authorized prescriber. It remains one of the highest-risk activities performed in pharmacy, as the risks of unlicensed medicines are combined with the inherent risks associated with the compounding of a formulation. The quality, safety and efficacy of compounded preparations are jeopardized by the lack of standardization of compounding practices, harmonization of formulations or information on stability.

'Specials' have a similar status but are usually made in larger volumes by licensed manufacturers and suitably licensed hospital units (the licence is issued by the appropriate regulatory authority to authorize manufacture, not the product). However, these products are not always subjected to full quality assurance test procedures, especially if they are not produced as a batch.

The preparation of the same drug as an unlicensed liquid medicine could range from crushing a tablet in a suspending agent with a 2-week shelf life to a sourced pure drug placed in a carefully formulated base with an extended shelf life. In all cases, however, bioequivalence of the liquid medicine compared with a tablet or capsule will not have been demonstrated, and therefore once a patient has been given and stabilized on a certain unlicensed product, it is preferable to always source the same product for that patient.

The main measure of quality of an unlicensed product is via the certificate with which it is supplied. A certificate of analysis is supplied when the special has been produced in a batch and the supplier has quality assured the final product by analysing the ingredients to confirm (quantitatively) the content of the active ingredient and excipients in the final product. A certificate of conformity basically confirms that in the making of a one-off product, the production formula and process was followed. Any problems with sourced ingredients will not be identified within such a process, nor will mistakes in production. Consequently, a certificate of analysis is always preferable to a certificate of conformity.

There might be an appropriate product with a license available in another country, which can be imported, yet remains unlicensed in the country of import. However, this option is not without logistic issues (product information provided in the local language, recall systems in place, time to obtain it, cost, etc.).

When sourcing and supplying unlicensed medicines, pharmacists need to be aware of their increased legal liability. Where licensed medicines are used within the terms of their license, liability for any subsequent patient harms reside with the manufacturer. If, however, a patient is harmed following receipt of an unlicensed medicine, the liability is shared between the prescriber and the supplier, with the actions of both being carefully considered in any subsequent legal action.

Whilst a small number of medicines are licensed for administration via enteral feed tubes, the administration of medicines via enteral tubes usually represents an unlicensed action, as most medicines have not been tested via this route. The practice of crushing or dispersing tablets, or opening capsules before administration, does not therefore significantly increase the legal liability associated with this activity.

Dosage form issues

Immediate-release film-coated tablets

Immediate-release film coats are placed on medicines for various reasons (see Chapter 32). These include:

- to mask the taste of the drug; and
- to prevent contact sensitization when the medicine is being handled.

In some cases (when the coat is nonfunctional and is there, for instance, only for colour recognition), damaging the film coat immediately before administration is unlikely to adversely affect patient care. Removing a taste-masking coating may decrease palatability, whilst film coats which protect against contact sensitization should not be disrupted.

Drugs that have a small therapeutic window can switch from being effective to causing adverse events just by small changes to their bioavailability. Crushing or dispersing digoxin tablets, which have a bioavailability of just less than 70%, could in theory increase the bioavailability to 100% and effectively increase the dose received in the patient by almost

50%. Where formulations of drugs with a small therapeutic window are manipulated, the clinical effects should be monitored to ensure that toxicity does not ensue.

Gastro-resistant (enteric) coated tablets

Gastro-resistant coats (see Chapters 31 and 32) are placed on tablets:

- to protect the stomach from the active ingredient within the medicine (e.g. naproxen, aspirin);
- to protect the active ingredient from the hostile environment of the stomach (e.g. omeprazole, lansoprazole); or
- to release the active ingredient beyond the stomach (e.g. sulfasalazine for local treatment within the colon).

It is never appropriate to recommend tampering with gastro-resistant coated formulations.

Modified-release products

Modified-release products are carefully designed to release the drug over an extended period so as to reduce the peak drug concentrations in the blood observed with immediate-release products, and reduce the required frequency of dosing (discussed further in Chapter 31). Reduction in peak plasma concentrations minimizes side effects (e.g. for nifedipine and theophylline), whereas reducing dosing frequency improves patient adherence.

Where a particular formulation is intended to extend the duration of drug release, a larger dose of the drug is incorporated compared with the dose in an immediate-release product. Consequently, anything that damages the designed release mechanism (such as crushing tablets) could increase the likelihood of adverse events in the patient resulting from a larger than usual dose dump (Fig. 45.3). Where dose dumping of this type occurs, elimination of the drug is quicker and thus the patient will experience a period between doses when drug levels are subtherapeutic (see Chapters 22 and 31). Consequently, tampering with any modified-release product is not recommended, unless the manufacturer clearly indicates that this is allowable. Modified-release morphine capsules (MXL®), for example, contain modified-release pellets which can be safely released from the outer shell of the capsule, providing they are not themselves tampered with or chewed, as this will affect their release properties.

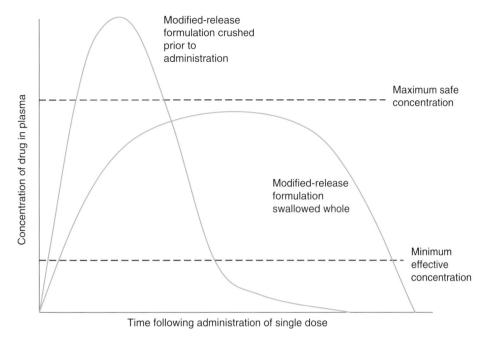

Fig. 45.3 • Theoretical release of drug from an intact modified-release formulation and from a modified-release formulation that has been crushed.

Dosage form administration issues

Administering medicines via enteral feed tubes

In extreme cases, where it is deemed no longer safe to administer medicines orally to elderly patients, enteral tubes which bypass the oral route may be inserted. Enteral tubes, which are primarily designed for the administration of foods and liquids, can be sited either through the nasal cavity to the exit site (see later) or directly into the stomach or jejunum through the abdominal wall.

Enteral feeding tubes are commonly used to maintain or supplement nutritional and fluid intake in patients with significant dysphagia. Within acute care, a nasogastric tube is most frequently used, the internal diameter usually being 1.5 mm to 2.5 mm. Enteral feeding tube external diameters (D) are typically measured in 'French units' or 'French gauge'. One French unit (Fr) equals 0.33 mm, thus D (mm) = French gauge/3 or French gauge = D (mm) × 3. In general, the range of small-bore tube sizes for paediatric use is 6 Fr to 10 Fr. A size of 6 Fr is used for standard feeds and 7 Fr is used for higher-density and fibre feeds. The tubes have a range of lengths, usually 550 mm, 750 mm or 850 mm. In intensive care neonatal and paediatric units, the tubes used are likely to be smaller in length and diameter.

Within the community, permanent gastrostomy devices are most commonly used as these have minimal risk of displacement. Additionally, these tubes are usually of slightly wider bore. Increasingly, jejunal tubes are being used in patients who also have delayed gastric emptying, gastroparesis or pancreatic disease.

Enteral tubes provide significant resistance during the administration of medicines, due to both their length and their internal diameter. Administration of inappropriate formulations of medicines via these tubes can cause tube blockage, which at the very least prevents the patient from accessing food and water until the tube is unblocked, and can in extreme cases result in rehospitalization of patients to have a new tube sited.

Advice for administration of medicines via this route is specialized and one can find it in Smyth (2010) and White & Bradnam (2015) or by contacting an appropriate medicines information centre. The main practical point associated with the administration of medicines via enteral tubes is, however, the need to flush the tube with a suitable volume of water before, in-between, and after drug administration. This should minimize the adherence of the drug to the tube and minimize the likelihood of tube blockage, which is the main concern. Whilst most guidance is for a flush volume of between 20 mL and 30 mL at each point, a small number of licensed products which have recently entered the UK market have recommended volumes which are more equivalent to the volume of the tube itself, i.e. 5 mL. As more medicines become licensed, and evidence as to the most appropriate flush volume is developed, the most important message is that the tube must be flushed at all points to prevent blockage. Research continually shows that the main error in the administration of medicines via this route is the lack of flushing by the administrator.

Several factors need to be considered when one is choosing a medicine and formulation for administration via an enteral feeding tube: the dimensions of the tube, the exit site, the excipients in the formulation and any possible interaction of the formulation with components of the enteral feed.

Because of the small internal diameter of these tubes, the risk of tube blockage from the administration of an inappropriate formulation is high. This is not just inappropriately crushed tablets, but also granular liquids, such as Ciproxin®, or dispersible tablets with a large particle size, e.g. Pentasa®. Even if the taste of dispersed or crushed mixtures is theoretically of less concern, patients with enteral tubes do report tasting medicines administered via this route.

For enteral tube administration, a solution is preferred. This will be administered via the tube, without resistance or blockage. Liquids with a high viscosity should be diluted immediately before use to facilitate administration. However, one should confirm the best approach to diluting a solution via the Summary of Product Characteristics (SPC/SmPC) or by contacting the manufacturer.

The exit site of the enteral feeding tube can potentially influence the bioavailability and tolerability of the medication. Medication delivered directly to the jejunum may be incompletely absorbed or result in a rapid peak in plasma concentration, depending on the site of drug absorption. In addition, liquid formulations with a high osmolarity (e.g.. syrup-based formulations) can have an osmotic laxative effect if delivered undiluted into the jejunum.

There are many clinically important interactions between enteral feeds and medicines. These are usually the result of the drug binding to the protein or electrolytes in the feed, or competition with amino acids for absorption. Significant interactions occur with phenytoin, theophylline, warfarin, L-dopa, quinolones, tetracyclines and rifampicin. Specific guidance should be given when these medications are supplied to minimize the effect of the interaction. This is usually achieved through administration of the medication during a break in the feeding regimen.

The practice of tablet splitting

To facilitate administration, sometimes tablets are cut into smaller segments, for instance to achieve a smaller dose for a child. The limitations described earlier with respect to coated tablets equally apply. Additionally, it should be checked that if a score line is present, it is appropriate and safe (i.e. clearly stated in the Summary of Product Characteristics for a particular product) for a part-tablet to be administered. If this is not the case, the manufacturer should be contacted to confirm content uniformity and stability of tablet segments.

Mixing medicines with food and beverages

Mixing of solid dosage forms with food and beverages can be undertaken either to facilitate administration to provide a pleasant vehicle or to try to reduce the poor taste of a medication. Dispersing crushed tablets or capsule contents in water, beverages or soft food is common in clinical paediatric practice, even if there is often very limited information to support this. There is a need to be pragmatic, but the effect of food on bioavailability should be checked, if data are available. Immediate potential incompatibilities, such as mixing the medicine with acidic food or drinks (e.g. orange juice), dairy products or warm/cold foodstuffs, need to be assessed. Decisions are often made with few evidence-based data, but by application of common sense, and where possible with the help of the pharmaceutical manufacturer.

Future developments in the formulation of paediatric and geriatric medicines

Considerations for a patient-centric approach in formulation development

The current provision for specifically designed and tested paediatric and geriatric medicines is poor.

However, there are moves to improve the present situation. The changes in the regulatory environment for paediatric medicines in the US and in Europe will ultimately increase the availability of medicines authorized for children, as well as increase the information available for the use of medicinal products in the paediatric population.

Children, especially those in the younger age groups, require age-appropriate formulations that pharmaceutical manufacturers should develop. The gold standard is that these formulations and presentations should allow both safe and accurate dose administration to children and adults of all groups.

The European Medicines Agency (2005, 2013) (reinforced by the World Health Organization, 2012) in support of the Make Medicines Child Size initiative has reviewed the various considerations for the pharmaceutical development of paediatric medicines. It advises that special attention should be paid to answer the following questions:

- What (will be administered)?
- Where (will it be given)?
- How (will it be administered)?
- When (for how long, from what age, how frequently)?

These questions lead to the following considerations:

- In addition to a consideration of the conventional biopharmaceutical properties of the drug substance, such as dose, solubility and permeability, other factors such as organoleptic properties, especially taste, should be considered early on in the product development process. This will help to avoid issues arising later when a product undergoes clinical trials in the target population.
- The age of the target group – not only physical age and stature but also developmental age in relation to pharmacokinetic and pharmacodynamic parameters, behaviour, activities (school, nursery, etc.).
- By whom and where the medicine will be administered and used, e.g. by the parents at home, by care assistants (e.g. in nursery or care home) or by the child himself or herself.
- The condition to be treated (e.g. short term or long term) and related patient characteristics of that condition (e.g. fluid restriction, presence of enteral tubing, concomitant drug administration, disability, critical illness symptoms and age-related conditions, such as dysphagia).
- The possible administration challenges, namely patient acceptability of the finished product. For example, if a solid dosage form is developed to be swallowed whole, the size, the shape and the number, if more than one is required, should be optimized. For liquid preparations, the volume of administration, whether parenteral or oral, should be minimal, including dilution if needed. The measuring device and vial size should be appropriate to avoid dosing errors. If food is used as a vehicle, either to facilitate administration or to improve palatability, its effect on bioavailability should be anticipated.
- The choice of excipients (qualitative and quantitative composition; Table 45.1) will depend on the availability of safety data for excipients relevant to the target age group(s). It is frequently the case that the available safety data are not as comprehensive as for adults.

On this basis, the most sensitive development aspects are likely to arise in paediatric medicines for long-term use in the most vulnerable patient groups (neonates, infants and young children). There is also an increased interest in elderly patients, particularly how their specific physiological and medical conditions are taken into account in the development and evaluation of new medicines so as to fill in for the lack of clinical trials in the (older) old, and the potential health impact of the extrapolation of research findings to this population. The European Medicines Agency has a geriatric medicines strategy and has established a geriatric expert group taking into consideration the expected increase in the geriatric population. These initiatives have paved the way towards ensuring safe and effective medicines for older patients (e.g. clinical data from geriatric patients should be presented and discussed in marketing authorization applications). However, the same level of scrutiny as is now occurring for the young has yet to be applied to rationalize formulation development for the elderly population.

Summary

Tablets and capsules, which are the most commonly prescribed dosage forms, may not be the most appropriate forms for individuals who have difficulties in swallowing, because of their young age, the ageing process or conditions associated with ageing. The extent of swallowing function should always be ascertained, if necessary by a speech and language therapist, as this will enable the most appropriate formulation to be identified.

A licensed formulation should be identified and recommended if it is suitable and available. Unlicensed medicines are used, but their quality can differ considerably and a certificate of analysis should always be obtained from a supplier where available, in preference to a certificate of conformity.

Sometimes, although quite prevalent for children, manipulation of an existing pharmaceutical product may be the only option available to meet the needs of a particular patient. However, the appropriateness of this approach should always be carefully considered, as certain formulations such as gastro-resistant coated or extended-release products should generally not be modified before administration. The purpose of a film coat for a particular product should be ascertained. Patients receiving drugs with a narrow therapeutic window from formulations which have been manipulated should be monitored for toxicity. Generally, modified-released products should never be crushed or tampered with before administration.

Enteral tubes, which have traditionally been used to bypass the swallow mechanism after surgery and for patients with significant trauma, are increasingly being used in the community setting. Primarily designed for the administration of liquids and food, they create an additional barrier to the administration of medicines. Incorrectly administered medicines can cause tube blockage and result in rehospitalization, and consequently specialist reference sources should be used to provide advice in these circumstances.

Excipient exposure needs to be ascertained for the most vulnerable patients.

It is expected that with international regulatory changes incentivizing the pharmaceutical industry to develop better medicines for children (Regulation (EC) No 1901/2006) and the growing focus on our increasingly ageing population, more appropriate dosage forms will be authorized soon to help health care professionals, parents and carers support the use of medicines in children and the elderly.

Please check your eBook at **https://studentconsult. inkling.com/** for self-assessment questions. See inside cover for registration details.

References

Ari, A., Fink, J.B., 2011. Guidelines for aerosol devices in infants, children and adults: which to choose, why and how to achieve effective aerosol therapy. Expert Rev. Respir. Med. 5, 561–572.

Asmus, M.J., Liang, J., Coowanitwong, I., et al., 2004. In vitro performance characteristics of valved holding chamber and spacer devices with a fluticasone metered-dose inhaler. Pharmacotherapy 24 (2), 159–166.

Breitkreutz, J., Tuleu, C., 2009. Pediatric and geriatric pharmaceutics and formulation. In: Florence, A.T., Siepmann, J. (Eds.), Modern Pharmaceutics, fifth ed. Informa Healthcare, New York.

European Medicines Agency, 2005. Reflection Paper on Formulations of Choice for the Paediatric Population. EMEA/196218/05. European Medicines Agency, London.

European Medicines Agency Committee for Medicinal Products

for Human Use, 2013. Guideline on Pharmaceutical Development of Medicines for Paediatric Use. EMA/CHMP/QWP/805880/2012 Rev. 2. European Medicines Agency, London.

International Conference on Harmonisation of Technical Requirements for Registration of Pharmaceuticals for Human Use, 1995. Note for Guidance on Studies in Support of Special Populations: Geriatrics. Questions and Answers. ICH topic E7. CPMP/ICH/379/95.

International Conference on Harmonisation of Technical Requirements for Registration of Pharmaceuticals for Human Use, Geneva.

International Conference on Harmonisation of Technical Requirements for Registration of Pharmaceuticals for Human Use, 1999. Clinical Investigation of Medicinal Products in the Paediatric

Population. ICH topic E11. CPMP/ICH/2711/99. International Conference on Harmonisation of Technical Requirements for Registration of Pharmaceuticals for Human Use, Geneva.

Smyth, J.A., 2010. The NEWT Guidelines for Administration of Medication to Patients with Enteral Feeding Tubes or Swallowing Difficulties. North East Wales NHS Trust, Wrexham.

White, R., Bradnam, V. (Eds.), 2015. Handbook of Drug Administration via Enteral Feeding Tubes, third ed. Pharmaceutical Press, London.

World Health Organization, 2012. Development of Paediatric Medicines: Points to Consider in Formulation. WHO Technical Report Series, no. 970, 2012, Annex 5. World Health Organization, Geneva.

Bibliography

European Medicines Agency, 2007. Guideline on the Role of Pharmacokinetics in the Paediatric Population. CHMP/EWP/147013/04. European Medicines Agency, London.

Tomlin, S., Cockerill, H., Costello, I., et al., 2009. Making Medicines Safer for Children – Guidance for the Use of Unlicensed Medicines in Paediatric Patients. Medendium Group Publishing, Berkhamsted, pp. 441–445.

Tuleu, C., 2007. Paediatric formulations in practice. In: Florence, A.T., Moffat, A.C. (Eds.), Paediatric Drug Handling. ULLA Postgraduate Pharmacy Series. Pharmaceutical Press, London.

Tuleu, C., Solomonidou, D., Breitkreutz, J., 2009. Paediatric formulations. In: Rose, K., van den Anker, J.N. (Eds.), Guide to Paediatric Clinical Research. Karger, Basel.

CHAPTER CONTENTS

KEY POINTS

- The pharmaceutical pack is as important as the packaged medicine. The pack provides containment, protection, presentation, identification, information, and convenience, and aids with patient adherence. In some cases, the pack is essential for the medicine's administration.
- The closure, such as a stopper, lid, top or cap, is an integral part of the pack.
- The primary pack (also called the container closure system) is in direct contact with the medicine. It must be compatible with the medicine, and must not change it in any way.
- A pack can be a single-unit pack (e.g. a sachet) or a multiple-unit pack (e.g. a bottle containing many tablets).
- Glass, plastics and metal are the most commonly used primary packaging materials. Paper is used mainly in the secondary packaging. The latter holds/covers the primary pack.
- Laminates – consisting of plies (layers) of different materials such as paper, plastic and metal – combine the advantages of the different materials, and are used, for example, in sachets.
- Packaging must be designed for the safe use of medicines.

Introduction

Packaging of medicines is crucial to their use. Without the packaging, dispensing and, for many medicines, administration would be almost impossible. Packaging contains, presents, protects and preserves the medicine, in addition to providing identification, information, tamper evidence, convenience and compliance during storage, distribution, display and use. Packaging enables a medicine's requirements of efficacy, safety, uniformity, reproducibility, integrity, purity and stability to be maintained throughout its shelf life. Furthermore, some pharmaceutical packaging is essential for the medicine's use, i.e. the pack is the delivery device. Examples of this are pressurized metered-dose inhalers and transdermal patches.

The role of packaging is expanding. It is seen as a key component to combat the increasing incidence of drug counterfeiting, which occurs even in countries where the supply chains are trustworthy. Packaging is also increasingly being used to facilitate medicine administration by health care practitioners and by patients (e.g. by the use of prefilled syringes). As for other goods, pharmaceutical packaging is a visual communication tool, and is being used to brand and promote products to the consumer, so much so that pharmaceutical companies sometimes get in trouble with regulators. Packaging that reminds patients to take their medicines and which tracks patient adherence will become more important in the future to reduce the costs of nonadherence with drug therapy. Furthermore, with the ageing population, and the increasing need to reduce health care costs, intelligent packaging can be a component of the 'Internet of things', which would enable greater home-centric (as opposed to hospital-centric) health care services. For example, systems where a biopatch (worn on the body) monitors various physiological parameters, such as blood pressure, and wirelessly transmits the information to a (remote) physician, who, for example, adjusts the drug dose and sends instructions back to the smart packaging, which then dispenses the correct medicine at the right dose and at the right time to the patient, have been trialled (Yang et al., 2014).

The pharmaceutical pack

The primary pack (e.g. a bottle and screw cap) contains the drug product and is in direct contact with it (this is also known as the container closure system). The secondary pack (e.g. a carton box for a glass bottle) contains the primary pack, as well as ancillary components, such as dispensing spoons and information leaflets. The tertiary packaging (e.g. a cardboard outer box) contains multiple secondary packs, facilitates handling and transport, and prevents damage associated with handling, transport and storage. Different aspects of the pharmaceutical pack are discussed in the following sections.

Primary packs

The wide range of pharmaceutical products, such as solid powders, granules, tablets, capsules, semisolids (e.g. creams, ointments, gels) and liquids (e.g. solutions, suspensions, emulsions), some of which are sterile, obviously requires a great diversity, both in primary pack design and in packaging materials. The latter include paper, glass, plastics, rubbers, and metal or combination materials such as laminates. Examples of primary packs include blister packs, strip packs, sachets, bottles, ampoules, vials, bags, tubes and prefilled syringes.

The primary pack may be a multiple-unit pack and contain many doses (e.g. a bottle containing many tablets) or a single-unit pack and contain a single dose (e.g. blister pack, sachet, single-unit dose eye drops). Examples of pharmaceutical primary packs are shown in Fig. 46.1. Multiple-unit packs may be more economical in terms of material; for example, one bottle containing 1 month's supply of tablets for one patient or a multidose vial of vaccines for administration to many patients. However, multidose containers rely on the user's practice, which may be faulty; for instance, changing the needle but reusing the same syringe when the contents of a multidose vial are used on multiple patients, which can lead to infection outbreaks. In addition, the remaining doses in the container are exposed to the environment every time a multidose container is opened, which can lead to contamination of the remaining product. Single-unit containers offer many advantages, such as protection of a dose from the environment until use, as the container is typically opened immediately before administration. Thus single-use containers offer greater product stability and assurance of sterility. They can also be used to package preservative-free preparations for people who are sensitive to preservatives used in multidose presentations (e.g. eye drops). In addition, as fewer steps are required to prepare a dose for a patient (e.g. for a prefilled syringe compared with a multidose vial), single-dose containers can reduce the incidence of errors such as the withdrawal of an incorrect dose, and hence improve patient safety.

Packaging for product stability

The primary pack must ensure product stability. It must be compatible with the product, and take nothing out of the product and add nothing to it. Sorption (absorption or adsorption) of the drug or other excipients, such as preservatives, into the container would reduce product potency and stability, whilst chemicals leaching out of the container and into the product could induce drug degradation. Solvent loss from a product can also occur if the

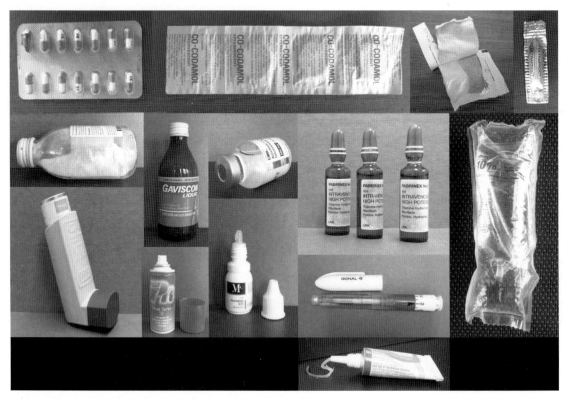

Fig. 46.1 • Examples of primary packaging, from *top left*, blister packaging, strip packaging, sachet, pouch for a suppository, glass bottle for solid powder for dispersion, glass bottle for liquid preparations, glass vial for parenteral preparations, glass ampoules, plastic bag for intravenous liquids, metal and plastic in a pressurized metered-dose inhaler (pMDI), metal canister, plastic eye drop bottle, prefilled syringe for injections and metal ointment tube.

container is permeable, which could result in drug and excipient precipitation.

In addition, the pack must protect the product against atmospheric factors, such as extremes of temperature, light, moisture, oxygen, carbon dioxide and particulates (e.g. dust, dirt), as well as biological hazards, such as microorganisms, insects and rodents. Drug molecules can undergo chemical reactions triggered by light, heat, moisture or atmospheric gases, such as oxygen (see Chapter 47 for more details). For example, heat can degrade a drug. Light can provide the energy necessary for a drug isomer to change its configuration. Oxygen can cause drug degradation via oxidation. Carbon dioxide can dissolve in the water in unbuffered aqueous products and lower their pH by forming carbonic acid. Moisture can cause drug degradation via hydrolysis. Moisture ingress into a product can also cause dilution of liquid products and wetting of solid products and can create an aqueous environment which may support microbial growth.

Protection of a medicine against these hazards is achieved by the judicious use of the packaging materials and the inclusion of substances which can remove the hazard. For example, opaque or amber-coloured containers reduce exposure to light. Containers which are produced from fairly impermeable materials, such as glass, minimize the egress of solvent from the product and the ingress of moisture and gases. Desiccants (e.g. silica gel, bentonite and activated carbon) and oxygen absorbers (such as iron oxide, StabilOx® and PharmaKeep®) may also be used. These are contained within sachets or canisters that are placed inside containers (e.g. integrated within the container closures). The absorbers may also be integrated within the container walls (e.g. in Oxy-Guard® barrier bottles). A combination of an impermeable container and a moisture/oxygen absorber sachet may also be used, the impermeable container protecting against degradation that could arise from ingress of moisture/oxygen from the atmosphere into the container and the sachet absorbing any moisture/oxygen present in the headspace (the air in a container above its contents).

Products that are heat-sensitive need to be kept within a narrow temperature range from the point of manufacture to the point of use. The cold chain is therefore crucial to ensure the product is effective when used. However, the cold chain cannot always be guaranteed, for example when the electricity supply is sporadic (as it is in many countries) or when someone fails to store the product correctly. In such cases, the incorrectly stored medicines are potentially degraded and hence wasted. To reduce wastage, temperature monitors may be attached to containers to record their exposure to heat. For example, the vaccine vial monitor is a heat-sensitive label that is placed on vaccine vials. The monitor changes colour as a function of temperature and time, allowing health care workers to determine, at a glance, if the vaccine in a vial is suitable for use.

Secondary and tertiary packaging also contribute to protection against atmospheric factors to some extent (e.g. against light). However, their major role is to provide protection against mechanical hazards during handling and storage, such as shock (e.g. when dropped), compression, vibration, abrasion and puncture.

Packaging for tamper resistance, tamper evidence, child resistance and access by older people

The primary pack must be tamper resistant and tamper evident to improve the product's security from pilferage and deliberate contamination, thereby safeguarding the product's legitimate user. Examples of tamper-evident (TE) approaches include TE bands incorporated into bottle caps, and TE shrink bands applied to the bottle neck and cap. Ideally, packs would be completely tamper-proof, although this is probably impossible to achieve against determined attempts.

Child-resistant packaging of medicines, introduced to reduce the accidental poisoning of children by medicines, has prevented thousands of poisonings, and may have saved many lives. The aim of child-resistant packaging is to make it difficult for children to open containers and access the medicine, while ensuring that adults can still open and close the packaging easily. However, easy access to the medicine by adults is not always the case. Older people, who are more likely to have impaired vision, hand strength

and dexterity, often have difficulties opening medicine packaging. Examples include difficulties removing tamper-evident screw caps and child-resistant closures, and removing medicines from push-through or peel-off blister packs, for instance when the metal/plastic is too firm, or when the pull tab is too small to grasp. Such difficulties accessing medicines can reduce medication adherence, and lead to poor disease control. Strategies to overcome the difficulties with opening medicine packs include asking someone else, using tools such as scissors, pliers, or a screw-cap opener, transferring the medicines to another container or not reclosing the container fully between administrations. The latter may compromise the product's stability, as well as increase the possibility of children accessing the medicine. Pharmacists and pharmacy staff can play a significant role in helping older patients take their medicines by questioning patients and carers, and offering solutions and packaging that are more senior-friendly.

Closures

A closure is a device (e.g. stopper, lid, top or cap) which is used to close a container, and is an integral part of the pack. The word 'pack' therefore covers both the container and the closure. Without the latter, the functions of the pack, such as containment, presentation, protection and convenience, cannot be fulfilled. Like the container, the closure must be inert, compatible with the contents, and protect the latter against environmental hazards, such as oxygen, light and moisture. Certain closures must also maintain sterility (e.g. in multiuse vials for parenteral products).

A good seal between the container and the closure prevents anything from leaking out of or gaining access into the pack, and is obtained by a snug fit between the inner face of the closure and the external face of the container. Resilient liners inside the closure are sometimes used to achieve a snug fit, although many plastic closures are internally moulded to achieve a good seal and are liner-free. The closure has to be user-friendly, allow easy opening by legitimate consumers and be easy to reclose (for multiunit packs), as well as being child resistant, tamper resistant and tamper evident. Closures may also include dispensing devices (e.g. a pump on bottles containing creams). The outer surface of the closure may also be ribbed to allow good grip when it is being opened by twisting. Pharmaceutical closures are mostly made of plastic (thermosets and thermoplastics), although metal is also used (e.g. on parenteral vials).

The word 'closure' does not always refer to a stopper-type device. Metal tubes have two closures: a cap at one end, whilst the other end of the tube is sealed by folding and crimping. Flexible packaging, such as pouches, sachets and blister packs, does not contain a closure as previously defined. It is instead sealed by heat and/or pressure, or with adhesives, and is not reclosable.

Packaging materials

Once the properties and functions of the desired packaging have been defined, the primary packaging material can be selected, taking into account the dosage form, the route of administration, product stability, any need for sterilization and for visual inspection of the packaged medicine, patient adherence and convenience, aesthetics, cost, marketing, environmental friendliness, etc.

Liquids, which are in constant intimate contact with the primary pack, as opposed to solids such as tablets and capsules, require greater quality from a pack so that they 'take nothing out of the product and add nothing to it'. Injectable liquids require even greater quality from the pack compared with oral liquids, to maintain sterility and freedom from other possible contaminants, such as extraneous particulates. Packaging for medicines which are terminally sterilized in their final packs needs to be made from materials that can withstand the sterilization procedure. Semisolid products need to be able to be dispensed from the container, under slight pressure (e.g. squeezing of a tube).

The packaging material is obviously very important, and the different materials are described next. Glass, metal and plastic are the materials most commonly used in primary packs; their properties with respect to their use in packaging are compared in Table 46.1.

Glass

Glass, believed to have been first discovered around 3000 BC in the East Mediterranean and which has been used for thousands of years, is widely used for packaging pharmaceuticals because of its excellent barrier properties, relative inertness and compatibility with pharmaceuticals. Its many advantages are shown in Table 46.1, and it has traditionally been the gold standard in pharmaceutical packaging.

Primarily consisting of silicon dioxide (silica), glass is produced by the heating together of various inorganic substances to form a molten mass, and then rapid cooling of the latter, which solidifies in a noncrystalline state. Sand (or more properly silicon dioxide, which is the main constituent of sand), limestone (calcium carbonate) and soda ash (sodium carbonate) are heated together to very high temperatures in a furnace. The ingredients melt and gradually react and form a homogeneous molten mass. The latter is then converted into glass containers by one of two basic methods: blow moulding or tubular glass fabrication. Blow moulding, the older method, is when a 'gob' (a small piece of highly viscous molten glass) of glass is moulded into a container. The second method involves conversion of the homogeneous molten glass mass into tubing as it moves out of the furnace. The tubing is cut to defined lengths, and the individual glass tubes are then converted into containers.

In addition to silica, soda ash and limestone, other compounds are added in trace amounts to achieve certain properties in the glass formed. For example:

- Alumina (Al_2O_3) increases the hardness, durability and clarity of the glass.
- Selenium or cobalt oxides improve clarity.
- Lead oxide gives clarity and sparkle (but makes glass soft).
- Boron compounds give low thermal expansion and high resistance to heat shock.
- Arsenic trioxide and sodium sulfate are added to reduce blisters in the glass.

Opacity and different colours are also achieved by the inclusion of compounds, as shown in Table 46.2. The different colours convey specific properties. For example:

- Amber glass is widely used to package pharmaceuticals susceptible to degradation by sunlight.
- Green glass is mostly used for packaging beverages.
- Blue glass makes white products appear whiter.
- Opaque white (opal) conveys prestige to upmarket toiletries and cosmetics.

Glass is not totally inert

Although glass is fairly inert, it is not totally inert. As described already, glass is composed principally of silicon dioxide, and various amounts of other oxides,

Table 46.1 Comparison of glass, metal and plastic as a function of packaging requirements

Property	Material used in primary packaging		
	Glass	Metal	Plastic
Compatibility with product	Inert to most chemicals. Can be used to package many different medicines	Can potentially interact with product. To prevent this, the metal surface is coated	Compatibility depends on the nature of the plastic
Weight	Heavy. Less acceptable to consumers and greater transport cost	Light because it is strong even when thin sections are used	Light
Permeability to gases and water vapour, odour	Prevents atmospheric gases, such as oxygen and carbon dioxide, from entering the container. Protects the packaged pharmaceutical product from potential degradation, such as oxidation and hydrolysis. Prevents volatile ingredients in the product from escaping into the atmosphere. Thus the pharmaceutical product is kept stable	Excellent barrier to gases and water vapour	Permeability depends on the nature of the plastic
Stability at high temperature	Stable. Allows hot filling of glass containers and sterilization by heat	Stable	Depends on the nature of the plastic
Clarity/opacity	Clear. Allows visualization of contents, which is especially important for parenteral products	Not clear. Opacity can be an advantage as contents are protected from light. Opacity is a disadvantage as contents cannot be visualized	Can be clear, translucent or opaque
Strength	Yes. Allows stacking during distribution	Yes. Its strength and durability means it can be used as the overcap on vials with a rubber closure	Depends on the nature of the plastic
Shatterproof	No. Glass is brittle, and broken glass is a hazard. There is a risk of product loss and of product contamination by broken glass. This makes glass less acceptable to consumers	Yes	Yes
Recyclable	Yes	Yes	Less easily recyclable than glass and metal
Cost	High	Less than glass	Some plastics are cheap, others are expensive

such as sodium, potassium, calcium, magnesium, aluminium, boron and iron. The basic structural network of glass is formed by the silicon dioxide tetrahedron. Whilst boric oxide will enter this structure (and thereby be held more strongly), the other oxides do not enter the silica tetrahedron and are only loosely bound, and are therefore free to migrate. Thus some of the glass components can leach out of the glass and into the contents of the container. For example, sodium oxide can leach out from the glass surface into water contained within the container. The leaching event is an ion-exchange process and involves the exchange of hydrogen ions (from the water) for the alkali ions (from the glass). As a result, the pH of the contents is increased. Another problem occurs when glass is stored at high temperature and high humidity or when ambient temperature and humidity conditions fluctuate greatly.

Table 46.2 Additives that are generally used to achieve different colours of glass

Colour	Possible additives
Amber	Iron oxides, manganese oxides, carbon oxides, sulfur compounds
Browns	Iron oxides, carbon oxides, sulfur compounds
Greens	Iron oxides
Yellow greens	Uranium oxides
Yellow	Lead with antimony
Deep blue	Cobalt oxide
Light blue	Copper compounds
Reds	Gold chloride, selenium compounds, copper compounds
Amethyst	Manganese oxides
Black	Mix of manganese, cobalt and iron
White	Tin compounds, antimony oxides

Salts in the glass migrate from the body of the glass and accumulate at its surface. This physical change is called blooming. Such problems are obviously unacceptable. To reduce leaching, the glass can be soaked in heated water or a dilute acid solution, which removes most of the surface-leachable salts. The inner surface of a glass container can also be treated (e.g. with a sulfur compound) to make it more resistant to water or acidic (but not alkaline) solutions. In addition to leaching of glass components from the glass into the container contents, glass can undergo delamination, i.e. dislodging of thin layers of glass called lamellae or flakes from the inner surface, as a result of dissolution by hydrolysis and leaching of glass components. The factors which influence delamination include the quality of the glass (discussed later), the nature of the contents, the glass manufacturing and any sterilization processes.

Pharmaceutical types of glass and containers

Glass containers for pharmaceutical use are produced from either borosilicate (neutral) glass or soda–lime–silica glass. The containers are classified in international pharmacopoeias according to their hydrolytic stability: the inner surface of the container or glass grains are made to contact water and the release of alkali ions from the glass into the water is measured. Accordingly,

the glass containers are classified as described in the following paragraphs:

Type I glass and containers. Type I glass is the highest pharmaceutical grade and is produced by addition of boric oxide to glass; hence this glass is also called borosilicate glass. It contains significant amounts of boric oxide, aluminium oxide and alkali and/or alkaline earth oxides in the glass network. It is the most inert glass, shows high hydrolytic resistance (i.e. low leaching of glass components into water), and high resistance to thermal shock because of the chemical composition of the glass itself. This glass can therefore be used during severe sterilization procedures. This glass is also the most expensive to produce. Type I glass containers are suitable for most parenteral and nonparenteral products.

Type II glass and containers. Type II glass containers are made from soda–lime–silica glass. This glass contains alkaline metal oxides, mainly sodium oxide, and alkaline earth oxides, mainly, calcium oxide, in the glass network. This glass itself has a moderate hydrolytic resistance because of its chemical composition. However, treatment of the inner surface of the glass container with sulfur dioxide increases the hydrolytic resistance of the container, as the sulfur dioxide reacts with the oxides found on the glass surface. For example, sodium oxide is converted to sodium sulfate, which can then be removed by washing of the glass. Thus such surface treatment reduces the amount of ions that can leach out of the glass, and type II glass is also referred to as treated soda–lime glass or dealkalized soda–lime glass. Type II glass containers are suitable for most acidic and neutral aqueous preparations for parenteral and nonparenteral uses. They are not used for alkaline solutions, as at higher pH the oxides in the glass more easily leach out.

Type III glass and containers. Type III glass is soda–lime–silica glass and has moderate hydrolytic resistance. Type III glass containers are suitable for nonparenteral preparations. Because of the moderate hydrolytic resistance, they are not generally used for aqueous parenteral products, although they may be used for nonaqueous preparations for parenteral administration and for certain powders for parenteral administration following reconstitution.

As mentioned already, treatment of the inner surface of glass containers produced with soda–lime–silica glass increases the hydrolytic resistance. The outer surface of glass containers may also be treated to reduce friction and for protection against abrasion and breakage.

Plastics

The versatility of plastics has led to their use in almost all aspects of our lives, and they are used to package a wide variety of domestic products. They are widely used as containers (e.g. bottles, trays), closures (e.g. screw tops), cling films, carrier bags, sacks, overwraps, etc. Plastics are also widely used to package medicines in a variety of ways, such as:

- bottles for solid and liquid products;
- tubes for creams, ointments and gels;
- pouches to contain individual suppositories;
- blister packs;
- bags to contain intravenous solutions and parenteral nutrition products;
- overwraps;
- bottle closures and closure liners; and
- tamper-evident films over bottle necks and stoppers.

Advantages and limitations of plastics

The use of plastics as a pharmaceutical packaging material is growing because of the significant advantages and consumer preference. Plastics are light and shatterproof and can be clear or opaque (clarity may be desired for product inspection; opacity may be desired to protect the contained medicine). Plastics are easily shaped and sealed, which gives great versatility in the design of the pack, and allows the inclusion of administration aids, such as a squeezable dropper. The many plastic materials, with a range of physical, chemical, optical and performance properties, enables great versatility.

Plastics do, however, have certain disadvantages compared with traditional packaging materials, such as glass and metal, which limit their use. They are not as chemically inert and impermeable (to environmental gases, such as oxygen) compared with type I glass. Plastics are less resistant to heat and long-term light exposure compared with glass and metal. Plastics are also liable to undergo stress cracking, where the presence of solvents, such as alcohols, acids or oils, causes a plastic pack to become brittle, crack and eventually fail over time. Certain components of the plastic packaging material can also leach out of the plastic and into the contained product. At the same time, drug and excipients can adsorb to or absorb into the plastic material.

Plastic chemistry

Plastics are polymeric materials. Many different types of polymers or polymer mixes are used in packaging.

Polymers, macromolecules of repeating units called monomers, are produced by addition or condensation reactions, where one chemical species reacts with another (or itself) to form a new and larger compound. Thus polymers may be copolymers (which consist of more than one type of monomer) or homopolymers (containing only one type of monomer). For example, ethylene can be polymerized into the homopolymer polyethylene, or can be made to react with a different species such as vinyl acetate to produce the copolymer ethylene vinyl acetate. Polymers may be linear, branched, or cross-linked and may contain amorphous and/or crystalline regions where the polymer chains are arranged in a random or highly ordered manner respectively (Fig. 46.2). A linear un-cross-linked polymeric material can be visualized as a bowl of spaghetti (Fig. 46.2a), where the individual spaghetti strands represent polymer chains. The molecular weights of the individual monomer parts in a polymer chain add up to the molecular weight of the polymer. The polymer chains in a polymeric material are of different lengths (i.e. contain different numbers of monomer units), and thus the polymeric material's molecular weight is not exact, but can be considered as the average of the molecular weights of all the strands contained within a sample. Common plastic polymers used in pharmaceutical packaging have molecular weights ranging from approximately 10 000 to 1 000 000. In contrast to the 'bowl of spaghetti', a cross-linked polymer can be considered as one very large molecule, where all the monomer parts and polymer chains are irreversibly linked (Fig. 46.2c).

Thermoplastic and thermosetting polymers

Plastics can be divided into two classes: thermoplastics and thermosetting plastics. In general, thermoplastics have linear and branched polymer chains, whilst thermoset polymers are cross-linked.

At high temperature, thermoplastic polymers melt and become liquid, the polymer chains flow and the material can be moulded into a variety of shapes, such as bottles, tubes and films. Softening and reshaping by the application of heat and mechanical force can be performed multiple times. Examples of thermoplastics include poly(vinyl chloride), polyethylene, polystyrene, polypropylene, nylon, polyester and polycarbonate. The properties and uses of the most commonly used plastics in pharmaceutical packaging are shown in Table 46.3.

Table 46.3 The different types of plastics used to package pharmaceutical products and their properties

	Plastic			
	PE HDPE LDPE 	PP 	PS 	PVC
General	PE is compatible with a wide variety of drug products. However, it sorbs other materials, e.g. preservatives. HDPE is the most widely used plastic in pharmaceutical packaging	PP has several advantages over PE. Contains less additives than PE. Has lower tendency than PE to sorb certain chemicals	PS is found in three different forms in packaging: (1) crystal PS (in cups, bottles); (2) high-impact PS (opaque, more resistant to impact); (3) PS foam – used as insulating and cushioning material	Has a long history in pharmaceutical packaging, although it is now being replaced by other plastics because of health and environment issues. Many additives are used in its manufacture
Cost	Low	Low	Low	Low
Use	HDPE is used when a rigid container is desired, e.g. bottles for dry solid dosage forms (not meant for constitution into solution). LDPE is used when a flexible pack is required, e.g. squeeze bottles, blister packs	Used when a rigid container is desired, e.g. bottles for dry solid and oral liquid dosage forms. PP films are used in blister packs. Also used for parenteral and ophthalmic preparations	Bottles for tablets and capsules	Intravenous bags for blood products, glucose, saline solutions, blister packs, bottles
Optical and physical properties	HDPE has a milky translucence. It is strong and stiff. LDPE is clear and flexible	Clear	Crystal PS is clear and rigid but brittle	Clear. Glossy appearance. Range from stiff material to flexible films
Resistance to heat	HDPE can be autoclaved	Resistant to heat – can be used in high heat sterilization procedures	Softens at low temperature, cannot be used in packaging requiring heat resistance	Heat sensitive
Barrier to moisture	HDPE has a good moisture barrier. LDPE has a poorer moisture barrier than HDPE	Excellent	Poor	Fair barrier
Barrier to gases (e.g. oxygen), odours, flavours	Permeable to oxygen. Cannot be used to package oxygen-sensitive products. Poor odour barrier	Better odour barrier than PE	Poor gas barrier	Poor to medium
Resistance to oils and other chemicals	Permeable to oils, e.g. volatile oils for aroma. Permeable to halogens. HDPE is more resistant to oils and chemicals than LDPE	More resistant to grease and oils than PE	Poor resistance	Excellent barrier to oils, fats, flavourings

HDPE, high-density polyethylene; *LDPE*, low-density polyethylene; *PE*, polyethylene; *PP*, polypropylene; *PS*, polystyrene; *PVC*, poly(vinyl chloride).

Poly(ethylene terephthalate) (PET). Common name polyester.	Poly(vinylidene chloride) copolymers (PVDC)	Fluoropolymer, e.g. polychlorotrifluoroethylene (PCTFE)
Has become the most widely used plastic for cough syrups and a wide variety of oral liquid products. It is the material of choice to replace PVC bottles	One of the most effective barrier materials. Their high cost means that they are not used on their own but are coextruded with less expensive materials. Or they are used in coatings applied to paper, cellophane, plastic films, or rigid plastic containers to add barrier properties to these	Used in pharmaceutical packaging because of its excellent moisture or water barrier properties. Its high cost means it is used as a thin layer (laminated to PVC) in blister packs
Medium, likely to decrease because of widespread use	High	High
Bottles for liquid products (not parenteral), e.g. cough syrups. Film used to make sterilizable pouches	Films. Coextruded with other materials as a barrier layer. Used in coatings (see above) and blister packs	Blister packs
Clear and strong	Clear, flexible	Clear
Resistant to high temperature – sterilization possible	High	High
Good barrier	Excellent	Excellent
Good barrier to gas	Excellent barrier to gases flavours, odours	Excellent gas barrier
Excellent barrier to grease and oils	Barrier to most organic liquids and water	Resistant

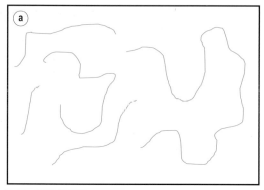

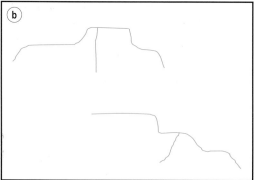

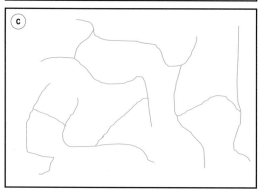

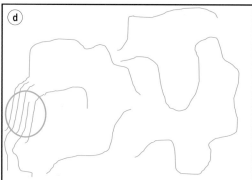

Fig. 46.2 • **(a)** Linear polymer consisting of polymer chains of different lengths. **(b)** Branched polymer. **(c)** Cross-linked polymer. **(d)** The *circle* shows a region of high order (crystallinity) in a polymeric material that is mostly amorphous (i.e. polymer chains are oriented in a random manner).

Thermoplastics are used in blow–fill–seal technology, which is used to produce liquid-filled plastic containers, with container formation, filling and sealing occurring in one continuous operation, which occurs over a period of less than a few seconds. In the container blowing step, pharmaceutical-grade plastic granules, most usually polypropylene or polyethylene, are melted at high temperature and extruded into a hollow tube, termed the 'parison'. The parison is cut to the desired length, then two halves of the container mould close around it, the lower end is sealed and then air is blown into the parison, causing it to expand to the shape of the container. This container is partially cooled, filled with liquid via a needle and sealed. The completed, filled containers are removed from the filling equipment, and excess plastic is removed. The ability to operate this process in a controlled environment without the intervention of operators makes this process particularly suitable for aseptic production of sterile pharmaceutical products (see Chapter 36 for more information).

In contrast to thermoplastics, thermoset polymers can be shaped only once following polymer formation, because the cross-linked polymer chains cannot flow. Further heating would lead to breakage of the bonds in the polymer and polymer degradation. Examples of thermoset polymers include urea formaldehyde, epoxides, urethanes, unsaturated polyesters and rubbers. These are mainly used to produce closures, as metal coatings, and as adhesives in the pharmaceutical packaging industry.

Process residues and additives in plastics

During polymer synthesis a variety of chemicals, such as solvents, catalysts, initiators and accelerators, are needed to assist the polymerization process. These chemicals are therefore present to some extent in the final product; they are then known as process residues. Unreacted monomers may also be present. When the polymer is subsequently made into a finished product (e.g. a bottle), further chemicals (additives and processing aids) are added to control or enhance the properties of the polymer/finished product, or to aid the manufacturing process. These chemicals include plasticizers, fillers, toughening agents, stabilizers, antioxidants, opacifiers, colourants, UV absorbers, lubricants, slip and antiblocking agents and internal release agents. The function of these additives and processing aids is shown in Table 46.4; their inclusion (or not) will depend on the plastic and the finished product.

Unreacted monomers, process residues, additives and processing aids present in a plastic pack may leach out of the plastic material and into the packaged product. For this reason, pharmaceutical grade polymers have strict limits on the amount of chemicals that can leach out of the plastic material.

Rubbers and elastomers

Rubber has many applications in pharmaceutical packaging; for example, closures for vials and bottles, and ports on plastic bags used to contain parenteral nutrition products. Elastomers are polymers that can be stretched (to more than twice their original length) and which return to their original length once the force is removed. Elastomers may be natural (extracted from rubber trees) or synthetic (derived from petrochemicals), and common pharmaceutical examples include butyl, chlorobutyl, natural and silicone elastomers. Rubbers are formulations of these elastomers, and in addition to the elastomer polymer, contain a number of substances (2–10) such as fillers, vulcanizing agents, cure accelerators, activators, plasticizers, lubricants, antioxidants and pigments.

To produce rubber formulations, the elastomer and other required materials are placed in a mixer, which breaks the materials into small fragments and produces a uniform dispersion. The latter, a viscous liquid, is placed in a heated mould, where heat and pressure promote polymer cross-linking and 'cure' the formulation, such that a strong, tough and elastic rubber is produced. The rubber is then trimmed and washed to remove residual materials that may have migrated to the surface during moulding. Residual materials may also be extracted from the rubber by different techniques, such as autoclaving. The rubber

Table 46.4 Process residues and additives in plastics

Additives and processing aids	Role	Examples
Plasticizer	Improve flow properties. Increase softness and flexibility	Phthalate ester
Filler, extender	Inert solid substance. May reduce plastic degradation. May be used to reduce cost	Talc
Toughening agent/impact modifier	Increase strength of brittle plastics	Rubber added to polystyrene
Stabilizer	Increase stability of plastic, to combat effects of heat and light	Calcium–zinc salts added to poly(vinyl chloride)
Antioxidant	Prevent or retard oxidative degradation of plastic	Cresols
UV absorber	To protect plastic or packaged product from UV degradation	Substituted phenols
Opacifier	Make plastic opaque	Titanium dioxide
Whitener	Give a 'whiter than white' appearance	Ultramarine
Colourant	Colour the plastic	Pigments and dyes
Lubricant	Prevent adhesion of plastic to metal parts during fabrication	Waxes, liquid paraffin
Internal release agent	Provide release from moulds	Metal stearates, silicone fluids
Antiblock or slip agent	Used for films made or used on high-speed equipment, where nonslip or film sticking together would interfere with processing	Amides, finely divided silica
Antistatic agent	Reduce static accumulation on plastic	Surfactants

surface may be treated with chlorine to produce a shiny glaze or coated with materials, such as silicon oils, to reduce the coefficient of friction.

Like other polymers, rubbers are not totally inert. They are permeable to some extent to gases and moisture; they may also sorb components of the packaged product, and residues and low molecular weight components may leach from them into the packaged contents. Other properties of rubber include its elasticity, hardness, pressure to puncture, tendency to fragment, coring and resealability (following puncture with a hypodermic needle used to remove the contents), break force and vacuum retention. For rubber closures in vials/bottles, the rubber should be hard enough to be firm yet allow easy insertion (and removal) of a needle through a vial closure. Appropriate elasticity will allow a good seal between the closure and the container, and permit resealing on removal of a hypodermic needle. The rubber should fragment minimally when pierced by a hypodermic needle.

Metal

Metal is widely used to package food, beverages, aggressive products, etc. Aluminium and tinplate (a sheet of steel that is coated with a thin deposit of tin) are the metals used in the packaging of pharmaceuticals. They are used in the form of cans (e.g. pressurized metered-dose inhaler [pMDI] containers), tubes (for creams, ointments, gels), pouches (for powders, granules, liquids, suppositories), blister packs and closures.

Metal has many advantages as a packaging material. It is mechanically strong and can withstand the high internal pressure in pMDI containers. It is shatterproof, lightweight (because it is strong even when thin layers are used), impermeable to gases and light and malleable. It can be tailored in hardness and flexibility with respect to the desired container. Both soft and hard forms of aluminium and tinplate are used in pharmaceutical packaging; hard material is used for its strength and durability in containers such as aerosol cans, whilst soft and malleable metal is used to produce collapsible tubes and flexible pouches and as the collar/overcap on parenteral vials with rubber stoppers. Malleability allows the metal collar/overcap to be crimped in place and flexible pouches and metal tubes to be crimped closed. The metal's malleability also means that when metal tubes are squeezed to expel the product (e.g. a cream), the tube does not spring back to its original shape and air is not sucked back into the container, which could otherwise react with the product or cause it to dry out.

Metal can, however, interact with the pharmaceutical product. To isolate the metal from the product, the metal surface is coated with vinyl-, acrylic- and epoxy-based resins. The outside of the metal container is also coated to enable printing.

Paper

Paper is one of the oldest pharmaceutical packaging materials. It has diverse applications, including labels and leaflets, collapsible and rigid cartons, bags and sacks, and sachets. Unlike the other packaging materials – glass, metal and plastic – paper is not usually used in the manufacture of the primary pack. An exception is the sachet, where the paper is separated from the product by a layer of another material.

Paper is defined as a matted or felted sheet usually composed of natural plant fibre. When the paper material weighs 250 g m^{-2} or more or is 300 μm or more in thickness, it is known as paperboard. Softwood from spruce, fir, pine and eucalyptus trees is now the most common source of fibre in papermaking, although bagasse (from sugar cane), cotton, straw, flax, bamboo, jute, hemp, grass, esparto, rags and sisal have also been used.

To produce paper, cellulose fibre is extracted from the wood by the pulping of the latter (mechanically and/or chemically). The pulp is then mechanically treated to break down any fibre bundles, to hydrate and break up the surface of the fibres, and this is then bleached if desired. A variety of nonfibrous additives are added to the treated pulp to control water and ink permeation (rosins), to increase strength (starches, gums, resins) and to improve the optical brightness and printing qualities (clay, talc, titanium dioxide). The mixture (consisting of 99% water, fibre and additives, known as 'furnish') is then fed to the papermaking machine, where most of the water is removed, and the solid material is turned into sheets of paper. The latter is pressed between multiple stacks of heavy rollers, which smooth out the surface of the paper and make it more suitable for printing. A number of coatings may then be applied to the paper to further improve its surface properties, such as to reduce its porosity and liquid penetration rate (using gelatin, starch, modified rosins or waxes) or increase its opacity, gloss, brightness and printability (using clay, calcium carbonate or titanium dioxide).

Advantages and disadvantages of paper as a packaging material

Paper has many advantages as a ready material, including:

- Its relatively low cost and ready availability.
- Its generally nontoxic origin.
- Its easy recyclability.
- It is readily torn or cut open, an advantage when paper is used in sachets.
- Its 'deadfold' (ability to hold a crease) allows the making of cartons and bags as well as its use for patient information leaflets;
- Its rigidity and strength allow its use in cartons. At the same time, it can act as a slight cushion to protect the primary pack.
- It is easily printed on and coated.
- The nature and properties of the finished paper can be controlled, such that paper may be tailor-made for specific applications. For example, its opacity and colour can be varied by the use of additives, and its porosity can be adjusted to allow diffusion of steam for sterilization while maintaining a barrier to microorganisms.

Paper does have certain disadvantages, and these result in it not generally being used on its own in the primary pack. These disadvantages include:

- The lack of barrier properties against moisture, gases and odours.
- It is moisture sensitive.
- It has no heat- or cold-seal properties and hence cannot be sealed without adhesives or special coatings.
- It has poor transparency and gloss compared with certain plastic films.

To overcome such disadvantages, paper can be combined with other materials. For example, paper can be further coated by polymers, or laminated to plastic or to aluminium foil to improve its barrier properties with regard to gases and moisture, and to create heat-sealing ability when it is used in the primary pack.

Laminates

A laminate is made by the bonding together of two or more plies (layers) of different materials, such as paper, plastic and metal. The aim is to combine the desirable properties of the different plies into a single packaging structure. A minimum amount of material is used, and the laminate is cost-effective.

Laminates are used to produce pharmaceutical packs such as sachets, blister packs, tubes and pouches. An example is a structure consisting of paper, metal foil and polythene plies, used for sachet packaging. The paper provides strength, printability and the ability to easily tear the package, the foil provides an excellent barrier to light, moisture and gases and the polythene provides heat sealability.

Packaging and regulatory bodies

Like the drug substance and drug product, the pharmaceutical packaging is subject to regulation and approval by government agencies, such as the US Food and Drug Administration, the European Medicines Agency and the UK's Medicines and Healthcare products Regulatory Agency. The packaging is considered part of the product, and manufacturers must submit large amounts of data to show that the packaging is safe, is efficacious and performs as claimed. The regulatory bodies produce guidance documents to assist manufacturers, such as on labelling, patient information leaflets, closures and the testing of containers. The *United States Pharmacopeia* includes requirements for containers, and many of the drug product monographs include the requirements for packaging, such as 'preserve in single-dose containers, preferably in Type I glass, protected from light'. Labelling and patient information leaflets are part of the pack and are also subject to regulation, although they are not covered in this chapter.

Repackaging

An original pack is one which is intended to be dispensed directly to the patient without modification except for the addition of appropriate labelling. Many medicines are packaged by the manufacturer into such packs which can be dispensed directly to the patient. Repackaging (i.e. the transfer of medicines from their original pack into different packs) is also fairly common in community and hospital pharmacy, for distribution to hospital wards, clinics and nursing homes or on patient request (e.g. by a patient who might struggle to open an original child-resistant pack).

The new primary container should be chosen with care, ensuring good containment and protection of the medicine, and compatibility between the product and the pack. The repacker must be aware of the issues regarding medicine repackaging, such as the potential for errors, the physical and chemical stability of drugs and medicines, cleanliness, cross-contamination, shelf life of repackaged products, legal aspects, and clear and full labelling. When multiple medicines are repackaged into multicompartment compliance aids (MCA), where more than one medication is present in each blister/compartment, special attention must be given to drug stabilities and compatibilities among the medications that are in contact with one another. Currently, there is little information in the published literature or from medicine manufacturers about medicine compatibilities and potential problems, despite the widespread use of MCAs. Pharmacists and health care workers must remain vigilant when using MCAs.

Designing packaging for safe medicine use

A quarter of medication errors – which are common and cause significant morbidity, mortality and cost – have been attributed to medicines which have similar names (similar looking and similar sounding names) or similar packaging (Emmerton & Rizk, 2012). For example, at least 15 children died following vaccination against measles in northern Syria in 2014, when atracurium was mistakenly used instead of sterile water. Both vials had a similar appearance, and the atracurium vials had been incorrectly added to vaccination packs (Pakenham-Walsh & Ana, 2014). Clearer packaging has to be 'designed in' to both primary and secondary packs to prevent such errors.

Actions that would result in clearer and safer packaging have been recommended by a number of researchers and institutions. Examples of good practice include:

- choosing medicine names that are least likely to be confused with the names of existing medicines;
- designing packaging that is easy to read (e.g. use of nonreflective foil on blister packs, large and clear fonts with a good contrast to the background);
- appropriately aligning text for easy reading;
- emphasizing the difference between look-alike or sound-alike (LASA) medicine names, with use of colour, font size or tall man lettering (e.g. chlorproPAMIDE and chlorproMAZINE), and between strengths of the same medicine;
- ensuring that company logos and images do not break the text;
- allocating space on packs for the dispensing label;
- matching the styles of primary and secondary packaging;
- using dispensing labels of sufficient size and attaching these to the medicine packs appropriately; and
- using dispensing bags to reinforce key safety messages.

Clearly pharmacists and pharmaceutical scientists can play a significant part in reducing packaging-related medication errors, given their roles in dispensing and labelling medicines, as well as in the pharmaceutical industry, including in packaging and marketing products.

Please check your eBook at **https://studentconsult. inkling.com/** for self-assessment questions. See inside cover for registration details.

References

Emmerton, L.M., Rizk, M.F.S., 2012. Look-alike and sound-alike medicines: risks and 'solutions'. Int. J. Clin. Pharm. 34 (1), 4–8.

Pakenham-Walsh, N., Ana, J., 2014. Confusing drug packaging contributes to death of 15 children. Lancet Glob. Health 2 (11), E634.

Yang, G., Xie, L., Mäntysalo, M., et al., 2014. A health-IoT platform based on the integration of intelligent packaging, unobtrusive bio-sensor, and intelligent medicine box. IEEE Trans. Industr. Inform. 10 (4), 2180–2191.

Bibliography

Bauer, E.J., 2009. Pharmaceutical Packaging Handbook. Informa Healthcare, New York.

Dean, D.A., Evans, E.R., Hall, I.H., 2000. Pharmaceutical Packaging Technology. Taylor and Francis, London.

Food and Drug Administration, 1999. Guidance for Industry. Container Closure Systems for Packaging Human Drugs and Biologics. Chemistry, Manufacturing and Controls Documentation. Available at http://www.fda.gov/downloads/Drugs/GuidanceComplianceRegulatory Information/Guidances/ ucm070551.pdf.

Jenkins, W.A., Osborn, K.R., 1993. Packaging Drugs and Pharmaceuticals. Technomic Publishing, Lancaster.

Lynch, B., Song, P., 2012. Vaccine packaging at the clinical interface of vaccine, healthcare worker, and patient. Biopharm International 25 (10), 34–36.

Medicines and Healthcare products Regulatory Agency, 2016. Medicines: packaging, labelling and patient information leaflets. https://www.gov.uk/guidance/medicines-packaging-labelling-and-patient-information-leaflets. (Accessed 5 January 2017).

National Patent Safety Agency, 2008. Design for Patient Safety: A Guide to Labelling and Packaging of Injectable Medicines. Available at http://www.nrls.npsa.nhs.uk/resources/collections/design-for-patient-safety/?entryid45=59831.

Rees, J.A., Smith, I., Watson, J., 2014. Pharmaceutical Practice, fifth ed. Churchill Livingstone, Edinburgh.

Soroka, W., Emblem, A., Emblem, H., 1996. Fundamentals of Packaging Technology. Institute of Packaging Professionals, Naperville.

47

Chemical stability in dosage forms

Andrew R. Barnes

KEY POINTS

- Chemical stability is often the critical factor that limits the shelf life of pharmaceutical products.
- Hydrolysis reactions are important degradation mechanisms for acids, amides and related compounds such as penicillins.
- Oxidation reactions tend to give complex mixtures of products and may involve free-radical mechanisms.
- Isomeric change may occur because of racemization or epimerization, or the formation of geometrical or structural isomers.
- Drugs that absorb the wavelengths of light present in sunlight or artificial light may undergo light-induced degradation.
- Chemical incompatibility occurs if drugs, or other ingredients present in the dosage form, react together.
- The amino acid residues of proteins may undergo oxidation, hydrolysis, deamidation or racemization, potentially leading to loss of the three-dimensional conformation of the protein and aggregation.

Introduction

Chemical degradation of the drug is often the critical factor that limits the shelf life of a pharmaceutical product. The degradation of other ingredients in the formulation, such as antimicrobial preservatives or antioxidants, may also be a critical factor.

The nature of the degradation products that form in the dosage form may be the factor that limits the shelf life of a product. This may be because the degradation products are toxic; for instance, the antifungal drug flucytosine degrades to fluorouracil, which is cytotoxic. The degradation products may alternatively give the product an unacceptable appearance. For instance, the oxidation products of adrenaline are highly coloured.

In general, drug molecules tend not to undergo spontaneous chemical degradation; the cause is usually some other reactive molecule within the dosage form. Often, this is due to the presence of water or molecular oxygen, but the drug may also react with other formulation constituents or react with other molecules of the same drug. Protection of the formulation from chemical degradation is one of the primary aims of dosage form design.

This chapter discusses the common types of chemical degradation that affect 'small-molecule' drugs and then looks at the specific stability issues affecting proteins and peptides.

Chemical degradation reactions

Hydrolysis

Hydrolysis is the breaking of a molecular bond by reaction with water. Water is common in pharmaceutical products, either as an ingredient or as a contaminant, and hydrolysis reactions are the most common cause of chemical degradation. Most hydrolysis reactions involve derivatives of carboxylic acids, such as esters and amides, which are frequently found in drug molecules.

The ester group hydrolyses to produce a carboxylic acid and an alcohol (Fig. 47.1a). The carbon of the ester carboxyl group is relatively electron deficient, owing to bond polarization caused by the adjacent oxygen atoms. Nucleophilic attack by water is therefore promoted at this carbon atom. For instance, the degradation of aspirin (acetylsalicylic acid) results in the formation of salicylic acid and acetic acid (Fig. 47.2). Aspirin is too unstable to allow the formulation of an aqueous aspirin product with a suitable shelf life.

Hydrolysis reactions of esters, amides and related molecules are catalysed by an acid and by a base. To use ester hydrolysis as an example, catalysis by a base involves nucleophilic attack by a hydroxyl ion at the electron-deficient carbon of the carbonyl group to produce a tetrahedral intermediate (Fig. 47.3a and b). This is followed by ejection of the alcohol (Fig. 47.3c). In this scheme, ionization of the

carboxylic acid in alkaline solution is ignored for clarity.

Catalysis by an acid involves protonation of the carbonyl group (Fig. 47.4a) to produce resonance structures (Fig. 47.4b and c). The positively charged carbon atom promotes nucleophilic attack by water (Fig. 47.4c) to produce a tetrahedral intermediate (Fig.47.4d). Transfer of H^+ within the molecule (Fig. 47.4e) results in loss of the alcohol portion (Fig. 47.4f).

Amides degrade to a carboxylic acid and an amine (Fig. 47.1b). Amides tend to be more stable to hydrolysis than the corresponding esters because the nitrogen atom is less electronegative than the oxygen atom in the corresponding ester. Examples of amide-containing drugs include lidocaine and paracetamol. The antimicrobial drug chloramphenicol is an

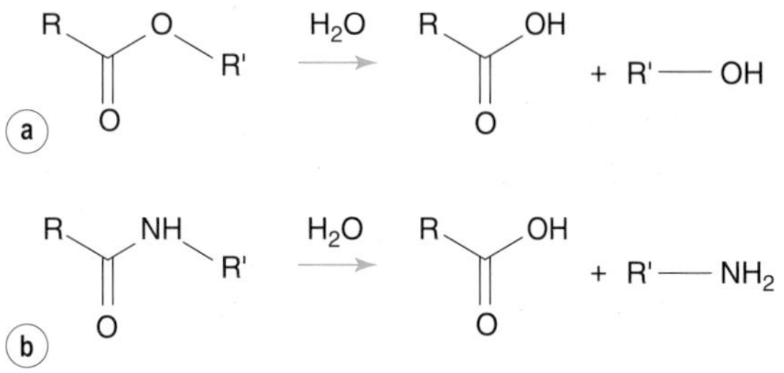

Fig. 47.1 • Hydrolysis reactions: **(a)** esters and **(b)** amides.

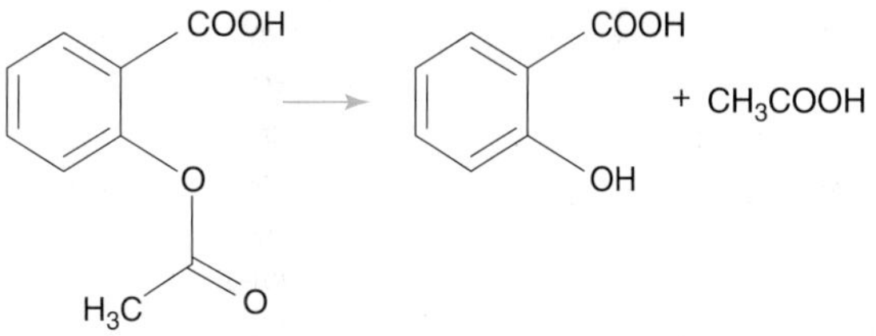

Fig. 47.2 • Hydrolysis of aspirin to salicylic acid and acetic acid.

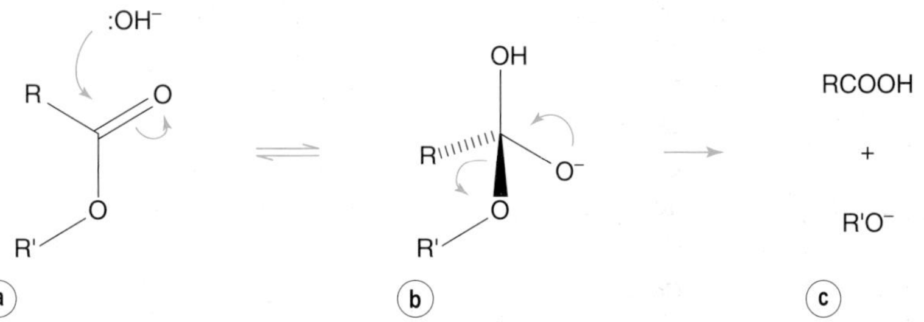

Fig. 47.3 • Base-catalysed ester hydrolysis.

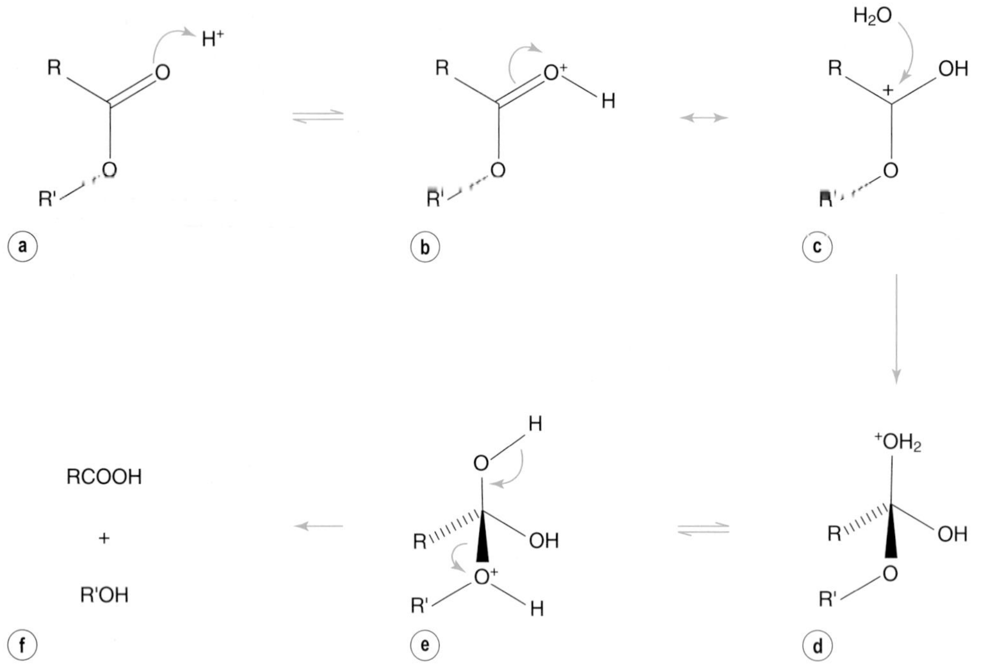

Fig. 47.4 • Acid-catalysed ester hydrolysis.

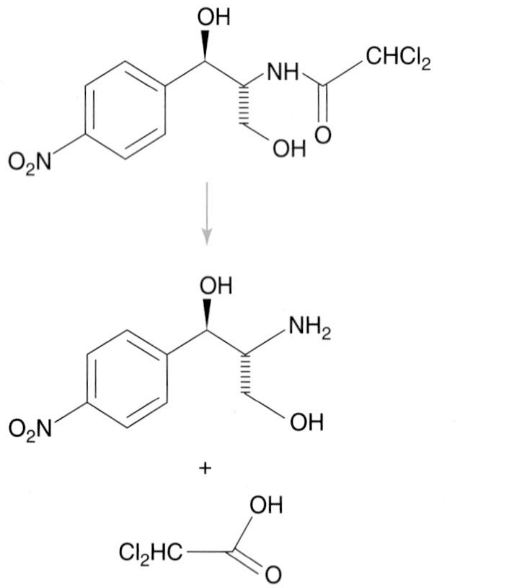

Fig. 47.5 • Hydrolysis of chloramphenicol to 2-amino-1-(4-nitrophenyl)propane-1.3-diol and dichloroacetic acid.

amide-containing drug that is relatively susceptible to hydrolysis compared with many amides (Fig. 47.5). This is due to a high degree of polarization of the amide bond by the highly electronegative chlorine substituents that are adjacent. Eye drop preparations

of chloramphenicol therefore must be stored in a refrigerator.

The lactam group, which is a cyclic amide, is important because it is present in penicillin and cephalosporin antibiotics, and this group is very susceptible to hydrolysis. This reactivity of the molecule is due to bond strain in the four-membered β-lactam ring. A variety of hydrolysis products are formed. For benzylpenicillin, a major hydrolysis product is benzylpenicilloic acid (Fig. 47.6). Penicillins have a side chain that possesses an amide group, but this is less susceptible to hydrolysis than the β-lactam ring. Benzylpenicillin cannot be administered by the oral route because it is hydrolysed rapidly by the acidic conditions in the stomach. Orally active penicillins such as amoxicillin are relatively less susceptible to hydrolysis.

Oxidation

Oxidation reactions involve an increase in the number of carbon–oxygen bonds in a molecule or a reduction in the number of carbon–hydrogen bonds. These reactions are a common cause of chemical instability of drugs. They are also responsible for the deterioration of vegetable oils, which may be used in

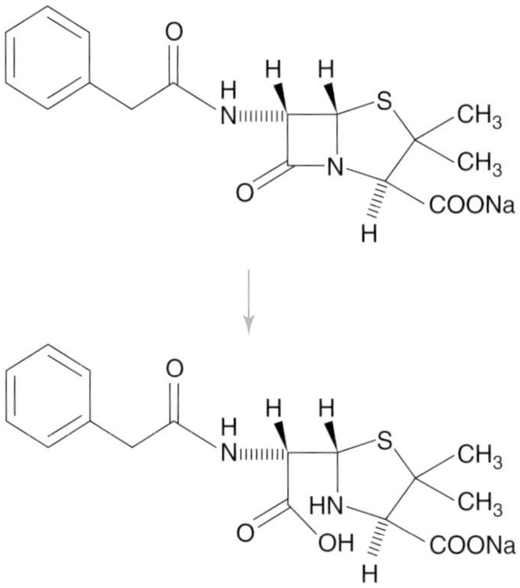

Fig. 47.6 • Hydrolysis of the β-lactam ring of benzylpenicillin to give benzylpenicilloic acid.

Table 47.1 Drug oxidation reactions

Functional group undergoing oxidation	Resulting oxidation product	Example drugs
Phenolic hydroxyl, catechols 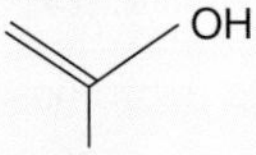	Carbonyl group 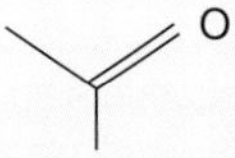	Propofol, adrenaline and related catecholamines
Phenolic hydroxyl 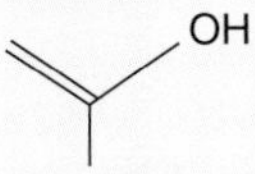	Dimeric product 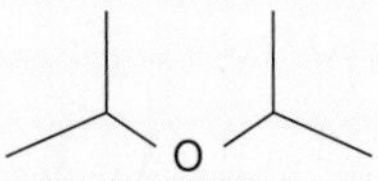	Morphine
Amine	N-Oxide	Morphine
Thioether	S-Oxide	Promethazine and related phenothiazines
Thiol 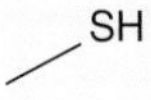	Disulfide 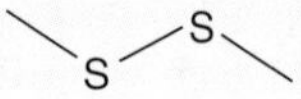	Captopril, 6-mercaptopurine

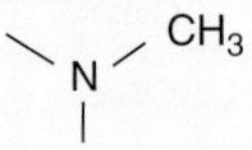

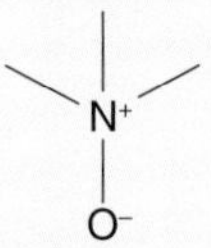

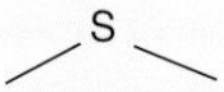

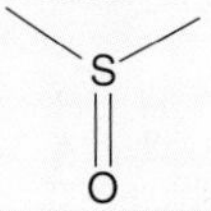

pharmaceutical products as a solvent or as an emollient in emulsions and creams. Oxidation reactions tend to be complex, giving a variety of degradation products. Table 47.1 summarizes common examples.

Oxidation that occurs at ambient temperature and involves molecular oxygen is known as *autoxidation*. Most such reactions involve free radicals, which are chemical species that possess an unpaired electron. Free-radical oxidations are often complex but involve three main phases. The following scheme is a representative summary of the oxidation of many drugs and of vegetable oils.

The *initiation phase* results in the formation of a low concentration of free radicals. For a drug, RH, the generation of free radicals can be represented as

$$RH \rightarrow R^+ + H\bullet$$

$$(47.1)$$

Initiation is promoted by light and the presence of heavy metals, which are inevitably found as trace contaminants of pharmaceutical products.

During the *propagation phase*, the concentration of free radicals increases greatly:

$$R\bullet + O_2 \rightarrow RO_2\bullet$$

$$(47.2)$$

$$RO_2\bullet + RH \rightarrow ROOH + R\bullet$$

$$(47.3)$$

The presence of oxygen results in the formation of hydroperoxides (ROOH), which react further to produce stable oxidation products. In this phase, degradation accelerates, with potentially disastrous results for the product.

In the *termination phase*, the availability of oxygen or drug diminishes, the rate of reaction slows and free radicals combine to produce unreactive end products. The stable reaction products formed in vegetable oils include carboxylic acids, which are responsible for the rancid smell formed when such oils deteriorate.

Oxidation of some drugs occurs rapidly in solution at room temperature. Ascorbic acid (vitamin C) undergoes a rapid oxidation in solution to dehydroascorbic acid (Fig. 47.7). This reaction is reversible but dehydroascorbic acid is rapidly and irreversibly hydrolysed at the ester linkage to form diketogulonic acid.

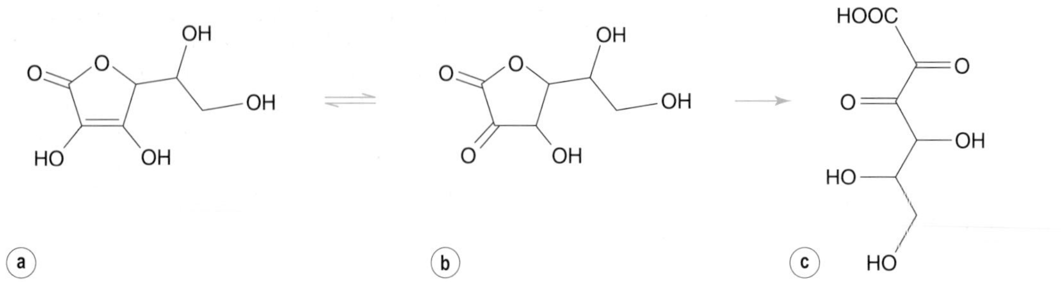

Fig. 47.7 • Oxidation of ascorbic acid **(a)** to dehydroascorbic acid **(b)** and subsequent hydrolysis to diketogulonic acid **(c)**.

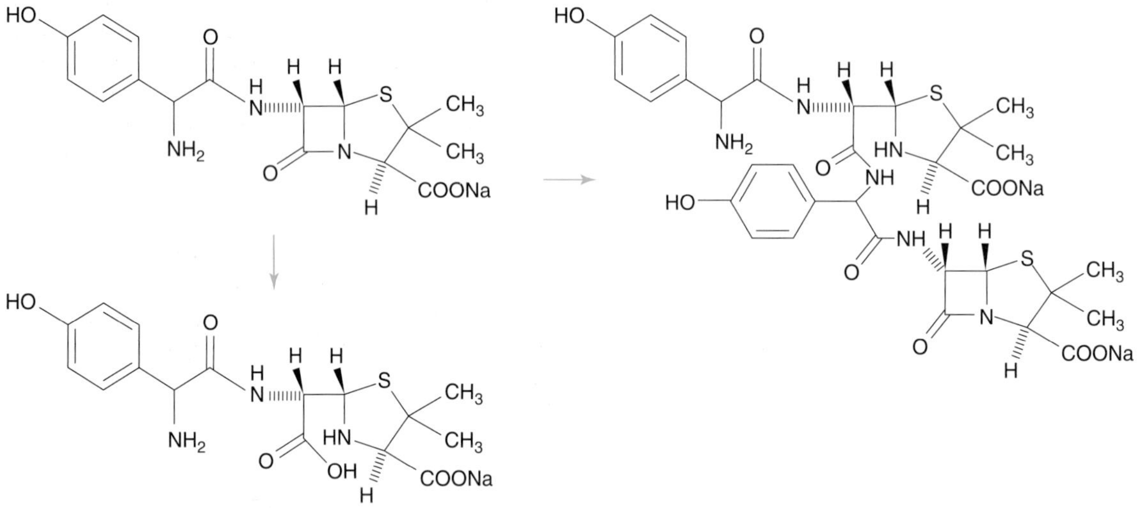

Fig. 47.8 • Amoxicillin degrades by both β-lactam ring hydrolysis and dimerization.

Dimerization and polymerization

Reaction of a drug molecule with another molecule of the same drug may result in the formation of a dimer or polymer. The penicillin antibiotic amoxicillin, besides undergoing hydrolysis of the β-lactam ring, undergoes dimerization by nucleophilic attack on the β-lactam ring by the amino group (Fig. 47.8), especially in more concentrated solutions. The reaction can continue to produce a trimer and tetramer.

Polymerization is a major mechanism of degradation of the disinfectant glutaraldehyde at alkaline pH (Fig. 47.9). Because glutaraldehyde undergoes keto–enol tautomerism, an aldol condensation reaction between the keto and enol forms of the molecule results in the production of a dimer. Further reaction to produce a polymer then occurs. To avoid polymerization on storage, glutaraldehyde solution needs to be formulated at an acidic pH, where polymerization does

not occur. Its disinfectant activity is optimal at a slightly alkaline pH, so an alkaline buffer is added immediately before use.

Hofmann elimination

The reaction of a quaternary amine with a base, known as Hofmann elimination, results in the elimination of a tertiary amine and formation of an alkene. This reaction is not a widespread mode of pharmaceutical degradation; however, it is of major interest because of its role in the metabolism of the neuromuscular blocking drug atracurium, and the related drug cisatracurium. To avoid the variable duration of action of other classes of neuromuscular blocking drugs, due to variability in liver function and enzymatic metabolism, the atracurium molecule was designed to undergo spontaneous chemical degradation after administration to the patient. Atracurium is relatively

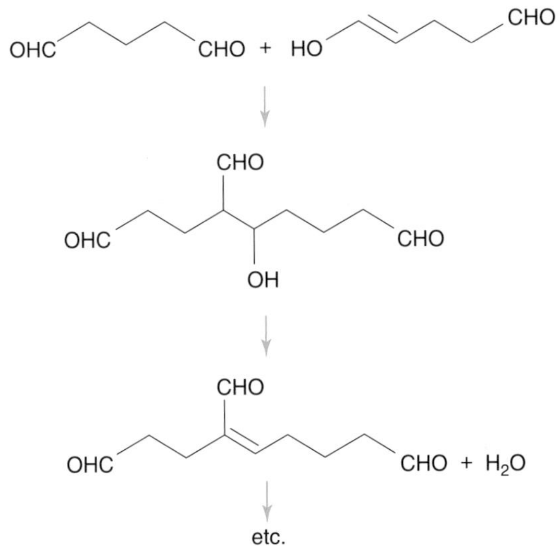

Fig. 47.9 • Polymerization reaction of glutaraldehyde. Two molecules of glutaraldehyde are shown in the keto and enol forms respectively.

stable when formulated as an injection at pH 3–4 and stored under refrigeration. When atracurium is injected into the patient, the higher pH of approximately 7.4 (and to some extent the higher temperature) causes rapid chemical degradation via Hofmann elimination, resulting in reproducible removal of the drug from the patient (Fig. 47.10).

Isomeric change

Different isomers of a drug often have differing pharmacological activity or toxicity.

Optically active molecules with one chiral centre are known as *enantiomers*. The conversion of one enantiomer into its mirror image is known as *racemization*. In addition to susceptibility to oxidation, adrenaline may also undergo racemization in aqueous solution. The reaction is acid and base catalysed and involves the formation of an alcoholate anion, which

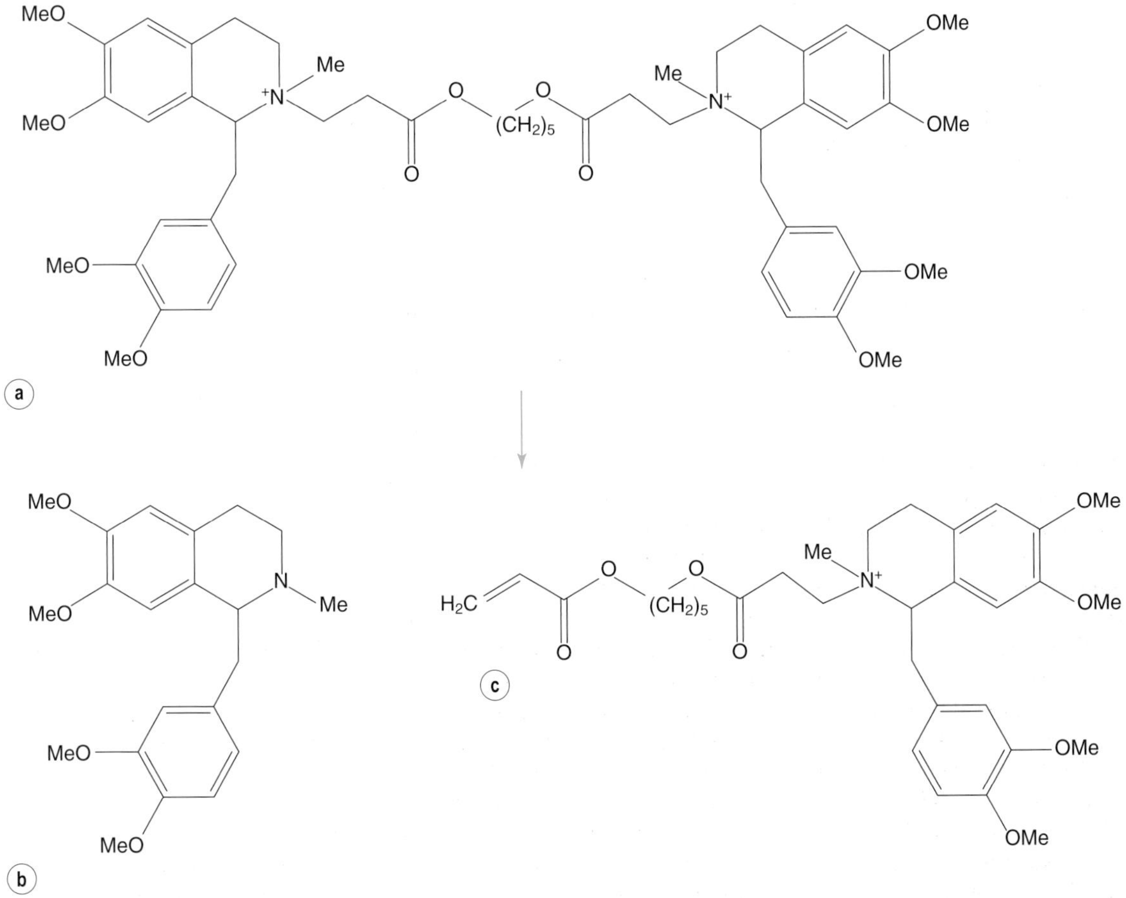

Fig. 47.10 • Atracurium degradation by Hofmann elimination. Degradation of atracurium **(a)** to give a tertiary amine **(b)** and an alkene **(c)**.

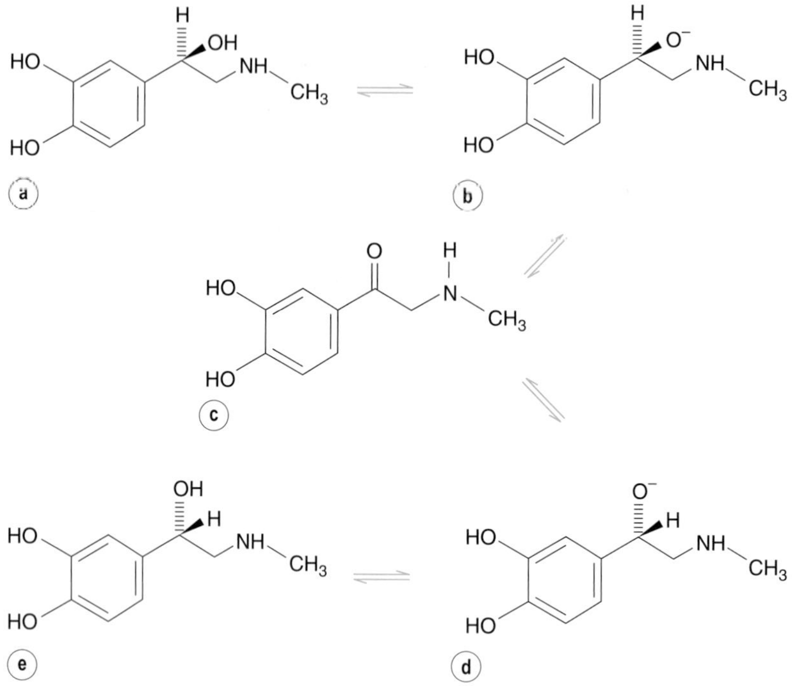

Fig. 47.11 • (R)-Adrenaline **(a)** converts to an alcoholate ion with the R configuration **(b)** and then to a carbonyl-containing intermediate **(c)**. This may revert to the original alcoholate ion with the R configuration **(b)** or to the alcoholate ion with the S configuration **(d)**, which can then form (S)-adrenaline **(e)**.

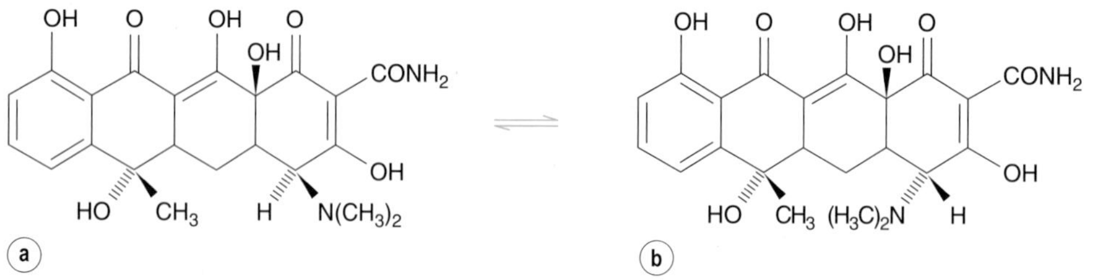

Fig. 47.12 • Epimerization of tetracycline **(a)** to 4-epitetracycline **(b)**.

reversibly forms a carbonyl-containing intermediate with no chiral centre (Fig. 47.11). Regeneration of the alcoholate anion in either of its isomeric forms is then possible. This reaction would eventually result in an equilibrium mixture of equal concentrations of each isomer. (R)-Adrenaline has much greater pharmacological activity than (S)-adrenaline. The reason for the difference in potency is that in (R)-adrenaline the amino and hydroxyl substituents are oriented on the same side of the molecule, allowing them both to form hydrogen bonds with the adrenaline receptor in vivo. However, in (S)-adrenaline only one of these substituents can bond with the receptor because they are on opposite sides of the molecule.

In drug molecules with more than one chiral centre (*diasteriomers*), racemization at one of the chiral centres is known as *epimerization*. The antibiotic tetracycline, for instance, forms the 4-epitetracycline epimer (Fig. 47.12), which is not active against microorganisms and is more toxic than tetracycline.

Geometrical isomers differ in the conformation of groups around a carbon–carbon double bond or a cyclic group. Retinol and all other related molecules, which together are known as vitamin A, contain an unsaturated hydrocarbon chain. In addition to making the molecule susceptible to oxidation, this also enables the molecule to undergo geometrical isomerization. The double bonds in the chain are all

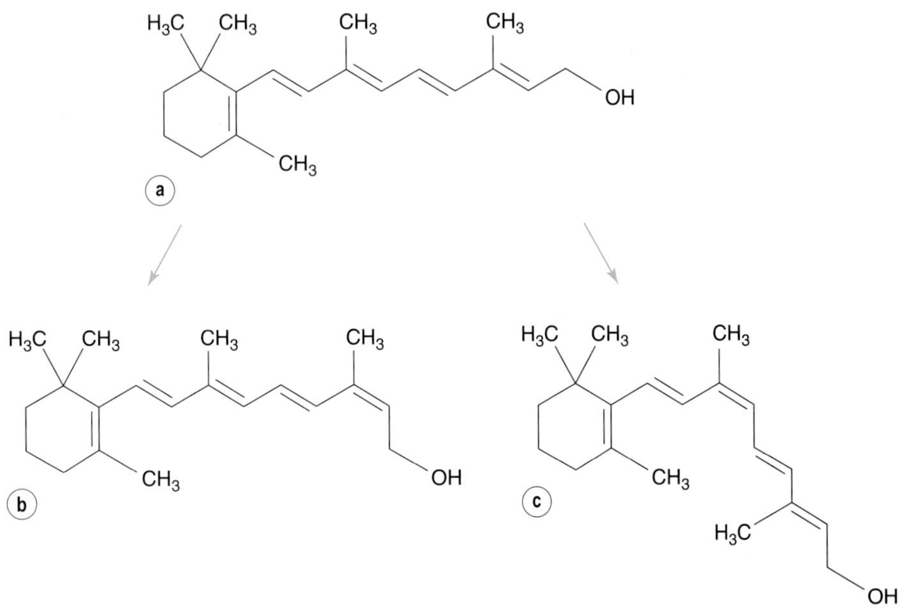

Fig. 47.13 • All-*trans*-retinol (a) undergoes thermal degradation to give 13-*cis*-retinol (b) and undergoes photodegradation to form 9-*cis*-retinol (c).

in the *trans* configuration. On storage of all-*trans*-retinol, or on subjecting it to heat, the molecule changes configuration at the double bond at the 13-position of the molecule, to form 13-*cis*-retinol (Fig. 47.13), which has no activity as a vitamin.

Structural isomers are sometimes formed as a result of drug degradation. The best known example of this is betamethasone 17-valerate, a potent corticosteroid. A major route of degradation of this drug is by migration of the valerate ester substituent to the side chain, forming betamethasone 21-valerate (Fig. 47.14). The mechanism is promoted by the close proximity of the hydroxyl group in the side chain to the ester substituent. This reaction is of concern where topical formulations of betamethasone 17-valerate are diluted with an inappropriate diluent.

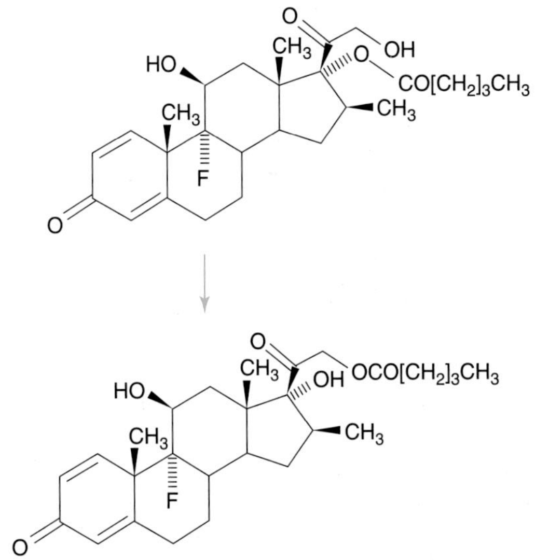

Photodegradation

Molecules that absorb the wavelengths of light associated with sunlight or artificial light may be susceptible to light-induced degradation (*photolysis*). The 300 nm to 400 nm wavelengths tend to be most damaging. Shorter wavelengths are also damaging but are not of practical concern because they are not present to a great extent in sunlight or artificial light.

Carbonyl, nitro, alkene, aryl chloride and phenolic compounds are most susceptible to photodegradation.

Fig. 47.14 • Degradation of betamethasone 17-valerate to betamethasone 21-valerate.

Many photolysis reactions involve oxidation mechanisms, although other mechanisms may occur. Photodegradation of retinol, as well as promoting oxidative reactions, results in the formation of 9-*cis*-retinol. In contrast, degradation occurring in the absence of light causes isomerization at position 13 (Fig. 47.13).

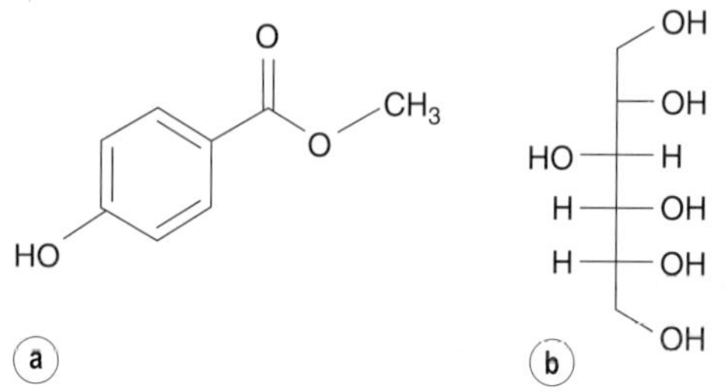

Fig. 47.15 • **(a)** Methyl hydroxybenzoate. **(b)** Sorbitol.

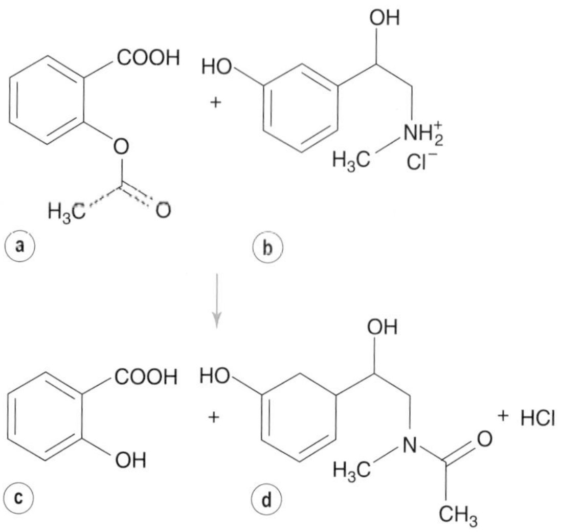

Fig. 47.16 • Transesterification reaction of aspirin **(a)** with phenylephrine hydrochloride **(b)** to give salicylic acid **(c)** and N-acetylphenylephrine **(d)**.

Chemical incompatibilities

Degradation of a drug may be caused by reaction with another drug present in the formulation or with a formulation excipient.

Hydroxybenzoate ester (parabens) antimicrobial preservatives undergo transesterification reactions with sugars and sugar alcohols, which may be present in a formulation as sweetening agents. For instance, methyl hydroxybenzoate undergoes reaction with sorbitol (Fig. 47.15) to produce a variety of sorbitol hydroxybenzoate esters by reaction with sorbitol's various hydroxyl groups.

A related reaction involves the interaction of aminophylline with suppository bases. Aminophylline is a complex, formed between theophylline and ethylenediamine, which has increased aqueous solubility compared with theophylline alone. On storage of aminophylline suppositories, the melting point of the base increases to above physiological temperature, preventing release of the drug. The mechanism for this is the formation of amide bonds between ethylenediamine and the carboxyl groups of fatty acids present in the suppository base. The reaction is the reverse of the amide hydrolysis reaction shown in Fig. 47.1b.

Transacetylation reactions have been reported for some drugs. For instance, in tablet formulations that contain aspirin and phenylephrine hydrochloride (a drug used as a nasal decongestant), the acetyl group is transferred from aspirin to phenylephrine (Fig. 47.16). A similar reaction occurs between aspirin and paracetamol. Aspirin also reacts with the polyethylene glycol base of suppository formulations, transferring the acetyl group to the polyethylene glycol.

The Maillard reaction involves a reducing sugar and an amine. Reducing sugars tautomerize to an open ring form, containing a reactive aldehyde or keto group. The reaction is responsible for the browning of cooked foods, where the amino group is provided by the protein present in the food. It may also occur between amine-containing drugs and lactose or other sugars used as a diluent in the formulation of solid dosage forms. This reaction results in yellowing of white tablets on storage. For example, lactose (Fig. 47.17a) tautomerizes to its aldehydic form (Fig. 47.17b), which reacts with an amine to produce, via several intermediate stages, a coloured l-amino-2-keto sugar (Fig. 47.17c). Other reducing sugars include glucose and fructose. Nonreducing sugars, which do not undergo this reaction, include sucrose and mannitol.

Sodium metabisulfite is commonly added to adrenaline injection as an antioxidant. However, it reacts with the drug to form adrenaline sulfonate (Fig. 47.18), and this is a significant degradation route for adrenaline.

Stability of proteins and peptides

Proteins and peptides have a long-established use as therapeutic agents, but are becoming increasingly important (along with other biopharmaceuticals) because of the opportunities offered by the use of recombinant DNA technology. This allows the production of molecules designed with specific properties

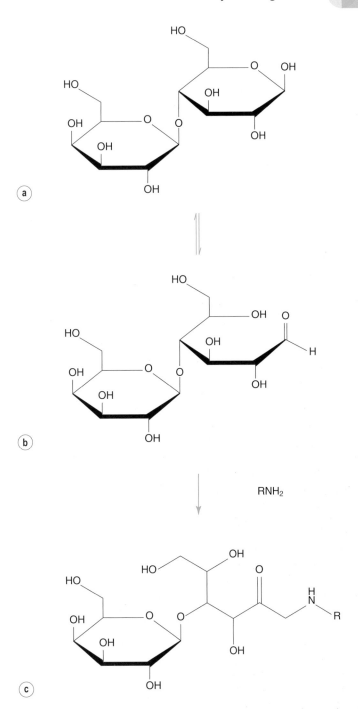

Fig. 47.17 • The Maillard reaction between lactose, via its open-ring tatutomer, and an amine drug. The Maillard reaction between lactose **(a)**, via its open-ring tautomer **(b)**, and an amine drug (RNH₂) to give a coloured 1-amino-2-keto sugar **(c)**.

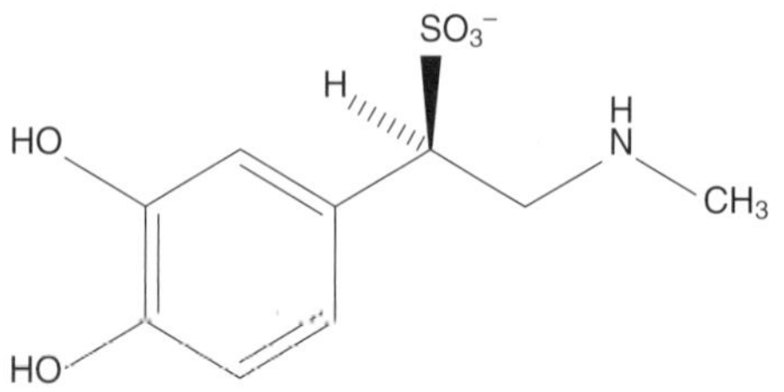

Fig. 47.18 • Adrenaline sulfonate.

(e.g. monoclonal antibodies). These products are discussed in detail in Chapter 43, whilst this section discusses specifically the stability issues associated with these complex molecules.

Physical stability of proteins

The biological activity of a protein is governed by its three-dimensional conformation, whereby the specific sequence of amino acid residues in the protein (its *primary structure*) results in it coiling (*secondary structure*) and folding (*tertiary structure*). There is a close interrelationship between the chemical and physical stability of proteins, so these aspects will be dealt with together.

A protein in its naturally folded (*native*) state adopts a conformation whereby hydrophobic regions of the molecule are located within its globular structure. This is its most energetically favourable conformation because these regions are hidden from the surrounding aqueous environment. As the protein unfolds (to its *non-native state*), the hydrophobic regions are exposed. These may then interact with surfaces, causing loss of protein from the solution by adsorption. However, a major mode of protein loss is for the hydrophobic regions on adjacent protein molecules to associate, forming *aggregates*. These aggregates initially remain in solution; however, the process can continue until a visible precipitate is formed.

Partially unfolded protein molecules may revert to the native state; however, aggregate formation is generally irreversible.

In addition to loss of therapeutic activity, aggregation of protein drugs can also result in an increase in the immunogenicity of the protein, potentially causing safety problems in clinical use.

Aggregation of proteins is caused by several factors:

- *Heat*. This prevents the use of heat sterilization processes for protein-based dosage forms.
- *Freezing* (during a freeze-drying process, or if a protein solution is inadvertently frozen during storage).
- *Shear stresses* arising from stirring or pumping protein solution during dosage form manufacture may also cause aggregation. In this case, an increase in the area of the air–liquid interface occurs and protein adsorbs at the interface with its hydrophobic regions exposed to the air. Hydrophobic interactions can then occur between adjacent molecules, resulting in aggregation.
- *Chemical degradation* of amino acid residues at specific positions in the protein chain, occurring during processing or storage, may cause changes in the tertiary or secondary structure, resulting in loss of biological activity.

Chemical aspects of protein stability

On storage, more than one position in a peptide or protein molecule may be subject to chemical change, sometimes by various modes of chemical reaction. The extent to which chemical change alters the protein's activity is variable and depends on the specific protein. The factors influencing reactivity are:

- *Amino acids*. Different amino acids differ in their susceptibility to chemical degradation.
- *Position in the amino acid sequence*. Some combinations of amino acids are highly susceptible to degradation.
- *Location within the protein tertiary structure*. Residues that are immobilized because of their being buried within the protein are protected from reaction with water, oxygen or other protein chains.

The most common chemical reactions are oxidation, disulfide bridge interchange, hydrolysis, deamidation and racemization.

Oxidation of amino acid residues

Reaction with atmospheric oxygen is a major route of protein degradation, both in solution and in freeze-dried formulations. Amino acids that are susceptible to oxidation are similarly susceptible to this form of degradation when incorporated into a peptide or protein. Methionine and cysteine residues are most susceptible. Methionine oxidizes to form methionine

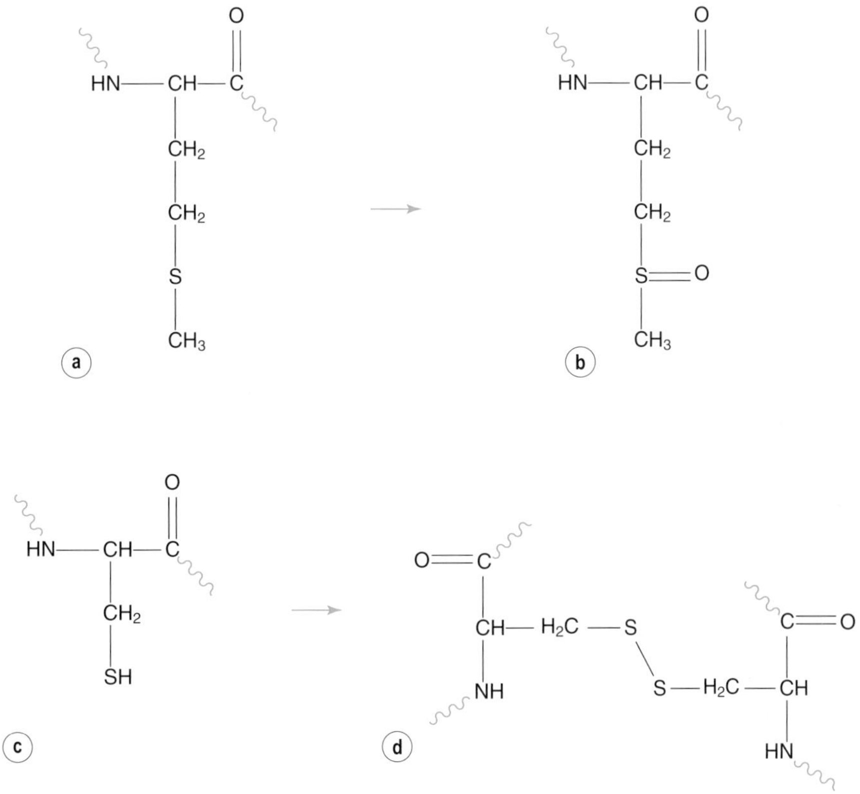

Fig. 47.19 • The methionine residue **(a)** oxidizes to methionine sulfoxide **(b)**. Cysteine **(c)** reacts with another cysteine residue to form a disulfide **(d)**.

sulfoxide (Fig. 47.19a and b). Two cysteine residues react together to form a disulfide bridge (Fig. 47.19c and d). Bridges between cysteine residues within the same molecule play a part in maintaining the native protein conformation. However, reaction between residues on different molecules may lead to aggregation. This reaction is thus more likely to cause change of the protein's conformation, and therefore aggregation, than oxidation of methionine residues.

Disulfide bond interchange

Disulfide bonds may break and reform between different cysteine residues, potentially destabilizing the protein's conformation.

Hydrolysis of proteins

Scission (division) of the amino acid chain by hydrolysis of the peptide bond between residues is possible. The asparagine–proline bond is most susceptible (Fig. 47.20).

Deamidation

Glutamate and asparagine residues degrade by reaction at their amide side chain. Asparagine–glycine sequences are especially susceptible. Deamidation at asparagine residues forms aspartate and its structural isomer isoaspartate (Fig. 47.21). The relatively minor change to the chemical structure caused by deamidation can result in substantial change to the protein conformation and hence bioactivity.

Six of the 51 amino acid residues that form insulin are susceptible to deamidation, especially the C-terminal asparagine residue.

Racemization of amino acid residues

Conversion of the amino acids within the protein chain from the naturally occurring L conformation to the D conformation may occur; this may change the protein's activity. Asparagine residues are most susceptible.

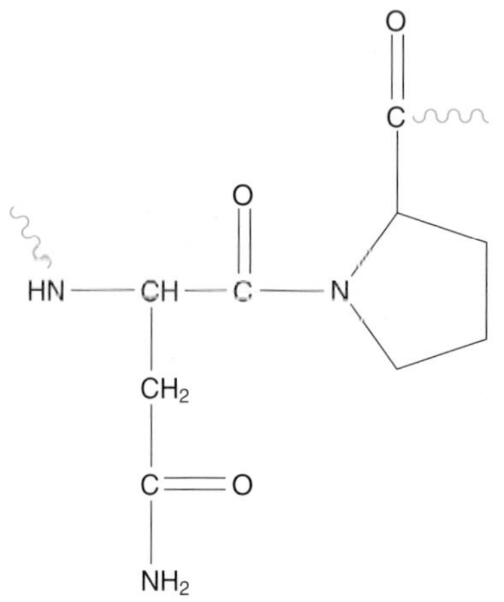

Fig. 47.20 • The asparagine–proline sequence.

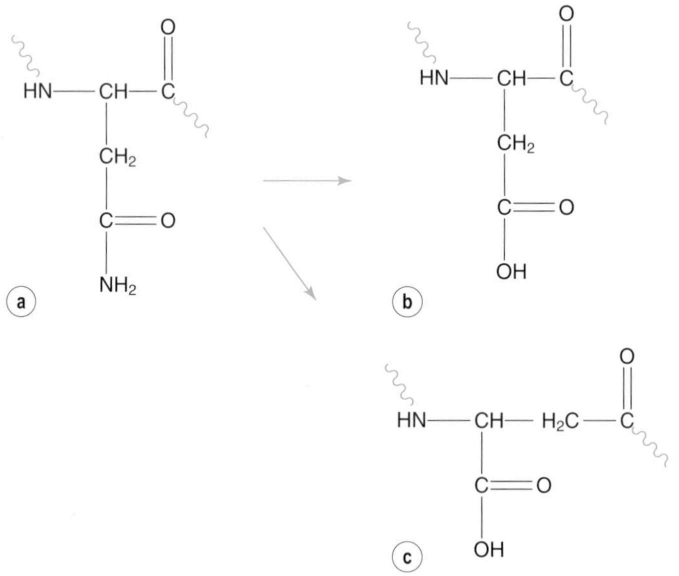

Fig. 47.21 • Deamidation of the asparagine residue **(a)** forms aspartate **(b)** and isoaspartate **(c)**.

Chemical modification of protein stability

Genetic manipulation may be used to improve the stability of a protein pharmaceutical by introducing selective mutations into specific sites in the protein.

Chemical stability may be increased by replacement of chemically reactive amino acid residues with less reactive ones.

Physical stability can also be directly increased. Substitutions that improve intramolecular interactions within the protein molecule, either between different regions of the molecule or within the structure of helical regions, will reduce flexibility of the protein chain, reducing the risk of unfolding.

For instance, selective replacement of cysteine or asparagine residues with the less reactive serine may increase chemical stability. However, insertion of additional cysteine residues may increase protein stability because of their ability to form disulfide bonds within the molecule. The stability of biopharmaceuticals, including proteins and peptides, and formulation strategies to reduce degradation are discussed in detail in Chapter 43.

Please check your eBook at **https://studentconsult. inkling.com/** for self-assessment questions. See inside cover for registration details.

Bibliography

Albini, A., Fasani, E., 1998. Drugs: Photochemistry and Photostability. Royal Society of Chemistry, Cambridge.

Banga, A.K., 2015. Therapeutic Peptides and Proteins: Formulation, Processing and Delivery Systems, third ed. CRC Press, Boca Raton.

Connors, K.A., Amidon, G.L., Stella, V.J., 1986. Chemical Stability of Pharmaceuticals: A Handbook for Pharmacists, second ed. Wiley, New York.

International Conference on Harmonisation of Technical Requirements for Registration of Pharmaceuticals for Human Use, 1995. Q5C Stability Testing of Biotechnological/Biological Products. International Conference on Harmonisation of Technical Requirements for Registration of Pharmaceuticals for Human Use, Geneva.

48

Microbial contamination, spoilage and preservation of medicines

Norman A. Hodges

KEY POINTS

- Medicines are vulnerable to contamination and spoilage by microorganisms. The words *contamination* and *spoilage* have different meanings; contamination is the *entry* of microorganisms into the product, whilst spoilage describes the product damage that results from microbial growth.

- Microorganisms should be excluded from medicines not only because they represent an infection hazard but also because they may degrade the active pharmaceutical ingredient, reduce the product's physical stability or make it unacceptable to the patient.

- Anhydrous medicines are not normally susceptible to spoilage because microbial reproduction will not occur in the absence of water. The amount of free water available for microbial growth in a product is determined by the water activity (A_w). Reducing the water activity of a product is therefore a means of protecting it against spoilage.

- Microbial contamination of medicines arises from three principal sources: the raw materials (particularly water), the manufacturing environment and personnel.

- Raw materials of animal, vegetable or mineral origin normally have a higher level of contamination than those made by chemical synthesis, where heat, extremes of pH or organic solvents tend to kill microorganisms.

- The 'Orange Guide' describes manufacturing practices that are designed to minimize both the contamination introduced into a product and the opportunities for those contaminants to reproduce while the product is being made.

- Preservative chemicals are required for most water-containing nonsterile products and for multidose sterile products.

- The range of available preservatives is quite limited, and they all suffer from one or more of the following faults: only possessing good activity against bacteria or fungi, but not both; exhibiting reduced antimicrobial activity in certain pH ranges – several only working well in acid conditions; causing skin sensitivity reactions; and interacting with other common excipients – several preservatives lose activity in the presence of surfactants.

The need to protect medicines against microbial spoilage

The need to protect foods against microbial spoilage is well appreciated because microbial growth results in obvious signs of deterioration. However, there is a much lower level of awareness among members of the general public of the need to similarly protect cosmetics, toiletries and medicines. Although most medicines present a less favourable environment for microbial growth than foods, a wide variety of potentially hazardous organisms are nevertheless capable of growing to high concentrations in unprotected products. The subject of preservation is therefore an important aspect of medicine formulation, simply because patients taking medicines are, by definition, unhealthy, and so quite possibly more vulnerable to infection.

It is important to distinguish between the words *contamination* and *spoilage* because they are sometimes used synonymously, which is incorrect.

Contamination, in this context, means the introduction of microorganisms into a product (i.e. it describes microbial ingress). Contaminating organisms can arise from many sources (considered later in this chapter) during the course of both product manufacture and subsequent use of the product. The procedures of good manufacturing practice (also considered later) are used to limit the first of these (Medicines and Healthcare products Regulatory Agency, 2017), but contamination arising from the patient is largely out of the control of the manufacturer except in the context of container design and labelling. It is now commonplace to adopt containers that minimize contact between the patient's body and the product; for example, collapsible tubes are used for creams and ointments rather than open-mouthed tubs or jars, into which fingers can be inserted, although the latter are still in use, particularly for products supplied in large volumes (e.g. Aqueous Cream BP). Similarly, single-dose eye drops may be preferred to bottles where the dropper can come into contact with an infected eye and then be placed again in the eye drop solution. Despite this, contamination by the patient is still a problem to be considered in container design and product preservation.

Spoilage follows contamination and describes the process and consequences of microbial growth in the product. Considering the potential for product spoilage and taking appropriate steps to minimize the risk of it occurring are very much the responsibility of the formulation scientist and the manufacturer.

There are three principal reasons why microorganisms should be excluded totally from medicines or their presence should be subjected to stringent limits set by pharmacopoeias and regulatory agencies, such as the US Food and Drug Administration (FDA), the European Medicines Agency (EMA) or the UK's Medicines and Healthcare products Regulatory Agency (MHRA):

- Products or raw materials contaminated with pathogenic organisms may be an infection hazard.
- Microorganisms may cause chemical or physical changes in the product that render it less potent or effective.
- Microbial growth is likely to make the product unacceptable to the patient or consumer even if there are no significant infection risks or loss of efficacy.

It is quite obvious that medicines should not contain pathogenic organisms that represent a source of infection. However, specifying the species and numbers of organisms representing an infection hazard is not straightforward. Certain pathogens are recognized as 'objectionable organisms' and must be totally excluded from particular raw materials or product types (see Chapter 14), but the risk of infection is influenced not just by the number of organisms and their type but by other factors too. For example, an organism may be present at a concentration that would be regarded as relatively harmless to a healthy individual but which may pose a problem for patients with impaired immunity.

Towards the end of the last century there were several reports in the pharmaceutical literature of infection occurring as a result of medicines containing pathogenic species (e.g. salmonellae, clostridia and *Pseudomonas aeruginosa*), but such reports became far less frequent with the adoption of more rigorous quality standards and regulatory control of manufacture. However, contaminated medicines are by no means a thing of the past. The FDA publishes details of product recalls on its website, and in 2015 there were eight such recalls due to concerns about potential or confirmed microbial contamination in the 'drugs' category of products, and a further 11 in the 'therapeutic biological products' category. It should be emphasized that there is the possibility of an infection arising from the use of a product contaminated with a concentration of organisms that is too low to be detectable by sight or smell. This situation is potentially much more hazardous than that of a patient confronted with a medicine in which microbial growth is clearly evident.

Quite apart from representing an infection hazard, microorganisms may damage the medicine by degrading either the active ingredient or one or more excipients, thus compromising the quality and fitness for use of the product.

Degradation is usually due to either hydrolysis or oxidation, but decarboxylation, racemization and other reactions may also occur. Active ingredients known to be susceptible to microbial attack include steroids, alkaloids, analgesics and antibiotics; several specific examples are given by Bloomfield (2007) and Baird (2011). The numbers and variety of excipients that have been reported to be degraded are at least as great as those of active ingredients. Thus most categories of excipients contain materials that have been shown to be susceptible to microbial enzymes, acids or other metabolic products.

Common examples of product instability or deterioration include emulsion phase separation due to surfactant degradation, loss of viscosity due to microbial effects on gums, mucilages and cellulose derivatives used as thickening agents, and alcohol and acid accumulation following fermentation of sugars. Despite the very purpose of their use being to restrict microbial growth, some preservatives are vulnerable to inactivation by microorganisms that, in exceptional cases, use them as a carbon and energy source. Nor should it be assumed that products whose very purpose is to kill microorganisms will necessarily be self-sterilizing: previous FDA product recalls have involved antiseptic wipes containing alcohol and iodine which were designed to decontaminate skin before injection or surgery, but the wipes were, themselves, sources of microbial contamination.

If microbial growth within the product is sufficiently extensive, it is possible for the presence of the organisms to be detectable by:

- their physical presence (cloudiness in liquid medicines, moulds on or in creams and syrups, or as discolouration of tablets stored in a damp environment);
- changes in colour (pigment production);
- smell (due, for example, to amines, acetic acid or other organic acids, or sulfides from protein breakdown); and
- gas accumulation without any obvious odour (bubbles of carbon dioxide following sugar fermentation).

Clearly, any product manifesting such changes would be unlikely to be used by the patient. This may result in short-term problems for the patient of obtaining alternative supplies and, possibly, longer-term problems for the manufacturer in terms of customer complaints, product recalls, adverse publicity and possible legal action.

Products and materials vulnerable to spoilage

Spoilage, in the sense of detectable physical or chemical change within a pharmaceutical product, nearly always follows growth and reproduction of the contaminating organisms. The pharmacopoeial and regulatory limits for the maximum permissible numbers of microorganisms in manufactured products or raw materials are typically not more than 100–1000 colony-forming units per millilitre or gram depending on the dosage form in question. Whilst these concentrations may allow some pathogens to initiate infections, they are not normally sufficient to cause detectable changes in chemical composition, physical appearance or stability. Bacteria and fungi are just the same as all other living organisms in requiring water for growth (although not necessarily for mere survival). This means that only products containing sufficient water to permit such growth are vulnerable to spoilage. Consequently, spoilage is not normally a problem in anhydrous products such as ointments and dry tablets or capsules, although hygroscopic materials such as gelatin and glycerol may absorb enough water from the atmosphere to enable moulds (but not normally bacteria) to grow. Similarly, cellulosic materials, particularly paper and other packaging, may show mould growth if stored in humid atmospheres (e.g. in tropical climates).

The fact that a product contains water and is obviously a liquid does not necessarily mean that the water is available to participate in chemical reactions and enable microorganisms to grow. Some of the water present in a solution is bound to the solute because of hydrogen bonding or other mechanisms. Thus, a parameter that indicates the proportion of 'free' or available water is a useful guide for the ease with which microorganisms might grow in the product. Such a parameter is *water activity* (A_w), which is the ratio of the water vapour pressure of a solution to the water vapour pressure of pure water at the same temperature. A_w is expressed on a scale from 0 to 1 with a value of 1 representing pure water. As the concentration of solute in a solution is increased, A_w falls proportionally, and the range of organisms able to grow in the solution progressively diminishes. Thus it is possible to construct a table indicating the minimum A_w values that permit the growth of different types of microorganism (Table 48.1).

To a certain extent, the values of A_w in Table 48.1 are reflective of the natural habitats of the organisms concerned; pseudomonads (species within the genus *Pseudomonas*) and other waterborne organisms therefore tend to require high A_w values for optimum growth, whilst skin organisms such as staphylococci and micrococci that exist in relatively high salt concentrations (from sweat glands) will tolerate significantly lower values. Pharmaceutical materials that have high solute concentrations (e.g. syrups) may to a large extent be self-preserving, just like salted foods. Syrup BP, for example, is 67% by weight sucrose, has an A_w value of 0.86 and so is not susceptible to *bacterial* growth, but may contain chemical preservatives to protect it from mould spoilage.

Variations in water activity may arise within a single container of a manufactured medicine by, for example, water evaporating from the bulk liquid during storage at high temperatures and that water vapour condensing on cool glass around the neck of a bottle as the storage temperature drops, then running back to dilute the surface layer of the product. It is for this reason that syrups should not be stored in conditions where the temperature fluctuates.

Table 48.1 Water activity (A_w) minima permitting growth of various organisms

Organism	Approximate minimum water activity
Many common waterborne or soil organisms and nonskin pathogens (e.g. *Pseudomonas aeruginosa*, clostridia, *Escherichia coli*)	0.95
Staphylococci and micrococci	0.87
Many yeasts (e.g. *Saccharomyces* and *Candida* spp.)	0.88–0.92
Many fungi (e.g. *Penicillium*, *Aspergillus*, *Mucor*)	0.8–0.9
Osmophilic yeasts (e.g. *Zygosaccharomyces rouxii*)	0.65

The possibility also exists for contaminants to grow and generate water from respiration and so produce localized increases in A_w which allow other less osmotolerant organisms to grow subsequently. Reducing the water activity of a product as a means of diminishing its susceptibility to spoilage is a formulation strategy that should not be overlooked. However, sugars and glycerol are the only common and acceptable ingredients that may be used in this way in oral products; alcohols and glycols may also be used in topical products.

Sources and control of microbial contamination

To manufacture medicines of acceptable microbiological quality, it is necessary to know the common sources of microbial contaminants in the manufacturing environment and the typical organisms that might arise from each source. It is also useful to know how quickly and to what concentration those organisms might grow in pharmaceutical materials so as to put in place good manufacturing procedures that will minimize contamination and spoilage.

Sources and types of contaminating organisms

Microbial contamination of medicines arises from three principal sources:

1. the raw materials, including water, from which the product is manufactured;
2. the manufacturing environment, including the atmosphere, equipment and work surfaces; and
3. manufacturing personnel.

The relative contributions of these three sources vary depending on the type of product in question. It has been noted (see Chapter 14) that raw materials of different origin may differ significantly in their extent of microbial contamination. 'Natural' materials originating from animals (e.g. gelatin), vegetables (starch, cellulose derivatives, alginates) or minerals (talc, kaolin, magnesium trisilicate, bentonite) usually have much higher bioburdens than synthesized chemicals, in which organisms are often killed by heat, extremes of pH or organic solvents. Despite the high levels of microorganisms to be found in locations where many natural materials arise (gelatin, for example, originates in the slaughterhouse, where faecal contamination of animal carcasses is not uncommon), the cleaning and purification procedures currently used mean that contamination levels are only one or two orders of magnitude higher than those for synthesized chemicals. This is reflected in the pharmacopoeial limit of not more than 10^4 colony-forming units of aerobic bacteria per gram for some oral products containing materials of natural origin compared with 10^2 colony-forming units per gram otherwise.

Generally, the types of contaminating organisms are reflective of the origins of the product and this, in turn, is reflected in the objectionable organisms that must be absent. For example, salmonellae and *Escherichia coli* might arise in faeces, so gelatin is subject to tests for the absence of these species. The same organisms might originate from natural fertilizers used on commercial crops, and so they must be absent too from vegetable drugs, starches, mucilages, etc. Both vegetable drugs and mined minerals may contain organisms originating from the soil (e.g. *Bacillus* and *Clostridium* species), usually as spores. Vegetable drugs may be contaminated with spores of fungal plant pathogens such as *Cladosporium* that rarely arise in other circumstances.

Water is the most commonly used raw material for manufacturing medicines. Not only is it obviously present in most liquid medicines, it may be added, then removed, during manufacture of dry products too (e.g. during tablet granulation). It is also used in the factory for cleaning equipment, work surfaces, mixing vessels and bottles or other product containers. As a consequence, the microbiological quality of both ingredients and cleaning water can have a profound effect on the final bioburden of the manufactured product. To those unfamiliar with methods of water purification, it is a paradox that pharmaceutical purified water is more likely to contain high levels of bacteria (particularly after storage) than the mains water that is used as the source material. This is simply a consequence of the fact that mains water (potable water) is chlorinated, and the chlorine, which acts as a preservative, is removed during purification. Despite this purification process, purified water still contains sufficient dissolved nutrients to support the growth of several species of Gram-negative bacteria to population levels well in excess of 10^5 per millilitre. Such levels may be attained within days rather than weeks of room-temperature storage after chlorine removal. The species commonly found are described as low-demand organisms (i.e. they are metabolically versatile and can efficiently utilize as nutrients low

concentrations of a diverse range of carbon-containing compounds). Pseudomonads (i.e. the organisms resembling the pathogen *Pseudomonas aeruginosa*) are good examples of low-demand Gram-negative bacteria, although organisms of other genera, such as *Flavobacterium* and *Alcaligenes*, also arise.

Product contaminants originating from the manufacturing environment all tend to have one characteristic in common: they survive well in dry conditions. The Gram-negative bacteria that are prevalent in water are rarely seen in this situation. Most of these environmental contaminants are spore-formers, both bacteria and fungi, or Gram-positive bacteria such as micrococci and staphylococci. All these can persist for long periods while attached to dust particles suspended in the atmosphere or settled on floors, work surfaces or equipment. Pharmaceutical factories are supplied with filtered air, so the level of particulate contamination in the atmosphere in a room where there is no activity (i.e. operators are absent) is usually very low. The main component of the dust in a manufacturing area that is in operation is skin scales shed by operational personnel. Humans replace skin constantly and are therefore continually shedding particles with attached skin bacteria; these particles are typically approximately 20 μm in size and cannot be seen with the naked eye. The extent to which skin scales are shed depends on many factors, such as the design and coverage of protective clothing, general health, personal hygiene and, in particular, levels of activity. People standing or sitting normally shed far fewer particles than those who are in motion. Statistics and estimates of the extent to which humans shed skin scales differ substantially, but approximately 10^9 per day is a commonly quoted value (Cosslett, 2007).

Swabbing with antiseptics or washing with bactericidal soap reduces the numbers of microorganisms on the skin, but is by no means totally effective. Fig. 48.1 shows a Petri dish of nutrient medium used to take 'finger dabs' from fingers treated in this way. In the upper left segment, bacterial colonies were cultured from an unwashed finger; the upper right shows the colonies from a finger washed with bactericidal soap and the bottom sector shows those from a finger swabbed for 1 minute with cotton wool soaked in antiseptic. It is clear that short periods of exposure to bactericidal soaps cannot be relied on to eliminate contamination, and a recognized antiseptic is far more effective.

The methods and equipment used for monitoring levels of contaminants arising from water, raw

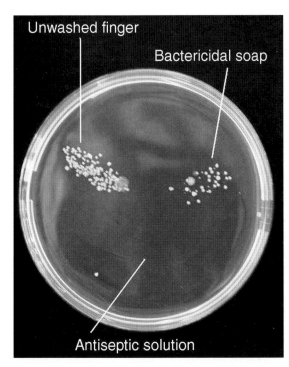

Fig. 48.1 • Colonies of bacteria resulting from 'finger dabs' onto agar: bacteria from an unwashed finger *(top left)*; bacteria from a finger washed with 'bactericidal' soap *(top right)*; no colonies arising from a finger swabbed with antiseptic solution *(bottom sector)*.

materials and the environment are described in Chapter 14.

Factors influencing the growth of spoilage organisms

In addition to water activity, which was considered earlier in this chapter, factors influencing the rate and extent of growth of a contaminant within a pharmaceutical raw material or manufactured medicine include:

- nutrient availability;
- temperature;
- pH;
- redox potential; and
- the presence and concentration of antimicrobial chemicals.

Microorganisms differ enormously in their metabolic capabilities. Some, such as *Escherichia coli*, *Pseudomonas aeruginosa* and several *Bacillus* species, can synthesize all the amino acids and vitamins they need from a variety of simple carbon and nitrogen sources. The minerals that they require are often present in sufficient concentration as impurities in the ingredients of the medicinal product. Thus, in the absence of antimicrobial chemicals, organisms of this type may grow to concentrations of 10^4 per millilitre or gram, or even higher in products such as syrups, linctuses and creams. Products containing glycerol, sugars, amino acids or proteins would clearly represent such ideal media for microbial growth that their preservation is sometimes difficult to achieve despite the addition of preservatives. Even in the absence of these nutritionally rich materials, many bacteria and fungi are still able to utilize other components of the formulation as food sources. Several of these have already been mentioned, but in addition to surfactants and various viscosity-raising agents, the volatile and fixed oils used as flavourings or emulsion components are particularly suitable as nutrients for microorganisms.

The rate of spoilage progression will vary with temperature, although the period for which a manufactured medicine is usually stored before use is normally so long that the difference in bacterial growth rate between, say, 15°C and 20°C may become insignificant in the context of a 2-year shelf life. However, there is the possibility of organisms growing during the course of manufacture, and so it is important for production scientists to be aware just how rapidly the population of contaminants may rise. Fig. 14.1 shows that the concentration of *Pseudomonas aeruginosa* rose 10000-fold in 44 hours at ambient room temperature in a multidose veterinary injection that was supposedly preserved with benzethonium chloride. Clearly, the potential for a rapid increase in numbers is even greater when there is no antimicrobial agent present at all.

Most bacteria have an optimum pH for growth that is near neutrality, but most fungi favour slightly acidic conditions and grow best at pH 5–6. Although the product pH may markedly influence the growth rate itself, it also has a bearing on the activity and stability of any antimicrobial chemicals present, so the magnitudes of these various effects may have to be considered at the product formulation stage, and a compromise value may have to be selected for the product pH. This is considered further in the next section.

Redox potential (oxidation–reduction potential; E_h) is a term that indicates whether oxidizing or reducing conditions exist in a liquid. It is expressed as a positive or negative value on a scale in millivolts.

Oxidizing conditions (favouring the growth of aerobic organisms) prevail in culture media or liquids with positive E_h values, and reducing conditions (favouring anaerobes) apply at negative values. Facultative anaerobic organisms, such as *Escherichia coli* and many similar intestinal pathogens, will grow under both conditions from +300 mV to −100 mV (Food and Drug Administration, 2015). Most pharmaceutical products possess positive redox potentials, and so anaerobic growth is not common, but there is the potential for aerobic primary contaminants to utilize the available dissolved oxygen and so render the product vulnerable to secondary spoilage by anaerobes.

Antimicrobial chemicals are usually added as preservatives in multidose sterile medicines and in nonsterile medicines. Their properties and the factors influencing their selection are considered later in this chapter. However, it is not uncommon for other ingredients of the product to possess antimicrobial activity or enhance the activity of recognized preservatives. Alcohols used as cosolvents are good examples: ethanol, 2-propanol, propylene glycol and glycerol all possess useful antimicrobial activity, although, with the exception of glycerol, their use tends to be limited to topical products. Ethylenediaminetetraacetic acid (EDTA) has a dual role in many pharmaceutical products. It is a chelating agent used to remove metal ions that may catalyse the oxidation of certain active ingredients and, although it possesses little antimicrobial activity in its own right, it may markedly potentiate the action of many established preservatives (see later). Indeed, EDTA is present in most proprietary multidose anti-inflammatory eye drops currently available in the UK. In every case, one of its functions is to potentiate the activity of benzalkonium chloride used as the preservative.

Control of contamination and spoilage during manufacture

Whilst product contamination during use is largely outside the manufacturer's control, there are many steps that can be taken to minimize contamination while the product is made, both by restricting the entry of new organisms into it and by limiting the opportunities for growth of organisms that are unavoidably present at the start, such as those from water or raw materials. Many of these procedures and precautions are described in *Rules and Guidance for Pharmaceutical Manufacturers and Distributors* (known as the 'Orange Guide'; Medicines and Healthcare products Regulatory Agency, 2017). That publication and other regulatory and pharmacopoeial requirements make it clear that use of good manufacturing practices to limit microbial contamination in the first place is the preferred strategy, rather than, for example, permitting contaminants to enter and proliferate in the product and then attempting to kill them by physical or chemical means.

The factors impacting on the hygienic manufacture of medicines are shown in Fig. 48.2. Much of this is

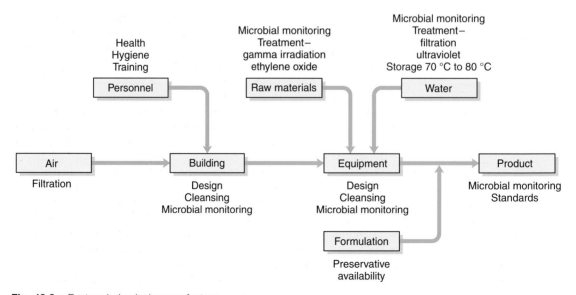

Fig. 48.2 • Factors in hygienic manufacture.

self-explanatory, although certain aspects merit more attention. Standards for atmospheric cleanliness in the manufacturing area apply not just for the production of sterile products but also for the production of nonsterile medicines. Thus the air supply is invariably high-efficiency particulate air (HEPA) filtered, and as air-conditioning plants often act as a breeding ground for microorganisms, filters need to be installed downstream of such equipment. The factors to be considered in the design of premises and equipment are detailed in the Orange Guide, as are the procedures for cleaning and disinfection. There is evidence that persistent use of a single disinfectant might predispose to the development of bacterial resistance to it, although this evidence is far less strong than that concerning antibiotics. Nevertheless, there is a requirement that disinfectants be used on a rotational basis to minimize this risk, and in aseptic areas where sterile products are manufactured, the disinfectant solutions are filter-sterilized because they may, themselves, be a source of contamination with resistant organisms.

Because humans are frequently the principal source of microbial contamination in the manufacturing environment, their health, hygiene, clothing and training may all have an impact on product contamination. The design of clothing for use in different areas is described in detail in the Orange Guide. Whilst it is an unacceptable practice to use heat, radiation or antimicrobial chemicals to 'clean up' a product which has been allowed to acquire a high level of contaminants that could have been avoided, it is acceptable to use these methods to reduce high bioburdens that are unavoidable (e.g. in raw materials of natural origin). Thus raw materials may be exposed to radiation or ethylene oxide for this purpose, and filtration units or ultraviolet (UV) light sources may be used to reduce the bioburden in water. If the water is to be used as an ingredient of an injectable product, filtration is preferable to exposure to UV light because it physically removes the contaminating Gram-negative bacteria that may act as a source of endotoxins, which could cause fever on injection. Although UV light kills the bacteria, the endotoxins remain because the lipopolysaccharide component of the bacterial outer membrane from which they are derived is not destroyed. Because of the ability of Gram-negative bacteria to grow readily in stored purified water, it is also common for the water to be maintained at a high temperature, typically 80 °C, whenever possible during the manufacturing process so as to prevent such growth.

The final factor shown in Fig. 48.2 to impact on hygienic manufacture is that of preservative availability. Whilst the inclusion of a preservative to protect the product from spoilage sounds simple in principle, there are several ways in which the preservative activity may be diminished or virtually abolished as a result of interaction with other components of the formulation or the container. These are considered later.

Selection and use of preservatives

The antimicrobial chemicals commonly used as preservatives in medicines are described in Chapter 15. The properties that are normally required in such a preservative include the following:

- a broad spectrum of antimicrobial activity covering Gram-positive and Gram-negative bacteria, yeasts and moulds, and no vulnerability to resistance development;
- low toxicity for humans, enabling it to be used in topical, oral and parenteral products;
- good solubility in water and low oil solubility;
- stable and effective over a wide pH range and compatible with common excipients; and
- nonvolatile, odourless and tasteless.

Not surprisingly, no single preservative satisfies all these criteria; if there were such an agent, it would be universally used to the exclusion of all others. Thus the selection of a preservative (or combination of preservatives) for a newly developed product is inevitably a compromise determined by the formulation characteristics and intended use of the product. Unfortunately, the list of available preservatives is diminishing rather than expanding. This is due to both the high cost of safety testing that would be a prerequisite for the introduction of an entirely new preservative and toxicity concerns resulting in the use of some agents being largely discontinued (e.g. phenylmercury salts and chloroform, which were formerly used in ophthalmic/parenteral products and in oral medicines respectively). Even parabens (p-hydroxybenzoates), which have been the most commonly used preservatives in medicines for many decades, are now viewed with some suspicion because of fears regarding their very weak oestrogenic action and their potential to stimulate proliferation of cultured breast cancer cells.

Because the function of a preservative is to kill, or at least prevent the growth of, microorganisms, it might be expected that the first item on the list would be a major determinant in preservative selection, but the intended use and route of administration of a product are usually the major factors limiting the choice. The range of potential preservatives is greatest for topical products, and becomes much more restricted when the toxicity considerations applying to oral and parenteral products are applied. Thus there are several preservatives whose use is restricted largely to topical medicines (e.g. bronopol, isothiazolones and imidazolidinyl ureas).

Despite the concerns regarding the toxicity of parabens, they remain by far the most frequently selected preservatives for topical and oral products, although sodium benzoate is also regularly chosen for oral medicines. Multidose injections are now rarely used in human medicine but are still used in veterinary practice. Again, parabens are used as preservatives, although their suitability for this product category is also now questioned; benzyl alcohol, phenol and chlorbutanol are common alternatives. Eye drops are usually, but not invariably, multidose products, which, although initially sterile, may require protection against patient-derived contaminants during use. Benzalkonium chloride, often with EDTA, is more common in eye drops intended for the UK market than all other preservatives put together. Despite this popularity, there is increasing concern about the potential for benzalkonium chloride to cause corneal irritation. Single-dose or unpreserved eye drops are also used. Hiom (2012) has tabulated the commonly used preservatives and their application in different dosage forms.

Because of the limited and diminishing range of acceptable preservatives, in recent years increasing attention has been paid to the possible benefits of using preservatives in combination. Not only is there scope for reducing the concentrations of the agents, which should confer the benefits of reduced toxicity or irritancy, but use of two or more preservatives together might also result in a broader spectrum of antimicrobial cover, a lower risk of resistance development and enhanced activity due to synergy. There are combinations in which each component fills a gap in the antimicrobial spectrum of the other (e.g. parabens and imidazolidinyl ureas, which, individually, have weak activity against *Pseudomonas aeruginosa* and fungi respectively). The practically useful examples of synergistic combinations have been considered by Hiom (2012). Generally, synergy is most likely

to be exhibited when the two agents have dissimilar modes of action. If two agents from the same chemical class or with the same target site in the microbial cell are combined, the result is commonly found to be additive. Care is required, however, in the investigation and reporting of synergy for two reasons:

- It is well established that synergy might arise only at selected combination ratios, so it is unwise to assume that the effects displayed at one ratio will be seen at other ratios.

- Synergy must be divorced from the effects of concentration exponents (see Chapter 15). It is tempting to assume that doubling the concentration of a preservative results in a doubling of its antimicrobial activity, and so two agents together producing more than twice the effect of either one alone must be synergy. This logic is incorrect however, because some agents that have high concentration exponents (e.g. phenols) exhibit a large change in activity for a small change in concentration. Combining two such agents can result in a dramatic increase in effect that might be erroneously interpreted as synergy, whereas the increase is only that to be expected from doubling the concentration of either component alone.

Preservative interactions with formulation components and containers

The adequacy with which a formulated medicine is protected from spoilage by the use of a preservative cannot easily be predicted from a study of the activity of the preservative in simple aqueous solutions. A person with limited knowledge of pharmaceutical microbiology might, for example, expect that it would be possible to confirm that a medicine was adequately preserved simply by conducting an assay for the preservative and showing it to be present at a concentration higher than that required to inhibit the growth of common contaminants (i.e. higher than minimum inhibitory concentrations quoted in reference books and explained in Chapter 14). Not infrequently, however, this logic does not apply, because the preservative activity is reduced as a result of it interacting with other components of the formulation or the container, or by a change in the environmental conditions within the product. As a consequence, it is necessary to measure preservative efficacy not by a chemical assay but by a pharmacopoeial preservative efficacy test where the manufactured medicine is inoculated with a range of test organisms whose death rate is measured over a 28-day period (see Chapter 14).

Contaminating microorganisms do not invariably grow uniformly throughout a medicine packed in its final market container; they may be concentrated near the surface as a result of the higher oxygen availability there or, in the case of an emulsion, they grow in the water phase rather than the oil phase. The concentration of preservative available at the site where the organisms are growing is therefore the principal determinant of how effectively the medicine is protected from spoilage, and the 'free' preservative concentration (that which is actually available to kill microorganisms) may be significantly lower than the calculated value. Fig. 48.3 shows the major factors that influence preservative activity.

Several groups of common preservatives are affected by pH. This may be a consequence of:

- a change in ionization of the preservative molecule which alters the relative proportions of its undissociated and dissociated forms, which possess different intrinsic antimicrobial potencies;
- an effect on cell surface charge influencing adsorption of preservative molecules onto the microbial cell; or
- a change in the solubility or stability of the preservative molecule.

The weak organic acids (e.g. benzoic and sorbic acids) are the most commonly cited examples of preservatives whose ionization and activity are pH dependent, but there are several others. These acids are effective in formulations that are naturally acidic or can be buffered to a low pH. This is because in these conditions they exist as the undissociated molecules, which are more lipid soluble and more effective than the ionized forms that predominate when the ambient pH exceeds the molecule's pK_a. Phenolic preservatives exhibit similar but less marked pH dependence. Parabens are also slightly affected in the same way.

This situation contrasts with that seen with quaternary ammonium compounds, which are most effective in neutral or slightly alkaline conditions. Bacterial cells are usually negatively charged, and a rise in pH increases the number of such charges and so promotes the binding of positively charged molecules such as quaternary ammonium compounds.

Even though many liquid medicines contain a buffer to restrict pH change, it is not uncommon for the product specification to quote a permissible pH range that is sufficiently large to have a significant impact on preservative activity and for the product pH to drift within that range during the shelf life, which may be 2 years or more. Slow precipitation during storage (e.g. parabens precipitating with falling pH) is a further problem that is not necessarily detected by chemical assays because the assay procedure may redissolve the precipitate.

The oil–water partition coefficient is another molecular property that can have a marked influence on preservatives when they are used in emulsions. As microorganisms grow in the aqueous phase or at the oil–water interface, a preservative that accumulates in the oil phase is essentially inactive, although again this will not necessarily be apparent because a chemical assay is likely to show that the correct

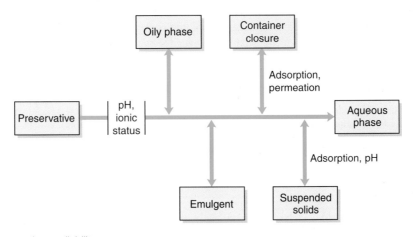

Fig. 48.3 • Preservative availability.

amount of preservative is present in a given weight or volume of a sample. This is a factor that makes parabens less useful choices as cream preservatives because they are usually a lot more soluble in vegetable oil than they are in water, although their partitioning might be reduced by substitution of mineral oil for vegetable oil. Again phenolics and some other preservatives are similarly affected, so when one is selecting preservatives for multiphase formulations, it is useful to consult publications such as the *Handbook of Pharmaceutical Excipients* (Rowe et al., 2016), where lists of solubilities and partition coefficients may indicate the likely extent of the problem.

Entrapment of preservatives within micelles of surfactants or emulsifying agents is a related phenomenon, where again the preservative is present but unavailable to inhibit microbial spoilage. Surfactants such as lecithin, polysorbate 80 and Lubrol W are so effective in removing preservative in this way that they are commonly used as inactivators (neutralizers) to prevent preservative carry-over and erroneous results in bioburden and preservative efficacy determinations (see Chapter 14). Dissolution and dialysis techniques together with mathematical models may provide some indication of the extent of preservative loss in such complex formulations. Complexation between anionic surfactants (e.g. sodium lauryl sulfate) and cationic preservatives (e.g. chlorhexidine and quaternary ammonium compounds) is also a potential problem in emulsion formulation.

Preservatives may be removed from solution by adsorption onto suspended solids, such as bentonite, kaolin, magnesium trisilicate and talc. In the case of bentonite, the potential to adsorb cationic drugs has been investigated as a means of retarding drug release to achieve a long-acting formulation. Antacid products, in particular, may prove difficult to protect because of preservative adsorption, and there have been several reports of products based on aluminium hydroxide,

magnesium trisilicate or kaolin being vulnerable to preservative inactivation. This is reflected in the *United States Pharmacopeia* (United States Pharmacopeial Convention, 2016), which specifies less stringent preservative performance criteria for antacids than for other oral products. The problems posed by adsorption are compounded by the fact that the phenomenon may also be pH dependent, so the most favourable pH for preservative activity itself may be one that promotes adsorption. Other hydrocolloids used as viscosity-raising agents in oral and topical products (e.g. alginates, tragacanth, cellulose derivatives and polyvinylpyrrolidone) may also reduce preservative activity. In some cases, this is simply a charge effect where an anionic polymer (e.g. alginate) complexes a cation (e.g. a quaternary ammonium compound).

Another major mechanism by which preservative activity may be compromised is interaction with the container or, in the case of volatile agents such as chlorbutanol, permeation through the container and loss by evaporation. Preservatives may adsorb onto the internal surface or penetrate into the material of the container itself. This problem has become more significant as plastic has tended to replace glass as a packaging material. Rubber stoppers in vials may also cause preservative loss. Most plastics, but particularly those commonly used for container manufacture such as polypropylene and polyethylene, have the potential to remove significant amounts of parabens and other common preservatives. The surface-to-volume ratio of the product in its container is likely to have a bearing on the magnitude of the problem; small containers have a relatively larger surface and may exhibit proportionately greater loss.

Please check your eBook at **https://studentconsult.inkling.com/** for self-assessment questions. See inside cover for registration details.

References

Baird, R.M., 2011. Microbial spoilage, infection risk and contamination control. In: Denyer, S.P., Hodges, N., Gorman, S.P., et al. (Eds.), Hugo and Russell's Pharmaceutical Microbiology, eighth ed. Wiley-Blackwell, Oxford.

Bloomfield, S.F., 2007. Microbial contamination: spoilage and hazard. In: Denyer, S., Baird, R. (Eds.), Guide to Microbiological Control in

Pharmaceuticals, second ed. CRC Press, London.

Cosslett, A.G., 2007. The design of controlled environments. In: Denyer, S., Baird, R. (Eds.), Guide to Microbiological Control in Pharmaceuticals, second ed. CRC Press, London.

Food and Drug Administration, 2015. Evaluation and definition of potentially hazardous foods -

chapter 3. factors that influence microbial growth. In: Safe Practices for Food Processors. US Food and Drug Administration, Silver Spring. Available at: http://www.fda.gov/Food/FoodScienceResearch/SafePracticesforFoodProcesses/ucm094145.htm.

Hiom, S., 2012. Preservation of medicines and cosmetics. In: Fraise, A.P., Maillard, J.-M.Sattar, S. (Eds.),

Principles and Practice of Disinfection, Preservation and Sterilization. Wiley-Blackwell, Oxford.

Medicines and Healthcare products Regulatory Agency, 2017. Rules and Guidance for Pharmaceutical Manufacturers and Distributors, tenth ed. Pharmaceutical Press, London.

Rowe, R.C., Sheskey, P.J., Cook, W.G., et al. (Eds.), 2016. Handbook of Pharmaceutical Excipients, eighth ed. Pharmaceutical Press, London.

United States Pharmacopeial Convention, 2016. 51 antimicrobial effectiveness testing. In: United States Pharmacopeia. US Pharmacopeial Convention, Rockville.

49

Product stability and stability testing

Paul Marshall

CHAPTER CONTENTS

KEY POINTS

- The stability of a pharmaceutical product is a critical aspect of the Quality Target Product Profile (QTPP).
- Stability is a relative concept, dependent on the protectiveness of the container closure system, the recommended storage conditions and the shelf life of the pharmaceutical product.
- Pharmaceutical products degrade over time by a variety of chemical, physical and/or microbiological mechanisms.
- Stabilization of a pharmaceutical product can be achieved in a number of ways, such as by control of the pH, moisture content and storage conditions (temperature, light and humidity).
- Careful selection of compatible excipients, the manufacturing process and the packaging materials used in the container closure system is crucial in ensuring a stable product.
- Stabilizing additives, such as antioxidants and antimicrobial preservatives, may be used but should not disguise a poorly formulated product, poor manufacturing practices, inadequate packaging or inappropriate storage conditions.
- Overages (of the active substance) in the manufacture of a drug product should not be used to compensate for degradation.
- Different types of stability studies may be undertaken during product development and throughout the lifecycle of the pharmaceutical product.
- Testing at elevated temperature and relative humidity can be used to elucidate the degradation pathway and predict the long-term stability of a product.
- Formal stability studies on the pharmaceutical product in the container closure system to be marketed are required to demonstrate that it remains safe, efficacious and of an acceptable quality throughout its shelf life.
- Stability data are used to establish the retest period of an active substance, the shelf life of a drug product and appropriate storage conditions.

Introduction

The stability of a pharmaceutical product is a relative concept, in that it is dependent on the protectiveness of the container closure system, the recommended storage conditions and the inherent stability of the active substance, excipients and the specific properties and aspects of the pharmaceutical dosage form. Stability can be defined as the ability of a pharmaceutical product to withstand physical, chemical or microbiological changes or decomposition when exposed to various environmental conditions. The product should be formulated and stored in a way that ensures it remains efficacious and safe, and be of an acceptable quality when used by health care professionals and patients – in short, the pharmaceutical product should be fit for purpose throughout its unopened and in-use shelf lives.

Shelf life is the term use by pharmacopoeias and regulatory authorities to delineate the period during which a drug product, following manufacture, remains suitable for its intended use by patients. Typical shelf lives are 2 or 3 years, but they may be significantly shorter or longer. The shelf life is established through rigorous stability testing and must always be qualified by the container closure system and storage conditions. Some degree of degradation may occur during the shelf life, but the duration is chosen so that an acceptable quantity of drug remains in the product, and any degradation products are at levels which do not pose a risk to the patient. If a pharmacopoeial monograph has been elaborated for the drug product, this will typically provide standardized shelf-life acceptance limits for drug assay (usually with a lower limit of at least 90% of the stated content) and for impurities throughout the shelf life of the product.

In the context of this chapter, 'pharmaceutical product' refers to both the active substance and the finished drug product, unless otherwise specified.

Mechanisms of degradation

Whenever the stability of pharmaceutical products is considered, it is important firstly to understand the various chemical and physical mechanisms of degradation.

Chemical stability

Active substances have diverse, and often complex, molecular structures and may therefore be susceptible to different and variable degradation pathways. Important chemical degradation reactions include hydrolysis, isomerization, polymerization, oxidation, photochemical reactions and other chemical interactions. The chemical basis for these reactions is described more fully in Chapter 47.

It is therefore beneficial to consider the likely pathways by which an active substance may degrade to assist the development of the formulation, the choice of manufacturing process, selection of the container closure system and the proposed storage conditions of the drug product so that chemical degradation is minimized.

Excipients may also degrade or change on storage. This may subsequently affect the function for which they are being included in the drug product. For example, hydrolysis of viscosity-modifying polymers can lead to a loss of viscosity; oxidation of preservatives may result in a loss of preservation; water absorption by hygroscopic excipients may induce dissolution. Excipients could also degrade to produce related substances that have toxicity issues.

It is very important to remember that degradation may not occur by only one mechanism; degradation may occur by multiple mechanisms that may interact, or even act as a catalysis, with each other.

Oxidation

Oxygen is abundant in the air, such that it is inevitable that a pharmaceutical product will be exposed to it during manufacture and storage. Oxidation is a well-known chemical degradation mechanism (see Chapter 47).

Oxidation may be prevented by removal of the available oxygen, although this is difficult to do completely in practice. Instead, an inert gas such as nitrogen or carbon dioxide can be used to displace the oxygen and afford protection to the product. For example, oxygen-sensitive products can be manufactured under a nitrogen shower or the headspace of containers can be flushed with argon or nitrogen before closure (e.g. as is the case with nicotine).

Alternatively, antioxidants may be included in the formulation. True antioxidants, such as ascorbic acid or sodium metabisulfite (both typically used in aqueous products), butylated hydroxytoluene (used in medicated chewing gums) and α-tocopherol (used in omega-3 oils), are thought to scavenge free radicals and block the subsequent chain reactions. Reducing agents (e.g. ascorbic acid) have a lower redox potential than the active substance and are thus preferentially oxidized rather than the active substance. Antioxidant synergists enhance the effects of antioxidants and chelate the trace metals that initiate oxidation (e.g. sodium edetate is used to stabilize penicillin-, adrenaline- and prednisolone-containing products). However, the inclusion of an antioxidant should not disguise a poorly formulated product or inadequate packaging, and must be fully and scientifically justified to the regulatory authorities. Likewise, it is not permissible to include an overage of the active substance (e.g. an amount above the labelled amount) to compensate for degradation.

Protecting the product from light, either by inclusion of a storage warning or by use of amber or opaque containers, may also prevent oxidation, as will storage at lower temperatures, typically refrigeration. In aqueous products, oxidation is generally promoted at high pH, and thus decreasing the pH as low as possible will afford some protection.

The container closure system can also provide protection against oxidation (see also Chapter 46). The oxygen transmission rate is a useful indicator of the protectiveness of the material. Glass and aluminium packaging offer the most protection against oxidation. Plastic packaging materials have different levels of protection depending on their composition and thickness.

Hydrolysis

Hydrolysis is another common degradation pathway for pharmaceutical products, and is typically the main degradation pathway for active substances having ester (e.g. benzocaine, aspirin and methylphenidate) and amide (e.g. β-lactam antibiotics and bupivacaine) moieties in their structure (see Chapter 47).

For most parenteral products and oral solutions, the active substance is formulated as an aqueous solution, and therefore the potential for hydrolysis is unavoidable. Suspensions are likely to be more stable than solutions because much of the active substance is protected within the insoluble particles. Solid dosage forms are not immune from the risk of hydrolysis. Water is often present in solid dosage forms as moisture, either resulting from the manufacturing process (e.g. when aqueous wet granulation or film coating are used) or inherently present in the excipients. The *European Pharmacopoeia* maximum limits for water in some common tablet fillers are 15% for maize and pregelatinized starch, 7% for microcrystalline cellulose and 4.5% to 5.5% for lactose. Gelatin capsule shells also contain water, typically up to 15%, as a plasticizer. Active substances (e.g. ethambutol, sodium valproate and ranitidine) and excipients (e.g. sorbitol, citric acid, sodium carboxymethylcellulose and polyvinylpyrrolidone)

may also exhibit hygroscopicity, by which they are able to absorb water from the atmosphere.

The strategies used to prevent hydrolysis centre around exclusion of water from the pharmaceutical product. For liquid dosage forms, stability can be considerably improved by formulation and storage of the product as a dry powder to be reconstituted before it is dispensed to the patient. Oral antibiotic solutions typically have a 2- or 3-year shelf life when stored as dry powders, but expire within 7–10 days once reconstituted into solutions. Freeze-drying of a solution to produce a solid lyophilized cake is also an alternative that is used for some parenteral injections (e.g. diacetylmorphine injections). Lyophilization (freeze-drying) (see Chapter 29) ensures the product dissolves rapidly during reconstitution, which is critical for a parenteral product.

For solid dosage forms, careful selection of excipients with low moisture content or predrying of excipients before manufacturing can reduce the likelihood of hydrolytic degradation. Replacing an aqueous solvent in a formulation with a nonaqueous one is also a potential means of avoiding hydrolysis. Choosing direct compression or dry granulation, rather than aqueous wet granulation, will also reduce the likelihood of hydrolysis.

Hygroscopic excipients that absorb moisture from the atmosphere should be avoided (e.g. non-hygroscopic mannitol could be used as a replacement for hygroscopic sorbitol). If the active substance is identified as hygroscopic early enough in the drug development stage, and if feasible, it may be possible to chemically modify the structure of the active substance to make it less hygroscopic. Manufacturing under controlled and reduced relative humidity (e.g. around 30–40% relative humidity) also reduces uptake of moisture by the product.

The container closure system can provide a moisture barrier for the pharmaceutical product (see Chapter 46). In Europe, solid oral dosage forms (e.g. tablets and capsules) are commonly packed in blister packs. The blister materials can have different compositions that provide differing levels of protection against moisture: poly (vinyl chloride) (PVC) < PVC–poly(vinylidene chloride) (PVdC) < PVC–polyethylene (PE)—PVdC < PVC–Aclar® laminates. Alternatively, aluminium–PVC or aluminium–polypropylene films may be used, and are generally regarded as having the highest moisture protection because of the aluminium layer. The level of moisture protection of a packaging material can be derived from the moisture vapour transmission rate, which

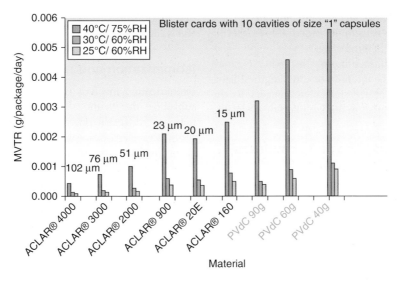

Fig. 49.1 • Moisture vapour transmission rates (MVTR) of plastic blister materials of differing thickness. *PVdC,* poly(vinylidene chloride), *RH,* relative humidity. From Dries, 2013.

is a function of the material composition and thickness (Fig. 49.1). The higher the moisture vapour transmission rate, the less protective is the packaging against moisture.

In contrast to European preferences for blister packs, US patients tend to prefer bottles, which can be manufactured from high-density polyethylene, low-density polyethylene, poly(ethylene terephthalate) or polypropylene (see Chapter 46). The relative moisture protection of these materials is as follows poly(ethylene terephthalate) < low-density polyethylene < polypropylene ≪ high-density polyethylene. Glass bottles or aluminium tubes offer the highest level of protection. A distinct disadvantage of bottles with respect to protection from moisture is that they are repeatedly opened by the patient during administration, exposing the product to atmospheric moisture. This can be mitigated by inclusion of a desiccant cartridge in the bottle, but this must have sufficient water-absorbing capacity for the proposed unopened and opened shelf life, and the risk of the patient accidentally swallowing the cartridge (e.g. in products used by dementia patients) should also be considered.

Hydrolysis is temperature dependent, so reduction of the storage temperature (e.g. by storing in a refrigerated 2 °C to 8 °C environment) may also slow down the rate of hydrolysis, for example, in the case of oral antibiotic mixtures. The acidity or alkalinity of a solution may affect hydrolysis, so control of the pH by use of a buffer system may reduce hydrolytic

reactions (e.g. borate in chloramphenicol eye and ear drops).

Photochemical reactions

Pharmaceutical products will be exposed to the light at some point during their manufacture, storage or use. Photochemical reactions are typically very complex and will be a concern if the product absorbs light within the range of natural UV–visible sunlight (290 nm to 700 nm), as photodegradants are strongly linked to safety of the product.

Photodegradation is perhaps more prevalent in solutions, where light can penetrate throughout the entire product; in the case of solid dosage forms, it is typically limited to the surface.

Prevention of photochemical reactions can be achieved by protection of the product from light with use of opaque container closure systems (see Chapter 46). Opaque primary packaging of parenteral products can make it difficult for health care professionals to see if the product has precipitated or contains particles, which may present a safety risk to the patient (Tran et al., 2006). Alternatively, opaque secondary packaging can be used; for example, ampoules can be packed in cardboard cartons. Opaque covers can be used to shroud syringe drivers or infusion bags, as well as the giving lines used during administration.

European regulatory authorities require photostability testing of the product to determine whether it is susceptible to photodegradation and whether the container closure system intended for marketing affords suitable light protection.

Decreasing the surface area of the product exposed to light, reducing the intensity or wavelength of light, or adding EDTA or free-radical scavengers to the drug product may also minimize photodegradation.

Formation of adducts and complexes

The drug product typically contains a number of excipients or additives, in addition to either one or more active substances, which may chemically or physically interact with each other, in addition to any degradation of the active substance. This may reduce the efficacy of the product as the active substance will not be available for absorption or the new complex/adduct may pose a safety concern in its own right. A complex is where two or more molecular entities are loosely associated. An adduct is a new chemical species formed by the direct combination of two molecular entities with no loss of atoms, in contrast to a chemical reaction. Active substances that contain primary or secondary amines (e.g. pramipexole and memantine) can undergo the Maillard reaction with reducing sugars. The levels of the memantine–lactose adduct is specifically controlled in the *United States Pharmacopeia* monograph for memantine tablets. Benzocaine in sugar-medicated lozenges can complex with glucose and fructose produced from the hydrolytic degradation of sucrose. Formulation of paracetamol with aspirin can lead to transacetylation of the paracetamol with aspirin, as well as direct hydrolysis of the paracetamol. Esterification of indometacin in polyoxyethylene (which is also known as polyethylene glycol) suppository bases has also been demonstrated.

Active substance–excipient adducts should be considered when one is developing analytical methods used in stability testing as they may be responsible for a lack of mass balance between levels of the active substance and total impurities. The active substance–excipient adduct may not be solubilized during sample preparation and thus will be unavailable for analysis. Conversely, any sample preparation should not degrade adducts into the original constituents, unless this occurs in vivo, otherwise testing may suggest the product is safer or more efficacious than it really is.

The importance of accurately determining the levels of any possible adducts is that they are considered in the same way as other related substances and degradation impurities, and should be controlled at levels that have been shown to be toxicologically safe.

Isomerization and polymerization

Isomerization involves the conversion of an active substance into its optical or geometric isomer, which may have different pharmacological or toxicological properties. For example, the loss of activity of adrenaline in parenteral products at low pH is attributed to the conversion from the active (*R*)-adrenaline to the inactive (*S*)-adrenaline. Tetracyclines undergo epimerization in acidic conditions to produce epitetracycline, which has a reduced therapeutic activity. Vitamin A is also known to be susceptible to *cis–trans* isomerization, with the *cis* isomer having less activity than the *trans* isomer.

Polymerization is where two or more molecules combine to form a complex molecule. Concentrated aqueous solutions of aminopenicillins, such as ampicillin and amoxicillin, are known to form dimers on storage, via the self-aminolysis of the β-lactam ring.

Temperature

Temperature appreciably influences the rate of degradation reactions, and may be described by the empirical equation proposed by Arrhenius in 1889 (see Chapter 7 for further information):

$$k = A \exp\left(\frac{-E_a}{RT}\right)$$

$$(49.1)$$

where k is the reaction rate, A is the pre-exponential frequency factor, E_a is the activation energy (in joules per mole), R is the universal gas constant and T is temperature (in kelvins)

Logarithmically transforming Eq. 49.1 produces a linear equation of the form $y = mx + c$:

$$\ln k = \ln A - \frac{E_a}{RT}$$

$$(49.2)$$

This equation can be used as a basis for a plot of the results from stress or forced degradation studies at elevated temperatures to extrapolate the rate constant at different temperatures. This interrelationship can then be used to gain an idea of the stability of the drug product.

There are a number of limitations to the use of the Arrhenius equation. Both the activation energy

(E_a) and the rate constant (k) are experimentally determined. These represent macroscopic reaction-specific parameters that are not related to threshold energies and individual molecular reactions involved in degradation.

Linear specific rates of change must be obtained at all temperatures used in the experimental study, which requires the rate of reaction to be constant over the period stability is evaluated. If the degradation kinetics vary, the specific rate that is assignable to the specific temperature is unable to be identified. If the reaction mechanism changes with temperature, this would also alter the slope of the reaction curve.

The activation energy must also be independent of the temperature of interest, which may not be the case if more than one reaction process is occurring. Some degradation reactions may be more significant at higher temperature than at lower temperature, and vice versa. Some primary degradation products may convert more rapidly to secondary degradation products at higher temperatures, leading to less accumulation, which may cause subsequent problems with analytical method development and impurity profile safety. Elevated temperatures can lead to less moisture in solid dosage forms, and thus less degradation. The amount of dissolved oxygen reduces with increasing temperature, which will decrease oxidative degradation and result in elevated temperature studies predicting better long-term stability than is the case. There is also a discontinuity between theoretical values calculated with the Arrhenius equation and experimental data around the glass transition temperature.

Consequently, the precision of the shelf-life estimates obtained with the Arrhenius equation can be poor, with studies typically yielding estimates with a wide range of uncertainty. However, from a practical perspective in the development of pharmaceutical products, the Arrhenius equation is a useful tool for estimating the real-time stability of a pharmaceutical product from elevated temperature studies. It is generally accepted that an increase in temperature by 10°C will increase the degradation rate by a factor of approximately two to three times. In other words, the Q_{10} temperature coefficient (which is a measure of the rate of change of a biological or chemical system as a consequence of the temperature being increased by 10°C) will be between 2 and 3.

For those products that are unstable at room temperature, refrigerated storage (2°C to 8°C) is an option to increase stability. However, this option should not be taken lightly as it increases the complexity and cost of the supply chain as refrigeration will need to be maintained at all times.

Cooling of the product to −20°C or even to −70°C to increase stability adds significantly greater complexity to the storage and distribution of drug products, and specialist distribution companies should be used. In the case of parenteral products, the product will need to be fully thawed to avoid injection of ice crystals into the patient. If heat is used to defrost the product, this may lead to the same degradation that freezing was used to avoid. Some chemicals and biopharmaceuticals are actually less stable when frozen.

The global pharmaceutical market must be considered when the stability of a pharmaceutical product is being evaluated with respect to temperature. Manufacturers of both active substances and drug products tend to be located in one geographical location (because of cost and expertise) and ship their products worldwide, rather than operate multiple manufacturing sites. It is critical that products are transported and stored in their recommended storage conditions, particularly if the products require cold-chain distribution, and this is a requirement of good manufacturing and distribution practice (Medicines and Healthcare products Regulatory Agency, 2017).

Corrosion

Corrosion is not considered a traditional degradation mechanism, but the numbers of drug–device combination products that may include electrical components are increasing. Drug–device combination products are now being developed to take advantage of new developments in device and electrical designs. The correct functioning of an electrical device is particularly critical where delivery of the active substance is device controlled. For instance, the drug containing hydrogel of a novel patient-controlled iontophoretic device for the transdermal delivery of fentanyl caused the printed electronic circuit boards to corrode, resulting in self-activation of the device and potential overdose. This was overcome by developing separate electronic controller and drug units that are assembled before use, thus avoiding moisture from the hydrogel corroding the circuits (European Medicines Agency, 2015).

Physical stability

The appearance, physical attributes and functionality of the pharmaceutical product are as important as chemical stability. There is a wide variety of finished drug products, and it is fair to say that the various pharmaceutical forms can each present different and unique stability challenges.

Appearance

The appearance, taste, smell and feel of a drug product should not change during its shelf life. Changes in appearance may be an early sign of chemical degradation and warrant further investigation. Examples of changes include discolouration of solutions, tablet coatings and gelatin capsules becoming tacky, mottled or even cracking (which may be critical for some modified-release or gastro-resistant tablets or capsules), aggregation of powders, cracking or creaming of creams and emulsions, ointments and gels becoming gritty, and the cracking of oral films.

The odour of a pharmaceutical product may also indicate degradation has occurred. The degradation of aspirin in products is accompanied by the characteristic vinegary smell of acetic acid.

The appearance of the packaging is also important for stability. For example, the distension of blister pockets can indicate that the active substance or the excipients have degraded releasing a gas as a degradation product (e.g. carbon dioxide in the case of effervescent tablets).

Polymorphic form

Polymorphic form is only a concern where the active substance exhibits polymorphism, is present in the solid form within the dosage form and the product safety, efficacy and performance may be affected by the polymorphic form (see Chapter 8). The same concern applies if the active substance exists in different solvates. Typically, polymorphism and solvate formation may affect the dissolution behaviour of solid dosage forms, either by increasing or decreasing the dissolution rate, which may in turn influence efficacy or safety.

Precipitation and particle size

Active substances or excipients in oral and parenteral solutions may precipitate during storage, particularly if the solution has been formulated near its saturation point or has become saturated through evaporation of the solvent. This will result in the poor appearance of the drug product but may also have more serious consequences with respect to efficacy and safety. Precipitation may cause the drug product to become inhomogeneous, leading to issues with dose uniformity and dissolution rate, and ultimately bioavailability. The presence of large numbers of particles in a parenteral product is a potentially life-threatening risk as it may result in vein irritation, phlebitis, clinically occult pulmonary granulomas, local tissue infarction, severe pulmonary dysfunction, occlusion of capillaries and arteries, anaphylaxis and death (Tran et al., 2006). Consequently, pharmacopoeial standards are in place to limit particulate matter in parenteral products. The change in particle size of the dose emitted from nasal sprays and inhalation products can also affect dose delivery and reduce the efficacy of the product.

Ostwald ripening may also occur (see Chapter 26), whereby larger crystals are formed from the dissolution of smaller crystals, leading to a gritty and coarse texture. In some products (e.g. paracetamol and pseudoephedrine solutions), large crystals in excess of 10 mm can form on storage.

Rheological properties

A change in the rheological properties of a liquid or semisolid drug product can affect the dosing and administration of a drug product. For example, a change in the viscosity of an oral solution may influence how easily and accurately the solution is drawn up into an oral syringe or is poured into a spoon. The rheological properties of a cream or ointment can influence how easily it is spread on the skin or mucous membranes, and whether application is painful or likely to cause further damage to the affected area (e.g. as is the case with haemorrhoid preparations).

Water content

The amount of water in a drug product may be important as it can facilitate chemical degradation (as described earlier) and microbial proliferation. However, it can also lead to other issues, such as a reduction in tablet hardness and increased tackiness of film coatings and capsules. The permeability of plastic packaging materials to moisture has been previously described; in addition to drug product absorbing moisture from the atmosphere through these plastic materials, the evaporation of water or solvents from solutions contained in plastic containers or bottles can also occur, leading to the active substance becoming more concentrated in the solution, and eventually precipitating.

Gelatin capsules contain approximately 15% water, and the capsule contents may absorb water from the capsule shell, particularly if the contents are hygroscopic or deliquescent.

Acidity and alkalinity

Preservative efficacy and protection against microbial spoilage may be influenced by changes in pH. Sodium benzoate is effective only in acidic conditions (pH 2–5); it is almost without effect in alkaline conditions. Benzyl alcohol has little activity above pH 8 and optimum activity below pH 5. In contrast, the *para*-hydroxybenzoates (parabens) are effective over a wide pH range (Rowe et al., 2016).

A change in the pH of parenteral solutions or products applied to mucous membranes (e.g. nasal, eye, vaginal and rectal) may result in adverse reactions, such as local irritation of the mucous membranes, pain on injection and phlebitis.

Resistance to crushing, friability, disintegration and dissolution

The resistance to crushing of a tablet can change on storage, the tablet becoming either less or more resistant. There are a number of mechanisms underpinning this change, such as absorption of water, which acts as a plasticizer for some of the excipients, and long-term elastic or plastic formative changes resulting from the energy applied to the tablet during compression. In addition to changes to the crushing resistance, there may be changes in friability, disintegration and dissolution. Tablets that become more friable can more easily break during handling, transportation (e.g. in a bottle) and removal from the packaging (e.g. when they are 'deblistered'), and this is a quality issue. Tablets that are more resistant to crushing may take longer to disintegrate and dissolve.

Gelatin capsules, including gelatin enrobing of tablets, may undergo irreversible cross-linking of the polymeric gelatin chains. These 'pellicles' are insoluble and may retard or even prevent dissolution of the dosage form.

Redispersibility and reconstitution

Suspensions (oral, parenteral or inhalation) may be prone to sedimentation and even caking on storage; this is where the suspended solid material falls out of suspension to form a compacted layer at the bottom of the container that is difficult to resuspend. The ability of the solid material to remain suspended or to redisperse easily on shaking is critical to ensure a uniform drug product and reproducible dosing (see Chapter 26). Caking may be problematic for drug products requiring reconstitution before administration, as it is difficult for the liquid to penetrate and suspend or dissolve the solid caked mass. This leads to dose uniformity issues (e.g. with oral antibiotic suspensions) and the increased likelihood of a large amount of particulate matter being injected (e.g. with powders for injection, such as diamorphine).

Functionality

Where pharmaceutical products have a physical, mechanical or electrical mechanism that allows the product to operate and deliver the active substance, its functionality should not change during storage. For example, transdermal patches can lose adhesiveness, resulting in the failure to adhere and remain in contact with skin, which can impact the delivery of the drug. Conversely, the adhesive can become so tacky that it is difficult to remove the release liner before administration of the patch onto the skin. The plungers of prefilled oral and injection syringes should remain easily moveable within the syringe barrel, without excessive plunger pressure being required, to ensure an accurate dose can be easily given; the plunger should not become completely seized within the barrel.

Absorption, adsorption and leaching

Pharmaceutical products, particularly liquid formulations, have the potential to either adsorb onto or absorb into the container closure system, leading, for example, to a loss of active substance or preservative. Non-polar molecules are susceptible to sorption to plastics and rubber. For instance, glyceryl trinitrate evaporates from tablets and may be lost by absorption/adsorption onto plastic packaging, and is typically packed in glass bottles with aluminium-lined caps to prevent this. Diazepam can be lost from solutions in contact with plastic packaging, as are some preservatives in contact with rubber closures. The pH of the solution may influence the extent of sorption if the active substance is ionizable, as the un-ionized form is more likely to undergo adsorption/absorption.

Where liquid products are stored in a plastic container closure system, there is the potential for the plasticizers or other components in the plastic to leach into the product over time, which may give rise to toxicity issues. This is normally investigated during product development, whereby the materials of the container closure system are stored in the liquid product (or simulated product) at extreme conditions to see what compounds can potentially be extracted from the container materials. It is critical to know what chemicals have been added to the plastic materials during manufacture so that the range of compounds for which analysis is performed can be narrowed. The study is then repeated at the recommended and elevated conditions to see whether the extractable compounds actually leach into the product from the container. These materials may then need to be monitored during formal stability studies. For example, paclitaxel injection may use a polyoxyethylated castor oil and ethanol solvent system, which can extract the plasticizer diethylhexyl phthalate from PVC containers.

Glass containers may release soluble mineral substances into aqueous products, which can be determined by measuring the hydrolytic resistance of the glass. The mineral substance can result in a change in the pH of the solution, which can then catalyse chemical degradation. The *European Pharmacopoeia* classifies glass containers depending on the composition of the glass, any surface treatment and its hydrolytic resistance. The *European Pharmacopoeia* provides corresponding recommendations of the types of products for which they are suitable (see Chapter 46).

Microbiological stability

Proliferation of bacteria, yeasts and moulds in a drug product can adversely affect the product itself, as well as pose a serious risk to patient safety. Pharmacopoeias lay down requirements for the microbial quality of both sterile and non-sterile products. Sterility of a product is assured by use of a suitably validated production process (manufacture and sterilization), good manufacturing practice (GMP) and the integrity of the container closure system. The microbiological quality of sterile products once they have been opened also needs consideration. Single-use sterile products, such as injections contained in glass or plastic ampoules or preservative-free eye drops, should be used immediately once they have been opened, with any unused product being discarded as the sterility and microbiological quality cannot be assured. Other injectable products, such as insulin vials, and eye drops may include a preservative system allowing

multiple use; however, in-use shelf life is typically limited to approximately 4 weeks. Microbial spoilage and the preservation of pharmaceutical products are considered in Chapter 48.

Stability testing of pharmaceutical products

The purpose of stability testing is to provide evidence on how the quality of a drug substance or drug product varies with time under the influence of a variety of environmental factors, such as temperature, humidity and light, and to establish a retest period for the drug substance or a shelf life for the drug product and recommended storage conditions.

The stability of a pharmaceutical product is a critical aspect of the Quality Target Product Profile (QTPP) and is investigated throughout the various stages of a product's development and lifecycle. With use of scientific first principles and knowledge of the mechanisms of degradation, together with previous experience gained from the stability testing of similar dosage forms, it is possible to develop a pharmaceutical product and its container closure system to avoid obvious stability issues and increase the likelihood of an acceptably long retest period or shelf life, and establish acceptable storage conditions.

The stability of a pharmaceutical product is complex, often being dependent on multiple physical, chemical and microbiological factors that may or may not interact with each other, such that an acceptable stability profile can never be fully predicted – in short, this complexity means that stability testing of a pharmaceutical product is a necessary part of any development programme.

The design of a stability study depends on the stage of product development and what knowledge about a product's stability profile is being sought.

Types of stability studies

Preformulation studies

In the preformulation stage, the physicochemical properties of the active substance are fully characterized (see Chapter 23). Stress testing or forced stability studies expose the active substance, both solid and solubilized forms, to extreme conditions over a short period (e.g. 14–28 days): elevated temperature (e.g. 50°C, 60°C or 70°C); elevated humidity (e.g.

60%, 75%, 85% or 90% relative humidity); acid and base hydrolysis (e.g. 0.01 N to 1 N acid/base); oxidation (e.g. 0.3% to 3% hydrogen peroxide) and photolysis (e.g. 1.2×10^6 lux hours). Regulatory or pharmacopoeial authorities do not prescribe formal conditions for stress testing. Conditions should be selected to obtain a degradation level of approximately 10%, although this level may vary from one company to another, and from one active substance to another.

The aim of these studies is to degrade the active substance to elucidate the likely degradation mechanisms and pathways, which is useful for the development of the container closure system and the formulation of the drug product. Of course, where an existing active substance is used, this information may be derived from published literature sources. Stress testing or forced stability studies are also used to validate and demonstrate that the analytical methods are stability indicating.

Binary mixes

Once the degradation pathway is known, this knowledge, together with any previous development experience and scientific first principles, can be used to carefully select suitable excipients to be formulated with the active substance in the drug product. Binary mixes of the active substance and excipient can then be used to confirm excipient compatibility. Binary mixes are usually a 1:1 ratio of the active substance and excipient in either a powder blend/compact or an aqueous slurry mixture (to investigate the effect of moisture), although it may be more scientific for the ratio to mimic the levels likely to be used in the formulation. Tertiary mixes, where an additional excipient is added to the binary mix, may also be used. These mixes are then subject to testing at accelerated conditions (e.g. 40 °C/75% relative humidity, 40 °C/85% relative humidity or 50 °C, and light) for a short period (1–3 months), with evaluation of the mixes for changes in appearance, content and degradation products. Alternatively, thermal methods, such as differential scanning calorimetry, can be used to detect interactions between the active substance and excipients. The benefit here is that there is no need for stability studies, so the cycle time and sample consumption are much reduced; however, the data can be difficult to interpret, false positives/negatives are frequently encountered and the outcome is sensitive to sample preparation.

Formulation and container development stability studies

A drug product may undergo several stages of formulation development. The first formulation stage may be for preclinical studies or phase I (first in humans) clinical trials, where the product may be a simple parenteral injection or an early prototype formulation. Formulation, manufacturing and container closure development studies may be performed further to develop the formulation and the container closure system for phase II (first in patients) clinical studies. The formulation, manufacturing process and container closure system are then further optimized to arrive at the final formulation and container closure system for the large-scale phase III (pivotal) clinical studies (the data from which form the basis for marketing authorization applications to regulatory authorities) and eventual commercialization.

Stability testing of the different formulations is performed at appropriate stages to support the development programme, as well as to provide stability data to support the clinical trial (regulatory authorities require demonstration that clinical trial supplies are appropriately stable and are safe to be administered to volunteers). The types of stability study can range from forced degradation or stress testing of the drug product (principally to validate the analytical methods as stability indicating, but can also provide useful information on potential interactions with excipients within a formulated product), accelerated testing (which can give an indication of the likely long-term stability of different development formulations) and long-term or real-time testing (on prototype laboratory-scale or small pilot scale development batches) to formal stability studies (Table 49.1) on the exact formulation and container closure system that is intended to be marketed.

Bulk intermediate and final drug product (i.e. before it is packaged into the marketed container closure system) stability also needs to be monitored to support holding times during product manufacture.

Temperature cycling studies (from less than 0 °C to 40 °C) should be performed for inhalation, nasal and transdermal products, as well as suspensions, creams and emulsions (even solutions, in some cases). Temperature fluctuations can encourage precipitation and/or particle growth, which can have a significant effect on the quality and efficacy of these products. The performance of inhalation and nasal products at low temperature also needs to be characterized.

Table 49.1 Example protocols for formal International Council for Harmonisation of Technical Requirements for Pharmaceuticals for Human Use (ICH) stability studies on the general case, semi-permeable containers, refrigerated products and frozen products

Storage condition	Time (months)							
	0	3	6	9	12	18	24	36
General case								
5 °C	Only if long-term stability results fail to meet predefined acceptance criteria							
25 °C/60% RH	P/C/M	P/C	P/C	P/C	P/C/M	P/C	P/C/M	P/C/M
30 °C/65% RH	(P/C/M)	(P/C)	(P/C)	(P/C)	(P/C/M)			
40 °C/75% RH	P/C/M	P/C	P/C/M					
Semipermeable containers								
5 °C	Only if long-term stability results fail to meet predefined acceptance criteria							
25 °C/40% RH	P/C/M	P/C	P/C	P/C	P/C/M	P/C	P/C/M	P/C/M
30 °C/65% RH	(P/C/M)	(P/C)	(P/C)	(P/C)	(P/C/M)			
40 °C/75% RH	P/C/M	P/C	P/C/M					
Storage in a refrigerator								
5 °C	P/C/M	P/C	P/C	P/C	P/C/M	P/C	P/C/M	P/C/M
25 °C/60% RH	P/C/M	P/C	P/C/M					
Storage in a freezer								
−20 °C	P/C/M	P/C	P/C	P/C	P/C/M	P/C	P/C/M	P/C/M
Good Manufacturing Practice (GMP) stability testing (non-ICH)								
25 °C/60% RH or 30 °C/65% RH[a]	P/C/M				P/C/M		P/C/M	P/C/M

Tests in parentheses are typically performed only if accelerated test results fail to meet predefined acceptance criteria.
[a]Whichever condition is consistent with the storage conditions.
C, chemical testing; M, microbiological testing; P, physical testing; RH, relative humidity.

The manufacturer must select the most appropriate type of study to gain the maximum amount of useful information on the stability of the drug product, while making the most efficient use of the formulation, manufacturing, analytical, stability cabinet storage, financial and time resources at its disposal. Stability testing forms a significant part of a development programme both financially and in time, so it is important to get it right first time.

Postauthorization stability studies

The licensing of a pharmaceutical product is not the end of stability testing. If stability studies on commercial-scale batches have not been provided during the licensing submission, regulatory authorities will require the manufacturer to provide a commitment to stability-test the first three commercial-scale batches to confirm the retest period/ shelf life once the product is commercialized. The manufacturer has to notify the authorities immediately if the commercial-scale stability data do not agree with those previously provided in the Marketing Authorisation application, and do not conform to the agreed shelf life and storage conditions.

Pharmaceutical products are likely to undergo many changes during their lifecycle. It is quite common for manufacturers to amend the drug product formulation or change the manufacturing process and equipment, change suppliers of active substances/ excipients, change the manufacturer of the drug product or change the container closure system. It is also common for manufacturers to change the retest period or shelf life and storage conditions to suit the marketing requirements of the product. All these changes will need to be submitted to the regulatory authorities and supported by stability studies if a variation is sought to the marketing authorization.

GMP and good distribution practice stability studies

GMP requires the stability of a marketed product to be monitored during its shelf-life to determine whether the product remains, and can be expected to remain, within its licensed specifications under its labelled storage conditions (Medicines and Healthcare products Regulatory Agency, 2017). This requires manufacturers to initiate an ongoing or rolling stability programme, in which at least one batch per year of product manufactured, of every strength and every primary packaging type is included, unless otherwise justified. The stability study design can be different from that used for licensing purposes, but must generate sufficient stability data to permit trend analysis so that changes in the stability profile can be detected.

The stability of the product during transportation from the manufacturer(s) to the wholesaler(s) and finally the pharmacy also needs be verified, as the recommended storage advice applies to both static and mobile (during transportation) storage (Medicines and Healthcare products Regulatory Agency, 2017). Certain pharmaceutical products may be susceptible to temperature 'spikes' (the temperature suddenly deviates from and quickly recovers to within the target range) or 'plateaus' (the temperature lies outside the range for an extended time before eventual recovery), which can have different effects. Products requiring 'cold-chain' transportation (i.e. refrigerated or frozen) are highly susceptible to temperature excursions. This may require simulated transportation studies, accelerated testing or temperature/humidity cycling studies to be performed if this information cannot be gleaned from development or formal stability studies.

Climatic zones

The pharmaceutical industry is a global business, and pharmaceutical products may be manufactured, transported and marketed in several countries and continents. Climatic conditions can differ between the different regions, and can change throughout the year. This can potentially result in a considerable amount of testing to evaluate the stability of the product in different regions. However, Schumacher (1972) and Grimm (1986, 1998) proposed reducing the number of long-term test conditions on the basis of the environmental conditions in just four climatic zones.

- *climatic zone I – temperate climate* (e.g. UK, northern Europe, Canada, New Zealand and Russia);
- *climatic zone II – subtropical and Mediterranean climate* (e.g. Japan, southern Europe, South Africa and USA);
- *climatic zone III – hot and dry climate* (e.g. Middle East, northern Africa, Argentina and Australia); and
- *climatic zone IV – hot and humid climate* (e.g. northern South America, Southeast Asia, China, parts of India and central Africa).

In 2005, the World Health Organization (WHO) Expert Committee on Specifications for Pharmaceutical Preparations recommended the subdivision of climatic zone IV (hot and humid) into two zones: climatic zone IVA (hot and humid) and climatic zone IVB (hot and very humid). The current proposed meteorological criteria for the different climatic zones are described in Table 49.2.

Mean kinetic temperature

The mean kinetic temperature (MKT) in any part of the world can be derived from climatic data, and is a simplified way of expressing the overall effect of temperature fluctuations during storage and transportation of pharmaceuticals (as well as other

Table 49.2 World Health Organization proposed criteria for the different climatic zones

Climatic zone		Meteorological criteria (mean annual temperature measured in the open air/mean annual partial water vapour pressure)
I	Temperate	≤ 15 °C / ≤ 11 hPa
II	Subtropical and Mediterranean	> 15 °C to 22 °C / > 11 to 18 hPa
III	Hot and dry	> 22 °C / ≤ 15 hPa
IVA	Hot and humid	> 22 °C / > 15 to 27 hPa
IVB	Hot and very humid	> 22 °C / > 27 hPa

Data from World Health Organization, 2006.

perishable goods, such as food). The MKT is a single calculated temperature at which the total amount of degradation over a particular period is equal to the sum of the individual degradations that would occur at various temperatures. It is higher than the arithmetic mean temperature, and takes into account the Arrhenius equation.

The MKT can be calculated as follow (Seevers et al., 2009):

$$T_K = \frac{\dfrac{-\Delta H}{R}}{\ln\left(\dfrac{e^{-\Delta H/RT_1} + e^{-\Delta H/RT_2} + \cdots + e^{-\Delta H/RT_n}}{n}\right)}$$

(49.3)

where ΔH is the heat of activation for the degradation reaction (assumed to be 83.144 kJ mol^{-1} unless more accurate information is available from experimental studies), R is the universal gas constant (8.3144 × 10^{-3} kJ K^{-1} mol^{-1}), T_1, T_2 and T_n are the average temperature (in kelvins) during the first, second, and nth periods, and n is the total number of temperatures recorded. The time interval between temperature measurements is assumed to be identical.

The concept of the MKT does permit excursions (i.e. minor variation) of the storage temperature. For example, the *United States Pharmacopeia* Controlled Room Temperature permits storage between 15 °C and 30 °C, providing the MKT is not more than 25 °C; transient spikes up to 40 °C are permitted if the manufacturer so instructs as long as their duration does not exceed 24 hours. However, the MKT should not be used to compensate for poor temperature control of storage and transportation facilities.

Stability test conditions

The evaluation of the different climatic conditions and the MKT by each of the 194 WHO member states resulted in the recommended storage conditions for long-term stability studies (Fig. 49.2). This results

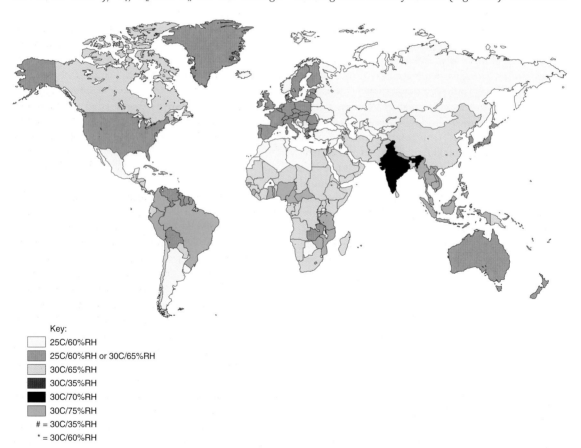

Key:
- 25C/60%RH
- 25C/60%RH or 30C/65%RH
- 30C/65%RH
- 30C/35%RH
- 30C/70%RH
- 30C/75%RH
- # = 30C/35%RH
- * = 30C/60%RH

Fig. 49.2 • World map of World Health Organization long-term storage conditions.

in some interesting discrepancies between the meteorological conditions and the regulatory requirements. For example, Canada is meteorologically in climatic zone I (temperate) but is in climatic zone IVA (hot and humid) from a stability testing perspective; northern Africa and the Middle East are typically hot and dry (climatic zone III) but the long-term testing conditions are more humid (climatic zone IVA). The WHO long term stability testing conditions do not necessarily correlate with climatic conditions, as the WHO conditions typically include a safety factor, but companies are required to use these conditions to license their products. Companies are allowed to use more harsh long-term testing conditions.

The intermediate storage condition is normally 30 °C/65% relative humidity, unless this is the long-term storage condition, in which case there is no intermediate condition. The accelerated storage condition is 40 °C/75% relative humidity.

These storage conditions describe the general case for testing pharmaceutical products. If the product is intended to be stored in a refrigerator, the long-term storage condition is 5 °C ± 3 °C and accelerated storage is 25 °C/65% relative humidity, 30 °C/65% relative humidity or 30 °C/75% relative humidity. Products intended for storage in a freezer have a long-term condition of −20 °C; products that need to be stored below −20 °C are treated on a case-by-case basis.

Where the drug product is stored in a semipermeable container closure system, long-term testing in lower humidity conditions (25 °C/40% relative humidity or 30 °C/35% relative humidity) should be performed to determine the propensity of the product to lose water vapour through the plastic packaging, particularly if the product is intended to be marketed in climatic zone III (hot and dry). Alternatively, a higher storage humidity can be used, and water loss at the reference relative humidity can be derived through calculation. At 40 °C, the calculated rate of water loss during storage at not more than 25% relative humidity is equal to the measured water loss rate at 75% relative humidity multiplied by 3.0. Where the packaging is impermeable (e.g. glass ampoules), relative humidity is not a concern.

Testing at accelerated and intermediate conditions

Accelerated conditions are designed to be a moderately more stressful temperature and relative humidity environment than the long-term storage conditions, with intermediate conditions somewhere in the middle. Accelerated conditions should be differentiated from stress testing, where more extreme conditions may be used.

Pharmaceutical products are generally stable (in the order of years) at long-term storage conditions, and thus stability testing over this period presents a practical problem for the manufacturer. Testing at accelerated or intermediate conditions can significantly reduce the time taken to generate stability data, giving an early indicator of the stability of the pharmaceutical product.

Accelerated or intermediate stability data can also be used in the extrapolation of the available long-term stability data to set longer retest periods or shelf lives than the period covered by the long-term data. It is for this reason primarily that it is recommended to initiate stability testing at accelerated and/or intermediate conditions, in addition to long-term conditions, in any formal stability study design.

The prediction of long-term stability from data obtained at accelerated conditions does have its limitations and it is acknowledged that shelf-life estimates may have a high degree of uncertainty. To reduce this uncertainty, the concepts of a moisture-corrected Arrhenius equation (Eqn. 49.4) and an isoconversion paradigm or model have been applied, together with a statistical design of experiment and analysis approach, to develop the Accelerated Stability Assessment Program (ASAP), which has improved the predictability of shelf life for a wide range of products (Waterman and Colgan, 2008; Waterman et al., 2007).

The 'isoconversion paradigm' is essentially a model where the amount of degradation is kept approximately the same by adjustment of the time that the product is exposed to different elevated temperature and humidity conditions (Table 49.3). This overcomes some of the limitations of the empirically (experimentally) derived Arrhenius equation being unable to accurately reflect the complex individual molecular reactions involved in degradation (as described earlier). For example, in a solid dosage form, active substance molecules can exist in an amorphous state or in crystalline domains, and may be adjacent to different excipients. Consequentially, the molecules may degrade at different rates as a function of the amount of degradation. Often, only a small amount of active substance is in a very reactive form that will degrade, with the rest being relatively stable. If the proportion of the reactive form changes with

Table 49.3 Typical conditions and duration of testing with the ASAP isoconversion model protocol for a solid dosage form of a drug substance with average temperature and relative humidity dependence

Temperature (°C)	Relative humidity (%)	Duration of testing (days)
50	75	14
60	40	14
70	5	14
70	75	1
80	40	2

Data from Waterman & Colgan, 2008.

Box 49.1

Worked example

By application of Eq. 49.4; if a product has a high B constant of 0.09 and the relative humidity (RH) of the storage condition is increased from 65% RH to 75% RH, then the shelf life will be reduced by an order of 2.46, i.e. a 24-month shelf life will be reduced to 9 months.

$$\frac{\ln k_{75\%RH}}{\ln k_{65\%RH}} = B(75 - 65) = 0.09 \times 10 = 0.9$$

$$\frac{k_{75\%RH}}{k_{65\%RH}} = \exp(0.9) = 2.46$$

temperature and/or humidity, this can result in the degradation kinetics becoming very complex. This exceeds the limitations of the Arrhenius equation, and thus can make prediction of stability at other conditions difficult.

If the amount of active substance converting to degradation products is kept the same, the proportions of the different reacting species remain the same (isoconversion), and this compensates for the complex reaction kinetics.

The moisture-corrected Arrhenius equation is (Waterman and Colgan, 2008)

$$\ln k = \ln A - \frac{E_a}{RT} + B \,(\text{relative humidity})$$

$$(49.4)$$

The influence of relative humidity on the degradation of an active substance can be understood in terms of the magnitude of the constant B, which can have values ranging from a low value of 0 to a high value of 0.09. There is an exponential relationship between relative humidity and drug reactivity, such that a small change in humidity will result in a large difference in stability and shelf-life prediction (Box 49.1).

It is postulated that the influence of relative humidity on the rate of degradation is attributed to water increasing the mobility of the reacting species rather than being a direct reactant (hydrolytic reactions are not more susceptible to relative humidity).

ASAP can provide improved predicted shelf-life estimates with as little as 14 days' stability testing, which is much faster than traditional accelerated

testing, and thus is attractive to manufacturers developing pharmaceutical products and container closure systems. The use of ASAP to set retest periods and shelf lives, and the associated storage conditions, is not currently accepted by regulatory authorities in Europe.

Long-term stability testing

A manufacturer must ensure that long-term stability testing is conducted on the product, as intended to be marketed, at conditions that represent the recommended storage conditions for the duration of the retest period or shelf life. If the data are not available at the time of submission, then the manufacturer will need to provide commitments to provide the data if requested by the regulatory authorities, typically by continuing the existing formal stability studies used in the initial regulatory submission. The GMP requirement to implement an ongoing long-term stability programme was discussed earlier.

Stability studies supporting marketing authorization submissions

The International Council for Harmonisation of Technical Requirements for Pharmaceuticals for Human Use (ICH) has published several quality or 'Q' guidelines for stability testing of active substances and drug products, e.g. ICH Q1A(R2), which can be accessed via the ICH website (http://www.ich.org; see also Table 49.4).

Table 49.4 International Council for Harmonisation of Technical Requirements for Pharmaceuticals for Human Use stability guidelines for chemical and biological products

Code	Guideline
Q1A(R2)	Stability Testing of New Drug Substances and Products (second revision 2003). This guideline provides recommendations on stability testing protocols including temperature, humidity and trial duration for climatic zones I and II. Furthermore, the revised document takes into account the requirements for stability testing in climatic zones III and IV so as to minimize the different storage conditions for submission of a global dossier
Q1B	Stability Testing: Photostability of New Drug Substances and Products (1996). This guideline forms an annex to Q1A(R2), and gives guidance on the basic testing protocol required to evaluate the light sensitivity and stability of new drugs and products
Q1C	Stability Testing for New Dosage Forms (1996). This guideline extends Q1A(R2) for new formulations of already approved medicines and defines the circumstances under which reduced stability data can be accepted
Q1D	Bracketing and Matrixing Designs for Stability Testing of New Drug Substances and Products (2002). This guideline describes general principles for reduced stability testing and provides examples of bracketing and matrixing designs
Q1E	Evaluation of Stability Data (2003). This guideline extends Q1A(R2) by explaining possible situations where extrapolation of retest periods/shelf lives beyond the real-time data may be appropriate. Furthermore, it provides examples of statistical approaches to stability data analysis
Q1F	Stability Data Package for Registration Applications in Climatic Zones III and IV. This guideline was withdrawn in 2006, leaving the definition of storage conditions in climatic zones III and IV to the respective regions and WHO
Q5C	Stability Testing of Biotechnological/Biological Products (1995). This document augments guideline Q1A, and deals with the particular aspects of stability test procedures needed to take account of the special characteristics of products in which the active components are typically proteins and/or polypeptides

R indicates that a guideline has been revised; hence R2 indicates a second revision.
WHO, World Health Organization.

The ICH Q guidelines aim to harmonize the quality and testing methods for pharmaceutical products, including conducting stability studies and evaluating the data. ICH is composed of the regulatory authorities of the EU, Japan, the USA, Switzerland and Canada, together with pharmaceutical industry representation from Europe, Japan, the USA and the rest of the world.

The Asia-Pacific Economic Cooperation (APEC), Association of Southeast Asian Nations (ASEAN), East African Community (EAC), Gulf Central Committee for Drug Registration (GCC), Pan-American Network for Drug Regulatory Harmonization (PANDRH) and Southern African Development Community (SADC) regional harmonization initiatives, and regulatory authorities from Australia, Brazil, China, Taiwan, India, the South Korea, Russia and Singapore are also involved in the ICH process for developing guidelines. The WHO also participates in the process as an observer.

In addition to ICH guidance, countries and regions may have specific additional or supplementary stability guidance which also needs to be taken into consideration when a product is being developed, e.g. Committee for Human Medicinal Products (CHMP) stability guidance (available from http://www.ema.europa.eu) and ASEAN stability guidance.

Stability guidelines essentially describe how formal stability studies on the active substance and the drug product should be conducted. Stability testing should be performed on at least three primary batches of the pharmaceutical product so as to measure any batch-to-batch variability. A primary batch should be at least pilot scale (typically 10% commercial manufacturing scale, or at least 100 000 units for tablets or capsules, whichever is larger) and should be representative of the commercial product (same synthetic process and critical control steps for active substances and same composition and manufacturing process for drug products). In certain situations, such as where the active substance is considered stable, the number of batches that need to be included in a stability study can be reduced.

The container closure system should simulate the commercial packaging for active substances and should be identical to that used for the drug product. Liquid products packaged in containers with separate closures will need to be stored inverted and laid on their side to allow any interaction between the product and the container closure to be monitored (e.g. sorption into a rubber vial closure).

Where there are multiple presentations of the drug product (e.g. different strengths or bottle pack sizes), stability testing will be required for each possible presentation. However, the concepts of bracketing and/or matrixing can be used to reduce the amount of testing. Bracketing is where only the samples on the extremes of certain factors (e.g. strength, container size and/or fill) are tested at every time point. Matrixing is where a selected subset of all the possible samples at a particular time point is tested. Reduced designs have pitfalls in that they may lead to shorter shelf-life estimation, or the stability studies have insufficient power to detect some main or interaction effects.

At least 12 months' long-term stability data (and/or intermediate data) and 6 months' accelerated data need to be provided to regulatory authorities by companies seeking a marketing authorization. However, in certain cases (e.g. generic products) the data requirement may be reduced to 6 months. ICH also provides guidance on the length of intervals between testing – a typical ICH stability study protocol is described in Table 49.1.

Photostability testing

Photostability of the active substance is initially studied as part of stress testing to elucidate degradation pathways, but can also be used to indicate whether there might be a need for light protection of the formulated product. Photostability testing of the drug product may be done during formulation and container closure development studies (using open and closed container studies).

Photostability studies of the pharmaceutical product and the container closure system intended to be marketed will need to be performed to confirm

the product is not affected by light exposure. This is typically achieved by an overall illumination of not less than 1.2×10^6 lux hours within a temperature-controlled light cabinet with use of light sources that replicate daylight (both visible and UV light). Typically, the product's appearance, assay and impurities are investigated, as are other Critical Quality Attributes (CQAs) that may be affected by light; for example, some polymers may cross-link in light, resulting in changes of viscosity.

The drug product may need to carry a label warning to advise that the product should be stored protected from light. This may also extend to its use by the health care professional or patient; for example, nitroprusside degrades to cyanide on exposure to light, therefore infusion bags need light-protecting over-bags and opaque giving sets should be used.

Stability specification

Before a stability study can be initiated, a stability specification that describes the CQAs (as derived from the Quality Target Product Profile, QTPP), analytical methods and acceptance criteria must be drawn up. This describes an acceptable level of quality for the pharmaceutical product, against which it is evaluated during stability testing.

There can be three different types of specification: release, shelf life and stability. The release and shelf-life specifications should include the same range of tests but may have different acceptance limits; for example, assay and impurity limits may be wider in the shelf-life specification to account for active substance degradation (acceptance limits for assay should relate to labelled content rather than the initial value). Regulatory authorities will use the shelf-life specification when testing products on the market (e.g. in the case of any dispute, adverse incident and market surveillance).

The stability specification typically contains only shelf-life specification tests for quality attributes that are susceptible to change over time, or are likely to have a critical impact on the quality, safety and/or efficacy of the product. An example of release, shelf-life and stability specifications and their differences is described in Table 49.5. ICH has published regulatory guidance on the setting of specifications (Table 49.6), and there may also be additional regional guidance. In Europe, there is a legislative requirement for the maximum acceptable deviation in the active substance content of the finished product not to

Table 49.5 Example of release, shelf-life and stability specifications for an oral immediate-release tablet containing 50 mg of active substance

Test	Reference to analytical methods	Acceptance limits		
		Release specification	Shelf-life specification	Stability specification
Appearance	Visual	White, biconvex, round tablet, 5 mm diameter	White, biconvex, round tablet, 5 mm diameter	White, biconvex, round tablet, 5 mm diameter
Identification	IR	Complies with reference	Complies with reference	Not tested[a]
Assay	HPLC method 1	95% to 105% of labelled content	93% to 105% of labelled content	93% to 105% of labelled content
Related substances:	HPLC method 2			
Impurity 1		0.2%	0.5%	0.5%
Impurity 2		0.2%	0.5%	0.5%
Impurity 3		0.2%	0.5%	0.5%
Single unknown		0.2%	0.2%	0.2%
Total		1.0%	2.0%	2.0%
Dissolution	Ph Eur apparatus 2 (paddle), HPLC method 3	$Q = 75\%$, 45 min	$Q = 75\%$, 45 min	$Q = 75\%$, 45 min
Uniformity of dosage units	Compendial method	Complies	Complies	Not tested
Microbial quality	Compendial method	Complies	Complies	Complies

[a]The active substance does not need to be identified as it is unlikely to change during the stability study.
HPLC, high-performance liquid chromatography; IR, infrared.

exceed ±5% at the time of manufacture, unless there is appropriate justification.

Pharmacopoeial requirements (e.g. *British Pharmacopoeia, European Pharmacopoeia, United States Pharmacopeia* and *Japanese Pharmacopoeia*) also need to be considered as the monographs are legally enforceable in the respective jurisdictions. Pharmacopoeial monographs are considered 'shelf-life' specifications.

Monographs may be general and thus apply to all products of that particular dosage form; for example, the *European Pharmacopoeia* monograph on tablets or the *European Pharmacopoeia* monograph on substances for pharmaceutical use. There are also specific monographs that apply only to a particular active substance (e.g. *European Pharmacopoeia* monograph for lisinopril dihydrate), excipient or drug product (e.g. *British Pharmacopoeia* monograph for lisinopril tablets). The *British Pharmacopoeia, United States Pharmacopeia* and *Japanese Pharmacopoeia* contain specific monographs for active substances, excipients and finished products, whereas the *European Pharmacopoeia* contains only specific monographs

for active substances and excipients, although the Ph. Eur. Commission has started elaborating product-specific monographs (e.g. *European Pharmacopoeia* monograph for sitagliptin tablets). Monographs undergo regular revision to ensure that they reflect the current technologies and quality of manufactured products placed on the market.

For lisinopril tablets marketed in the UK, the product shelf-life specification must comply with the specific *British Pharmacopoeia* product monograph tests and acceptance limits for identification, dissolution, related substance or impurities and assay, in addition to the test and acceptance limits for uniformity of dosage units, dissolution and disintegration described in the *European Pharmacopoeia* general monograph for tablets. The test for disintegration is usually waived when dissolution is performed. The specific and general monographs have different acceptance limits for dissolution, and the specification must comply with the limits described in the specific monograph.

The types of tests to be included in a specification are described in Table 49.7 – not all tests will be

Table 49.6 International Council for Harmonisation of Technical Requirements for Pharmaceuticals for Human Use guidelines that should be considered for setting specifications

Code	Guideline
Q3A(R2)	Impurities in New Drug Substances (2006). The guideline addresses the chemistry and safety aspects of impurities, including the listing of impurities in specifications, and defines the thresholds for reporting, identification and qualification
Q3B(R2)	Impurities in New Drug Products (2006). This guideline complements Q3A(R2) and provides advice regarding impurities in products containing new, chemically synthesized drug substances. The guideline specifically deals with those impurities which might arise as degradation products of the drug substance or arising from interactions between the drug substance and excipients or components of primary packaging materials. The guideline sets out a rationale for the reporting, identification and qualification of such impurities based on a scientific appraisal of likely and actual impurities observed, and of the safety implications, following the principles elaborated in the parent guideline. Threshold values for the reporting and control of impurities are proposed, based on the maximum daily dose of the drug substance administered in the product
Q3C(R6)	Impurities: Guideline for Residual Solvents (2016). This guideline recommends the use of less toxic solvents in the manufacture of drug substances and dosage forms, and sets pharmaceutical limits for residual solvents (organic volatile impurities) in drug products
Q3D	Guideline for Elemental Impurities (2014). This guideline aims to provide a global policy for limiting metal impurities qualitatively and quantitatively in drug products and ingredients. The Q3A(R2) guideline classifies impurities as organic, inorganic, and residual solvents. The Q3A(R2) and Q3B(R2) guidelines effectively address the requirements for organic impurities. An additional guideline, Q3C(R6), was developed to provide clarification of the requirements for residual solvents. The proposed new guideline, Q3D, would provide similar clarification of the requirements for metals, which are included in the ICH inorganic impurities classification
Q6A	Specifications: Test Procedures and Acceptance Criteria for New Drug Substances and New Drug Products: Chemical Substances (1999). This guideline addresses the process of selecting tests and methods and setting specifications for the testing of drug substances and dosage forms. Account has been taken of the considerable guidance and background information which are present in existing regional documents
Q6B	Specifications: Test Procedures and Acceptance Criteria for Biotechnological/Biological Products (1999). This guideline provides guidance on justifying and setting specifications for proteins and polypeptides which are derived from recombinant or nonrecombinant cell cultures. The scope is initially limited to well-characterized biotechnological products, although the concepts may be applicable to other biologicals as appropriate. In view of the nature of the products, the topic of specifications includes in-process controls, bulk drug, final product and stability specifications and gives guidance for a harmonized approach to determining appropriate specifications based on safety, process consistency, purity, analytical method, product administration and clinical data considerations

R indicates that a guideline has been revised; hence R2 indicates a second revision and R6 indicates a sixth revision.
ICH, International Council for Harmonisation of Technical Requirements for Pharmaceuticals for Human Use.

relevant to the dosage form under investigation. Data from development stability studies, the QTPP, pharmacopoeial requirements, guidance or legislation can be used to support the setting of acceptance criteria.

Analytical test procedures

The analytical procedures used to test pharmaceutical products should be 'state of the art' and suitable for their intended use; for example, thin-layer chromatography has increasingly been superseded by high-performance liquid chromatography and is no longer accepted by regulatory authorities.

Analytical procedures should be appropriately validated for specificity, accuracy, precision (repeatability and intermediate precision or reproducibility), limits of detection and quantitation, linearity and range, depending on the type of procedure. Robustness of the method should also be validated at an appropriate stage in the development of the analytical

Table 49.7 Critical Quality Attributes (CQA) that may be included in a specification

General quality attributes to be included in a specification	
Active substance	Appearance, identification, assay and related substances/impurities
Drug product	Appearance, identification, assay and related substances/impurities

Specific quality attributes to be included in a specification	
Active substance	Physicochemical properties, particle size distribution, polymorphic form, chirality, water content, inorganic impurities and microbial quality
Tablets and capsules	Dissolution, disintegration, hardness/friability (capsule brittleness), uniformity of dosage units, water content and microbial quality
Oral liquids (solutions, emulsions and suspensions)	Uniformity of dosage units, pH, microbial quality, antioxidant content, antimicrobial preservative content, extractables and leachables, alcohol content, dissolution, precipitation/particle size distribution, polymorphic form, phase separation, redispersibility, reconstitution time, rheological properties and water content
Parenteral products	Uniformity of dosage units, pH, sterility, endotoxins/pyrogens, particulate matter, water content (for nonaqueous products), antimicrobial preservative content, antioxidant content, extractables and leachables, functionality of delivery system (e.g. for prefilled syringes), osmolality/osmolarity, particle size distribution, redispersibility, reconstitution time and rheological properties
Inhalation and nasal products	Moisture content, mean delivered dose, delivered dose uniformity, uniformity of dosage units, fine particle mass, particle/droplet size distribution, leak rate, agglomeration, microbial quality, sterility, extractables and leachables, antimicrobial preservative, number of actuations per container, delivery rate, water content, spray pattern, foreign particulate matter and examination of the valve components/container corrosion/gasket deterioration
Topical	Homogeneity, pH, suspendability (for lotions), consistency, rheological properties, particle size distribution (for suspensions, when relevant), microbial quality and weight loss
Ophthalmic and otic preparations	In addition to the requirements for topical products, the requirements for ophthalmic or otic products should include sterility, particulate matter and extractable volume
Suppositories and pessaries	Softening range, disintegration and dissolution
Transdermal patches	In vitro dissolution, peel/adhesive properties of the patch and crystal formation
Drug–device combinations	Functioning of the device

Adapted from the recommendations of Word Health Organization, International Council for Harmonisation of Technical Requirements for Pharmaceuticals for Human Use and European Medicines Agency.

procedure, to determine the sensitivity of the procedure to foreseen and unforeseen changes. Test methods described in pharmacopoeial monographs have been validated against these criteria during the elaboration of the monograph and typically do not need further validation.

In addition to the already-mentioned validation studies, the test procedure should be *stability indicating* (i.e. it should be able to measure the desired analyte without interference from degradation products). Stress testing or forced stability studies are used to confirm the analytical procedure is stability indicating.

Evaluation of stability data

The analytical results from testing of the formal stability testing batches should be evaluated against the predefined acceptance criteria in the stability specification. The data should be analysed for any out-of-specification (OOS) values, increasing or decreasing trends (which may result in an OOS) and the degree of variability, all of which affect the confidence that a future manufactured batch will remain within the acceptance limits throughout its retest period or shelf life.

A systematic approach should be adopted in the presentation and evaluation of the stability data to facilitate easy review, trend analysis and identification of OOS results. The data should be presented in a tabulated format, supplemented by graphical representations to illustrate trends or OOS results (if appropriate). Quantitative values for the quality attributes should be reported, rather than a simple 'complies' conclusion, to allow trend/statistical analysis and extrapolation.

Extrapolation is where the known stability data are used to predict future stability behaviour beyond the period covered by long-term data. Variability of the stability data, their rate of change, and the stability of the pharmaceutical product at intermediate or accelerated conditions all affect the extent to which extrapolation of the long-term data can be done. Extrapolation is limited to no more than twice the period covered by long-term data or 12 months, whichever is shorter (ICH Q1E). Extrapolation is not permitted for biological or biotechnological products: these products will need to have long-term stability data covering the shelf life (ICH Q5C).

Statistical analysis is usually not required if the stability data show little change and variability. Where the data do change and/or are variable, statistical analysis of the stability data may be useful in setting a retest period or shelf life. ICH Q1E describes some approaches to the statistical analysis of stability data, e.g. linear regression, pooling of data ('poolability') and statistical modelling, although other methods are acceptable if suitably justified.

Linear regression is the most commonly used predictive analysis, consisting of finding the best-fitting straight line through scattered plots of the data. It can also be used with two-sided (for upper *and* lower acceptance limits) or one-sided (for upper *or* lower acceptance limit) 95% confidence limits to account for batch-to-batch and analytical variability. The confidence limits are used to define a region within which there is a 95% probability that the true regression line lies. Fig. 49.3 shows a typical linear regression of 12-month assay data and the calculated two-sided 95% confidence limits – note that the 95% limits do not run parallel to the line of best fit. With use of the acceptance limits for assay described in Table 49.5 (93.0% to 105.0%), the linear regression line of the data suggests that the assay values will fail to meet shelf-life specification limits after 32 months. However, if the variability of future batches as predicted with use of the 95% confidence limits is taken into account, assay is likely to fail to meet the

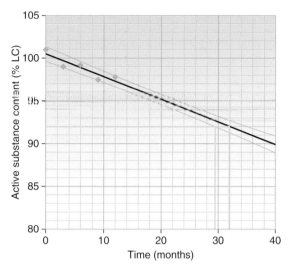

Fig. 49.3 • Linear regression analysis of assay values and the calculated 95% confidence limits. *LC*, label claim.

specification after approximately 29 months. Therefore the shelf life should be set at no more than 29 months, although manufacturers may set a shorter shelf life (e.g. 24 months) to build in a safety factor additional to that already present in the statistical model.

It is generally assumed that certain quantitative quality attributes of a pharmaceutical product will change over time following linear zero-order kinetics; however, some degradation mechanisms may follow first-order or second-order rate reactions and thus the data may need mathematical transformation (e.g. logarithmic transformation) before linear regression can be performed (see Chapter 7 for a full discussion of rates of reaction)

Pooling of data from different batches can be used to increase the number of data points used in the linear regression analysis, improving the estimation of the 95% confidence limits and reducing the width of the region. This can potentially give a longer shelf life than if the batches are individually considered. Pooling of data may be done only if the regression lines from different batches have a common slope and time-zero intercept, which can be determined by analysis of covariance or other suitable methods.

Stability studies supporting clinical trials

The regulatory requirements for investigational medicinal products (IMPs) tend to be more relaxed and flexible than those for a marketing authorization application, but depend on the stage of clinical development. The number of available batches and stability data may be limited for a phase I trial compared with a phase II or phase III trial, and this is reflected in the requirements. Specification limits are typically more generous than for a marketing authorization, but are based on batches that have been toxicologically characterized and/or have undergone clinical evaluation to assure safety of the product. The limits are expected to become more stringent as the product progresses through development. Analytical methods should be confirmed as suitable for phase I trials, but summary validation data need to be provided for phase II and phase III trials. Shelf lives can be extended by four times the period covered by long-term stability data for chemical investigational medicinal products but only by twice the period covered by long-term data for biological investigational medicinal products (up to a maximum of 12 months). Stability studies should be initiated and conducted in parallel with the clinical trial and throughout its entire duration, particularly for phase I. Stability studies on modified comparator/reference product and placebos may also need to be conducted, depending on the type of product.

Concluding comments

The stability of a pharmaceutical product is a critical aspect of the QTPP – it is important to ensure the product is safe and efficacious, and of an acceptable quality for patients. Stability of a pharmaceutical product is a relative concept that is dependent on the inherent stability of the active substance, excipients and dosage form, plus the protectiveness of the container closure system and the recommended storage conditions. Pharmaceutical products degrade on storage by a variety of physical, chemical and/or microbiological mechanisms, although it is possible to stabilize products by careful selection of compatible excipients, the manufacturing process and packaging materials. Whilst stabilizing additives, such as antioxidants or antimicrobial preservatives, may be included, they should not be used to disguise a poorly formulated product, poor manufacturing practices, inadequate packaging or inappropriate storage conditions. Overages (of the active substance) should not be used to compensate for degradation.

Different types of stability studies may be performed to investigate the stability of the pharmaceutical product, ranging from stress testing/forced degradation of the active substance, compatibility of binary mixes of active substance and excipients, accelerated (longer-term) testing of prototype formulations, longer-term testing of the product used in clinical studies to formal long-term and accelerated testing to support shelf-life and storage recommendations as part of a regulatory submission and commitments. Stability testing is likely to continue throughout the lifecycle of the pharmaceutical product, either as part of GMP commitments to ensure the product continues to remain stable or to support postapproval changes, such as the extension of shelf life and changes in the manufacturing and supply chain.

Please check your eBook at **https://studentconsult.** **inkling.com/** for self-assessment questions. See inside cover for registration details.

References

Dries, T., 2013. Presentation on best practice in pack stability trials. Testing of Pharmaceuticals. Informa, London.

European Medicines Agency, 2015. European Public Assessment Report on Ionsys, procedure EMEA/H/C/002715/0000. EMA/801150/2015. European Medicines Agency, London.

Grimm, W., 1986. Storage conditions for stability testing (part 2). Drugs Made Ger. 29, 39–47.

Grimm, W., 1998. Extension of the International Conference on Harmonisation tripartite guideline for stability testing of new drug substances and products to countries of Climatic Zones III and IV. Drug Dev. Ind. Pharm. 24, 313–325.

Medicines and Healthcare products Regulatory Agency, 2017. Rules and Guidance for Pharmaceutical Manufacturers and Distributors, tenth ed. Pharmaceutical Press, London.

Rowe, R.C., Sheskey, P.J., Cook, W.G., et al., 2016. Handbook of Pharmaceutical Excipients, 8th ed. Pharmaceutical Press, London.

Schumacher, P., 1972. Über eine für die Haltbarkeit von Arzneimitteln maßgebliche Klimaeinteilung (The impact of climate classification on the stability of medicines). Die Pharm. Ind. 34, 481–483.

Seevers, R.H., Hofer, J., Harber, P., et al., 2009. The use of mean kinetic temperature (MKT) in the handling, storage, and distribution of temperature sensitive pharmaceuticals. Pharm. Outsourcing May/June, 12–17.

Tran, T., Kupiec, T.C., Trissel, L.A., 2006. Particulate matter in injections: what is it and what are the concerns? Int. J. Pharm. Compd 10 (3), 202–204.

Waterman, K.C., Carella, A.J., Gumkowski, M.J., et al., 2007. Improved protocol and data analysis for accelerated shelf-life estimation of solid dosage forms. Pharm. Res. 24 (4), 780–790.

Waterman, K.C., Colgan, S.T., 2008. A science based approach to setting expiry dating for solid drug products. Reg. Rapp. 5 (7), 9–14.

World Health Organization, 2006. WHO Expert Committee on Specifications for Pharmaceutical Preparations. Fortieth Report. WHO Technical Report Series 937. World Health Organization, Geneva.

Bibliography

Chen, Y., 2009. Packaging selection for solid oral dosage forms. In: Qiu, Y., Chan, Y., Zhang, C.G., et al. (Eds.), Developing Solid Oral Dosage Forms: Pharmaceutical Theory & Practice. Academic Press, New York.

Connors, K.A., Amidon, G.L., Stella, V.J., 1986. Chemical Stability of Pharmaceuticals: A Handbook for Pharmacists, 2nd ed. John Wiley & Sons, New York.

International Conference on Harmonisation of Technical Requirements for Registration of Pharmaceuticals for Human Use, 1995. Q5C Stability testing of Biotechnological/Biological Products. International Conference on Harmonisation of Technical Requirements for Registration of Pharmaceuticals for Human Use. Geneva.

International Conference on Harmonisation of Technical Requirements for Registration of Pharmaceuticals for Human Use, 1996. Q1B Stability Testing: Photostability of New Drug Substances and Products. International Conference on Harmonisation of Technical Requirements for Registration of Pharmaceuticals for Human Use. Geneva.

International Conference on Harmonisation of Technical Requirements for Registration of Pharmaceuticals for Human Use, 1996. Q1C Stability Testing for New Dosage Forms. International Conference on Harmonisation of Technical Requirements for Registration of Pharmaceuticals for Human Use. Geneva.

International Conference on Harmonisation of Technical Requirements for Registration of

Pharmaceuticals for Human Use, 1999. Q6A Specifications: Test Procedure and Acceptance Criteria for New Drug Substances and Products. International Conference on Harmonisation of Technical Requirements for Registration of Pharmaceuticals for Human Use. Geneva.

International Conference on Harmonisation of Technical Requirements for Registration of Pharmaceuticals for Human Use, 1999. Q6B Specifications: Test Procedures and Acceptance Criteria for Biotechnological/Biological Products. International Conference on Harmonisation of Technical Requirements for Registration of Pharmaceuticals for Human Use. Geneva.

International Conference on Harmonisation of Technical Requirements for Registration of Pharmaceuticals for Human Use, 2002. Q1D Bracketing and Matrixing Designs for Stability Testing of New Drug Substances and Products. International Conference on Harmonisation of Technical Requirements for Registration of Pharmaceuticals for Human Use. Geneva.

International Conference on Harmonisation of Technical Requirements for Registration of Pharmaceuticals for Human Use, 2003. Q1A(R2) Stability Testing of New Drug Substances and Products. International Conference on Harmonisation of Technical Requirements for Registration of Pharmaceuticals for Human Use. Geneva.

International Conference on Harmonisation of Technical Requirements for Registration of

Pharmaceuticals for Human Use, 2003. Q1E Evaluation of Stability Data. International Conference on Harmonisation of Technical Requirements for Registration of Pharmaceuticals for Human Use. Geneva.

International Conference on Harmonisation of Technical Requirements for Registration of Pharmaceuticals for Human Use, 2006. Q1F Stability Data Package for *Registration* Applications in Climatic Zones III & IV. International Conference on Harmonisation of Technical Requirements for Registration of Pharmaceuticals for Human Use. Geneva.

International Conference on Harmonisation of Technical Requirements for Registration of Pharmaceuticals for Human Use, 2006. Q3A(R2) Impurities in New Drug Substances. International Conference on Harmonisation of Technical Requirements for Registration of Pharmaceuticals for Human Use. Geneva.

International Conference on Harmonisation of Technical Requirements for Registration of Pharmaceuticals for Human Use, 2006. Q3B(R2) Impurities in New Drug Products. International Conference on Harmonisation of Technical Requirements for Registration of Pharmaceuticals for Human Use. Geneva.

International Conference on Harmonisation of Technical Requirements for Registration of Pharmaceuticals for Human Use, 2009. Q8 Pharmaceutical Development. International Conference on Harmonisation of Technical Requirements for

Registration of Pharmaceuticals for Human Use. Geneva.

International Conference on Harmonisation of Technical Requirements for Registration of Pharmaceuticals for Human Use, 2011. Q3C(R5) Impurities: Guideline for Residual Solvents. International Conference on Harmonisation of Technical Requirements for Registration of Pharmaceuticals for Human Use. Geneva.

International Conference on Harmonisation of Technical

Requirements for Registration of Pharmaceuticals for Human Use, 2014. Q3D Guideline for Elemental Impurities. International Conference on Harmonisation of Technical Requirements for Registration of Pharmaceuticals for Human Use. Geneva.

Snape, T.J., Astles, A.M., Davies, J., 2010. Understanding the chemical basis of drug stability and degradation. Pharm. J. 285, 416.

Yoshioka, S., Stella, V.J., 2002. Stability of Drugs and Dosage Forms. Kluwer

Academic Publishers, New York.

Zhan, M., 2009. Global stability practice. In: Huynh-Ba, K. (Ed.), Handbook of Stability Testing in Pharmaceutical Development. Springer, New York.

Zahn, M., Kållberg, P.W., Slappendel, G.M., et al., 2006. A risk-based approach to establish stability testing conditions for tropical countries. J. Pharm. Sci. 95, 946–965. Erratum published J. Pharm. Sci. 2007, 96, 2177.

Index

Page numbers followed by "*f*" indicate figures, "*t*" indicate tables, and "*b*" indicate boxes.